Lippincott's Illustrated Reviews: Pharmacology

2nd edition

Lippincott's Illustrated Reviews: Pharmacology

Mary J. Mycek, Ph.D.
Department of Pharmacology and Toxicology
University of Medicine and Dentistry of New Jersey–
New Jersey Medical School
Newark, New Jersey

Richard A. Harvey, Ph.D.
Department of Biochemistry
University of Medicine and Dentistry of New Jersey–
Robert Wood Johnson Medical School
Piscataway, New Jersey

Pamela C. Champe, Ph.D.
Department of Biochemistry
University of Medicine and Dentistry of New Jersey–
Robert Wood Johnson Medical School
Piscataway, New Jersey

Clinical Consultant (Antimicrobials):
Bruce D. Fisher, M.D.
Department o f Medical Education
Muhlenberg Regional Medical Center
Plainfield,

Computer graphics:
Michael Cooper
Cooper Graphics
48 Van Syckel Road
Hampton, New Jersey

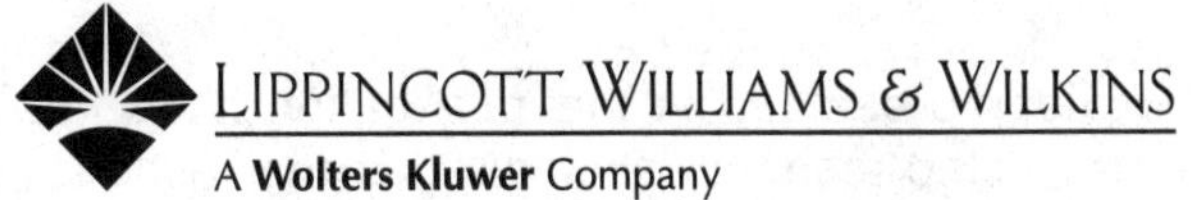

Philadelphia • Baltimore • New York • London
Buenos Aires • Hong Kong • Sydney • Tokyo

Acquisitions Editor: Richard Winters
Sponsoring Editor: Mary Beth Murphy
Production Manager: Janet Greenwood

9 8 7

Library of Congress Cataloging-in-Publication Data

Mycek, Mary Julia
Pharmacology/Mary J. Mycek, Richard A. Harvey, Pamela C. Champe; clinical consultant (antimicrobials), Bruce Fisher; computer graphics, Michael Cooper.—2nd ed.
p. cm —(Lippincott's Illustrated Reviews)
Rev. ed. of: Pharmacology/editors, Richard A. Harvey, Pamela C. Champe. c1992
Includes bibliographic references and index.
ISBN 0-7817-2413-9 (alk. paper)
1. Pharmacology—Outlines, syllabi, etc. 2. Pharmacology—Examinations, questions, etc. I. Harvey, Richard A. II. Champe, Pamela C. III. Pharmacology. IV. Title. V. Series
[DNLM: 1. Pharmacology—examination questions. 2. Pharmacology—outlines. QV 18.2 M995p 1997]
RM301.14.P47 1997
615'.1'076—dc20
DNLM/DLC
for Library of Congress 96-9180
CIP

Care has been taken to confirm the accuracy of the information presented and to describe generally accepted practices. However, the author, editors, and publisher are not responsible for errors of omission or for any consequences from application of the information in this book and make no warranty, express or implied, with respect to the contents of the publication.

The authors, editors, and publisher have exerted every effort to ensure that drug selection and dosage set forth in this text are in accordance with current recommendations and practice at the time of publication. However, in view of ongoing research, changes in government regulations, and the constant flow of information relating to drug therapy and drug reactions, the reader is urged to check the package insert for each drug for any change in indications and dosage and for added warnings and precautions. This is particularly important when the recommended agent is a new or infrequently employed drug.

Some drugs and medical devices presented in this publication have Food and Drug Administration (FDA) clearance for limited use in restricted research settings. It is the responsibility of the health care provider to ascertain the FDA status of each drug or device planned for use in their clinical practice.

Contributors:

Henry Brezenoff, Ph.D.
Department of Pharmacology and Toxicology
University of Medicine and Dentistry of New Jersey–
New Jersey Medical School
Newark, New Jersey

Rachel Giuliano, Ph.D.
Department of Pharmacology and Toxicology
University of Medicine and Dentistry of New Jersey–
New Jersey Medical School
Newark, New Jersey

Richard Howland, Ph.D.
Department of Pharmacology and Toxicology
University of Medicine and Dentistry of New Jersey–
New Jersey Medical School
Newark, New Jersey

Joseph McArdle, Ph.D.
Department of Pharmacology and Toxicology
University of Medicine and Dentistry of New Jersey–
New Jersey Medical School
Newark, New Jersey

Victor Radice, R. Ph.
B.S. Columbia University
Consulting Pharmacist
Wayne, New Jersey

Student Contributors :

Darah Biddle
College of Pharmacy
Rutgers University
New Brunswick, New Jersey

Richard F. Eschle
College of Pharmacy
Rutgers University
New Brunswick, New Jersey

Preface

Who will find this book useful

Lippincott's Illustrated Reviews: Pharmacology integrates and summarizes the essentials of medical pharmacology for (1) students in the health-related professions who are preparing for licensure examination [for example, the United States Medical Licensure Examination (USMLE) Step 1], and (2) professionals who wish to review or update their knowledge in this rapidly expanding area of biomedical science. The *Illustrated Review* uses an information-intensive, outline format along with summary figures and practice questions to teach this complex material.

How to use this book

OUTLINE TEXT *Lippincott's Illustrated Reviews: Pharmacology* uses a unique expanded outline format which allows the rapid review and assimilation of facts and concepts. The current knowledge in the field of medical pharmacology has been "predigested" and the relevant information has been recast in a hierarchical organization. Important topics are shown in bold print, whereas the names of drugs are featured in an italic typeface. This organization enables the reader to readily scan a page to locate specific information or to find a particular drug. A phonetic pronunciation guide for drug names assures that the reader will have a conversational familiarity with the therapeutic agents described in the book. Each chapter starts with a chart that lists and classifies the drugs to be discussed in that chapter. This permits the reader to immediately understand and remember the significant relationships among the facts and concepts.

ILLUSTRATIONS *Lippincott's Illustrated Reviews:Pharmacology* contains more than 400 original illustrations, each carefully crafted to compliment and amplify the text. This volume features a new kind of diagram in which pharmacologic processes are illustrated with a blend of graphics and explanations. This marriage of words and art allows the reader to integrate a body of knowledge without the distraction of constantly shifting from text to illustrations. For example, to sort out the intricacies of neurotransmitter synthesis and release in an ordinary textbook would require repeated skipping from text to figures. By contrast, the *Illustrated Review* (see for example, Figure 4.3, p.37) reveals the major steps and their significance at a glance.

CROSS-REFERENCES WITHIN THIS BOOK *Lippincott's Illustrated Review:Pharmacology* not only permits the easy assimilation of pharmacologic facts and concepts but also provides an extensive network of more than 400 cross-references to other relevant information in the volume. Thus, when readers encounter a new block of information, they are immediately directed by page citations to related material that reinforces and expands the original information. This elaborate matrix of references provides a cross fertilization that increases learning and retention. The student ends up with the "the big picture."

CROSS-REFERENCES TO OTHER BOOKS IN THE SERIES A unique feature of this volume is the large number of references to *Lippincott's Illustrated Reviews: Biochemistry*, which is the biochemistry volume in the Lippincott series. Designated as InfoLink references, they are located at the end of each chapter. This permits a reader with an interest in learning additional information related to a particular topic to readily locate relevant material covered in the biochemistry review. InfoLink also emphasizes the interrelationships between these biomedical disciplines—a skill that is increasingly being tested by the USMLE, Step I.

QUESTIONS AND ANSWERS A total of more than 200 practice questions (of the types used by the National Board of Medical Examiners and other standardized test writers) are included at the end of each chapter so that readers can check their progress in mastering the material. Answers with explanations are provided so that the reader knows both the correct answer and also why the distractors in the multiple choice questions are incorrect. These answers and their explanations are juxtaposed with the original questions in a special section at the end of the book. Thus readers can confirm the correct answers to a group of study questions without the disorientation of flipping from page to page.

FINDING INFORMATION An extensive index of more than 4000 entries permits the reader to instantly locate specific information. The index includes commonly used trade-names of drugs.

Readers should thumb through this carefully coordinated review of therapeutically useful agents . . . . they may be surprised that learning pharmacology can be so enjoyable!

Acknowledgments

We are grateful to the many friends and colleagues who generously contributed their time and effort to help us make this book as accurate and as useful as possible. We would like to acknowledge the contributions of Drs. Zigmund Kaminski, Edward J. Flynn, Lester A Sultatos, Uri Lopatin and Kafui DeMasio who provided many helpful comments. We would particularly like to express our thanks to Dr. Bruce Fisher whose clinical insights and suggestions were invaluable in clarifying confusing concepts. We highly value the additional support of our other colleagues at Robert Wood Johnson Medical School and in New Jersey Medical School. We (RAH and PCC) owe a special thanks to our Chairman, Dr. Masayori Inouye, who has encouraged us in this and other teaching projects. We would also like to thank Dr. Victor Gruber, the Director of the National Medical School Review, for sharing his insights into educational mechanisms for effectively integrating the biomedical sciences.

Without talented artists, an Illustrated Review would be impossible, and we have been particularly fortunate in working with Michael Cooper throughout this project. His artistic sense and computer graphics expertise have greatly added to our ability to bring alive pharmacology "stories" for our readers. We also wish to thank Jo Gershman, who was a contributing artist.

The editors and production staff of the Lippincott William & Wilkins were a constant source of encouragement and discipline. We particularly want to acknowledge the tremendously helpful, supportive, creative contributions of our editor, Richard Winters, whose imagination and positive attitude helped us out of the valleys. Final editing and assembly of the book has been greatly enhanced through the efforts of Janet Greenwood and Mary Beth Murphy. Finally, the authors give thanks to Drs. Marilyn Schorin and Sewell Champe for their unfailing personal and professional support of this project, and to the late John Mycek for his encouragement.

Contents

UNIT I: Introduction to Pharmacology

Chapter 1: Absorption, Distribution, and Elimination of Drugs **1**
Chapter 2: Pharmacokinetics and Drug Receptors **17**

UNIT II: Drugs Affecting the Autonomic Nervous System

Chapter 3: The Autonomic Nervous System **27**
Chapter 4: Cholinergic Agonists **35**
Chapter 5: Cholinergic Antagonists **45**
Chapter 6: Adrenergic Agonists **55**
Chapter 7: Adrenergic Antagonists **71**

UNIT III: Drugs Affecting the Central Nervous System

Chapter 8: Treatment of Parkinson's Disease **81**
Chapter 9: Anxiolytic and Hypnotic Drugs **89**
Chapter 10: CNS Stimulants **99**
Chapter 11: Anesthetics **107**
Chapter 12: Antidepressant Drugs **119**
Chapter 13: Neuroleptic Drugs **127**
Chapter 14: Opioid Analgesics and Antagonists **133**
Chapter 15: Drugs Used to Treat Epilepsy **143**

UNIT IV: Drugs Affecting the Cardiovascular System

Chapter 16: The Treatment of Congestive Heart Failure **151**
Chapter 17: Antiarrhythmic Drugs **163**
Chapter 18: Antianginal Drugs **175**
Chapter 19: Antihypertensive Drugs **179**
Chapter 20: Drugs Affecting Blood **193**
Chapter 21: Antihyperlipidemic Drugs **207**

UNIT V: Drugs Affecting Other Organ Systems

Chapter 22: Drugs Affecting the Respiratory System **217**
Chapter 23: Diuretic Drugs **223**
Chapter 24: Gastrointestinal and Antiemetic Drugs **235**
Chapter 25: Hormones of the Pituitary and Thyroid **247**
Chapter 26: Insulin and Oral Hypoglycemic Drugs **255**
Chapter 27: Steroid Hormones **263**

UNIT VI: Chemotherapeutic Drugs

Chapter 28: Principles of Antimicrobial Therapy **279**
Chapter 29: Folate Antagonists **289**
Chapter 30: Inhibitors of Cell Wall Synthesis **297**
Chapter 31: Protein Synthesis Inhibitors **311**
Chapter 32: Quinolones and Urinary Tract Antiseptics **323**
Chapter 33: Antimycobacterial Drugs **331**
Chapter 34: Antifungal Drugs **337**
Chapter 35: Antiprotozoal Drugs **345**
Chapter 36: Anthelmintic Drugs **359**
Chapter 37: Antiviral Drugs **363**
Chapter 38: Anticancer Drugs **373**

UNIT VII: Anti-Inflammatory Drugs and Autacoids
Chapter 39: Anti-inflammatory Drugs **401**
Chapter 40: Autacoids and Autacoid Antagonists **419**

Appendix: Illustrated Case Studies **429**

Pharmacology Update
Chapter 8: Treatment of Parkinson's Disease **443**
Chapter 15: Drugs Used to Treat Epilepsy **445**
Chapter 20: Drugs Affecting Blood **446**
Chapter 21: Antihyperlipidemic Drugs **449**
Chapter 22: Drugs Affecting the Respiratory System **450**
Chapter 26: Insulin and Oral Hypoglycemic Drugs **452**
Chapter 27: Steroid Hormones **454**
Chapter 32: Quinolones and Urinary Tract Antiseptics **456**
Chapter 37: Antiviral Drugs **457**
Chapter 38: Anticancer Drugs **463**
Chapter 39: Anti-inflammatory Drugs **466**
Chapter 40: Autacoids and Autacoid Antagonists **470**

Chapter 41: Immunosuppressants **470**
Chapter 42: Drugs Used to Treat Obesity **474**
Chapter 43: Drug Used to Treat Osteoporosis **476**
Chapter 44: Miscellaneous Drugs **477**

Index **479**

Lippincott's Illustrated Reviews: Pharmacology

2nd edition

UNIT I:
Introduction to Pharmacology

Absorption, Distribution, and Elimination of Drugs

1

I. OVERVIEW

The aim of drug therapy is to prevent, cure, or control various disease states. To achieve this goal, adequate drug doses must be delivered to the target tissues so that therapeutic, yet nontoxic levels are obtained. The clinician must recognize that the speed of onset of drug action, the intensity of the drug's effect, and the duration of the drug action are controlled by four fundamental pathways of drug movement and modification in the body (Figure 1.1). First, drug absorption from the site of administration permits entry of the therapeutic agent (either directly or indirectly) into plasma (input). Second, the drug may then reversibly leave the blood stream and distribute into the interstitial and intracellular fluids (distribution). Third, the drug may be metabolized by the liver, kidney, or other tissues. Finally, the drug and its metabolites are eliminated from the body (output) in urine, bile, or feces. Chapters 1 and 2 describe how knowledge of these processes influences the clinician's decision as to the route of administration, drug loading, and dosing interval.

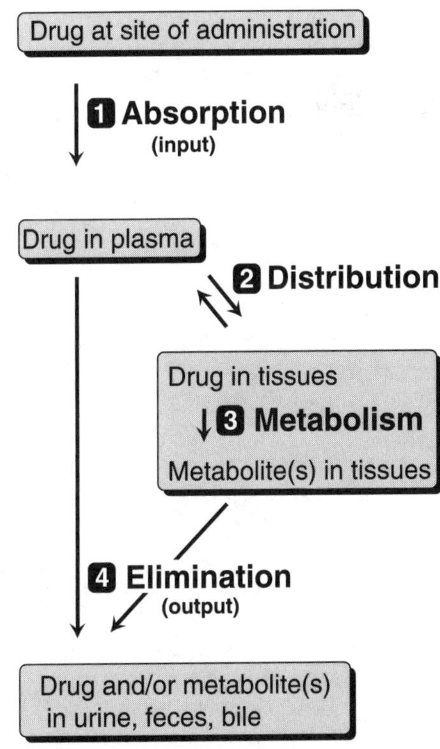

Figure 1.1
Schematic representation of drug absorption, distribution, metabolism and elimination.

II. ROUTES OF DRUG ADMINISTRATION

The route of administration is determined primarily by the properties of the drug (such as water or lipid solubility, ionization, etc.) and by the therapeutic objectives (for example, the desirability of a rapid onset of action or the need for long-term administration or restriction to a local site). There are two major routes of drug administration, enteral and parenteral. (Figure 1.2 illustrates the subcategories of these routes as well as other methods of drug administration.)

Lippincott's Illustrated Reviews: Pharmacology, Second Edition.
by Mary J. Mycek, Richard A. Harvey and Pamela C. Champe.
Lippincott Williams & Wilkins, Philadelphia, PA © 2000.

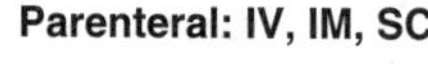

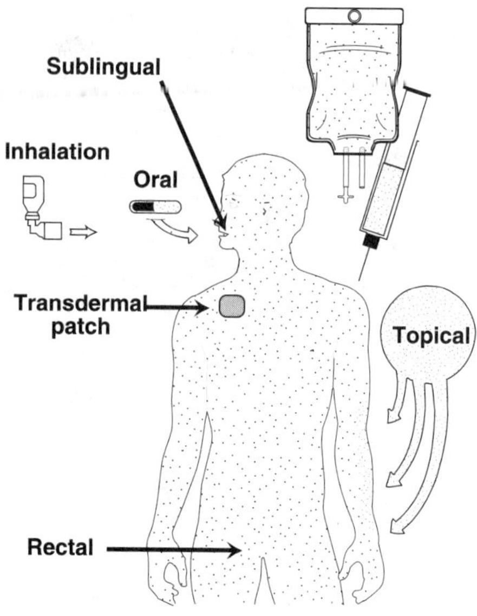

Figure 1.2
Commonly used routes of drug administration. (IV=intravenous; IM=intramuscular; SC=subcutaneous).

A. Enteral

1. **Oral:** Giving a drug by mouth is the most common route of administration, but it is also the most variable, and requires the most complicated pathway to the tissues. Some drugs are absorbed from the stomach; however, the duodenum is often the major site of entry to the systemic circulation because of its larger absorptive surface. [Note: Most drugs absorbed from the gastrointestinal (GI) tract enter the portal circulation and encounter the liver before they are distributed in the general circulation (Figure 1.3). First-pass metabolism by the intestine or liver limits the efficacy of many drugs when taken orally. For example, more than 90% of *nitroglycerin* is cleared during a single passage through the liver.] Ingestion of drugs with food can influence absorption. The presence of food in the stomach delays gastric emptying time so that drugs that are destroyed by acid, for example, *penicillin*, become unavailable for absorption (see p. 302). [Note: Enteric coating of a drug protects it from the acidic environment and may prevent gastric irritation. Depending on the formulation, the release of the drug may be prolonged, producing a sustained-release preparation.]

2. **Sublingual:** Placement under the tongue allows the drug to diffuse into the capillary network and therefore to enter the systemic circulation directly. Administration of an agent by this route has the advantage that the drug bypasses the intestine and liver and is not inactivated by metabolism.

3. **Rectal:** Fifty percent of the drainage of the rectal region bypasses the portal circulation; thus the biotransformation of drugs by the liver is minimized. Both the sublingual and the rectal routes of administration have the additional advantage that they prevent the destruction of the drug by intestinal enzymes or by low pH in the stomach. The rectal route is also useful if the drug induces vomiting when given orally or if the patient is already vomiting. [Note: The rectal route also is commonly used to administer antiemetic agents.]

B. Parenteral

Parenteral administration is used for drugs that are poorly absorbed from the gastrointestinal (GI) tract, and for agents such as *insulin* that are unstable in the GI tract. Parenteral administration is also used for treatment of unconscious patients and under circumstances that require a rapid onset of action. Parenteral administration provides the most control over the actual dose of drug delivered to the body. The three major parenteral routes are intravascular (intravenous or intra-arterial), intramuscular, and subcutaneous (see Figure 1.2). Each has its advantages and drawbacks.

1. **Intravascular:** Intravenous (IV) injection is the most common parenteral route. For drugs that are not absorbed orally, there is often no other choice. With IV administration, the drug avoids the GI tract and, therefore, first-pass metabolism by the liver. This route permits a rapid effect and a maximal degree of control over the circulating levels of the drug. However, unlike drugs present in the GI tract, those that are injected cannot be recalled by

strategies such as emesis or binding to activated charcoal. Intravenous injection of some drugs may introduce bacteria through contamination, induce hemolysis, or cause other adverse reactions by the too rapid delivery of high concentrations of drug to the plasma and tissues. Therefore, the rate of infusion must be carefully controlled. Similar concerns apply to intra-arterially (IA) injected drugs.

2. **Intramuscular (IM):** Drugs administered intramuscularly can be aqueous solutions or specialized depot preparations—often a suspension of drug in a nonaqueous vehicle, such as ethylene glycol or peanut oil. Absorption of drugs in aqueous solution is fast, whereas that from depot preparations is slow. As the vehicle diffuses out of the muscle, the drug precipitates at the site of injection. The drug then dissolves slowly, providing a sustained dose over an extended period of time. An example is sustained-release *haloperidol decanoate* (see p. 130), whose slow diffusion from the muscle produces an extended neuroleptic effect.

3. **Subcutaneous (SC):** This route of administration, like that of IM injection, requires absorption and is somewhat slower than the IV route. SC injection minimizes the risks associated with intravascular injection. [Note: Minute amounts of *epinephrine* are sometimes combined with a drug to restrict its area of action. *Epinephrine* acts as a local vasoconstrictor and decreases removal of a drug, such as *lidocaine*, from the site of administration.] Other examples of drugs utilizing SC administration include solids such as silastic capsules containing the contraceptive *levonorgestrel* that are implanted for long-term activity (see p. 268), and also programmable mechanical pumps that can be implanted to deliver *insulin* in some diabetics.

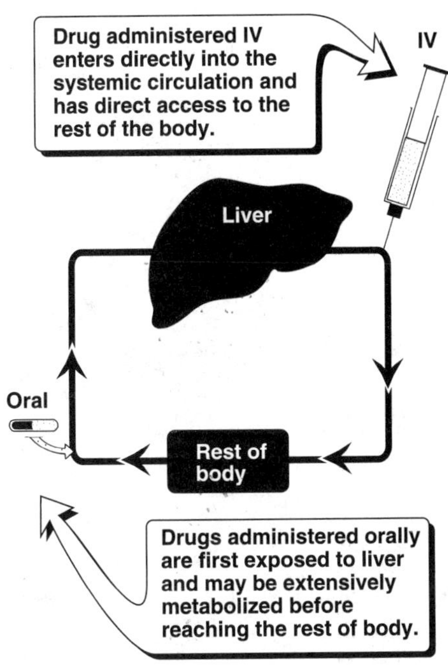

Drug administered IV enters directly into the systemic circulation and has direct access to the rest of the body.
IV
Liver
Oral
Rest of body
Drugs administered orally are first exposed to liver and may be extensively metabolized before reaching the rest of body.

Figure 1.3
First-pass metabolism can occur with orally administered drugs. (IV = intravenous).

C. Other

1. **Inhalation:** Inhalation provides the rapid delivery of a drug across the large surface area of the mucous membranes of the respiratory tract and pulmonary epithelium, producing an effect almost as rapidly as by intravenous injection. This route of administration is used for drugs that are gases (for example, some anesthetics), or those that can be dispersed in an aerosol. The route is particularly effective and convenient for patients with respiratory complaints (for example, asthma or chronic obstructive pulmonary disease) as drug is delivered directly to the site of action and systemic side effects are minimized (see p. 219).

2. **Intranasal:** *Desmopressin* is administered intranasally in the treatment of diabetes insipidus; salmon *calcitonin*, a peptide hormone used in the treatment of of osteoporosis, is available as a nasal spray. The abused drug, *cocaine*, is generally taken by sniffing.

3. **Intrathecal/Intraventricular:** It is sometimes necessary to introduce drugs directly into the cerebrospinal fluid (CSF), such as *methotrexate* in acute lymphocytic leukemia (see p. 379).

4. **Topical:** Topical application is used when a local effect of the drug is desired. For example, *clotrimazole* (see p. 343) is applied as a

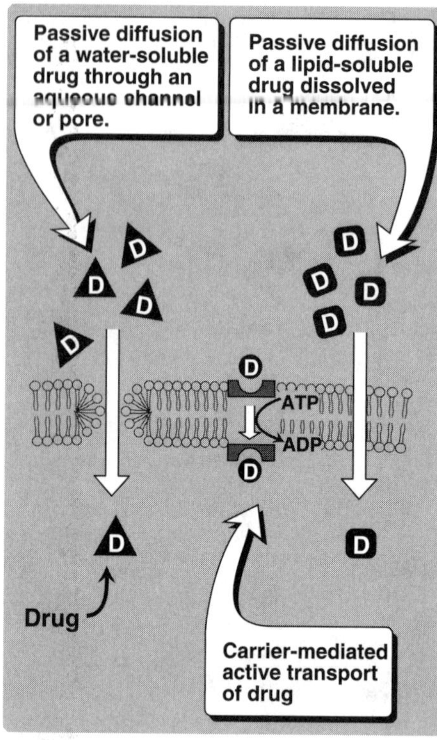

Figure 1.4
Schematic representation of drugs crossing cell membrane of epithelial cell of gastrointestinal tract.

cream directly to the skin in the treatment of dermatophytosis, and *atropine* (see p. 47) is instilled directly into the eye to dilate the pupil and permit measurement of refractive errors.

5. **Transdermal:** This route of administration achieves systemic effects by application of drugs to the skin, usually via a transdermal patch. The rate of absorption can vary markedly depending upon the physical characteristics of the skin at the site of application. This route is most often used for the sustained delivery of drugs, such as the antianginal drug, *nitroglycerin* (see p. 175).

III. ABSORPTION OF DRUGS

Absorption is the transfer of a drug from its site of administration to the blood stream. The rate and efficiency of absorption depend on the route of administration. For intravenous delivery, absorption is complete, that is, the total dose of drug reaches the systemic circulation. Drug delivery by other routes may result in only partial absorption and thus lower bioavailability. For example, the oral route requires that a drug dissolve in the gastrointestinal fluid and then penetrate the epithelial cells of the intestinal mucosa; disease states or the presence of food may affect this process.

A. Transport of drug from the GI tract

Depending on their chemical properties, drugs may be absorbed from the GI tract by either passive diffusion or active transport.

1. **Passive diffusion:** The driving force for passive absorption of a drug is the concentration gradient across a membrane separating two body compartments, that is, the drug moves from a region of high concentration to one of lower concentration. Passive diffusion does not involve a carrier, is not saturable, and shows a low structural specificity. The vast majority of drugs gain access to the body by this mechanism. Lipid-soluble drugs readily move across most biological membranes, whereas water-soluble drugs penetrate the cell membrane through aqueous channels (Figure 1.4).

2. **Active transport:** This mode of drug entry involves specific carrier proteins that span the membrane. A few drugs that closely resemble the structure of naturally occurring metabolites are actively transported across cell membranes using these specific carrier proteins. Active transport is energy-dependent and is driven by the hydrolysis of adenosine triphosphate (see Figure 1.4). It is capable of moving drugs against a concentration gradient, that is, from a region of low drug concentration to one of higher drug concentration. The process shows saturation kinetics for the carrier, much in the same way that an enzyme-catalyzed reaction shows a maximal velocity at high substrate levels when binding to the enzyme is maximal.[1]

B. Effect of pH on drug absorption

Most drugs are either weak acids or weak bases. Acidic drugs (HA) release a H^+ causing a charged anion (A^-) to form:[2]

[1,2]See p. 16 for Infolink references to other books in this series.

$$HA \rightleftarrows H^+ + A^-$$

Weak bases (BH^+) can also release a H^+; however, the protonated form of basic drugs is usually charged, and loss of a proton produces the uncharged base (B).

$$BH^+ \rightleftarrows B + H^+$$

1. **Passage of an uncharged drug through a membrane:** A drug passes through membranes more readily if it is uncharged (Figure 1.5). Thus, for a weak acid, the uncharged HA can permeate through membranes, and A^- cannot. For a weak base, the uncharged form, B, penetrates through the cell membrane, but BH^+ does not. Therefore, the effective concentration of the permeable form of each drug at its absorption site is determined by the relative concentrations of the charged and uncharged forms. The ratio between the two forms is, in turn, determined by the pH at the site of absorption and by the strength of the weak acid or base, which is represented by the pK_a (Figure 1.6). [Note: The pK_a is a measure of the strength of the interaction of a compound with a proton. The lower the pK_a of a drug, the stronger the acid. Conversely, the higher the pK_a, the stronger the base.] Distribution equilibrium is achieved when the permeable form of drug achieves an equal concentration in all body water spaces. Highly lipid-soluble drugs rapidly cross membranes and often enter tissues at a rate determined by blood flow.

2. **Determination of how much drug will be found on either side of a membrane:** The relationship of pK_a and the ratio of acid-base concentrations to pH is expressed by the Henderson-Hasselbalch equation[3]:

$$pH = pK_a + \log \frac{[\text{non-protonated species}]}{[\text{protonated species}]}$$

$$\text{For acids: } pH = pK_a + \log \frac{[A^-]}{[HA]}$$

$$\text{For bases: } pH = pK_a + \log \frac{[B]}{[BH^+]}$$

This equation is useful in determining how much drug will be found on either side of a membrane that separates two compartments that differ in pH, for example, stomach (pH 1.0 to 1.5) and blood plasma (pH 7.4). [Note: The lipid solubility of the nonionized drug directly determines its rate of equilibration.]

C. Physical factors influencing absorption

1. **Blood flow to the absorption site:** Blood flow to the intestine is much greater than the flow to the stomach; thus absorption from the intestine is favored over that from the stomach. [Note: Shock

A Weak acid

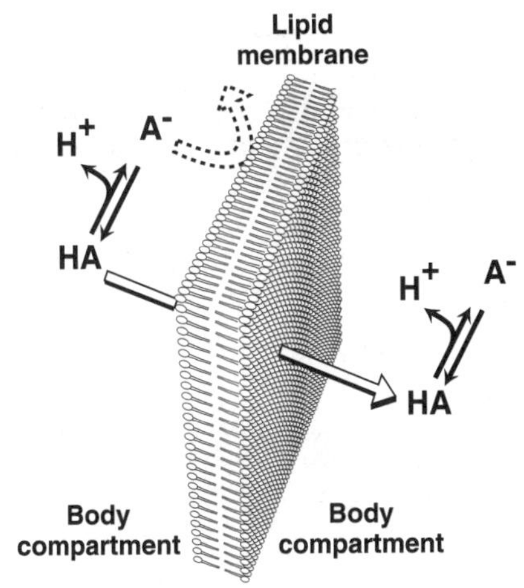

B Weak base

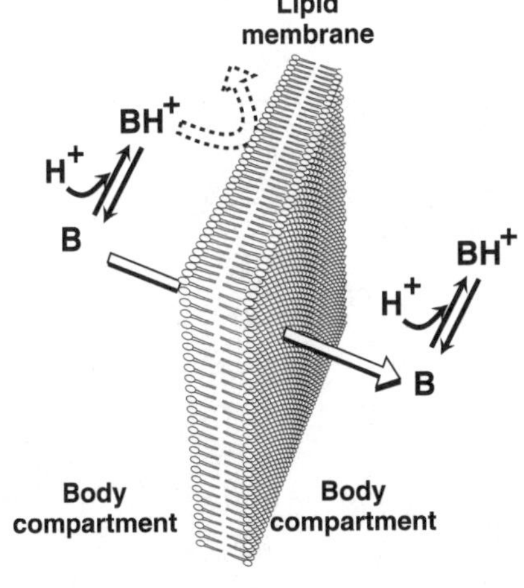

Figure 1.5
A. Diffusion of non-ionized form of a weak acid through lipid membrane; B. Diffusion of non-ionized form of a weak base through lipid membrane.

[3]See p. 16 for Infolink references to other books in this series.

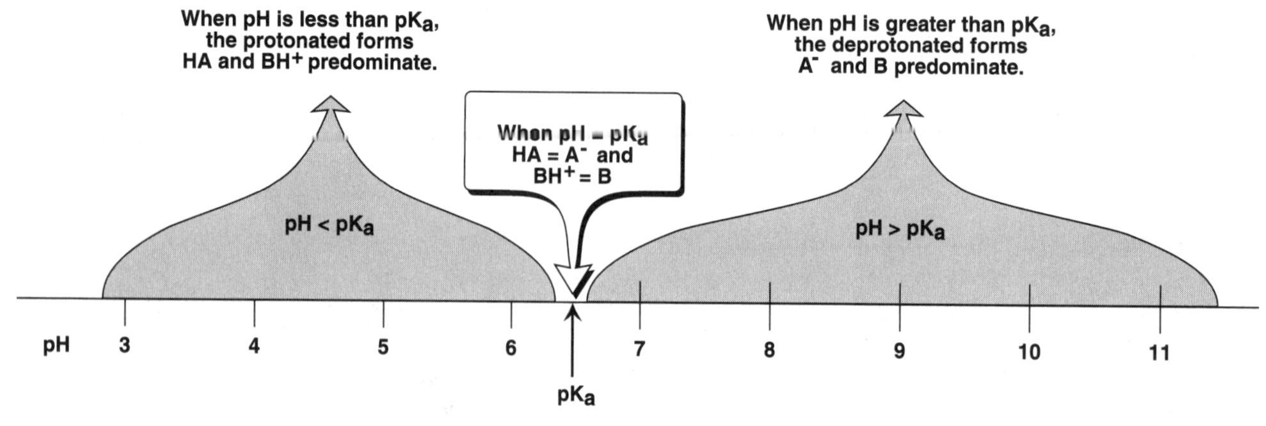

Figure 1.6
The distribution of a drug between its ionized and un-ionized form depends on the ambient pH and pK_a of the drug. For illustrative purposes, the drug has been assigned a pK_a of 6.5.

severely reduces blood flow to cutaneous tissues, thus minimizing the absorption from subcutaneous administration.]

2. **Total surface area available for absorption:** Because the intestine has a surface rich in microvilli, it has a surface area about 1,000 times that of the stomach; thus absorption of the drug across the intestine is more efficient.

3. **Contact time at the absorption surface:** If a drug moves through the GI tract very quickly, as in severe diarrhea, it is not well absorbed. Conversely, anything that delays the transport of the drug from the stomach to the intestine delays the rate of absorption of the drug. [Note: Parasympathetic input increases the rate of gastric emptying, whereas sympathetic input (prompted, for example, by exercise or stressful emotions) prolongs gastric emptying. Also, the presence of food in the stomach both dilutes the drug and slows gastric emptying. Therefore, a drug taken with a meal is generally absorbed more slowly.]

IV. BIOAVAILABILITY

Bioavailability is the fraction of administered drug that reaches the systemic circulation. Bioavailability is expressed as the fraction of administered drug that gains access to the systemic circulation in a chemically unchanged form. For example, if 100 mg of a drug is administered orally and 70 mg of this drug is absorbed unchanged, the bioavailability is 70%.

A. Determination of bioavailability

Bioavailability is determined by comparing plasma levels of a drug after a particular route of administration (for example, oral administration) with plasma drug levels achieved by IV injection, in which all of the agent enters the circulation. When the drug is given orally, only part of the administered dose appears in the plasma. By plotting plasma concentrations of the drug versus time, one can measure the area under the curve (AUC). This curve reflects the extent of absorption of the drug. [Note: By definition this is 100% for drugs delivered intravenously.] Bioavailability of a drug administered orally is the ratio of the area calculated for oral administration compared with the area calculated for IV injection (Figure 1.7).

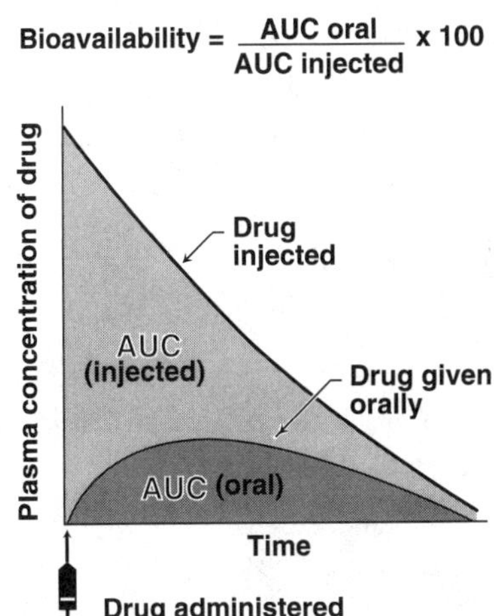

Figure 1.7
Determination of the bioavailability of a drug. (AUC = area under curve.)

B. Factors that influence bioavailability

1. **First-pass hepatic metabolism:** When a drug is absorbed across the GI tract, it enters the portal circulation before entering the systemic circulation (see Figure 1.3). If the drug is rapidly metabolized by the liver, the amount of unchanged drug that gains access to the systemic circulation is decreased. Many drugs, such as *propranolol* or *lidocaine*, undergo significant biotransformation during a single passage through the liver.

2. **Solubility of drug:** Very hydrophilic drugs are poorly absorbed because of their inability to cross the lipid-rich cell membranes. Paradoxically, drugs that are extremely hydrophobic are also poorly absorbed, because they are totally insoluble in the aqueous body fluids and, therefore, cannot gain access to the surface of cells. For a drug to be readily absorbed it must be largely hydrophobic yet have some solubility in aqueous solutions.

3. **Chemical instability:** Some drugs, such as *penicillin G* (see p. 302), are unstable in the pH of the gastric contents. Others, such as *insulin* (see p. 258), may be destroyed in the GI tract by degradative enzymes.

4. **Nature of the drug formulation:** Drug absorption may be altered by factors unrelated to the chemistry of the drug. For example, particle size, salt form, crystal polymorphism, and the presence of excipients (such as binders and dispersing agents) can influence the ease of dissolution and, therefore, alter the rate of absorption.

C. Bioequivalence

Two related drugs are bioequivalent if they show comparable bioavailability and similar times to achieve peak blood concentrations. Two related drugs with a significant difference in bioavailability are said to be bioinequivalent.

D. Therapeutic equivalence

Two similar drugs are therapeutically equivalent if they have comparable efficacy and safety. [Note: Clinical effectiveness often depends both on maximum serum drug concentrations and the time after administration required to reach peak concentration. Therefore, two drugs that are bioequivalent may not be therapeutically equivalent.]

V. DRUG DISTRIBUTION

Drug distribution is the process by which a drug reversibly leaves the blood stream and enters the interstitium (extracellular fluid) and/or the cells of the tissues. The delivery of a drug from the plasma to the inter-

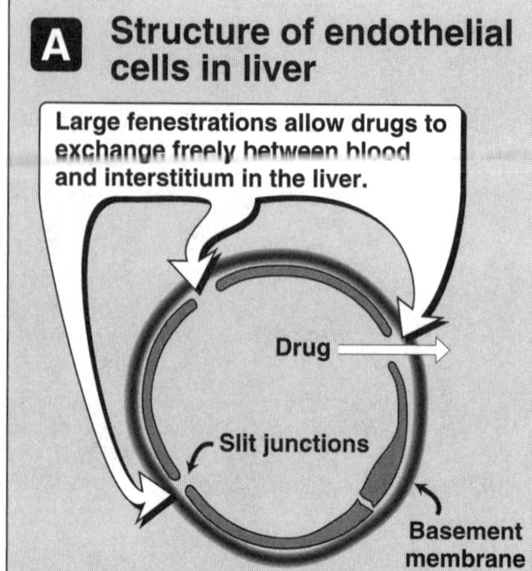

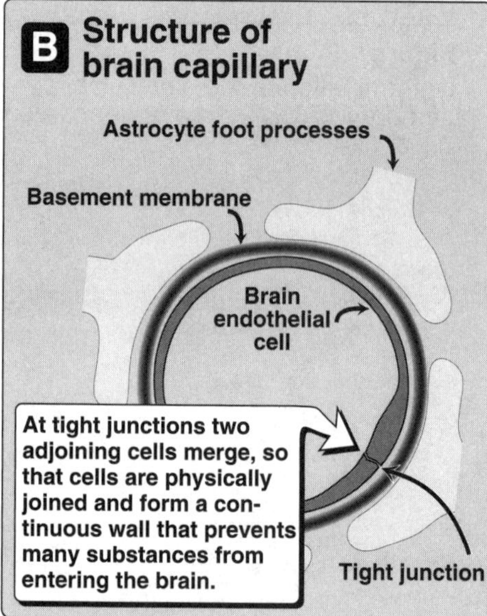

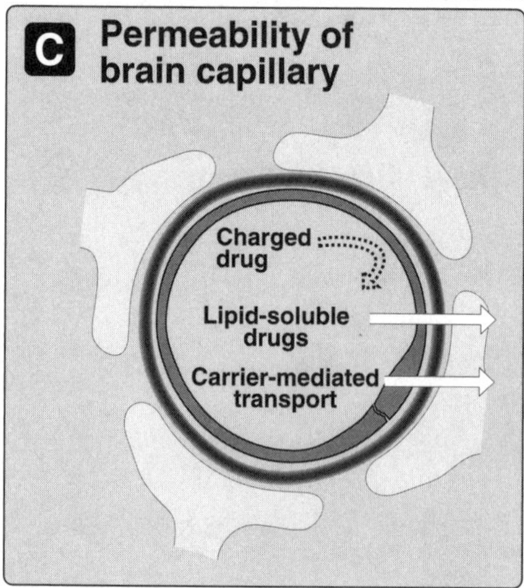

Figure 1.8
Cross section of liver and brain capillaries.

stitium primarily depends on blood flow, capillary permeability, the degree of binding of the drug to plasma and tissue proteins, and the relative hydrophobicity of the drug.

A. Blood flow

The rate of blood flow to the tissue capillaries varies widely as a result of the unequal distribution of cardiac output to the various organs. Blood flow to the brain, liver, and kidney is greater than that to the skeletal muscles, whereas adipose tissue has a still lower rate of blood flow.

B. Capillary permeability

Capillary permeability is determined by capillary structure and by the chemical nature of the drug.

1. **Capillary structure:** Capillary structure varies widely in terms of the fraction of the basement membrane that is exposed by slit (tight) junctions between endothelial cells. In the brain, the capillary structure is continuous, and there are no slit junctions (Figure 1.8). This contrasts with the liver and spleen, where a large part of the basement membrane is exposed due to large discontinuous capillaries, through which large plasma proteins can pass.

   a. **Blood-brain barrier:** In order to enter the brain, drugs must pass through the endothelial cells of the capillaries of the central nervous system (CNS) or be actively transported. For example, the large neutral amino acid carrier transports *levodopa* into the brain. Lipid-soluble drugs readily penetrate into the CNS, since they can dissolve in the membrane of the endothelial cells. Ionized or polar drugs generally fail to enter the CNS, since they are unable to pass through the endothelial cells of the CNS, which have no slit junctions. These tightly juxtaposed cells form tight junctions that constitute the so-called blood-brain barrier (Figure 1.8).

2. **Drug structure:** The chemical nature of the drug strongly influences its ability to cross cell membranes. Hydrophobic drugs, which have a uniform distribution of electrons and no net charge, readily move across most biological membranes. These drugs can dissolve in the lipid membranes and therefore permeate the entire cell's surface. The major factor influencing the hydrophobic drug's distribution is the blood flow to the area. By contrast, hydrophilic drugs, which have either a nonuniform distribution of electrons or a positive or negative charge, do not readily penetrate cell membranes and must go through the slit junctions (see Figure 1.8).

C. Binding of drugs to proteins

Reversible binding to plasma proteins sequesters drugs in a non-diffusible form and slows their transfer out of the vascular compartment. Binding is relatively non-selective as to chemical structure and takes place at sites on the protein to which endogenous compounds such as bilirubin, normally attach. Plasma albumin is the major drug-binding protein and may act as a drug reservoir, for example, as the concentration of the free drug decreases due to elimination by metabolism or excretion, the bound drug dissociates from the protein. This maintains the free drug concentration as a constant fraction of the total drug in the plasma. (See p. 11 for further discussion of drug binding by proteins.)

VI. VOLUME OF DISTRIBUTION

The volume of distribution (V_d) is a hypothetical volume of fluid into which the drug is disseminated. Although the volume of distribution has no physiological or physical basis, it is sometimes useful to compare the distribution of a drug with the volumes of the water compartments in the body (Figure 1.9).

A. Water compartments in the body

Once a drug enters the body, from whatever route of administration, it has the potential to distribute into any one of three functionally distinct compartments of body water, or to become sequestered in some cellular site.

1. **Plasma compartment:** If a drug has a very large molecular weight or binds extensively to plasma proteins, it is too large to move out through the endothelial slit junctions of the capillaries and thus is effectively trapped within the plasma (vascular) compartment. As a consequence, the drug distributes in a volume (the plasma) that is about 6% of the body weight or, in a 70-kg individual, about 4 L of body fluid. Aminoglycoside antibiotics (see p. 314) show this type of distribution.

2. **Extracellular fluid:** If the drug has a low molecular weight but is hydrophilic, it can move through the endothelial slit junctions of the capillaries into the interstitial fluid. However, hydrophilic drugs cannot move across the membranes of cells to enter the water phase inside the cell. Therefore, these drugs distribute into a volume that is the sum of the plasma water and the interstitial fluid, which together constitute the extracellular fluid. This is about 20% of the body weight, or about 14 L in a 70-kg individual.

3. **Total body water:** If the drug has a low molecular weight and is hydrophobic, it can not only move into the interstitium through the slit junctions, but can also move through the cell membranes into the intracellular fluid. The drug therefore distributes into a volume of about 60% of body weight, or about 42 L in a 70-kg individual.

4. **Other sites:** In pregnancy, the fetus may take up drugs and thus increase the V_d. Drugs such as *thiopental* (see p. 115), which are stored in fat, may also have unusually high volumes of distribution.

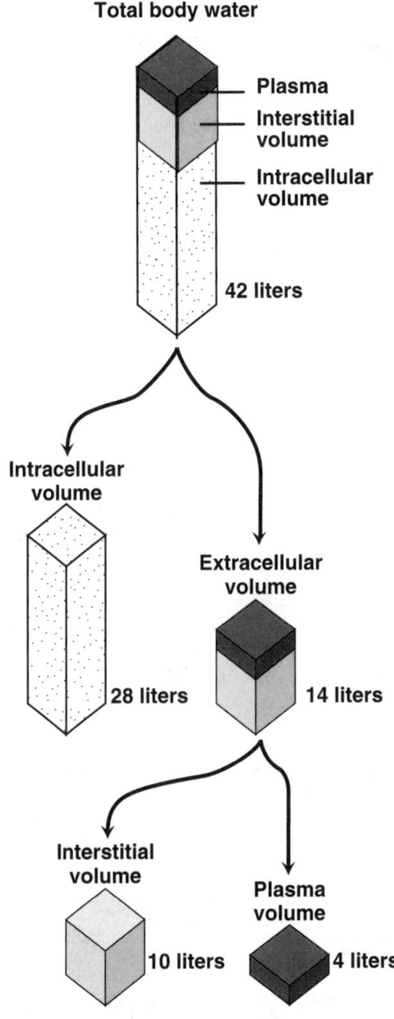

Figure 1.9
Relative size of various distribution volumes within a 70-kg individual.

B. The apparent volume of distribution

A drug rarely associates exclusively with only one of the water compartments of the body. Instead, the vast majority of drugs distribute into several compartments, often avidly binding cellular components, for example, lipids (abundant in adipocytes and cell membranes), proteins (abundant in plasma and within cells), or nucleic acids (abundant in the nuclei of cells). Therefore, the volume into which drugs distribute is called the apparent volume of distribution or V_d.

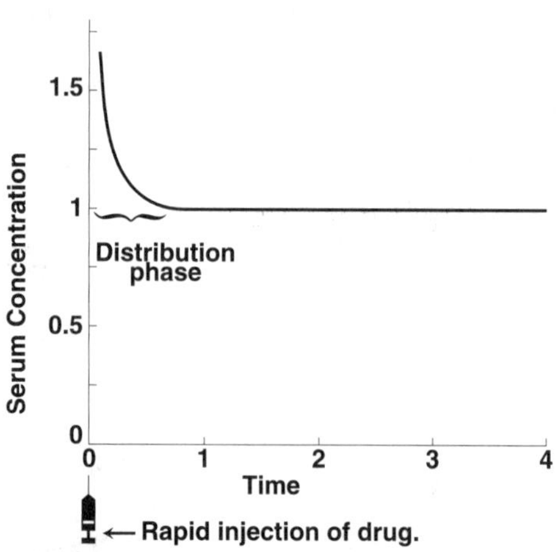

Figure 1.10
Drug concentrations in serum after a single injection of drug at time = 0. Assume that drug distributes but is not eliminated.

1. Determination of V_d

a. Distribution of drug in the absence of elimination: The apparent volume into which a drug distributes, V_d, is determined by injection of a standard dose of drug, which is initially contained entirely in the vascular system. The agent may then move from the plasma into the interstitium and into cells, causing the plasma concentration to decrease with time. Assume for simplicity that the drug is not eliminated from the body; the drug then achieves a uniform concentration that is sustained with time (Figure 1.10). The concentration within the vascular compartment is the total amount of drug administered divided by the volume into which it distributes, V_d:

$$C = D/V_d \quad \text{or} \quad V_d = D/C$$

C = Plasma concentration of drug
D = Total amount of drug in the body

For example, if 25 mg of a drug (D = 25 mg) is administered, and the plasma concentration is 1.0 mg/L, then the V_d = 25 mg/1.0 mg/L = 25 L.

b. Distribution of drug when elimination is present: In reality, drugs are eliminated from the body, and a plot of plasma concentration versus time shows two phases. The initial decrease in plasma concentration is due to a rapid distribution phase in which the drug is transferred from the plasma into the interstitium and the intracellular water. This is followed by a slower elimination phase during which the drug leaves the plasma compartment and is lost from the body, for example, by renal or biliary elimination or hepatic biotransformation (Figure 1.11). The rate at which the drug is eliminated is usually proportional to the concentration of drug (C), that is, the rate with most drugs is first order and shows a linear relationship with time if ln C (rather than C) is plotted versus time (Figure 1.12).

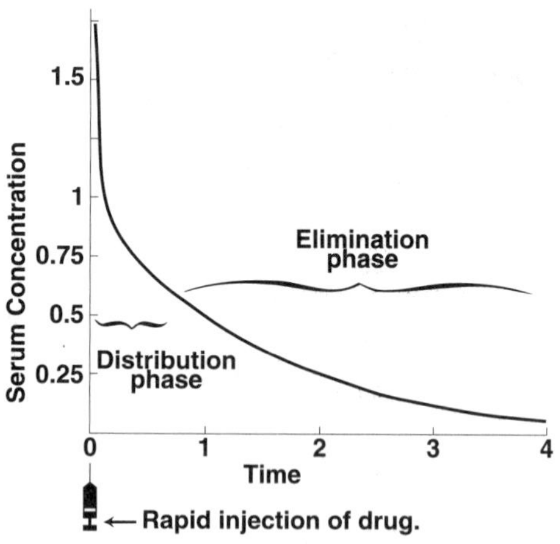

Figure 1.11
Drug concentrations in serum after a single injection of drug at time = 0. Assume that drug distributes and is subsequently eliminated.

c. Calculation of drug concentration if distribution were instantaneous: Assume that the elimination process began at the time of injection and continued throughout the distribution phase. Then the concentration of drug in the plasma, C, can be extrapolated back to zero time (the time of injection) to determine C_0, which is the concentration of drug that would have been achieved if the distribution phase had occurred instantly. For example, if 10 mg of drug is injected into a patient and the plasma concentration extrapolated to zero time concentration is C_0 = 1.0 mg/L (from graph shown in Figure 1.12), then V_d = 10 mg/1.0 mg/L = 10 L.

d. Uneven drug distribution between compartments: The apparent volume of distribution assumes that the drug distributes uniformly in a single compartment. However, most drugs distribute unevenly in several compartments and the volume of distribution does not describe a real, physical volume but rather reflects the ratio of drug in the extraplasmic spaces relative to the plasma space. Nonetheless, V_d is useful since it can be used to calculate the amount of drug needed to achieve a desired plasma concentration. For example, assume the arrhythmia of a cardiac patient is not well controlled due to inadequate plasma levels of *digitalis*. Suppose the concentration of the drug in the plasma is C_1 and the desired level of *digitalis* (known from clinical studies) is a higher concentration, C_2. The clinician needs to know how much additional drug should be administered to bring the circulating level of drug from C_1 to C_2.

$V_d \bullet C_1$ = amount of drug initially in body

$V_d \bullet C_2$ = amount of drug in the body needed to achieve the desired plasma concentration

The difference between the two values is the additional dosage needed, which equals $V_d(C_2 - C_1)$.

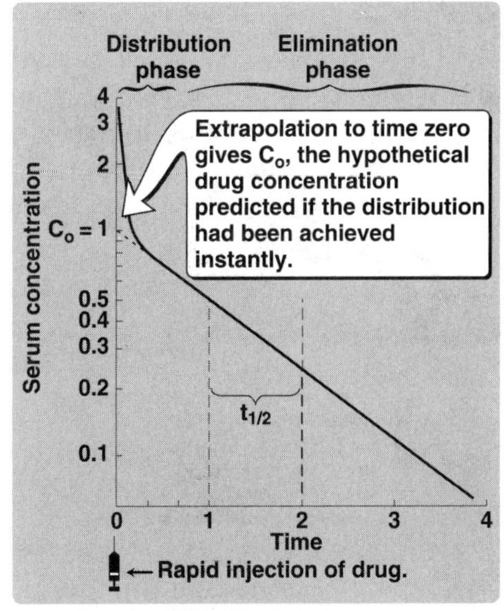

Figure 1.12
Drug concentrations in serum after a single injection of drug at time = 0. Data plotted on log scale.

2. **Effect of a large V_d on the half-life of a drug:** A large V_d has an important influence on the half-life of a drug, since drug elimination depends on the amount of drug delivered to the liver or kidney (or other organs where metabolism occurs) per unit of time. Delivery of drug to the organs of elimination depends not only on blood flow but also on the fraction of the drug in the plasma. If the V_d for a drug is large, most of the drug is in the extraplasmic space and is unavailable to the excretory organs. Therefore, any factor that increases the volume of distribution can lead to an increase in the half-life and extend the duration of action of the drug. [Note: An exceptionally large V_d indicates considerable sequestration of the drug in some organ or compartment.]

VII. BINDING OF DRUGS TO PLASMA PROTEINS

Drug molecules may bind to plasma proteins (usually albumin). Bound drugs are pharmacologically inactive; only the free, unbound drug can act on target sites in the tissues and elicit a biological response. Thus, by binding to plasma proteins, drugs become "trapped" and, in effect, inactive. [Note: Hypoalbuminemia may alter the level of free drug.]

A. Binding capacity of albumin

The binding of drugs to albumin is reversible and may show low capacity (one drug molecule per albumin molecule) or high capacity (a number of drug molecules binding to a single albumin molecule). Drugs can also bind with varying affinities. Albumin has the strongest affinity for anionic drugs (weak acids) and hydrophobic drugs. Most hydrophilic drugs and neutral drugs do not bind to albumin. [Note: Many drugs are hydrophobic by design, since this property permits absorption after oral administration.]

B. Competition for binding between drugs

When two drugs are given, each with high affinity for albumin, they compete for the available binding sites. The drugs with high affinity for albumin can be divided into two classes, depending on whether the dose of drug (the amount of drug found in the body under conditions used clinically) is greater than or less than the binding capacity of albumin (the number of millimoles of albumin multiplied by the number of binding sites, Figure 1.13).

A **Class I drugs: Dose less than available binding sites**

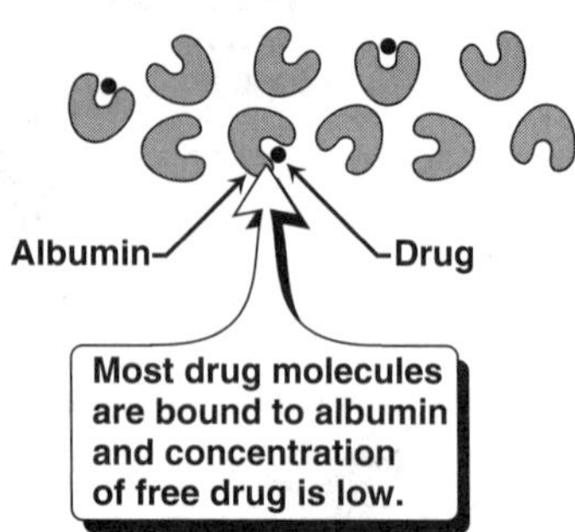

Albumin
Drug
Most drug molecules are bound to albumin and concentration of free drug is low.

B **Class II drugs: Dose greater than available binding sites**

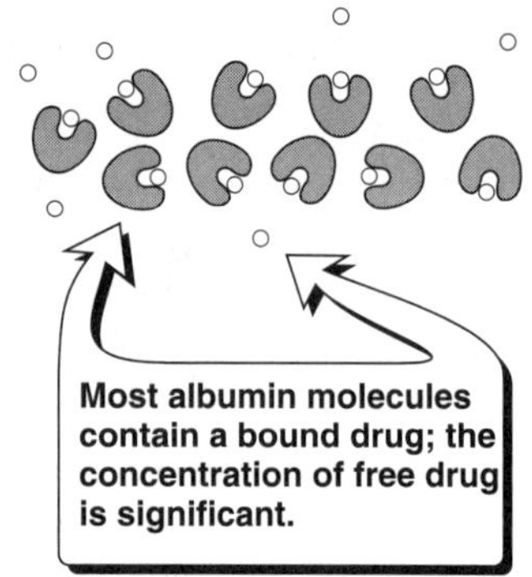

Most albumin molecules contain a bound drug; the concentration of free drug is significant.

C **Administration of a Class I and a Class II drug.**

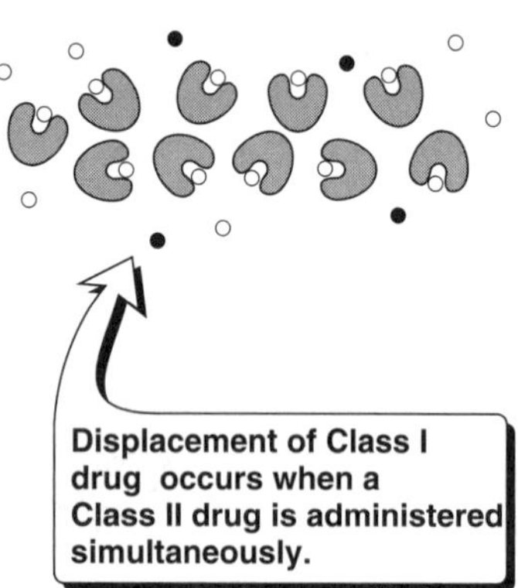

Displacement of Class I drug occurs when a Class II drug is administered simultaneously.

Figure 1.13
Binding of Class I and Class II drugs to albumin when drugs are administered alone (A,B), or together (C).

1. **Class I drugs:** If the dose of drug is less than the binding capacity of albumin, then the dose/capacity ratio is low. The binding sites are in excess of the available drug, and the drug fraction bound is high. This is the case for Class I drugs, which includes the majority of clinically useful agents.

2. **Class II drugs:** These drugs are given in doses that greatly exceed the number of albumin binding sites. The dose/capacity ratio is high, and a relatively high proportion of the drug exists in the free state, not bound to albumin.

3. **Clinical importance of drug displacement:** This assignment of drug classification assumes importance when a patient who is taking a Class I drug, such as *tolbutamide*, is given a Class II drug, such as a sulfonamide antibiotic. The *tolbutamide* is normally 95% bound, and only 5% is free. This means that most of the drug is sequestered on albumin and is inert in terms of exerting pharmacologic actions. If a sulfonamide is administered, it displaces *tolbutamide* from albumin, leading to a rapid increase in the concentration of free *tolbutamide* in plasma, because almost 100% is now free compared with the initial 5%. [Note: The *tolbutamide* concentration does not remain elevated since the drug moves out of the plasma into the interstitial fluid and achieves a new equilibrium.]

C. Relationship of drug displacement to V_d

The impact of drug displacement from albumin depends on both V_d and the therapeutic index of the drug. If the V_d is large, the drug displaced from the albumin distributes to the periphery and the change in free drug concentration in the plasma is not significant. If the V_d is small, the newly displaced drug does not move into the tissues as much, and the increase in free drug in the plasma is more profound. If the therapeutic index (see p. 22) of the drug is small, this increase in drug concentration may have significant clinical consequences. [Note: Clinically, drug displacement from albumin is one of the most significant sources of drug interactions.]

VIII. DRUG METABOLISM

Drugs are most often eliminated by biotransformation and/or excretion into the urine or bile. The liver is the major site for drug metabolism, but specific drugs may undergo biotransformation in other tissues. [Note: Some agents are initially administered as inactive compounds (prodrugs) and must be metabolized to their active forms.]

A. Kinetics of metabolism:

1. **First-order kinetics:** The metabolic transformation of drugs is catalyzed by enzymes, and most of the reactions obey Michaelis-Menten kinetics.[4]

$$v = \text{rate of drug metabolism} = \frac{V_{max}\,[C]}{K_m + [C]}$$

In most clinical situations the concentration of the drug, [C], is much less than the Michaelis constant, K_m, and the Michaelis-Menten equation reduces to

$$v = \text{rate of drug metabolism} = \frac{V_{max}\,[C]}{K_m}$$

that is, the rate of drug metabolism is directly proportional to the concentration of free drug, and first order kinetics are observed (Figure 1.14). This means that a constant fraction of drug is metabolized per unit time.

2. **Zero-order kinetics:** With a few drugs, such as *aspirin* (see p. 407), *ethanol* and *phenytoin* (see p. 146), the doses are very large, so the [C] is much greater than K_m, and the velocity equation becomes:

$$v = \text{rate of drug metabolism} = \frac{V_{max}\,[C]}{[C]} = V_{max}$$

The enzyme is saturated by a high free-drug concentration, and the rate of metabolism remains constant over time. This is called zero order kinetics (or sometimes referred to clinically as non-linear kinetics). A constant amount of drug is metabolized per unit time.

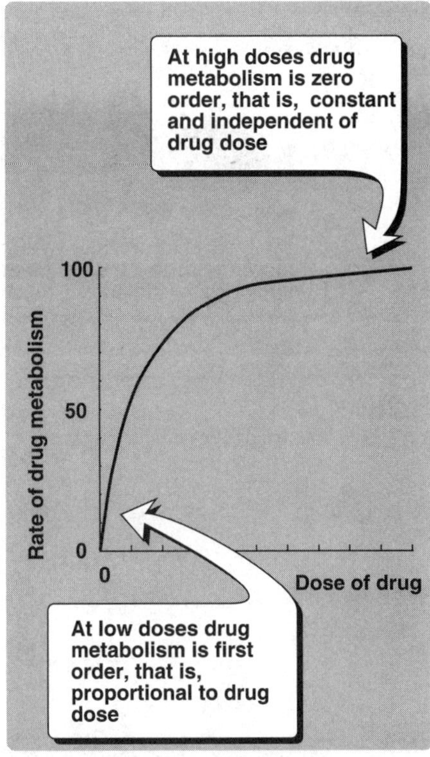
At high doses drug metabolism is zero order, that is, constant and independent of drug dose
100
50
0
Rate of drug metabolism
0
Dose of drug
At low doses drug metabolism is first order, that is, proportional to drug dose

Figure 1.14
Effect of drug dose on the rate of metabolism.

B. Reactions of drug metabolism

The kidney cannot efficiently eliminate lipophilic drugs that readily cross cell membranes and are reabsorbed in the distal tubules (see p. 23). Therefore, lipid-soluble agents must first be metabolized in the liver using two general sets of reactions, called Phase I and Phase II (Figure 1.15).

1. **Phase I:** Phase I reactions function to convert lipophilic molecules into more polar molecules by introducing or unmasking a polar functional group, such as –OH, or $-NH_2$. Phase I metabolism may increase, decrease, or leave unaltered the drug's pharmacologic activity.

   a. **Phase I reactions utilizing the P-450 system:** The Phase I reactions most frequently involved in drug metabolism are catalyzed by the cytochrome P-450 system (also called microsomal mixed function oxidase).

$$\text{Drug} + O_2 + \text{NADPH} + H^+ \rightarrow \text{Drug}_{\text{modified}} + H_2O + \text{NADP}^+$$

[4]See p. 16 for Infolink references to other books in this series.

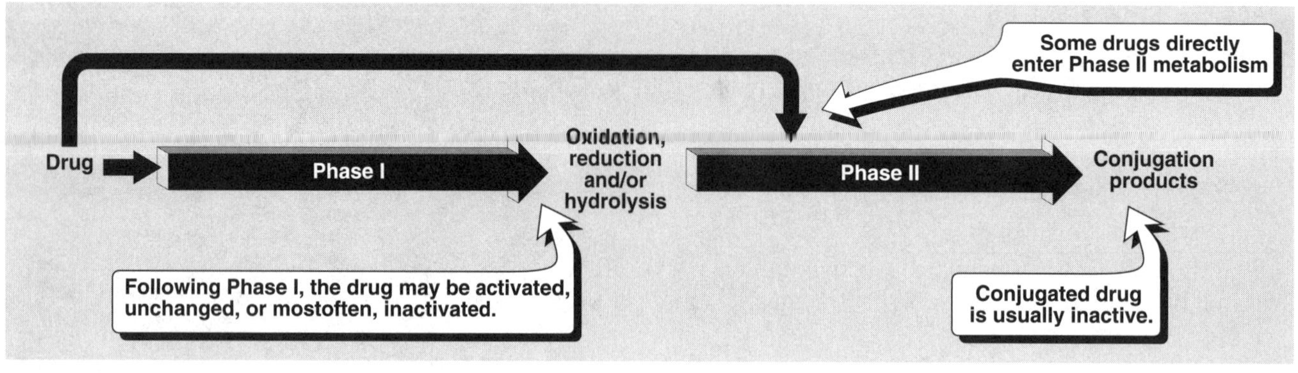

Figure 1.15
The biotransformations of drugs.

Isozyme: CYP2C9/10

COMMON SUBSTRATES	INDUCERS
Warfarin Phenytoin Ibuprofen Tolbutamide	Phenobarbital Rifampin

Isozyme: CYP2D6

COMMON SUBSTRATES	INDUCERS
Desipramine Imipramine Haloperidol Propanolol	

Isozyme: CYP3A4/5

COMMON SUBSTRATES	INDUCERS
Carbamazepine Cyclosporine Erythromycin Nifedipine Verapamil	Carbamazepine Dexamethasone Phenobarbital Phenytoin Rifampin

Figure 1.16
Some representative P-450 isozymes.

The oxidation proceeds by the drug binding to the oxidized form of cytochrome P-450, and then oxygen is introduced through a reductive step coupled to NADPH:cytochrome P-450 oxidoreductase.

b. **Summary of the P-450 system:** The P-450 system is important for the metabolism of many endogenous compounds (steroids, lipids, etc.), and for the detoxication of exogenous substances. Cytochrome P-450, designated as CYP, is composed of many families of heme-containing isozymes that are located in most cells, but mainly those in the liver and intestinal tract. [Note: The term, P-450, originates from the spectral peak produced at or near 450 nm when the isozyme (in its reduced state) is treated with carbon monoxide.] The family name is indicated by a number followed by a capital letter for the subfamily (e.g., CYP3A). Another number is added to indicate the specific isozyme (CYP3A4). Each of the isozymes has a broad and overlapping specificity (see Figure 1.16). Some drugs can induce the synthesis of many different isozymes, thereby accelerating the clearance of substrates of those metabolic pathways and decreasing their levels. Conversely, clearance of substances can by lowered and their levels elevated by inhibition of their biotransformation. The interplay of these processes is responsible for many drug-drug interactions.

c. **Phase I reactions not involving the P-450 system:** These include amine oxidation (for example, oxidation of catecholamines or histamine, alcohol dehydrogenation (for example, ethanol oxidation), and hydrolysis (for example, of procainamide).

2. **Phase II:** This phase consists of conjugation reactions. If the metabolite from Phase I metabolism is sufficiently polar, it can be excreted by the kidneys. However, many metabolites are too lipophilic to be retained in the kidney tubules. A subsequent conjugation reaction with an endogenous substrate, such as glucuronic acid, sulfuric acid, acetic acid or an amino acid results in polar, usually more water-soluble compounds that are most often therapeutically inactive. Glucuronidation is the most common and the most important conjugation reaction. Neonates are deficient in

this conjugating system making them particularly vulnerable to drugs such as *chloramphenicol* (see p. 321). [Note: Drugs already possessing an –OH, –HN2, or –COOH group may enter Phase II directly, and become conjugated without prior Phase I metabolism.] The highly polar drug conjugates may then be excreted by the kidney.

3. **Reversal of order of the Phases:** Not all drugs undergo Phase I and II reactions in that order. For example, *isoniazid* (see p. 332) is first acetylated (a Phase II reaction) and then hydrolyzed to isonicotinic acid (a Phase I reaction).

Study Questions

Choose the ONE best answer.

1.1 Which one of the following statements is CORRECT?

A. Weak bases are absorbed efficiently across the epithelial cells of the stomach.
B. Coadministration of atropine speeds the absorption of a second drug.
C. Drugs showing large V_d can be efficiently removed by dialysis of the plasma.
D. Stressful emotions can lead to a slowing of drug absorption.
E. If the V_d for a drug is small, most of the drug is in the extraplasmic space.

> Correct answer = D. Both exercise and strong emotions prompt sympathetic output, which slows gastric emptying. In the stomach a weak base is primarily in the protonated, charged form, which does not readily cross the epithelial cells of the stomach. Atropine is a parasympathetic blocker and slows gastric emptying. This delays the rate of drug absorption. A large V_d indicates that most of the drug is outside the plasma space and dialysis would not be effective. A small V_d indicates extensive binding to plasma proteins.

1.2 Which one of the following is TRUE for a drug whose elimination from plasma shows first-order kinetics?

A. The half-life of the drug is proportional to the drug concentration in plasma.
B. The amount eliminated per unit time is constant.
C. The rate of elimination is proportional to the plasma concentration.
D. Elimination involves a rate-limiting enzymic reaction operating at its maximal velocity (V_m).
E. A plot of drug concentration versus time is a straight line.

> Correct answer = C. The direct proportionality between concentration and rate is the definition of first-order. The half-life of a drug is a constant. For first-order reactions, the fraction of the drug eliminated is constant, not the amount. A rate limiting reaction operating at V_m would show zero-order kinetics. First order kinetics show a linear plot of log [drug concentration] versus time.

1.3 All of the following statements are true EXCEPT:

A. Aspirin (pK_a = 3.5) is 90% in its lipid-soluble, protonated form at pH = 2.5.
B. The basic drug promethazine (pK_a = 9.1) is more ionized at pH = 7.4 than at pH = 2.
C. Absorption of a weakly basic drug is likely to occur faster from the intestine than from the stomach.
D. Acidification of the urine accelerates the secretion of a weak base, pK_a = 8.
E. Uncharged molecules more readily cross cell membranes than charged molecules.

> Correct choice = B. As the pH of the solution becomes less than the pK_a, the ratio $[BH^+]/[B]$ increases; thus $[BH^+]$ is greater at pH = 2. At one pH unit on the acid side of pK_a, the $[HA]/[A^-]$ = 10, or 90% is in form HA, the protonated form of aspirin. Weak bases are more charged in the acidic gastric juice and are not readily absorbed. The drug which is a weak base is more ionized in acidified urine and less able to be reabsorbed. Uncharged molecules have a greater solubility in the lipid bilayer of membranes, and thus more readily cross membranes.

1.4 A patient is treated with drug A, which has a high affinity for albumin and is administered in amounts that do not exceed the binding capacity of albumin. A second drug, B, is added to the treatment regimen. Drug B also has a high affinity for albumin but is administered in amounts that are 100 times the binding capacity of albumin. Which of the following occurs after administration of drug B?

A. An increase in the tissue concentrations of drug A.
B. A decrease in the tissue concentrations of drug A.
C. A decrease in the volume of distribution of drug A.
D. A decrease in the half-life of drug A.
E. Addition of more drug A significantly alters the serum concentration of unbound drug B.

Correct answer = **A.** Drug A is largely bound to albumin and only a small fraction is free. Most of drug A is sequestered on albumin and is inert in terms of exerting pharmacologic actions. If drug B is administered, it displaces drug A from albumin, leading to rapid increase in the concentration of free drug A in plasma, because almost 100% is now free. Drug A moves out of the plasma into the interstitial water and the tissues. The V_d of drug A increases, providing less drug to the organ of excretion, and prolonging the overall lifetime of the drug. Since drug B is already in 100-fold excess of its albumin-binding capacity, dislodging some of drug B from albumin does not significantly affect its serum concentration.

1.5 The addition of glucuronic acid to a drug

A. decreases its water solubility.
B. usually leads to inactivation of the drug.
C. is an example of a Phase I reaction.
D. occurs at the same rate in adults and the newborn.
E. involves cytochrome P-450.

Correct answer = **B.** The addition of glucuronic acid prevents recognition of the drug by its receptor. Glucuronic acid is charged, and the drug conjugate has increased water solubility. Conjugation is a Phase II reaction. Neonates are deficient in the conjugating enzymes. Cytochrome P-450 is involved in Phase I reactions.

1.6 Drugs showing zero-order kinetics of elimination

A. are more common that those showing first order kinetics.
B. decrease in concentration exponentially with time.
C. have a half-life independent of dose.
D. show a plot of drug concentration versus time that is linear.
E. show a constant fraction of the drug eliminated per unit time.

Correct answer = D. Drugs with zero-order kinetics of elimination show a linear relationship between drug concentration and time. In most clinical situations the concentration of a drug is much less than the Michaelis-Menten constant (K_m). A decrease in drug concentration is linear with time. The half-life of the drug increases with dose. A constant amount of drug is eliminated per unit time.

1.7 A drug, given as a 100 mg single dose, results in a peak plasma concentration of 20 µg/ml. The apparent volume of distribution is (assume a rapid distribution and negligible elimination prior to measuring the peak plasma level):

A. 0.5 L.
B. 1 L.
C. 2 L.
D. 5 L.
E. 10 L.

Correct answer = **D.** V_d = D/C, where D = total amount of drug in the body and C = plasma concentration of drug. Thus V_d = 100mg/20 µg/ml = 100 mg/20 mg/L = 5 L.

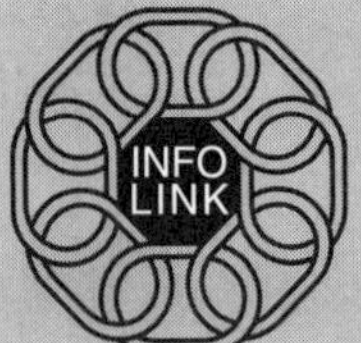

[1]See p. 52 in **Biochemistry** (2nd ed.) for a discussion of effect of substrate levels on reaction velocity.

[2]See p. 6 in **Biochemistry** (2nd ed.) for a discussion of acid-base chemistry.

[3]See p. 8 in **Biochemistry** (2nd ed.) for a discussion of Henderson-Hasselbalch equation.

[4]See p. 52 in **Biochemistry** (2nd ed.) for a discussion of Michaelis-Menten kinetics.

Pharmacokinetics and Drug Receptors

2

I. OVERVIEW

Pharmacokinetics is defined as the quantitative, time-dependent changes of both the plasma drug concentration and the total amount of drug in the body, following the drug's administration by various routes (the two most common of these routes being intravenous infusion and oral fixed-dose, fixed-time interval regimens—for example, "one tablet every four hours"). The interactions of the processes described in Chapter 1 determine the pharmacokinetic profile of a drug. The significance of identifying the pharmacokinetics of a drug lies not only in defining the factors that influence its levels and persistence in the body, but also in tailoring the therapeutic use of drugs that have a high toxic potential. [Note: The following discussion assumes that the administered drug distributes into a single body compartment. In actuality, most drugs equilibrate between two or three compartments and thus display complex kinetic behavior. However, the simpler model suffices to demonstrate the concepts.]

II. KINETICS OF INTRAVENOUS INFUSION

With continuous intravenous infusion, the rate of drug entry into the body is constant. In the majority of cases, the elimination of a drug is first-order, that is, a constant fraction of the agent is cleared per unit time. Therefore, the rate of drug exit from the body increases proportionately as the plasma concentration increases and at every point in time is proportional to the plasma concentration of the drug.

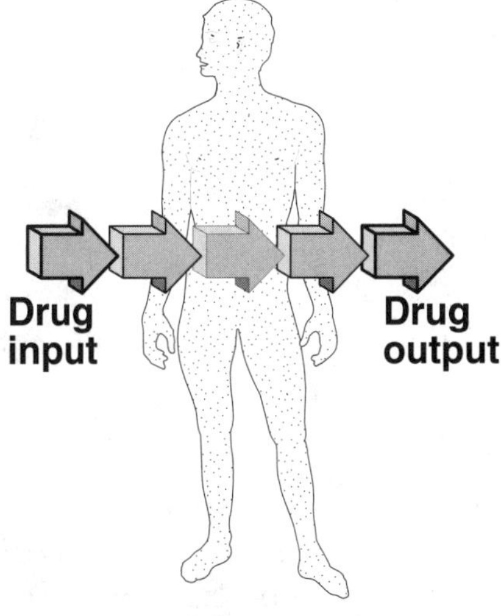

Figure 2.1
At steady state, input (rate of infusion) equals output (rate of elimination).

A. Steady-state drug levels in blood

Following the initiation of an intravenous infusion, the plasma concentration of drug rises until the rate of drug eliminated from the body precisely balances the input rate. Thus a steady-state is achieved in which the plasma concentration of drug remains constant. [Note: The rate of drug elimination from the body = $(CL_t)(C)$, where CL_t is total body clearance (see p 24), and C is the plasma concentration of drug.] Two questions can be asked about achieving the steady-state. First, what is the relationship between the rate of drug infusion and the plasma concentration of drug achieved at the

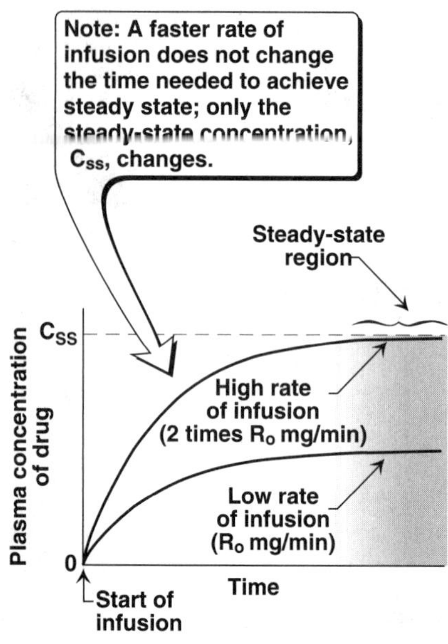

Figure 2.2
Effect of infusion rate on the steady-state concentration of drug in plasma. (R_o = rate of infusion of drug.)

plateau, or steady state? Second, what length of time is required to reach the steady-state drug concentration?

B. Influence of the rate of drug infusion on the steady-state

A steady-state plasma concentration of drug occurs when the rate of drug elimination is equal to the rate of administration (Figure 2.1), as described by the equation:

$$C_{ss} = R_o/k_eV_d = R_o/CL_t$$

where C_{ss} = the steady state concentration of drug

R_o = the infusion rate (for example, mg/min)

k_e = first-order rate constant for drug elimination from the total body

V_d = volume of distribution

CL_t = total body clearance (see p. 24)

Since k_e, CL_t, and V_d are constant for most drugs showing linear kinetics, C_{ss} is directly proportional to R_o, that is, the steady-state plasma concentration is directly proportional to the infusion rate. For example, if the infusion rate is doubled, the plasma concentration ultimately achieved at the steady state is doubled (Figure 2.2). Furthermore, the steady-state concentration is inversely proportional to the clearance of the drug, CL_t. Thus, any factor that decreases clearance, such as liver or kidney disease, increases the steady-state concentration of an infused drug (assuming V_d remains constant).

C. Time required to reach the steady state drug concentration

The concentration of drug rises from zero at the start of the infusion to its ultimate steady-state level, C_{ss} (Figure 2.3). The fractional rate of approach to a steady state is achieved by a first-order process.

1. **Exponential approach to steady state:** The rate constant for attainment of steady state is the rate constant for total body elimination of the drug, k_e. Thus, 50% of the final steady-state concentration of drug is observed after time elapsed since the infusion, t, is equal to $t_{1/2}$, where $t_{1/2}$ (or half-life) is the time required for the drug concentration to change by 50%. Waiting another half-life allows the drug concentration to approach 75% of C_{ss} (see Figure 2.3). The drug concentration is 90% of the final steady-state concentration in 3.3 times $t_{1/2}$. For convenience, therefore, one can assume that a drug will reach steady state in about 4 half-lives.

2. **Effect of the rate of drug infusion:** The sole determinant of the rate that a drug approaches steady state is the $t_{1/2}$ or k_e, and this rate is influenced only by the factors that affect the half-life. The rate of approach to steady state is not affected by the rate of drug infusion. Although increasing the rate of infusion of a drug increases the rate at which any given concentration of drug in the plasma is achieved, it does not influence the time required to reach the ultimate steady-state concentration. This is because the steady-state concentration of drug rises directly with the infusion rate (see Figure 2.2).

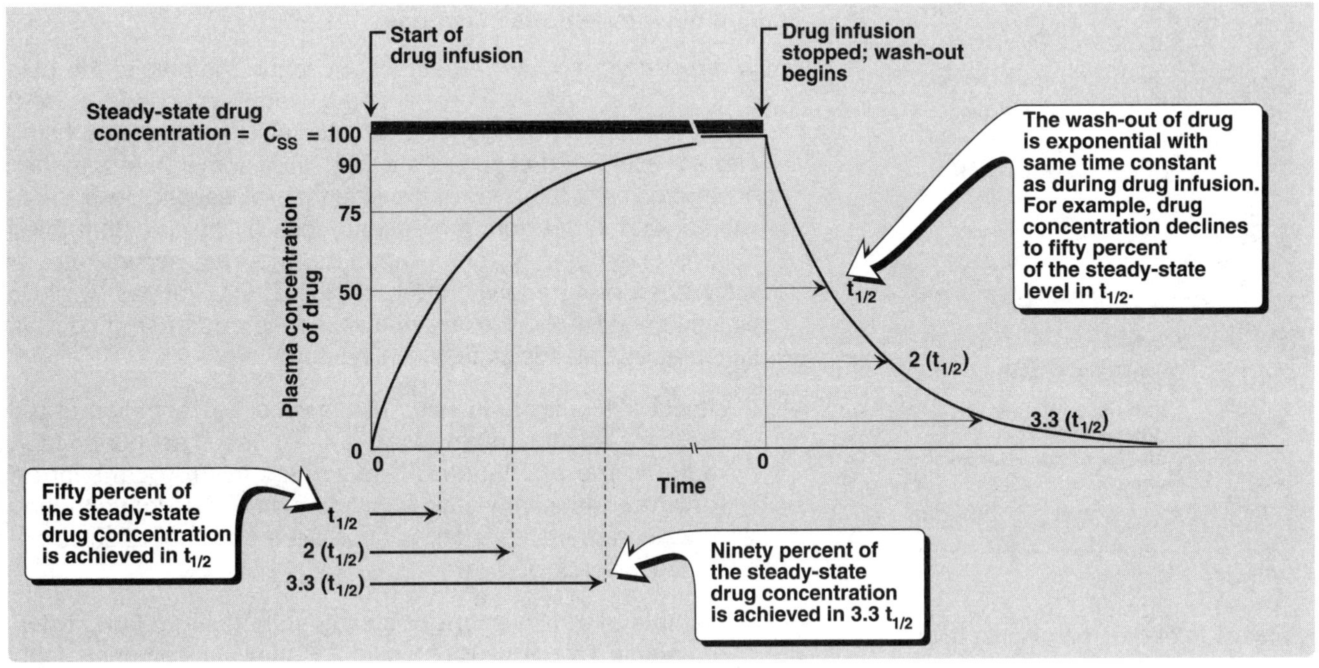

Figure 2.3
Rate of attainment of steady-state concentration of drug in plasma.

3. **Rate of drug decline when the infusion is stopped:** When the infusion is stopped, the plasma concentration of a drug declines (washes out) to zero with the same time course observed in approaching the steady state (see Figure 2.3).

4. **Loading dose:** A delay in achieving the desired plasma levels of drug may be clinically unacceptable. Therefore, a "loading dose" of drug can be injected as a single dose to achieve the desired plasma level rapidly, followed by an infusion to maintain the steady state (maintenance dose). In general, the loading dose can be calculated as:

Loading dose = (V_d) (desired steady-state plasma concentration)

III. KINETICS OF FIXED-DOSE, FIXED-TIME-INTERVAL REGIMENS

Administration of a drug by fixed doses rather than by continuous infusion is often more convenient. However, fixed doses, given at fixed-time intervals, result in time-dependent fluctuations in the circulating level of drug.

A. Single intravenous injection

For simplicity, assume the injected drug rapidly distributes into a single compartment. Since the rate of elimination is usually first order in regard to drug concentration, the circulating level of drug decreases exponentially with time (Figure 2.4). [Note: The $t_{1/2}$ does not depend on the dose of drug administered.]

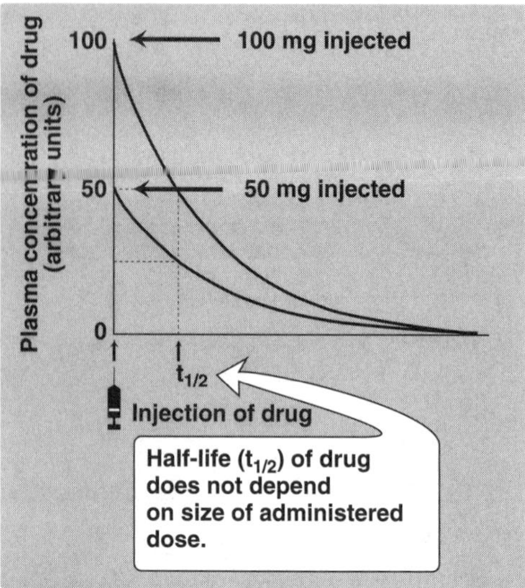

Figure 2.4
Effect of dose of single intravenous injection of drug on plasma levels.

B. Multiple intravenous injections

When a drug is given repeatedly at regular intervals, the plasma concentration increases until a steady state is reached (Figure 2.5). Because most drugs are given at intervals shorter than 5 half-lives and are eliminated exponentially with time, some drug from the first dose remains in the body at the time that the second dose is administered, and some from the second dose at the time that the third dose is given and so forth. Therefore, the drug accumulates until, within the dosing interval, the rate of drug loss (driven by elevated plasma concentration) exactly balances the rate of drug administration, that is, a steady state is achieved.

1. **Effect of dosing frequency:** The plasma concentration of a drug oscillates about a mean. Using smaller doses at shorter intervals reduces the amplitude of the swings in drug concentration. However, the steady-state concentration of the drug and the rate at which the steady state is approached are not affected by the frequency of dosing.

2. **Example of achievement of steady state using different dosage regimens:** The curve B of Figure 2.5 shows the amount of drug in the body when one gram of drug is administered intravenously to a patient, and the dose is repeated at a time interval that corresponds to the half-life of the drug. At the end of the first dosing interval, 0.50 units of drug remain from the first dose when the second dose is administered. At the end of the second dosing interval, 0.75 units are present when the third dose is taken. The minimal amount of drug during the dosing interval progressively increases and approaches a value of 1.00 unit, whereas the maximal value immediately following drug administration progressively approaches 2.00 units. Therefore, at the steady state, 1.00 unit of drug is lost during the dosing interval, which is exactly matched by the rate at which the drug is administered, that is, the "rate in" equals the "rate out." As in the case for intravenous infusion (see p. 18), 90% of the steady-state value is achieved in 3.3 times $t_{1/2}$.

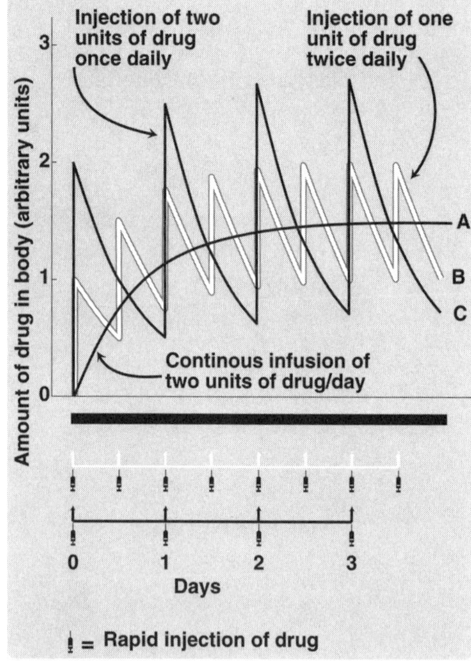

Figure 2.5
Predicted plasma concentrations of a drug given by infusion (A), twice daily injection (B), or once daily injection (C). Model assumes rapid mixing in a single body compartment and a $t_{1/2}$ of 12 hours.

C. Orally administered drugs

Most drugs that are administered on an outpatient basis are taken orally on a fixed-dose fixed-time interval regimen, for example, a specific dose, taken one, two or three times daily. In contrast to intravenous injection, orally administered drugs may be absorbed slowly, and the plasma concentration of the drug is influenced by both the rate of absorption and the rate of drug elimination (Figure 2.6).

IV. DOSE-RESPONSE QUANTITATION

A. Drug receptors

A drug receptor is a specialized target macromolecule, present on the cell surface or intracellularly, that binds a drug and mediates its pharmacologic actions. Drugs may interact with enzymes (for example, inhibition of dihydrofolate reductase by *trimethoprim,* p. 294), nucleic acids (for example, blockade of transcription by *dactinomycin,* p. 384) or membrane receptors (for example, alteration of membrane permeability by acetylcholine). In each case, the formation of the drug-receptor complex leads to a biologic response, and the magnitude of the response is proportional to the number of drug-receptor complexes:

$$\text{Drug} + \text{Receptor} \rightarrow \text{Drug-receptor complex} \rightarrow \text{Effect}$$

This concept is closely related to the formation of complexes between enzyme and substrate[1] or antigen and antibody; these interactions have many common features, perhaps the most noteworthy being specificity. However, the receptor not only has the ability to recognize a ligand (drug), but can also couple or transduce this binding into a response by causing a conformational change or a biochemical effect. [Note: For most drugs, the nature of the target molecule is unknown. The actions of a few drugs are not mediated by specific receptors, but depend on nonspecific chemical or physical interactions. For example, anesthetic gases (see p. 112) are thought to alter the structure of the membrane.]

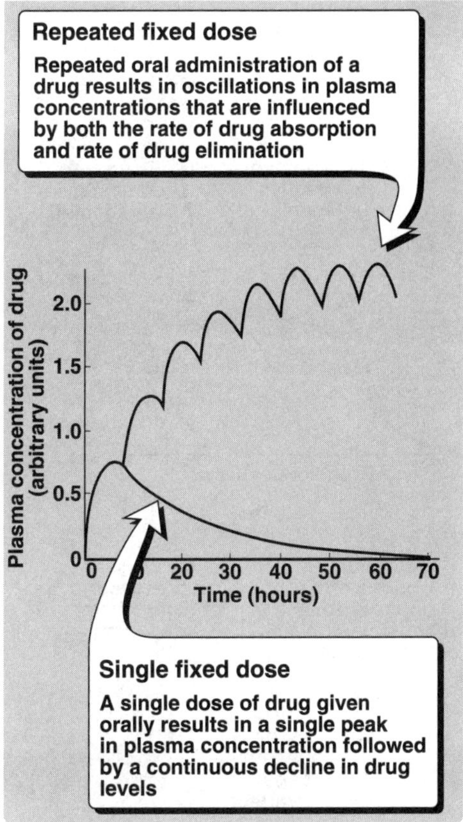

Figure 2.6
Predicted plasma concentrations of a drug given by repeated oral administrations.

B. Graded dose-response curve

An agonist is defined as an agent that can bind to a receptor and elicit a response. The magnitude of the drug effect depends on its concentration at the receptor site, which in turn is determined by the dose of drug administered and by factors characteristic of the drug, such as rate of absorption, distribution, and metabolism. The effect of a drug is most easily analyzed by plotting the magnitude of the response versus the log of the drug dose, thus obtaining a graded dose-response curve (Figure 2.7).

1. **Efficacy:** Efficacy is the maximal response produced by a drug. It depends on the number of drug-receptor complexes formed and the efficiency with which the activated receptor produces a cellular action (see Figure 2.7). Efficacy is analogous to maximal velocity for an enzyme catalyzed reaction[2]. [Note: A compound may bind to the receptor and not elicit a response. It is thus said to have zero efficacy, and may act as an antagonist.]

2. **Potency:** Potency, also termed effective dose concentration, is a measure of how much drug is required to elicit a given response. The lower the dose required for a given response, the more potent the drug. Potency is most often expressed as the dose of drug that gives 50% of the maximal response, ED_{50} (see Figure 2.7). A drug with a low ED_{50} is more potent than a drug with a larger ED_{50}. The affinity (K_d) of the receptor for a drug is an important factor in determining the potency. However, efficacy is more important than potency since it focuses on the effectiveness of the drug. (For example, a more potent drug may not reach its receptor in sufficient concentrations due to some pathologic condition.)

3. **Slope of the dose-response curve:** The slope of the midportion of the dose-response curve varies from drug to drug. A steep slope indicates that a small increase in drug dosage produces a large change in response.

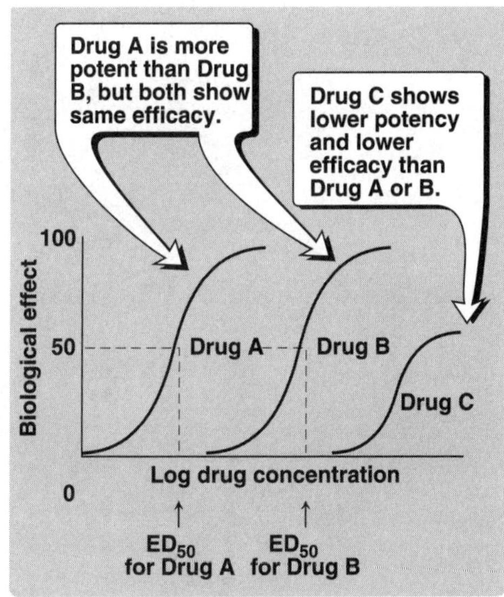

Figure 2.7
Typical dose response curve for drugs showing differences in potency and efficacy. ED_{50} = drug dose that shows 50% of maximal response.

[1,2]See p. 26 for Infolink references to other books in this series.

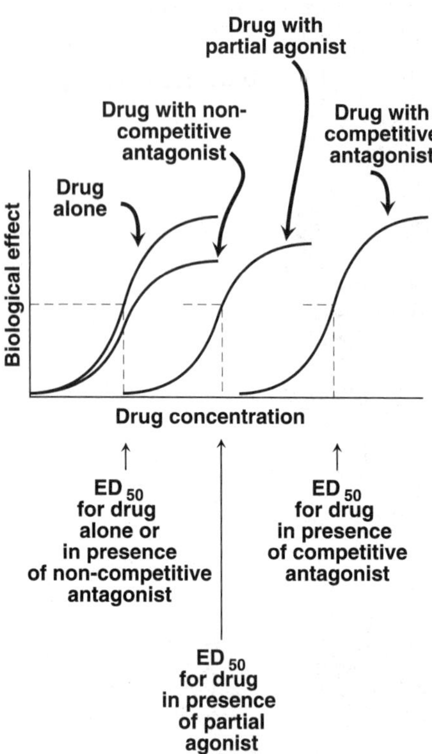

Figure 2.8
Effects of drug antagonists.

C. Reversible antagonists

1. **Competitive:** These agents interact with receptors at the same site as the agonist and, thus, compete for binding of the agonist (Figure 2.8). A competitive antagonist shifts the dose-response curve to the right, causing the drug to behave as if it were less potent. This behavior is analogous to a competitive inhibitor for an enzyme-catalyzed reaction.[3]

2. **Noncompetitive:** These agents either prevent the binding of the agonist or prevent the agonist from activating the receptor. A noncompetitive antagonist decreases the maximal response and is analogous to a noncompetitive inhibitor for an enzyme-catalyzed reaction.[4]

3. **Partial agonist:** Partial agonists block the agonist binding site but cause less response than a full agonist. A partial agonist may have an affinity for the receptor that is increased, decreased, or equivalent to that of an agonist.

V. THERAPEUTIC INDEX

The therapeutic index of a drug is the ratio of the dose that produces toxicity to the dose that produces a clinically desired or effective response in a population of individuals.

Therapeutic index = toxic dose/effective dose

The therapeutic index is thus a measure of the drug's safety, since a large value indicates that there is a wide margin between doses that are effective and doses that are toxic.

A. Determination of therapeutic index

The therapeutic index is determined by measuring the frequency of desired response and toxic response at various doses of drug. For example, Figure 2.9 shows the response to *warfarin* (see p. 199), an oral anticoagulant with a narrow therapeutic index, and *penicillin* (see p. 297), an antimicrobial drug with a large therapeutic index.

1. **Warfarin (example of a drug with a small therapeutic index):** As the dose of *warfarin* is increased, a greater fraction of the patients respond (for this drug, the desired response is a two-fold increase in prothrombin time) until eventually all patients respond (see Figure 2.9A). However, at higher doses of *warfarin*, a toxic response occurs, namely a high degree of anticoagulation that results in hemorrhage. Note that when the therapeutic index is low, it is possible to have a range of concentrations where the effective and toxic responses overlap, that is, some patients hemorrhage while others achieve the desired two-fold prolongation of prothrombin time. Variation in patient response is therefore most likely to occur with a drug showing a narrow therapeutic index, since the effective and toxic concentrations are similar.

[4]See p. 26 for Infolink references to other books in this series.

Agents with a low therapeutic index, that is, drugs in which dose is critically important, are those drugs in which bioinequivalence is likely to result in a therapeutic consequence (see p. 7).

2. **Penicillin (example of a drug with a large therapeutic index):** For drugs with a large therapeutic index, such as *penicillin* (see Figure 2.9B), it is safe and common to give doses in excess (often about ten-fold excess) of that which is minimally required to achieve a desired response. In this case, the bioavailability does not critically alter the therapeutic effects.

VI. DRUG ELIMINATION

Removal of a drug from the body may occur via a number of routes, the most important being through the kidney into the urine. Other routes include the bile, intestine, lung, or milk in nursing mothers. A patient in renal failure may undergo extracorporeal dialysis, which will remove small molecules such as drugs.

A. Renal elimination of a drug

1. **Glomerular filtration:** Drugs enter the kidney through renal arteries, which divide to form a glomerular capillary plexus. Free drug (not bound to albumin) flows through the capillary slits into Bowman's space as part of the glomerular filtrate (Figure 2.10). The glomerular filtration rate (GFR = 125 ml/min) is normally about 20% of the renal plasma flow (RPF = 600 ml/min). Lipid solubility and pH do not influence the passage of drugs into the glomerular filtrate.

2. **Proximal tubular secretion:** Drug that was not transferred into the glomerular filtrate leaves the glomeruli through efferent arterioles, which divide to form a capillary plexus surrounding the nephric lumen in the proximal tubule. Secretion primarily occurs in the proximal tubules by two energy-requiring active transport systems, one for anions (for example, deprotonated forms of weak acids) and one for cations (protonated forms of weak bases). Each of these transport systems shows a low specificity and can transport many compounds; thus, competition between drugs for the carriers can occur within each transport system (for example, see *probenecid*, p. 417). [Note: Premature infants and neonates have incompletely developed tubular secretory mechanism and thus may retain certain drugs.]

3. **Distal tubular reabsorption:** As a drug moves toward the distal convoluted tubule, its concentration increases and exceeds that of the perivascular space. The drug, if uncharged, may diffuse out of the nephric lumen back into the systemic circulation. Manipulating the pH of the urine to increase the ionized form of the drug in the lumen may be used to minimize the amount of back diffusion and hence increase the clearance of an undesirable drug. For example, a patient presenting with a *phenobarbital* overdose can be given bicarbonate, which alkalinizes the urine and keeps the drug ionized, thereby decreasing its reabsorption.

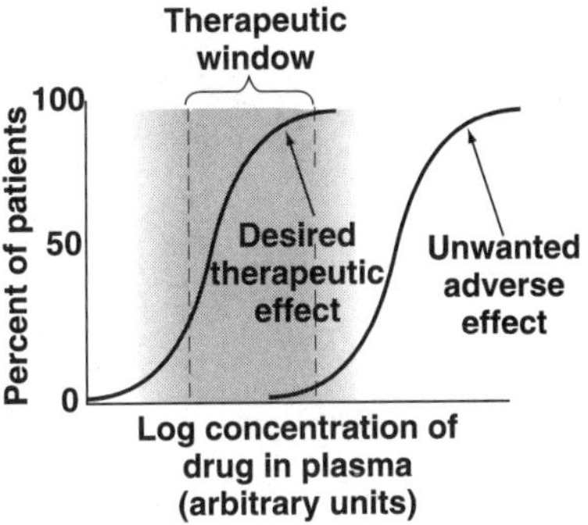

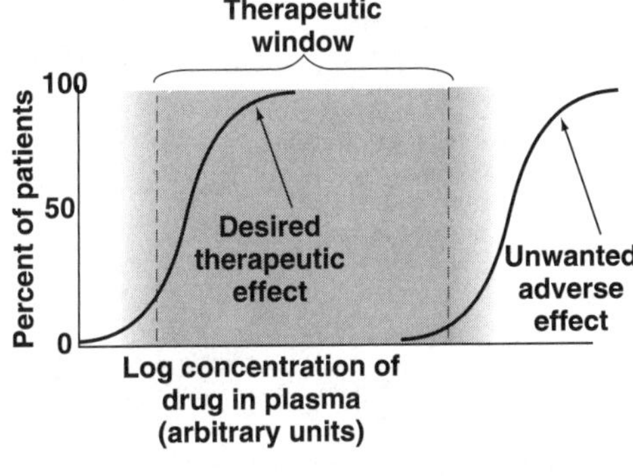

Figure 2.9
Cumulative percent of patients responding to plasma levels of drug.

If the drug is a weak base, acidification of the urine with NH_4Cl leads to protonation of the drug and an increase in its clearance. This process is called "ion trapping."

4. **Role of drug metabolism:** Most drugs are lipid soluble and diffuse out of the kidney's tubular lumen when the drug concentration in the filtrate becomes greater than that in the perivascular space. In order to minimize this reabsorption, drugs are modified by the body to be more polar using two types of reactions: Phase I reactions (see p. 13) that involve either the addition of hydroxyl groups or the removal of blocking groups from hydroxyl, carboxyl or amino groups, or Phase II reactions (see p. 14) that use conjugation with sulfate, glycine, or glucuronic acid to increase drug polarity. The conjugates are ionized, and the charged molecules cannot back-diffuse out of the kidney lumen (Figure 2.11).

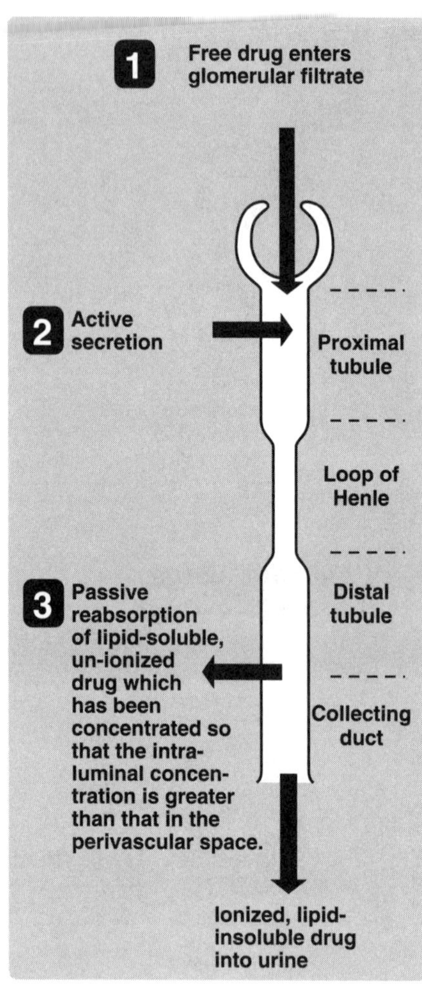
1 Free drug enters glomerular filtrate
2 Active secretion
Proximal tubule
Loop of Henle
Distal tubule
3 Passive reabsorption of lipid-soluble, un-ionized drug which has been concentrated so that the intra-luminal concentration is greater than that in the perivascular space.
Collecting duct
Ionized, lipid-insoluble drug into urine

Figure 2.10
Drug elimination by the kidney.

B. Quantitative aspects of renal drug elimination

Plasma clearance is expressed as the volume of plasma from which all drug appears to be removed in a given time, for example, as ml/min. Clearance equals the amount of renal plasma flow multiplied by the extraction ratio, and since these are normally invariant over time, clearance is constant.

1. **Extraction ratio:** This ratio is the decline of drug concentration in the plasma from the arterial to the venous side of the kidney. The drugs enter the kidneys at concentration C_1 and exit the kidneys at concentration C_2. The extraction ratio = C_2/C_1

2. **Excretion rate:**

$$\underset{\text{mg/min}}{\text{Excretion rate}} = \underset{\text{ml/min}}{(\text{clearance})}\ \underset{\text{mg/ml}}{(\text{plasma concentration})}$$

The elimination of a drug usually follows first order kinetics, and the concentration of drug in plasma drops exponentially with time. This may be used to determine the half-life of the drug (the time during which the concentration of the drug decreases from C to $\frac{1}{2}$C).

$$t_{1/2} = \ln 0.5/k_e = 0.693\ V_d/CL$$

C. Total body clearance

The total body (systemic) clearance (CL_{total}) is the sum of the clearances from the various drug metabolizing and drug-eliminating organs. The kidney is often the major organ of excretion; however, the liver also contributes to drug loss through metabolism and/or excretion into the bile. A patient in renal failure may sometimes benefit from a drug that is excreted by this pathway into the intestine and feces, rather than through the kidney. Some drugs may also be reabsorbed through the enterohepatic circulation, thus prolonging their half-life. Total clearance can be calculated by using the following equation:

$$CL_{total} = CL_{hepatic} + CL_{renal} + CL_{pulmonary} + CL_{other}$$

It is not possible to measure and sum these individual clearances. However, total clearance can be derived from the steady state equation (see p. 18):

$$CL_{total} = k_e V_d$$

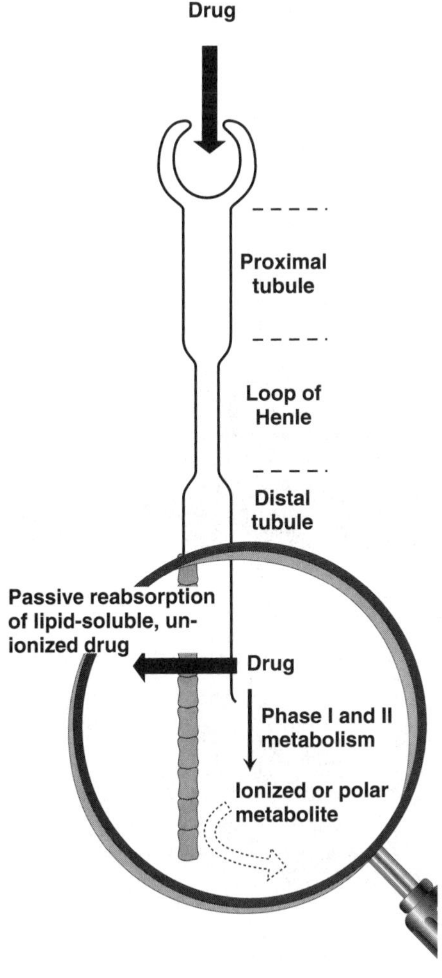

Figure 2.11
Effect of drug metabolism on reabsorption in the distal tubule.

D. Volume of distribution and the half-life of a drug

The half-life of a drug is inversely related to its clearance and directly proportional to its volume of distribution.

$$t_{1/2} = 0.693\ V_d/CL_{total}$$

This equation shows that as the volume of distribution increases, the half-life of a drug becomes longer. The larger the volume of distribution, the more drug is outside the plasma compartment and is unavailable for excretion by the kidney or metabolism by the liver.

E. Clinical situations resulting in increased drug half-life

When a patient has an abnormality that alters the half-life of a drug, adjustment in dosage is required. It is important to be able to predict in which patients a drug is likely to have a longer half-life. The half-life of a drug is increased by:

1. diminished renal plasma flow, for example, in cardiogenic shock, heart failure, or hemorrhage.
2. addition of a second drug that displaces the first from albumin and, hence, increases the volume of distribution of the drug.
3. decreased extraction ratio, for example, as seen in renal disease.
4. decreased metabolism, for example, when another drug inhibits its biotransformation, or hepatic insufficiency as with cirrhosis.

Study Questions

Choose the ONE best answer.

2.1 A drug with a half-life of 12 hours is administered by continuous intravenous infusion. How long will it take for the drug to reach 90% of its final steady-state level?

A. 18 hours.
B. 24 hours.
C. 30 hours.
D. 40 hours.
E. 90 hours.

Correct answer = D. One approaches 90% of the final steady-state in 3.3 times $t_{1/2}$ = 3.3 • 12 ~ 40 hours.

2.2 Which of the following results in a doubling of the steady-state concentration of a drug?

A. Doubling the rate of infusion.

B. Maintaining the infusion rate, but doubling the loading dose.

C. Doubling the rate of infusion and doubling the concentration of the infused drug.

D. Tripling the rate of infusion.

E. Quadrupling the rate of infusion.

Correct answer = A. The steady-state concentration of a drug is directly proportional to the infusion rate. Increasing the loading dose provides a transient increase in drug level, but the steady-state level remains unchanged. Doubling both the rate of infusion and concentration of the infused drug leads to a 4-fold increase in the steady-state drug concentration. Tripling or quadrupling the rate of infusion leads to either a 3-fold or 4-fold increase in the steady-state drug concentration.

2.3 Which of the following statements is correct?

A. If 10 mg of drug A produces the same response as 100 mg of drug B, drug A is more efficacious than drug B.

B. The greater the efficacy, the greater the potency of a drug.

C. In selecting a drug, potency is usually more important than efficacy.

D. A competitive antagonist increases ED_{50}.

E. Variation in response to a drug among different individuals is most likely to occur with a drug showing a large therapeutic index.

Correct answer = D. In the presence of a competitive antagonist, a higher concentration of drug is required to elicit a given response. Efficacy and potency can vary independently, and the maximal response obtained is often more important than the amount of drug needed to achieve it. For example, in Choice A, no information is provided about the efficacy of drug A, so all one can say is that drug A is more potent than drug B. Variability between patients in the pharmacokinetics of a drug is most important clinically when the effective and toxic doses are not very different, as is the case with a drug that shows a small therapeutic index.

2.4 Which of the following most closely describes the clearance rate of a drug that is infused at a rate of 4 mg/min and produces a steady-state concentration of 6 mg/L in the plasma?

A. 67 ml/min.

B. 132 ml/min.

C. 300 ml/min.

D. 667 ml min.

E. 1,200 ml/min.

Correct answer = D. Clearance is the volume of plasma from which all drug is removed in a given time (in this case per minute). At steady state, the excretion rate = infusion rate = 4 mg/min. Thus, clearance (ml/min) = excretion rate (mg/ml)/plasma concentration (mg/ml) = (4 mg/ml)/(0.006 mg/ml) = 667 ml/min.

2.5 The antimicrobial drug, tetracycline, is found to be therapeutically effective when 250 mg of drug are present in the body. The $t_{1/2}$ of tetracycline is 8 hours. What is the correct rate of infusion?

A. 7 mg/hr.

B. 12 mg/hr.

C. 22 mg/hr.

D. 37 mg/hr.

E. 45 mg/hr.

Correct answer = C. The correct rate of infusion is $R=K_dV_dC$, where $K_d = 0.69/t_{1/2} = 0.69/8$ hours = 0.086 hr^{-1}; therefore, the instantaneous rate of loss of the tetracycline is 8.6 % per hr of whatever amount of drug is present in the body. (V_dC = the total amount of drug in the body.) When 250 mg of tetracycline are present in the body, the rate of drug loss is 250 mg x 8.6 %/hour = 250 x 0.086 hr^{-1} = 21.5 mg/hr.

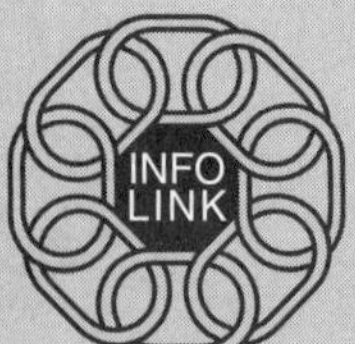

[1]See p. 48 in **Biochemistry** (2nd ed.) for a discussion of the interaction of enzyme with substrate.

[2]See p. 53 in **Biochemistry** (2nd ed.) for a discussion of maximal velocity for an enzyme catalyzed reaction.

[3]See p. 54-56 in **Biochemistry** (2nd ed.) for a discussion of competitive and noncompetitive inhibition of an enzyme catalyzed reaction.

UNIT II: Drugs Affecting the Autonomic Nervous System

The Autonomic Nervous System

3

I. OVERVIEW

The autonomic nervous system, along with the endocrine system, coordinates the regulation and integration of body functions. The endocrine system sends signals to target tissues by varying the levels of blood-borne hormones. In contrast, the nervous system exerts its influence by the rapid transmission of electrical impulses over nerve fibers that terminate at effector cells, where specific effects are caused due to the release of a neuromediator substance. Drugs that produce their primary therapeutic effect by mimicking or altering the functions of the autonomic nervous system are called autonomic drugs and are discussed in the following four chapters. These autonomic agents act either by stimulating portions of the autonomic nervous system or by blocking the action of the autonomic nerves. This chapter outlines the fundamental physiology of the autonomic nervous system and describes the role of neurotransmitters in the communication between extracellular events and chemical changes within the cell.

II. INTRODUCTION TO THE NERVOUS SYSTEM

The nervous system is divided into two anatomical divisions, the central nervous system (CNS), which is composed of the brain and spinal cord, and the peripheral nervous system, which includes neurons located outside the brain and spinal cord, that is, any nerves that enter or leave the CNS (Figure 3.1). The peripheral nervous system can be further divided into the efferent division, whose neurons carry signals away from the brain and spinal cord to the peripheral tissues, and the afferent division, whose neurons bring information from the periphery to the CNS.

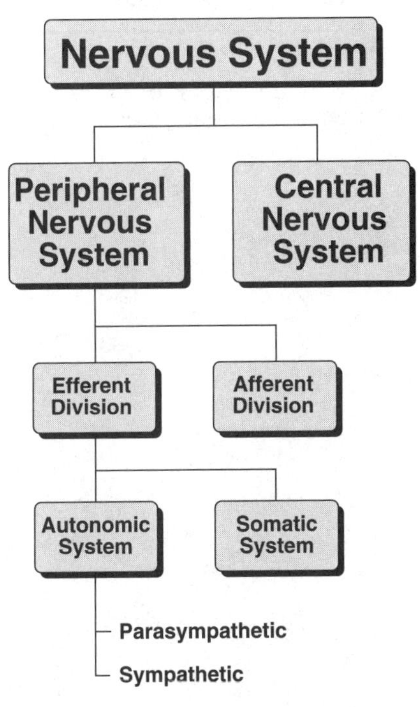

Figure 3.1
Organization of the nervous system.

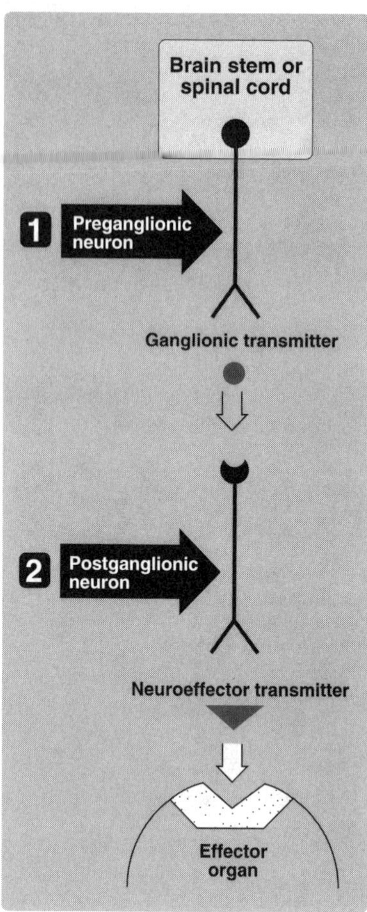

Figure 3.2
Efferent neurons of the autonomic nervous system.

A. Functional divisions within the nervous system

The efferent portion of the peripheral nervous system can be further divided into two major functional subdivisions, the somatic and autonomic systems (see Figure 3.1). The somatic efferents are involved in voluntarily controlled functions such as contraction of the skeletal muscles in locomotion. The autonomic system functions involuntarily to regulate the everyday needs and requirements of the body without the conscious participation of the mind. It is composed primarily of visceral motor (efferent) neurons that innervate smooth muscle of the viscera, cardiac muscle, vasculature and the exocrine glands.

B. Anatomy of the autonomic nervous system

1. **Efferent neurons:** The autonomic nervous system carries nerve impulses from the CNS to the effector organs by way of two types of efferent neurons (Figure 3.2). The first nerve cell is called a **preganglionic neuron** and its cell body is located within the CNS. Preganglionic neurons emerge from the brain stem or spinal cord and make a synaptic connection in ganglia (an aggregation of nerve cell bodies located in the peripheral nervous system). These ganglia function as relay stations between the preganglionic neuron and a second nerve cell, the **postganglionic neuron**. The latter neuron has a cell body originating in the ganglion. It is generally nonmyelinated and terminates on effector organs such as smooth muscles of the viscera, cardiac muscle, and the exocrine glands (Figure 3.2).

2. **Afferent neurons:** The afferent neurons (fibers) of the autonomic nervous system are important in the reflex regulation of this system, for example, by sensing pressure in the carotid sinus and aortic arch and signaling the CNS to influence the efferent branch of the system to respond (see below).

3. **Sympathetic neurons:** The efferent autonomic nervous system is divided into the sympathetic and the parasympathetic nervous systems (see Figure 3.1). The preganglionic neurons of the sympathetic system come from thoracic and lumbar regions of the spinal cord and synapse in two cord-like chains of ganglia that run in parallel on each side of the spinal cord. Axons of the postganglionic neuron extend from these ganglia to the glands and viscera. [Note: The adrenal medulla, like the sympathetic ganglia, receives preganglionic fibers from the sympathetic system. Lacking axons, the adrenal medulla, in response to stimulation by neurotransmitters, influences other organs by secreting the hormone epinephrine, also known as adrenaline (and lesser amounts of norepinephrine) into the blood.]

4. **Parasympathetic neurons:** The parasympathetic preganglionic fibers arise from the cranial and sacral areas of the spinal cord and synapse in ganglia near or on the effector organs. In both the sympathetic and parasympathetic systems, postganglionic fibers extend from the ganglia to effector organs.

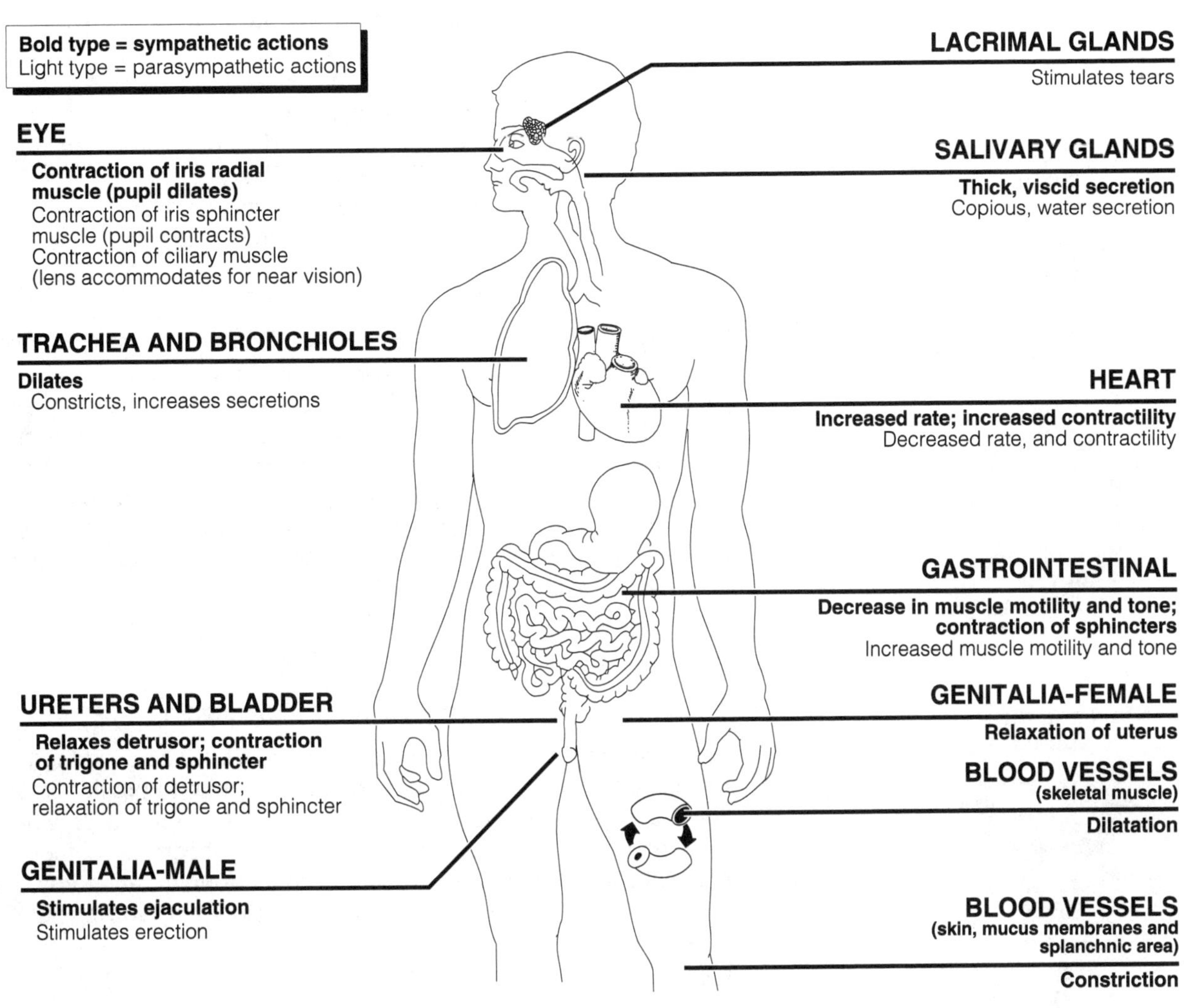

Figure 3.3
Action of sympathetic **(bold type)** and parasympathetic (light type) nervous systems on effector organs.

C. Functions of the sympathetic system

Though continually active to some degree (for example, in maintaining the tone of vascular beds), the sympathetic division has the property of adjusting in response to stressful situations, such as trauma, fear, hypoglycemia, cold, or exercise.

1. **Effects of stimulation of the sympathetic division:** The effect of sympathetic output is to increase heart rate and blood pressure, to mobilize energy stores of the body, and to increase blood flow to skeletal muscles and heart while diverting flow from the skin and internal organs. Sympathetic stimulation also results in dilation of the pupils and the bronchioles (Figure 3.3).

2. **Fight or flight response:** The changes experienced by the body during emergencies have been referred to as the "fight or flight" response (Figure 3.4). These reactions are triggered both by direct sympathetic activation of the effector organs and by stimulation of the adrenal medulla to release epinephrine and lesser

amounts of norepinephrine. These hormones enter the blood stream and promote responses in effector organs that contain adrenergic receptors (see Figure 6.6, p. 60). The sympathetic nervous system tends to function as a unit and often discharges as a complete system, for example, during severe exercise or in reactions to fear (see Figure 3.4). This system, with its diffuse distribution of postganglionic fibers, is involved in a wide array of physiologic activities, but it is not essential for life.

"Fight or flight" stimuli

Sympathetic output (diffuse)

"Rest and digest" stimuli

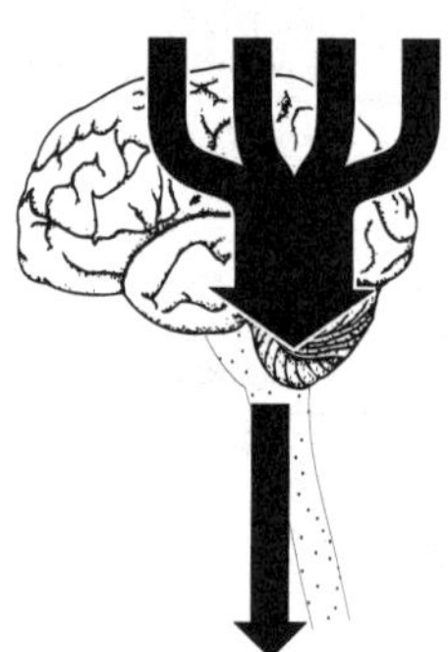

Parasympathetic output (discrete)

Sympathetic and parasympathetic actions often oppose each other

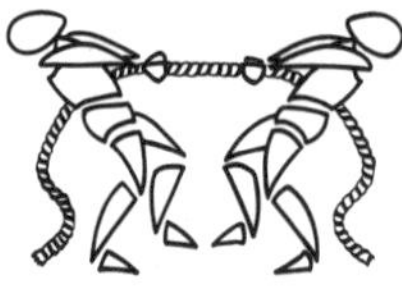

Figure 3.4
Sympathetic and parasympathetic actions are elicited by different stimuli.

D. Functions of the parasympathetic system:

The parasympathetic division maintains essential bodily functions, such as digestive processes and elimination of wastes, and is required for life (see Figure 3.3). It usually acts to oppose or balance the actions of the sympathetic division and is generally dominant over the sympathetic system in "rest and digest" situations (see Figure 3.4). The parasympathetic system is not a functional entity as such and never discharges as a complete system. If it did, it would produce massive, undesirable, and unpleasant symptoms. Instead, discrete parasympathetic fibers are activated separately, and the system functions to affect specific organs, such as the stomach or eye.

E. Role of the CNS in autonomic control of viscera

Although the autonomic nervous system is a motor system, it does require sensory input from peripheral structures to provide information on the state of affairs in the body. This feed-back is provided by streams of afferent impulses, arising in the viscera and other autonomically innervated structures, that travel to integrating centers in the CNS—the hypothalamus, medulla oblongata, and spinal cord. These centers respond to the stimuli by sending out efferent reflex impulses via the autonomic nervous system (Figure 3.5).

1. **Reflex arcs:** Most of the afferent impulses are translated into reflex responses without involving consciousness. For example, a fall in blood pressure causes pressure-sensitive neurons (baroreceptors in the heart, vena cava, aortic arch, and carotid sinuses) to send fewer impulses to cardiovascular centers in the brain. This prompts a reflex response of increased sympathetic output to the heart and vasculature, and decreased parasympathetic output to the heart, which results in a compensatory rise in blood pressure and tachycardia (see Figure 3.5).

2. **Emotions and the autonomic nervous system:** Stimuli that evoke feelings of strong emotion, such as rage, fear, or pleasure, can modify the activity of the autonomic nervous system.

F. Innervation by the autonomic nervous system

1. **Dual innervation:** Most organs in the body are innervated by both divisions of the autonomic nervous system. Thus, the heart has vagal parasympathetic innervation that slows rate of contraction, and sympathetic innervation that speeds contraction. Despite this dual innervation, one system usually predominates in controlling the activity of a given organ. For example, in the heart, the vagus is the predominant controlling factor for rate.

2. **Organs receiving only sympathetic innervation:** Although most tissues receive dual innervation, some effector organs, such as the adrenal medulla, kidney, pilomotor muscles, and sweat glands, receive innervation only from the sympathetic system. The control of blood pressure is also mainly a sympathetic activity, with essentially no participation by the parasympathetic system.

G. Somatic nervous system

The efferent somatic nervous system differs from the autonomic system in that a single myelinated motor neuron, originating in the CNS, travels directly to skeletal muscle without the mediation of ganglia. As noted earlier, the somatic nervous system is under voluntary control, whereas the autonomic is an involuntary system.

III. CHEMICAL SIGNALING BETWEEN CELLS

Neurotransmission in the autonomic nervous system is an example of the more general process of chemical signaling between cells. In addition to neurotransmission, other types of chemical signaling are the release of local mediators and the secretion of hormones.

A. Local mediators

Most cells in the body secrete chemicals that act locally, that is, they act on cells in their immediate environment. These chemical signals are rapidly destroyed or removed; thus, they do not enter the blood and are not distributed throughout the body. Histamine (see p. 420) and prostaglandins (see p. 419) are examples of local mediators.

B. Hormones

Specialized endocrine cells secrete hormones into the blood stream, where they travel throughout the body exerting effects on broadly distributed target cells in the body. (Hormones are described in Chapters 25-27.)

C. Neurotransmitters

Each neuron is a distinct anatomic unit, and no structural continuity exists between most neurons. Communication between nerve cells—and between nerve cells and effector organs—occurs through the release of specific chemical signals, called neurotransmitters, from the nerve terminals. This release depends on processes that are triggered by Ca^{++} uptake and regulated by phosphorylation of synaptic proteins. The neurotransmitters rapidly diffuse across the synaptic cleft or gap (synapse) between nerve endings and combine with specific receptors on the postsynaptic (target) cell (see pp. 37 and 57).

1. **Membrane receptors:** All neurotransmitters and most hormones and local mediators are too hydrophilic to penetrate the lipid bilayer of target-cell plasma membranes; instead, their signal is mediated by binding to specific receptors on the cell surface of target organs. [Note: A receptor is defined as a recognition site for a substance. It shows a binding specificity and is coupled to processes that eventually evoke a response. Most receptors are proteins. They need not be located in the membrane.]

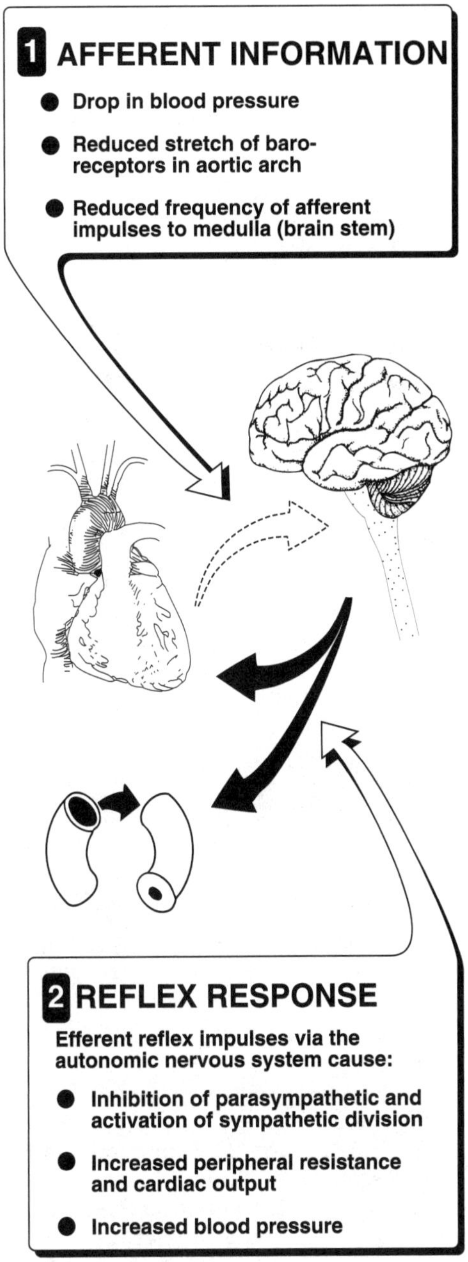

1 AFFERENT INFORMATION

- Drop in blood pressure
- Reduced stretch of baroreceptors in aortic arch
- Reduced frequency of afferent impulses to medulla (brain stem)

2 REFLEX RESPONSE

Efferent reflex impulses via the autonomic nervous system cause:

- Inhibition of parasympathetic and activation of sympathetic division
- Increased peripheral resistance and cardiac output
- Increased blood pressure

Figure 3.5
Baroreceptor reflex arc responds to a decrease in blood pressure.

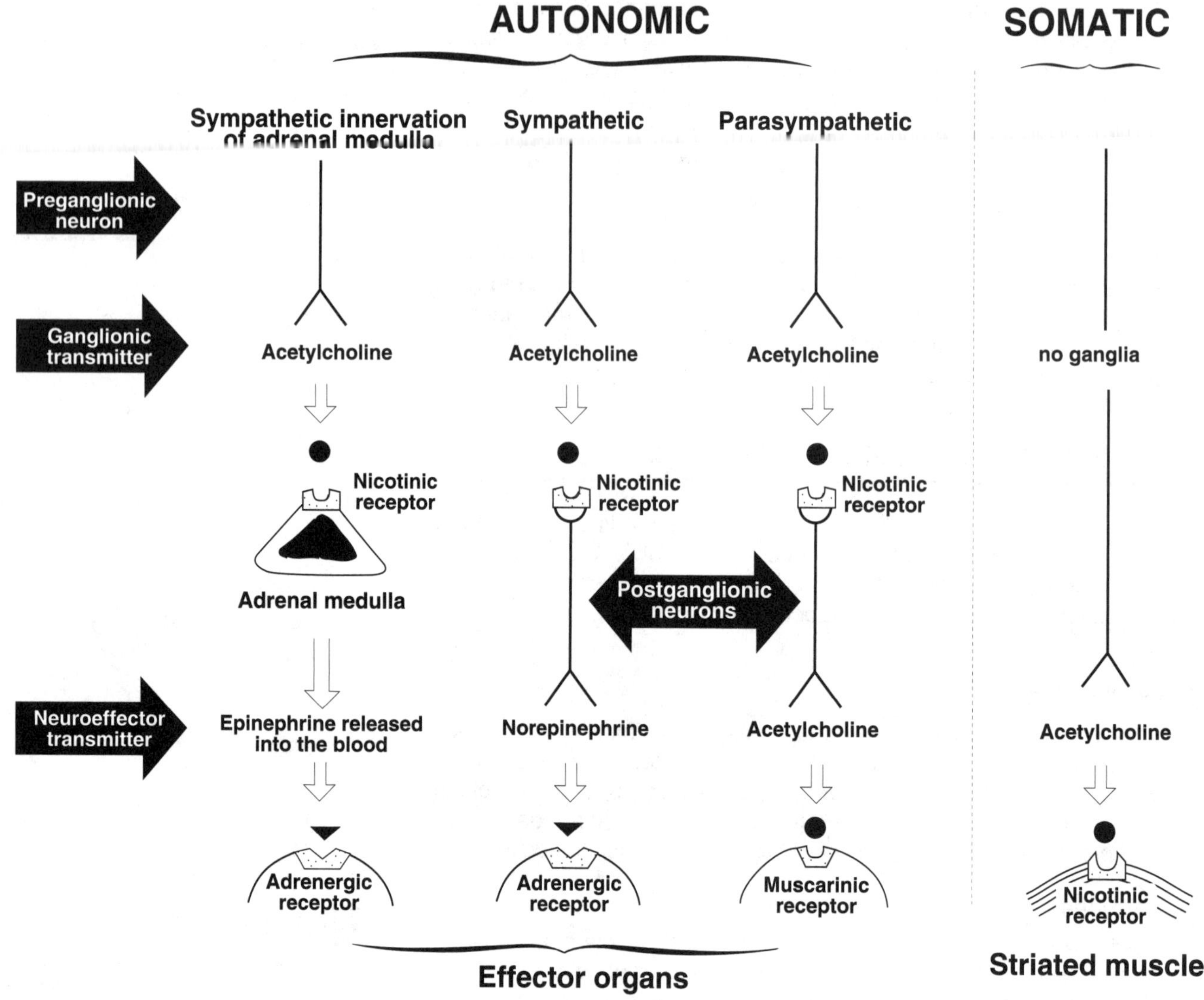

Figure 3.6
Summary of the neurotransmitters released and the types of receptors found within the autonomic and somatic nervous systems. [Note: This schematic diagram does not show that the parasympathetic ganglia are close to or on the surface of the effector organs and that the postganglionic fibers are usually shorter than the preganglionic fibers.]

2. **Types of neurotransmitters:** Although over 50 chemical signal molecules in the nervous system have tentatively been identified, 6 signal compounds—norepinephrine (and the closely related epinephrine), acetylcholine, dopamine, serotonin, histamine, and γ-aminobutyric acid—are most commonly involved in the actions of therapeutically useful drugs. Each of these chemical signals binds to a specific family of receptors. Cholinergic and adrenergic neurotransmitters are the primary chemical signals in the autonomic nervous system, whereas a wide variety of neurotransmitters function in the CNS.

a. Acetylcholine: The autonomic nerve fibers can be classified into two groups based on the chemical nature of the neurotransmitter released. If transmission is mediated by acetylcholine, the neuron is termed **cholinergic**. Acetylcholine mediates the transmission of nerve impulses across autonomic ganglia in both the sympathetic and parasympathetic nervous systems (Figure 3.6). It is the neurotransmitter at the adrenal medulla. Transmission from the autonomic postganglionic nerves to the effector organs in the parasympathetic system also involves the release of acetylcholine. In the somatic nervous system, transmission at the neuromuscular junction (that is, between nerve fibers and voluntary muscles) is also cholinergic.

b. Norepinephrine and epinephrine: If norepinephrine or epinephrine is the transmitter, the fiber is called **adrenergic** (adrenaline being another name for epinephrine). In the sympathetic system, norepinephrine mediates the transmission of nerve impulses from autonomic postganglionic nerves to effector organs. Norepinephrine and adrenergic receptors are discussed in Chapters 6 and 7. A summary of the neuromediators released and the type of receptors within the peripheral nervous system is shown in Figure 3.6. [Note: A few sympathetic fibers, such as those involved in sweating, are cholinergic; for simplicity, they are not shown on Figure 3.6.]

IV. SECOND MESSENGER SYSTEMS IN INTRACELLULAR RESPONSE

The binding of chemical signals to receptors activates enzymatic processes within the cell membrane that ultimately result in a cellular response, such as the phosphorylation of intracellular proteins or changes in the conductivity of ion channels. A neurotransmitter can be thought of as a signal, and a receptor as a signal detector and transducer. "Second messenger" molecules, produced in response to neurotransmitter binding to a receptor, translate the extracellular signal into a response that may be further propagated or amplified within the cell. Each component serves as a link in the communication between extracellular events and chemical changes within the cell.

A. Actions of membrane receptors

Neurotransmitter receptors are membrane proteins that provide a binding site that recognizes and responds to neurotransmitter molecules. Some receptors, such as the postsynaptic receptors of nerve or muscle, are directly linked to membrane ion channels; thus, binding of the neurotransmitter occurs rapidly (within fractions of a millisecond) and directly affects ion permeability (Figure 3.7A). The effect of neurotransmitters on these chemically gated ion channels is discussed on p. 82.

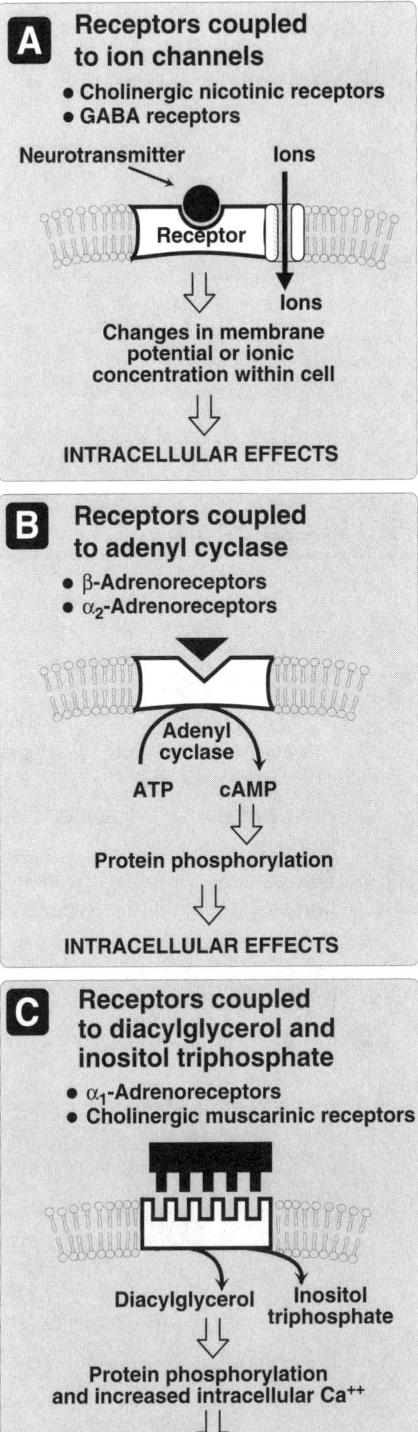

Figure 3.7
Three mechanisms whereby binding of a neurotransmitter leads to a cellular effect.

B. Regulation involving second messenger molecules

Some receptors are not directly coupled to ion gates. Rather, the receptor signals its recognition of a bound neurotransmitter by initiating a series of reactions, which ultimately results in a specific intracellular response. "Second messenger" molecules—so named because they intervene between the original message (the neurotransmitter or hormone) and the ultimate effect on the cell—are part of the cascade of events that translates neurotransmitter binding into a cellular response. The two most widely recognized second messengers are the adenylyl cyclase system and the calcium/phosphatidylinositol system (Figure 3.7B and C).

Study Questions

Choose the ONE best answer

3.1. All of the following statements concerning the autonomic nervous system are true EXCEPT for which one?

A. The autonomic nervous system is composed entirely of efferent neurons.

B. The sympathetic division is activated in response to stressful situations.

C. The parasympathetic division originates from cell bodies in the central nervous system.

D. The control of blood pressure is mainly a sympathetic activity, with essentially no participation of the parasympathetic system.

E. The parasympathetic nervous system is not required for life.

> Correct choice = E. The parasympathetic nervous system is essential for life. Visceral motor (efferent) neurons innervate smooth muscle of the viscera, cardiac muscle, and the exocrine glands. The afferent neurons of the autonomic nervous system are important in the reflex regulation, for example, by sensing pressure in the carotid sinus and aortic arch and signaling the CNS to influence the efferent branch of the system to respond. Conditions such as trauma, fear, hypoglycemia, cold, or exercise activate the sympathetic neurons. Both sympathetic and parasympathetic neurons emerge from the brain stem or spinal cord. Blood pressure is regulated largely by sympathetic control of vascular tone.

3.2. Which one of the following statements concerning the parasympathetic nervous system is CORRECT?

A. The parasympathetic system uses norepinephrine as a neurotransmitter.

B. The parasympathetic system often discharges as a single, functional system.

C. The parasympathetic division is involved in accommodation of near vision, movement of food, and urination.

D. The postganglionic fibers of the parasympathetic division are long, compared to those of the sympathetic nervous system.

E. The parasympathetic system controls the secretion of the adrenal medulla.

> Correct answer = C. The parasympathetic system maintains essential bodily functions, such as vision, movement of food, and urination. It uses acetylcholine, not norepinephrine, as a neurotransmitter, and discharges as discrete fibers that are activated separately. The postganglionic fibers of the parasympathetic system are short compared to the sympathetic division. The adrenal medulla is under control of the sympathetic system.

3.3. Which one of the following is characteristic of parasympathetic stimulation?

A. Decrease in intestinal motility.

B. Inhibition of bronchial secretion.

C. Contraction of sphincter muscle in the iris of the eye (miosis).

D. Contraction of sphincter of urinary bladder.

E. Increase in heart rate.

> Correct answer = C.

Cholinergic Agonists

4

I. OVERVIEW

Drugs affecting the autonomic nervous system are divided into two subgroups according to the type of neuron involved in their mechanism of action. The cholinergic drugs, which are described in this and the following chapter, act on receptors that are activated by acetylcholine. The second group—the adrenergic drugs (discussed in Chapters 6 and 7)—act on receptors that are stimulated by norepinephrine or epinephrine. Both the cholinergic and adrenergic drugs act either by stimulating or blocking neurons of the autonomic nervous system. Figure 4.1 summarizes the cholinergic agonists discussed in this chapter.

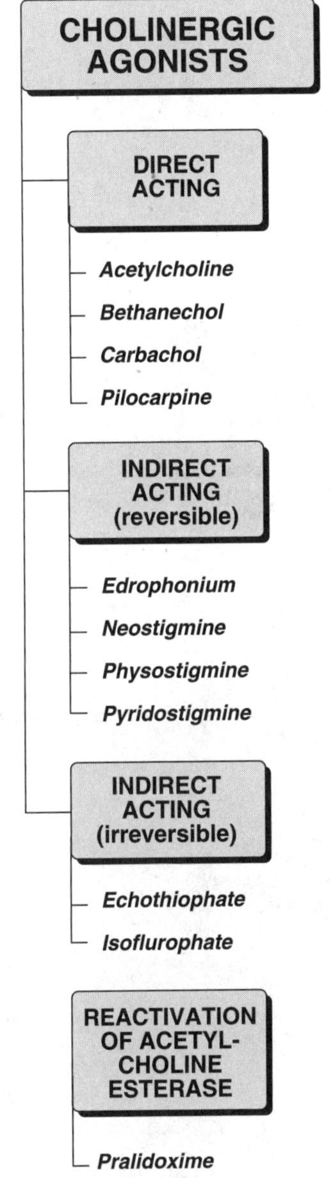

Figure 4.1
Summary of cholinergic agonists.

II. THE CHOLINERGIC NEURON

The preganglionic fibers terminating in the adrenal medulla, the autonomic ganglia (both parasympathetic and sympathetic), and the postganglionic fibers of the parasympathetic division use acetylcholine as a neurotransmitter (Figure 4.2). Cholinergic neurons innervate voluntary muscles of the somatic system and are also found in the CNS.

A. Neurotransmission at cholinergic neurons

Neurotransmission in cholinergic neurons involves six steps. The first four, synthesis, storage, release and binding of the acetylcholine to a receptor, are followed by the fifth step, degradation of the neurotransmitter in the synaptic gap (that is, the space between the nerve endings and adjacent receptors located on nerves or effector organs), and the sixth step, the recycling of choline (Figure 4.3).

1. **Synthesis of acetylcholine:** Choline is transported from the extracellular fluid into the cytoplasm of the cholinergic neuron by a carrier system that cotransports sodium and can be inhibited by the drug *hemicholinium*. Choline acetyltransferase (CAT) catalyzes the reaction of choline with acetyl CoA to form acetylcholine in the cytosol.

2. **Storage of acetylcholine in vesicles:** The acetylcholine is packaged into vesicles by an active transport process coupled to the efflux of protons. The mature vesicle not only contains acetylcholine but also adenosine triphosphate and proteoglycan. The function of the latter substances in the nerve terminal is unknown.

3. **Release of acetylcholine:** When an action potential propagated by the action of voltage-sensitive sodium channels arrives at a nerve ending, voltage-sensitive calcium channels in the presynaptic membrane open, causing an increase in the concentration of intracellular calcium. Elevated calcium levels promote the fusion of synaptic vesicles with the cell membrane and release of acetylcholine into the synapse. This release is blocked by botulinum toxin. By contrast, black widow spider venom causes all of the cellular acetylcholine stored in synaptic vesicles to spill into the synaptic gap.

4. **Binding to receptor:** Acetylcholine released from the synaptic vesicles diffuses across the synaptic space and binds to either postsynaptic receptors on the target cell or to presynaptic receptors in the membrane of the neuron that released the acetylcholine.

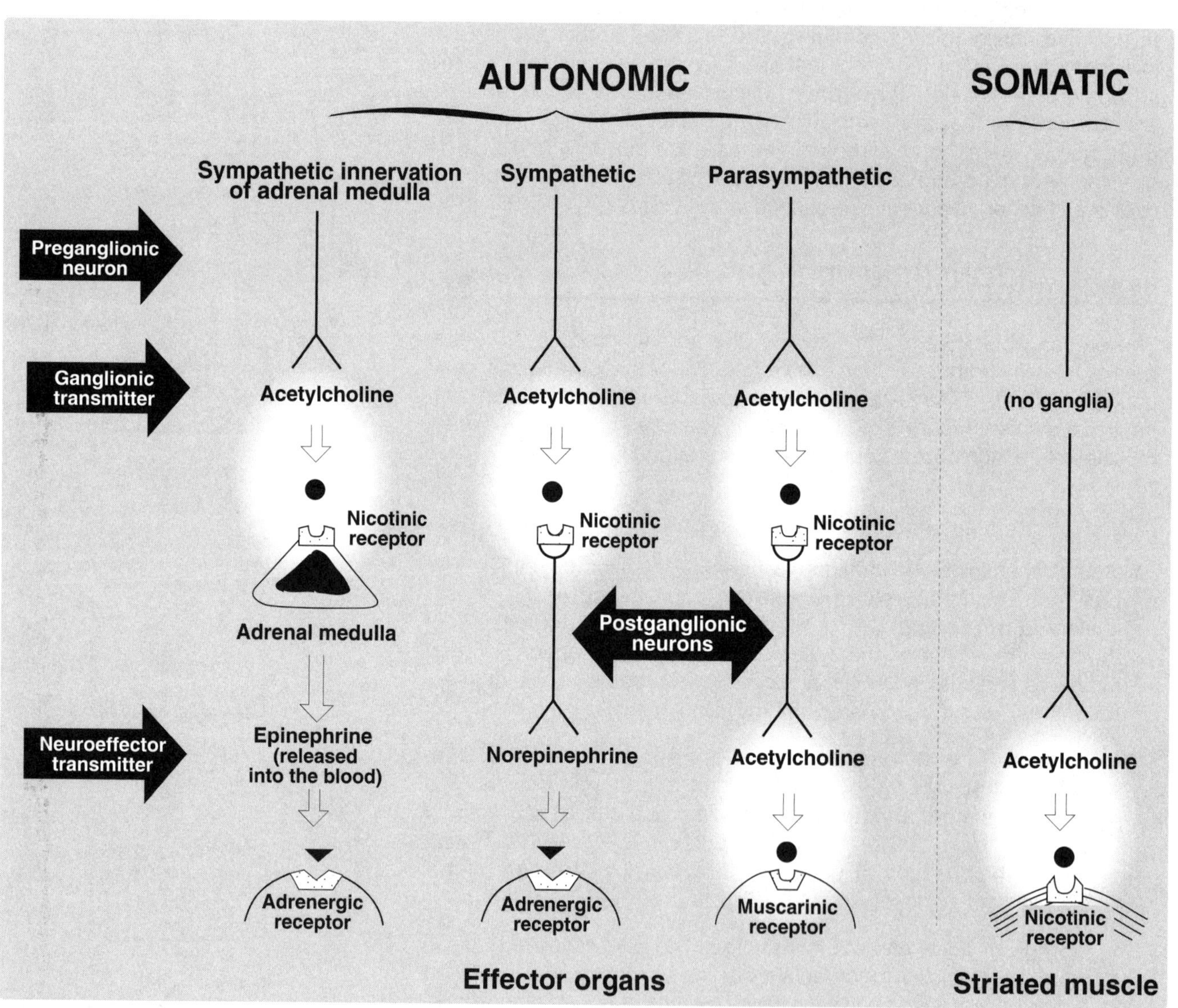

Figure 4.2
Sites of actions of cholinergic agonists in the autonomic and somatic nervous systems.

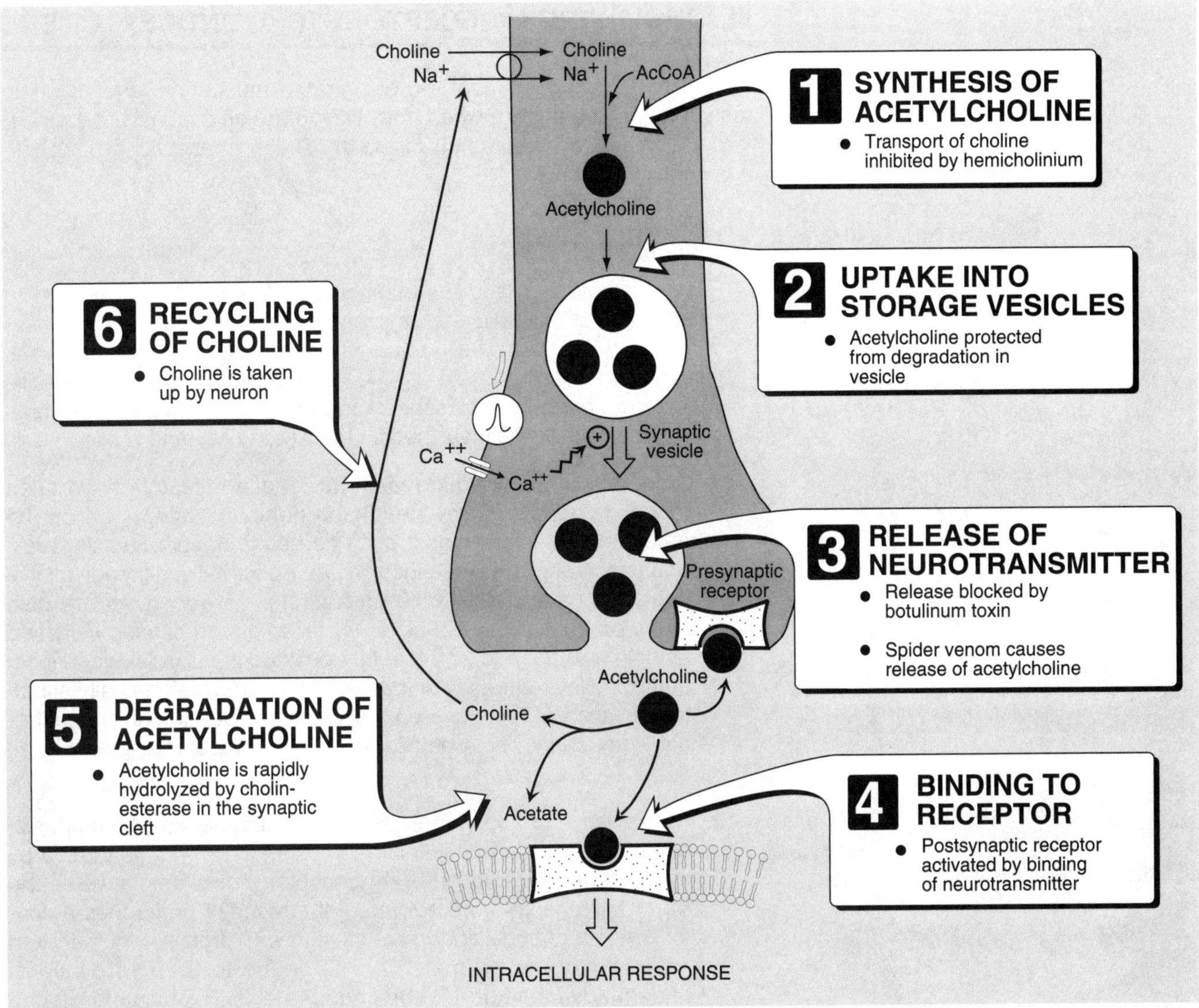

Figure 4.3
Synthesis and release of acetylcholine from the cholinergic neuron.

Binding to the receptor leads to a biological response within the cell such as the initiation of a nerve impulse in a postganglionic fiber or activation of specific enzymes in effector cells as mediated by second messenger molecules (see p. 33 and below).

5. **Degradation of acetylcholine:** The signal at the postjunctional effector site is rapidly terminated. This occurs in the synaptic cleft where acetylcholinesterase cleaves acetylcholine to choline and acetate (see Figure 4.3).

6. **Recycling of choline:** Choline may be recaptured by a sodium-coupled high affinity uptake system that transports the molecule back into the neuron, where it is acetylated and stored until released by a subsequent action potential.

III. CHOLINERGIC RECEPTORS (CHOLINOCEPTORS)

Two families of cholinoceptors, designated muscarinic and nicotinic receptors, can be distinguished from each other on the basis of their different affinities for agents that mimic the action of acetylcholine (cholinomimetic agents).

A. Muscarinic receptors

These receptors, in addition to binding acetylcholine, also recognize muscarine, an alkaloid that is present in certain poisonous mushrooms. By contrast, the muscarinic receptors show only a weak affinity for nicotine (Figure 4.4). Using binding studies and specific inhibitors, several subclasses of muscarinic receptors have been pharmacologically distinguished as M_1, M_2, M_3, M_4, and M_5.

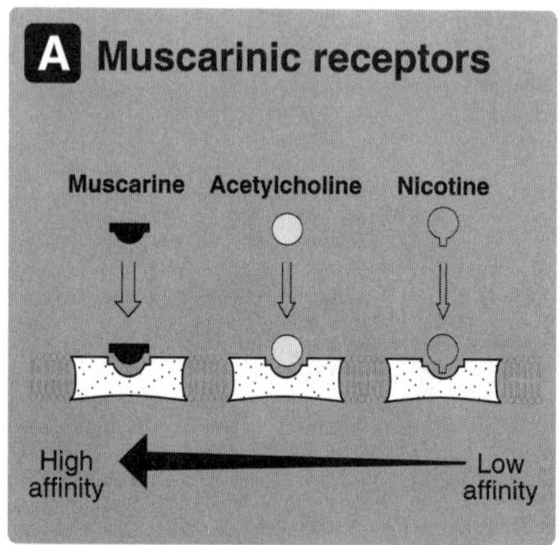

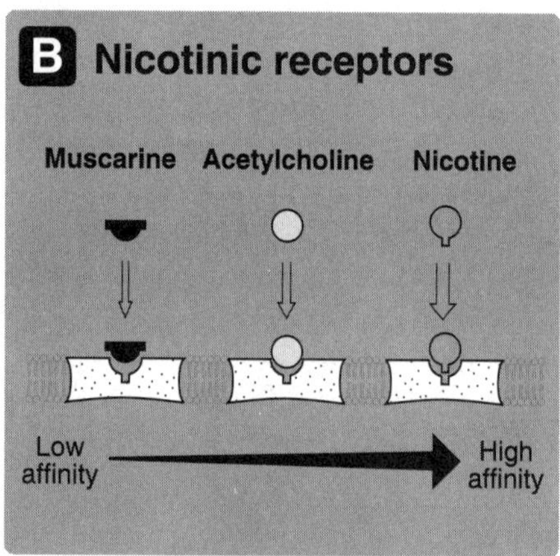

Figure 4.4
Types of cholinergic receptors.

1. **Locations of muscarinic receptors:** These receptors have been found on ganglia of the peripheral nervous system and on the autonomic effector organs, such as heart, smooth muscle, brain and exocrine glands (see Figure 4.2). Specifically, although all five subtypes have been found on neurons, M_1 receptors are also found on gastric parietal cells, M_2 receptors on cardiac cells and smooth muscle, and M_3 receptors on exocrine glands and smooth muscle. [Note: Drugs with muscarinic actions preferentially stimulate muscarinic receptors on these tissues, but at high concentration may show some activity at nicotinic receptors (see Figure 4.4).]

2. **Mechanisms of acetylcholine signal transduction:** A number of different molecular mechanisms transmit the signal generated by acetylcholine occupation of the receptor. For example, when the M_1 or M_3 receptors are activated, the receptor undergoes a conformational change and interacts with a G protein, which in turn activates phospholipase C. This leads to the hydrolysis of phoshatidylinositol-(4,5)-bisphosphate (PIP_2) to yield diacylglycerol (DAG) and inositol (1,4,5)-trisphosphate (IP_3), which cause an increase in intracellular Ca^{++}. This cation can then interact to stimulate or inhibit enzymes, or cause hyperpolarization, secretion or contraction.[1] In contrast, activation of the M_2 subtype on the cardiac muscle stimulates a G protein that inhibits adenylyl cyclase and increases K^+ conductance, to which the heart responds with a decrease in rate and force of contraction.

3. **Muscarinic agonists and antagonists:** Attempts are currently underway to develop muscarinic agonists and antagonists that are directed against specific receptor subtypes. For example, *pirenzepine*, a tricyclic anticholinergic drug, selectively inhibits M_1 muscarinic receptors, such as in the gastric mucosa. At therapeutic doses, *pirenzepine* does not cause many of the side effects seen with the non-subtype-specific drugs. Therefore, *pirenzepine* may be useful in the treatment of gastric and duodenal ulcers (see p. 239). [Note: At the present time there are no clinically important agents that interact with the M_4 and M_5 receptors.]

[1]See p. 44 for Infolink references to other books in this series.

4. **Nicotinic receptors:** These receptors, in addition to binding acetylcholine, also recognize nicotine but show only a weak affinity for muscarine (see Figure 4.4). Nicotine initially stimulates and then blocks the receptor. Nicotinic receptors are located in the CNS, adrenal medulla, autonomic ganglia, and the neuromuscular junction (see Figure 4.2). Drugs with nicotinic action stimulate the nicotinic receptors located on these tissues. The nicotinic receptors of autonomic ganglia differ from those of the neuromuscular junction. For example, ganglionic receptors are selectively blocked by *hexamethonium*, whereas neuromuscular junction receptors are specifically blocked by *tubocurarine* (see p. 50).

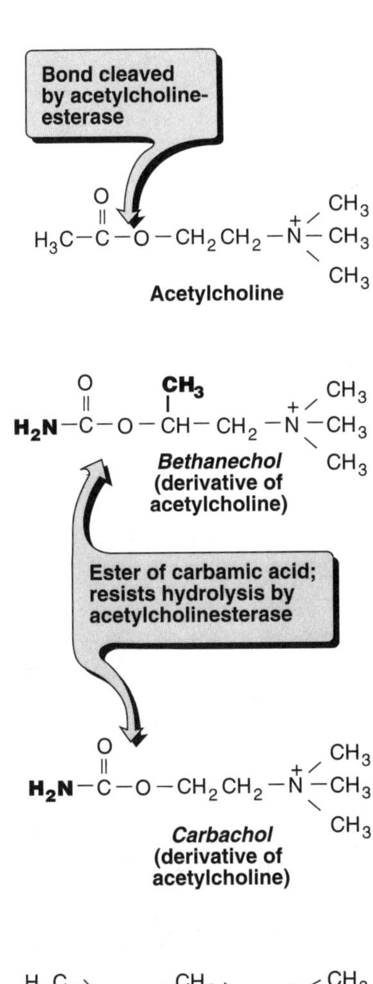

Figure 4.5
Comparison of the structures of some cholinergic agonists.

IV. DIRECT-ACTING CHOLINERGIC AGONISTS

Cholinergic agonists mimic the effects of acetylcholine by binding directly to cholinoceptors. These agents are synthetic esters of choline, such as *carbachol* and *bethanechol*, or naturally occurring alkaloids, such as *pilocarpine* (Figure 4.5). All of the direct-acting cholinergic drugs have longer durations of action than acetylcholine. Some of the more therapeutically useful drugs (*pilocarpine* and *bethanechol*) preferentially bind to muscarinic receptors and are sometimes referred to as muscarinic agents. [Note: Muscarinic receptors are located primarily, but not exclusively, at the neuroeffector junction of the parasympathetic nervous system.] However, as a group, the direct-acting agonists show little specificity in their actions, which limits their clinical usefulness.

A. Acetylcholine

Acetylcholine [a se teel KOE leen] is a quarternary ammonium compound that cannot penetrate membranes. Although it is the neurotransmitter of parasympathetic and cholinergic nerves, it is therapeutically of no importance because of its multiplicity of actions and its rapid inactivation by acetylcholinesterase. Acetylcholine has both muscarinic and nicotinic activity. Its actions include:

1. **Decrease in heart rate and cardiac output:** The actions of acetylcholine on the heart mimic the effects of vagal stimulation. For example, acetylcholine, if injected intravenously, produces a brief decrease in cardiac rate and stroke volume as a result of a reduction in the rate of firing at the sinoatrial (SA) node. [Note: It should be remembered that normal vagal activity regulates the heart by the release of acetylcholine at the SA node.]

2. **Decrease in blood pressure:** Injection of acetylcholine causes vasodilation and the lowering of blood pressure. Although no innervation of the vasculature by the parasympathetic system exists, there are cholinergic receptors on the blood vessels that respond by causing vasodilation. The vasodilation is due to an acetylcholine-induced rise in intracellular Ca^{++}—caused by the phosphatidylinositol system—that results in the formation of nitric oxide (NO) from arginine in endothelial cells.[2] [Note: NO is also known as endothelium-derived relaxing factor (EDRF).] (See p. 176 for more detail on nitric oxide.) In the absence of adminis-

[2]See p. 44 for Infolink references to other books in this series.

tered cholinergic agents, the vascular receptors have no known function, since acetylcholine is never released into the blood in any significant quantities. *Atropine* (see p. 45) blocks these muscarinic receptors and prevents acetylcholine from producing vasodilation.

3. **Other actions:** In the gastrointestinal tract, acetylcholine increases salivary secretion, and stimulates intestinal secretions and motility. Bronchiolar secretions are also stimulated. In the genitourinary tract, the tone of the detrusor urinae muscle is increased. In the eye, acetylcholine is involved in stimulating ciliary muscle contraction for near vision and in the constriction of the pupillae sphincter muscle, causing miosis (marked constriction of the pupil).

B. Bethanechol

Bethanechol [be THAN e kole] is structurally related to acetylcholine; the acetate is replaced by carbamate and the choline is methylated (see Figure 4.5). Hence, it is not hydrolyzed by acetylcholinesterase, although it is inactivated through hydrolysis by other esterases. It has little or no nicotinic actions but does have strong muscarinic activity. Its major actions are on the smooth musculature of the bladder and gastrointestinal tract. It has a duration of action of about 1 hour.

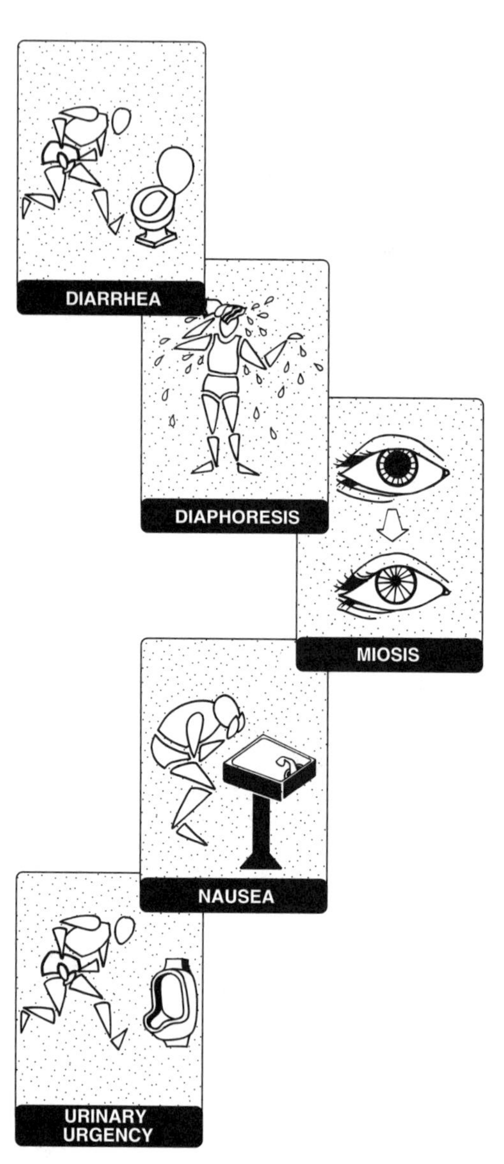

Figure 4.6
Some adverse effects observed with cholinergic drugs.

1. **Actions:** *Bethanechol* directly stimulates muscarinic receptors, causing increased intestinal motility and tone, and it also stimulates the detrusor muscles of the bladder while the trigone and sphincter are relaxed, causing expulsion of urine.

2. **Therapeutic applications:** In urologic treatment, *bethanechol* is used to stimulate the atonic bladder, particularly in postpartum or postoperative nonobstructive urinary retention.

3. **Adverse effects:** *Bethanechol* causes the actions of generalized cholinergic stimulation (Figure 4.6). These include sweating, salivation, flushing, decreased blood pressure, nausea, abdominal pain, diarrhea, and bronchospasm.

C. Carbachol (Carbamylcholine)

Carbachol [KAR ba kole] has both muscarinic as well as nicotinic actions. Like *bethanechol*, *carbachol* is an ester of carbamic acid and a poor substrate for acetylcholinesterase (see Figure 4.5). It is biotransformed by other esterases but at a much slower rate. A single administration can last as long as one hour.

1. **Actions:** *Carbachol* has profound effects on both the cardiovascular system and the gastrointestinal system because of its ganglion-stimulating activity and may first stimulate and then depress these systems. It can cause release of *epinephrine* from the adrenal medulla by its nicotinic action. Locally instilled into the eye, it mimics the effects of acetylcholine, causing miosis.

2. **Therapeutic uses:** Because of its high potency and relatively long duration of action, *carbachol* is rarely used therapeutically, except in the eye as a miotic agent to cause contraction of the pupil and a decrease in intraocular pressure.

3. **Adverse effects:** At doses used ophthalmologically, there are little to no side effects.

D. Pilocarpine

The alkaloid *pilocarpine* [pye loe KAR peen] is a tertiary amine and is stable to hydrolysis by acetylcholinesterase (see Figure 4.5). Compared with acetylcholine and its derivatives, it is far less potent. *Pilocarpine* exhibits muscarinic activity and is primarily used in ophthalmology.

1. **Actions:** Applied topically to the cornea, *pilocarpine* produces a rapid miosis and contraction of the ciliary muscle. The eye undergoes a spasm of accommodation, and vision is fixed at some particular distance, making it impossible to focus (Figure 4.7). [Note the opposing effects of *atropine*, a muscarinic blocker, on the eye (see p. 45).] *Pilocarpine* is one of the most potent stimulators of secretions such as sweat, tears, and saliva, but it is not used for this purpose.

2. **Therapeutic use in glaucoma:** *Pilocarpine* is the drug of choice in the emergency lowering of intraocular pressure of both narrow-angle (also called closed-angle) and wide-angle (also called open-angle) glaucoma. *Pilocarpine* is extremely effective in opening the trabecular meshwork around Schlemm's canal, causing an immediate drop in intraocular pressure as a result of the increased drainage of aqueous humor. This action lasts up to 1 day and can be repeated. Cholinesterase inhibitors, such as *isoflurophate* and *echothiophate*, have longer durations of action. [Note: Carbonic anhydrase inhibitors, such as *acetazolamide* (see p. 226), *epinephrine* (see p. 61), and the β adrenergic blocker, *timolol* (see p. 76), are effective in treating glaucoma chronically but are not used for the emergency lowering of intraocular pressure.]

3. **Adverse effects:** *Pilocarpine* can enter the brain and cause CNS disturbances. It stimulates profuse sweating and salivation.

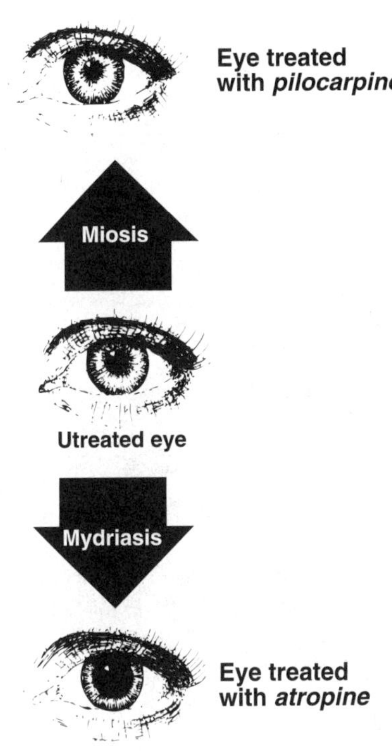

Figure 4.7
Actions of *pilocarpine* and *atropine* on the iris and ciliary muscle of the eye.

V. ANTICHOLINESTERASES (REVERSIBLE)

Acetylcholinesterase is an enzyme that specifically cleaves acetylcholine to acetate and choline. It is located both pre-and post-synaptically in the nerve terminal, where it is membrane bound. Inhibitors of acetylcholinesterase indirectly provide a cholinergic action by prolonging the lifetime of acetylcholine produced endogenously at the cholinergic nerve endings. This results in the accumulation of acetylcholine in the synaptic space (Figure 4.8). These drugs can thus provoke a response at all cholinoceptors in the body, including both muscarinic and nicotinic receptors of the autonomic nervous system as well as the neuromuscular junction and the brain.

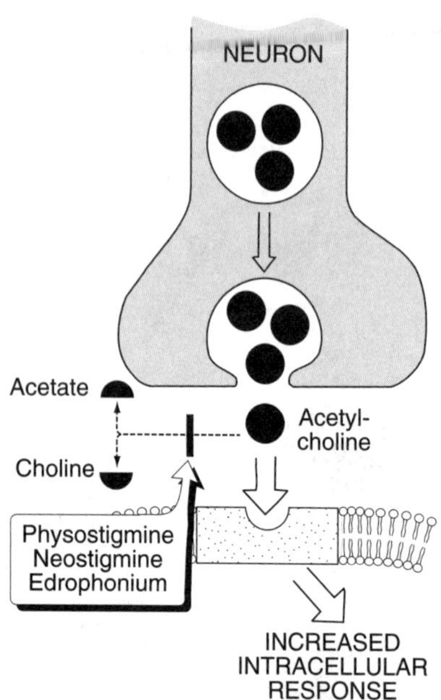

Figure 4.8
Mechanisms of action of indirect (reversible) cholinergic agonists.

A. Physostigmine

Physostigmine [fi zoe STIG meen] is an alkaloid (a nitrogenous compound found in plants) and a tertiary amine. It is a substrate for acetylcholinesterase, and forms a relatively stable enzyme-substrate intermediate that reversibly inactivates acetylcholinesterase. The result is potentiation of cholinergic activity throughout the body.

1. **Actions:** *Physostigmine* has a wide range of actions because it stimulates not only muscarinic and nicotinic sites of the autonomic nervous system but also the nicotinic receptors of the neuromuscular junction. Its duration of action is about 2–4 hours. *Physostigmine* can enter and stimulate the CNS.

2. **Therapeutic uses**: The drug increases intestinal and bladder motility, which serve as its therapeutic action in atony of either organ. Placed topically in the eye, it produces miosis and spasm of accommodation and a lowering of intraocular pressure. It is used to treat glaucoma, but *pilocarpine* is more effective. *Physostigmine* is also used in the treatment of overdoses of drugs with anticholinergic actions such as *atropine* (see p. 45), *phenothiazines* (see p. 127), and tricyclic antidepressants (see p. 119).

3. **Adverse effects:** The effects of *physostigmine* on the CNS may lead to convulsions when high doses are used. Bradycardia may also occur. Inhibition of acetylcholinesterase at the skeletal neuromuscular junction causes the accumulation of acetylcholine and ultimately results in paralysis of skeletal muscle. However, these effects are rarely seen with therapeutic doses.

B. Neostigmine

Neostigmine [nee oh STIG meen] is a synthetic compound that reversibly inhibits acetylcholinesterase as does *physostigmine*. Unlike *physostigmine*, *neostigmine* is more polar and therefore does not enter the CNS. Its effect on skeletal muscle is greater than that of *physostigmine*, and it can stimulate contractility before it paralyzes. *Neostigmine* has a moderate duration of action, usually 2–4 hours. It is used to stimulate the bladder and GI tract, and is also used as an antidote for *tubocurarine* and other competitive neuromuscular blocking agents (see p. 50). *Neostigmine* has found use in symptomatic treatment of myasthenia gravis, an autoimmune disease caused by antibodies to the nicotinic receptor that bind to the acetylcholine receptors of neuromuscular junctions. This causes their degradation, and thus makes fewer receptors available for interaction with the neurotransmitter. Adverse effects of *neostigmine* include the actions of generalized cholinergic stimulation, such as salivation, flushing, decreased blood pressure, nausea, abdominal pain, diarrhea, and bronchospasm.

C. Pyridostigmine:

Pyridostigmine [peer id doe STIG meen] is another cholinesterase inhibitor that is used in the chronic management of myasthenia gravis. Its duration of action (3–6 hours) is longer than that of *neostigmine* (2–4 hours).

D. Edrophonium

The actions of *edrophonium* [ed roe FOE nee um] are similar to those of *neostigmine*, except that it is more rapidly absorbed and has a short duration of action (10–20 minutes). *Edrophonium* is a quarternary amine and is used in the diagnosis of myasthenia gravis. Intravenous injection of *edrophonium* leads to a rapid increase in muscle strength. Care must be taken since excess drug may provoke a cholinergic crisis. *Atropine* is the antidote.

VI. ANTICHOLINESTERASES (IRREVERSIBLE)

A number of synthetic organophosphate compounds have the capacity to bind covalently to acetylcholinesterase. The result is a long lasting increase in acetylcholine at all sites where it is released. Many of these drugs are extremely toxic and were developed by the military as nerve agents. Related compounds such as parathion are employed as insecticides.

A. Isoflurophate

1. **Mechanism of action:** *Isoflurophate* [eye soe FLURE oh fate] (diisopropylfluorophosphate, DFP) is an organophosphate that covalently binds to a serine-OH at the active site of acetylcholinesterase (Figure 4.9). Once this occurs, the enzyme is permanently inactivated, and restoration of acetylcholinesterase activity requires the synthesis of new enzyme molecules. Following covalent modification of acetylcholinesterase, the phosphorylated enzyme slowly releases one of its isopropyl groups (Figure 4.9). The loss of an alkyl group, which is called aging, makes it impossible for chemical reactivators, such as *pralidoxime* (see below), to break the bond between the remaining drug and the enzyme. Newer nerve agents, available to the military, age in minutes or seconds. DFP ages in 6–8 hours.

2. **Actions:** Actions include generalized cholinergic stimulation, paralysis of motor function (causing breathing difficulties), and convulsions. *Isoflurophate* produces intense miosis and thus has found therapeutic use. *Atropine* in high dosage can reverse many of the muscarinic and central effects of *isoflurophate*.

3. **Therapeutic uses:** An ophthalmic ointment of the drug is used topically in the eye for the chronic treatment of open-angle glaucoma. The effects may last for up to one week after a single administration. [Note: *Echothiophate* [ek oe THI oh fate] is a newer drug that covalently bonds to acetylcholinesterase. Its use is the same as *isoflurophate*.]

4. **Reactivation of acetylcholinesterase:** *Pralidoxime* (PAM) is a synthetic pyridinium compound that can reactivate inhibited acetylcholinesterase. The presence of a charged group allows it to approach an anionic site on the enzyme where it essentially displaces the organophosphate and regenerates the enzyme. If given before aging of the alkylated enzyme occurs, it can reverse the effects of *isoflurophate* except for those in the CNS. With the newer nerve agents, which produce aging of the enzyme complex within seconds, *pralidoxime* is less effective.

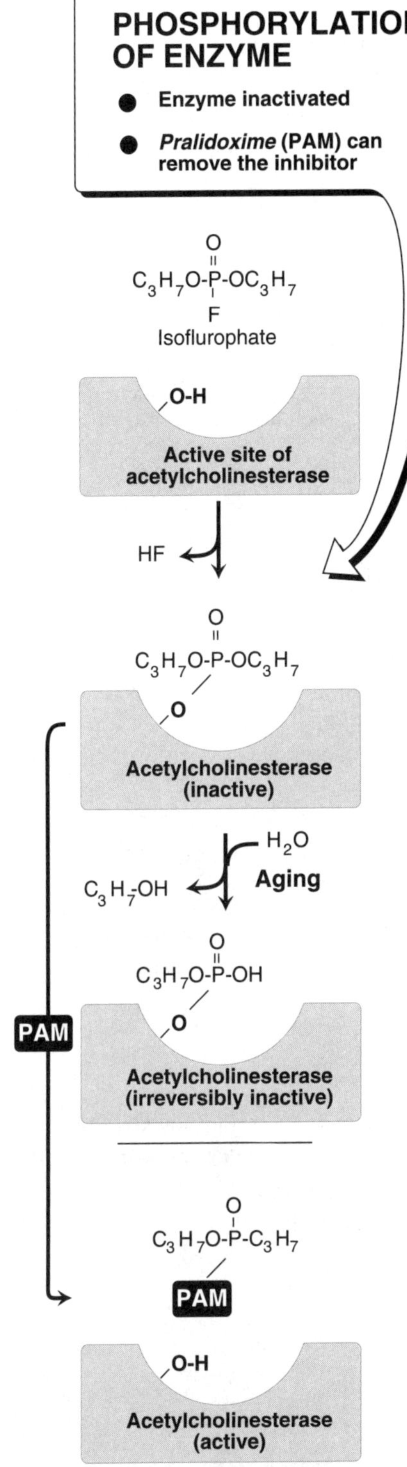

Figure 4.9
Covalent modification of acetylcholinesterase by isoflurophate; also shown is the reactivation of the enzyme with *pralidoxime*.

Choose the ONE best answer

4.1. Which of the following is NOT an expected symptom of poisoning with isoflurophate?

A. Paralysis of skeletal muscle
B. Increased bronchial secretions
C. Miosis
D. Tachycardia
E. Convulsions

Correct answer = D. Bradycardia (rather than tachycardia) and decreased cardiac output result from increased parasympathetic stimulation. Since isoflurophate inhibits acetylcholinesterase and increases the concentration of acetylcholine at the synapse, it mimics (parasympathetic) stimulation.

4.2. Which of the following INCORRECTLY matches a cholinergic agonist with a pharmacologic action?

A. Bethanechol: stimulates atonic bladder.
B. Carbachol: induces release of epinephrine from the adrenal medulla.
C. Acetylcholine: decreases heart rate and cardiac output.
D. Pilocarpine: reduces intraocular pressure.
E. Physostigmine: decreases intestinal motility.

Correct answer = E. Physostigmine potentiates cholinergic activity throughout the body and therefore it increases intestinal and bladder motility.

4.3. Pilocarpine:

A. is used to lower intraocular pressure in glaucoma.
B. is cleaved by acetylcholinesterase.
C. selectively binds to nicotinic receptors.
D. inhibits secretions such as sweat, tears, and saliva.
E. cannot enter the brain.

Correct answer = A. Pilocarpine is used in glaucoma where it is the treatment of choice for the acute attack. It is not cleaved by acetylcholinesterase. It binds mainly to muscarinic receptors, and can enter the brain. Pilocarpine is a potent stimulator of secretions.

4.4 Neostigmine:

A. is contraindicated in glaucoma.
B. has a shorter duration of action than edrophonium.
C. decreases the acetylcholine concentration at the neuromuscular junction.
D. may result in bowel hypermotility, salivation, and sweating.
E. exacerbates tubocurarine poisoning.

Correct answer = D. Neostigmine stimulates muscarinic receptors. It has a longer duration of action than edrophonium, lasting for 2–4 hours, compared to 10–20 minutes for the latter drug. Neostigmine increases the acetylcholine concentration at the neuromuscular junction, making this drug useful in treating myasthenia gravis. It can also be used to lower intraocular pressure, but pilocarpine is more effective.

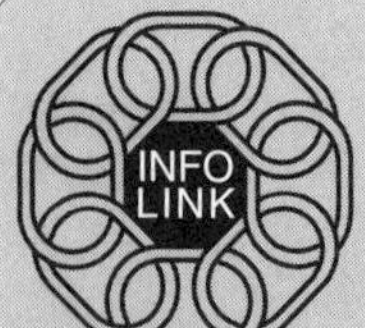

[1]See p. 83 in **Biochemistry** (2nd ed.) for a discussion of Ca^{++} as a regulatory signal.

[2]See p. 85 in **Biochemistry** (2nd ed.) for a discussion of nitric oxide as a regulatory signal.

Cholinergic Antagonists

5

I. OVERVIEW

The cholinergic antagonists (also called cholinergic blockers or anti-cholinergic drugs) bind to cholinoceptors but do not trigger the usual receptor-mediated intracellular effects. The most useful of these agents selectively block the muscarinic synapses of the parasympathetic nerves. The effects of parasympathetic innervation are thus interrupted, and the actions of sympathetic stimulation are left unopposed. A second group of drugs, the ganglionic blockers, show a preference for the nicotinic receptors of the sympathetic and parasympathetic ganglia. A third family of compounds, the neuromuscular blocking agents, interfere with transmission of efferent impulses to skeletal muscles. Figure 5.1 summarizes the cholinergic antagonists discussed in this chapter.

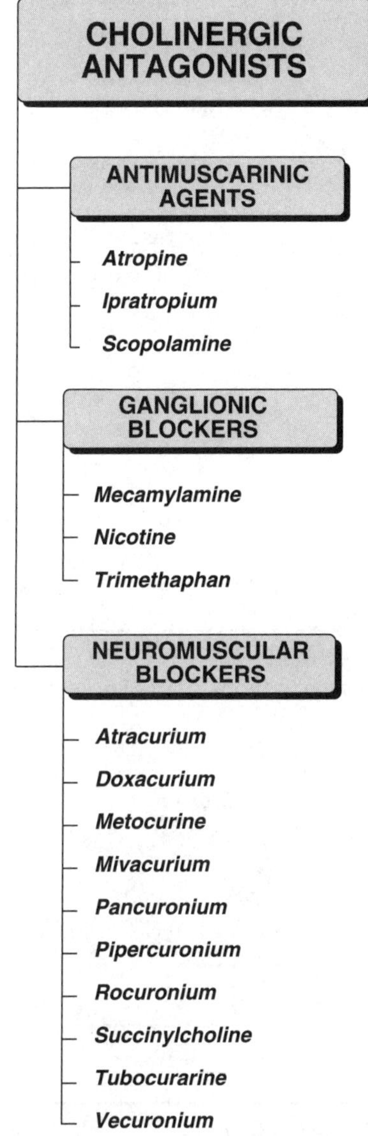

Figure 5.1
Summary of cholinergic antagonists

II. ANTIMUSCARINIC AGENTS

These agents, for example, *atropine* and *scopolamine,* block muscarinic receptors (Figure 5.2) causing inhibition of all muscarinic functions. In addition, these drugs block the few exceptional sympathetic neurons that are cholinergic, such as those innervating sweat glands. In contrast to the cholinergic agonists, which have limited usefulness therapeutically, the cholinergic blockers are beneficial in a variety of clinical situations. Because they do not block nicotinic receptors, the antimuscarinic drugs have little or no action at skeletal neuromuscular junctions or autonomic ganglia.

A. Atropine

Atropine [A troh peen], a belladonna alkaloid, has a high affinity for muscarinic receptors, where it binds competitively, preventing acetylcholine from binding to that site (Figure 5.3). *Atropine* is both a central and peripheral muscarinic blocker. Its general actions last about 4 hours except when placed topically in the eye, where the action may last for days.

1. Actions:

a. Eye: *Atropine* blocks all cholinergic activity on the eye, resulting in mydriasis (dilation of the pupil; see Figure 4.6), unresponsiveness to light and cycloplegia (inability to focus for near vision). In patients with glaucoma, intraocular pressure may rise dangerously.

Lippincott's Illustrated Reviews: Pharmacology, Second Edition.
by Mary J. Mycek, Richard A. Harvey and Pamela C. Champe.
Lippincott Williams & Wilkins, Philadelphia, PA © 2000.

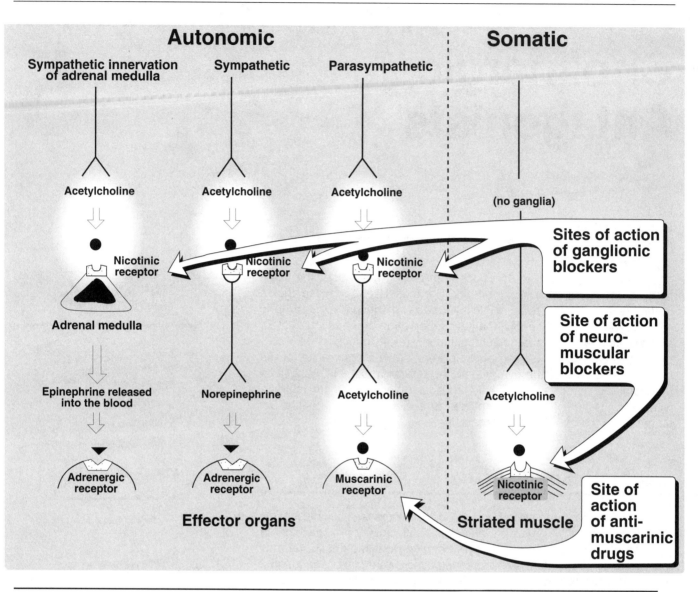

Figure 5.2
Sites of actions of cholinergic antagonists.

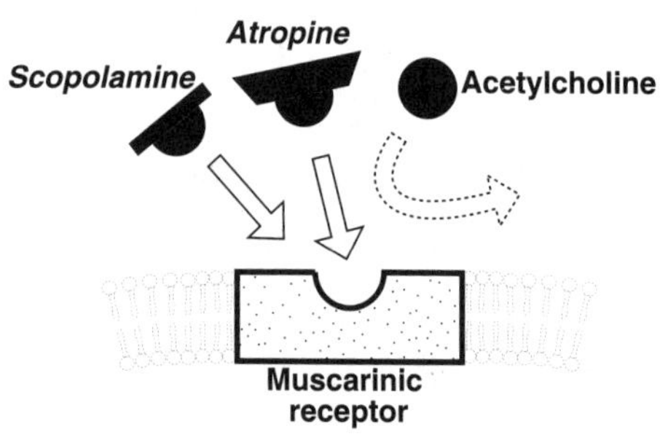

Figure 5.3
Competition of *atropine* and *scopolamine* with acetylcholine for the muscarinic receptor.

b. Gastrointestinal (GI): *Atropine* can be used as an antispasmodic to reduce activity of the GI tract. *Atropine* and *scopolamine* (which is discussed in the next section) are probably the most potent drugs available that produce this effect. Although gastric motility is reduced, hydrochloric acid production is not significantly affected. Thus, the drug is not effective in promoting healing of peptic ulcer. [Note: *Pirenzepine* (see p. 239), an M_1-muscarinic antagonist, does reduce gastric acid secretion at doses that do not antagonize other systems.]

c. Urinary system: *Atropine* is also employed to reduce hypermotility states of the urinary bladder. It is still occasionally used in enuresis (involuntary voiding of urine) among children but α-adrenergic agonists may be more effective with fewer side effects.

d. **Cardiovascular:** *Atropine* produces divergent effects on the cardiovascular system, depending on the dose (Figure 5.4). At low doses the predominant effect is a decreased cardiac rate (bradycardia). Originally thought to be due to central activation of vagal efferent outflow, newer data indicate that the effect results from blockade of the M_1 receptors on the inhibitory prejunctional neurons, thus permitting increased acetylcholine release. With higher doses of *atropine*, the cardiac receptors on the SA node are blocked, and the cardiac rate increases modestly (tachycardia). This generally requires at least 1 mg of *atropine*, which is a higher dose than ordinarily given. Arterial blood pressure is unaffected but at toxic levels, *atropine* will dilate the cutaneous vasculature.

e. **Secretions:** *Atropine* blocks the salivary glands to produce a drying effect on the oral mucous membranes (xerostomia). The salivary glands are exquisitely sensitive to *atropine*. Sweat and lacrimal glands are also affected. Inhibition of secretions by the former can cause elevated body temperature.

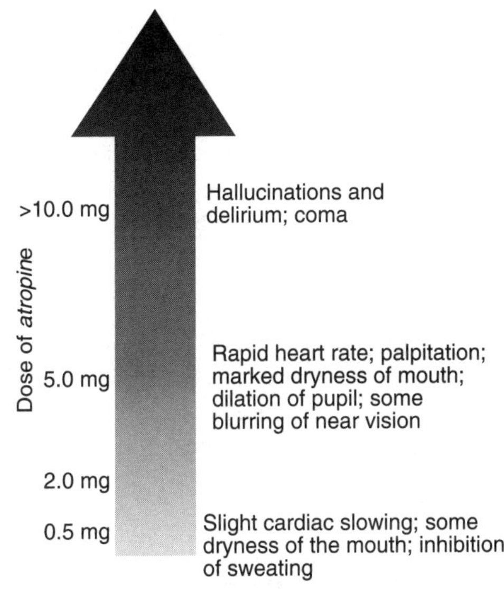

Figure 5.4
Dose-dependent effects of *atropine*.

2. **Therapeutic uses:**

a. **Ophthalmic:** In the eye, topical *atropine* exerts both mydriatic and cycloplegic effects and permits the measurement of refractive errors without interference by the accommodative capacity of the eye. [Note: *Phenylephrine* (see p. 66), or similar α-adrenergic drugs, are preferred for pupillary dilation if cycloplegia is not required. Also, individuals 40 years of age and older have decreased ability to accommodate, and drugs are not necessary for an accurate refraction.] *Atropine* may induce an attack in individuals with narrow angle glaucoma.

b. **Antispasmodic agent:** *Atropine* is used as an antispasmodic agent to relax the gastrointestinal tract and bladder.

c. **As antidote for cholinergic agonists:** *Atropine* is used for the treatment of overdoses of organophosphate (contained in certain insecticides) and some types of mushroom poisoning (certain mushrooms contain cholinergic substances). Its ability to enter the central nervous system (CNS) is of particular importance. *Atropine* blocks the effects of excess acetylcholine that results from inhibition of acetylcholinesterase by drugs such as *physostigmine* (see p. 42).

d. **Antisecretory agent:** The drug is sometimes used as an antisecretory agent to block secretions in the upper and lower respiratory tracts prior to surgery.

3. **Pharmacokinetics:** *Atropine* is readily absorbed, partially metabolized by the liver, and is eliminated primarily in the urine. It has a half-life of about 4 hours

4. **Adverse effects:** Depending on the dose, *atropine* may cause dry mouth, blurred vision, "sandy eyes", tachycardia, and constipation. Effects on the CNS include restlessness, confusion, halluci-

nations, and delirium, which may progress to depression, collapse of the circulatory and respiratory systems and death. In older individuals, the use of *atropine* to induce mydriasis and cycloplegia is considered too risky since it may exacerbate an attack of glaucoma in someone with a latent condition.

B. Scopolamine

Scopolamine [skoe POL a meen], another belladonna alkaloid, produces peripheral effects similar to those of *atropine*. However, *scopolamine* has greater action on the CNS and a longer duration of action in comparison to those of *atropine*. It has some special actions indicated below.

1. **Actions:** *Scopolamine* is one of the most effective anti-motion sickness drugs available (Figure 5.5). *Scopolamine* also has the unusual effect of blocking short-term memory. In contrast to *atropine, scopolamine* produces sedation, but at higher doses can instead produce excitement.

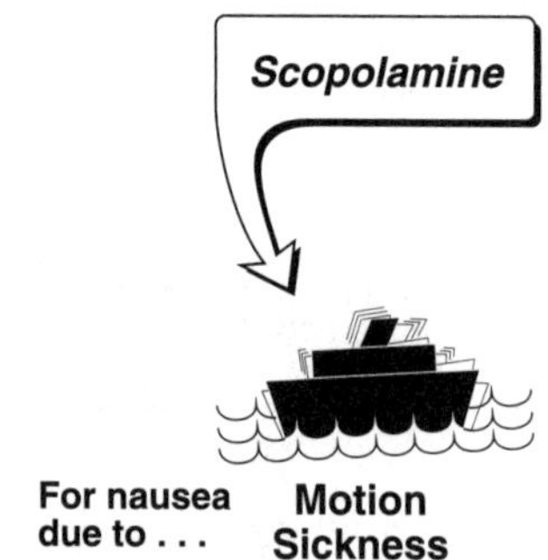

Figure 5.5
Scopolamine is an effective anti-motion sickness agent.

2. **Therapeutic uses:** Though similar to *atropine*, its therapeutic use is limited to prevention of motion sickness (for which *scopolamine* is particularly effective) and blocking of short-term memory. [Note: As with all such drugs used for this condition, it is much more effective prophylactically than for treating motion sickness after it occurs. The amnesic action of *scopolamine* is sometimes made use of in anesthetic procedures.]

3. **Pharmacokinetics and adverse effects:** These aspects are similar to those of *atropine*.

C. Ipratropium

Inhaled *ipratropium* [i pra TROE pee um], a quaternary derivative of *atropine* (see Figure 22.5, p. 220), is useful in treating asthma and chronic obstructive pulmonary disease in patients unable to take adrenergic agonists. *Ipratropium* is also used in the management of chronic obstructive pulmonary disease (see p. 222). Important characteristics of the muscarinic antagonists are summarized in Figure 5.6.

III. GANGLIONIC BLOCKERS

Ganglionic blockers specifically act on the nicotinic receptors, probably by blocking the ion channels of the autonomic ganglia (see Figure 5.2). These drugs show no selectivity toward the parasympathetic or sympathetic ganglia and are not effective as neuromuscular antagonists (see p. 50). Thus, these drugs block the entire output of the autonomic nervous system at the nicotinic receptor. The responses observed are complex and unpredictable, making it impossible to achieve selective actions. Therefore, ganglionic blockade is rarely used therapeutically today. However, they often serve as tools in experimental pharmacology.

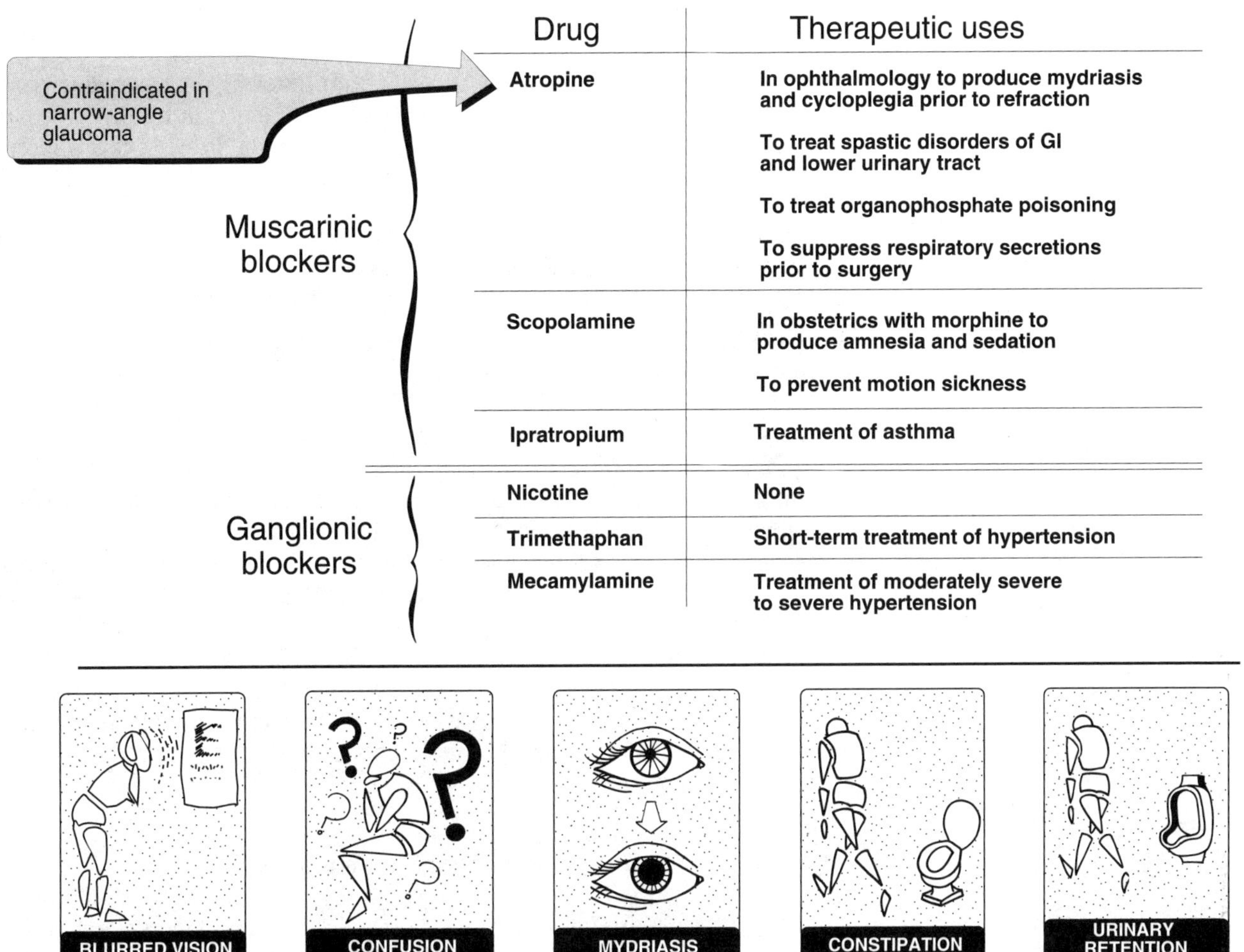

Drug
Therapeutic uses
Contraindicated in narrow-angle glaucoma
Muscarinic blockers
Atropine
In ophthalmology to produce mydriasis and cycloplegia prior to refraction
To treat spastic disorders of GI and lower urinary tract
To treat organophosphate poisoning
To suppress respiratory secretions prior to surgery
Scopolamine
In obstetrics with morphine to produce amnesia and sedation
To prevent motion sickness
Ipratropium
Treatment of asthma
Ganglionic blockers
Nicotine
None
Trimethaphan
Short-term treatment of hypertension
Mecamylamine
Treatment of moderately severe to severe hypertension
BLURRED VISION
CONFUSION
MYDRIASIS
CONSTIPATION
URINARY RETENTION
Adverse effects commonly observed with cholinergic antagonists

Figure 5.6
Summary of cholinergic antagonists.

A. Nicotine

A component of cigarette smoke, *nicotine* [NIC o teen] has many undesirable actions. Depending on the dose, *nicotine* depolarizes ganglia, resulting first in stimulation of and followed by paralysis of all ganglia. The stimulatory effects are complex, including an increase in blood pressure and cardiac rate (due to release of transmitter from adrenergic terminals and from the adrenal medulla), and increased peristalsis and secretions. At higher doses, the blood pressure falls because of ganglionic blockade, and activity both in the GI tract and bladder musculature ceases. See p. 100 for a full discussion of *nicotine*.

B. Trimethaphan

Trimethaphan [trye METH a fan] is a short-acting, competitive nicotinic ganglionic blocker that must be given by intravenous infusion. Today, the drug is used for the emergency lowering of blood pressure, for example, in hypertension caused by pulmonary edema or dissecting aortic aneurysm when other agents cannot be used.

C. Mecamylamine

Mecamylamine [mek a MILL a meen] produces a competitive nicotinic block of the ganglia. The duration of action is about 10 hours after a single administration. The uptake of the drug via oral absorption is good in contrast to *trimethaphan*.

IV. NEUROMUSCULAR BLOCKING DRUGS

This section presents drugs that block cholinergic transmission between motor nerve endings and the nicotinic receptors on the neuromuscular end-plate of skeletal muscle (see Figure 5.2). These neuromuscular blockers are structural analogs of acetylcholine and act either as antagonists (nondepolarizing type) or agonists (depolarizing type) at the receptors on the end-plate of the neuromuscular junction. Neuromuscular blockers are clinically useful during surgery to produce complete muscle relaxation, without having to employ higher anesthetic doses to achieve comparable muscular relaxation. A second group of muscle relaxants, the central muscle relaxants, are used to control spastic muscle tone. These drugs include *diazepam* (which binds at GABA receptors, see p. 90), *dantrolene* (which acts directly on muscles by interfering with the release of calcium from the sarcoplasmic reticulum), and *baclofen* (which probably acts at GABA receptors in the central nervous system).

A. Nondepolarizing (competitive) blockers

The first drug that was found capable of blocking the skeletal neuromuscular junction was curare, which the native hunters of the Amazon in South America used to paralyze game. The drug *tubocurarine* [too boe kyoo AR een] was ultimately purified and introduced into clinical practice in the early 1940s. The neuromuscular blocking agents have significantly increased the safety of anesthesia, since less anesthetic is required to produce muscle relaxation.

1. Mechanism of action

a. At low doses: Nondepolarizing neuromuscular blocking drugs combine with the nicotinic receptor and prevent the binding of acetylcholine (Figure 5.7). These drugs thus prevent depolarization of the muscle cell membrane and inhibit muscular contraction. Because these agents compete with acetylcholine at the receptor, they are called competitive blockers. Their action can be overcome by increasing the concentration of acetylcholine in the synaptic gap, for example, by administration of cholinesterase inhibitors such as *neostigmine* (see p. 42) or *edrophonium* (see p. 43). Anesthesiologists often employ this strategy to shorten the duration of the neuromuscular blockade.

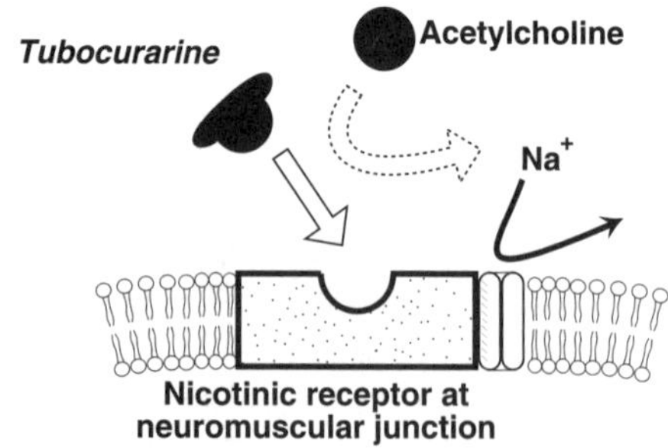

Figure 5.7
Mechanism of action of competitive neuromuscular blocking drugs.

b. At high doses: Nondepolarizing blockers block the ion channels of the end-plate. This leads to further weakening of neuromuscular transmission and reduces the ability of acetylcholinesterase inhibitors to reverse the actions of nondepolarizing muscle relaxants.

2. **Actions:** Not all muscles are equally sensitive to blockade by competitive blockers. Small, rapidly contracting muscles of the face and eye are most susceptible and are paralyzed first, followed by the fingers. Thereafter the limbs, neck, and trunk muscles are paralyzed, then the intercostal muscles are affected, and lastly, the diaphragm muscles are paralyzed.

3. **Therapeutic uses:** These blockers are used therapeutically as adjuvant drugs in anesthesia during surgery to relax skeletal muscle.

4. **Pharmacokinetics:** All neuromuscular blocking agents are injected intravenously since their uptake via oral absorption is minimal. They penetrate membranes very poorly and do not enter cells or cross the blood-brain barrier. Many of the drugs are not metabolized; their actions are terminated by redistribution. For example, *tubocurarine*, *pancuronium, mivacurium*, *metocurine* , and *doxacurium* are excreted in the urine unchanged. *Atricurium* is degraded spontaneously in the plasma and by ester hydrolysis.The aminosteroid drugs (*vecuronium* and *rocuronium* are deacetylated in the liver, and their clearance may be prolonged in patients with hepatic disease. These drugs are also excreted unchanged in the bile. The onset and duration of action of the neuromuscular blocking drugs are shown in Figure 5.8.

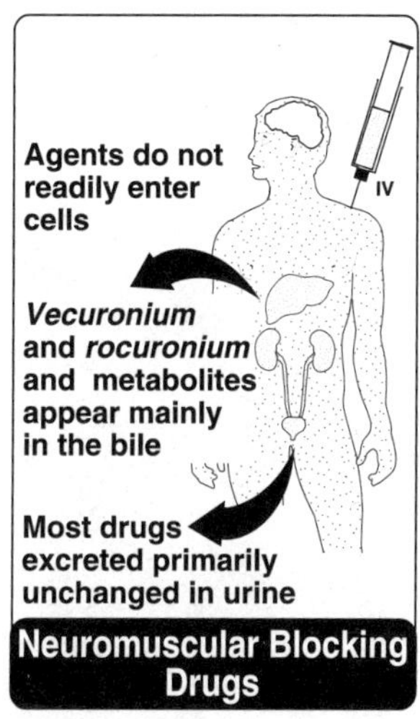
Agents do not readily enter cells
IV
Vecuronium and *rocuronium* and metabolites appear mainly in the bile
Most drugs excreted primarily unchanged in urine
Neuromuscular Blocking Drugs

5. **Adverse effects:** The effects of the neuromuscular blocking drugs are shown in Figure 5.8.

6. **Drug Interactions**

   a. **Cholinesterase inhibitors:** Drugs such as *neostigmine*, *physostigmine*, and *edrophonium* (see p. 42) can overcome the action of nondepolarizing neuromuscular blockers, but with increased dosage, cholinesterase inhibitors can cause a depolarizing block as a result of elevated acetylcholine concentrations at the end-plate membrane.

   b. **Halogenated hydrocarbon anesthetics:** Drugs such as *halothane* (see p. 113) act to enhance neuromuscular blockade by exerting a stabilizing action at the neuromuscular junction.

   c. **Aminoglycoside antibiotics:** Drugs like *gentamicin or tobramycin* (see p. 315) inhibit acetylcholine release from cholinergic nerves by competing with calcium ions. They synergize with *tubocurarine* and other competitive blockers, enhancing the blockade.

   d. **Calcium channel blockers:** These agents may increase the neuromuscular block of *tubocurarine* and other competitive blockers as well as depolarizing blockers.

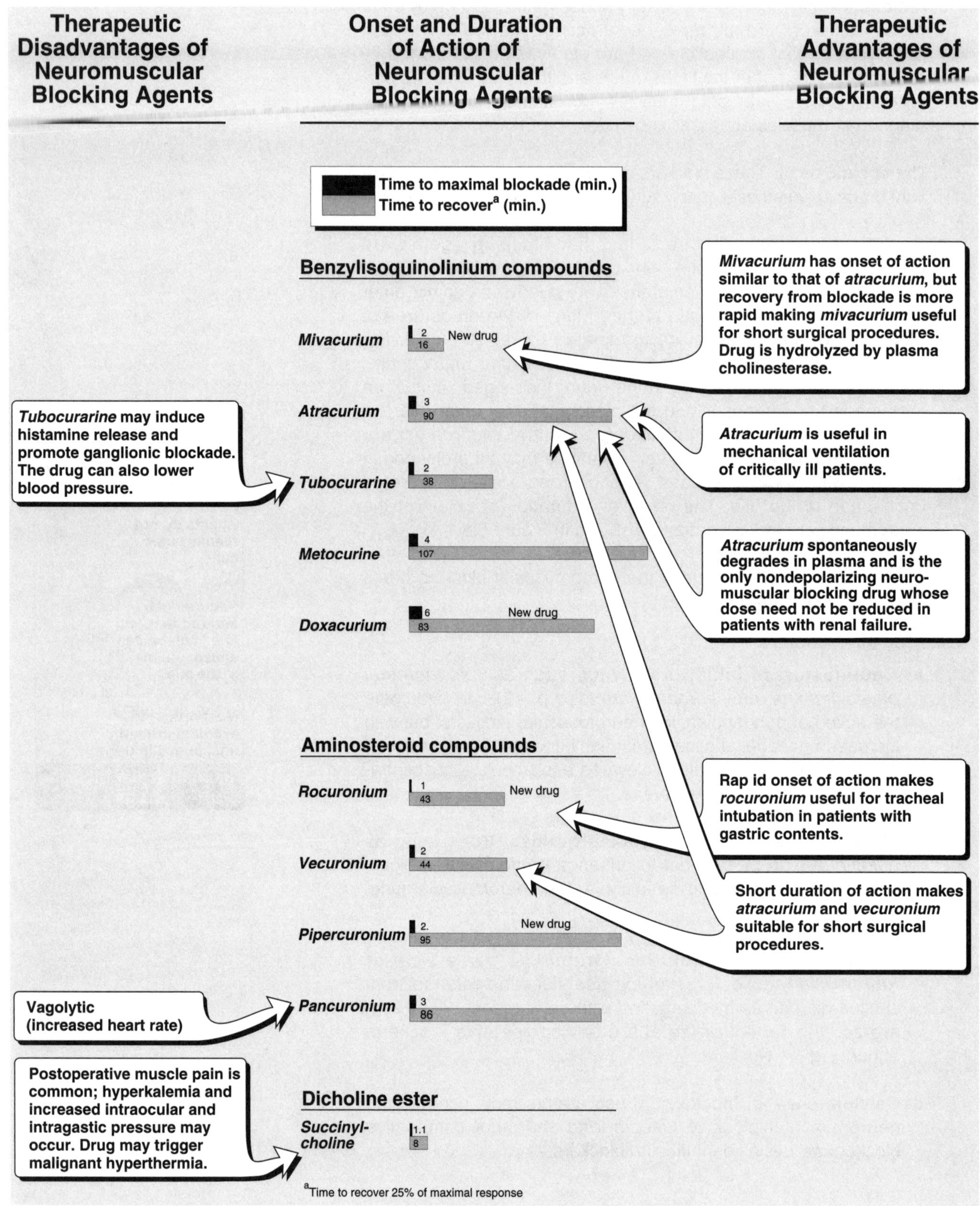

Figure 5.8
Onset and duration of action of neuromuscular blocking drugs (center column); summary of therapeutic considerations. [Note: "New drug" indicates drug approved after 1992.]

B. Depolarizing agents

1. **Mechanism of action:** The depolarizing neuromuscular blocking drug, *succinylcholine* [suk sin ill KOE leen], attaches to the nicotinic receptor and acts like acetylcholine to depolarize the junction (Figure 5.9). Unlike acetylcholine, which is instantly destroyed by acetylcholinesterase, the depolarizing agent persists at high concentrations in the synaptic cleft, remaining attached to the receptor for a relatively long time, and providing a constant stimulation of the receptor. The depolarizing agent first causes the opening of the sodium channel associated with the nicotinic receptors, which results in depolarization of the receptor (Phase I). This leads to a transient twitching of the muscle (fasciculations). The continued binding of the depolarizing agent renders the receptor incapable of transmitting further impulses. With time, the continuous depolarization gives way to gradual repolarization as the sodium channel closes or is blocked. This causes a resistance to depolarization (Phase II) and a flaccid paralysis.

2. **Actions:** The sequence of paralysis may be slightly different, but as is seen with the competitive blockers, the respiratory muscles are paralyzed last. *Succinylcholine* initially produces short-lasting muscle fasciculations, followed within a few minutes by paralysis. The drug does not produce a ganglionic block, except in high doses, although it does have weak histamine-releasing action. Normally, the duration of action of *succinylcholine* is extremely short, since this drug is rapidly broken down by plasma cholinesterase.

3. **Therapeutic uses:** Because of its rapid onset and short duration of action, *succinylcholine* is useful when rapid endotracheal intubation is required during the induction of anesthesia (a rapid action is essential if aspiration of gastric contents is to be avoided during intubation). It is also employed during electroconvulsive shock treatment.

4. **Pharmacokinetics:** *Succinylcholine* is injected intravenously. Its brief duration of action (several minutes) results from rapid hydrolysis by plasma cholinesterase. It is therefore usually given by continuous infusion.

5. **Adverse effects:**

   a. **Hyperthermia:** When *halothane* (see p. 113) is used as an anesthetic, administration of *succinylcholine* has occasionally caused malignant hyperthermia (with muscular rigidity and hyperpyrexia) in genetically susceptible people (Figure 5.8). This is treated by rapidly cooling the patient and by administration of *dantrolene*, which blocks release of Ca^{++} from the sarcoplasmic reticulum of muscle cells, thus reducing heat production and relaxing muscle tone.

   b. **Apnea:** A genetically related deficiency of plasma cholinesterase or presence of an atypical form of the enzyme can lead to apnea due to paralysis of the diaphragm.

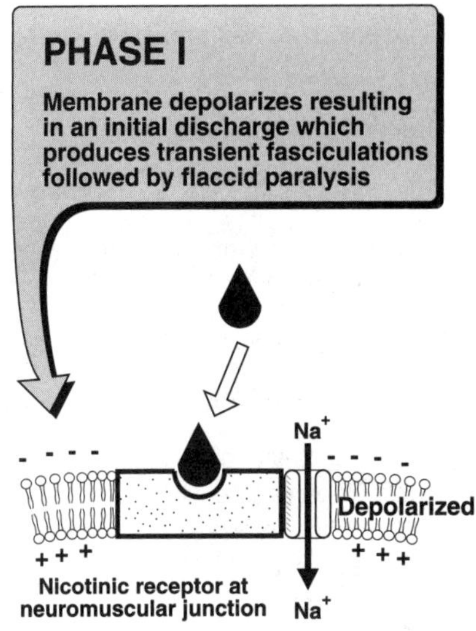

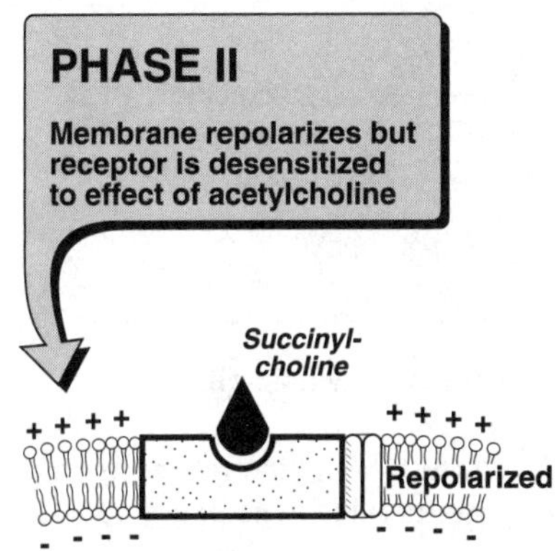

Figure 5.9
Mechanism of action of depolarizing neuromuscular blocking drugs.

Questions 5.1 to 5.6

For each description (below) select the most appropriate drug (A to I).

5.1 Depolarizes neuromuscular end plate

5.2 Reverses the effects of nondepolarizing blockers, such as tubocurarine

5.3 May cause the release of histamine

5.4 Acts at peripheral and central muscarinic cholinergic receptors

5.5 Used as adjunctive therapy in treating asthma

5.6 Degraded spontaneously in the plasma

A. Succinylcholine
B. Neostigmine
C. Tubocurarine
D. Scopolamine.
E. Carbachol
F. Atracurium
G. Atropine
H. Ipratropium

Correct answers

5.1 A: Succinylcholine
5.2 B: Neostigmine
5.3 C: Tubocurarine
5.4 D: Scopolamine
5.5 H: Ipratropium
5.6 I: Atricurium

Choose the ONE best answer.

5.7. Which ONE of the following drugs most closely resembles atropine in its pharmacologic actions?

A. Scopolamine
B. Trimethaphan
C. Physostigmine
D. Acetylcholine
E. Carbachol

The correct answer = A. Scopolamine has effects similar to those of atropine. Trimethaphan is a ganglionic blocker affecting nicotinic receptors; atropine affects primarily muscarinic receptors. Physostigmine, an anticholinesterase drug, is the antidote for an excess of atropine. Atropine blocks the effects of acetylcholine and direct-acting agonists, such as carbachol.

5.8. Which ONE of the following drugs does NOT produce miosis (marked constriction of the pupil)?

A. Carbachol
B. Isoflurophate
C. Atropine
D. Pilocarpine
E. Neostigmine

Correct answer = C. On the eye, atropine blocks all cholinergic activity resulting in mydriasis (dilation of the pupil). Carbachol (a direct acting cholinergic agonist), isoflurophate (an indirect-acting cholinergic agonist), pilocarpine (a direct-acting cholinergic agonist), and neostigmine (an indirect-acting cholinergic agonist) all mimic the effect of parasympathetic stimulation and produce miosis.

5.9. Which ONE of the following drugs would be useful in the long-term treatment of myasthenia gravis?

A. Edrophonium
B. Atropine
C. Neostigmine
D. Scopolamine
E. Bethanechol

Correct answer = C. Neostigmine provides symptomatic treatment of myasthenia gravis by inhibiting acetylcholinesterase and thereby increasing acetylcholine. In contrast, edrophonium, an indirect cholinergic agonist, is useful in the diagnosis of myasthenia gravis, but its duration of action is too short for effective long-term treatment. Atropine and scopolamine block the action of acetylcholine on the cholinergic receptors of the neuromuscular junction. Bethanechol is not effective at the neuromuscular junction.

5.10 A 50-year-old male farm worker is brought to the emergency room. He was found confused in the orchard and since then has lost consciousness. His heart rate is 45 and his blood pressure is 80/40 mm Hg. He is sweating and salivating profusely. Which of the following treatments is indicated?

A. Physostigmine
B. Norepinephrine
C. Trimethaphan
D. Atropine
E. Edrophonium

The correct answer = D. The patient is exhibiting signs of cholinergic stimulation. Since he is a farmer, insecticide poisoning is a likely diagnosis. Thus either intravenous or intramuscular doses of atropine are indicated to antagonize the muscarinic symptoms. Physostigmine and edrophonium are cholinesterase inhibitors and would exacerbate the problem. Norepinephrine would not be effective in combatting the cholinergic stimulation. Trimethaphan being a ganglionic blocker would also worsen the condition.

Adrenergic Agonists

6

I. OVERVIEW

The adrenergic drugs affect receptors that are stimulated by *norepinephrine* or *epinephrine*. Some adrenergic drugs act directly on the adrenergic receptor (adrenoceptor) by activating it and are said to be sympathomimetic. Others, which will be dealt with in Chapter 7, block the action of the neurotransmitters at the receptors, while still other drugs affect adrenergic function by interrupting the release of *norepinephrine* from adrenergic neurons. This chapter describes agents that either directly or indirectly stimulate the adrenoceptor (Figure 6.1).

II. THE ADRENERGIC NEURON

Adrenergic neurons release *norepinephrine* as the neurotransmitter. These neurons are found in the central nervous system (CNS), and also in the sympathetic nervous system where they serve as links between ganglia and the effector organs. The adrenergic neurons and receptors located either presynaptically on the neuron or post-synaptically on the effector organ are the sites of action of the adrenergic drugs (Figure 6.2).

A. Neurotransmission at adrenergic neurons

Neurotransmission in adrenergic neurons closely resembles that already described for the cholinergic neurons (p. 37), except that *norepinephrine* is the neurotransmitter instead of acetylcholine. Neurotransmission takes place at numerous beadlike enlargements called varicosities; the process involves five steps: the synthesis, storage, release, and receptor binding of the *norepinephrine*, followed by removal of the neurotransmitter from the synaptic gap (Figure 6.3).

1. **Synthesis of norepinephrine:** Tyrosine is transported by a Na^+-linked carrier into the axoplasm of the adrenergic neuron, where it is hydroxylated to dihydroxyphenylalanine (DOPA) by tyrosine hydroxylase[1]. This is the rate-limiting step in the formation of *norepinephrine*. DOPA is decarboxylated to form *dopamine*.

ADRENERGIC AGONISTS

DIRECT-ACTING

- ***Albuterol***
- ***Clonidine***
- ***Dobutamine****
- ***Dopamine****
- ***Epinephrine****
- ***Isoproterenol****
- ***Metaproterenol***
- ***Methoxamine***
- ***Norepinephrine****
- ***Phenylephrine***
- ***Ritodrine***
- ***Terbutaline***

INDIRECT-ACTING

- ***Amphetamine***
- ***Tyramine***

DIRECT and INDIRECT ACTING (mixed action)

- ***Ephedrine***
- ***Metaraminol***

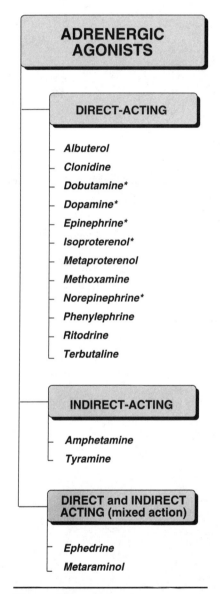

Figure 6.1
Summary of adrenergic agonists. Agents marked with an asterisk (*) are catecholamines.

[1]See p. 70 for Infolink references to other books in this series.

Lippincott's Illustrated Reviews: Pharmacology, Second Edition.
by Mary J. Mycek, Richard A. Harvey and Pamela C. Champe.
Lippincott Williams & Wilkins, Philadelphia, PA © 2000.

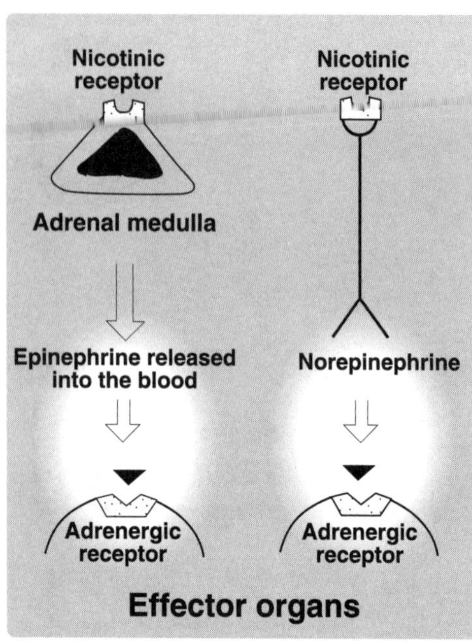

Figure 6.2
Sites of actions of adrenergic agonists.

2. **Storage of norepinephrine in vesicles:** *Dopamine* is transported into synaptic vesicles by an amine transporter system that is also involved in the re-uptake of preformed *norepinephrine*. This carrier system is blocked by *reserpine* (see p. 78). *Dopamine* is hydroxylated to form *norepinephrine* by the enzyme, *dopamine* β-hydroxylase. Synaptic vesicles contain dopamine or *norepinephrine* plus adenosine triphosphate and the β-hydroxylase. Not all of the *norepinephrine* is packaged in vesicles; some exists in a cytoplasmic pool that can be displaced. In the adrenal medulla, *norepinephrine* is methylated to yield *epinephrine*; both are stored in chromaffin cells. On stimulation, the adrenal medulla releases about 85% *epinephrine* and 15% *norepinephrine*.

3. **Release of norepinephrine:** An action potential arriving at the nerve junction triggers an influx of calcium ions from the extracellular fluid into the cytoplasm of the neuron. The increase in calcium causes vesicles inside the neuron to fuse with the cell membrane and expel their contents into the synapse. This release is blocked by drugs such as *guanethidine* (see p. 78).

4. **Binding by receptor:** *Norepinephrine* released from the synaptic vesicles diffuses across the synaptic space and binds to either postsynaptic receptors on the effector organ or to presynaptic receptors on the nerve ending (see Figure 6.3). The recognition of *norepinephrine* by the membrane receptors triggers a cascade of events within the cell, resulting in the formation of intracellular second messengers that act as links (transducers) in the communication between the neurotransmitter and the action generated within the effector cell. Adrenergic receptors use both the cyclic adenosine monophosphate (cAMP) second messenger system and the phosphoinositide cycle, described on p. 33, to transmit the signal into an effect.

5. **Removal of norepinephrine:** *Norepinephrine* may (1) diffuse out of the synaptic space and enter the general circulation, (2) be metabolized to O-methylated derivatives by post-synaptic cell membrane-associated catechol O-methyltransferase (COMT) in the synaptic space, or (3) be recaptured by an uptake system that pulls the *norepinephrine* back into the neuron. The uptake by the neuronal membrane involves a sodium-potassium activated ATPase that can be inhibited by tricyclic antidepressants such as *imipramine* (see p. 119), or by *cocaine* (see Figure 6.3).

6. **Potential fates of recaptured norepinephrine:** Once *norepinephrine* reenters the cytoplasm of the adrenergic neuron it may be taken up into adrenergic vesicles via the amine transporter system and be sequestered for release by another action potential or persist in a protected pool. Alternatively, *norepinephrine* can be oxidized by monoamine oxidase (MAO) present in neuronal mitochondria. The inactive products of *norepinephrine* metabolism are excreted in the urine as vanillylmandelic acid (VMA), metanephrine and normetanephrine.

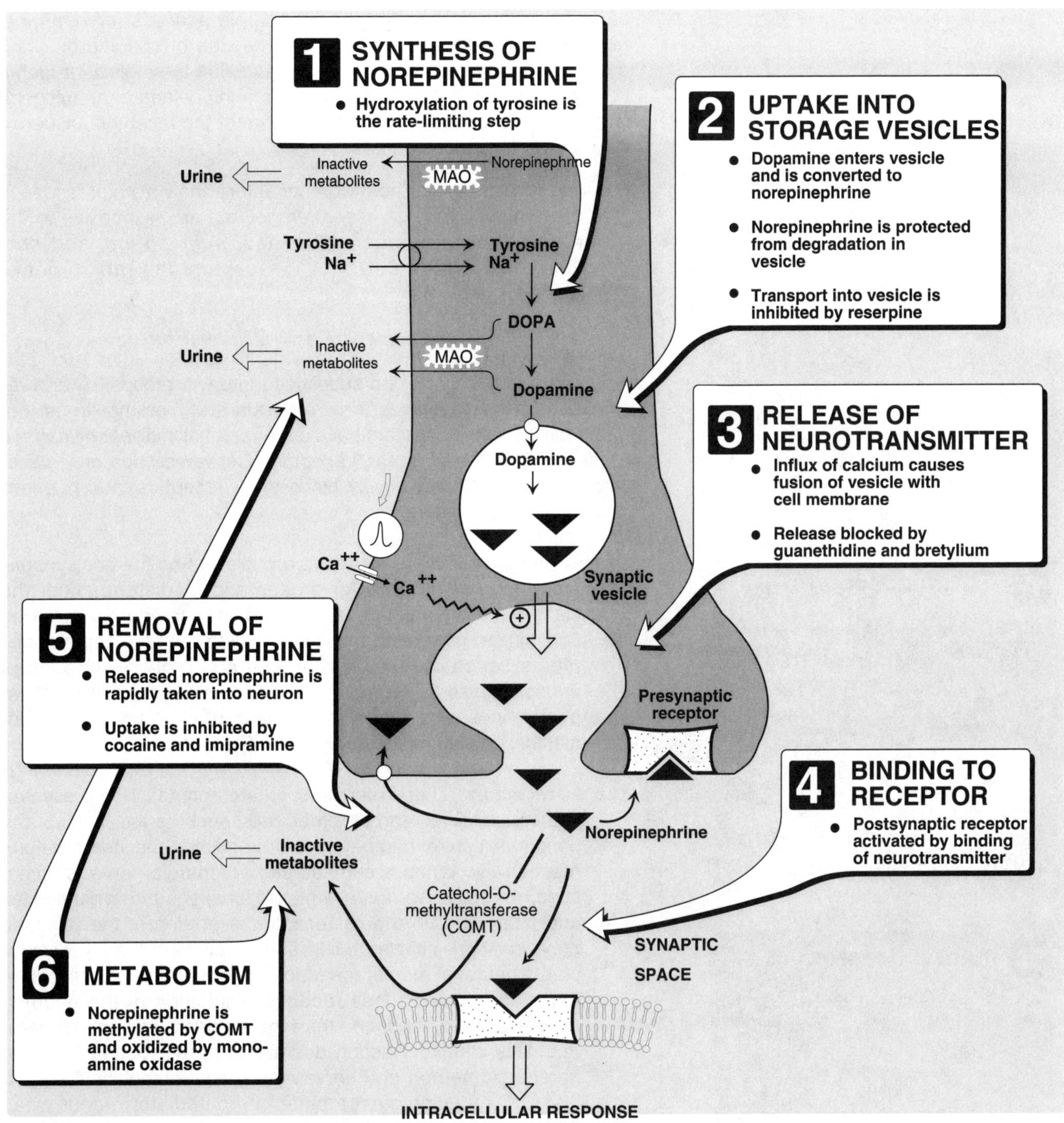

Figure 6.3
Synthesis and release of norepinephrine from the adrenergic neuron.

B. Adrenergic receptors (adrenoceptors)

In the sympathetic nervous system, several classes of adrenoceptors can be distinguished pharmacologically. Two families of receptors, designated "α" and "β", were initially identified on the basis of their responses to the adrenergic agonists, *epinephrine*, *norepinephrine*, and *isoproterenol*. The use of specific blocking drugs and the cloning of genes have revealed the molecular identities of a number of subtypes. These proteins belong to a multigene family. Alterations in the primary structure of the receptors influence their affinity for various agents.

1. **α_1 and α_2 receptors:** The α adrenoceptors show a weak response to the synthetic agonist, *isoproterenol*, but are responsive to the naturally occurring catecholamines, *epinephrine*, and *norepinephrine* (Figure 6.4). For α receptors the rank order of potency is:

   epinephrine ≥ *norepinephrine* >> *isoproterenol*

   The α adrenoceptors are subdivided into two groups, α_1 and α_2, based on their affinities for α agonists and blocking drugs. For example, the α_1 receptors have a higher affinity for *phenylephrine* (see p. 66) than do the α_2 receptors. Conversely, the drug *clonidine* (see p. 67) selectively binds to α_2 receptors, and has less effect on α_1 receptors.

   a. **α_1 receptors:** These receptors are present on the postsynaptic membrane of the effector organs and mediate many of the classic effects, originally designated as α-adrenergic, involving constriction of smooth muscle. Activation of α_1 receptors initiates a series of reactions through a G-protein activation of phospholipase C, resulting in the generation of IP_3 from phosphatidylinositol, causing the release of Ca^{++} from the endoplasmic reticulum into the cytosol[2] (Figure 6.5).

   b. **α_2 receptors:** These receptors, located primarily on presynaptic nerve endings and on other cells, such as the β cell of the pancreas, control adrenergic neuromediator and insulin output, respectively. When a sympathetic adrenergic nerve is stimulated, the released *norepinephrine* traverses the synaptic cleft and interacts with the α_1 receptor. A portion of the released *norepinephrine* "circles back" and reacts with the α_2 receptor on the neuronal membrane (see Figure 6.5). The stimulation of the α_2 receptor causes feedback inhibition of the ongoing release of *norepinephrine* from the stimulated adrenergic neuron. This inhibitory action decreases further output from the adrenergic neuron and serves as a local modulating mechanism for reducing sympathetic neuromediator output when there is high sympathetic activity. In contrast to α_1 receptors, the effects of binding at α_2 receptors are mediated by inhibition of adenylyl cyclase and a fall in the levels of intracellular cAMP.

2. **β receptors:** β receptors exhibit a set of responses different from those of the α receptors. These are characterized by a strong response to *isoproterenol*, with less sensitivity to *epinephrine* and *norepinephrine* (see Figure 6.4). For β receptors, the rank order of potency is:

   isoproterenol > *epinephrine* > *norepinephrine*

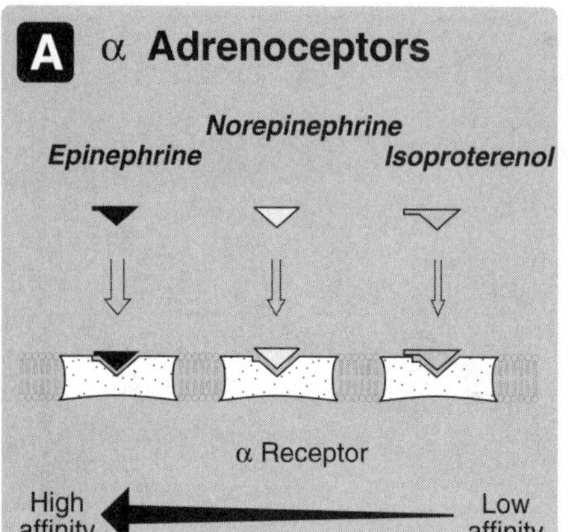

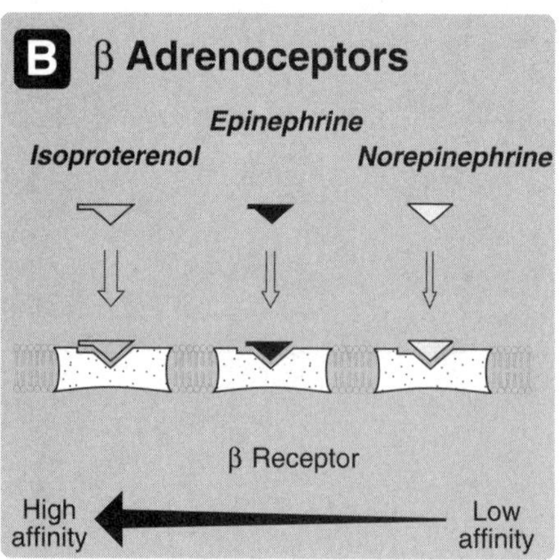

Figure 6.4
Types of adrenergic receptors.

[2]See p. 70 for Infolink references to other books in this series.

The β adrenoceptors can be subdivided into two major groups, β_1 and β_2, based on their affinities for adrenergic agonists and antagonists although several others have been identified by gene cloning. β_1 Receptors have approximately equal affinities for *epinephrine* and *norepinephrine*, whereas β_2 receptors have a higher affinity for *epinephrine* than for *norepinephrine*. Thus, tissues with a predominance of β_2 receptors (such as the vasculature of skeletal muscle) are particularly responsive to the hormonal effects of circulating *epinephrine* released by the adrenal medulla. Binding of a neurotransmitter at the β_1 or β_2 receptor results in activation of adenylyl cyclase and therefore increased concentrations of cAMP within the cell.

3. **Distribution of receptors:** Adrenergically innervated organs and tissues tend to have a predominance of one type of receptor. For example, tissues such as the vasculature to skeletal muscle have both α_1 and β_2 receptors, but the β_2 receptors predominate. Other tissues may have one type of receptor exclusively, with practically no significant numbers of other types of adrenergic receptors. For example, the heart contains predominantly β_1 receptors.

4. **Characteristic responses mediated by adrenoceptors:** It is useful to organize the physiologic responses to adrenergic stimulation according to receptor type, since many drugs preferentially stimulate or block one type of receptor. Figure 6.6 summarizes the most prominent effects mediated by the adrenoceptors. As a generalization, stimulation of α_1 receptors characteristically produces vasoconstriction (particularly in skin and abdominal viscera) and an increase in total peripheral resistance and blood pressure. Conversely, stimulation of β_1 receptors characteristically causes cardiac stimulation, while β_2 produces vasodilation (in skeletal vascular beds), and bronchiolar relaxation.

5. **Desensitization of receptors:** Prolonged exposure to the catecholamines reduces the responsivity of these receptors, a phenomenon known as desensitization. Three mechanisms have been suggested to explain this phenomenon: (1) sequestration of the receptors so that they are unavailable for interaction with the ligand; (2) down-regulation, that is, a disappearance of the receptor either by destruction or decreased synthesis; and (3) inability to couple to G-protein because the receptor has been phosphorylated on the cytoplasmic side by either protein kinase A or β adrenergic receptor kinase (βARK).

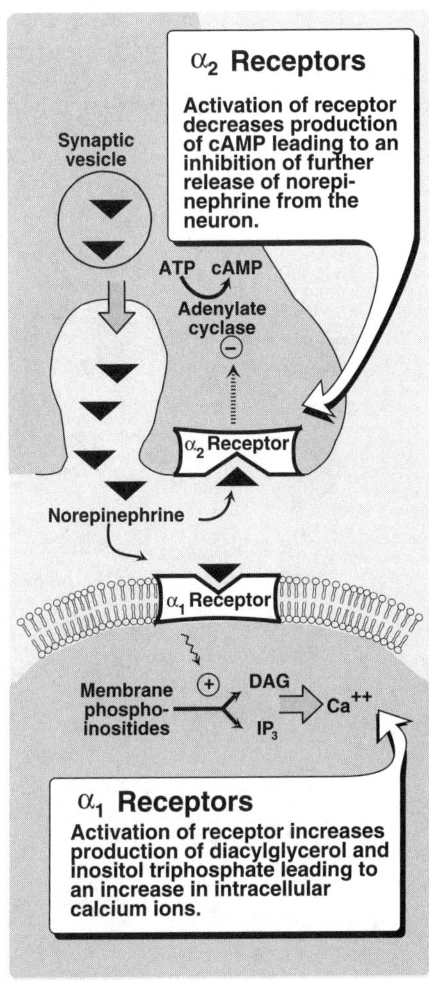

Figure 6.5
Second messengers mediate the effects of α receptors. DAG = diacylglcerol; IP_3 = inositol triphosphate.

III. CHARACTERISTICS OF ADRENERGIC AGONISTS

Most of the adrenergic drugs are derivatives of β-phenylethylamine (Figure 6.7). Substitutions on the benzene ring or on the ethylamine side chains produce a great variety of compounds with varying abilities to differentiate between α and β receptors and to penetrate the CNS. Two important structural features of these drugs are the number and location of OH substitutions on the benzene ring and the nature of the substituent on the amino nitrogen.

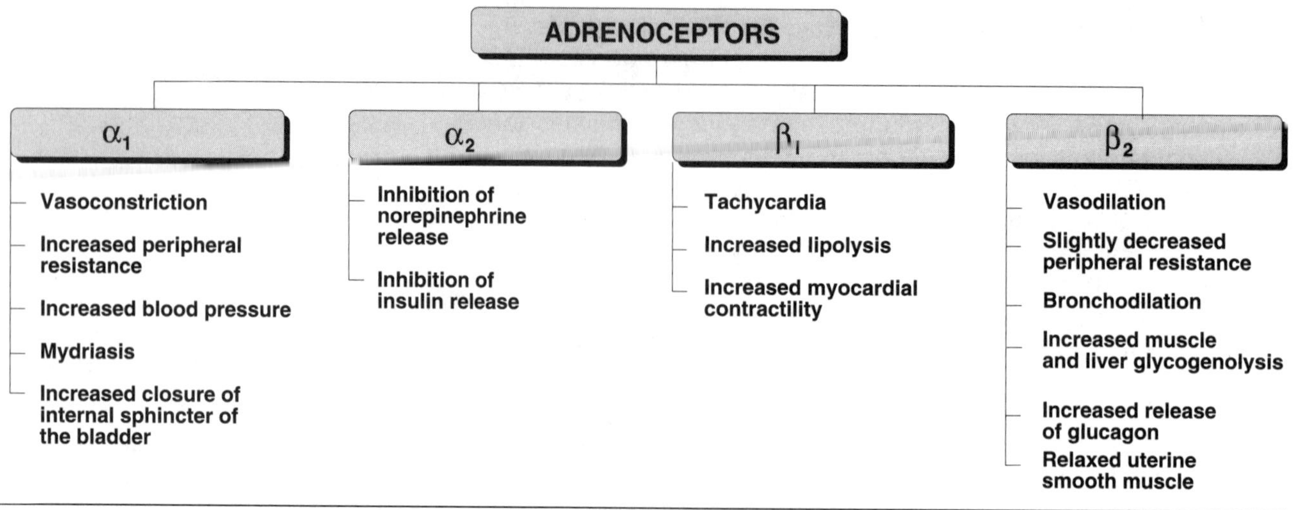

Figure 6.6
Major effects mediated by α– and β–adrenoceptors.

A. Catecholamines

Sympathomimetic amines that contain the 3,4-dihydroxybenzene group (such as, *epinephrine*, *norepinephrine*, *isoproterenol*, and *dopamine*) are called catecholamines. [Note: 1,2-dihydroxybenzene is catechol, Figure 6.7.] These compounds share the following properties:

1. **High potency:** Drugs that are catechol derivatives (with –OH groups in the 3 and 4 positions on the benzene ring) show the highest potency in activating α or β receptors.

2. **Rapid inactivation:** Not only are the catecholamines metabolized by COMT postsynaptically and by MAO intraneuronally, but they are also metabolized in other tissues. For example, COMT is in the gut wall and MAO is in the liver and gut wall. Thus catecholamines have only a brief period of action when given parenterally, and are ineffective when administered orally because of inactivation.

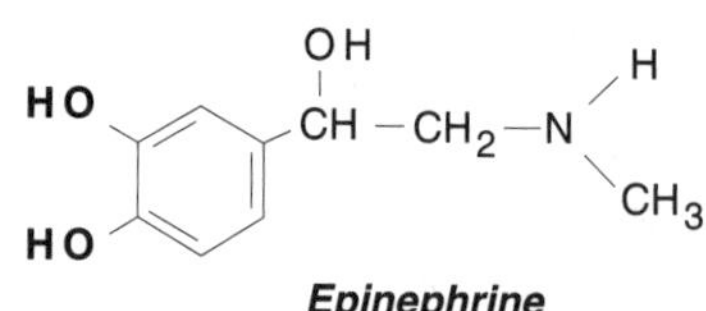

Epinephrine

3. **Poor penetration into the CNS:** Catecholamines are polar and therefore do not readily penetrate into the CNS. Nevertheless, most of these drugs have some clinical effects (anxiety, tremor, headaches) that are attributable to action on the CNS.

Phenylephrine

B. Non-catecholamines

Compounds lacking the catechol hydroxyl groups have longer half-lives, since they are not inactivated by COMT. These include *phenylephrine, ephedrine,* and *amphetamine. Phenylephrine*, an analog of *epinephrine*, has only a single OH at position 3 on the benzene ring, whereas *ephedrine* lacks hydroxyls on the ring but has a methyl substitution at the α-carbon. These are poor substrates for MAO and thus show a prolonged duration of action, since MAO is an important route of detoxification. Increased lipid solubility of many of the non-catecholamines permits greater access to the CNS. These compounds may act indirectly by causing the release of stored catecholamines.

Ephedrine

C. Substitution on amine nitrogen

The nature and bulk of the substituent on the amine nitrogen is important in determining the β selectivity of the adrenergic agonist. For example, *epinephrine* with a $-CH_3$ substituent on the amine nitrogen is more potent at β receptors than *norepinephrine*, which has an unsubstituted amine. Similarly, *isoproterenol* with an isopropyl substituent $-CH(CH_3)_2$ on the amine nitrogen (see Figure 6.7), is a strong β agonist with little α activity (see Figure 6.4).

D. Mechanism of action of adrenergic agonists

1. **Direct-acting agonists:** These drugs act directly on α or β receptors, producing effects similar to those that occur following stimulation of sympathetic nerves or release of the hormone *epinephrine* from the adrenal medulla (Figure 6.8). Examples of direct-acting agonists include *epinephrine, norepinephrine, isoproterenol,* and *phenylephrine.*

2. **Indirect-acting agonists:** These agents, which include *amphetamine* and *tyramine*, are taken up into the presynaptic neuron and cause the release of *norepinephrine* from the cytoplasmic pools or vesicles of the adrenergic neuron (see Figure 6.8). As with neuronal stimulation, the *norepinephrine* then traverses the synapse and binds to the α or β receptors.

3. **Mixed-action agonists:** Some agonists, such as *ephedrine* and *metaraminol*, have the capacity both to directly stimulate adrenoceptors and to release *norepinephrine* from the adrenergic neuron (see Figure 6.8).

IV. DIRECT-ACTING ADRENERGIC AGONISTS

Direct-acting agonists bind to adrenergic receptors without interacting with the presynaptic neuron. The activated receptor initiates synthesis of second messengers and subsequent intracellular signals. As a group these agents are widely used clinically.

A. Epinephrine

Epinephrine [ep ee NEF rin] is one of five catecholamines—*epinephrine, norepinephrine, dopamine, dobutamine,* and *isoproterenol*—commonly used in therapy. The first three catecholamines occur naturally, the latter two are synthetic compounds (see Figure 6.7). *Epinephrine* is synthesized from tyrosine in the adrenal medulla and released, along with small quantities of *norepinephrine*, into the blood stream. *Epinephrine* interacts with both α and β receptors. At low doses, β effects (vasodilation) on the vascular system predominate, whereas at high doses, α effects (vasoconstrictor) are strongest.

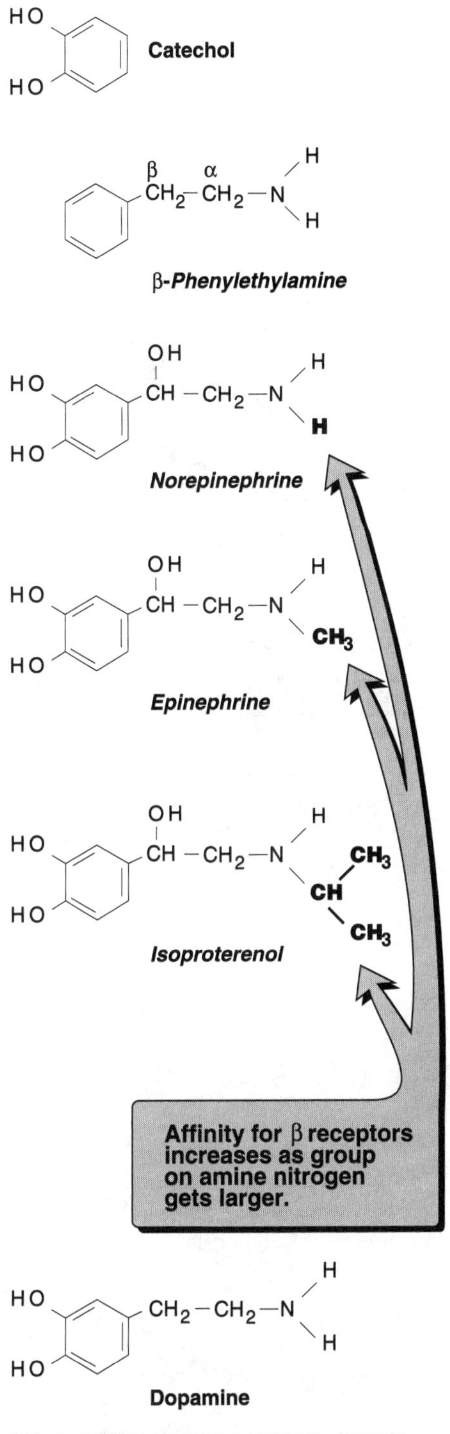

Figure 6.7
Structures of several important adrenergic agonists.

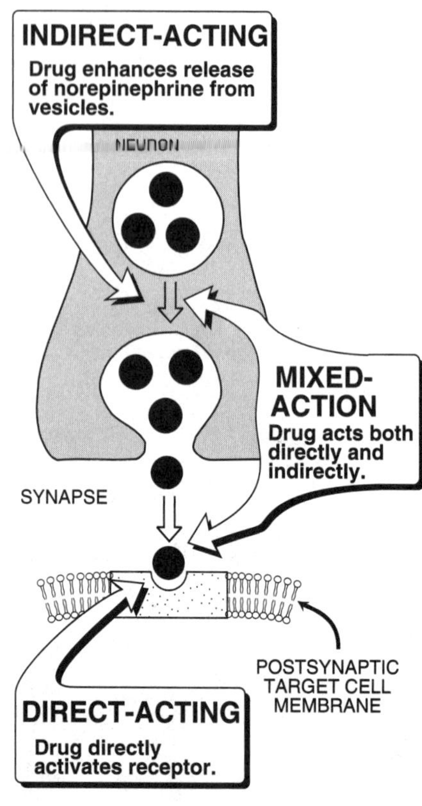

Figure 6.8
Sites of action of direct-, indirect- and mixed-acting adrenergic agonists.

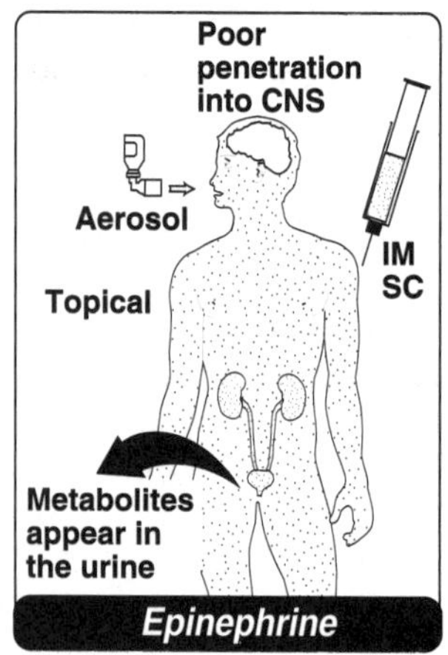

1. **Actions:**

   a. **Cardiovascular:** The major actions of *epinephrine* are on the cardiovascular system. *Epinephrine* strengthens the contractility of the myocardium (positive inotropic: β_1 action) and increases its rate of contraction (positive chronotropic: β_1 action). Cardiac output therefore increases. With these effects comes increased oxygen demands on the myocardium. *Epinephrine* constricts arterioles in the skin, mucous membranes, and viscera (α effects) and dilates vessels going to the liver and skeletal muscle (β_2 effects). Renal blood flow is decreased. The cumulative effect, therefore, is an increase in systolic blood pressure, coupled with a slight decrease in diastolic pressure (Figure 6.9) that can result in a reflex slowing of the heart.

   b. **Respiratory:** *Epinephrine* causes powerful bronchodilation by acting directly on bronchial smooth muscle (β_2 action). This action relieves all known allergic- or histamine-induced bronchoconstriction. In the case of anaphylactic shock, this can be life-saving. In individuals suffering from an acute asthmatic attack, *epinephrine* rapidly relieves the dyspnea (labored breathing) and increases the tidal volume (volume of gases inspired and expired).

   c. **Hyperglycemia:** *Epinephrine* has a significant hyperglycemic effect because of increased glycogenolysis in liver (β_2 effect), increased release of glucagon (β_2 effect), and a decreased release of insulin (α_2 effect). These effects are mediated via the cyclic AMP mechanism.

   d. **Lipolysis:** *Epinephrine* initiates lipolysis through its agonist activity on the β receptors of adipose tissue, which upon stimulation, activate adenylyl cyclase to increase cyclic AMP levels. Cyclic AMP stimulates a hormone-sensitive lipase, which hydrolyzes triacylglycerols to free fatty acids and glycerol.[3]

2. **Biotransformations:** *Epinephrine*, like the other catecholamines, is metabolized by two enzymatic pathways: COMT, which has S-adenosylmethionine as a cofactor, and MAO (see Figure 6.3). The final metabolites found in the urine are metanephrine and vanillylmandelic acid. [Note: Urine also contains normetanephrine, a product of *norepinephrine* metabolism.]

3. **Therapeutic uses**

   a. **Bronchospasm:** *Epinephrine* is the primary drug used in the emergency treatment of any condition of the respiratory tract where the presence of bronchoconstriction has resulted in diminished respiratory exchange. Thus, in treatment of acute asthma and anaphylactic shock, *epinephrine* is the drug of choice; within a few minutes after subcutaneous administration, greatly improved respiratory exchange is observed. Administration may be repeated after a few hours. However, selective β_2 agonists, such as *terbutaline*, are presently favored in the chronic treatment of asthma because of a longer duration of action and minimal cardiac stimulatory effect.

[3]See p. 70 for Infolink references to other books in this series.

b. **Glaucoma:** In ophthalmology, a 2% *epinephrine* solution may be used topically to reduce intraocular pressure in open-angle glaucoma. It reduces the production of aqueous humor by vasoconstriction of the ciliary body blood vessels.

c. **Anaphylactic shock:** *Epinephrine* is the drug of choice for the treatment of Type I hypersensitivity reactions in response to allergens.

d. **In anesthetics:** Local anesthetic solutions usually contain 1:100,000 parts *epinephrine* (p. 118). The effect of the drug is to greatly increase the duration of the local anesthesia. It does this by producing vasoconstriction at the site of injection, thereby allowing the local anesthetic to persist at the site before being absorbed into the circulation and metabolized. Very weak solutions of *epinephrine* (1:100,000) can also be used topically to vasoconstrict mucous membranes to control oozing of capillary blood.

4. **Pharmacokinetics:** *Epinephrine* has a rapid onset but brief duration of action. In emergency situations *epinephrine* is given intravenously for the most rapid onset of action; it may also be given subcutaneously, by endotracheal tube, by inhalation, or topically to the eye. Oral administration is ineffective, since *epinephrine* and the other catecholamines are inactivated by intestinal enzymes. Only metabolites are excreted in the urine.

5. **Adverse effects:**

a. **CNS disturbances:** *Epinephrine* can produce adverse CNS effects that include anxiety, fear, tension, headache, and tremor.

b. **Hemorrhage:** The drug may induce cerebral hemorrhage as a result of a marked elevation of blood pressure.

c. **Cardiac arrhythmias:** *Epinephrine* can trigger cardiac arrhythmias, particularly if the patient is receiving *digitalis* (see p. 157).

d. **Pulmonary edema:** *Epinephrine* can induce pulmonary edema.

6. **Interactions**

a. **Hyperthyroidism:** *Epinephrine* may have enhanced cardiovascular actions in patients with hyperthyroidism. If *epinephrine* is required in such an individual, the dose must be reduced. The mechanism appears to involve increased production of adrenergic receptors on the vasculature of the hyperthyroid individual leading to a hypersensitive response.

b. **Cocaine:** In the presence of *cocaine*, *epinephrine* produces exaggerated cardiovascular actions. This is due to the ability of *cocaine* to prevent re-uptake of catecholamines into the adrenergic neuron; thus, like *norepinephrine*, *epinephrine* remains at the receptor site for longer periods of time (see Figure 6.3).

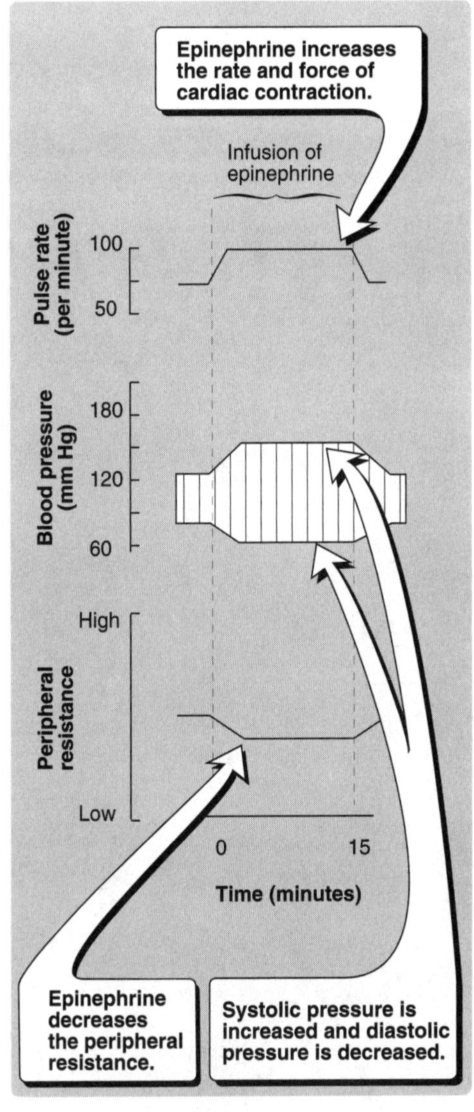

Figure 6.9
Cardiovascular effects of intravenous infusion of low doses of epinephrine.

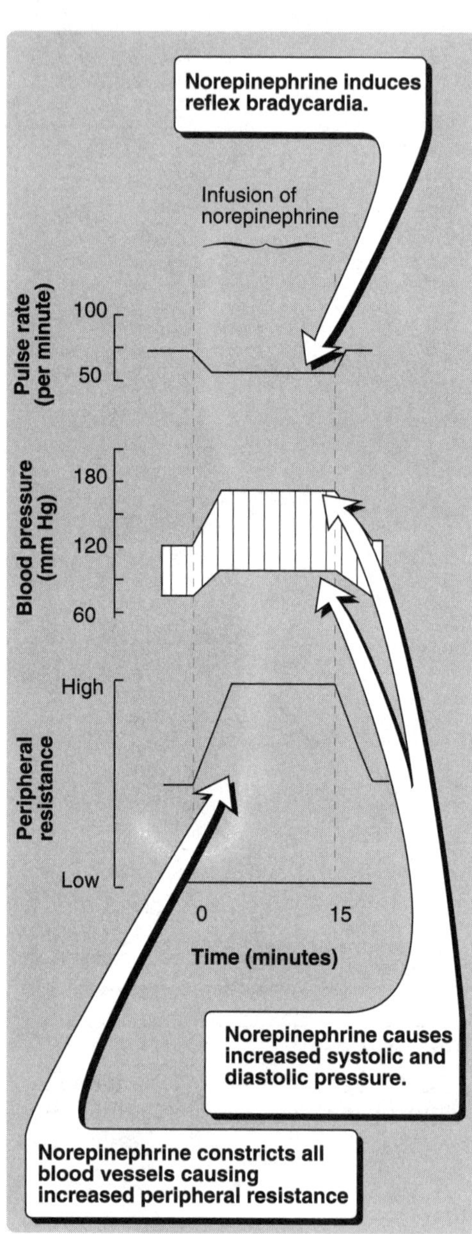

Figure 6.10
Cardiovascular effects of intravenous infusion of norepinephrine.

B. Norepinephrine

Since *norepinephrine* [nor ep ee NEF rin] is the neuromediator of adrenergic nerves, it should theoretically stimulate all types of adrenergic receptors. In practice, when the drug is given in therapeutic doses to humans, the α-adrenergic receptor is most affected.

1. Cardiovascular Actions

a. **Vasoconstriction:** *Norepinephrine* causes a rise in peripheral resistance due to intense vasoconstriction of most vascular beds, including the kidney (an α_1-receptor effect). Both systolic and diastolic blood pressures increase (Figure 6.10).

b. **Baroreceptor reflex:** In isolated cardiac tissue *norepinephrine* stimulates cardiac contractility; however, in vivo, little if any cardiac stimulation is noted. This is due to the increased blood pressure that induces a reflex rise in vagal activity by stimulating the baroreceptors. This bradycardia is sufficient to counteract the local actions of *norepinephrine* on the heart although the reflex compensation does not affect the positive inotropic effects of the drug (Figure 6.10).

c. **Effect of atropine pretreatment:** If *atropine* (which blocks the transmission of vagal effects, see p. 45) is given before *norepinephrine*, then *norepinephrine* stimulation of the heart is evident as tachycardia.

2. Therapeutic uses:

Norepinephrine is used to treat shock because it increases vascular resistance and, therefore, increases blood pressure; however, *dopamine* (see p. 65) is better, because it does not reduce blood flow to the kidney as does *norepinephrine*. Other actions of *norepinephrine* are not considered clinically significant. It is never used for asthma. [Note: When *norepinephrine* is used as a drug, it is sometimes called *levarterenol* [leev are TER a nole].]

C. Isoproterenol

Isoproterenol [eye soe proe TER a nole] is a direct-acting synthetic catecholamine that predominantly stimulates both β_1 and β_2 adrenergic receptors. Its non-selectivity is one of its drawbacks. Its action on α receptors is insignificant. Its chemical structure is given in Figure 6.7.

1. Actions

a. **Cardiovascular:** *Isoproterenol* produces intense stimulation of the heart to increase its rate and force of contraction, causing increased cardiac output (Figure 6.11). It is as active as *epinephrine* in this action and is therefore useful in the treatment of atrioventricular block or cardiac arrest. *Isoproterenol* also dilates the arterioles of skeletal muscle (β_2), resulting in a decreased peripheral resistance. Because of its cardiac stimulatory action, it may increase systolic blood pressure slightly, but it greatly reduces mean arterial and diastolic blood pressure (Figure 6.11).

b. **Pulmonary:** A profound and rapid bronchodilation is produced by the drug (β_2 action, Figure 6.12). *Isoproterenol* is as active as *epinephrine* and rapidly alleviates an acute attack of asthma, when taken by inhalation (which is the recommended route). This action lasts about one hour and may be repeated by subsequent doses.

c. **Other effects:** Other actions on β receptors, such as increases in blood sugar and increased lipolysis can be demonstrated, but are not clinically significant.

2. **Therapeutic uses:** *Isoproterenol* is now rarely used as a bronchodilator in asthma. It can be employed to stimulate the heart in emergency situations.

3. **Pharmacokinetics:** *Isoproterenol* can be absorbed systemically by the sublingual mucosa but is more reliably absorbed when given parenterally or as an inhaled aerosol. It is a marginal substrate for COMT and is stable to MAO action.

4. **Adverse effects:** *Isoproterenol's* adverse effects are similar to those of *epinephrine*.

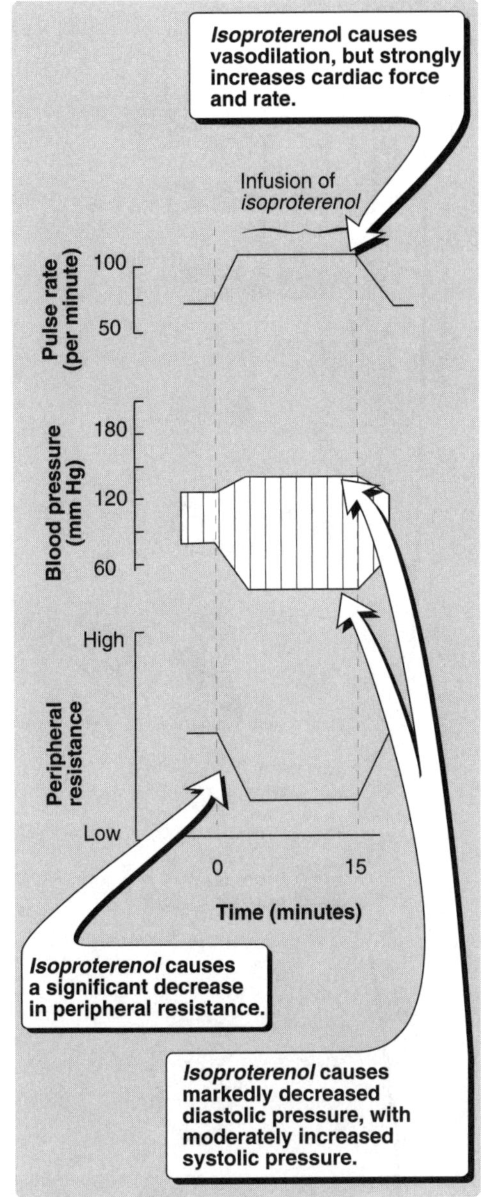

Figure 6.11
Cardiovascular effects of intravenous infusion of *isoproterenol*.

D. Dopamine

Dopamine [DOE pa meen], the immediate metabolic precursor of *norepinephrine*, occurs naturally in the CNS in the basal ganglia where it functions as a neurotransmitter as well as in the adrenal medulla. *Dopamine* can activate α- and β-adrenergic receptors. For example, at higher doses it can cause vasoconstriction by activating α receptors, whereas at lower doses, it stimulates β_1 cardiac receptors. In addition, D_1 and D_2 dopaminergic receptors, distinct from the α- and β-adrenergic receptors, occur in the peripheral mesenteric and renal vascular beds, where binding of *dopamine* produces vasodilatation. D_2 receptors are also found on presynaptic adrenergic neurons, where their activation interferes with *norepinephrine* release.

1. **Actions**

a. **Cardiovascular:** *Dopamine* exerts a stimulatory effect on the β_1 receptors of the heart, having both inotropic and chronotropic effects (Figure 6.12). At very high doses, *dopamine* activates α receptors on the vasculature, resulting in vasoconstriction.

b. **Renal and visceral:** *Dopamine* dilates renal and splanchnic arterioles by activating dopaminergic receptors, thus increasing blood flow to the kidneys and other viscera (see Figure 6.12). These receptors are not affected by α- or β-blocking drugs. Therefore, *dopamine* is clinically useful in the treatment of shock, in which significant increases in sympathetic activity might compromise renal function. [Note: Similar *dopamine* receptors are found in the autonomic ganglia and in the CNS.]

2. **Therapeutic uses**

a. **Shock:** *Dopamine* is the drug of choice for shock and is given by continuous infusion. It raises the blood pressure by stimulating

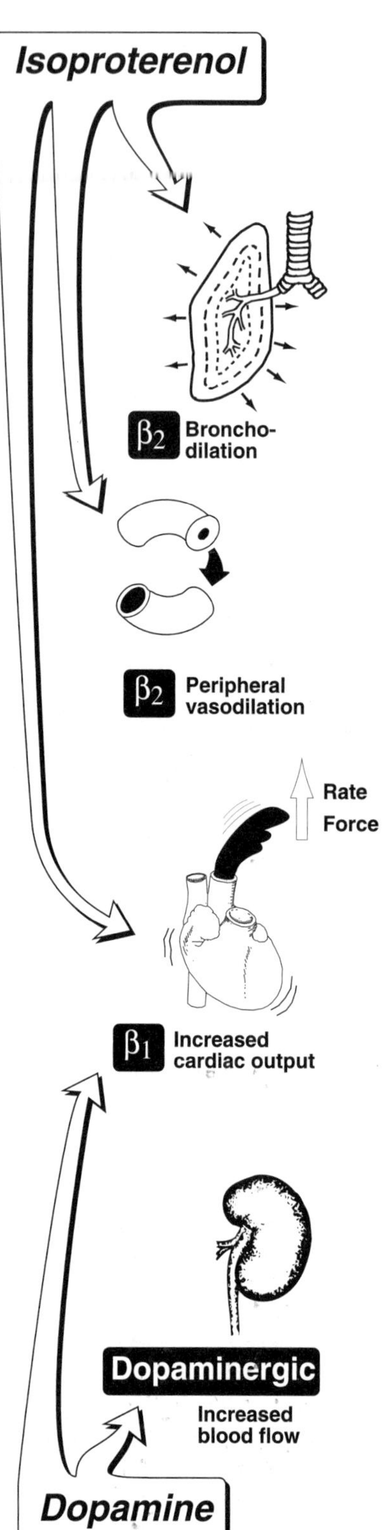

Figure 6.12
Clinically important actions of *isoproterenol* and *dopamine*.

the heart (β_1 action). In addition, it enhances perfusion to the kidney and splanchnic areas, as described above. An increased blood flow to the kidney enhances the glomerular filtration rate and causes sodium diuresis. In this regard, *dopamine* is far superior to *norepinephrine*, which diminishes the blood supply to the kidney and may cause kidney shutdown.

3. **Adverse effects:** An overdose of *dopamine* produces the same effects as sympathetic stimulation. *Dopamine* is rapidly metabolized to homovanillic acid, and its adverse effects (nausea, hypertension, arrhythmias) are therefore short-lived.

E. Dobutamine

1. **Actions:** *Dobutamine* [doe BYOO ta meen] is a synthetic, direct-acting catecholamine that is a β_1-receptor agonist. It is available as a racemic mixture. One of the stereoisomers has a stimulatory activity. It increases cardiac rate and output with few vascular effects.

2. **Therapeutic uses:** *Dobutamine* is used to increase cardiac output in congestive heart failure (p. 161). The drug increases cardiac output with little change in the heart rate and does not significantly elevate oxygen demands of the myocardium—a major advantage over other sympathomimetic drugs.

3. **Adverse effects:** *Dobutamine* should be used with caution in atrial fibrillation, since the drug increases atrioventricular conduction. Other adverse effects are the same as those for *epinephrine*. Tolerance may develop on prolonged use.

F. Phenylephrine

Phenylephrine [fen ill EF rin] is a direct-acting, synthetic adrenergic drug that binds primarily to α receptors and favors α_1 receptors over α_2 receptors. It is not a catechol derivative and therefore not a substrate for COMT. *Phenylephrine* is a vasoconstrictor that raises both systolic and diastolic blood pressures. It has no effect on the heart itself but induces reflex bradycardia when given parenterally. It is often used topically on the nasal mucous membranes and in ophthalmic solutions for mydriasis. *Phenylephrine* acts as a nasal decongestant (p. 221), and produces prolonged vasoconstriction. The drug is used to raise blood pressure and to terminate episodes of supraventricular tachycardia (rapid heart action arising both from the atrioventricular junction and atria). Large doses can cause hypertensive headache and cardiac irregularities.

G. Methoxamine

Methoxamine [meth OX a meen] is a direct-acting synthetic adrenergic drug that binds primarily to α receptors, with α_1 receptors favored over α_2 receptors. *Methoxamine* raises blood pressure by stimulating α_1 receptors in the arterioles, causing vasoconstriction. This causes an increase in total peripheral resistance. Because of its effects on the vagus, *methoxamine* is used clinically to relieve attacks of paroxysmal supraventricular tachycardia. It is also used to overcome hypotension during surgery involving *halothane* anesthetics. In contrast to most other adrenergic drugs, *methoxamine* does not tend to trigger cardiac arrhythmias in the heart that is sensitized by these general anesthetics. Adverse effects include hypertensive headache and vomiting.

H. Clonidine

Clonidine [KLOE ni deen] is an α_2 agonist that is used in essential hypertension to lower blood pressure because of its action in the CNS (see p. 189). It can be used to minimize the symptoms that accompany withdrawal from opiates or benzodiazepines. *Clonidine* acts centrally to produce inhibition of sympathetic vasomotor centers. Recently, an endogenous substance, agmantine, which appears to be the natural ligand at clonidine binding sites, has been identified.

I. Metaproterenol

Metaproterenol [met a proe TER a nole], although chemically similar to *isoproterenol*, is not a catecholamine and is resistant to methylation by COMT. It can be administered orally or by inhalation. The drug acts primarily at β_2 receptors, producing little effect on the heart. *Metaproterenol* produces dilation of the bronchioles and improves airway function. The drug is useful as a bronchodilator in the treatment of asthma and to reverse bronchospasm (Figure 6.13).

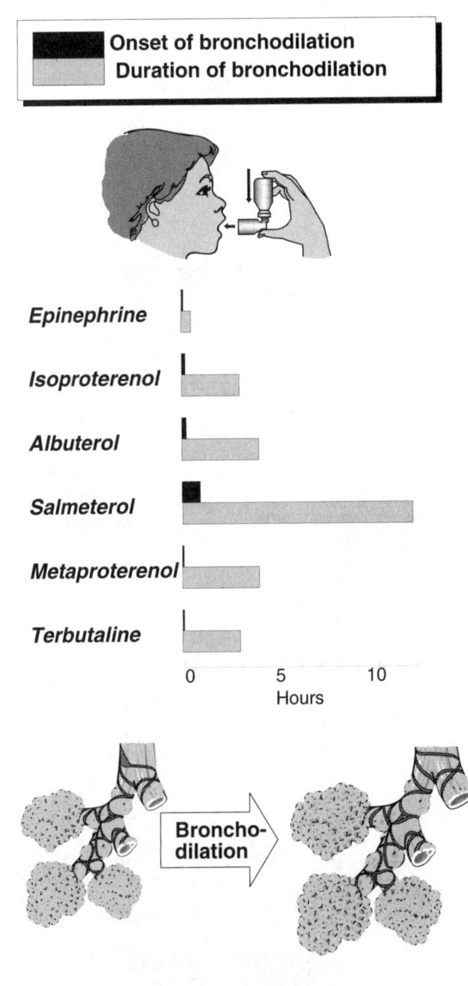

Figure 6.13
Onset and duration of broncho-dilation effects of inhaled adrenergic agonists.

J. Terbutaline

Terbutaline [ter BYOO te leen] is a β_2 agonist with more selective properties than *metaproterenol* and a longer duration of action. *Terbutaline* can be administered either orally or subcutaneously. It is used as a bronchodilator and to reduce uterine contractions in premature labor.

K. Albuterol

Albuterol [al BYOO ter ole] is a selective β_2 agonist with properties similar to those of *terbutaline*. The drug is widely used as an inhalant to relieve bronchospasm.

V. INDIRECT-ACTING ADRENERGIC AGONISTS

Indirect-acting adrenergic agonists cause *norepinephrine* release from presynaptic terminals (see Figure 6.8). They potentiate the effects of *norepinephrine* produced endogenously, but these agents do not directly affect postsynaptic receptors.

A. Amphetamine

Amphetamine's [am FET a meen] marked central stimulatory action is often mistaken by drug abusers as its only action. However, the drug can increase blood pressure significantly by α-agonist action on the vasculature as well as β- stimulatory effects on the heart. Its

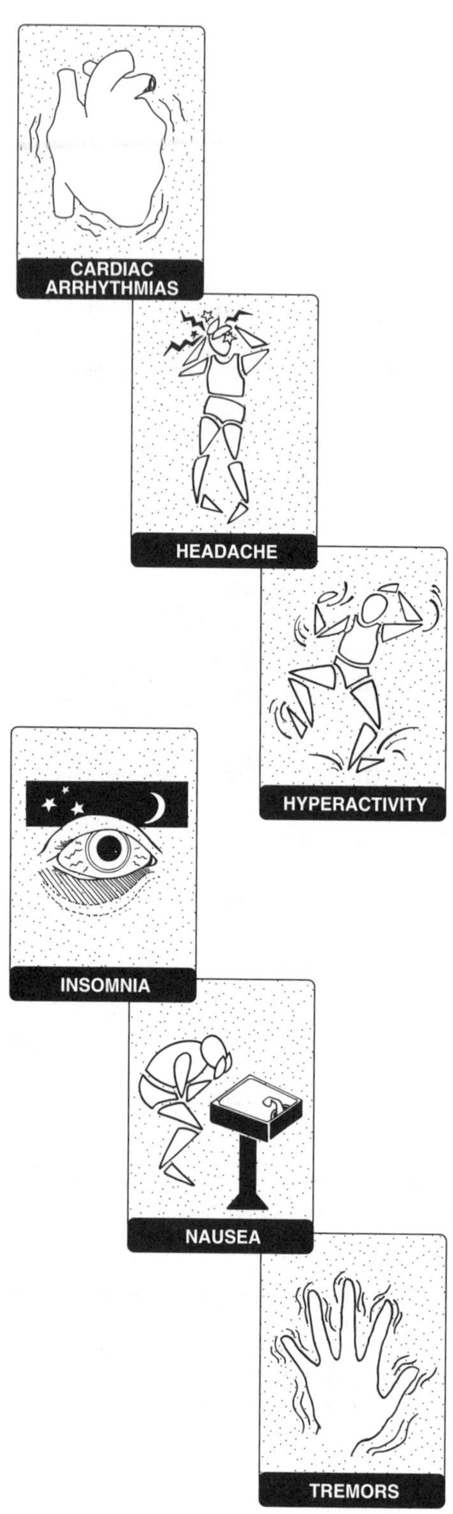

Figure 6.14
Some adverse effects observed with adrenergic agonists.

peripheral actions are mediated primarily through the cellular release of stored catecholamines; thus, *amphetamine* is an indirect-acting adrenergic drug. The actions and uses of amphetamines are discussed under stimulants of the CNS (see p. 103).The CNS stimulant effects of *amphetamine* and its derivatives have led to their use in the therapy of depression, hyperactivity in children, narcolepsy, and appetite control. Its use in pregnancy should be avoided because of adverse effects on the development of the fetus.

B. Tyramine

Tyramine [teye ra meen] is not a clinically useful drug, but it is found in fermented foods, such as ripe cheese and Chianti wine (see MAO inhibitors, p. 123). It is a normal by-product of tyrosine metabolism. Normally, it is oxidized by MAO, but if the patient is taking MAO inhibitors, it can precipitate serious vasopressor episodes. Like *amphetamine, tyramine* can enter the nerve terminal and displace stored *norepinephrine.* The released catecholamine acts on adrenoceptors.

VI. MIXED-ACTION ADRENERGIC AGONISTS

Mixed-action drugs induce the release of *norepinephrine* from presynaptic terminals and activate adrenergic receptors on the postsynaptic membrane (see Figure 6.8).

A. Ephedrine

Ephedrine [e FED rin], a plant alkaloid, is now made synthetically. The drug is a mixed-action adrenergic agent. It not only releases stored *norepinephrine* from nerve endings (Figure 6.8) but also directly stimulates both α and β receptors. Thus, a wide variety of adrenergic actions ensue that are similar to those of *epinephrine,* although less potent. *Ephedrine* is not a catechol and is a poor substrate for COMT and MAO; thus, the drug has a long duration of action. *Ephedrine* has excellent absorption orally and penetrates into the central nervous system. It is eliminated unchanged in the urine. *Ephedrine* raises systolic and diastolic blood pressures by vasoconstriction and cardiac stimulation. *Ephedrine* produces bronchodilation, but it is less potent than *epinephrine* or *isoproterenol* in this regard and produces its action more slowly. It is therefore sometimes used prophylactically in chronic treatment of asthma to prevent attacks, rather than to treat the acute attack. *Ephedrine* enhances contractility and improves motor function in myasthenia gravis, particularly when used in conjunction with anticholinesterases (see p. 43). *Ephedrine* produces a mild stimulation of the CNS. This increases alertness, decreases fatigue, and prevents sleep. It also improves athletic performance. *Ephedrine* has been used to treat asthma, as a nasal decongestant (due to its local vasoconstrictor action), and to raise blood pressure. [Note: the clinical use of *ephedrine* is declining due to the availability of better, more potent agents which cause fewer adverse effects.]

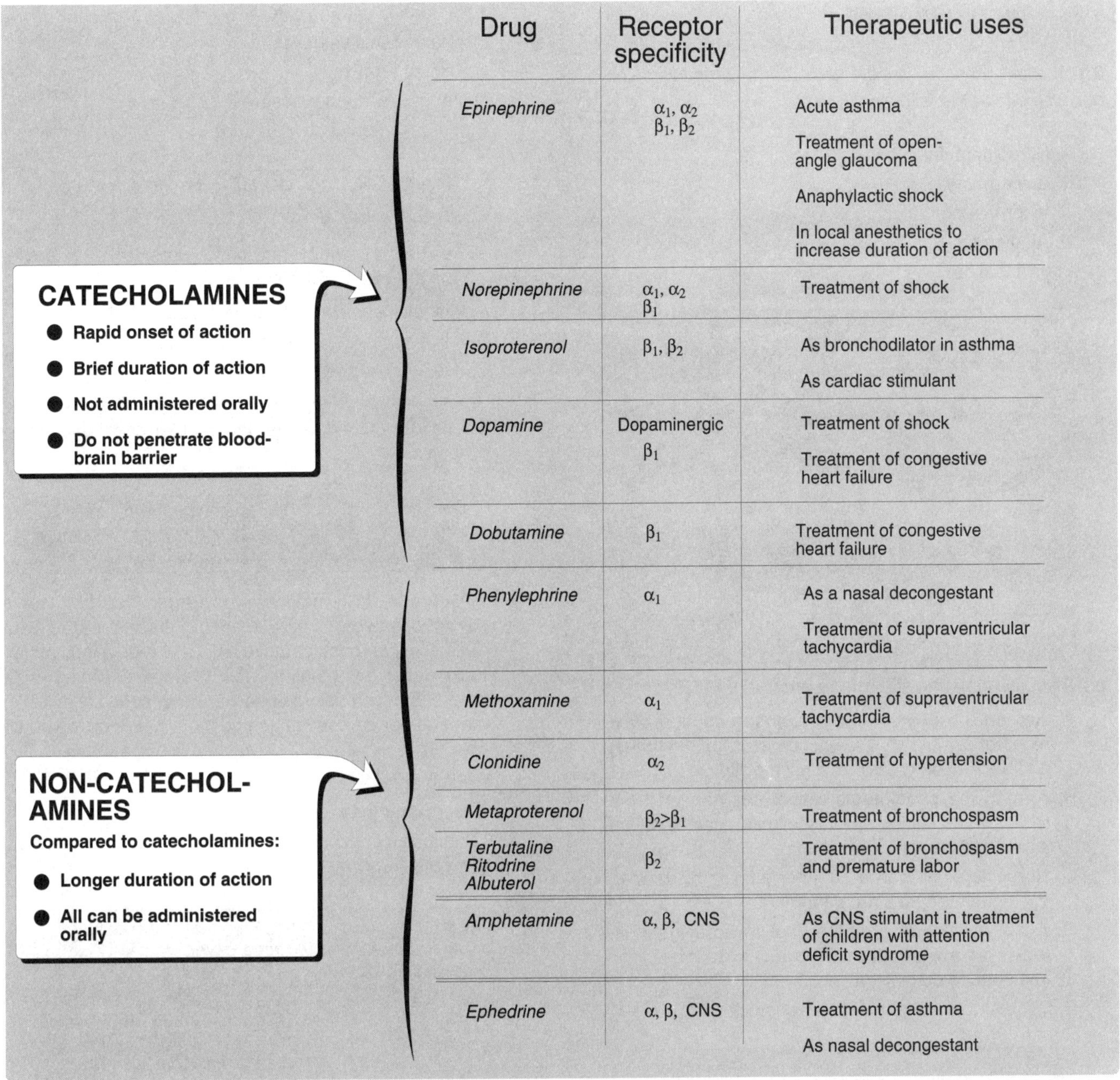

CATECHOLAMINES
- Rapid onset of action
- Brief duration of action
- Not administered orally
- Do not penetrate blood-brain barrier

NON-CATECHOLAMINES
Compared to catecholamines:
- Longer duration of action
- All can be administered orally

Drug	Receptor specificity	Therapeutic uses
Epinephrine	α_1, α_2, β_1, β_2	Acute asthma Treatment of open-angle glaucoma Anaphylactic shock In local anesthetics to increase duration of action
Norepinephrine	α_1, α_2, β_1	Treatment of shock
Isoproterenol	β_1, β_2	As bronchodilator in asthma As cardiac stimulant
Dopamine	Dopaminergic, β_1	Treatment of shock Treatment of congestive heart failure
Dobutamine	β_1	Treatment of congestive heart failure
Phenylephrine	α_1	As a nasal decongestant Treatment of supraventricular tachycardia
Methoxamine	α_1	Treatment of supraventricular tachycardia
Clonidine	α_2	Treatment of hypertension
Metaproterenol	β_2>β_1	Treatment of bronchospasm
Terbutaline *Ritodrine* *Albuterol*	β_2	Treatment of bronchospasm and premature labor
Amphetamine	α, β, CNS	As CNS stimulant in treatment of children with attention deficit syndrome
Ephedrine	α, β, CNS	Treatment of asthma As nasal decongestant

Figure 6.15
Summary of the adrenergic agonists.

B. Metaraminol

Metaraminol [met a RAM i nole] is a mixed-action adrenergic drug with actions similar to *norepinephrine.* This agent has been used in the treatment of shock (when an infusion of *norepinephrine* or *dopamine* is not possible) and to treat acute hypotension. It is given parenterally as a single injection. It enhances cardiac activity and produces mild vasoconstriction.

The important characteristics of the adrenergic agonists are summarized in Figures 6.14 and 6.15.

Choose the ONE best answer.

6.1 Diastolic pressure is increased after the administration of which one of the following drugs?

A. Norepinephrine
B. Epinephrine
C. Isoproterenol
D. Albuterol
E. Terbutaline

> Correct answer = A. Norepinephrine produces intense vasoconstriction and thereby increases peripheral resistance, so that both systolic and diastolic blood pressures increase. Epinephrine increases cardiac output, constricts arterioles in the skin and viscera (α effects), and dilates vessels going to skeletal muscle (β_2 effects); the overall result is an increase in systolic pressure. Isoproterenol is a β-specific agonist that increases cardiac output and decreases peripheral resistance; this causes a slight increase in systolic blood pressure and a significant decrease in diastolic blood pressure. Albuterol and terbutaline are vasodilators that act primarily at β_2 receptors.

6.2 All of the following statements are true EXCEPT:

A. Among the physiologic responses caused by α-receptor stimulation are vasoconstriction, mydriasis, and decreased gastrointestinal motility.
B. Among the physiologic responses caused by β-receptor stimulation are vasodilation, cardiac stimulation, and bronchial relaxation.
C. Norepinephrine has a stronger affinity for α receptors compared to β receptors.
D. Administration of atropine prior to norepinephrine leads to an increase in heart rate after norepinephrine administration.
E. Dobutamine is a potent vasoconstrictor.

> Correct choice = E. Dobutamine acts primarily at β_2 receptors and has little effect on vascular resistance.

6.3 Dopamine causes all but which one of the following actions?

A. Increases cardiac output
B. Dilates renal vasculature
C. Dilates bronchi
D. Increases blood pressure
E. Increases production of urine

> Correct choice = C. Dopamine has little effect of the β_2 receptors of the lung.

6.4 All of the following statements concerning phenylephrine are true EXCEPT:

A. It is an α agonist that causes vasoconstriction.
B. It is a synthetic, direct-acting agonist.
C. It is used to prevent bronchospasm.
D. It causes mydriasis when introduced into the eye.
E. It is often found in over-the-counter nasal decongestants.

> Correct choice = C. Phenylephrine is a synthetic, direct-acting α agonist. It does not affect alveolar smooth muscle, which contains primarily β_2 receptors.

6.5 A 58-year-old female has undergone surgery for a necrotic bowel. Despite having been treated with antibiotics, on postoperative day 5, she develops symptoms (fever, hypotension, tachycardia, declining urine output, and confusion) consistent with septic shock. To manage her care, what hemodynamic support would be helpful?

A. Fluid administration
B. Dopamine infusion
C. Antibiotic administration
D. Fluids and Dopamine

> Correct answer = D. It is important to increase the cardiac output to improve oxygen delivery and thus minimize anaerobic metabolism and improve CNS and renal perfusion. Since this patient apparently does not have a heart condition, such as congestive heart failure, she could benefit from fluid therapy. An inotropic agent, such as dopamine, would lead to an increased cardiac output and dilation of the renal vasculature. [Note: At high doses, however, it may constrict the renal beds due to interaction on α receptors.] Antibiotic administration is also important but will not improve the patient's hemodynamics.

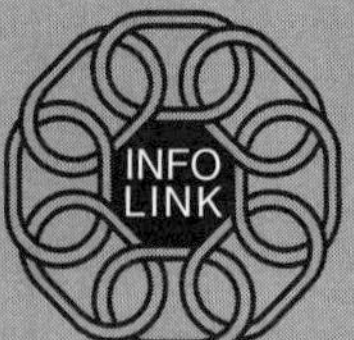

[1]See p. 267 in **Biochemistry** (2nd ed.) for a discussion of the synthesis DOPA from tyrosine.

[2]See p. 267 in **Biochemistry** (2nd ed.) for a discussion of the synthesis and actions of IP_3.

[3]See p. 267 in **Biochemistry** (2nd ed.) for a discussion of hormone-sensitive lipase.

Adrenergic Antagonists

7

I. OVERVIEW

The adrenergic antagonists (also called blockers) bind to adrenoceptors but do not trigger the usual receptor-mediated intracellular effects. These drugs act by either reversibly or irreversibly attaching to the receptor, thus preventing its activation by endogenous catecholamines. Like the agonists, the adrenergic antagonists are classified according to their relative affinity for α or β receptors in the peripheral nervous system. [Note: Antagonists that block dopamine receptors are most important in the central nervous system and will be considered in that section (see p. 127.] The receptor-blocking drugs discussed in this chapter are summarized in Figure 7.1.

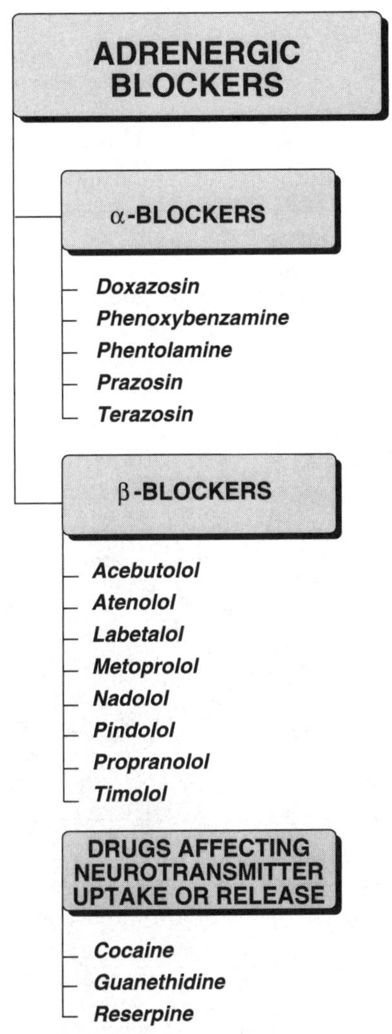

Figure 7.1
Summary of blocking agents and drugs affecting neurotransmitter uptake or release.

II. α-ADRENERGIC BLOCKING AGENTS

Drugs that block α adrenoceptors profoundly affect blood pressure. Since normal sympathetic control of the vasculature occurs in large part through agonist actions on α-adrenergic receptors, blockade of these receptors reduces the sympathetic tone of the blood vessels, resulting in decreased peripheral vascular resistance. This induces a reflex tachycardia resulting from the lowered blood pressure. [Note: β receptors, including β_1 adrenoceptors on the heart, are not affected by α blockade.] *Phenoxybenzamine* and *phentolamine* have limited clinical applications.

A. Phenoxybenzamine

Phenoxybenzamine [fen ox ee BEN za meen], a drug related to the nitrogen mustards, is non-selective, linking covalently to both α_1-postsynaptic and α_2-presynaptic receptors (Figure 7.2). The block is irreversible and noncompetitive; the only mechanism the body has to overcome the block is to synthesize new adrenoceptors, which requires a day or more. Therefore, the actions of *phenoxybenzamine* last about 24 hours after a single administration. After the drug is injected, a delay of a few hours occurs before a blockade develops, since the molecule must undergo biotransformation to the active form.

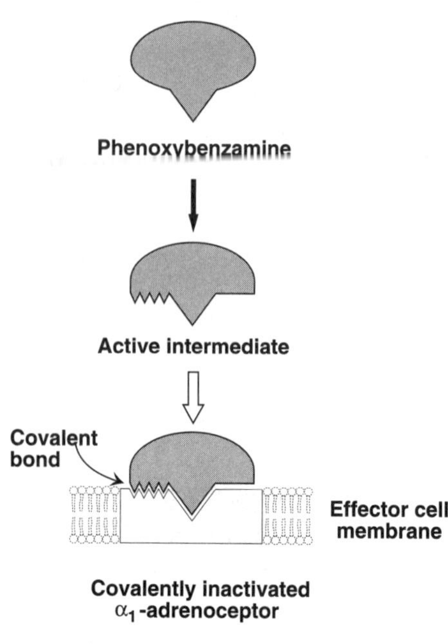

Figure 7.2
Covalent inactivation of α_1 adrenoceptor by phenoxybenzamine.

1. **Actions:**

   a. **Cardiovascular effects:** By blocking α receptors, *phenoxybenzamine* prevents vasoconstriction of peripheral blood vessels by endogenous catecholamines. The decreased peripheral resistance provokes a reflex tachycardia. Furthermore, the ability to block presynaptic α_2 receptors in the heart can contribute to an increased cardiac output. Thus the drug has been unsuccessful in maintaining lowered blood pressure in hypertension and has been discontinued for this purpose.

   b. **Epinephrine reversal:** All α-adrenergic blockers reverse the α-agonist actions of *epinephrine*. For example, the vasoconstrictive action of *epinephrine* is interrupted, but vasodilation of other vascular beds caused by stimulation of β-receptors is not blocked. Therefore, the systemic blood pressure decreases in response to *epinephrine* given in the presence of *phenoxybenzamine* (Figure 7.3). [Note: The actions of *norepinephrine* are not reversed but diminished, since *norepinephrine* lacks significant β-agonist action on the vasculature.] *Phenoxybenzamine* has no effect on the actions of *isoproterenol*, which is a pure β agonist (Figure 7.3).

2. **Therapeutic uses:** *Phenoxybenzamine* is used in the treatment of pheochromocytoma, a catecholamine-secreting tumor of cells derived from the adrenal medulla. Prior to surgical removal of the tumor, patients are treated with *phenoxybenzamine* to preclude hypertensive crisis that can result from manipulation of the tissue. This drug also finds use in the chronic management of these tumors, particularly when the catecholamine-secreting cells are diffuse and therefore inoperable. *Phenoxybenzamine* or *phentolamine* are sometimes effective in treating Raynaud's disease. Autonomic hyperreflexia which predisposes paraplegics to strokes can be managed with *phenoxybenzamine.*

3. **Adverse effects:** *Phenoxybenzamine* can cause postural hypotension, nasal stuffiness, and nausea and vomiting. It can inhibit ejaculation. The drug also may induce tachycardia, mediated by the baroreceptor reflex and is contraindicated in patients with decreased coronary perfusion.

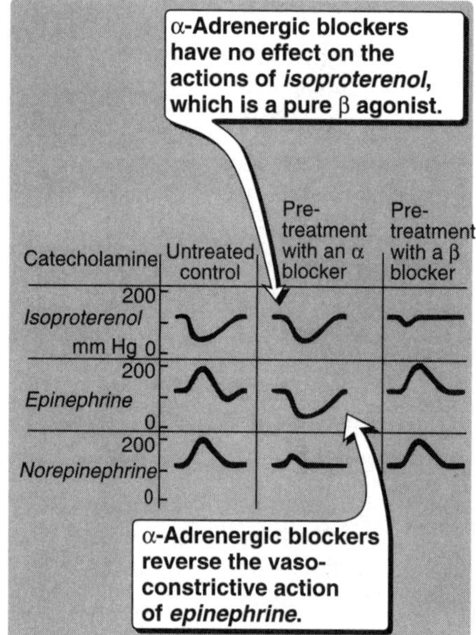

Figure 7.3
Summary of effects of adrenergic blockers on the changes in blood pressure induced by *isoproterenol*, *epinephrine*, and *norepinephrine*.

B. Phentolamine

In contrast to *phenoxybenzamine*, *phentolamine* [fen TOLE a meen] produces a competitive block of α_1 and α_2 receptors. The drug's action lasts for approximately 4 hours after a single administration. Like *phenoxybenzamine*, it produces postural hypotension and causes *epinephrine* reversal. *Phentolamine* had been used in the diagnosis of pheochromocytoma and in other clinical situations associated with excess release of catecholamines. *Phentolamine*-induced reflex cardiac stimulation and tachycardia are mediated by the baroreceptor reflex and by blocking the α_2 receptors of the cardiac sympathetic nerves. The drug can also trigger arrhythmias and anginal pain and is contraindicated in patients with decreased coronary perfusion.

C. Prazosin, terazosin and doxazosin

Prazosin [PRAY zoe sin], *terazosin* [ter AY zoe sin] and *doxazosin* [dox AY zoe sin] are selective competitive blockers of the α_1 receptor. In contrast to *phenoxybenzamine* and *phentolamine*, these drugs are useful in the treatment of hypertension. Metabolism leads to inactive products that are excreted in the urine, except for those of *doxazosin* which appear in the feces. *Doxazosin* is longest acting.

1. **Cardiovascular effects:** *Prazosin* and *terazosin* decrease peripheral vascular resistance and lower arterial blood pressure by causing the relaxation of both arterial and venous smooth muscle. These drugs, unlike *phenoxybenzamine* and *phentolamine*, cause minimal changes in cardiac output, renal blood flow, and glomerular filtration rate.

2. **Therapeutic uses:** Individuals with elevated blood pressure who have been treated with *prazosin* or *terazosin* do not become tolerant to its action (see p. 189). However, the first dose of these drugs produces an exaggerated hypotensive response that can result in syncope (fainting). This action, termed a "first-dose" effect, may be minimized by adjusting the first dose to one third or one fourth of the normal dose, and by giving the drug at bed time. The α_1 antagonists have been used as an alternative to surgery in patients with symptomatic benign prostatic hypertrophy. Blockade of the α receptors decreases tone in the smooth muscle of the bladder neck and prostate and improves urine flow. [Note: *Finasteride*, which inhibits dihydrotestosterone synthesis, has been approved for treatment of benign prostatic hypertrophy, but its effects are not evident for several weeks.]

3. **Adverse effects:** *Prazosin* and *terazosin* may cause dizziness, a lack of energy, nasal congestion, headache, drowsiness, and orthostatic hypotension (although to a lesser degree than that observed with *phenoxybenzamine* and *phentolamine*). An additive antihypertensive effect occurs when *prazosin* is given with either a diuretic or a β-blocker, thereby necessitating a reduction in its dose. Due to a tendency to retain sodium and fluid, *prazosin* is frequently used along with a diuretic. Male sexual function is not as severely affected by these drugs as it is by *phenoxybenzamine* and *phentolamine*. Figure 7.4 summarizes some adverse effects observed with α-blockers.

ORTHOSTATIC HYPOTENSION

TACHYCARDIA

VERTIGO

SEXUAL DYSFUNCTION

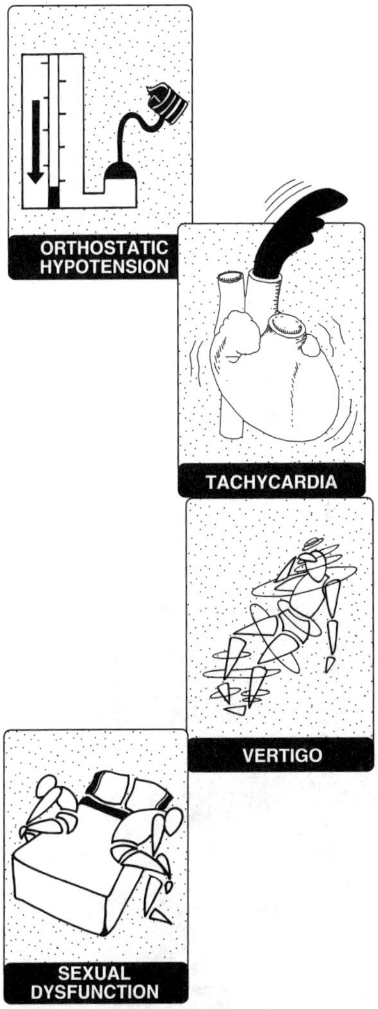

Figure 7.4
Some adverse effects commonly observed with α blockers.

III. β-ADRENERGIC BLOCKING AGENTS

All the clinically available β-blockers are competitive antagonists. Nonselective β-blockers act at both β_1 and β_2 receptors, whereas cardioselective β-antagonists primarily block β_1 receptors. These drugs also differ in intrinsic sympathomimetic activity, in central nervous system (CNS) effects, and in pharmacokinetics (Figure 7.5). Although all β-blockers lower blood pressure in hypertension, they do not induce postural hypotension because the α-adrenoceptors remain functional; therefore, normal sympathetic control of the vasculature is maintained. β-blockers are also effective in treating angina, cardiac arrhythmias, myocardial infarction, and glaucoma, as well as serving in the prophylaxis of migraine headaches. [Note: The names of all β-blockers end in "-olol", except for *labetalol*, which has a component of α_1-blocking actions.]

A. Propranolol: a nonselective β-antagonist

Propranolol [proe PRAN oh lole] is the prototype β-adrenergic antagonist and blocks both β_1 and β_2 receptors. Sustained release preparations for once-a-day dosing are available.

1. Actions

a. **Cardiovascular:** *Propranolol* diminishes cardiac output, having both negative inotropic and chronotropic effects (Figure 7.6). It directly depresses sino-auricular and atrioventricular activity. The resulting bradycardia usually limits the dose of the drug. Cardiac output, work, and oxygen consumption are decreased by blockade of β_1 receptors; these effects are useful in the treatment of angina (see p. 176). The β-blockers are effective in attenuating supraventricular cardiac arrhythmias but are generally not effective against ventricular arrhythmias (except those induced by exercise).

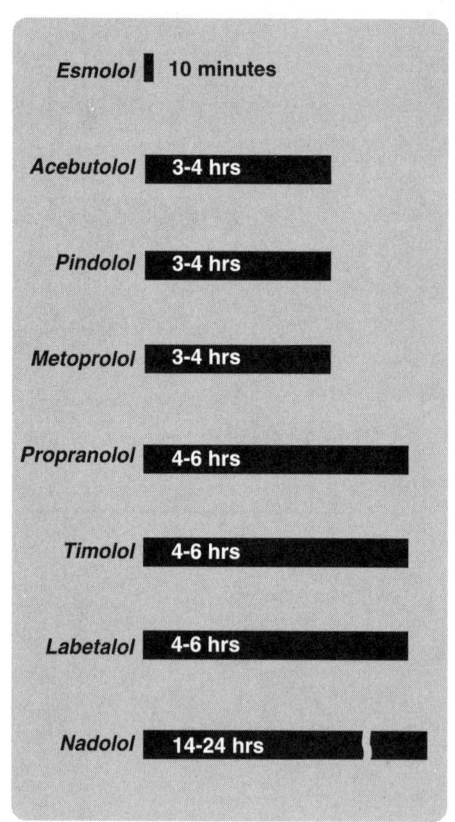

Figure 7.5
Elimination half-lives for some β blockers.

b. **Peripheral vasoconstriction:** Blockade of β receptors prevents β_2-mediated vasodilation (see Figure 7.6). The reduction in cardiac output leads to decreased blood pressure. This hypotension triggers a reflex peripheral vasoconstriction, which is reflected in reduced blood flow to the periphery. On balance, there is a gradual reduction of both systolic and diastolic blood pressures in hypertensive patients. No postural hypotension occurs, since the α_1-adrenergic receptors that control vascular resistance are unaffected.

c. **Bronchoconstriction:** Blocking β_2 receptors in the lungs of susceptible patients causes contraction of the bronchiolar smooth muscle (see Figure 7.6). This can precipitate a respiratory crisis in patients with chronic obstructive pulmonary disease or asthma. β-Blockers are thus contraindicted in patients with asthma.

d. **Increased Na^+ retention:** Reduced blood pressure causes a decrease in renal perfusion, resulting in an increase in Na^+ retention and plasma volume (see Figure 7.6). In some cases this compensatory response tends to elevate the blood pressure. For these patients, β-blockers are often combined with a diuretic to prevent Na^+ retention.

e. **Disturbances in glucose metabolism:** β blockade leads to decreased glycogenolysis and decreased glucagon secretion. Therefore, if an *insulin*-dependent diabetic is to be given *propranolol*, very careful monitoring of blood glucose is essential, since pronounced hypoglycemia may occur after *insulin* injection. β-Blockers also attenuate the normal physiologic response to hypoglycemia.

f. Blocks action of isoproterenol: All β-blockers, including *propranolol*, have the ability to block the actions of *isoproterenol* on the cardiovascular system. Thus, in the presence of a β-blocker, *isoproterenol* does not produce either the typical reductions in mean arterial pressure and diastolic pressure, nor cardiac stimulation (see Figure 7.3). [Note: In the presence of a β-blocker, *epinephrine* no longer lowers diastolic blood pressure nor stimulates the heart, but its vasoconstrictive action (mediated by α-receptors) remains unimpaired. The actions of *norepinephrine* on the cardiovascular system are primarily mediated by α receptors and are, therefore, unaffected.]

2. Therapeutic effects

a. Hypertension: *Propranolol* lowers blood pressure in hypertension by decreasing cardiac output (see p. 176).

b. Glaucoma: *Propranolol* and other β-blockers, particularly *timolol* (see p. 76), are effective in diminishing intraocular pressure in glaucoma. This occurs by decreasing the secretion of aqueous humor by the ciliary body. Many patients with glaucoma have been maintained with these drugs for years. They neither affect the ability of the eye to focus for near vision, nor change pupil size, as do the cholinergic drugs. However, in an acute attack of glaucoma, *pilocarpine* (see p. 41) is still the drug of choice.The β-blockers are only used to treat this disease chronically.

c. Migraine: *Propranolol* is also effective in reducing migraine episodes (see p. 427). The value of the β-blockers is in the treatment of chronic migraine in which the drug decreases the incidence and severity of the attacks. The mechanism may depend on the blockade of catecholamine-induced vasodilation in the brain vasculature. [Note: During an attack, the usual therapy with *sumatripan* (see p. 427) or other drugs is used.]

d. Hyperthyroidism: *Propranolol* and other β-blockers are effective in blunting the widespread sympathetic stimulation that occurs in hyperthyroidism. In acute hyperthyroidism (thyroid storm), β-blockers may be lifesaving in protecting against serious cardiac arrhythmias.

e. Angina pectoris: *Propranolol* decreases the oxygen requirement of heart muscle and therefore is effective in reducing the chest pain on exertion that is common in angina (see p. 176). *Propranolol* is therefore useful in the chronic management of stable angina (not for acute treatment). Tolerance to moderate exercise is increased and this is noticeable by improvement in the electrocardiogram. However, treatment with *propranolol* does not allow strenuous physical exercise, such as tennis.

f. Myocardial infarction: *Propranolol* and other β-blockers have a protective effect on the myocardium. Thus, patients who have had one myocardial infarction appear to be protected against a second heart attack by prophylactic use of β-blockers. In addition, administration of a β-blocker immediately following a

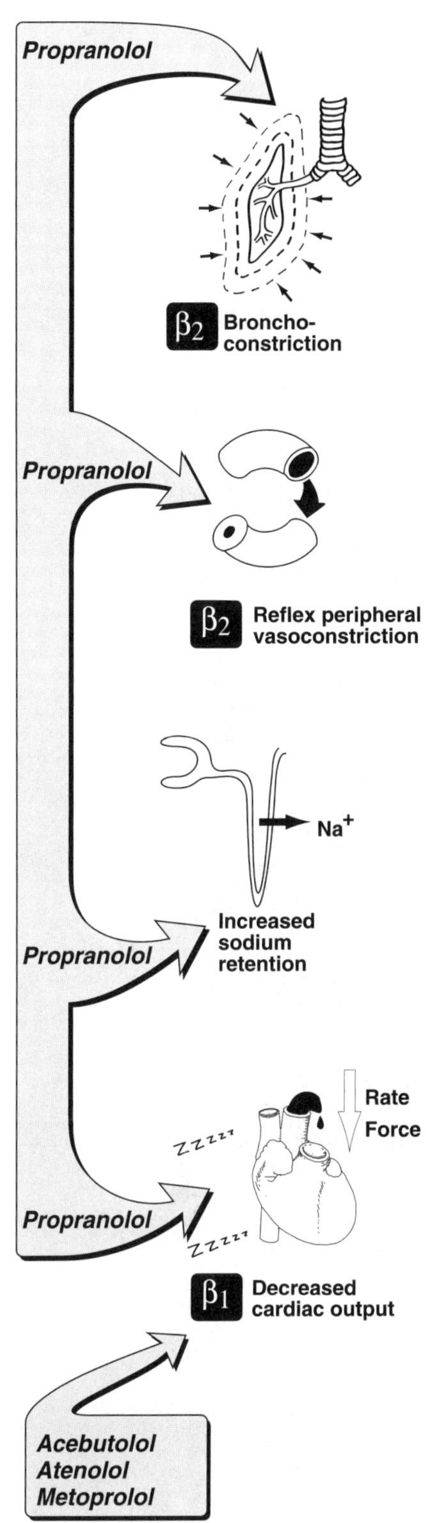

Figure 7.6
Actions of *propranolol* and other β_1 blockers.

myocardial infarction reduces infarct size and hastens recovery. The mechanism for these effects may be blocking of the actions of circulating catecholamines, which would increase the oxygen demand in an already ischemic heart muscle. *Propranolol* also reduces the incidence of sudden arrhythmic death after myocardial infarction (see p. 171).

3. Adverse effects:

a. Bronchoconstriction: *Propranolol* has a serious and potentially lethal side effect when administered to an asthmatic (Figure 7.7). An immediate contraction of the bronchiolar smooth muscle prevents air from entering the lungs. Deaths by asphyxiation have been reported for asthmatics who were inadvertently administered the drug. Therefore, *propranolol* must never be used in treating any individual with obstructive pulmonary disease.

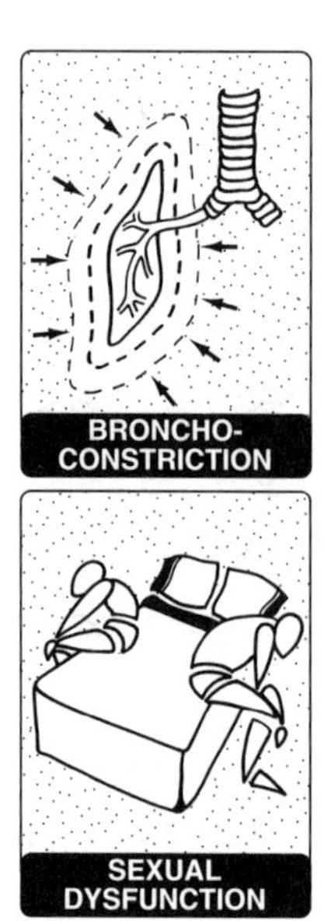

Figure 7.7
Adverse effects commonly observed in individuals treated with *propranolol.*

b. Arrhythmias: Treatment with the β-blockers must never be stopped quickly because of the risk of precipitating cardiac arrhythmias, which may be severe. The β-blockers must be tapered off gradually for 1 week. Long-term treatment with a β-antagonist leads to up-regulation of the β-receptor. On suspension of therapy, the increased receptors can worsen angina or hypertension.

c. Sexual impairment: Since sexual function in the male occurs through α-adrenergic activation, β-blockers do not affect normal ejaculation nor the internal bladder sphincter function. On the other hand, some men do complain of impaired sexual activity. The reasons for this are not clear and may be independent of β-receptor blockade.

d. Disturbances in metabolism: β Blockade leads to decreased glycogenolysis and decreased glucagon secretion. Fasting hypoglycemia may occur. [Note: Cardioselective β-blockers are preferred in treating *insulin*-dependent asthmatics. (see below).]

e. Drug interactions: Drugs that interfere with the metabolism of *propranolol*, such as *cimetidine* (see p. 236), *furosemide* (see p. 227), and *chlorpromazine* (see p. 127), may potentiate its antihypertensive effects. Conversely, those that stimulate its metabolism, such as barbiturates (see p. 94), *phenytoin* (see p. 146) and *rifampin* (see p. 333), can mitigate its effects.

B. Timolol and nadolol: nonselective β-antagonists

Timolol [TIM o lole] and *nadolol* [NAH doh lole] also block β_1 and β_2 adrenoceptors and are more potent than *propranolol. Nadolol* has a very long duration of action (see Figure 7.5). *Timolol* reduces the production of aqueous humor in the eye and is used topically in the treatment of chronic open-angle glaucoma, and occasionally for systemic treatment of hypertension.

C. Acebutolol, atenolol, metoprolol and esmolol: selective β1 antagonists

Drugs that preferentially block the β_1 receptors have been developed to eliminate the unwanted bronchoconstrictor effect (β_2) of *propranolol* seen among asthmatic patients. Cardioselective β-blockers, such as *acebutolol* [a se BYOO toe lole], *atenolol* [a TEN oh lole], and *metoprolol* [me TOE proe lole], antagonize β_1 receptors at doses 50 to 100 times less than those required to block β_2 receptors. This cardioselectivity is thus most pronounced at low doses and is lost at high drug doses. [Note: *Acebutolol* has some intrinsic agonist activity.]

1. **Actions:** These drugs lower blood pressure in hypertension and increase exercise tolerance in angina (see Figure 7.6). *Esmolol* [EZ moe lole] has a very short lifetime (see Figure 7.5) due to metabolism of an ester linkage. It is only given intravenously if required during surgery or diagnostic procedures (for example, cystoscopy). In contrast to *propranolol*, the cardiospecific blockers have relatively little effect on pulmonary function, peripheral resistance, and carbohydrate metabolism. Nevertheless, asthmatics treated with these agents must be carefully monitored to make certain that respiratory activity is not compromised.

2. **Therapeutic use in hypertension:** The cardioselective β-blockers are useful in hypertensive patients with impaired pulmonary function. Since these drugs have less effect on peripheral vascular β_2 receptors, coldness of extremities, a common side effect of β-blocker therapy, is less frequent. Cardioselective β-blockers are useful in diabetic hypertensive patients who are receiving *insulin* or oral hypoglycemic agents.

D. Pindolol and acebutolol: antagonists with partial agonist activity

1. **Actions:**

   a. **Cardiovascular:** *Acebutolol* and *pindolol* [PIN doe lole] are not pure blockers; instead they have the ability to weakly stimulate both β_1 and β_2 receptors (Figure 7.8) and are said to have intrinsic sympathomimetic activity (ISA). These partial agonists stimulate the β-receptor to which they are bound, yet they inhibit stimulation by the more potent endogenous catecholamines, *epinephrine* and *norepinephrine*. The result of these opposing actions is a much diminished effect on cardiac rate and cardiac output, compared to β-blockers without ISA.

   b. **Decreased metabolic effects:** Blockers with ISA minimize the disturbances of lipid and carbohydrate metabolism seen with other β-blockers.

2. **Therapeutic use in hypertension:** β-blockers with ISA are effective in hypertensive patients with moderate bradycardia, since a further decrease in heart rate is less pronounced with these drugs. Carbohydrate metabolism is less affected with *acebutolol* and *pindolol* than it is with *propranolol,* making them valuable in the treatment of diabetics.

A Agonists
(for example, *epinephrine*)

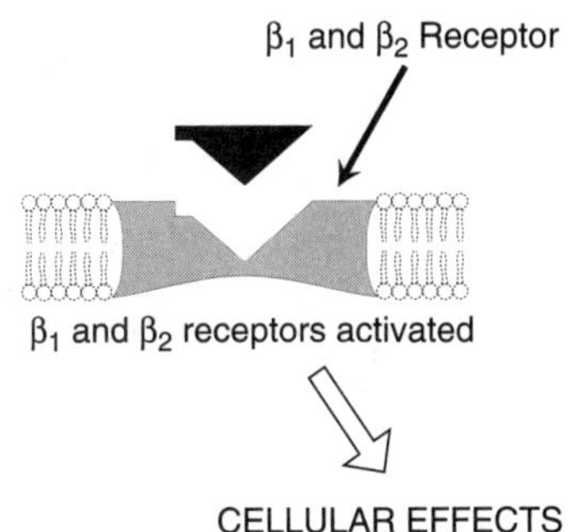
β1 and β2 Receptor
β1 and β2 receptors activated
CELLULAR EFFECTS

B Antagonists
(for example, *propranolol*)

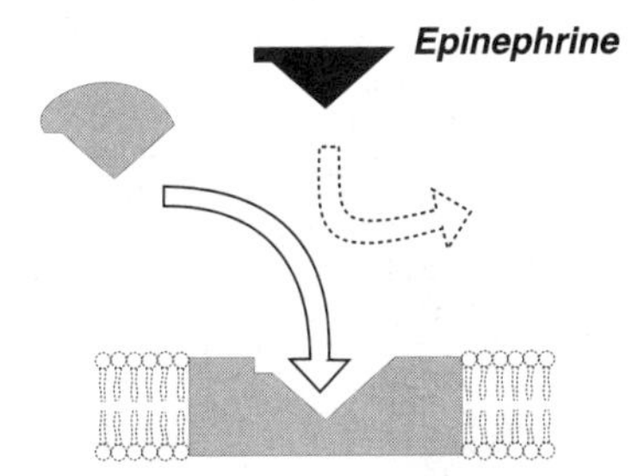
Epinephrine
β1 and β2 receptors blocked, but not activated

C Partial agonists
(for example, *pindolol* and *acebutolol*)

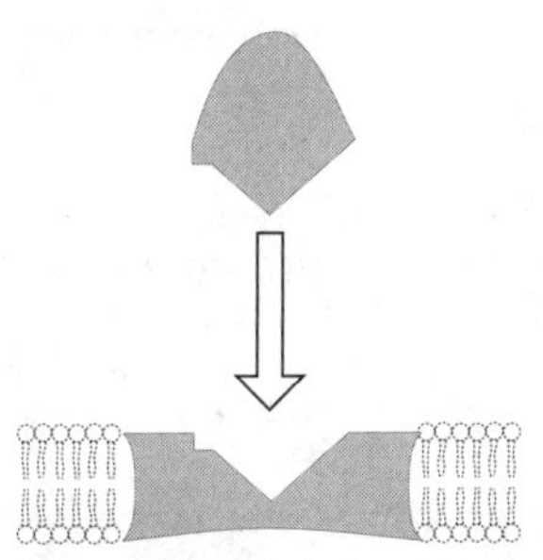
β1 and β2 receptors partially activated but unable to respond to more potent catecholamines
DECREASED CELLULAR EFFECTS

Figure 7.8
Comparison of agonists, antagonists, and partial agonists of β adrenoceptors.

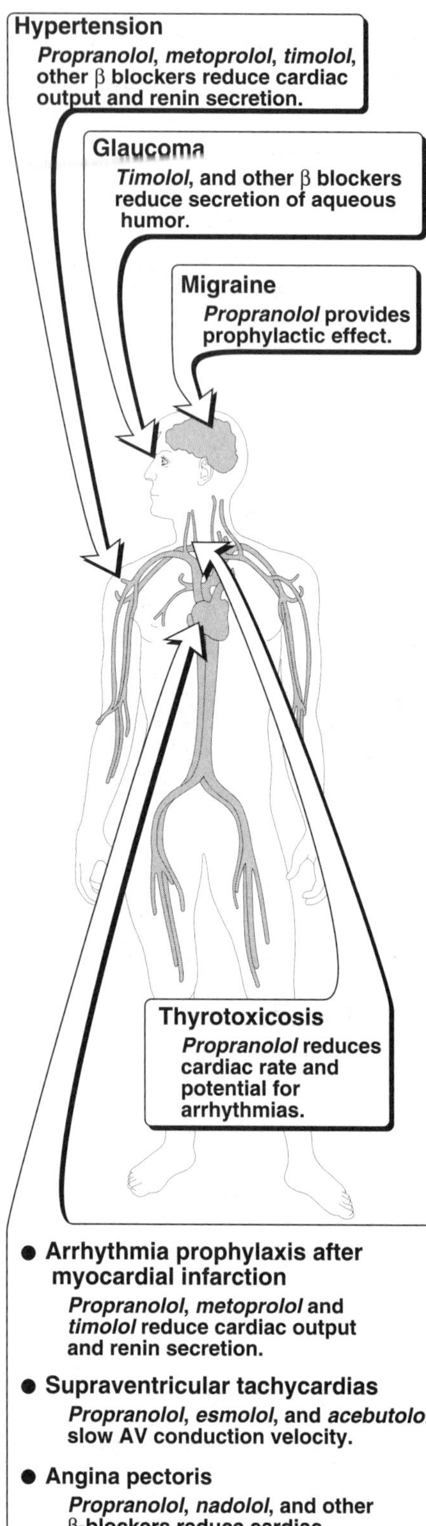

Hypertension
Propranolol, metoprolol, timolol, other β blockers reduce cardiac output and renin secretion.
Glaucoma
Timolol, and other β blockers reduce secretion of aqueous humor.
Migraine
Propranolol provides prophylactic effect.
Thyrotoxicosis
Propranolol reduces cardiac rate and potential for arrhythmias.
• Arrhythmia prophylaxis after myocardial infarction
Propranolol, metoprolol and timolol reduce cardiac output and renin secretion.
• Supraventricular tachycardias
Propranolol, esmolol, and acebutolol slow AV conduction velocity.
• Angina pectoris
Propranolol, nadolol, and other β-blockers reduce cardiac rate and force.

Figure 7.9
Some clinical applications of β-blockers.

E. Labetalol: an α and β-blocker

1. **Actions:** *Labetalol* [lay BET a lole] is a reversible β-blocker with concurrent α_1-blocking actions that produce peripheral vasodilation, thereby reducing blood pressure. *Labetalol* thus contrasts with the other β-blockers that produce peripheral vasoconstriction, and it is therefore useful in treating hypertensive patients for whom increased peripheral vascular resistance is undesirable. Labetalol does not alter serum lipid or blood glucose levels.

2. **Therapeutic use in hypertension:** *Labetalol* is useful for treating the elderly or black hypertensive patient in whom increased peripheral vascular resistance is undesirable. [Note: In general black hypertensive patients are not well controlled with β-blockers.] *Labetalol* may be employed as an alternative to *hydralazine* in the treatment of pregnancy-induced hypertension (PIH).

3. **Adverse affects:** Orthostatic hypotension and dizziness are associated with α_1 blockade. Figure 7.9 summarizes some of the indications for β-blockers.

IV. DRUGS AFFECTING NEUROTRANSMITTER RELEASE OR UPTAKE

As was noted on p. 68, some agonists, such as *amphetamine* and *tyramine*, do not act directly on the adrenoceptor. Instead, they exert their effects indirectly on the adrenergic neuron by causing the release of neurotransmitter from storage vesicles. Similarly, some agents act on the adrenergic neuron, to either interfere in neurotransmitter release or alter the uptake of the neurotransmitter into the adrenergic nerve.

A. Reserpine

Reserpine [re SER peen], a plant alkaloid, blocks the Mg^{++}/adenosine triphosphate (ATP)-dependent transport of biogenic amines, *norepinephrine*, *dopamine* and *serotonin*, from the cytoplasm into storage vesicles in the adrenergic nerves of all body tissues (see p. 57). This causes an ultimate depletion of *norepinephrine* levels in the adrenergic neuron, since monoamine oxidase can degrade the *norepinephrine* in the cytoplasm. Sympathetic function, in general, is impaired because of decreased release of *norepinephrine*. Hypertensive patients taking the drug show a gradual decline in blood pressure with a concomitant slowing of the cardiac rate. The drug has a slow onset of action and a long duration of action. When one stops taking the drug, the actions persist for many days.

B. Guanethidine

Guanethidine [gwahn ETH i deen] inhibits the response of the adrenergic nerve to stimulation or to indirectly-acting sympathomimetic amines. *Guanethidine* acts by blocking the release of stored *norepinephrine*. This results in a gradual lowering of blood pressure in hypertensives, and a decrease in cardiac rate. [Note:

There is also an accentuation of parasympathetic tone of the gastrointestinal tract.] *Guanethidine* also displaces *norepinephrine* from storage vesicles (thus producing a transient increase in blood pressure). This leads to gradual depletion of *norepinephrine* in nerve endings except those in the CNS. *Guanethidine* is now rarely used in the treatment of hypertension. *Guanethidine* commonly causes orthostatic hypotension and interferes with male sexual function. Supersensitivity to norepinephrine due to depletion of the amine can result in hypertensive crises in patients with pheochromocytoma. Due to supersensitivity patients taking cold preparations containing *phenylpropanolamine* also may have an exaggerated hypertensive response.

C. Cocaine

Cocaine [koe KANE] is unique among local anesthetics in having the ability to block the Na^+-K^+-activated ATPase (required for cellular uptake of norepinephrine) across the cell membrane of the adrenergic neuron. Consequently, norepinephrine accumulates in the synaptic space, resulting in enhancement of sympathetic activity and potentiation of the actions of epinephrine and norepinephrine. Therefore, small doses of the catecholamines produce greatly magnified effects in an individual taking *cocaine* as compared to one who is not. In addition, the duration of action of epinephrine and norepinephrine is increased. [Note: *Cocaine* as a CNS stimulant and drug of abuse is discussed on p. 101.]

Figure 7.10 summarizes the β-adrenergic antagonists.

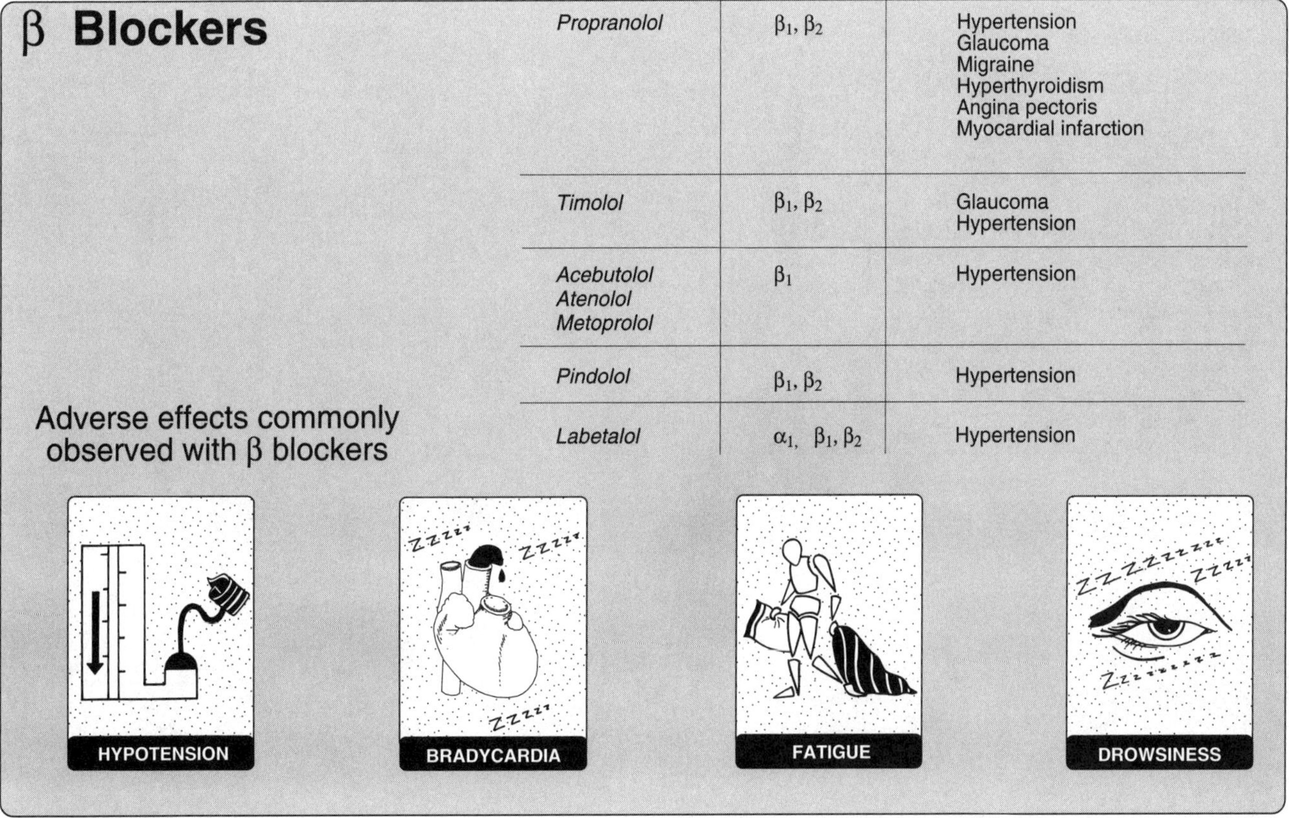

Propranolol	β_1, β_2	Hypertension Glaucoma Migraine Hyperthyroidism Angina pectoris Myocardial infarction
Timolol	β_1, β_2	Glaucoma Hypertension
Acebutolol *Atenolol* *Metoprolol*	β_1	Hypertension
Pindolol	β_1, β_2	Hypertension
Labetalol	α_1, β_1, β_2	Hypertension

Figure 7.10
Summary of β- adrenergic antagonists.

Choose the ONE best answer.

7.1 Systolic pressure is decreased after the injection of which of following drugs?

A. Phenylephrine
B. Dopamine
C. Ephedrine
D. Reserpine
E. Norepinephrine

Correct answer = D. Reserpine blocks the uptake of norepinephrine into intracellular storage vesicles, resulting in depletion of norepinephrine and gradual decline in blood pressure. Phenylephrine is a pure vasoconstrictor and raises systolic and diastolic blood pressures. Dopamine raises systolic and diastolic blood pressures by stimulating the heart and (at high doses) causing vasoconstriction. Ephedrine raises systolic and diastolic blood pressures by vasoconstriction and cardiac stimulation. Norepinephrine has a pressor effect.

7.2 Which one of the following drugs is useful in treating tachycardia?

A. Phenoxybenzamine
B. Isoproterenol
C. Phentolamine
D. Propranolol
E. Prazosin

Correct answer = D. Propranolol is a nonspecific β blocker that interferes with β_1 receptors on the heart, causing bradycardia, that is, a slowing of the heart rate. Phenoxybenzamine blocks α receptors and prevents vasoconstriction of peripheral blood vessels by endogenous catecholamines. This leads to a decrease in blood pressure and peripheral resistance, which causes a reflex tachycardia. Isoproterenol is a potent β agonist that promotes tachycardia. Phentolamine is an α blocker that causes hypotension, which may set off reflex tachycardia. Prazosin is not indicated for tachycardia.

7.3 A 60-year-old asthmatic man comes in for a check-up and complains that he is having some difficulty in "starting to urinate". Physical examination indicates that the man has a blood pressure of 160/100 mm Hg and a slightly enlarged prostate. Which of the following medications would be useful in treating both of these conditions?

A. Doxazosin
B. Labetalol
C. Phentolamine
D. Propranolol
E. Isoproterenol

The correct answer = A. Doxazosin is an competitive blocker at the α_1 receptor and lowers blood pressure. In addition it blocks the α receptors in the smooth muscle of the bladder neck and prostate to improve urine flow. Labetalol and propranolol, while effective for treating the hypertension, are contraindicated in an asthmatic. They would not improve urine flow. Phentolamine has too many adverse effects to be used as an hypertensive agent. Isoproterenol is a β agonist and is not employed as an hypertensive nor would it affect urinary function.

UNIT III: Drugs Affecting the Central Nervous System

Treatment of Parkinson's Disease

8

I. OVERVIEW OF CNS

Most drugs that affect the central nervous system (CNS) act by altering some step in the neurotransmission process. Drugs affecting the CNS may act presynaptically by influencing the production, storage, or termination of action of neurotransmitters. Other agents may activate or block postsynaptic receptors. This chapter provides an overview of the CNS with a focus on those neurotransmitters that are involved in the actions of the clinically useful CNS drugs. These concepts are useful in understanding the etiology of and the treatment strategies for Parkinson's disease—a disorder caused by the death of a group of brain cells whose actions are mediated by the neurotransmitter dopamine. Figure 8.1 shows the drugs used in the treatment of Parkinson's disease.

ANTIPARKINSON'S DRUGS

- *Amantadine*
- Antimuscarinic agents
- *Bromocriptine*
- *Carbidopa*
- *Deprenyl (Selegiline)*
- *Levodopa*
- *Pramipexole*[1]
- *Ropinirole*[1]
- *Tolcapone*[1]

Figure 8.1
Summary of agents used in the treatment of Parkinson's disease.
[1]Described in Pharmacology update, p. 443.

II. NEUROTRANSMISSION IN THE CNS

In many ways, the basic functioning of neurons in the CNS is similar to that of the autonomic nervous system described in Chapter 3. For example, transmission of information in the CNS and in the periphery both involve the release of neurotransmitters that diffuse across the synaptic space to bind to specific receptors on the postsynaptic neuron. In both systems, the recognition of the neurotransmitter by the membrane receptor of the postsynaptic neuron triggers intracellular changes (see p. 33). Several major differences exist between neurons in the peripheral autonomic nervous system and those of the CNS. The circuitry of the CNS is much more complex than the autonomic nervous

A Receptor empty (no agonists)

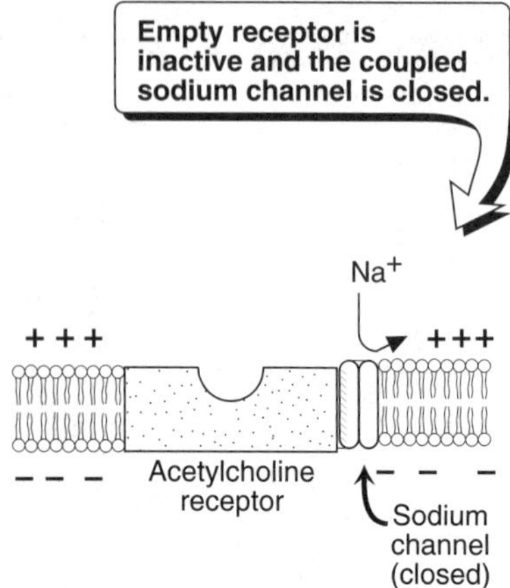
Empty receptor is inactive and the coupled sodium channel is closed.
Na+
+++
+++
– – –
– – –
Acetylcholine receptor
Sodium channel (closed)

B Receptor binding of excitatory neurotransmitter

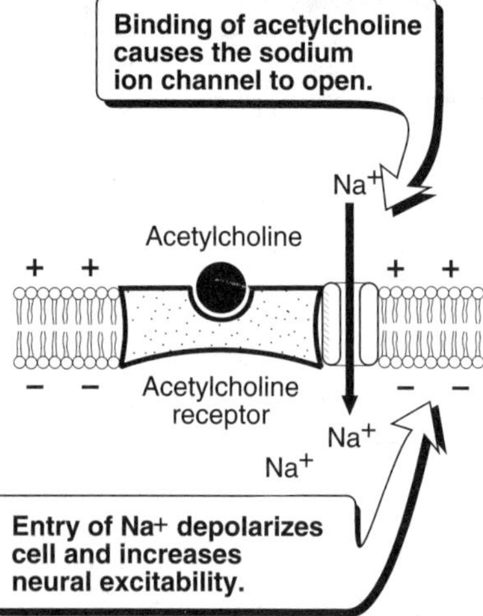
Binding of acetylcholine causes the sodium ion channel to open.
Na+
Acetylcholine
+ +
+ +
– –
– –
Acetylcholine receptor
Na+
Na+
Entry of Na+ depolarizes cell and increases neural excitability.

Figure 8.2
Binding of excitatory neurotransmitter, acetylcholine, causes depolarization of neuron.

system, and the number of synapses in the CNS is far greater. The CNS, unlike the peripheral autonomic nervous system, contains powerful networks of inhibitory neurons that are constantly active in modulating the rate of neuronal transmission. In addition, the CNS communicates through the use of more than 10 (and perhaps as many as 50) different neurotransmitters. In contrast, the autonomic system uses only two primary neurotransmitters, acetylcholine and norepinephrine.

III. SYNAPTIC POTENTIALS

In the CNS, receptors at most synapses are coupled to ion channels, that is, binding of the neurotransmitter to the postsynaptic membrane receptors results in a rapid but transient opening of ion channels. Open channels allow ions inside and outside the cell membrane to flow down their concentration gradients. The resulting change in the ionic composition across the membrane of the neuron alters the postsynaptic potential, producing either depolarization or hyperpolarization of the postsynaptic membrane, depending on the specific ions that move and the direction of their movement.

A. Excitatory pathways

Neurotransmitters can be classified as excitatory or inhibitory, depending on the nature of the action they elicit. Stimulation of excitatory neurons causes a movement of ions that results in a depolarization of the postsynaptic membrane. These excitatory postsynaptic potentials (EPSP) are generated by the following: (1) Stimulation of an excitatory neuron causes the release of neurotransmitter molecules, such as norepinephrine or acetylcholine, which bind to receptors on the postsynaptic cell membrane. This causes a transient increase in the permeability of sodium (Na^+) ions. (2) The influx of Na^+ causes a weak depolarization or excitatory postsynaptic potential (EPSP). (3) If the number of excitatory fibers stimulated increases, more excitatory neurotransmitter is released, finally causing the EPSP depolarization of the postsynaptic cell to pass a threshold, and an all-or-none action potential is generated. [Note: The generation of a nerve impulse typically reflects the activation of synaptic receptors by thousands of excitatory neurotransmitter molecules released from many nerve fibers.] (See Figure 8.2 for an example of an excitatory pathway.)

B. Inhibitory pathways

Stimulation of inhibitory neurons causes movement of ions that results in a hyperpolarization of the postsynaptic membrane. These inhibitory postsynaptic potentials (IPSP) are generated by the following: (1) Stimulation of inhibitory neurons releases neurotransmitter molecules, such as γ-aminobutyric acid (GABA) or glycine, which bind to receptors on the postsynaptic cell membrane. This causes a transient increase in the permeability of specific ions, such as, potassium and chloride ions. (2) The influx of chloride (Cl^-) and efflux of potassium (K^+) cause a weak hyperpolarization or inhibitory postsynaptic potential (IPSP) that moves the postsynaptic potential away from its firing threshold. This diminishes the generation of action potentials. (See Figure 8.3 for an example of an inhibitory pathway.)

C. Combined effects of the EPSP and IPSP

Most neurons in the CNS receive both EPSP and IPSP input. Thus, several different types of neurotransmitters may act on the same neuron, but each binds to its own specific receptor. The overall resultant action is due to the summation of the individual actions of the various neurotransmitters on the neuron. The neurotransmitters are not uniformly distributed in the CNS but are localized in specific clusters of neurons whose axons may synapse with specific regions of the brain. Many neuronal tracts thus seem to be chemically coded, and this may offer greater opportunity for selective modulation of certain neuronal pathways.

IV. OVERVIEW OF PARKINSON'S DISEASE

Parkinsonism is a progressive neurologic disorder of muscle movement, characterized by tremors, muscular rigidity, bradykinesia (slowness in initiating and carrying out voluntary movements), and postural and gait abnormalities. Parkinson's disease is the fourth most common neurologic disorder among the elderly, affecting 500,000 people in the United States alone. Most cases involve people over the age of 65 among whom the incidence is about 1:100 individuals.

A. Etiology

The cause of Parkinson's disease is unknown for most patients. The disease is correlated with a reduction in the activity of inhibitory dopaminergic neurons in the substantia nigra and corpus striatum—parts of the brain's basal ganglia system that are responsible for motor control. Genetic factors do not play a dominant role in the etiology of Parkinson's disease, although they may exert some influence on an individual's susceptibility to the disease. It appears increasingly likely that an unidentified environmental factor may play a role in the loss of dopaminergic neurons.

1. **Substantia nigra:** The substantia nigra, part of the extrapyramidal system, is the source of dopaminergic neurons that terminate in the striatum (Figure 8.4). Each dopaminergic neuron makes thousands of synaptic contacts within the striatum and therefore modulates the activity of a large number of cells. These dopaminergic projections from the substantia nigra fire tonically, rather than in response to specific muscular movements or sensory input. Thus, the dopaminergic system appears to serve as a tonic, sustaining influence on motor activity, rather than participating in specific movements.

2. **Striatum:** Normally, the striatum is connected to the substantia nigra by neurons that secrete the inhibitory transmitter GABA at their termini in the substantia nigra. In turn, cells of the substantia

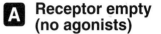

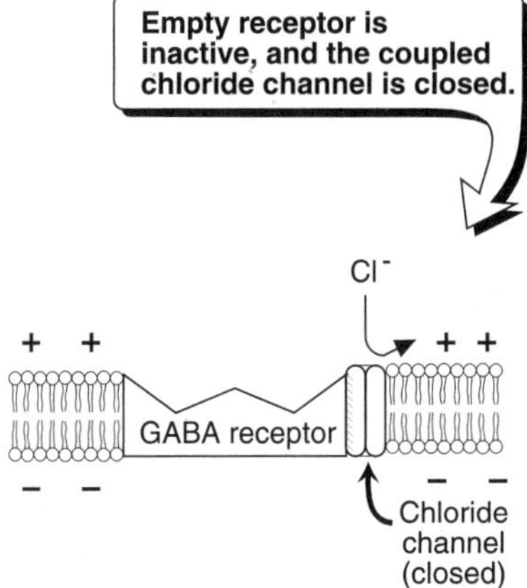

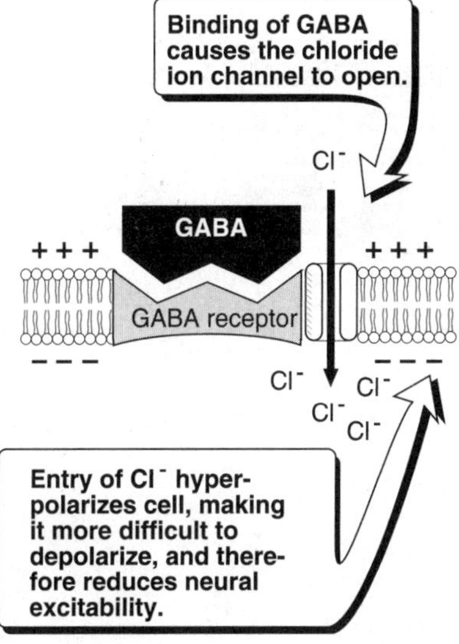

B Receptor binding of inhibitory neurotransmitter
Binding of GABA causes the chloride ion channel to open.
Cl⁻
GABA
+ + +
+ + +
Empty receptor is inactive, and the coupled chloride channel is closed.
GABA receptor
Chloride channel (closed)
– – –
– – –
Cl⁻
Cl⁻
Cl⁻
Cl⁻
Entry of Cl⁻ hyperpolarizes cell, making it more difficult to depolarize, and therefore reduces neural excitability.

Figure 8.3
Binding of inhibitory neurotransmitter, γ-aminobutyric acid (GABA), causes hyperpolarization of neuron.

nigra send neurons back to the striatum, secreting the inhibitory transmitter dopamine at their termini. This mutual inhibitory pathway normally maintains a degree of inhibition of the two separate areas. Nerve fibers from the cerebral cortex and thalamus secrete acetylcholine in the neostriatum, causing excitatory effects that initiate and regulate gross intentional movements of the body. In Parkinson's disease, destruction of cells in the substantia nigra results in the degeneration of neurons responsible for secreting dopamine in the neostriatum. Thus the normal modulating inhibitory influence of dopamine on the neostriatum is significantly diminished, resulting in the parkinsonian degeneration of the control of muscle movement (see Figure 8.4).

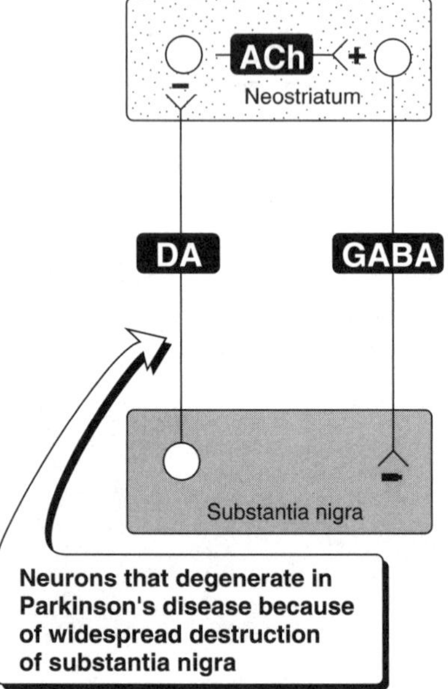
Sites of inhibition (-) or excitation (+) in the striatum and substantia nigra
ACh
+
-
Neostriatum
DA
GABA
Substantia nigra
-
Neurons that degenerate in Parkinson's disease because of widespread destruction of substantia nigra

Figure 8.4
Location of dopaminergic neurons deficient in Parkinson's disease. DA=dopamine; GABA= γ-aminobutyric acid; ACh=Acetylcholine.

3. **Secondary parkinsonism:** Parkinsonian symptoms infrequently follow viral encephalitis or multiple small vascular lesions. Drugs such as the phenothiazines and *haloperidol* (see p. 127), whose major pharmacologic action is blockade of dopamine receptors in the brain, may also produce parkinsonian symptoms. These drugs should not be used in parkinsonian patients.

B. Strategy of treatment

In addition to an abundance of inhibitory dopaminergic neurons, the neostriatum is also rich in excitatory cholinergic neurons that oppose the action of dopamine (see Figure 8.4). Many of the symptoms of parkinsonism reflect an imbalance between the excitatory cholinergic neurons and the greatly diminished number of inhibitory dopaminergic neurons. Therapy is aimed at restoring dopamine in the basal ganglia and antagonizing the excitatory effect of cholinergic neurons, thus reestablishing the correct dopamine/acetylcholine balance.

V. DRUGS USED IN PARKINSON'S DISEASE

Currently available drugs offer temporary relief from the symptoms of the disorder, but do not arrest or reverse the neuronal degeneration caused by the disease.

A. Levodopa (L-dopa) and carbidopa

Levodopa is a metabolic precursor of dopamine. It restores dopamine levels in the extrapyramidal centers (substantia nigra) that atrophy in parkinsonism. In patients with early disease, the number of residual dopaminergic neurons in the substantia nigra (typically about 20% of normal) is adequate for conversion of *levodopa* to dopamine. Thus, in new patients the therapeutic response to *levodopa* is consistent and the patient rarely complains that the drug effects "wear off." Unfortunately, with time the number of neurons decreases and there are fewer cells capable of taking up exogenously administered *levodopa* and converting it to dopamine for subsequent storage and release. Consequently motor control fluctuation develops. Relief provided by *levodopa* is only symptomatic and lasts only while the drug is present in the body.

1. **Mechanism of action**

a. **Levodopa:** Since parkinsonism results from insufficient dopamine in specific regions of the brain, attempts have been made to replenish the dopamine deficiency. Dopamine itself does not cross the blood-brain barrier, but its immediate precursor *levodopa* [lee voe DOE pa] is readily transported into the CNS and is converted to dopamine in the brain (Figure 8.5). Large doses of *levodopa* are required because much of the drug is decarboxylated to dopamine in the periphery (Figure 8.5), resulting in peripheral side effects (nausea, vomiting, cardiac arrhythmias, hypotension).

b. **Carbidopa:** The effects of *levodopa* on the CNS can be greatly enhanced by coadministering *carbidopa* [kar bi DOE pa], a dopamine decarboxylase inhibitor that does not cross the blood-brain barrier. *Carbidopa* diminishes the metabolism of *levodopa* in the GI tract and peripheral tissues; thus, it increases the availability of *levodopa* to the CNS. The addition of *carbidopa* lowers the dose of *levodopa* needed by 4- to 5-fold and, consequently, decreases the severity of the side effects of peripherally formed dopamine.

2. **Actions:** *Levodopa* decreases the rigidity, tremors, and other symptoms of parkinsonism.

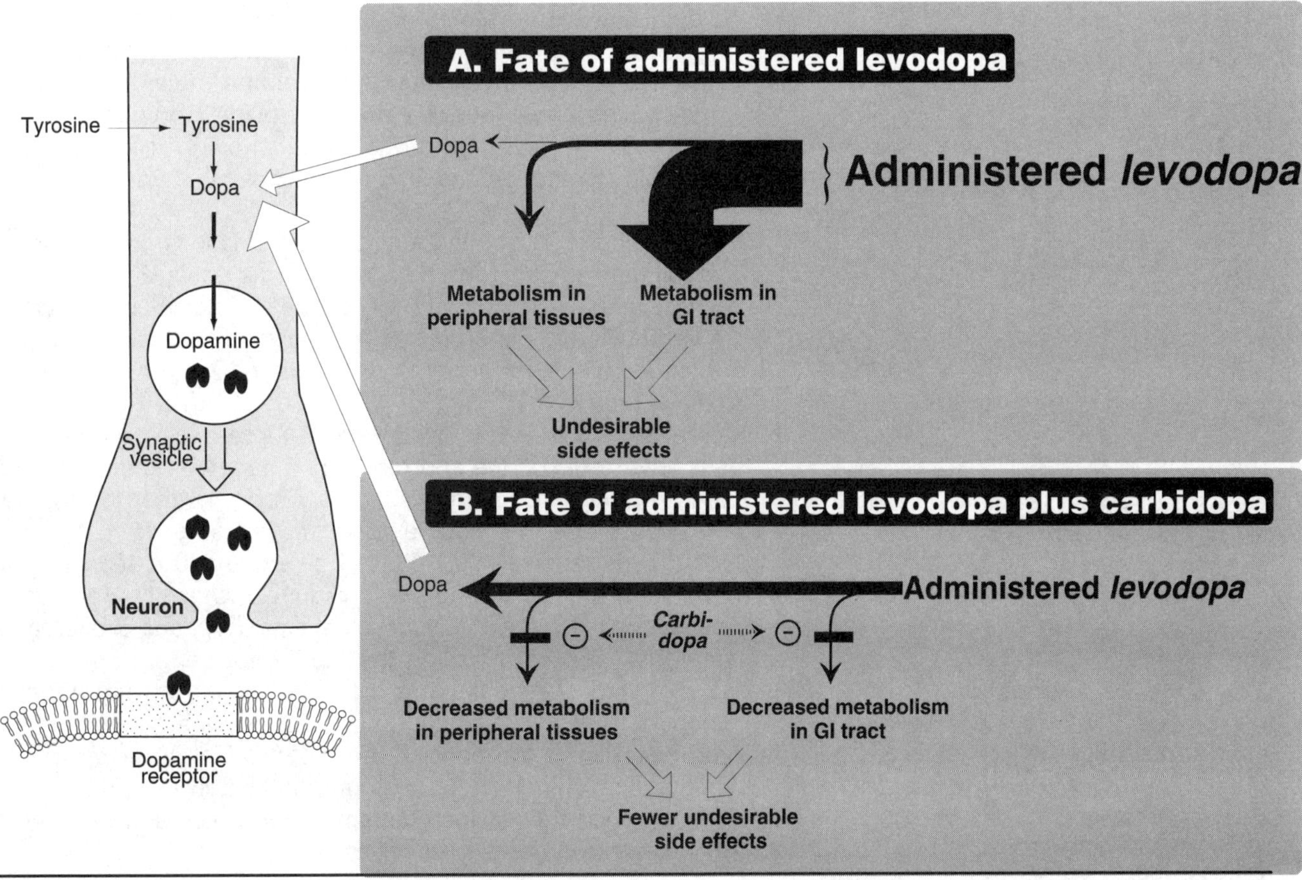

Figure 8.5
Synthesis of dopamine in the absence and presence of *carbidopa*, an inhibitor of dopamine decarboxylase in the peripheral tissues.

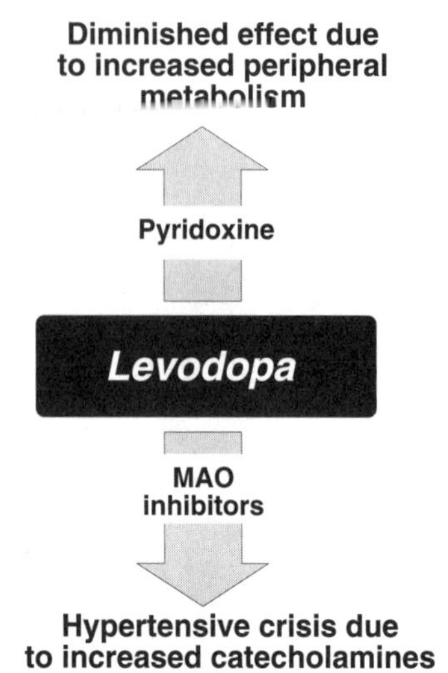

Figure 8.6
Some drug interactions observed with *levodopa.*

3. **Therapeutic uses:** *Levodopa* in combination with *carbidopa* is a potent and efficacious drug regimen currently available to treat Parkinson's disease. In approximately two thirds of patients with Parkinson's disease, *levodopa/carbidopa* treatment substantially reduces the severity of the disease for the first few years of treatment. Patients then typically experience a decline in response during the third to fifth year of therapy.

4. **Absorption and metabolism:** The drug is absorbed rapidly from the small intestine (when empty of food). *Levodopa* has an extremely short half-life (1 to 2 hours), which causes fluctuations in plasma concentration. This may produce fluctuations in motor response ("on-off" phenomenon), which may cause the patient to suddenly lose normal mobility and experience tremors, cramps, and immobility. Ingestion of meals, particularly if high in protein content, interferes with the transport of *levodopa* into the CNS. Large, neutral amino acids (for example, leucine and isoleucine) compete with *levodopa* for absorption from the gut and for transport across the blood-brain barrier. Thus *levodopa* should be taken on an empty stomach, typically 45 minutes before a meal. Withdrawal from the drug must be gradual.

5. **Adverse effects**

   a. **Peripheral effects:** Anorexia, nausea, and vomiting occur because of stimulation of the emetic center. Tachycardia and ventricular extrasystoles result from dopaminergic action on the heart. Hypotension may also develop. Adrenergic action on the iris causes mydriasis, and in some individuals, blood dyscrasias and a positive reaction to the Coombs' test are seen. Saliva and urine are a brownish color because of the melanin pigment produced from catecholamine oxidation.

   b. **CNS effects:** Visual and auditory hallucinations and abnormal involuntary movements (dyskinesia) may occur. These CNS effects are the opposite of parkinsonian symptoms and reflect the overactivity of dopamine at receptors in the basal ganglia. *Levodopa* can also cause mood changes, depression, and anxiety.

6. **Interactions:** The vitamin pyridoxine (B_6) increases the peripheral breakdown of *levodopa* and diminishes its effectiveness (Figure 8.6). Concomitant administration of *levodopa* and monoamine oxidase (MAO) inhibitors, such as *phenelzine* (see p. 124), can produce a hypertensive crisis caused by enhanced catecholamine production; therefore, caution is required when they are used simultaneously. In many psychotic patients, *levodopa* exacerbates symptoms, possibly through the buildup of central amines. In patients with glaucoma, the drug can cause an increase in intraocular pressure. Cardiac patients should be carefully monitored because of the possible development of cardiac arrhythmias. Antipsychotic drugs are contraindicated in parkinsonian patients, since these block dopamine receptors and produce a parkinsonian syndrome themselves.

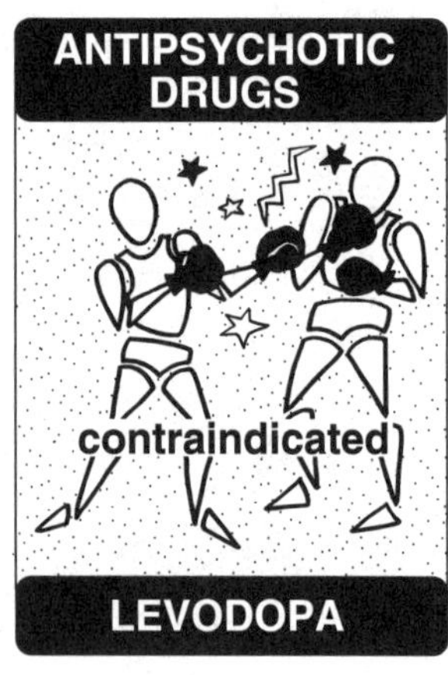

B. Bromocriptine

Bromocriptine [broh moh KRIP teen], an ergotamine (an alkaloid with vasoconstrictor action) derivative, is a dopamine receptor agonist. The drug produces little response in patients who do not react to *levodopa*, but it is often used with *levodopa* in patients responding to drug therapy. The dose is increased gradually during a period of 2 to 3 months. Side effects severely limit the utility of the dopamine agonists (Figure 8.7). The actions of *bromocriptine* are similar to those of *levodopa*, except that hallucinations, confusion, delirium, nausea, and orthostatic hypotension are more common, whereas dyskinesia is less prominent. In psychiatric illness, *bromocriptine* causes the mental condition to worsen. Serious cardiac problems may develop, particularly in patients with a history of myocardial infarction. In patients with peripheral vascular disease, a worsening of the vasospasm occurs, and in patients with peptic ulcer, there is a worsening of the ulcer.

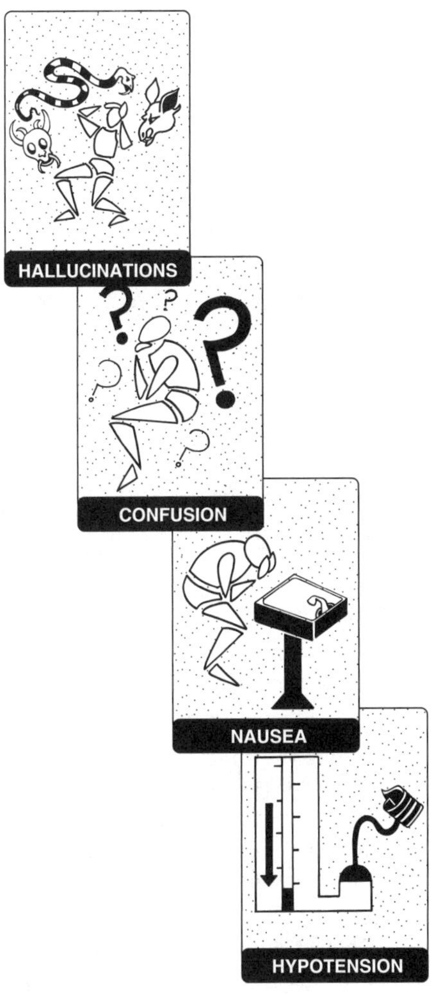

Figure 8.7
Some adverse effects of *bromocriptine*.

C. Amantadine

It was accidentally discovered that the antiviral drug, *amantadine* [a MAN ta deen], effective in the treatment of influenza (see p. 363), has antiparkinsonism action. It appears to enhance the synthesis, release, or re-uptake of dopamine from the surviving neurons. [Note: If dopamine release is already at a maximum, *amantadine* has no effect.] The drug may cause restlessness, agitation, confusion, and hallucinations, and at high doses it may induce acute toxic psychosis. Orthostatic hypotension, urinary retention, peripheral edema, and dry mouth also may occur. *Amantadine* is less efficacious than *levodopa* and tolerance develops more readily, but it has fewer side effects. The drug has little effect on tremor but is more effective than the anticholinergics against rigidity and bradykinesia.

D. Deprenyl

Deprenyl [DE pren ill], also called *selegiline* [se LE ge leen] selectively inhibits monoamine oxidase B (which metabolizes dopamine), but does not inhibit monoamine oxidase A (which metabolizes norepinephrine and serotonin). By thus decreasing the metabolism of dopamine, *deprenyl* has been found to increase dopamine levels in the brain (Figure 8.8). Therefore, it enhances the actions of *levodopa*, and when these drugs are administered together, *deprenyl* substantially reduces the required dose of *levodopa*. Unlike nonselective MAO inhbitors, *deprenyl* at recommended doses has little potential for causing hypertensive crises. However, if *deprenyl* is administered at high doses, the selectivity of the drug is lost and the patient is at risk for severe hypertension. Recent data suggest that early use of *deprenyl* may actually prolong the period before severe symptoms set in by as much as 50%, possibly by reducing the formation of free radicals.

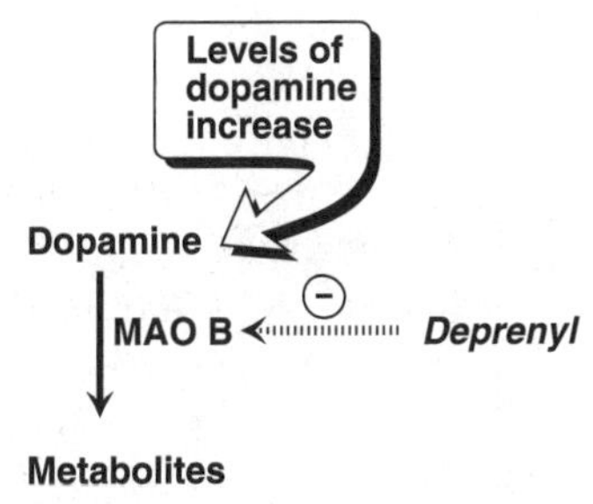

Figure 8.8
Action of *deprenyl* in dopamine metabolism.

E. Antimuscarinic agents

The antimuscarinic agents are much less efficacious than *levodopa* and play only an adjuvant role in antiparkinsonism therapy. The actions of *benztropine*, *trihexyphenidyl*, and *biperiden* are similar, although individual patients may respond more favorably to one drug. All these drugs can induce mood changes and produce xerostomia (dryness of the mouth) and visual problems, as do all muscarinic blockers. They interfere with gastrointestinal peristalsis and cannot be used in patients with glaucoma, prostatic hypertrophy, or pyloric stenosis. Blockage of cholinergic transmission produces effects similar to augmentation of dopaminergic transmission (again, because of the creation of an imbalance in the dopamine/acetylcholine ratio). Adverse effects are similar to those caused by high doses of *atropine* (see p. 45), for example, pupillary dilation, confusion, hallucination, urinary retention, and dry mouth.

See pp. 443-444 for a description of the newly approved drugs, *pramipexol*, *ropinirole* and *tolcapone*.

Study Questions

Choose the ONE best answer.

8.1 Which one of the following statements is correct?

A. Chlorpromazine is indicated in treating the nausea of levodopa treatment.

B. Vitamin B_6 increases the effectiveness of levodopa.

C. Administration of dopamine is an effective treatment of Parkinson's disease.

D. Levodopa-induced nausea is reduced by carbidopa.

E. Nonspecific MAO-inhibitors, such as phenelzine, are a useful adjunct to levodopa therapy.

> Correct answer = D. Carbidopa inhibits the peripheral decarboxylation of levodopa, permitting lower dosage. Chlorpromazine blocks the dopamine receptor site in the brain and therefore blocks the beneficial effects of levodopa. Vitamin B_6 enhances the peripheral decarboxylation of levodopa. Dopamine does not itself cross the blood-brain barrier. Phenelzine inhibits the metabolism of norepinephrine and serotonin and may produce a hypertensive crisis.

8.2 Which one of the following statements is INCORRECT?

A. Parkinsonian patients are characterized by an increased ratio of dopaminergic/cholinergic activity in the neostriatum.

B. Overtreatment of Parkinson's disease can result in the symptoms of psychosis.

C. Diets rich in protein may decrease the effects of levodopa.

D. Dyskinesia is the most important side effect of levodopa.

E. Treatment with deprenyl can delay the onset of parkinsonian symptoms.

> Correct choice = A. Parkinsonian patients show a deficiency of dopaminergic neurons, without a decrease in cholinergic actions. Elevated levels of dopamine can lead to behavorial disorders. Levodopa and large, neutral amino acids share a transport system that is needed to enter the brain; thus high protein diets may lead to elevated levels of circulating amino acids, resulting in a decrease in levodopa uptake. Dyskinesia is usually seen with longer-term therapy and is dose-related and reversible. The mechanism of action of deprenyl is not understood.

8.3 All of the following statements are correct EXCEPT:

A. Atropine blocks the cholinergic pathway in the neostriatum.

B. Deprenyl inhibits monoamine oxidase B and increases dopamine levels in the brain.

C. Bromocriptine directly activates dopaminergic receptors.

D. Amantadine inhibits the metabolism of levodopa.

E. Antimuscarinic agents are generally less efficacious then levodopa in the treatment of Parkinson's disease.

> Correct choice = D. The mechanism of action in parkinsonism of amantadine is unclear. It does not affect the metabolism of levodopa. The other statements are true.

Anxiolytic and Hypnotic Drugs

9

I. OVERVIEW

Anxiety is an unpleasant state of tension, apprehension, or uneasiness—a fear that seems to arise from an unknown source. Disorders involving anxiety are the most common mental disturbances. The symptoms of severe anxiety are similar to those of fear (such as, tachycardia, sweating, trembling, palpitations) and involve sympathetic activation. Episodes of mild anxiety are common life experiences and do not warrant treatment. However, the symptoms of severe, chronic, debilitating anxiety may be treated with antianxiety drugs (sometimes called anxiolytic or minor tranquilizers), and/or some form of psycho- or behavioral therapy. Since all of the antianxiety drugs also cause some sedation, the same drugs often function clinically as both anxiolytic and hypnotic (sleep-inducing) agents. Figure 9.1 summarizes the anxiolytic and hypnotic agents.

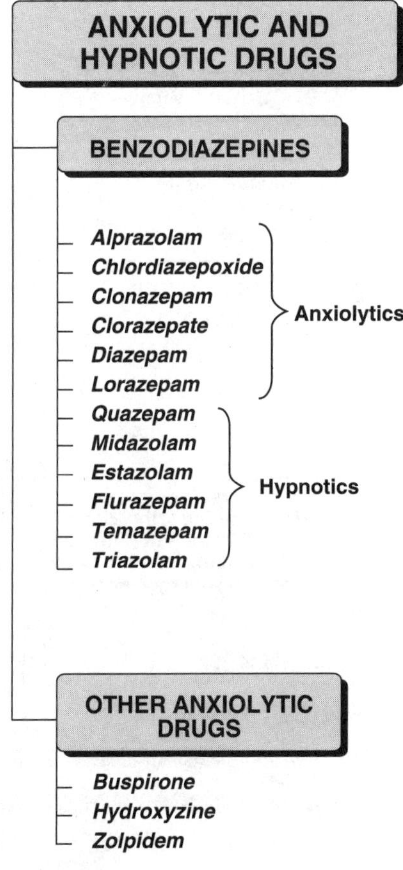

Figure 9.1
Summary of anxiolytic and hypnotic drugs.
(Figure continues on next page.)

II. BENZODIAZEPINES

Benzodiazepines are the most widely used anxiolytic drugs. They have largely replaced barbiturates and *meprobamate* in the treatment of anxiety, since the benzodiazepines are more effective and safer (Figure 9.2). Approximately 20 benzodiazepine derivatives are currently available.

A. Mode of action

Binding of γ-aminobutyric acid (GABA) to its receptor on the cell membrane triggers an opening of a chloride channel, which leads to an increase in chloride conductance (Figure 9.3). The influx of chloride ions causes a small hyperpolarization that moves the postsynaptic potential away from its firing threshold and thus inhibits the formation of action potentials (see p. 82). Benzodiazepines bind to specific, high affinity sites on the cell membrane, which are separate from but adjacent to the receptor for GABA. The benzodiazepine receptors are found only in the central nervous system (CNS), and their location parallels that of the GABA neurons. The binding of benzodiazepines enhances the affinity of GABA receptors for this neurotransmitter, resulting in a more frequent opening of adjacent chloride channels (see Figure 9.3). This in turn results in enhanced hyperpolarization and further inhibition of neuronal firing. [Note:

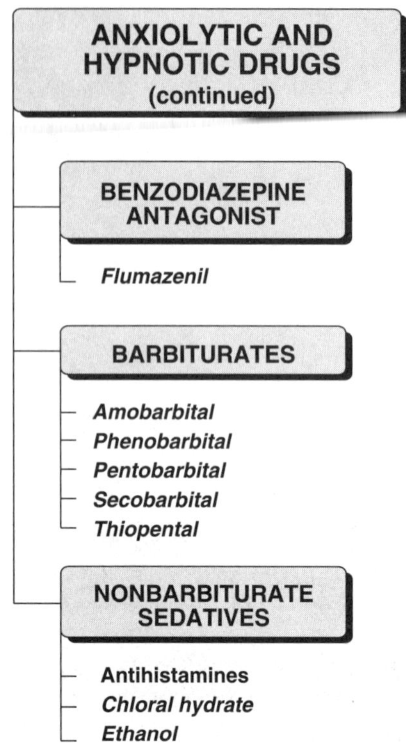

Figure 9.1 (continued)
Summary of anxiolytic and hypnotic drugs.

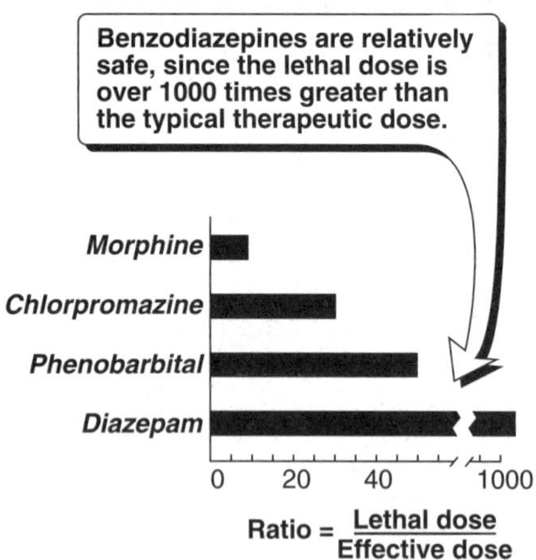

Figure 9.2
Ratio of lethal dose to effective dose for *morphine* (an opioid, Chapter 14), *chlorpromazine* (a neuroleptic, Chapter 13), and the anxiolytic, hypnotic drugs, *phenobarbital* and *diazepam*.

Benzodiazepines and GABA mutually increase the affinity of their binding sites without actually changing the total number of sites.] The clinical effects of the various benzodiazepines correlate well with each drug's binding affinity for the GABA receptor-chloride ion channel complex.

B. Actions

The benzodiazepines have no antipsychotic activity, nor any analgesic action and do not affect the autonomic nervous system. All of the benzodiazepines exhibit the following actions to a greater or lesser extent:

1. **Reduction of anxiety:** At low doses, the benzodiazepines are anxiolytic. They are thought to reduce anxiety by selectively inhibiting neuronal circuits in the limbic system of the brain.

2. **Sedative and hypnotic actions:** All of the benzodiazepines used to treat anxiety have some sedative properties. At higher doses, certain benzodiazepines produce hypnosis (artificially-produced sleep).

3. **Anticonvulsant:** Several of the benzodiazepines have anticonvulsant activity and are used to treat epilepsy and other seizure disorders.

4. **Muscle relaxant:** The benzodiazepines relax the spasticity of skeletal muscle, probably by increasing presynaptic inhibition in the spinal cord.

C. Therapeutic uses

The individual benzodiazepines show small differences in their relative anxiolytic, anticonvulsant, and sedative properties. However, the duration of action varies widely among this group, and pharmacokinetic considerations are often important in choice of drug.

1. **Anxiety disorders:** The benzodiazepines are useful in treating the anxiety that accompanies some forms of depression and schizophrenia. These drugs should not be used to alleviate the normal stress of everyday life, but should be reserved for continued severe anxiety, and then should only be used for short periods of time because of addiction potential. The longer acting agents such as *diazepam* [dye AZ e pam], are often preferred in those patients with anxiety that may require treatment for prolonged periods of time. The antianxiety effects of the benzodiazepines are less subject to tolerance than the sedative and hypnotic effects. For panic disorders, *alprazolam* [al PRAY zoe lam] is effective for short- and long-term treatment, although it may cause withdrawal reactions in about 30% of sufferers.

2. **Muscular disorders:** *Diazepam* is useful in the treatment of skeletal muscle spasms such as occur in muscle strain, and in treating spasticity from degenerative disorders, such as multiple sclerosis and cerebral palsy.

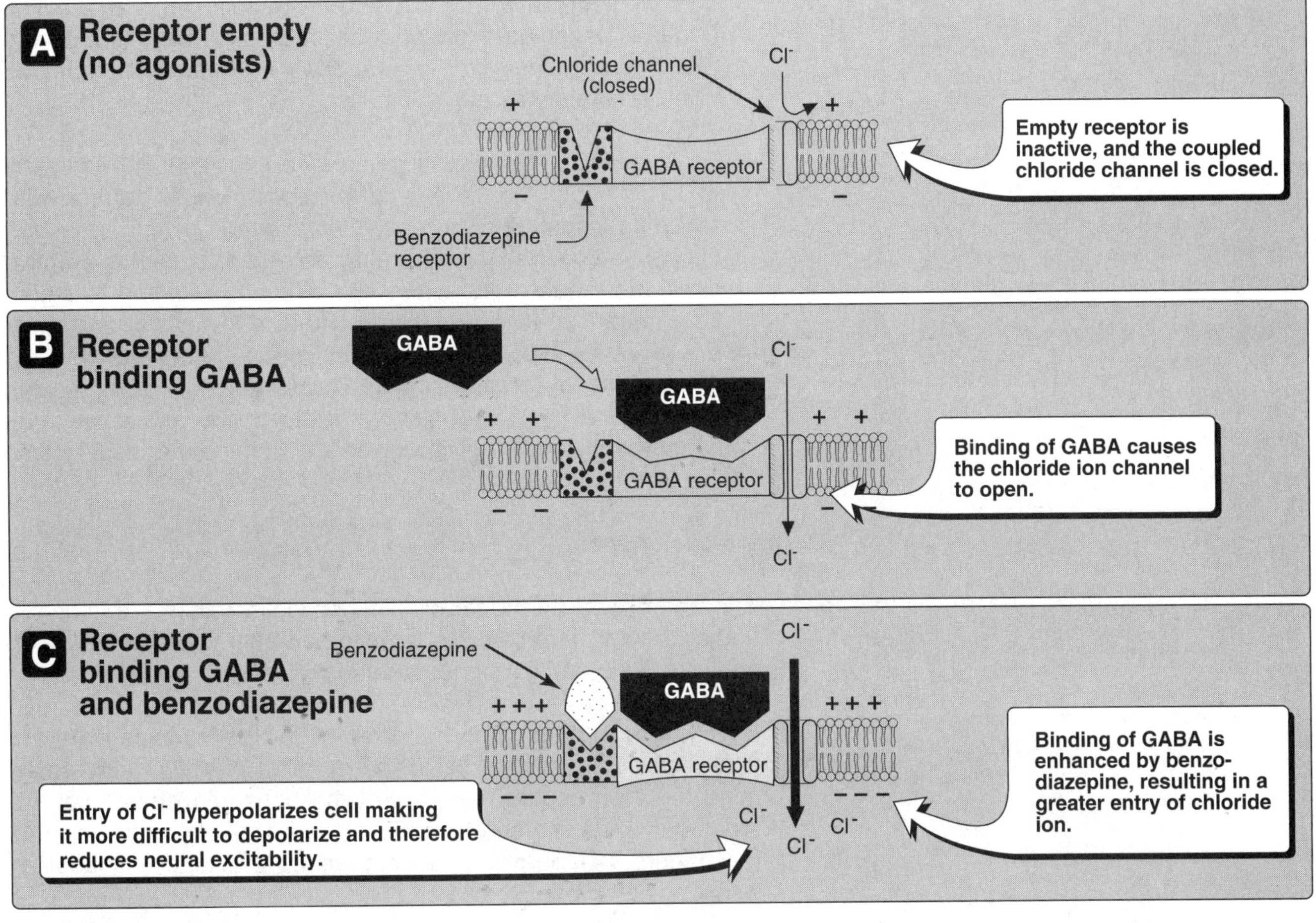
A Receptor empty (no agonists)
Chloride channel (closed)
Cl-
GABA receptor
Benzodiazepine receptor
Empty receptor is inactive, and the coupled chloride channel is closed.
B Receptor binding GABA
GABA
GABA receptor
Cl-
Binding of GABA causes the chloride ion channel to open.
C Receptor binding GABA and benzodiazepine
Benzodiazepine
GABA
GABA receptor
Cl-
Binding of GABA is enhanced by benzodiazepine, resulting in a greater entry of chloride ion.
Entry of Cl- hyperpolarizes cell making it more difficult to depolarize and therefore reduces neural excitability.

Figure 9.3
Schematic diagram of benzodiazepine-GABA-chloride ion channel complex. GABA= γ-aminobutyric acid.

3. **Seizures:** *Clonazepam* [kloe NA ze pam] is useful in the chronic treatment of epilepsy, whereas *diazepam* is the drug of choice in terminating grand mal epileptic seizures and status epilepticus (see p. 149). *Chlordiazepoxide* [klor di az e POX ide], *clorazepate* [klor AZ e pate], *diazepam*, and *oxazepam* [ox A ze pam] are useful in the acute treatment of alcohol withdrawal.

4. **Sleep disorders:** Not all of the benzodiazepines are useful as hypnotic agents, although all have sedative or calming effects. The three most commonly prescribed benzodiazepines for sleep disorders are long-acting *flurazepam* [flure AZ e pam], intermediate-acting *temazepam* [tem AZ e pam] and short-acting *triazolam* [trye AY zoe lam].

   a. **Flurazepam:** This long-acting benzodiazepine significantly reduces both sleep-induction time and the number of awakenings, and increases the duration of sleep. *Flurazepam* has a long-acting effect (Figure 9.4) and causes little rebound insomnia. With continued use, the drug has been shown to maintain its effectiveness for up to 4 weeks. *Flurazepam* and its active metabolites have a half-life of appoximately 85 hours, which may result in daytime sedation and accumulation of the drug.

b. **Temazepam:** This drug is useful in patients who experience frequent wakening. However, the peak sedative effect occurs two to three hours after an oral dose, and therefore it may be given several hours before bedtime.

c. **Triazolam:** This benzodiazepine has a relatively short duration of action and is therefore used to induce sleep in patients with recurring insomnia. Whereas *temazepam* is useful for insomnia caused by the inability to stay asleep, *triazolam* is effective in treating individuals who have difficulty in going to sleep. Tolerance frequently develops within a few days, and withdrawal of the drug often results in rebound insomnia, leading the patient to demand another prescription. Therefore, this drug is best used intermittently rather than daily. In general, hypnotics should be given for only a limited time, usually less than 2 to 4 weeks.

DURATION OF ACTION OF BENZODIAZEPINES

Long-acting

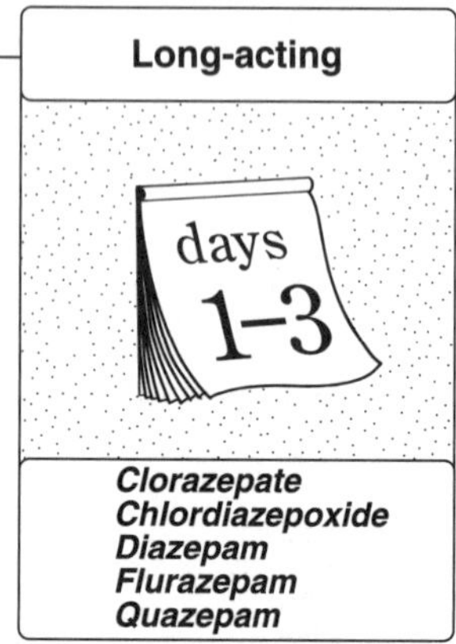

Clorazepate
Chlordiazepoxide
Diazepam
Flurazepam
Quazepam

Intermediate-acting

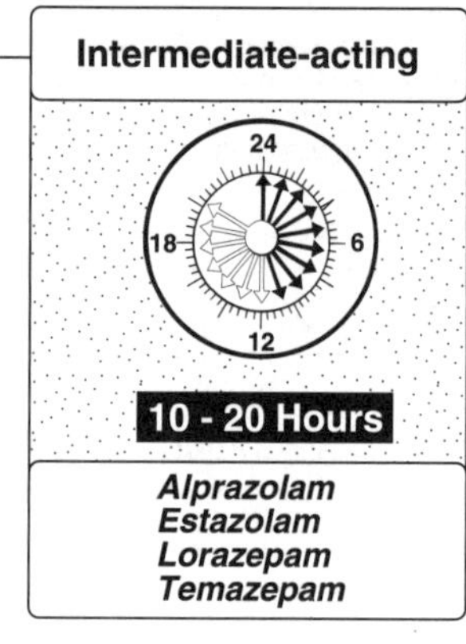

Alprazolam
Estazolam
Lorazepam
Temazepam

Short-acting

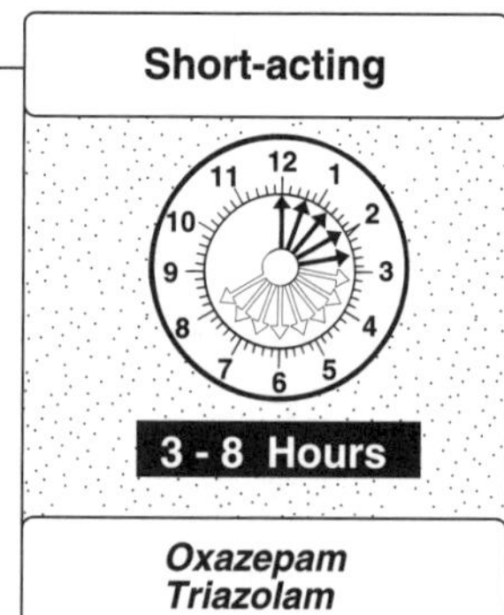

Oxazepam
Triazolam

Figure 9.4
Comparison of the durations of action of the benzodiazepines.

D. Pharmacokinetics

1. **Absorption and distribution:** The benzodiazepines are lipophilic and are rapidly and completely absorbed after oral administration and are distributed throughout the body.

2. **Duration of actions:** The half-lives of the benzodiazepines are very important clinically, since the duration of action may determine the therapeutic usefulness. The benzodiazepines can be roughly divided into short-, intermediate- and long-acting groups (see Figure 9.4). The longer acting agents form active metabolites with long half-lives.

3. **Fate:** Most benzodiazepines, including *chlordiazepoxide* and *diazepam*, are metabolized by the hepatic microsomal metabolizing system (see p. 14) to compounds that are also active. For these benzodiazepines, the apparent half-life of the drug represents the combined actions of the parent drug and its metabolites. The benzodiazepines are excreted in urine as glucuronides or oxidized metabolites.

E. Dependence

Psychological and physical dependence on benzodiazepines can develop if high doses of the drug are given over a prolonged period. Abrupt discontinuation of the benzodiazepines results in withdrawal symptoms, including confusion, anxiety, agitation, restlessness, insomnia, and tension. Because of the long half-lives of some of the benzodiazepines, withdrawal symptoms may not occur until a number of days after discontinuation of therapy. Benzodiazepines with a short elimination half-life, such as *triazolam*, induce more abrupt and severe withdrawal reactions than those seen with drugs that are slowly eliminated, such as *flurazepam* (Figure 9.5).

F. Adverse effects

1. **Drowsiness and confusion:** These effects are the two most common side effects of the benzodiazepines. Ataxia occurs at high

doses and precludes activities that require fine motor coordination, such as driving an automobile. Cognitive impairment (decreased long-term recall and acquisition of new knowledge) can occur with use of benzodiazepines. *Triazolam*, the benzodiazepine with the most rapid elimination, often shows a rapid development of tolerance, early morning insomnia and daytime anxiety, along with amnesia and confusion.

2. **Precautions:** Use benzodiazepines cautiously in treating patients with liver disease. They potentiate alcohol and other CNS depressants. Benzodiazepines are, however, considerably less dangerous than other anxiolytic and hypnotic drugs. As a result, a drug overdose is seldom lethal, unless other central depressants, such as alcohol, are taken concurrently.

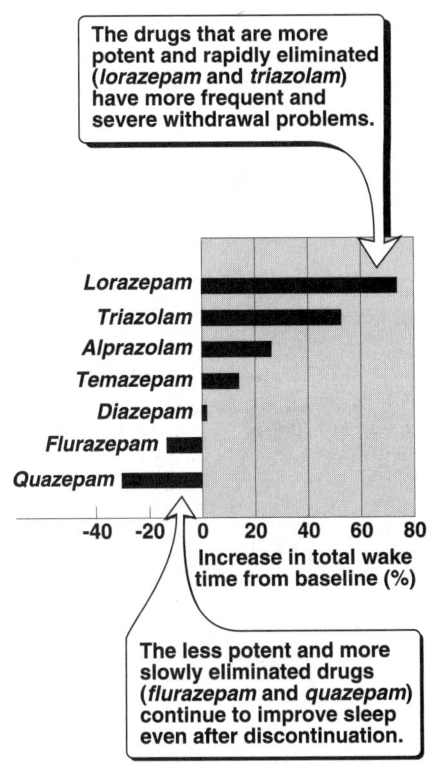

The drugs that are more potent and rapidly eliminated (*lorazepam* and *triazolam*) have more frequent and severe withdrawal problems.
Lorazepam
Triazolam
Alprazolam
Temazepam
Diazepam
Flurazepam
Quazepam
-40 -20 0 20 40 60 80
Increase in total wake time from baseline (%)
The less potent and more slowly eliminated drugs (*flurazepam* and *quazepam*) continue to improve sleep even after discontinuation.

Figure 9.5
Frequency of rebound insomnia resulting from discontinuation of benzodiazepine therapy.

III. OTHER ANXIOLYTIC AND HYPNOTIC AGENTS

A. Zolpidem

Although the hypnotic *zolpidem* [ZOL pih dem] is not a benzodiazepine, it acts on a subset of the benzodiazepine receptor family. *Zolpidem* has no anticonvulsant or muscle relaxing properties. It shows no withdrawal effects, exhibits minimal rebound insomnia and little or no tolerance occurs with prolonged use. *Zolpidem* is rapidly absorbed from the gastrointestinal tract, and has a rapid onset of action and short elimination half-life (about 3 hours). Adverse effects of *zolpidem* include nightmares, agitation, headache, gastrointestinal upset, dizziness, and daytime drowsiness. Although *zolpidem* potentially has advantages over the benzodiazepines, clinical experience with the drug is still limited.

B. Buspirone

Buspirone [byoo SPYE rone] is useful in the treatment of generalized anxiety disorders and has an efficacy comparable to the benzodiazepines. The actions of *buspirone* appear to be mediated by serotonin (5-HT_{1A}) receptors, although other receptors could be involved, since *buspirone* displays some affinity for DA_2 dopamine receptors and 5-HT_2 serotonin receptors. The mode of action thus differs from that of the benzodiazepines. Further, *buspirone* lacks anticonvulsant and muscle-relaxant properties of the benzodiazepines and causes only minimal sedation. The frequency of adverse effects is low, the most common effects being headaches, dizziness, nervousness, and lightheadness. Sedation and psychomotor and cognitive dysfunction are minimal, and dependence is unlikely. *Buspirone* has the disadvantage of a slow onset of action. Figure 9.6 compares some of the common adverse effects of *buspirone* and the benzodiazepine, *alprazolam.*

C. Hydroxyzine

Hydroxyzine [hye DROX i zeen] is an antihistamine with antiemetic activity. It has a low tendency for habituation; thus it is useful for patients with anxiety, who have a history of drug abuse. It is also often used for sedation prior to dental procedures or surgery.

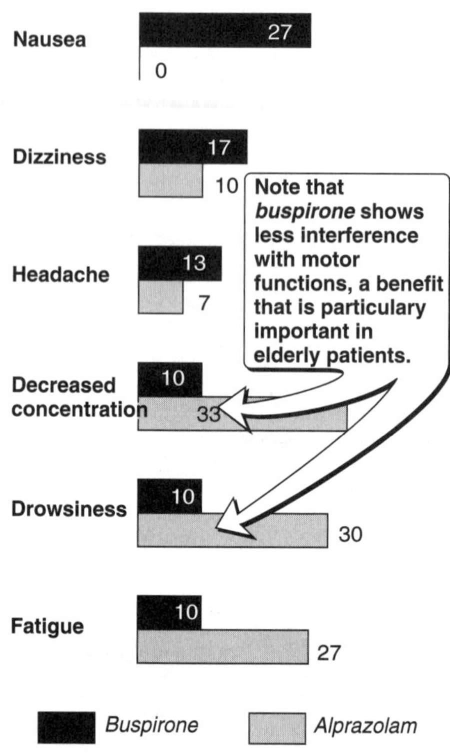

Figure 9.6
Comparison of common adverse effects of *buspirone* and *alprazolam*. Results are expressed as percent of patients showing each symptom.

IV. BENZODIAZEPINE ANTAGONIST

Flumazenil [floo MAZ eh nill] is a GABA receptor antagonist that can rapidly reverse the effects of benzodiazepines. The drug is available by IV administration only. Onset is rapid but duration is short, with a half-life of about one hour. Frequent administration may be necessary to maintain reversal of a long-acting benzodiazepine. Administration of *flumazenil* may precipitate withdrawal in dependent patients or may cause seizures if a benzodiazepine is used to control seizure activity. Dizziness, nausea, vomiting, and agitation are the most common side effects.

V. BARBITURATES

The barbiturates were formerly the mainstay of treatment used to sedate the patient or to induce and maintain sleep. Today, they have been largely replaced by the benzodiazepines, mainly because barbiturates induce tolerance, drug-metabolizing enzymes, physical dependence, and very severe withdrawal symptoms. Foremost is their ability to cause coma in toxic doses. Certain barbiturates, such as the very short-acting *thiopental*, are still used to induce anesthesia (see p. 115).

A. Mode of action

Barbiturates are thought to interfere with sodium and potassium transport across cell membranes. This leads to inhibition of the mesencephalic reticular activating system. Polysynaptic transmission is inhibited in all areas of the CNS. Barbiturates also potentiate GABA action on chloride entry into the neuron, although they do not bind at the benzodiazepine receptor.

B. Actions

Barbiturates are classified according to their duration of action (Figure 9.7). For example, *thiopental* [thye oh PEN tal], which acts within seconds and has a duration of action of about 30 minutes, is used in the intravenous induction of anesthesia. By contrast, *phenobarbital* [fee noe BAR bi tal], which has a duration of action greater than a day, is useful in the treatment of seizures (see p. 148). *Pentobarbital* [pen toe BAR bi tal], *secobarbital* [see koe BAR bi tal] and *amobarbital* [am oh BAR bi tal] are short-acting barbiturates, which are effective as sedative and hypnotic (but not antianxiety) agents.

1. **Depression of CNS:** At low doses, the barbiturates produce sedation (calming effect, reducing excitement). At higher doses, the drugs cause hypnosis, followed by anesthesia (loss of feeling or sensation), and finally coma and death. Thus, any degree of depression of the CNS is possible, depending on the dose. Barbiturates do not raise the pain threshold and have no analgesic properties. They may even exacerbate pain.

2. **Respiratory depression:** Barbiturates suppress the hypoxic and chemoreceptor response to CO_2, and overdosage is followed by respiratory depression and death.

3. **Enzyme induction:** Barbiturates induce P-450 microsomal enzymes in the liver (see p. 14). Therefore, chronic barbiturate administration diminishes the action of many drugs that are dependent on P-450 metabolism to reduce their concentration.

C. Therapeutic uses

1. **Anesthesia:** Selection of a barbiturate is strongly influenced by the desired duration of action. The ultra-short-acting barbiturates, such as *thiopental*, are used intravenously to induce anesthesia.

2. **Anticonvulsant:** *Phenobarbital* is used in long-term management of tonic-clonic seizures, status epilepticus, and eclampsia. *Phenobarbital* has been regarded as the drug of choice for treatment of young children with recurrent febrile seizures. However, *phenobarbital* can depress cognitive performance in children, and the drug should be used cautiously. *Phenobarbital* has specific anticonvulsant activity that is distinguished from the nonspecific CNS depression.

3. **Anxiety:** Barbiturates have been used as mild sedatives to relieve anxiety, nervous tension, and insomnia. Most have been replaced by the benzodiazepines.

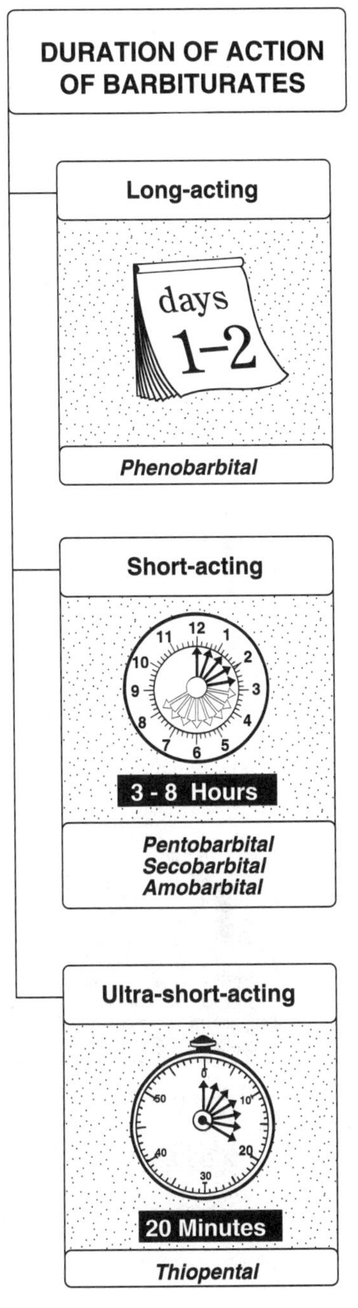

Figure 9.7
Barbiturates classified according to their duration of actions.

D. Pharmacokinetics

Barbiturates are absorbed orally and distributed widely throughout the body. All barbiturates redistribute in the body from the brain to the splanchnic areas, to skeletal muscle, and finally to adipose tissue. This movement is important in causing the short duration of action of *thiopental* and similar short-acting derivatives (see p. 115). Barbiturates are metabolized in the liver, and inactive metabolites are excreted in the urine.

E. Adverse effects

1. **CNS:** Barbiturates cause drowsiness, impaired concentration, and mental and physical sluggishness.

2. **Drug hangover:** Hypnotic doses of barbiturates produce a feeling of tiredness well after the patient awakes. This drug hangover leads to impaired ability to function normally for many hours after waking. Occasionally, nausea and dizziness occur.

3. **Precautions:** As noted previously, barbiturates induce the P-450 system and therefore may decrease the effect of drugs that are metabolized by these hepatic enzymes. Barbiturates increase porphyrin synthesis, and are contraindicated in patients with acute intermittent porphyria.

4. **Addiction:** Abrupt withdrawal from barbiturates may cause tremors, anxiety, weakness, restlessness, nausea and vomiting, seizures, delirium, and cardiac arrest. Withdrawal is much more severe than that associated with opiates and can result in death.

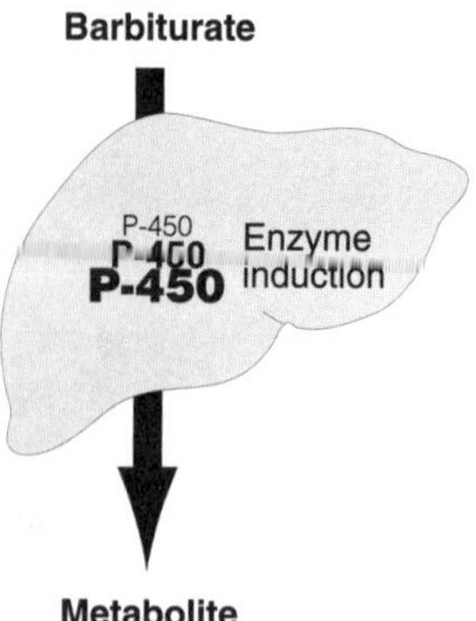

5. **Poisoning:** Barbiturate poisoning has been a leading cause of death among drug overdoses for many decades. Severe depression of respiration is coupled with central cardiovascular depression, and results in a shock-like condition with shallow, infrequent breathing. Treatment includes artificial respiration and purging the stomach of its contents if the drug has been recently taken. Hemodialysis may be necessary if large quantities have been taken. Alkalinization of the urine often aids in the elimination of *phenobarbital* (see p. 24).

VI. NONBARBITURATE SEDATIVES

A. Chloral hydrate

Chloral hydrate [KLOR al HYE drate] is a trichlorinated derivative of acetaldehyde that is converted to trichloroethanol in the body. The drug is an effective sedative and hypnotic that induces sleep in about 30 minutes and lasts about 6 hours. *Chloral hydrate* is irritating to the gastrointestinal tract and causes epigastric distress. It also produces an unusual, unpleasant taste sensation.

B. Antihistamines

Nonprescription antihistamines with sedating properties, such as *diphenhydramine* and *doxylamine* (see p. 422), are effective in treating mild types of insomnia. However, these drugs are usually ineffective for all but the milder form of situational insomnia. Further, they have numerous undesirable side effects that make them less useful than the benzodiazepines. These sedative antihistamines are marketed in numerous over-the-counter products.

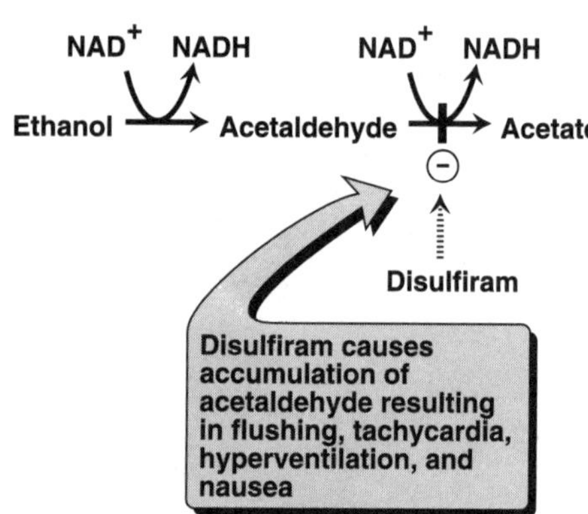

Figure 9.8
Metabolism of ethanol.

C. Ethanol

Ethanol (ethyl alcohol) has antianxiety and sedative effects, but its toxic potential outweighs its benefits. *Ethanol* [ETH an ol] is a CNS depressant, producing sedation and ultimately hypnosis with increasing dosage. *Ethanol* has a shallow dose-response curve; therefore, sedation occurs over a wide dosage range. Alcohol synergizes with many other sedative agents and can produce severe CNS depression with antihistamines or barbiturates.

1. **Disulfiram:** *Ethanol* is metabolized primarily in the liver, first to acetaldehyde by alcohol dehydrogenase, and then to acetate by aldehyde dehydrogenase. *Disulfiram* [dye SUL fi ram] blocks the oxidation of acetaldehyde to acetic acid by inhibiting aldehyde dehydrogenase (Figure 9.8). This results in the accumulation of acetaldehyde in the blood, causing flushing, tachycardia, hyperventilation, and nausea. *Disulfiram* has found some use in the patient seriously desiring to stop alcohol ingestion. A conditioned avoidance response is induced so that the patient abstains from alcohol to prevent the unpleasant effects of *disulfiram*-induced acetaldehyde accumulation.

Figure 9.9 summarizes the therapeutic disadvantages and advantages of some of the anxiolytic and hypnotic drugs.

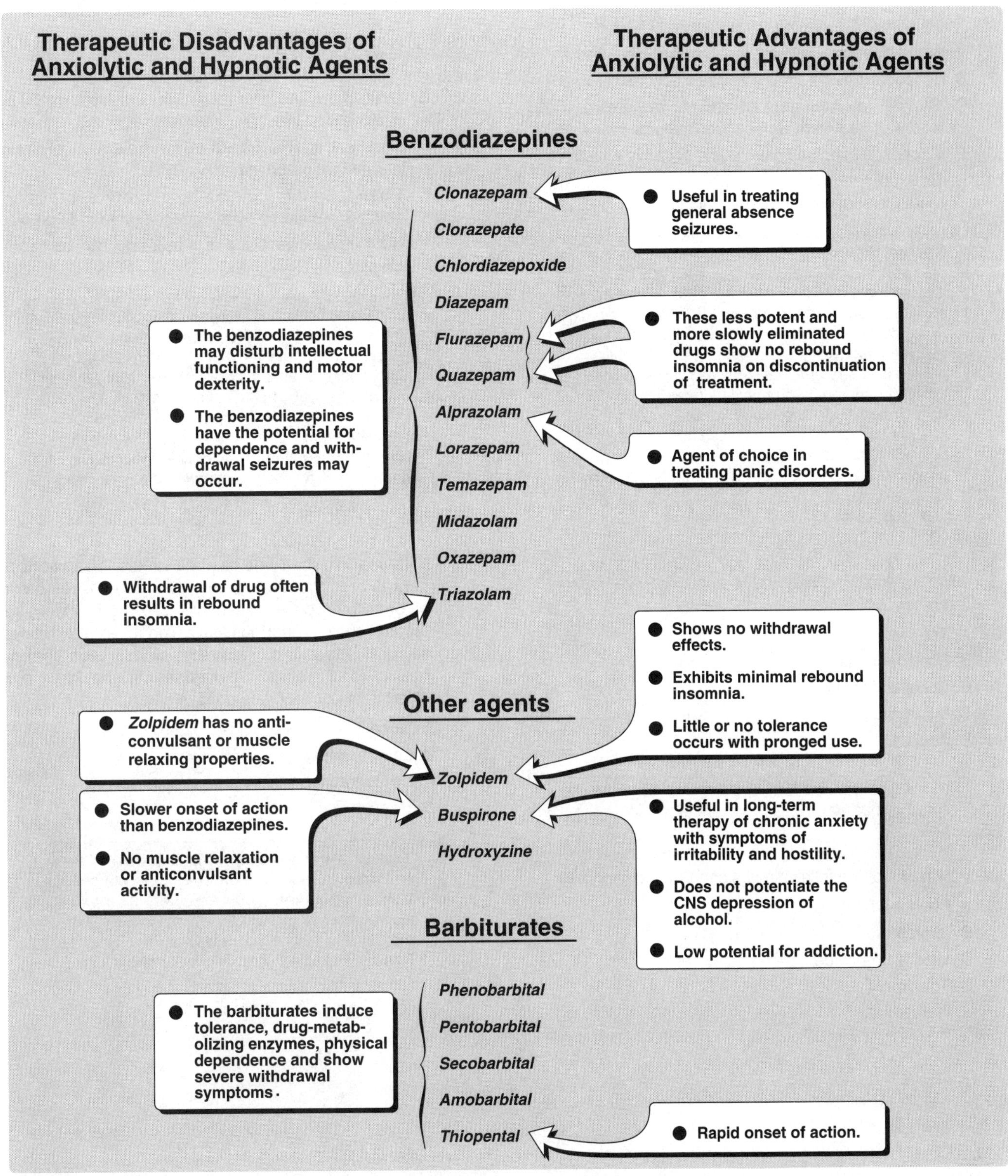

Figure 9.9
Therapeutic disadvantages and advantages of some anxiolytic and hypnotic agents.

Choose the ONE best answer.

9.1 Which one of the following statements is CORRECT?

A. Benzodiazepines directly open chloride channels.

B. Benzodiazepines show analgesic actions.

C. Clinical improvement of anxiety requires 2 to 4 weeks of treatment with benzodiazepines.

D. All benzodiazepines have some sedative effects.

E. Benzodiazepines, like other CNS depressants, readily produce general anesthesia.

Correct answer = D. Although all benzodiazepines can cause sedation, the drugs labeled "benzodiazepine hypnotics" in Figure 9.1 are promoted for the treatment of sleep disorder. Benzodiazepines enhance the binding of GABA to its receptor, which increases the permeability of chloride. The benzodiazepines do not relieve pain but may reduce the anxiety associated with pain. Unlike the tricyclic antidpressants and the MAO-inhibitors, the benzodiazepines are effective within hours of administration. Benzodiazepines do not produce general anesthesia and are, therefore, relatively safe drugs with a high therapeutic index.

9.2 All of the following respond to treatment with benzodiazepines EXCEPT:

A. Tetanus.

B. Schizophrenia.

C. Epileptic seizure.

D. Insomnia.

E. Anxiety.

Correct choice = B. Benzodiazepines have no antipsychotic activity.

9.3 Which one of the following is a short-acting hypnotic?

A. Phenobarbital

B. Diazepam

C. Chlordiazepoxide

D. Thiopental

E. Flurazepam

Correct answer = D. Thiopental is an ultra-short-acting drug used as an adjuvant to anesthesia.

9.4 Which one of the following statements is CORRECT?

A. Phenobarbital shows analgesic properties.

D. Diazepam and phenobarbital induce the P-450 enzyme system.

C. Phenobarbital is useful in the treatment of acute intermittent porphyria.

D. Phenobarbital induces respiratory depression, which is enhanced by the consumption of ethanol.

E. Buspirone has actions similar to the benzodiazepines.

Correct answer = D. Barbiturates and ethanol are a potentially lethal combination. Phenobarbital is unable to alter the pain threshold. Only phenobarbital strongly induces the synthesis of the hepatic cytochrome P-450 drug metabolizing system. Phenobarbital is contraindicated in the treatment of acute intermittent porphyria. Buspirone lacks the anticonvulsant and muscle-relaxant properties of the benzodiazepines and causes only minimal sedation.

9.5 A 45-year-old man who has been injured in a car accident is brought into the emergency room. His blood alcohol level on admission is 275 mg/dL. Hospital records show a prior hospitalization for alcohol related seizures. His wife confirms that he has been drinking heavily for 3 weeks. What treatment should be provided to the patient if he goes into withdrawal?

A. None

B. Lorazepam

C. Pentobarbital

D. Phenytoin

The correct answer = B. It is important to treat the seizures associated with alcohol withdrawal. Benzodiazepines, such as chlordiazepoxide, diazepam or or the shorter-acting lorazepam, are effective in controlling this problem. They are less sedating than pentobarbital or phenytoin.

CNS Stimulants

10

I. OVERVIEW

This chapter describes two groups of drugs that act primarily to stimulate the central nervous system (CNS) (Figure 10.1). The first group, the psychomotor stimulants, cause excitement and euphoria, decrease feelings of fatigue, and increase motor activity. The second group, psychotomimetic drugs or hallucinogens, produce profound changes in thought patterns and mood, with little effect on the brainstem and spinal cord. As a group, the CNS stimulants have few clinical uses, but they are important as drugs of abuse, along with the CNS depressants described in Chapter 9, and the narcotics described in Chapter 14 (Figure 10.2).

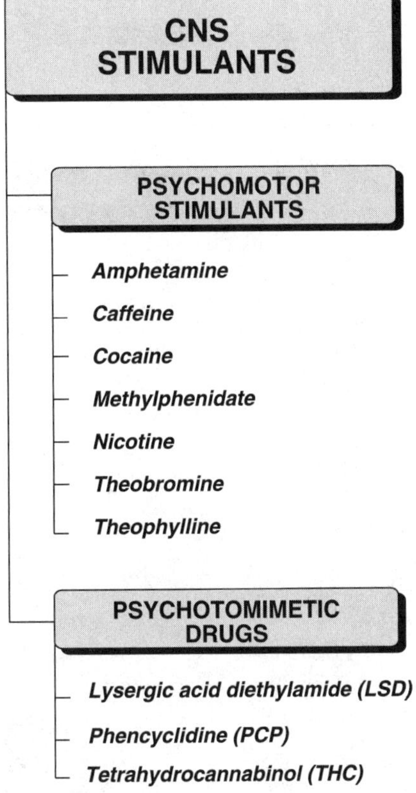

Figure 10.1
Summary of CNS stimulants.

II. PSYCHOMOTOR STIMULANTS

A. Methylxanthines

Methylxanthines include *theophylline* [thee OFF i lin] found in tea, *theobromine* [thee o BRO min] found in cocoa, and *caffeine* [kaf EEN]. *Caffeine*, the most widely consumed stimulant in the world, is found in highest concentration in coffee but is also present in tea, cola drinks, chocolate candy, and cocoa.

1. **Mechanism of action:** The methylxanthines may act by several mechanisms, including translocation of extracellular calcium, increase in cyclic adenosine monophosphate (cAMP) and cyclic guanosine monophosphate (cGMP) caused by inhibition of phosphodiesterase, and blockade of adenosine receptors.

2. **Actions:**

   a. **Central nervous system:** The *caffeine* contained in one to two cups of coffee (100 to 200 mg) causes a decrease in fatigue and increased mental alertness as a result of stimulating the cortex and other areas of the brain. Consumption of 1.5 grams of *caffeine* (12 to 15 cups of coffee) produces anxiety and tremors. The spinal cord is stimulated only by very high doses (2 to 5 g) of *caffeine*.

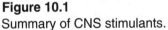

Lippincott's Illustrated Reviews: Pharmacology, Second Edition.
by Mary J. Mycek, Richard A. Harvey and Pamela C. Champe.
Lippincott Williams & Wilkins, Philadelphia, PA © 2000.

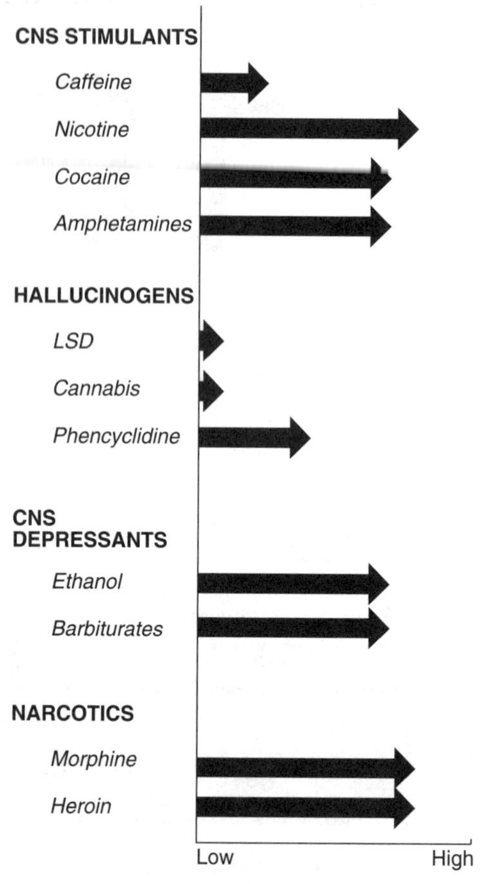

Figure 10.2
Relative potential for dependence for commonly abused substances.

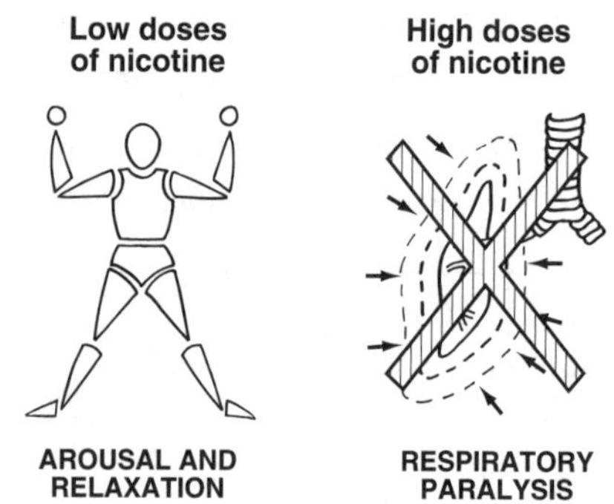

Figure 10.3
Actions of nicotine on the central nervous system.

b. **Cardiovascular system:** A high dose of *caffeine* has positive inotropic and chronotropic effects on the heart. [Note: Increased contractility can be harmful to patients with angina pectoris. Accelerated heart rate can trigger premature ventricular contractions in others.]

c. **Diuretic action:** *Caffeine* has a mild diuretic action that increases urinary output of sodium, chloride, and potassium.

d. **Gastric mucosa:** Since all methylxanthines stimulate secretion of hydrochloric acid (HCl) from the gastric mucosa, individuals with peptic ulcers should avoid beverages containing methylxanthines.

3. **Therapeutic uses:** *Caffeine* and its derivatives relax the smooth muscles of the bronchioles. Previously the main-stay of asthma therapy, *theophylline* has been largely replaced with β-agonists and corticosteroids (see p. 220).

4. **Pharmacokinetics:** The methylxanthines are well absorbed orally. *Caffeine* distributes throughout the body, including the brain. The drugs cross the placenta to the fetus and are secreted into the mother's milk. All the methylxanthines are metabolized in the liver, and the metabolites are then excreted in the urine.

5. **Adverse effects:** Moderate doses of *caffeine* cause insomnia, anxiety, and agitation. A high dosage is required to show toxicity, which is manifested by emesis and convulsions. The lethal dose is about 10 g for *caffeine* (about 100 cups of coffee), which induces cardiac arrhythmias; death from *caffeine* is thus highly unlikely. Lethargy, irritability, and headache occur in users who have routinely consumed more than 600 mg of *caffeine* per day (roughly 6 cups of coffee/day) and then suddenly stop.

B. Nicotine

Nicotine [NIC o teen] is the active ingredient in tobacco. Although this drug is not currently used therapeutically (except in smoking cessation therapy, see p. 101), *nicotine* remains important because it is second only to *caffeine* as the most widely used CNS stimulant and is second to alcohol as the most abused drug. In combination with the tars and carbon monoxide found in cigarette smoke, *nicotine* represents a serious risk factor for lung and cardiovascular disease, various cancers, as well as other illnesses.

1. **Mechanism of action:** In low doses, *nicotine* causes ganglionic stimulation by depolarization. At high doses, *nicotine* causes ganglionic blockade (see p. 49). *Nicotine* receptors exist in the CNS where similar actions occur. (See nicotinic receptors, p. 39.)

2. **Actions:**

a. **CNS:** *Nicotine* is highly soluble in lipid and readily crosses the blood-brain barrier. Cigarette smoking or administration of low doses of *nicotine* produces some degree of euphoria, and arousal, as well as relaxation, and improves attention, learning, problem solving, and reaction time. High doses of *nicotine* result in central respiratory paralysis and severe hypotension caused by medullary paralysis (Figure 10.3).

b. **Peripheral effects:** The peripheral effects of *nicotine* are complex. Stimulation of sympathetic ganglia as well as the adrenal medulla increases blood pressure and heart rate. Thus use of tobacco is particularly harmful in hypertensive patients. Many patients with peripheral vascular disease experience an exacerbation of symptoms with smoking. For example, *nicotine*-induced vasoconstriction can decrease coronary blood flow, adversely affecting the patient with angina. Stimulation of parasympathetic ganglia also increases motor activity of the bowel. At higher doses, blood pressure falls and activity ceases in both the gastrointestinal tract and bladder musculature as a result of a *nicotine*-induced block of parasympathetic ganglia.

3. **Pharmacokinetics:** *Nicotine* is highly-lipid soluble. Thus, absorption readily occurs via the oral mucosa, lungs, gastrointestinal mucosa, and skin. *Nicotine* crosses the placental membrane and is secreted in the milk of lactating women. Most cigarettes contain 6 to 8 mg of *nicotine*; the acute lethal dose is 60 mg. Over 90% of *nicotine* inhaled in smoke is absorbed. Clearance of *nicotine* involves metabolism in the lung and the liver, and urinary excretion. Tolerance to the toxic effects of *nicotine* develops rapidly, often within days after beginning usage.

4. **Adverse effects:** The CNS effects of *nicotine* include irritability and tremors. *Nicotine* may also cause intestinal cramps, diarrhea, and increased heart rate and blood pressure. In addition, cigarette smoking increases the rate of metabolism of a number of drugs. [Note: It is not known which of the over 3,000 components of cigarette smoke are responsible for this phenomenon, although the benzopyrenes have been implicated.]

5. **Withdrawal syndrome:** As with the other drugs in this class, *nicotine* is an addictive substance; physical dependence on *nicotine* develops rapidly and is severe. Withdrawal is characterized by irritability, anxiety, restlessness, difficulty in concentrating, headaches, and insomnia. Appetite is affected and gastrointestinal pain often occurs. [Note: Smoking cessation programs that combine pharmacologic and behavioral therapy are the most successful in helping individuals to stop smoking. The transdermal patch and chewing gum containing *nicotine* have been shown to reduce *nicotine*-withdrawal symptoms and to help smokers stop smoking. For example, the blood concentration of *nicotine* obtained from chewing gum is typically about one-half of the peak level observed with smoking (Figure 10.4).]

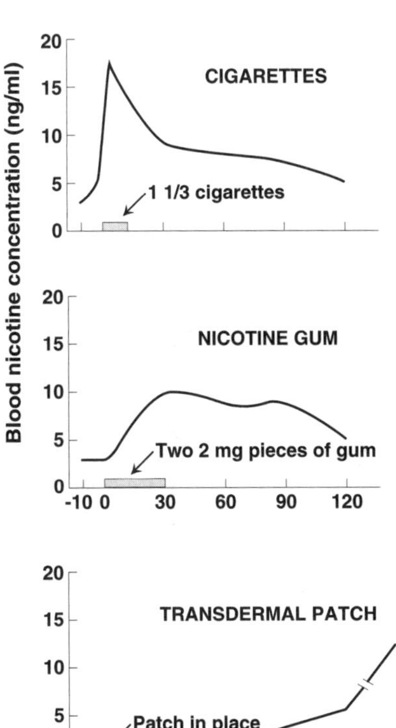

Figure 10.4
Blood concentrations of nicotine in individuals who smoked cigarettes, chewed nicotine gum or received nicotine by transdermal patch.

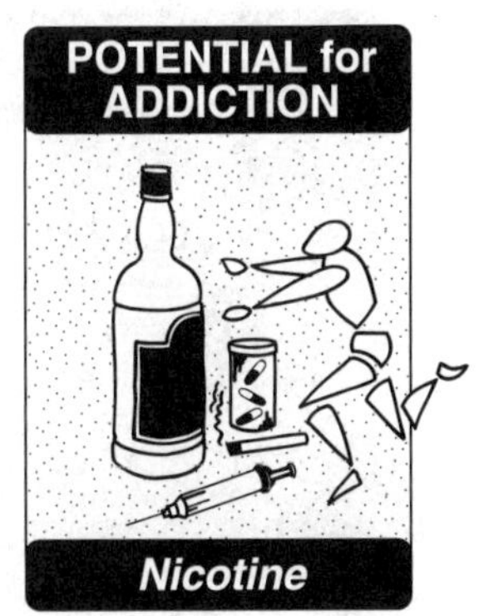

C. Cocaine

Cocaine [koe KANE] is an inexpensive, widely available, and highly addictive drug that is currently abused daily by over 3 million people in the United States.

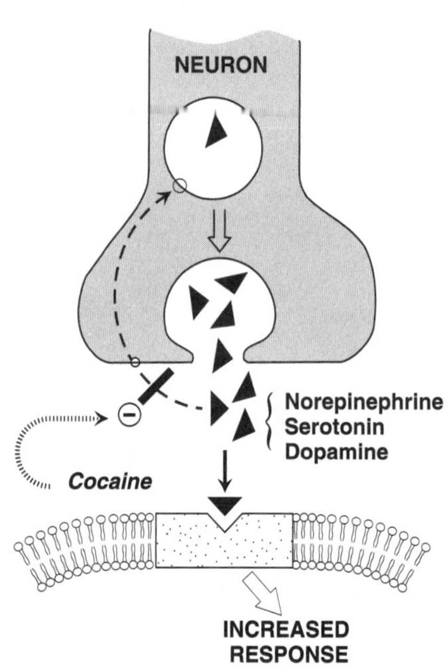

Figure 10.5
Mechanism of action of *cocaine*.

1. **Mechanism of action:** The primary mechanism of action underlying *cocaine*'s central and peripheral effects is blockade of norepinephrine, serotonin, and dopamine re-uptake into the presynaptic terminals from which these transmitters are released (Figure 10.5). This block potentiates and prolongs the CNS and peripheral actions of these catecholamines. In particular, the prolongation of dopaminergic effects in the brain's pleasure system (limbic system), produces the intense euphoria that *cocaine* initially causes. Chronic intake of *cocaine* depletes dopamine. This depletion triggers the vicious cycle of craving for *cocaine* that temporarily relieves severe depression.

2. **Actions:**

   a. **Central nervous system:** The behavioral effects of *cocaine* result from powerful stimulation of the cortex and brainstem. *Cocaine* acutely increases mental awareness and produces a feeling of well-being and euphoria that is similar to that caused by *amphetamine*. Like *amphetamine*, *cocaine* can produce hallucinations, delusions, and paranoia. *Cocaine* increases motor activity, and at high doses causes tremors and convulsions, followed by respiratory and vasomotor depression.

   b. **Sympathetic nervous systems:** Peripherally, *cocaine* potentiates the action of norepinephrine and produces the "fight or flight" syndrome characteristic of adrenergic stimulation. This is associated with tachycardia, hypertension, pupillary dilation, and peripheral vasoconstriction.

3. **Therapeutic uses:** *Cocaine* has a local anesthetic action that represents the only current rationale for the therapeutic use of *cocaine*; *cocaine* is applied topically as a local anesthetic during eye, ear, nose, and throat surgery. While the local anesthetic action of *cocaine* is due to a block of voltage-activated sodium channels, an interaction with potassium channels may contribute to *cocaine's* ability to cause cardiac arrhythmias. [Note: *Cocaine* is the only local anesthetic that causes vasoconstriction. This effect is responsible for the necrosis and perforation of the nasal septum seen in association with chronic inhalation of *cocaine* powder.]

4. **Pharmacokinetics:** *Cocaine* is self-administered by chewing, intranasal snorting, smoking, and intravenous (IV) injection. Peak effect occurs at 15 to 20 minutes after intranasal intake of *cocaine* powder, and the high disappears in 1 to 1.5 hours. Rapid but short-lived effects are achieved following IV injection of *cocaine*, or by smoking the free base form of the drug ("crack"). Because the onset of action is most rapid, the potential for overdosage and dependence is greatest with IV injection and crack smoking.

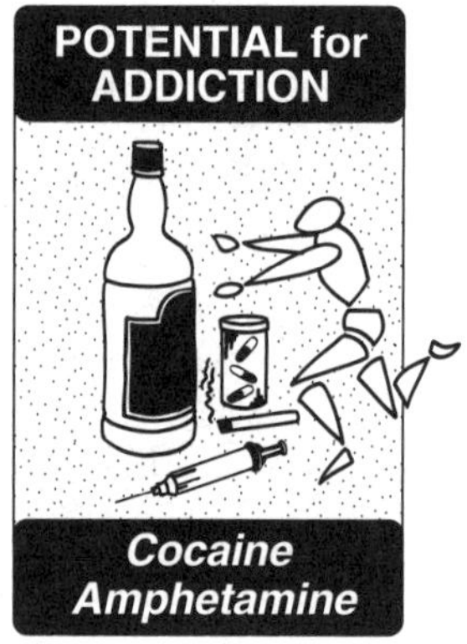

5. **Adverse effects:**

   a. **Anxiety:** The toxic response to acute *cocaine* ingestion can precipitate an anxiety reaction that includes hypertension, tachycardia, sweating, and paranoia.

b. Depression: Like all stimulant drugs, *cocaine* stimulation of the CNS is followed by a period of mental depression. Addicts withdrawing from *cocaine* exhibit physical and emotional depression as well as agitation. These symptoms can be treated with benzodiazepines (see p. 89) or phenothiazines (see p. 127).

c. Heart disease: *Cocaine* can induce seizures as well as fatal cardiac arrhythmias (Figure 10.6). Intravenous *diazepam* (see p. 89) and *propranolol* (see p. 74) may be required to control *cocaine*-induced seizures and cardiac arrhythmias, respectively. The incidence of myocardial infarction in *cocaine* users is unrelated to dose, to duration of use, or to route of administration. There is no marker to identify those individuals who may have life-threatenting cardiac effects after taking *cocaine*.

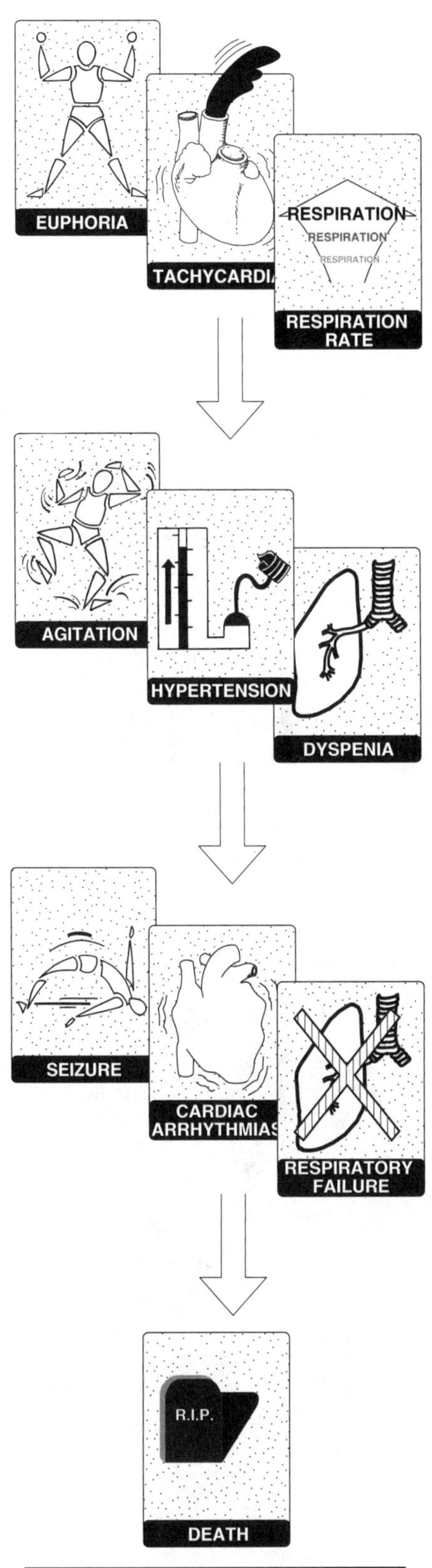

Figure 10.6
Major effects of *cocaine* use.

D. Amphetamine

Amphetamine shows neurologic and clinical effects that are quite similar to those of *cocaine*.

1. **Mechanism of action:** As with *cocaine*, the effects of *amphetamine* on the CNS and peripheral nervous system are indirect; that is, they depend upon an elevation of the level of catecholamine transmitters in synaptic spaces. *Amphetamine*, however, achieves this effect by releasing intracellular stores of catecholamines (Figure 10.7). Since *amphetamine* also blocks monoamine oxidase (MAO), high levels of catecholamines are readily released into synaptic spaces. Despite different mechanisms of action, the behavioral effects of *amphetamine* are similar to those of *cocaine*.

2. **Actions:**

   a. Central nervous system: The major cause of the behavioral effects of *amphetamines* is probably due to release of dopamine rather than release of norepinephrine. *Amphetamine* stimulates the entire cerebrospinal axis, cortex, brain stem, and medulla. This leads to increased alertness, decreased fatigue, depressed appetite, and insomnia. In high doses, convulsions can ensue. These CNS stimulant effects of *amphetamine* and its derivatives have led to their use in the therapy of depression, hyperactivity in children, narcolepsy, and appetite control.

   b. Sympathetic nervous system: In addition to its marked action on the CNS, *amphetamine* acts on the adrenergic system, indirectly stimulating the receptors through norepinephrine release (see p. 68).

3. **Therapeutic uses:** Factors that limit the therapeutic usefulness of *amphetamine* include psychological and physiological dependence similar to those with *cocaine*, and the development of tolerance to the euphoric and anorectic effects with chronic use. [Note: Less tolerance to the toxic CNS effects (for example, convulsions) develops.]

A No *amphetamine*

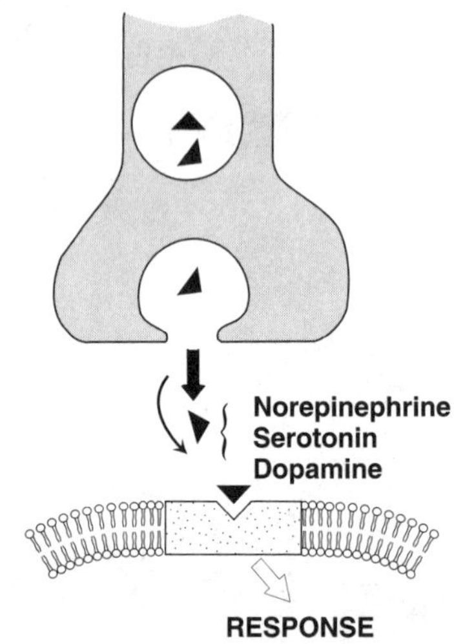

B With *amphetamine*

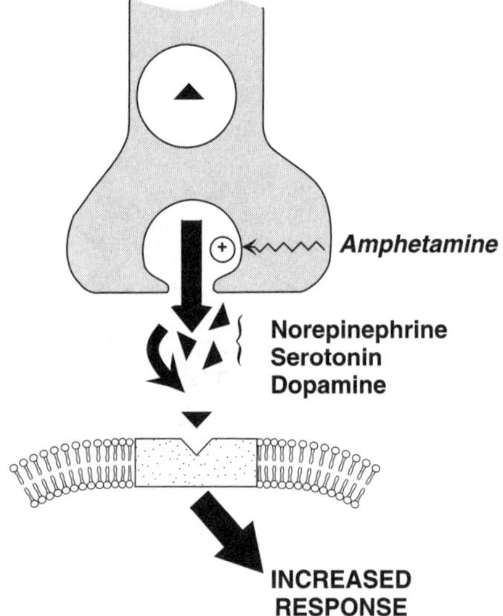

Figure 10.7
Mechanism of action of *amphetamine*.

a. **Attention deficit syndrome:** Some young children are hyperkinetic and lack the ability to be involved in any one activity for longer than a few minutes. *Amphetamine,* and more recently the *amphetamine* derivative *methylphenidate* [meth ill FEN i date], alleviate many of the behavioral problems associated with this syndrome, and reduce the hyperkinesia that the children demonstrate. Their attention is thus prolonged, allowing them to function better in a school atmosphere.

b. **Narcolepsy:** *Methylphenidate* is used to treat narcolepsy, a disorder marked by an uncontrollable desire for sleep.

4. **Pharmacokinetics:** Amphetamines are completely absorbed from the gastrointestinal tract, metabolized by the liver, and excreted in the urine. Amphetamine abusers often administer the drugs by intravenous injection and by smoking. The euphoria caused by *amphetamine* lasts 4 to 6 hours, or 4 to 8 times longer than the effects of *cocaine*. The amphetamines produce addiction—dependence, tolerance and drug-seeking behavior.

5. **Adverse effects:**

a. **Central effects:** Undesirable side effects of *amphetamine* usage include insomnia, irritability, weakness, dizziness, tremor, and hyperactive reflexes (Figure 10.8). *Amphetamine* can also cause confusion, delirium, panic states, and suicidal tendencies, especially in mentally ill patients. Chronic *amphetamine* use produces a state of "*amphetamine* psychosis" that resembles an acute schizophrenic attack. While *amphetamine* is associated with psychic and physical dependence, tolerance to its effects may occur within a few weeks. Overdoses of *amphetamine* are treated with *chlorpromazine* (see p. 127), which relieves the CNS symptoms as well as the hypertension because of its α-blocking effects.

b. **Cardiovascular effects:** In addition to its CNS effects, *amphetamine* causes palpitations, cardiac arrhythmias, hypertension, anginal pain, and circulatory collapse. Headache, chills, and excessive sweating may also occur. Because of its cardiovascular effects, *amphetamine* should not be given to patients with cardiovascular disease or those receiving MAO inhibitors.

c. **Gastrointestinal system effects:** *Amphetamine* acts on the gastrointestinal system, causing anorexia, nausea, vomiting, abdominal cramps, and diarrhea.

III. HALLUCINOGENS

A few drugs have as their primary action the ability to induce altered perceptual states reminiscent of dreams. Many of these altered states are accompanied by bright, colorful changes in the environment and by a plasticity of constantly changing shapes and color. The individual under the influence of these drugs is incapable of normal decision making, since the drug interferes with rational thought. These compounds are known as hallucinogens or psychotomimetic drugs.

A. Lysergic acid diethylamide (LSD)

Multiple sites in the CNS are affected by *LSD*. The drug shows serotonin (5-HT) agonist activity at presynaptic receptors in the midbrain, binding to both 5-HT_1 and 5-HT_2 receptors. Activation of the sympathetic nervous system occurs, which causes pupillary dilation, increased blood pressure, piloerection, and increased body temperature. Taken orally, low doses of *LSD* can induce hallucinations with brilliant colors, and mood alteration occurs. Tolerance and physical dependence have occurred, but true dependence is rare. Adverse effects include hyperreflexia, nausea, and muscular weakness. Sometimes high doses produce long-lasting psychotic changes in susceptible individuals. *Haloperidol* (see p. 127) and other neuroleptics can block the hallucinatory action of *LSD* and quickly abort the syndrome.

B. Tetrahydrocannabinol

The main alkaloid contained in marijuana is *dronabinol* [droe NAB i nol], also called Δ^9-*tetrahydrocannabinol* [tet ra hi dro can NAB i nol] (*THC*). *Dronabinol* produces euphoria that is followed by drowsiness and relaxation, depending on the social situation. *THC* impairs short-term memory and mental activity. It decreases muscle strength and impairs highly skilled motor activity, such as that required to drive a car. It increases appetite, causes xerostomia, visual hallucinations, delusions, and enhancement of sensory activity. Although THC-receptors have been identified in the CNS, the mechanism of action of *THC* is unknown. *THC* effects show immediately after smoking, but maximal effects take about 20 minutes. By 3 hours, the effects largely disappear. Adverse effects include an increased heart rate, decreased blood pressure, and a reddening of the conjunctiva. At high doses, a toxic psychosis develops. Tolerance and mild physical dependence occur with continued frequent use of the drug. *THC* is sometimes given for the severe emesis caused by some cancer chemotherapeutic agents (see p. 243).

C. Phencyclidine (PCP)

Phencyclidine [fen SYE kli deen] ("angel dust") inhibits the re-uptake of dopamine, 5-HT, and norepinephrine. It also has anticholinergic activity, but surprisingly produces hypersalivation. *Phencyclidine*, an analog of *ketamine* (see p. 117), causes dissociative anesthesia (insensitivity to pain, without loss of consciousness) and analgesia. In this state, it produces numbness of extremities, staggered gait, slurred speech, and muscular rigidity. Sometimes hostile and bizarre behavior occurs. In increased dosage, anesthesia, stupor, or coma result, but strangely, the eyes may remain open. Increased sensitivity to external stimuli exists, and the CNS actions may persist for a week. Tolerance often develops with continued use.

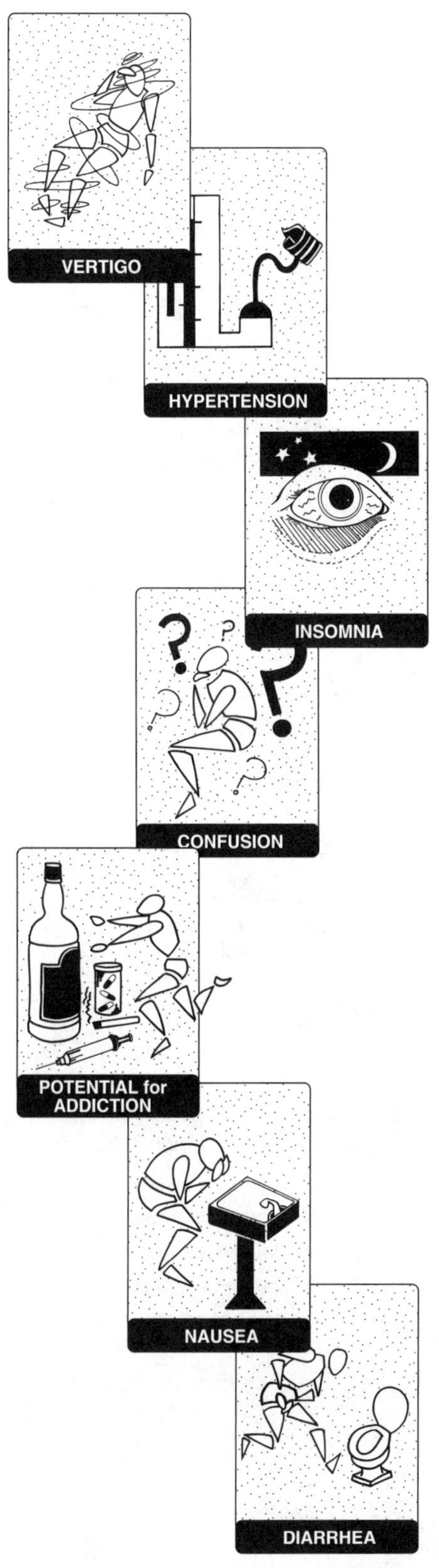

Figure 10.8
Adverse effects of amphetamines.

Choose the ONE best answer.

10.1 Which of the following is NOT characteristic of cocaine overdosage?

A. Dilation of the pupil.
B. Euphoria.
C. Tachycardia.
D. Peripheral vasodilation.
E. Hallucinations.

Correct choice = D. Cocaine causes peripheral vasoconstriction.

10.2 Which of the following statements about amphetamine is INCORRECT?

A. Overdosage of amphetamine can be managed with chlorpromazine.
B. Amphetamine is used as an adjunct with MAO inhibitors in the treatment of depression.
C. Amphetamine has a longer duration of action than cocaine.
D. Amphetamine depresses the hunger center in the hypothalamus.
E. Amphetamine acts on α- and β-adrenergic presynaptic terminals.

Correct choice = B. Amphetamines should not be used in patients receiving MAO inhibitors, since amphetamine itself weakly inhibits MAO. Chlorpromazine relieves the CNS symptoms and the hypertension because of its α-blocking effects. The euphoria caused by amphetamine lasts 4 to 6 hours, or 4 to 8 times longer than the effects of cocaine.

10.3 Which of the following statements concerning tetrahydrocannabinol (THC) is CORRECT?

A. THC decreases heart rate.
B. THC increases muscle strength.
C. THC decreases appetite.
D. THC causes hypotension.
E. THC has antiemetic action.

Correct answer = E. THC is sometimes used to treat the severe emesis caused by cancer chemotherapeutic agents.

10.4 Which one of the following drugs is INCORRECTLY paired with its toxic effects?

A. Amphetamine: Paranoid psychosis
B. Nicotine (low dose): Decreased heart rate and blood pressure
C. Cocaine: Anxiety and depression
D. LSD: Hallucinations
E. Caffeine: Insomnia and agitation

Correct answer = B. Nicotine activates the sympathetic nervous system and causes hypertension and tachycardia.

10.5 A very agitated young male was brought to the emergency room by the police. Psychiatric examination revealed that he had snorted cocaine several times in the past few days, the last time being 10 hours previously. He was given a drug which sedated him and he fell asleep. The drug very likely used to counter this patient's apparent cocaine withdrawal was:

A. Phenobarbital
B. Lorazepam
C. Cocaine
D. Hydroxyzine
E. Fluoxetine

Correct answer = B. The anxiolytic properties of benzodiazepines, such as lorazepam, make them the drugs of choice in treating the anxiety and agitation of cocaine withdrawal. Lorazepam also has hypnotic properties. Phenobarbital has hypnotic properties but it's anxiolytic properties are inferior to those of the benzodiazepines. Cocaine itself could counteract the agitation of withdrawal but its use would not be proper therapy. Hydroxyzine, an antihistaminic, is effective as an hypnotic and is sometimes used to deal with anxiety especially if emesis is a problem. Fluoxetine is an antidepressant with no immediate effects on anxiety.

Anesthetics

11

I. OVERVIEW

General anesthesia is essential to surgical practice because it renders patients analgesic, amnesic, and unconscious while causing muscle relaxation and suppression of undesirable reflexes. No single drug is capable of achieving these effects rapidly and safely. Rather, several different categories of drugs are utilized to produce "balanced anesthesia" (Figure 11.1). For example, adjuncts to anesthesia consist of preanesthetic medication and skeletal muscle relaxants. Preanesthetic medication serves to calm the patient, relieve pain, and protect against undesirable effects of the subsequently administered anesthetic or the surgical procedure. Skeletal muscle relaxants facilitate intubation and suppress muscle tone to the degree required for surgery. Potent general anesthetics are delivered via inhalation or intravenous injection. With the exception of *nitrous oxide*, modern inhaled anesthetics are all volatile, halogenated hydrocarbons that derive from early research and clinical experience with *diethyl ether* and *chloroform*. On the other hand, intravenous general anesthetics consist of a number of chemically unrelated drug types that are commonly used for the rapid induction of anesthesia. For some patients and surgical procedures, co-administration of local anesthetics and low doses of general anesthetics produces discreet analgesia, while minimizing the undesirable actions of the less selective agents.

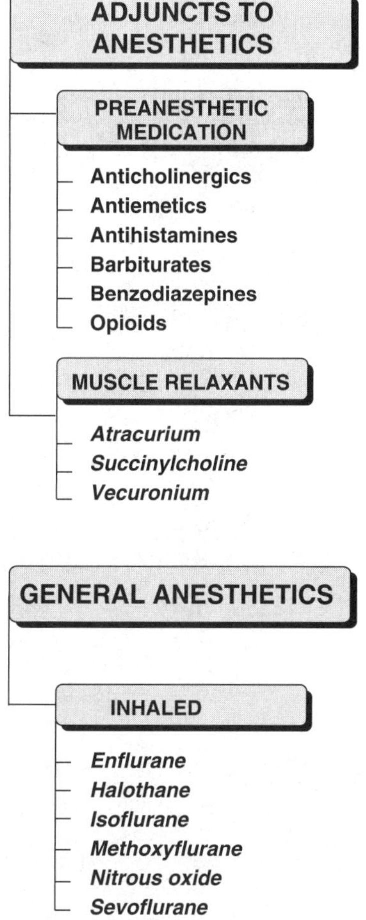

Figure 11.1
Summary of anesthetics.
(Figure continues on next page.)

II. PATIENT FACTORS IN SELECTION OF ANESTHESIA

During the preoperative phase, the anesthesiologist selects drugs that provide a safe and efficient anesthetic regimen based on the nature of the surgical procedure as well as the patient's physiologic and pharmacologic state.

A. Status of organ systems

1. **Liver and kidney:** Since the liver and kidney not only influence the long-term distribution and clearance of anesthetic agents, but also

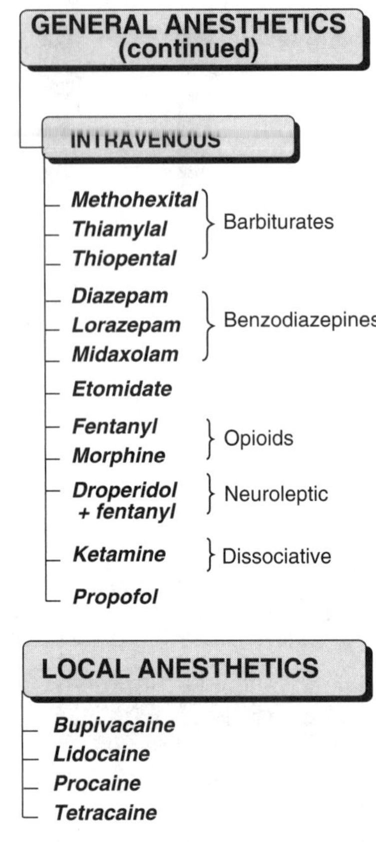

Figure 11.1 (continued)
Summary of anesthetics.

frequently serve as the target organs for toxic effects, the physiologic status of these organs must be considered. Of particular concern, release of fluoride, bromide, and other metabolic products of halogenated hydrocarbons can affect these organs, especially if these metabolites accumulate with repeated anesthetic administration.

2. **Respiratory system:** The condition of the respiratory system must be considered if inhalation anesthetics are indicated. For example, asthma, or ventilation or perfusion abnormalities complicate control of an inhalation anesthetic.

3. **Cardiovascular system:** While the hypotensive effect of most anesthetics is sometimes desirable, ischemic injury of tissues could follow reduced perfusion pressure. Should a hypotensive episode during a surgical procedure necessitate treatment, a vasoactive substance must be selected after considering the possibility that the anesthetic present may sensitize the heart to the arrhythmogenic effects of sympathomimetic agents.

4. **Nervous system:** The existence of neurologic disorders (for example, epilepsy, myasthenia gravis) influences the selection of an anesthetic. So, too, would a patient history suggestive of a genetically-determined sensitivity to halogenated hydrocarbon-induced malignant hyperthermia (see p. 113).

B. Concomitant use of drugs

1. **Multiple adjunct agents:** Quite often, surgical patients receive one or more of the following preanesthetic medications: benzodiazepines (for example, *diazepam*, see p. 89) to relieve anxiety and facilitate amnesia; barbiturates (for example, *pentobarbital*, see p. 94) for sedation; antihistamines for prevention of allergic reactions (for example, *diphenhydramine*, see p. 422) or to reduce gastric acidity (*cimetidine*, see p. 236); antiemetics (for example, *droperidol*, see p. 242); opioids (for example, *fentanyl*, see p. 139) for analgesia; and/or anticholinergics (for example, *scopolamine*, see p. 48) to prevent bradycardia and secretion of fluids into the respiratory tract (Figure 11.2). These agents facilitate smooth induction of anesthesia, and when continuously administered, they also lower the dose of anesthetic required to maintain the desired level of surgical (Stage III) anesthesia. However, such co-administration can also enhance undesirable anesthetic effects (for example, hypoventilation) and may produce negative effects not observed when the same drugs are given alone.

2. **Concomitant use of additional nonanesthetic drugs:** Surgery patients may be chronically exposed to agents for the treatment of the underlying disease, as well as to drugs of abuse that alter the response to anesthetics. For example, alcoholics have elevated levels of hepatic microsomal enzymes involved in the metabolism of barbiturates, and drug abusers may be overly tolerant of the anesthetic, since drugs of abuse and anesthetics can act on the same biochemical pathway(s).

III. INDUCTION, MAINTENANCE AND RECOVERY FROM ANESTHESIA

Anesthesia can be divided into three stages: induction, maintenance, and recovery. Induction is defined as the period of time from onset of administration of the anesthetic to the development of effective surgical anesthesia in the patient. Maintenance provides a sustained surgical anesthesia. Recovery is the time from discontinuation of administration of anesthesia until consciousness is regained. Induction of anesthesia depends on how fast effective concentrations of the anesthetic drug reach the brain; recovery is the reverse of induction and depends on how fast the anesthetic drug is removed from the brain.

A. Induction

During induction it is essential to avoid the dangerous excitatory phase (Stage II delirium) characterizing the slow onset of action of some anesthetics (see below). Thus, general anesthesia is normally induced with an intravenous anesthetic like *thiopental*; unconsciousness results within 25 seconds after injection. At that time, additional inhalation or intravenous drugs comprising the selected anesthetic may be given to produce the desired depth of surgical (Stage III) anesthesia. [Note: This often includes co-administration of an intravenous skeletal muscle relaxant to facilitate intubation and relaxation. Currently used muscle relaxants include *vecuronium*, *atracurium*, and *succinylcholine* (see p. 52).]

B. Maintenance of anesthesia

Maintenance is the time during which the patient is surgically anesthetized. After administering the selected anesthetic mixture, the anesthesiologist monitors the patient's vital signs and response to various stimuli throughout the surgical procedure in order to carefully balance the amount of drug inhaled and/or infused with the depth of anesthesia. Anesthesia is usually maintained by the administration of gases or volatile anesthetics, since these agents offer good minute-to-minute control over the depth of anesthesia.

C. Recovery

Postoperatively, the anesthesiologist withdraws the anesthetic mixture and monitors the immediate return of the patient to consciousness. For most anesthetic agents, recovery is the reverse of induction; that is, redistribution from the site of action rather than metabolism underlies recovery. The anesthesiologist continues to monitor the patient to be sure that there are no delayed toxic reactions, for example, diffusion hypoxia for *nitrous oxide*, and hepatotoxicity with halogenated hydrocarbons.

D. Depth of anesthesia

The depth of anesthesia can be divided into a series of four sequential stages; each is characterized by increased CNS depression that is caused by accumulation of the anesthetic drug in the brain. With

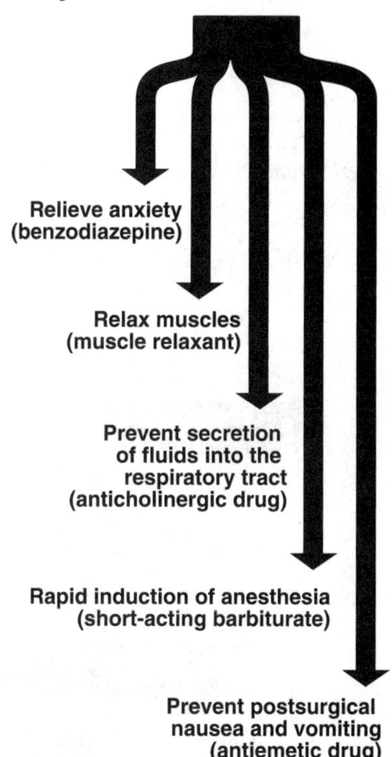
Some functions of adjuncts to anesthesia
Relieve anxiety (benzodiazepine)
Relax muscles (muscle relaxant)
Prevent secretion of fluids into the respiratory tract (anticholinergic drug)
Rapid induction of anesthesia (short-acting barbiturate)
Prevent postsurgical nausea and vomiting (antiemetic drug)

Figure 11.2
Components of balanced anesthesia.

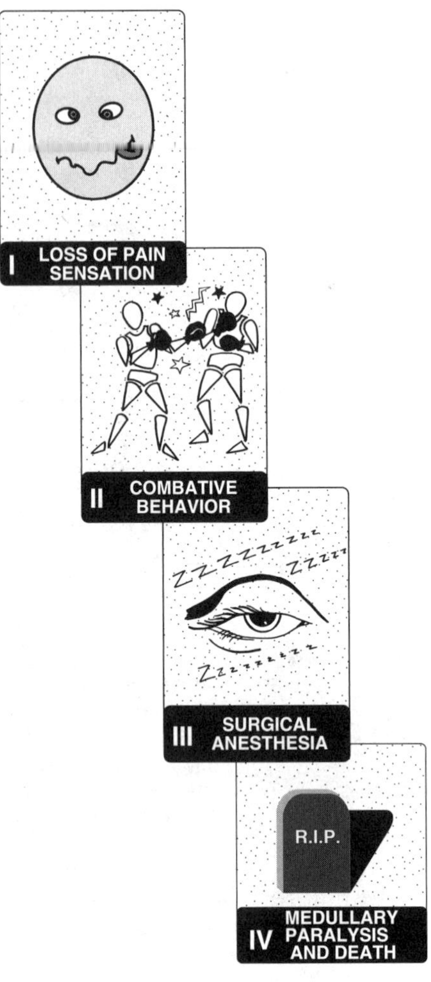
I LOSS OF PAIN SENSATION
II COMBATIVE BEHAVIOR
III SURGICAL ANESTHESIA
R.I.P.
IV MEDULLARY PARALYSIS AND DEATH

Figure 11.3
Stages of anesthesia.

ether, which produces a slow onset of anesthesia, all the stages are discernible (Figure 11.3). However, with *halothane* and many other commonly used anesthetics, the stages are difficult to clearly characterize because of the rapidity of onset of anesthesia.

1. **Stage I—analgesia:** Loss of pain sensation results from interference with sensory transmission in the spinothalamic tract. The patient is conscious and conversational. A reduced awareness of pain occurs as Stage II is approached.

2. **Stage II—excitement:** The patient experiences delirium and violent combative behavior. There is a rise and irregularity in blood pressure. The respiratory rate may be increased. To avoid this stage of anesthesia, a short-acting barbiturate, such as *sodium pentothal*, is given intravenously before inhalation anesthesia is administered.

3. **Stage III—surgical anesthesia:** Regular respiration and relaxation of the skeletal muscles occur in this stage. Eye reflexes decrease progressively, until the eye movements cease and the pupil is fixed. Surgery may proceed during this stage.

4. **Stage IV—medullary paralysis:** Severe depression of the respiratory center and vasomotor center occur during this stage. Death can rapidly ensue.

IV. INHALATION ANESTHETICS

Inhaled gases are the mainstay of anesthesia and are primarily used for the maintenance of anesthesia after administration of an intravenous agent. Inhalation anesthetics have a benefit that is not available with intravenous agents, since the depth of anesthesia can be rapidly altered by changing the concentration of the inhaled anesthetic. Because most of these agents are rapidly eliminated from the body, they do not cause postoperative respiratory depression.

A. Common features of inhaled anesthestics

Modern inhalation anesthetics are nonexplosive agents that include the gas *nitrous oxide* as well as a number of volatile halogenated hydrocarbons. As a group, these agents decrease cerebrovascular resistance, resulting in increased perfusion of the brain. They cause bronchodilation and decrease minute ventilation. Their clinical potency cannot be predicted by their chemical structure, but potency does correlate with their solubility in lipid. The movement of these agents from the lungs to the different body compartments depends upon their solubility in blood and various tissues. Recovery from their effects is due to redistribution from the brain.

B. Potency

The potency of inhaled anesthetics is defined quantitatively as the minimum alveolar concentration (MAC), which is the concentration of anesthetic gas needed to eliminate movement among 50% of patients challenged by a standardized skin incision. The MAC is usually expressed as the percent of gas in a mixture required to achieve the effect. Numerically, MAC is small for potent anesthetics, such as *halothane*, and large for less potent agents, such as *nitrous oxide*. Therefore, the inverse of MAC is an index of potency of the anesthetic. The MAC values are useful in comparing pharmacologic effects of different anesthetics (Figure 11.4). The more lipid-soluble an anesthetic, the lower the concentration of anesthetic needed to produce anesthesia.

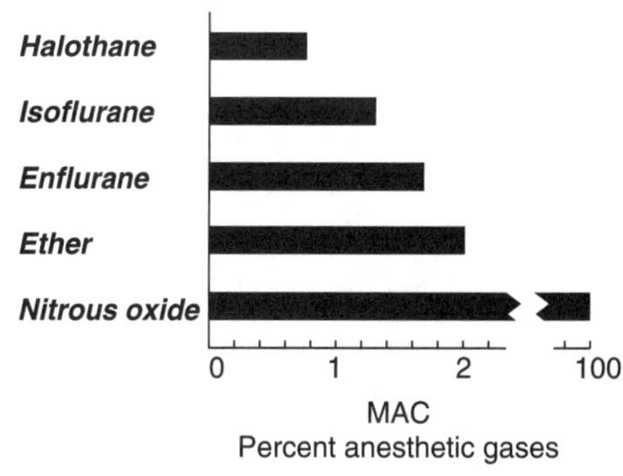

Figure 11.4
Minimal alveolar concentrations (MAC) for anesthetic gases.

C. Uptake and Distribution of Inhalation Anesthetics

The partial pressure of an anesthetic gas at the origin of the respiratory pathway is the driving force that moves the anesthetic into the alveolar space and thence into the blood, which delivers the drug to the brain and various other body compartments. Since gases move from one compartment to another within the body according to partial pressure gradients, a steady state is achieved when the partial pressure in each of these compartments is equivalent to that in the inspired mixture. The time course for attaining this steady state is determined by the following three factors:

1. **Alveolar wash-in:** This term refers to the replacement of the normal lung gases with the inspired anesthetic mixture. The time required for this process is directly proportional to the functional residual capacity of the lung, and inversely proportional to the ventilatory rate; it is independent of the physical properties of the gas. Once the partial pressure builds within the lung, anesthetic uptake from the lung begins.

2. **Solubility in blood:** The first compartment that the anesthetic gas encounters is the blood. Solubility in blood is determined by a physical property of the anesthetic molecule called the blood/gas partition coefficient, which is the ratio of the total amount of gas in the blood relative to the gas equilibrium phase (Figure 11.5). Drugs with low versus high solubility in blood differ in their speed of induction of anesthesia. For example, when an anesthetic gas with low blood solubility, such as *nitrous oxide*, diffuses from the alveoli into the circulation, little of the anesthetic dissolves in the blood. Therefore, the equilibrium between the inhaled anesthetic and arterial blood occurs rapidly, and relatively few additional molecules of anesthetic are required to raise arterial tension (that is, steady-state is rapidly achieved). In contrast, an anesthetic gas with high blood solubility, such as *halothane*, dissolves more completely in the blood, and greater amounts of the anesthetic and longer periods of time are required to raise arterial tension. This results in increased times of induction and recovery, and slower changes in the depth of anesthesia in response to changes in the concentration of the inhaled drug.

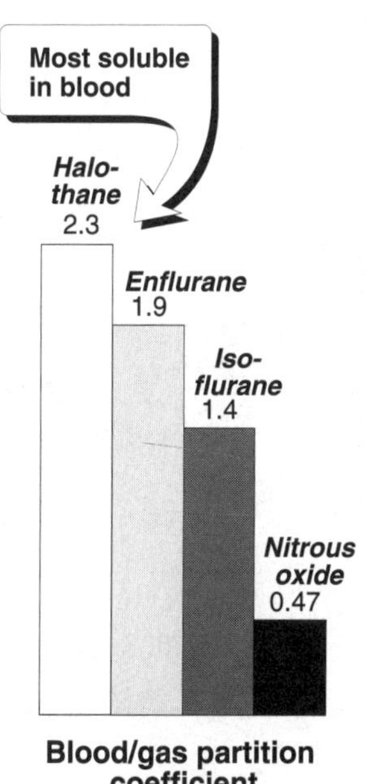

Figure 11.5
Blood/gas partition coefficients for the inhalation anesthetics.

3. **Tissue uptake:** The arterial circulation distributes the anesthetic to various tissues, and the pressure gradient drives free anesthetic gas into tissues. The time required for a particular tissue to achieve a steady-state with the partial pressure of an anesthetic gas in the inspired mixture is inversely proportional to the blood flow to that tissue (faster flow results in a more rapidly achieved steady-state), and directly proportional to the capacity to store anesthetic (larger

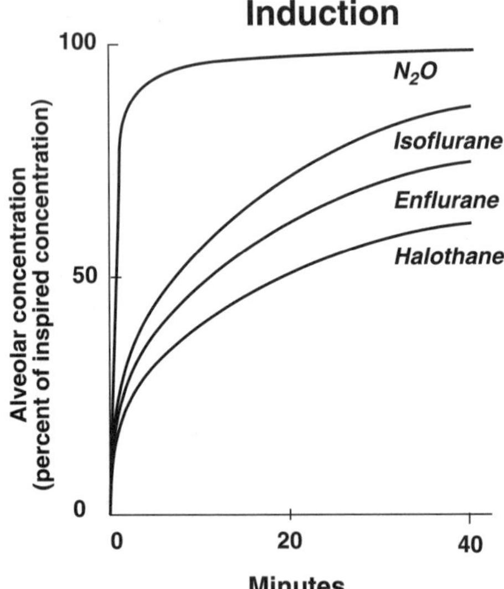

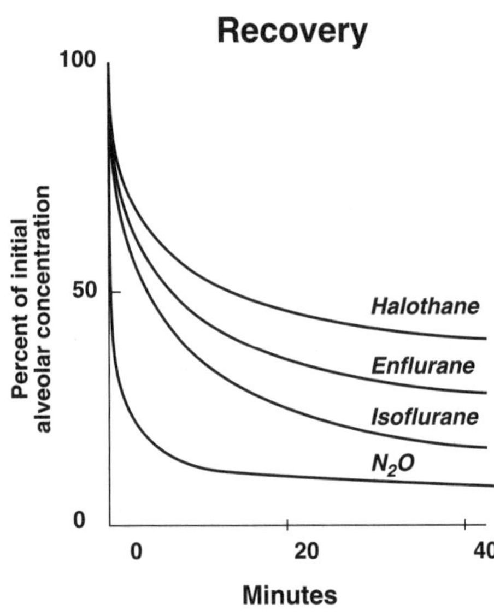

Figure 11.6
Changes in the alveolar blood concentration of the inhalation anesthetics with time.

capacity results in a longer time to achieve steady-state). Capacity, in turn, is directly proportional to the tissue's volume, and the tissue/blood solubility coefficient of the anesthetic molecule. On the basis of these considerations, four major compartments determine the time course of anesthetic uptake:

a. **Brain, heart, liver, kidney, endocrine glands:** These highly perfused tissues rapidly attain a steady-state with the partial pressure of the anesthetic in blood.

b. **Skeletal muscles:** These are poorly perfused during anesthesia. This and the fact that they have a large volume, prolong the time required to achieve steady-state.

c. **Fat:** This tissue is also poorly perfused. However, potent general anesthetics are very lipid soluble. Therefore, fat has a large capacity to store anesthetic. This combination of slow delivery to a high capacity compartment prolongs the time required to achieve steady state.

d. **Bone, ligaments, and cartilage:** These are poorly perfused and have a relatively low capacity to store anesthetic. Therefore, these tissues have only a slight impact on the time course of anesthetic distribution in the body.

4. **Return of gas-depleted blood to the lung:** As the venous circulation returns blood depleted of anesthetic to the lung, more gas moves into the blood from the lung according to the partial pressure difference. Over time, the partial pressure in the alveolar space closely approximates the partial pressure in the inspired mixture; that is, there is no further anesthetic uptake from the lung.

5. **Uptake curves for inhaled anesthetics:** Figure 11.6 illustrates the uptake curves for four inhalation anesthetics. The solubility in blood, as well as tissues, is in the following order: *halothane* > *enflurane* > *isoflurane* > *nitrous oxide*. Because of its low solubility, the partial pressure of *nitrous oxide* in the inspired mixture and the body most rapidly achieves a steady-state.

6. **Washout:** When the administration of an inhalation anesthetic is discontinued, the body now becomes the "source" that drives the anesthetic into the alveolar space. The same factors that influence attainment of steady-state with an inspired anesthetic determine the time course of clearance of the drug from the body. Thus, *nitrous oxide* exits the body faster than *halothane*.

C. Mechanism of Action

Inhalation anesthetics are nonselective in their action. That is, in addition to their clinically important effect on the central nervous system (CNS), they also alter the function of various peripheral cell types. The fact that chemically unrelated molecules produce a state of general anesthesia argues against a specific anesthetic receptor. Further, whereas anesthetics alter the function of receptors for neurotransmitters (for example, γ-aminobutyric acid, glutamate), they do so nonselectively. Thus, the fact that CNS regions, like the reticular activating system and cortex, represent important sites of anesthetic action is apparently unrelated to the presence of a specific receptor in a particular region, but rather to the role of the CNS in controlling the overall state of consciousness and response to sensory stimuli.

D. Specific inhalation anesthetics

Each of the halogenated gases has characteristics beneficial for selected clinical applications. No one anesthetic is superior to another under all circumstances. [Note: In a very small population of patients, all of the halogenated hydrocarbon anesthetics have the potential to induce malignant hyperthermia. While the etiology of this condition is unknown, it appears to be inherited. Thus, asking whether a family member responded adversely to gaseous anesthesia could provide the warning needed to avoid a rare encounter with this pathology. Should a patient exhibit the hyperthermia and muscle rigidity characteristic of malignant hyperthermia, *dantrolene* is given as the anesthetic mixture is withdrawn.]

1. **Halothane:** This agent is the prototype to which newer agents in this series of anesthetics are compared. While *halothane* [hal loe thane] is a potent anesthetic, it is a relatively weak analgesic. Thus, *halothane* is usually co-administered with *nitrous oxide*, opioids, or local anesthetics. Like other halogenated hydrocarbons, *halothane* is vagomimetic and will cause *atropine*-sensitive bradycardia. In addition, *halothane* has the undesirable property of causing cardiac arrhythmias. These are especially serious if hypercapnia (increased arterial carbon dioxide tension) develops due to reduced alveolar ventilation, or if the plasma concentration of catecholamines increases. The latter fact is of particular significance since *halothane* produces hypotension. Should it become necessary to counter excessive hypotension during *halothane* anesthesia, it is recommended that a direct-acting vasoconstrictor (for example, *phenylephrine*, see p. 66) be given. *Halothane* is oxidatively metabolized in the body to tissue-toxic hydrocarbons (for example, trifluroethanol) and bromide ion. These substances may be responsible for the toxic reactions that some patients (especially females) develop after *halothane* anesthesia. This reaction begins as fever, anorexia, nausea, and vomiting, and patients may exhibit signs of hepatitis. Although the incidence of this reaction is low—approximately 1 in 10,000 individuals—50% of such patients will die of hepatic necrosis. To avoid this condition, a *halothane* anesthesia is not repeated at intervals less than 2 to 3 weeks. [Note: *Halothane* is not hepatotoxic in pediatric patients and that, combined with its pleasant odor, make it the agent of choice in children.]

2. **Enflurane:** This gas is less potent than *halothane*, but it produces rapid induction and recovery. About 2% of the agent is metabolized to fluoride ion, which is excreted by the kidney. Therefore, *enflurane* [EN floo rane] is contraindicated in patients with kidney failure. *Enflurane* anesthesia exhibits the following differences from *halothane*: fewer arrhythmias, less sensitization of the heart to catecholamines, and greater potentiation of muscle relaxants

due to a more potent "curare-like" effect. A disadvantage of *enflurane* is that it causes CNS excitation at twice the MAC and at lower doses if hyperventilation reduces the pCO_2.

3. **Isoflurane:** This is a newer halogenated anesthetic that has low biotransformation and low organ toxicity. Unlike the other halogenated anesthetic gases, *isoflurane* [ey soe FLURE ane] does not induce cardiac arrhythmias and does not sensitize the heart to the action of catecholamines. *Isoflurane* is a very stable molecule that undergoes little metabolism, as a result of which, less fluoride is produced. *Isoflurane* is not currently believed to be tissue toxic.

4. **Methoxyflurane:** This agent is the most potent inhalation anesthetic because of its high solubility in lipid. Prolonged administration of *methoxyflurane* [meth ox ee FLURE ane] is associated with the metabolic release of fluoride, which is toxic to the kidneys. Therefore, *methoxyflurane* is rarely used outside of obstetric practice. It finds use in child-birth because it does not relax the uterus when briefly inhaled.

5. **Nitrous oxide:** Whereas *nitrous oxide* [nye truss OX ide] (N_2O or "laughing gas") is a potent analgesic, it is a weak general anesthetic. Thus, it is frequently combined with other more potent agents. Because it moves very rapidly into and out of the body, *nitrous oxide* can increase the volume (pneumothorax) or pres-

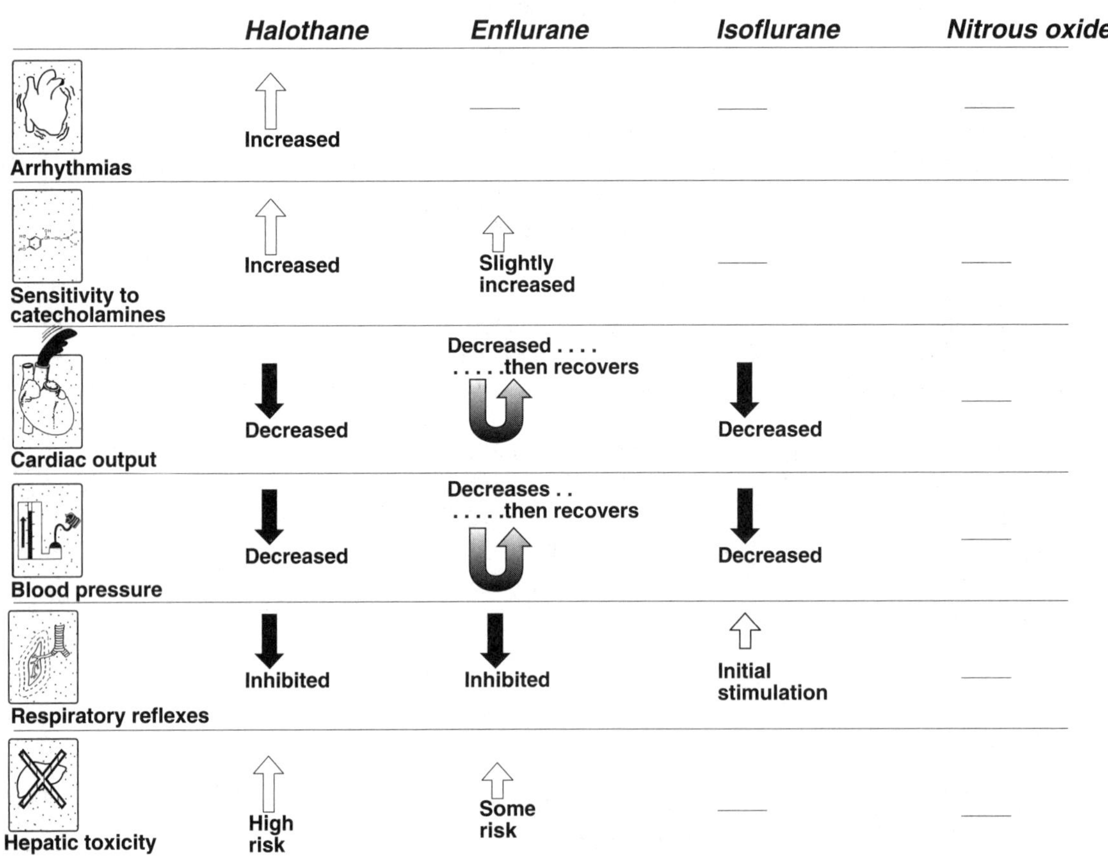

	Halothane	*Enflurane*	*Isoflurane*	*Nitrous oxide*
Arrhythmias	Increased	—	—	—
Sensitivity to catecholamines	Increased	Slightly increased	—	—
Cardiac output	Decreased	Decreased . . . . .then recovers	Decreased	—
Blood pressure	Decreased	Decreases . . . . . . .then recovers	Decreased	—
Respiratory reflexes	Inhibited	Inhibited	Initial stimulation	—
Hepatic toxicity	High risk	Some risk	—	—

Figure 11.7
Characteristics of some inhalation anesthetics.

sure (sinuses) within closed body compartments. Furthermore, its speed of movement allows *nitrous oxide* to retard oxygen uptake during recovery, thus causing diffusion hypoxia. This anesthetic does not depress respiration nor does it produce muscle relaxation. It also has the least effect on the cardiovascular system and on increasing cerebral blood flow, and is the least hepatotoxic of the inhalation anesthetics. It is therefore probably the safest of these anesthetics, provided that at least 20% oxygen is always administered at the same time. [Note: *Nitrous oxide* at 80% (without other adjunct agents) cannot produce surgical anesthesia.] *Nitrous oxide* is often employed at concentrations of 30% in combination with oxygen for analgesia, particularly in dental surgery.

6. **Sevoflurane:** This fluorocarbon has recently been approved for induction and maintenance of general anesthesia. *Sevoflurane* has low pungency, allowing rapid uptake without irritating the airway during induction and making it suitable for induction through a mask in children. The drug has low solubility in blood and shows a rapid uptake and excretion. Some characteristics of the inhaled anesthetics are summarized in Figure 11.7

V. INTRAVENOUS ANESTHETICS

Intravenous anesthetics are often used for the rapid induction of anesthesia, which is then maintained with an appropriate inhalation agent. They rapidly induce anesthesia, and must therefore be injected slowly. Recovery from intravenous anesthestics is due to redistribution from sites in the CNS.

A. Barbiturates

Thiopental (see p. 94) is a potent anesthetic and a weak analgesic. It is the most widely used intravenously administered general anesthetic. It is an ultra-short-acting barbiturate and has a high lipid solubility. When agents such as *thiopental*, *thiamylal* [thye AM i lal], and *methohexital* [meth oh HEX i tal] are administered intravenously, they quickly enter the CNS and depress function, often in less than 1 minute. However, diffusion out of the brain can occur very rapidly as well, because of redistribution of the drug to other body tissues, including skeletal muscle and ultimately adipose tissue (Figure 11.8). This latter site serves as a reservoir of drug from which the agent slowly leaks out and is metabolized and excreted. The short duration of anesthetic action is due to the decrease of its concentration in the brain to a level below that necessary to produce anesthesia. These drugs may remain in the body for relatively long periods of time after their administration, since only about 15% of the dose of barbiturate entering the circulation is metabolized by the liver per hour. Thus, metabolism of *thiopental* is much slower than tissue redistribution. The barbiturates are not significantly analgesic and require some type of supplementary analgesic administration during anesthesia, otherwise objectionable changes in blood pressure and autonomic function may ensue. *Thiopental* has minor effects on the

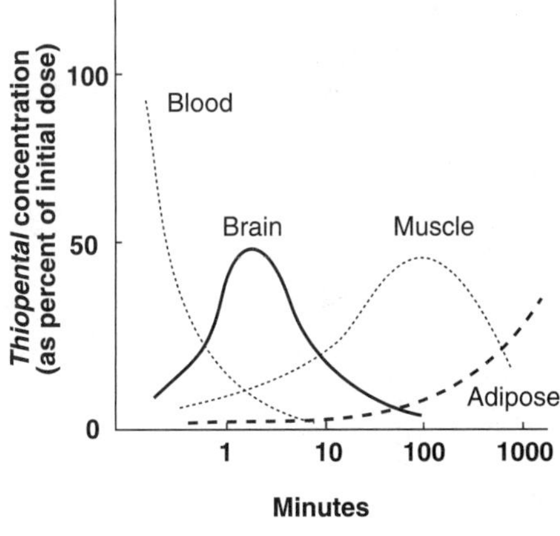

Figure 11.8
Redistribution of *thiopental* from brain to muscle and adipose tissue.

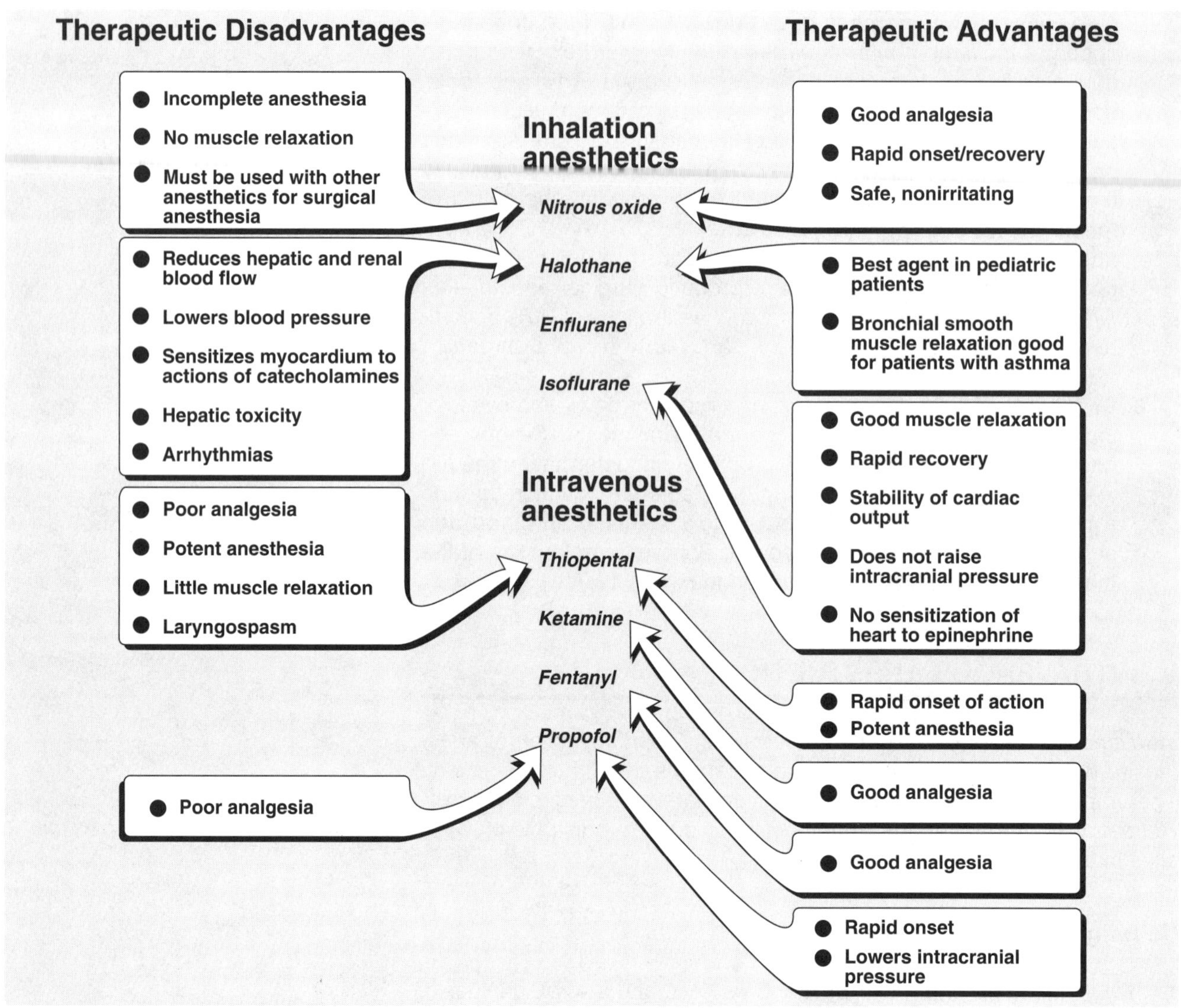

Figure 11.9
Therapeutic disadvantages and advantages of some anesthetic agents.

cardiovascular system, but it may contribute to severe hypotension in hypovolemic or shock patients. All barbiturates can cause apnea, coughing, chest wall spasm, laryngospasm, and bronchospasm; this is a concern for asthmatic patients. Barbiturates are contraindicated in patients with acute intermittent or variegate porphyria.

B. Benzodiazepines

Although *diazepam* (see p. 89) is the prototype benzodiazepine, *lorazepam* and *midazolam* are more potent. All three facilitate amnesia while causing sedation. *Etomidate* [e TOE mi date] is a hypnotic substance lacking analgesic properties that can cause uncontrolled skeletal muscle activity.

C. Opioids

Because of their analgesic property, opioids are frequently used together with other anesthetics; for example, the combination of *morphine* (see p. 135) and *nitrous oxide* provide good anesthesia for cardiac surgery. However, opioids are not good amnesics and they can all cause hypotension, respiratory depression, and muscle rigidity as well as postanesthetic nausea and vomiting. *Fentanyl* (see p. 139) is more frequently used than *morphine.* Opioid effects can be antagonized by *naloxone* (see p. 141).

D. Neuroleptanesthesia

The combination of *droperidol* and *fentanyl* is a fixed ratio preparation called INNOVAR. Since *droperidol* is a neuroleptic substance, INNOVAR is said to produce neurolept analgesia; if combined with a more potent anesthetic, INNOVAR produces neuroleptic anesthesia. A neuroleptic has adrenergic blocking as well as sedative, antiemetic, and anticonvulsant properties. Since INNOVAR can cause extrapyramidal muscle movements, it is contraindicated in Parkinson's patients.

E. Ketamine

Ketamine [KET a meen], a short-acting nonbarbiturate anesthetic, induces a dissociated state in which the patient appears awake but is unconscious and does not feel pain. This dissociative anesthesia provides sedation, amnesia, and immobility. *Ketamine* stimulates the central sympathetic outflow, which in turn, causes stimulation of the heart and increased blood pressure and cardiac output. It also increases plasma catecholamine levels and increases blood flow. *Ketamine* is therefore used when circulatory depression is undesirable. On the other hand, these effects mitigate against the use of *ketamine* in hypertensive or stroke patients. The drug is lipophilic and enters the brain circulation very quickly, but like the barbiturates, it can redistribute to other organs and tissues. It is metabolized in the liver, but small amounts can be excreted unchanged. *Ketamine* is employed mainly in children and young adults for short procedures, but it is not widely used, because it increases cerebral blood flow and induces postoperative hallucinations ("nightmares").

F. Propofol

Propofol [pro POF ol] is an IV sedative/hypnotic used in the induction or maintenance of anesthesia. Onset is smooth and occurs within about 40 seconds of administration. Supplemenation with narcotics for analgesia is required. While *propofol* facilitates depression in the CNS, high plasma levels can cause excitation. *Propofol* decreases blood pressure without depressing the myocardium. It also reduces intracranial pressure.

Some therapeutic advantages and disadvantages of the anesthetic agents are summarized in Figure 11.9.

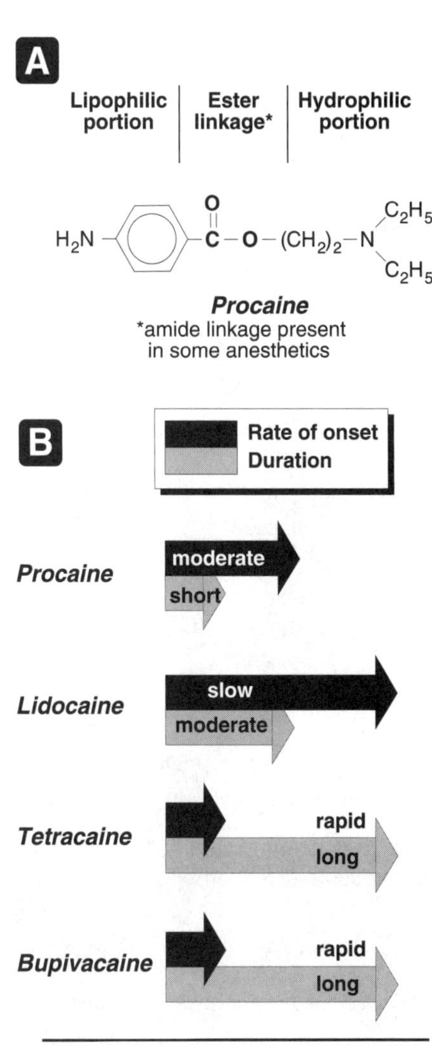

Figure 11.10
A. Structural formula of *procaine*.
B. Pharmacokinetic properties of local anesthetics.

VI. LOCAL ANESTHETICS

These drugs are applied locally and block nerve conduction of sensory impulses from the periphery to the CNS. Local anesthetics abolish sensation (and in higher concentrations, motor activity) in a limited area of the body without producing unconsciousness. They inhibit sodium channels of the nerve membrane. The small, unmyelinated nerve fibers, that conduct impulses for pain, temperature, and autonomic activity, are most sensitive to actions of local anesthetics. All of the local anesthetics consist of a hydrophilic amino group linked through a connecting group of variable length to a lipophilic aromatic residue (Figure 11.10). Both potency and toxicity of the local anesthetics increase as the connecting group becomes longer. Adverse effects result from systemic absorption of toxic amounts of the locally applied anesthetic. Seizures are the most significant of these systemic effects. By adding the vasoconstrictor *epinephrine* to the local anesthetic, the rate of absorption is decreased (see p. 63). This both minimizes systemic toxicity and increases the duration of action.

Study Questions

Questions 11.1 – 11.7

Given the following drugs:

A. Methoxyflurane
B. Succinylcholine
C. Diazepam
D. Halothane
E. Nitrous oxide
F. Thiopental
G. Innovar®
H. Ketamine
I. Etomidate
K. Isoflurane

Match the most appropriate anesthetic or adjunct from the list above with the following descriptions:

11.1 Acts at the neuromuscular junction to cause initial muscle excitation.

> Correct answer = B (Succinylcholine).

11.2 Contains tissue toxic bromide.

> Correct answer = D (Halothane).

11.3 Potent analgesic; weak anesthetic.

> Correct answer = E (Nitrous oxide).

11.4 Potent anesthetic; weak analgesic.

> Correct answer = F (Thiopental).

11.5 Drug combination producing neurolept analgesia.

> Correct answer = G (Innovar®).

11.6 Used solely in obstetric practice.

> Correct answer = A (Methoxyflurane).

11.7 Facilitates surgical amnesia.

> Correct answer = C (Diazepam).

Choose the ONE best answer

11.8 Which one of the following is most likely to require administration of a muscle relaxant?

A. Ethyl ether
B. Halothane
C. Methoxyflurane
D. Benzodiazepines
E. Nitrous oxide

> Correct answer = E. Nitrous oxide has virtually no muscle relaxing properties. Ether, methoxyflurane, and benzodiazepine produce good muscle relaxation; halothane produces moderate muscle relaxation.

Antidepressant Drugs

12

I. OVERVIEW

Major depresssion and bipolar disorder are pervasive mood altering illnesses affecting energy, sleep, appetite, libido and the ability to function. Depression is different from schizophrenia, which produces disturbances in thought. The symptoms of depression are intense feelings of sadness, hopelessness, despair, and the inability to experience pleasure in usual activities. Mania is characterized by the opposite behavior, that is, enthusiasm, rapid thought and speech patterns, and extreme self-confidence and impaired judgment. All clinically useful antidepressant drugs (also called thymoleptics) potentiate, either directly or indirectly, the actions of norepinephrine, dopamine, and/or serotonin in the brain. (See Figure 12.1 for a summary of the antidepressant agents.) This, along with other evidence, led to the biogenic amine theory, which proposes that depression is due to a deficiency of monoamines such as norepinephrine and serotonin at certain key sites in the brain. Conversely, mania is envisioned as caused by an overproduction of these neurotransmitters.The amine theory of depression is probably overly simplistic, since it is now known that the antidepressant drugs, particularly the tricyclic antidepressants, affect many biological systems in addition to neurotransmitter uptake. It is not known which of these neurochemical systems is most responsible for the antidepressant activity.

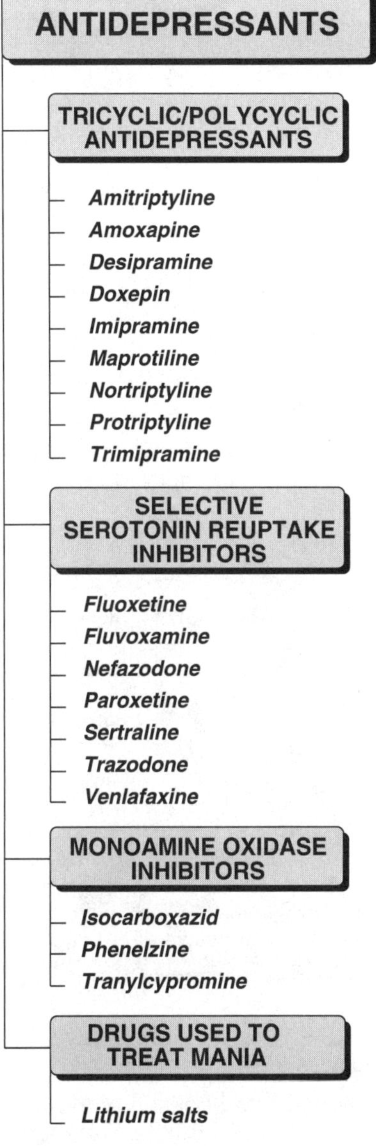

Figure 12.1
Summary of antidepressants.

II. TRICYCLIC/POLYCYCLIC ANTIDEPRESSANTS

The tricyclic and polycyclic antidepressants block norepinephrine, and serotonin uptake into the neuron. Prolonged therapy probably leads to alterations in selected central nervous system (CNS) receptors. The important drugs in this group are *imipramine* ([im IP ra meen], the prototype), *amitriptyline* [a mee TRIP ti leen], *desipramine* ([dess IP ra meen], a demethylated derivative of *imipramine*), *nortriptyline* [nor TRIP ti leen], *protriptyline* [proe TRIP te leen], and *doxepin* [DOX e pin]. *Amoxapine* [a MOX a peen] and *maprotiline* [ma PROE ti leen] are termed "second generation" to distinguish them from the older tricyclic antidepressants. [Note: These second generation drugs have actions similar to *imipramine*, although they exhibit slightly different pharmacokinetics.] All the tricyclic antidepressants (TCAs) have similar therapeutic efficacy, and the choice of drug depends on tolerance of side effects and duration of action. Patients who do not respond to one TCA may benefit from a different drug in this group.

Lippincott's Illustrated Reviews: Pharmacology, Second Edition.
by Mary J. Mycek, Richard A. Harvey and Pamela C. Champe.
Lippincott Williams & Wilkins, Philadelphia, PA © 2000.

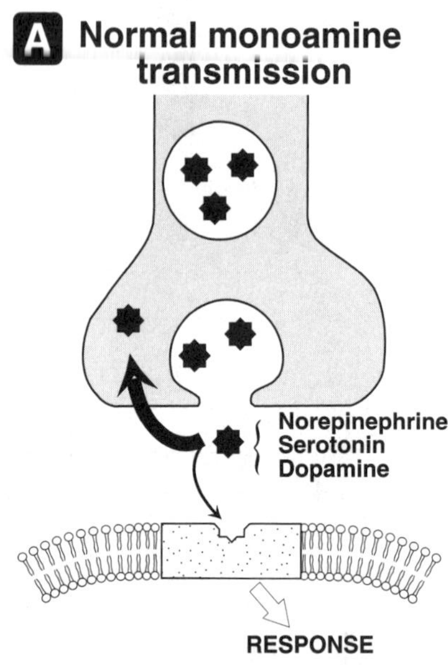

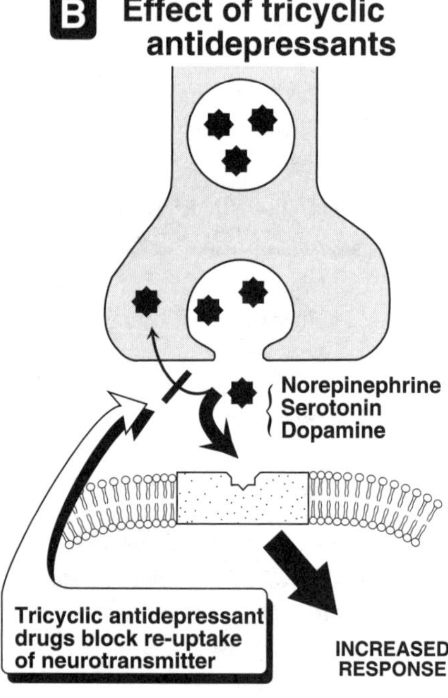

Figure 12.2
Mechanisms of action of tricyclic and polycyclic antidepressant drugs.

A. Mode of action

1. **Inhibition of neurotransmitter uptake:** TCAs inhibit the neuronal reuptake of norepinephrine, and serotonin into presynaptic nerve terminals (Figure 12.2). By blocking the major route of neurotransmitter removal, the TCAs lead to increased concentrations of monoamines in the synaptic cleft, resulting in antidepressant effects. This theory has been discounted by some because of several observations. For example, the potency of the TCA in blocking neurotransmitter uptake often does not correlate with clinically observed antidepressant effects. Further, blockade of reuptake of neurotransmitter occurs immediately after administration of the drug, but the antidepressant effect of the TCA requires several weeks of continued treatment. This suggests that decreased uptake of neurotransmitter is only an initial event that may not be related to the antidepressant effects. It has been suggested that monoamine receptor densities in the brain may change over a 2 to 4 week period with drug use and may be important in the onset of activity.

2. **Blocking of receptors:** The TCAs also block serotonergic, α-adrenergic, histamine, and muscarinic receptors (Figure 12.3). It is not known which, if any, of these accounts for the therapeutic benefit.

B. Actions

TCAs elevate mood, improve mental alertness, increase physical activity, and reduce morbid preoccupation in 50 to 70% of individuals with major depression. The onset of the mood-elevation is slow, requiring 2 weeks or longer (Figure 12.4). These drugs do not produce CNS stimulation or mood elevation in normal individuals. Tolerance to the anticholinergic properties of the TCAs develops within a short time. Some tolerance to the autonomic effects of TCAs develops. Physical and psychological dependence have been reported. The drugs can be used for prolonged treatment of depression without loss of effectiveness.

C. Therapeutic uses

The tricyclic antidepressants are effective in treating severe major depression. Some panic disorders also respond to TCAs. *Imipramine* has been used to control bed-wetting in children (older than 6 years) by causing contraction of the internal sphincter of the bladder. At present it is used cautiously, because of the inducement of cardiac arrhythmias and other serious cardiovascular problems.

D. Pharmacokinetics

1. **Absorption and distribution:** The TCAs are well absorbed upon oral administration, and because of their lipophilic nature, are widely distributed and readily penetrate into the CNS. This lipid solubility also causes these drugs to have long half-lives, for example, 4 to 17 hours for *imipramine*. As a result of their variable first pass metabolism in the liver, TCAs have low and inconsistent bioavailability. Therefore the patient's response is

DRUG	UPTAKE INHIBITION		RECEPTOR AFFINITIES		
	Norepinephrine	Serotonin	Muscarinic	Histaminergic	Adrenergic
Tricyclic antidepressant *Imipramine*	++	+++	++	+	+
Selective serotonin reuptake inhibitor *Fluoxetine*	0	++++	0	0	0

Figure 12.3
Relative receptor specificity of some antidepressant drugs.

used to adjust dosage. The initial treatment period is typically 4 to 8 weeks. The dosage can be gradually reduced unless relapse occurs.

2. **Fate:** These drugs are metabolized by the hepatic microsomal system (see p. 14) and conjugated with glucuronic acid. Ultimately, the TCAs are excreted as inactive metabolites via the kidney.

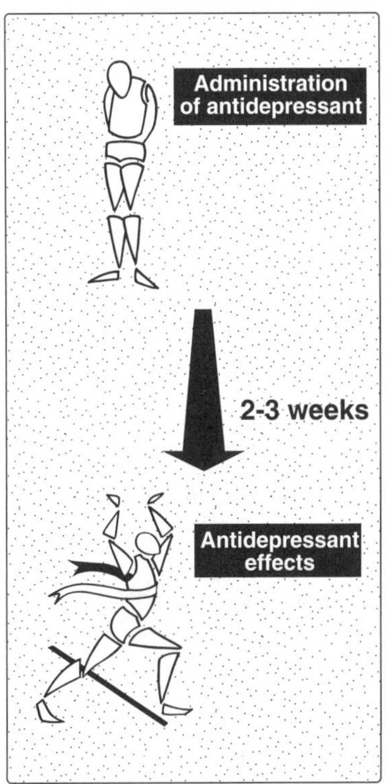

Figure 12.4
Onset of therapeutic effects of the major antidepressant drugs (tricyclic antidepressants, serotonin reuptake inhbitors, and monoamine oxidase inhibitors) requires several weeks.

E. Adverse effects

1. **Antimuscarinic effects:** Blockade of acetylcholine receptors leads to blurred vision, xerostomia (dry mouth), urinary retention, constipation, and aggravation of glaucoma and epilepsy.

2. **Cardiovascular:** Increased catecholamine activity results in cardiac overstimulation, which can be life-threatening if an overdose of one of the drugs is taken. The slowing of atrioventricular conduction among depressed elderly patients is of particular concern.

3. **Orthostatic hypotension:** TCAs block α-adrenergic receptors, causing orthostatic hypotension and reflex tachycardia. In clinical practice this is the most serious problem in the elderly.

4. **Sedation:** Sedation may be prominent, especially during the first several weeks of treatment.

5. **Precautions:** The tricyclic antidepressants should be used with caution in manic-depressive patients, since they may unmask manic behavior. The tricyclic antidepressants have a narrow therapeutic index; for example, 5 to 6 times the maximal daily dose of *imipramine* can be lethal. Depressed patients who are suicidal should be given only limited quantities of these drugs and should be monitored closely. Drug interactions with the tricyclic antidepressants are shown in Figure 12.5.

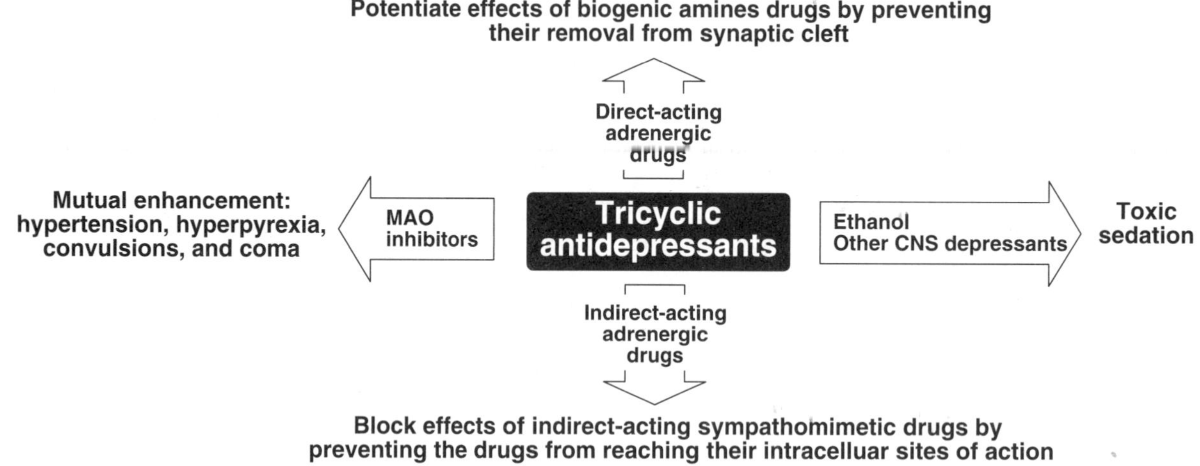

Figure 12.5
Drugs interacting with tricyclic antidepressants.

III. SELECTIVE SEROTONIN-REUPTAKE INHIBITORS

The selective serotonin-reuptake inhibitors (SSRI) are a new group of chemically unique antidepressant drugs that specifically inhibit serotonin reuptake (see Figure 12.3). This contrasts with the tricyclic antidepressants that nonselectively inhibit the uptake of norepinephrine, and serotonin, and block muscarinic, H_1-histaminic and α_1-adrenergic receptors. Compared with tricyclic antidepressants, the SSRIs cause fewer anticholinergic effects and lower cardiotoxicity. However, the newer serotonin reuptake inhibitors should be used cautiously until their long-term effects have been evaluated.

Neuroleptic drugs (for example, *haloperidol*)
Tricyclic antidepressants
Some β-adrenergic antagonists
Some antiarrhythmic drugs
P-450
Fluoxetine
Metabolites

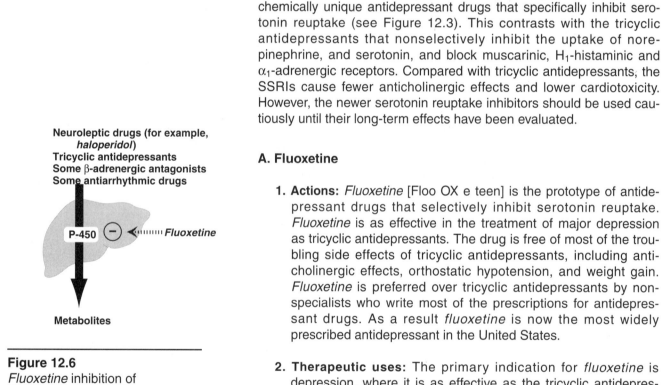

Figure 12.6
Fluoxetine inhibition of P-450 drug metabolism.

A. Fluoxetine

1. **Actions:** *Fluoxetine* [Floo OX e teen] is the prototype of antidepressant drugs that selectively inhibit serotonin reuptake. *Fluoxetine* is as effective in the treatment of major depression as tricyclic antidepressants. The drug is free of most of the troubling side effects of tricyclic antidepressants, including anticholinergic effects, orthostatic hypotension, and weight gain. *Fluoxetine* is preferred over tricyclic antidepressants by nonspecialists who write most of the prescriptions for antidepressant drugs. As a result *fluoxetine* is now the most widely prescribed antidepressant in the United States.

2. **Therapeutic uses:** The primary indication for *fluoxetine* is depression, where it is as effective as the tricyclic antidepressants. *Fluoxetine* is effective in treating bulimia nervosa and obsessive-compulsive disorder. The drug has been used for a variety of other indications, including anorexia nervosa, panic disorder, pain associated with diabetic neuropathy, and for premenstrual syndrome.

3. **Pharmacokinetics:** *Fluoxetine* is available therapeutically as a mixture of the R and the more active S enantiomers. Both com-

pounds are demethylated to the active metabolite, norfluoxetine. *Fluoxetine* and norfluoxetine are slowly cleared from the body, with a 1 to 10 day half-life for the parent compound, and 3 to 30 days for the active metabolite. *Fluoxetine* is administered orally; with a constant dose, a steady-state plasma concentration of the drug is achieved after several weeks of treatment. *Fluoxetine* is a potent inhibitor of a hepatic cytochrome P-450 isoenzyme responsible for the elimination of tricyclic antidepressant drugs, neuroleptic drugs, and some antiarrhythmic and β-adrenergic anatagonist drugs (Figure 12.6). [Note: About 7% of the white population lack this P-450 enzyme and therefore metabolize *fluoxetine* very slowly.]

4. **Adverse affects:** Commonly observed adverse effects of *fluoxetine* are summarized in Figure 12.7. Loss of libido, delayed ejaculation and anorgasmia are probably under-reported side effects often noted by clinicians but are not prominently featured in the list of standard side effects. Overdoses of *fluoxetine* do not cause cardiac arrhythmias but can cause seizures. For example, in a report of patients who took an overdose of *fluoxetine* (up to 1200 mg compared with 20 mg/day as a therapeutic dose) about half of the patients had no symptoms.

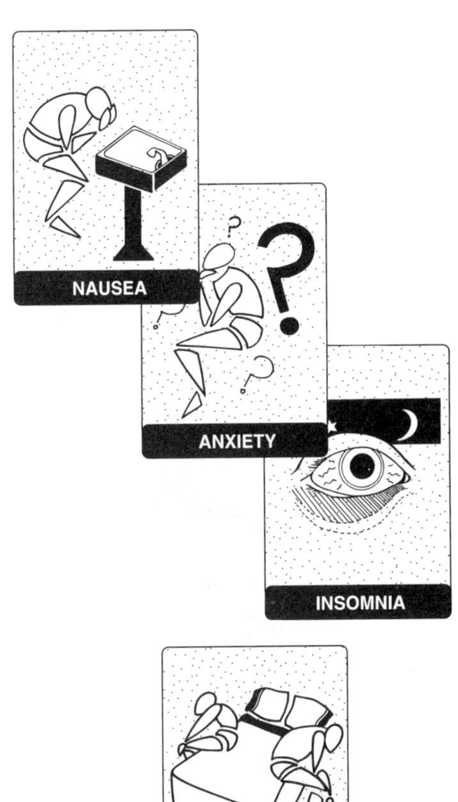

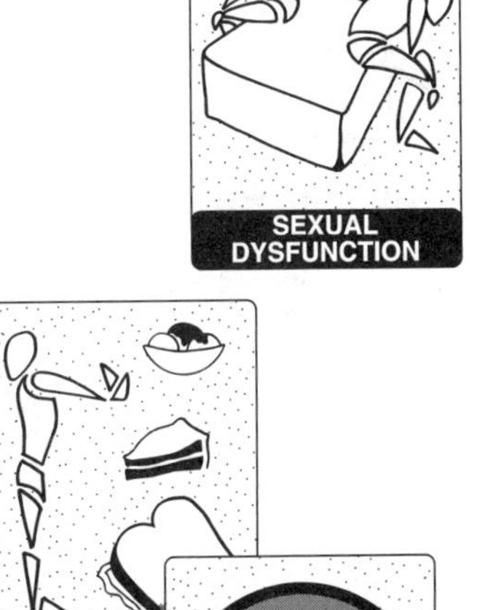

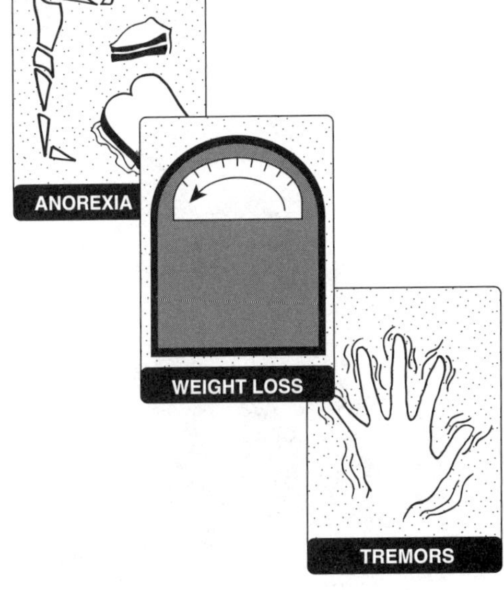

Figure 12.7
Some commonly oberved adverse effect of *fluoxetine*.

B. Other selective serotonin reuptake inhibitors

Other antidepressant drugs that primarily affect serotonin reuptake include *trazodone* [TRAZ oh done], *fluvoxamine* [floo VOX a meen], *nefazodone* [ne FAZ oh don], *paroxetine* [pah ROX a teen], *sertraline* [SIR trah leen], and *venlafaxine* [vin lah FACKS in]. These SSRIs differ from *fluoxetine* in their relative effects on the reuptake of serotonin and norepinephrine. They do not seem to be more efficacious than *fluoxetine,* but their profiles of side effects are somewhat different. There is a high variability among patients in the rate of elimintion of these drugs (including *fluoxetine*), and failure to tolerate one drug should not preclude a trial of another SSRI.

IV. MONOAMINE OXIDASE INHIBITORS

Monoamine oxidase (MAO) is a mitochondrial enzyme found in neural and other tissues, such as the gut and liver. In the neuron, MAO functions as a "safety valve" to oxidatively deaminate and inactivate any excess neurotransmitter molecules (norepinephrine, dopamine, and serotonin) that may leak out of synaptic vesicles when the neuron is at rest. The MAO inhibitors may irreversibly or reversibly inactivate the enzyme, permitting neurotransmitter molecules to escape degradation and therefore to both accumulate within the presynaptic neuron and to leak into the synaptic space. This causes activation of norepinephrine and serotonin receptors, and may be responsible for the antidepressant action of these drugs. Three MAO inhibitors are currently available for treatment of depression: *phenelzine* [FEN el zeen], *isocarboxazid* [eye soe kar BOX a zid], and *tranylcypromine* [tran ill SIP roe meen]; no one drug is a prototype. Use of MAO inhibitors is now limited because of the complicated dietary restrictions required of patients taking MAO inhibitors.

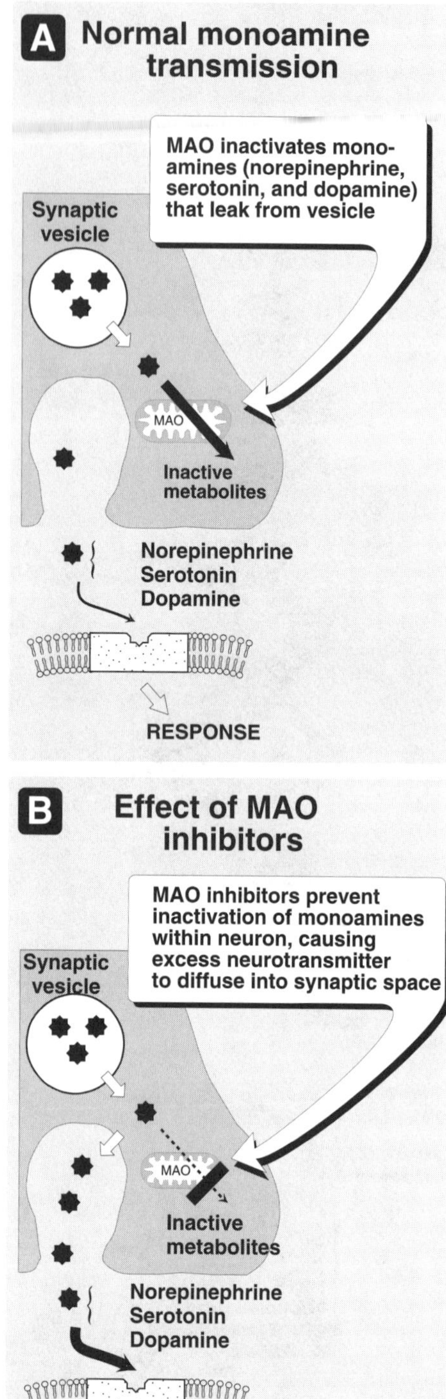

Figure 12.8
Mechanism of action of MAO inhibitors.

A. Mode of action

Most MAO inhibitors, such as *isocarboxazid*, form stable complexes with the enzyme, causing irreversible inactivation. This results in increased stores of norepinephrine, serotonin and dopamine within the neuron, and subsequent diffusion of excess neurotransmitter into the synaptic space (Figure 12.8).These drugs inhibit not only MAO in brain, but oxidases that catalyze oxidative deamination of drugs and potentially toxic substances, such as tyramine, which is found in certain foods. The MAO inhibitors therefore show a high incidence of drug-drug and drug-food interactions (see "Adverse effects").

B. Actions

Although MAO is fully inhibited after several days of treatment, the antidepressant action of the MAO inhibitors, like that of the TCAs (see p. 119), is delayed several weeks. *Phenelzine* and *tranylcypromine* have a mild amphetamine-like stimulant effect.

C. Therapeutic uses

MAO inhibitors are indicated for depressed patients who are unresponsive or allergic to tricyclic antidepressants or who experience strong anxiety. Patients with low psychomotor activity may benefit from the stimulant properties of MAO inhibitors. These drugs are also useful in the treatment of phobic states. A special subcategory of depression, called atypical depression, may respond to MAOIs. Atypical depresssion is characterized by labile mood, rejection sensitivity and appetite disorders.

D. Pharmacokinetics

These drugs are well absorbed on oral administration, but antidepressant effects require 2 to 4 weeks of treatment. Enzyme regeneration, when irreversibly inactivated, varies but usually occurs several weeks after termination of the drug. Thus, when switching antidepressant agents, a minimum of 2 weeks delay must be allowed after termination of MAO-inhibitor therapy. MAO inhibitors are metabolized and excreted rapidly in the urine.

E. Adverse effects

Severe and often unpredictable side effects limit the widespread use of MAO inhibitors. For example, tyramine, contained in certain foods, such as aged cheeses, chicken liver, beer, and red wines, is normally inactivated by MAO in the gut. Individuals receiving a MAO inhibitor are unable to degrade tyramine obtained from the diet. Tyramine causes the release of large amounts of stored catecholamines from nerve terminals, resulting in headache, tachycardia, nausea, hypertension, cardiac arrhythmias, and stroke. Patients must therefore be educated to avoid tyramine-containing foods. *Phentolamine* (see p. 72) or *prazosin* (see p. 73) are helpful in the management of tyramine-induced hypertension. [Note: Treatment with MAO inhibitors may be dangerous in severely depressed patients with suicidal tendencies. Purposeful consumption of tyramine-containing foods is a possibility.] Other possible side effects of treatment with MAO inhibitors include drowsiness, orthostatic hypotension, blurred vision, dryness of the mouth, dysuria, and constipation. MAO inhibitors and SSRIs should not be co-administered due to the risk of life-threatening "serotonin-syndrome". Both drugs require washout periods of 6 weeks before administering the other

V. LITHIUM SALTS

Lithium salts are used prophylactically in treating manic-depressive patients and in the treatment of manic episodes. They are also effective in treating 60 to 80% of patients exhibiting mania and hypomania. Although many cellular processes are altered by treatment with *lithium salts*, the mode of action is unknown. [Note: It is currently proposed that *lithium* acts by altering the cellular concentration of the second messenger, inositol triphosphate (IP_3), see p. 33).] *Lithium* is given orally, and the ion is excreted by the kidney. *Lithium salts* are very toxic. Their safety factor and therapeutic index are extremely low—comparable to those of *digitalis* (see p.161). Adverse effects include ataxia, tremors, confusion, and convulsions. *Lithium* causes no noticeable effect on normal individuals. It is not a sedative, euphoriant or depressant. Figure 12.9 summarizes the therapeutic disadvantages and advantages of the antidepressant drugs.

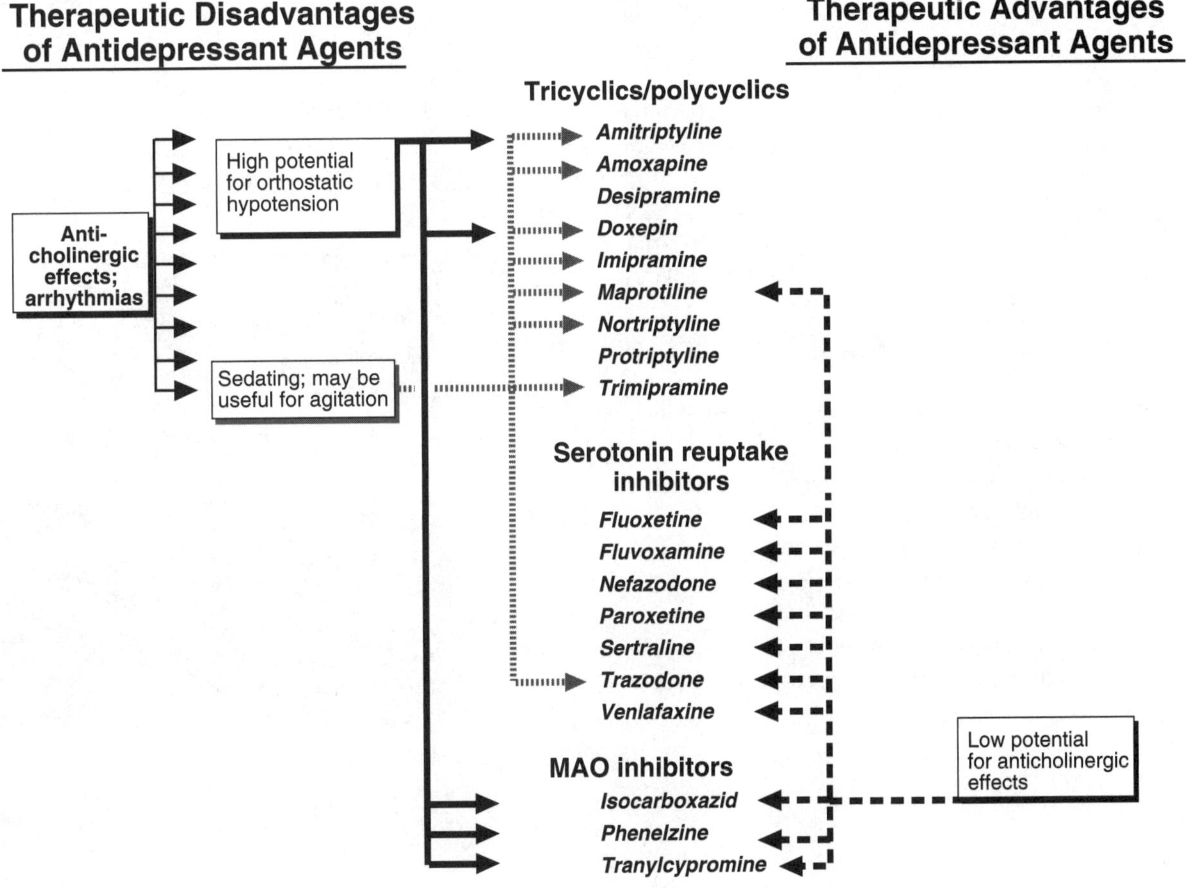

Figure 12.9
Therapeutic disadvantages and advantages of some drugs used to treat depression.

Choose the ONE best answer.

12.1 Which one of following is an appropriate therapeutic use for imipramine?

A. Insomnia
B. Epilepsy
C. Bed-wetting in children
D. Glaucoma
E. Mania

Correct answer = C. Imipramine can be used with caution to contract the internal sphincter of the bladder.

12.2 MAO inhibitors are contraindicated with all of the following EXCEPT:

A. indirect adrenergic agents, such as ephedrine.
B. tricyclic antidepressants.
C. beer and cheese.
D. aspirin.
E. dopamine.

Correct answer = D. MAO inhibitors and aspirin can be taken concurrently. Hypertensive crisis may result from use (concurrently or within 2 weeks) of MAO inhibitors and indirect sympathomimetic amines, such as ephedrine. Concomitant use of MAO inhibitors and tricyclic antidepressants may result in mutual enhancement of effects with the possibility of hyperpyrexia, hypertension, seizures and death. Tyramine-containing foods, such as aged cheeses and beer, may precipitate a hypertensive crisis because of the accumulation and release of stored catecholamines from nerve endings. MAO inhibitors may lead to an exaggerated response to dopamine.

12.3 Which of the following statements concerning tricyclic antidepressants is correct?

A. All of the tricyclic antidepressants show similar therapeutic efficacy.
B. Hypertension is a common adverse effect.
C. The tricyclic antidepressants selectively inhibit uptake of norepinephrine into the neuron.
D. These drugs show an immediate therapeutic effect.
E. These drugs must be administered intramuscularly.

Correct choice = A. The choice of tricyclic antidepressants depends on the tolerance of side effects and the desired duration of action. Orthostatic hypotension (not hypertension) is a side effect of the tricyclic drugs. The tricyclic antidepressants nonspecifically block the uptake of norepinephrine and serotonin; the onset of action requires 2 weeks or longer. These drugs are usually given orally.

12.4 Which of the following is common to the tricyclic antidepressants and MAO inhibitors?

A. They can produce sedation.
B. They produce physical dependence.
C. They show strong interaction with certain foods.
D. They can produce postural hypotension.
E. They decrease availability of epinephrine and serotonin in the synaptic cleft

Correct answer = D.

12.5 Which of the following antidepressant agents exhibits an amphetamine-like CNS stimulation?

A. Imipramine
B. Doxepin
C. Tranylcypromine
D. Trazodone
E. Lithium salts

Correct answer = C.

12.6 A very upset mother brings in her 10 year old son to ask help in dealing with his bed-wetting. Which of the following drugs might alleviate this problem?

A. Fluoxetine
B. Imipramine
C. Tranylcypromine
D. Trazodone

The correct answer = B The tricyclic antidepressants and especially imipramine are effective in this condition because it contracts the internal sphincter of the bladder. Fluoxetine and trazodone act at serotonin receptors and have no effect on bladder function. Tranylcypromine is an MAO inhibitor with serious side effects.

Neuroleptic Drugs

13

I. OVERVIEW

Neuroleptic drugs (also called antischizophrenic drugs, antipsychotic drugs, or major tranquilizers) are used primarily to treat schizophrenia but are also effective in other psychotic states, such as manic states and delirium. The traditional neuroleptic drugs are competitive inhibitors at a variety of receptors, but their antipsychotic effects reflect competitive blocking of dopamine receptors. These drugs vary in their potency, but no one drug is clinically more effective than another. In contrast, the newer "atypical" antipsychotic drugs appear to owe their unique activity to blockade of serotonin receptors. Therapy has tended toward the use of high potency drugs, such as *thiothixene* [thye oh THIX een], *haloperidol* [ha loe PER i dole], and *fluphenazine* [floo FEN a zeen]. *Chlorpromazine* [klor PROE ma zeen], the prototype of the neuroleptic agents, is used infrequently because of its high incidence of serious side effects. Neuroleptic drugs are not curative and do not eliminate the fundamental thinking disorder, but often do permit the psychotic patient to function in a supportive environment.

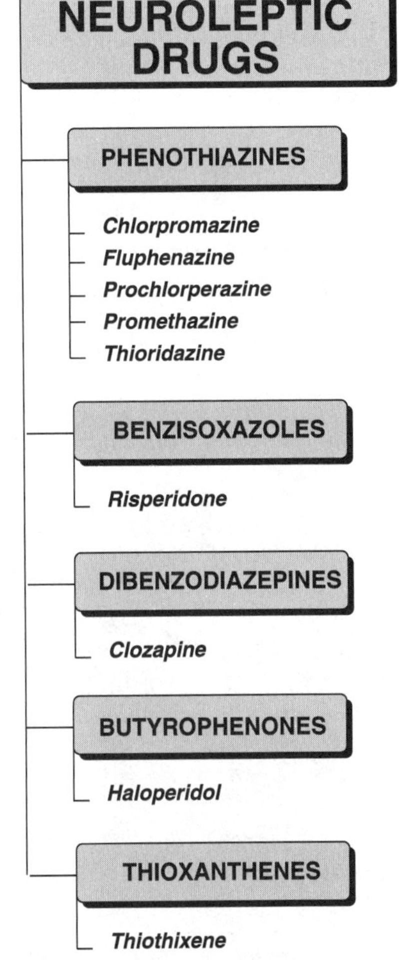

Figure 13.1
Summary of neuroleptic agents.

II. SCHIZOPHRENIA

Schizophrenia is a particular type of psychosis, that is, a mental disorder caused by some inherent dysfunction of the brain. It is characterized by delusions, hallucinations (often in the form of voices), and thinking or speech disturbances. This mental disorder is a common affliction, occurring among about 1% of the population, or at about the same incidence as diabetes mellitus. The illness often initially affects people during adolescence and is a chronic and disabling disorder. Schizophrenia has a strong genetic component and probably reflects some fundamental biochemical abnormality, possibly an overactivity of the mesolimbic dopaminergic neurons.

III. NEUROLEPTIC DRUGS

The neuroleptic drugs can be divided into five major classifications based on the structure of the drug (Figure 13.1). This classification is of modest importance, because within each chemical group, different side chains have profound effects on the potencies of the drugs. The management of

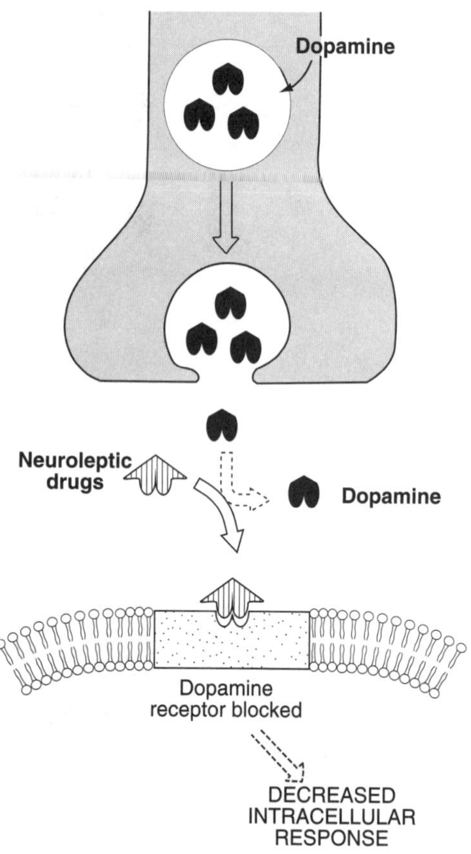

Figure 13.2
Dopamine-blocking actions of neuroleptic drugs.

psychotic disorders can typically be achieved by familiarity with the effects of one or two drugs in each class.

A. Mode of action

1. **Dopamine receptor-blocking activity in brain:** All of the neuroleptic drugs block dopamine receptors in the brain and in the periphery (Figure 13.2). Five types of dopamine receptors have been identified: D_1 and D_5 receptors activate adenylyl cyclase, whereas D2, D_3 and D_4 receptors inhibit adenylyl cyclase. The neuroleptic drugs bind to these receptors to varying degrees; however, the clinical efficacy of the traditional neuroleptic drugs correlates closely with their relative ability to block D_2 receptors in the mesolimbic system of the brain. The actions of the neuroleptic drugs are antagonized by agents that raise dopamine concentration, for example, *L-dopa* (see p. 84) and amphetamines (see p. 103).

2. **Serotonin receptor-blocking activity in brain:** The newer "atypical" agents appear to exert part of their unique action through inhibition of serotonin (S) receptors. Thus, *clozapine* [KLOE za peen] has high affinity for D_1 and D_4, S_2, muscarinic and α-adrenergic receptors, but it is also a dopamine D_2-receptor antagonist. Another new agent, *risperidone* [ris PEER i dohn], blocks S_2 receptors to a greater extent than it does D_2 receptors. Both of these drugs exhibit a low incidence of extrapyramidal side effects.

B. Actions

The antipsychotic actions of neuroleptic drugs reflect blockade at dopamine and/or serotonin receptors. However, many of these agents also block cholinergic, adrenergic, and histamine receptors, causing a variety of side effects (Figure 13.3).

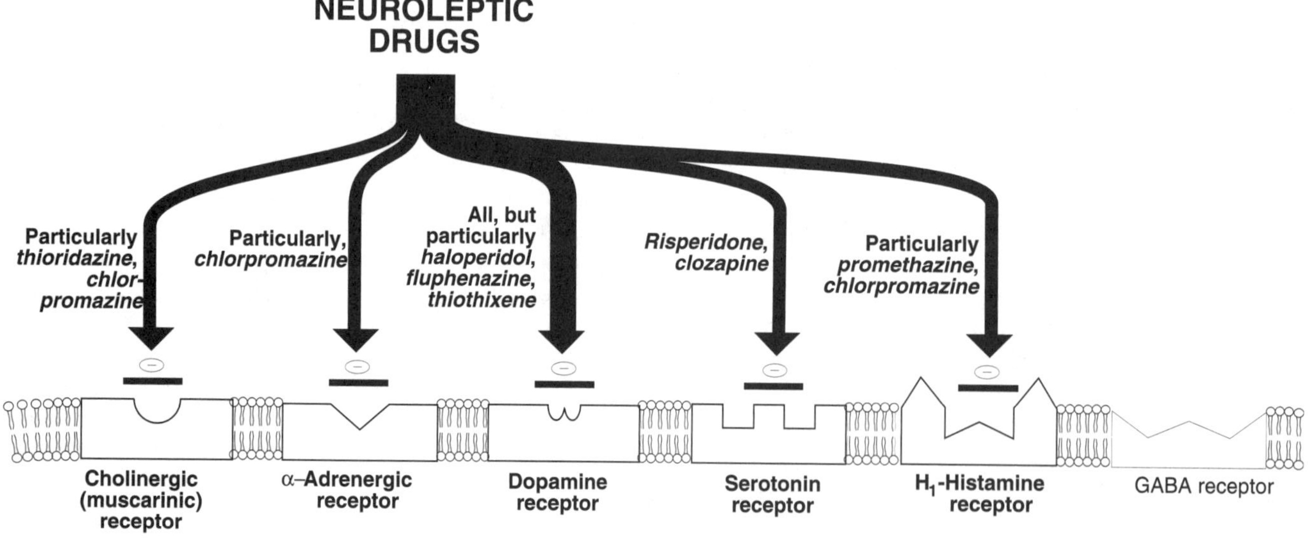

Figure 13.3
Neuroleptic drugs block at dopaminergic and serotonergic receptors as well as at adrenergic, cholinergic, and histamine-binding receptors. GABA = γ-aminobutyric acid.

1. **Antipsychotic actions:** The neuroleptic drugs reduce the hallucinations and agitation associated with schizophrenia by blocking dopamine receptors in the mesolimbic system of the brain. These drugs also have a calming effect and reduce spontaneous physical movement. In contrast to the central nervous system (CNS) depressants, such as barbiturates, the neuroleptics do not depress intellectual function of the patient, and motor incoordination is minimal. The antipsychotic effects usually take several weeks to occur, suggesting that the therapeutic effects are related to secondary changes in the corticostriatal pathways.

2. **Extrapyramidal effects:** Parkinsonian symptoms, akathisia (motor restlessness), and tardive dyskinesia (inappropriate postures of the neck, trunk, and limbs) occur with chronic treatment. Blocking of dopamine receptors in the nigrostriatal pathway probably causes these unwanted parkinsonian symptoms. *Clozapine* and *risperidone* exhibit a low incidence of these symptoms.

3. **Antiemetic effect:** With the exception of *thioridazine* [thye oh RID a zeen], most of the neuroleptic drugs have antiemetic effects that are mediated by blocking D_2 dopaminergic receptors of the chemoreceptor trigger zone of the medulla (see p. 241 for a discusssion of emesis). Figure 13.4 summarizes the antiemetic uses of neuroleptic agents, along with the therapeutic applications of other drugs that combat nausea.

4. **Antimuscarinic effects:** All of the neuroleptics, particularly *thioridazine* and *chlorpromazine*, cause anticholinergic effects, including blurred vision, dry mouth, sedation, confusion, and inhibition of gastrointestinal and urinary smooth muscle, leading to constipation and urinary retention.

5. **Other effects:** Blockade of α-adrenergic receptors causes orthostatic hypotension and lightheadedness. The neuroleptics also alter temperature-regulating mechanisms and can produce poikilothermia (body temperature varies with the environment). In the pituitary, neuroleptics block D_2 receptors, leading to an increase in prolactin release.

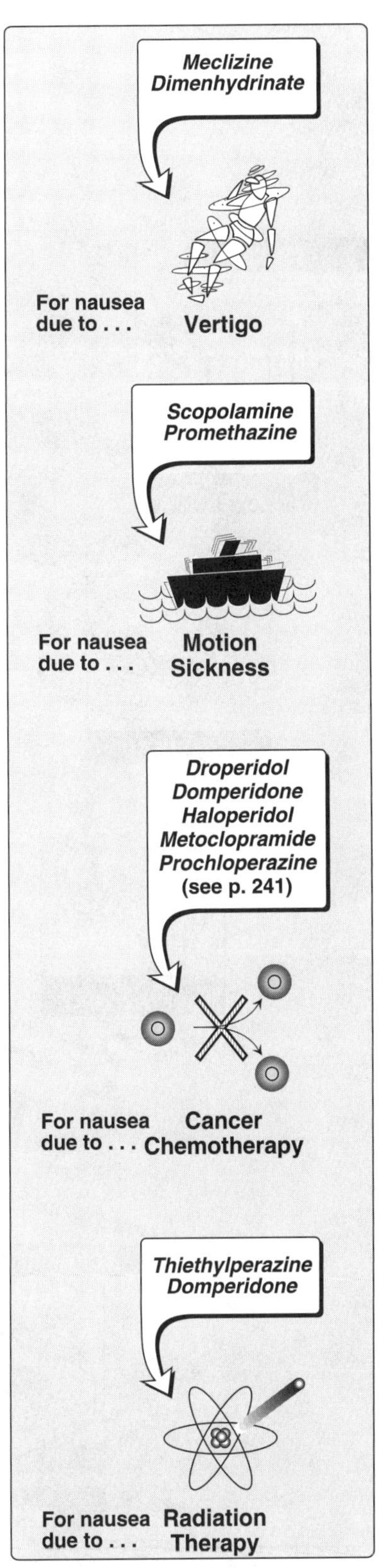

Figure 13.4
Therapeutic application of antiemetic agents.

C. Therapeutic uses

1. **Treatment of schizophrenia:** The neuroleptics are the only efficacious treatment for schizophrenia. Not all patients respond, and complete normalization of behavior is seldom achieved. The traditional neuroleptics are most effective in treating positive symptoms of schizophrenia (delusions, hallucinations and thought disorders). The newer agents with serotonin blocking activity are effective in many patients resistant to the traditional agents, especially in treating negative symptoms of schizophrenia (withdrawal, blunted emotions, reduced ability to relate to people).

2. **Prevention of severe nausea and vomiting:** The neuroleptics, (most commonly *prochlorperazine*), are useful in the treatment of drug-induced nausea (see p. 241). Nausea arising from emotion

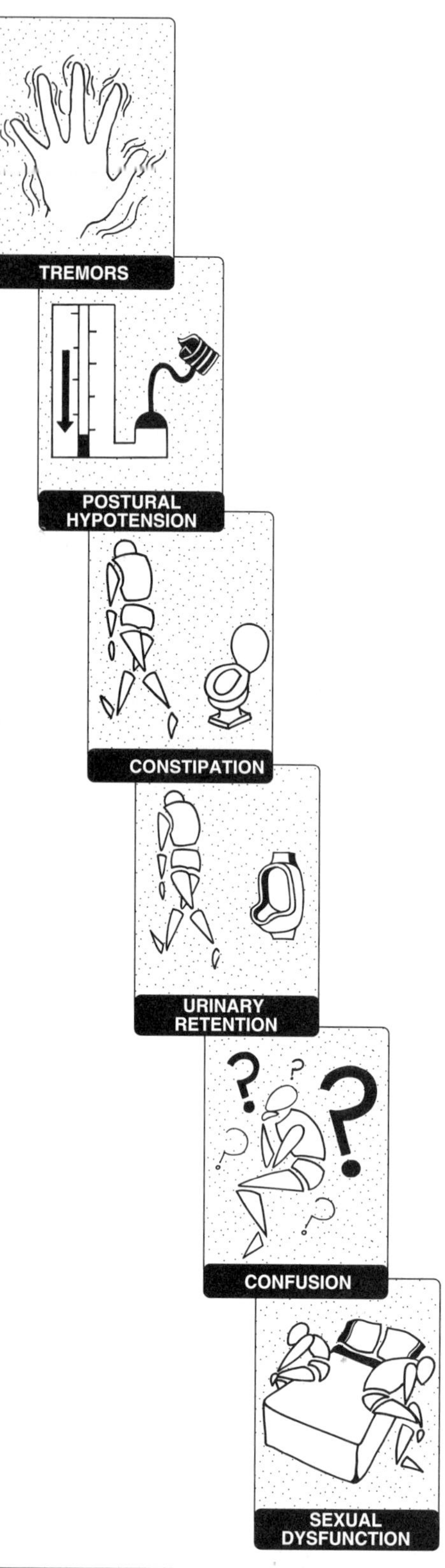

Figure 13.5
Adverse effects commonly observed in individuals treated with neuroleptic drugs.

should be treated with sedatives and antihistamines, rather than with these powerful drugs. *Scopolamine* (see p. 48) is the drug of choice for treatment of motion sickness.

3. **Other uses:** The neuroleptic drugs may be used as tranquilizers to manage agitated and disruptive behavior. Neuroleptics are used in combination with narcotic analgesics for treatment of chronic pain with severe anxiety. *Chlorpromazine* is used to treat intractable hiccups. *Droperidol* [droe PER i dole] is a component of neuroleptanesthesia (see p. 117). *Promethazine* [proe METH a zeen] is not a good antipsychotic drug, but the agent is used in treating pruritus because of its antihistaminic properties (see p. 422).

D. Absorption and metabolism

The neuroleptics show variable absorption after oral administration. These agents readily pass into the brain, have a large volume of distribution, bind well to plasma proteins, and are metabolized to many different substances by the P-450 system in the liver. *Fluphenazine decanoate* and *haloperidol decanoate* are slow release (up to 3 weeks) formulations of neuroleptics, administered by intramuscular injection. These drugs are increasingly used in treating outpatients and individuals who are noncompliant. However, about 30% of these patients develop extrapyramidal symptoms. The neuroleptic drugs produce some tolerance but little physical dependence.

E. Adverse effects

Adverse effects of the neuroleptic drugs occur in practically all patients and are significant in about 80% (Figure 13.5). Although antipsychotic drugs have an array of adverse effects, their therapeutic index is high.

1. **Parkinsonian effects:** The inhibitory effects of dopaminergic neurons are normally balanced by the excitatory actions of cholinergic neurons. Blocking dopamine receptors alters this balance, causing a relative excess of cholinergic influence and resulting in extrapyramidal motor effects.

   a. **Effect of anticholinergic drugs:** If cholinergic activity is also blocked, a new, more nearly normal balance is restored, and extrapyramidal effects are minimized. This can be achieved by administration of an anticholinergic drug, such as *benztropine*. The therapeutic tradeoff is fewer extrapyramidal effects in exchange for the side effects of parasympathetic blockade. [Note: Often, the parkinsonian actions persist, despite the anticholinergic drugs.] Those drugs that exhibit strong anticholinergic activity, such as *thioridazine*, show few extrapyramidal disturbances, since the cholinergic activity is strongly dampened. This contrasts with *haloperidol* and *fluphenazine*, which have low anticholinergic activity and produce extrapyramidal effects because of the preferential blocking of dopaminergic transmission without the blocking of cholinergic activity.

b. **Clozapine and risperidone:** These drugs have a low potential for causing extrapyramidal symptoms and lower risk of tardive dyskinesia. These drugs appear to be superior to *haloperidol* and *chlorpromazine* in treating the symptoms of schizophrenia, especially the negative symptoms. *Risperidone* should be included among the first-line antipsychotic drugs, whereas *clozapine* should be reserved for severely schizophrenic patients who are refractory to traditional therapy. *Clozapine* can produce bone marrow suppression and cardiovascular side effects. The risk of severe agranulocytosis necessitates frequent monitoring of white blood cell count. Figure 13.6 summarizes the receptor-binding properties of *clozapine*, *chlorpromazine*, and *haloperidol*.

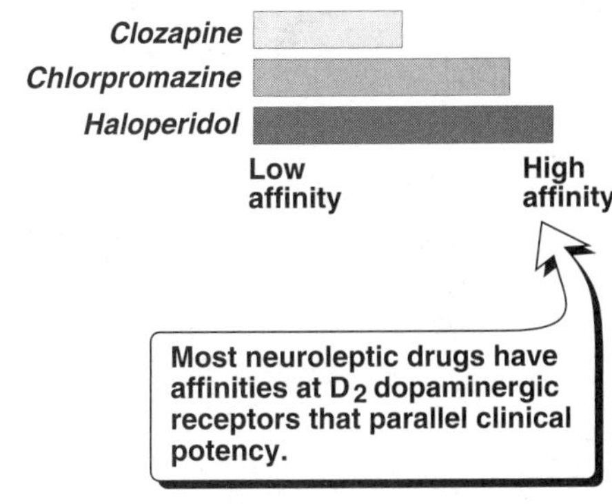

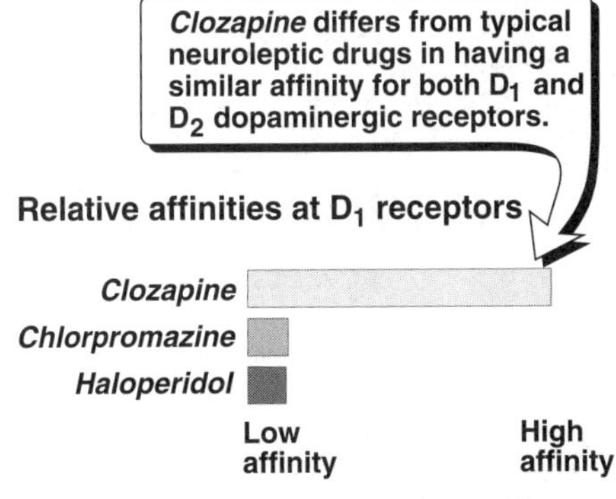

Figure 13.6
Relative affinity of *clozapine, chlorpromazine* and *haloperidol* at D_1 and D_2 dopaminergic receptors

2. **Tardive dyskinesia:** Long-term treatment with neuroleptics can cause this motor disorder. Patients display involuntary movements, including lateral jaw movements and "fly-catching" motions of the tongue. A prolonged holiday from neuroleptics may cause the symptoms to diminish or disappear within 3 months. However, in many individuals, dyskinesia is irreversible and persists after discontinuation of therapy. Tardive dyskinesia is postulated to result from an increased number of dopamine receptors that are synthesized in response to long-term dopamine receptor blockade. This makes the neuron supersensitive to the actions of dopamine and allows the dopaminergic input to this structure to overpower the cholinergic input, causing excess movement in the patient.

3. **Other effects:** Drowsiness occurs due to CNS depression, usually during the first 2 weeks of treatment. Confusion is sometimes encountered.The neuroleptics often produce dry mouth, urinary retention, constipation, and loss of accommodation. They block α-adrenergic receptors, resulting in lowered blood pressure and orthostatic hypotension. The neuroleptics depress the hypothalamus, causing amenorrhea, galactorrhea, infertility, and impotence.

4. **Cautions and contraindications:** Acute agitation accompanying withdrawal from alcohol or other drugs may be aggravated by the neuroleptics. Stabilization with a simple sedative, such as a benzodiazepine (see p. 89), is the preferred treatment. *Chlorpromazine* is contraindicated in patients with seizure disorders, since this drug can lower seizure threshold. The neuroleptics can also aggravate epilepsy. The high incidence of agranulocytosis with *clozapine* may limit its use to patients resistant to other drugs.

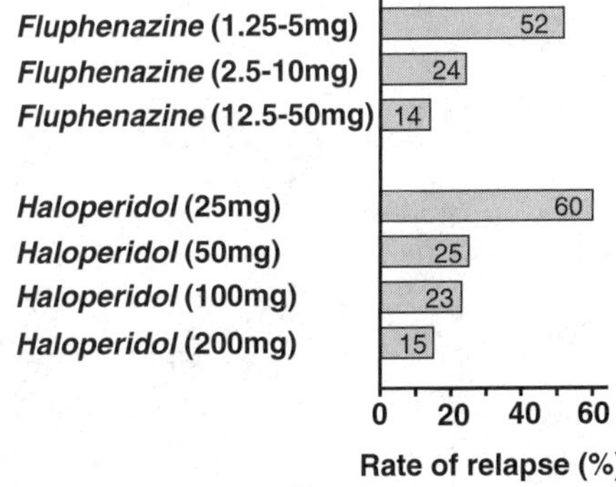

Figure 13.7
Cumulative rates of relapse among patients with schizophrenia after one year of maintenance therapy with either *fluphenazine* or *haloperidol*.

F. Maintenance treatment

Patients who have had two or more schizophrenic episodes should receive maintenance therapy for at least five years, and some experts prefer indefinite therapy. Low doses of antipsychotic drugs are not as effective in preventing relapse as higher dose maintenance therapy (Figure 13.7). Figure 13.8 summarizes the therapeutic uses of the neuroleptic drugs.

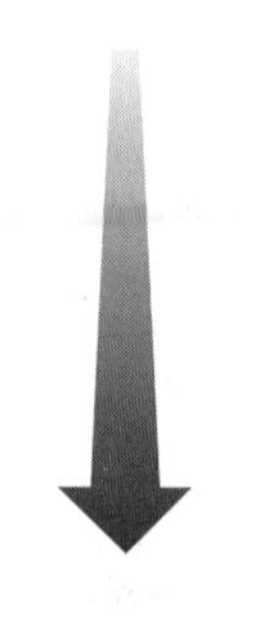

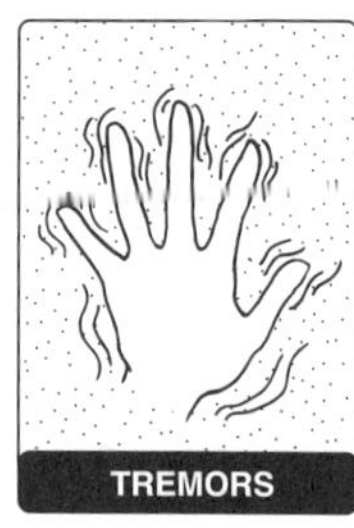

Drug	Therapeutic notes
Haloperidol	Little adrenergic or muscarinic activity. Available as slow release depot form
Fluphenazine	Available as slow release depot form
Thiothixene	
Thioridazine	Strong muscarinic antagonist
Chlorpromazine	Used infrequently because of adverse effects
Clozapine	Few extrapyramidal effects; causes a potentially fatal agranulcytosis in 1-2% of patients.
Risperidone	Minimal sedation, low potential for extrapyramidal effects.

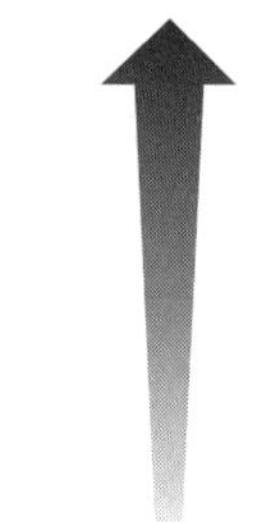

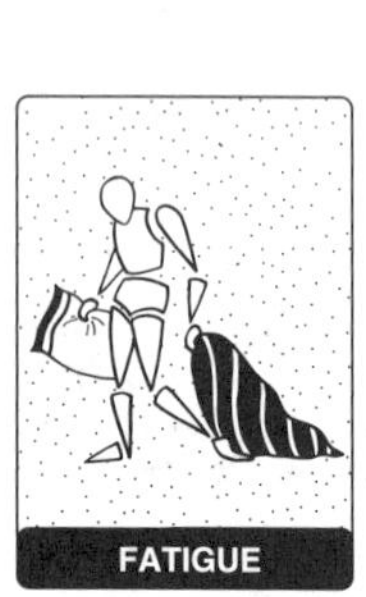

Sedation and cardiovascular effects commonly seen with agents in the lower portion of table

Parkinsonian effects commonly seen with agents in the upper portion of table

Figure 13.8
Summary of neuroleptic agents.

Study Questions

Choose the ONE best answer.

13.1 The neuroleptic drugs:

A. are equally effective against the positive and negative symptoms of schizophrenia.
B. can cause blurred vision, urinary retention and other signs of muscarinic blockade.
C. bind selectively to D_2-dopaminergic receptors.
D. have antiparkinsonism effects similar to levodopa.
E. have a rapid onset of antipsychotic action.

> Correct answer = B. The traditional neuroleptics are most effective in treating positive symptoms of schizophrenia (delusions, hallucinations and thought disorders). The newer agents with serotonin blocking activity are effective in many patients resistant to the traditional agents, especially in treating negative symptoms of schizophrenia (withdrawal, blunted emotions, reduced ability to relate to people). Most of the neuroleptic drugs block both D_1 and D_2 dopaminergic receptors. Most neuroleptic drugs cause parkinsonism effects. The antipsychotic effects occur after several weeks of administration.

13.2 All of the following statements about the extrapyramidal effects of neuroleptics are correct EXCEPT:

A. They are caused by blockade of dopamine receptors.
B. They are less likely to be produced by clozapine than by fluphenazine.
C. They can be countered to some degree by antimuscarinic drugs.
D. Haloperidol does not cause extrapyramidal disturbances.
E. Neuroleptics may cause tardive dyskinesia.

> Correct choice = D. Tardive dyskinesia appears to be produced to the same degree and frequency by all the neuroleptic drugs when used in equieffective antipsychotic doses.

13.3 All of the following are observed in patients taking neuroleptic agents EXCEPT:

A. sexual dysfunction.
B. increased blood pressure.
C. altered endocrine function.
D. constipation.
E. orthostatic hypotension.

> Correct choice = B. The neuroleptics block α-adrenergic receptors resulting in lowered blood pressure and orthostatic hypotension.

Opioid Analgesics and Antagonists

14

I. OVERVIEW

Opioids are natural or synthetic compounds that produce morphine-like effects. The term opiates is reserved for drugs, such as *morphine* and *codeine*, obtained from the juice of the opium poppy. All drugs in this category act by binding to specific opioid receptors in the central nervous system (CNS) to produce effects that mimic the action of endogenous peptide neurotransmitters, the opiopeptins (for example, the endorphins, and the enkephalins). Although the opioids have a broad range of effects, their primary use is to relieve intense pain and the anxiety that accompanies it, whether it be from surgery or as a result of injury or a disease, such as cancer. However, their widespread availability has led to abuse of those opioids with euphoric properties. Antagonists that can reverse the actions of opioids are also very important clinically in cases of overdose. (See Figure 14.1 for a summary of the opioid agonists and antagonists.)

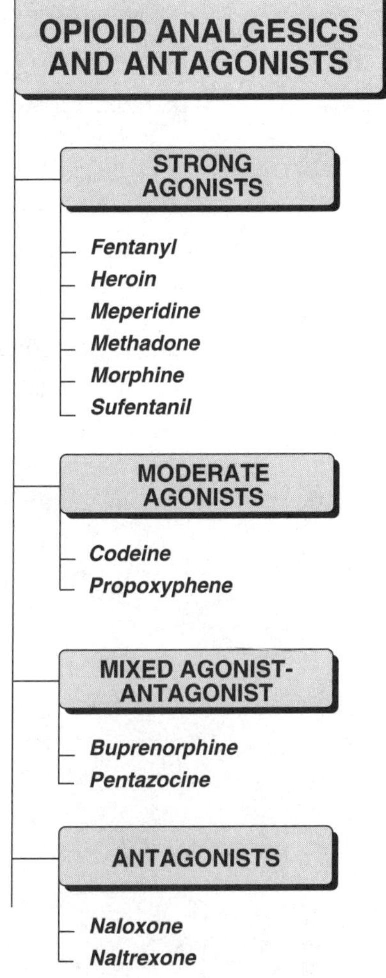

OPIOID ANALGESICS AND ANTAGONISTS
STRONG AGONISTS
Fentanyl
Heroin
Meperidine
Methadone
Morphine
Sufentanil
MODERATE AGONISTS
Codeine
Propoxyphene
MIXED AGONIST-ANTAGONIST
Buprenorphine
Pentazocine
ANTAGONISTS
Naloxone
Naltrexone

Figure 14.1
Summary of opioid analgesics and antagonists.

II. OPIOID RECEPTORS

Opioids interact stereospecifically with protein receptors on the membranes of certain cells in the CNS, on nerve terminals in the periphery, and on cells of the gastrointestinal tract. The major effects of the opioids are mediated by 4 families of receptors, designated by the Greek letters, μ, κ, σ and δ, each of which exhibits a different specificity for the drug(s) it binds (Figure 14.2). In general, binding potency correlates with analgesia. The analgesic properties of the opioids are primarily mediated by the μ receptors; however, the κ receptors in the dorsal horn also contribute. The enkephalins interact more selectively with the δ receptors in the periphery. Other receptors for the opioids, such as the σ receptor, have been shown to be less specific; for example, the σ receptor also binds nonopioid agents, such as the hallucinogen *phencyclidine* (see p. 105). The σ receptor may be responsible for the hallucinations and dysphoria sometimes associated with opioids. [Note: *Naloxone* [nal OX own] does not antagonize binding at this receptor as it does at the others.] All opioid receptors are coupled to inhibitory G proteins, and inhibit adenylyl cyclase. They may also be associated with ion channels to increase K^+ efflux (hyperpolarization) or reduce Ca^{++} influx, thus impeding neuronal firing and transmitter release.

Lippincott's Illustrated Reviews: Pharmacology, Second Edition.
by Mary J. Mycek, Richard A. Harvey and Pamela C. Champe.
Lippincott Williams & Wilkins, Philadelphia, PA © 2000.

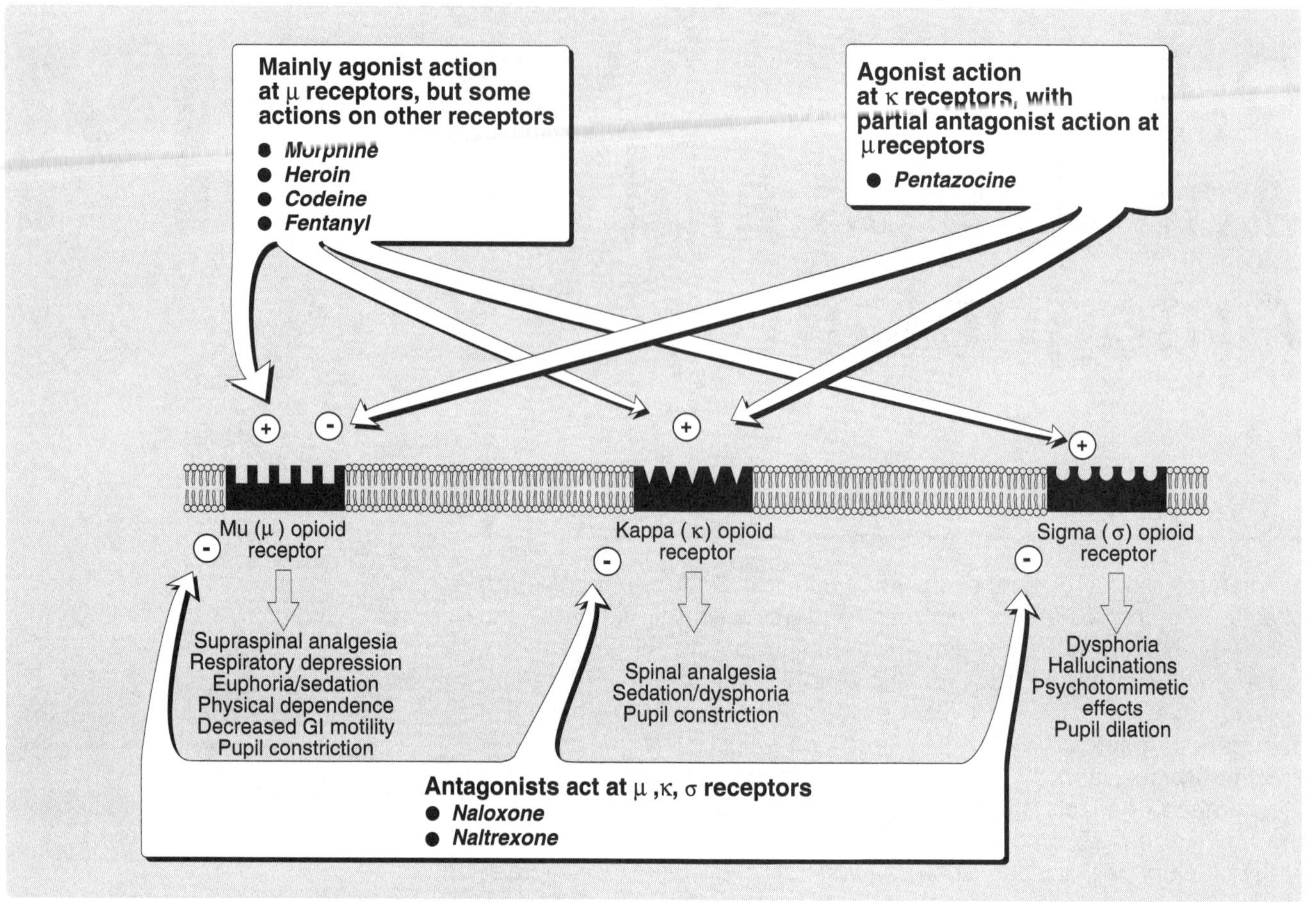

Figure 14.2
Actions of agonists and antagonists at opioid receptors.

A. Distribution of receptors

High densities of opioid receptors are present in five general areas of the CNS known to be involved in integrating information about pain. These pathways descend from the periacqueductal gray (PAG) through the dorsal horn of the spinal cord. They have also been identified in the periphery.

1. **Brainstem:** Opioid receptors mediate respiration, cough, nausea and vomiting, maintenance of blood pressure, pupillary diameter, and control of stomach secretions.

2. **Medial thalamus:** This area mediates deep pain that is poorly localized and emotionally influenced.

3. **Spinal cord:** Receptors in the substantia gelatinosa are involved with the receipt and integration of incoming sensory information, leading to the attenuation of painful afferent stimuli.

4. **Hypothalamus:** Receptors here affect neuroendocrine secretion.

5. **Limbic system:** The greatest concentration of opiate receptors in the limbic system is located in the amygdala. These receptors probably do not exert analgesic action, but they may influence emotional behavior.

6. **Periphery:** Opioids also bind to peripheral sensory nerve fibers and their terminals. As in the CNS, they inhibit Ca^{++}-dependent release of excitatory, proinflammatory substances (for example, substance P) from these nerve endings. It has been suggested that this may contribute to the antiinflammatory effects of opioids.

7. **Immune cells:** Opioid-binding sites have also been found on immune cells. The role of these receptors in nociception (response or sensitivity to painful stimuli) has not been determined.

III. STRONG AGONISTS

Morphine [MOR feen] is the major analgesic drug contained in crude opium and is the prototype agonist. *Codeine* [KOE deen] is present in lower concentrations and is inherently less potent. These drugs show a high affinity for μ receptors, varying affinities for δ and κ receptors, and low affinity for σ receptors.

A. Morphine

1. **Mechanism of action:** Opioids exert their major effects by interacting with opioid receptors in the CNS and the gastrointestinal tract. Opioids cause hyperpolarization of nerve cells, inhibition of nerve firing, and presynaptic inhibition of transmitter release. *Morphine* acts at μ receptors in lamina I and II of the substantia gelatinosa of the spinal cord, and decreases the release of substance P, which modulates pain perception in the spinal cord. *Morphine* also appears to inhibit the release of many excitatory transmitters from nerve terminals carrying nociceptive (painful) stimuli.

2. **Actions:**

   a. **Analgesia:** *Morphine* causes analgesia (relief of pain without the loss of consciousness). Opioids relieve pain both by raising the pain threshold at the spinal cord level, and more importantly, by altering the brain's perception of pain. Patients treated with *morphine* are still aware of the presence of pain, but the sensation is not unpleasant. The maximum analgesic efficacy and the potential for addiction for representative agonists is shown in Figure 14.3.

   b. **Euphoria:** *Morphine* produces a powerful sense of contentment and well-being. Euphoria may be caused by stimulation of the ventral tegmentum.

   c. **Respiration:** *Morphine* causes respiratory depression by reduction of the sensitivity of respiratory center neurons to carbon dioxide. This occurs with ordinary doses of *morphine* and

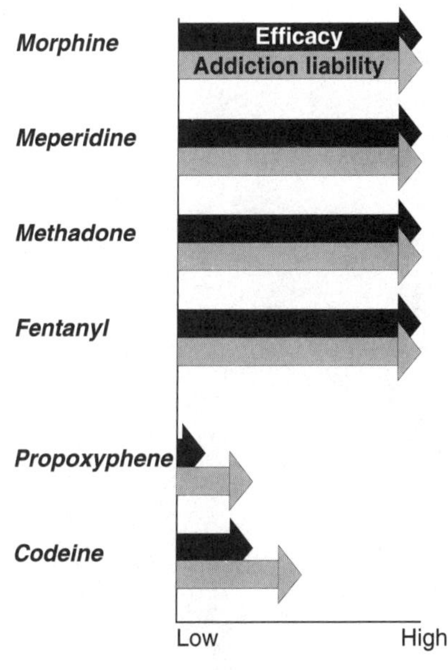

Figure 14.3
A comparison of the maximum efficacy and addiction/abuse liability of commonly used narcotic analgesics.

is accentuated as the dose increases until, ultimately, respiration ceases. Respiratory depression is the most common cause of death in acute opioid overdose.

d. **Depression of cough reflex:** *Morphine* and *codeine* have antitussive properties. In general, cough suppression does not correlate closely with analgesic and respiratory depressant properties of opioid drugs. The receptors involved in the antitussive action appear to be different than those involved in analgesia.

e. **Miosis:** The pinpoint pupil, characteristic of *morphine* use, results from stimulation of μ and κ receptors. *Morphine* excites the Edinger-Westphal nucleus of the oculomotor nerve, which causes enhanced parasympathetic stimulation to the eye. There is little tolerance to the effect, and all addicts demonstrate pin-point pupils. This is important diagnostically, because most other causes of coma and respiratory depression produce dilation of the pupil.

f. **Emesis:** *Morphine* directly stimulates the chemoreceptor trigger zone in the area postrema that causes vomiting. However, the emesis does not produce unpleasant sensations.

g. **Gastrointestinal tract:** *Morphine* relieves diarrhea and dysentery. It decreases motility of smooth muscle and increases tone. It increases pressure in the biliary tract. *Morphine* also increases the tone of the anal sphincter. Overall, *morphine* produces constipation, with little tolerance developing.

h. **Cardiovascular:** *Morphine* has no major effects on the blood pressure or heart rate except at large doses, when hypotension and bradycardia may occur. Because of respiratory depression and carbon dioxide retention, cerebral vessels dilate and increase the cerebrospinal fluid (CSF) pressure. Therefore, *morphine* is usually contraindicated in individuals with severe brain injury.

i. **Histamine release:** *Morphine* releases histamine from mast cells, causing urticaria, sweating, and vasodilation. Because it can cause bronchoconstriction, asthmatics should not receive the drug.

j. **Hormonal actions:** *Morphine* inhibits release of gonadotropin-releasing hormone and corticotropin-releasing hormone and decreases the concentration of luteinizing hormone, follicle-stimulating hormone, adrenocorticotropic hormone, and β-endorphin. Testosterone and cortisol levels decrease. *Morphine* increases prolactin and growth hormone release by diminishing dopaminergic inhibition. It increases antidiuretic hormone (ADH) and thus leads to urinary retention.

3. Therapeutic uses:

a. Analgesia: Despite intensive research, few other drugs have been developed that are as effective in the treatment of pain. Opioids induce sleep, and in clinical situations when pain is present and sleep is necessary, opiates may be used to supplement the sleep-inducing properties of benzodiazepines, such as *flurazepam* (see p. 89) [Note: The sedative-hypnotic drugs are not usually analgesic, and may have diminished sedative effect in the presence of pain.]

b. Treatment of diarrhea: *Morphine* decreases the motility of smooth muscle and increases tone.

c. Relief of cough: *Morphine* suppresses the cough reflex; however, *codeine* or *dextromethorphan* (see p. 222) are more widely used. *Codeine* has greater antitussive action than *morphine*.

4. Pharmacokinetics:

a. Administration: Absorption of *morphine* from the gastrointestinal tract is slow and erratic, and the drug is usually not given orally. *Codeine*, by contrast, is well absorbed when given by mouth. Significant first pass metabolism of *morphine* occurs in the liver; therefore, intramuscular, subcutaneous, or intravenous injections produce the most reliable responses. Opiates have been commonly taken for nonmedical purposes by inhalation of the smoke from burning crude opium, which provides a rapid onset of drug action.

b. Distribution: *Morphine* rapidly enters all body tissues, including the fetuses of pregnant women, and should not be used for analgesia during labor. Infants born of addicted mothers show physical dependence on opiates and exhibit withdrawal symptoms if opioids are not administered. Only a small percentage of *morphine* crosses the blood-brain barrier, since *morphine* is the least lipophilic of the common opioids. This contrasts with the more fat-soluble opioids, such as *fentanyl* and *heroin*, which readily penetrate into the brain and rapidly produce an intense "rush" of euphoria.

c. Fate: *Morphine* is metabolized in the liver to glucuronides. Morphine-6-glucuronide is a very potent analgesic, whereas the conjugate at the 3-position is inactive. The conjugates are excreted primarily in the urine, with small quantities appearing in the bile. The duration of action of *morphine* is 4 to 6 hours in naive individuals. [Note: Due to the low conjugating capacity in neonates, they should not receive *morphine*.]

5. Adverse effects: Severe respiratory depression occurs. Other effects include vomiting, dysphoria, and allergy-enhanced hypotensive effects (Figure 14.4). The elevation of intracranial pressure, particularly in head injury, can be serious. *Morphine* enhances cerebral and spinal ischemia. In prostatic hypertrophy, *morphine* may cause acute urinary retention. A serious action is stoppage of

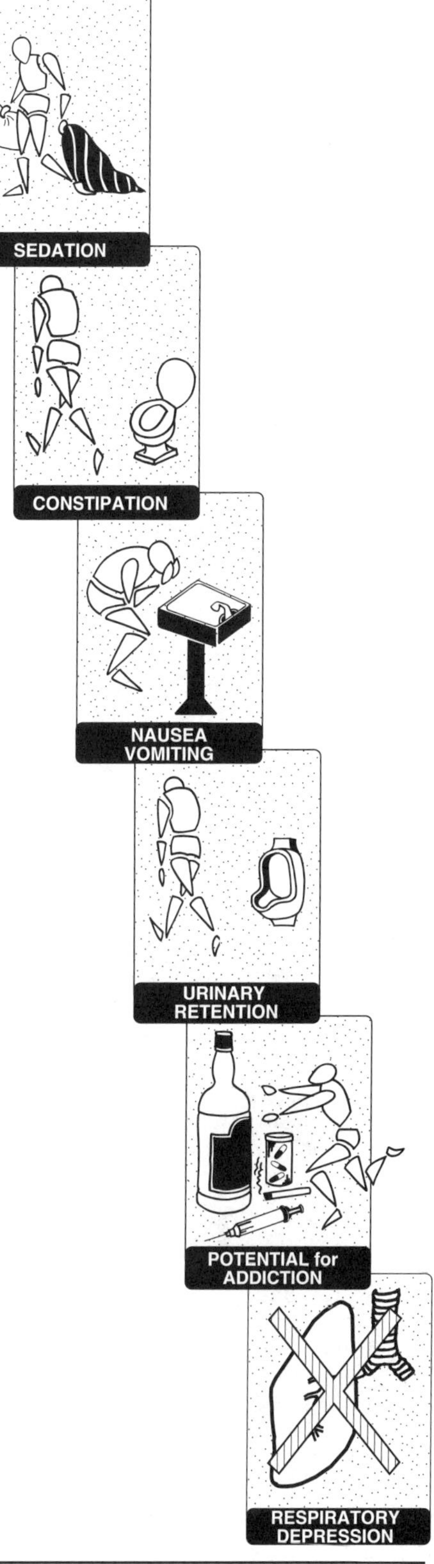

Figure 14.4
Adverse effects commonly observed in individuals treated with opioids.

respiratory exchange in emphysema or cor pulmonale patients. If employed in such individuals, respiration must be carefully watched. Patients with adrenal insufficiency or myxedema may experience extended and increased effects from the opioids.

6. **Tolerance and physical dependence:** Repeated use produces tolerance to the respiratory depressant, analgesic, euphoric, and sedative effects of *morphine*. However, tolerance usually does not develop to the pupil-constricting and constipating effects of the drug. Physical and psychologic dependence readily occur with *morphine* and with some of the other agonists to be described (see Figure 14.3). Withdrawal produces a series of autonomic, motor and psychological responses that incapacitate the individual and causes serious, almost unbearable symptoms. However, it is very rare that the effects are so profound as to cause death.

7. **Drug interactions:** The depressant actions of *morphine* are enhanced by phenothiazines (see p. 127), monoamine oxidase inhibitors (see p.123), and tricyclic antidepressants (see p. 119 and Figure 14.5). Low doses of *amphetamine* (see p. 103) strangely enhance analgesia. *Hydroxyzine* (see p. 422) also enhances analgesia.

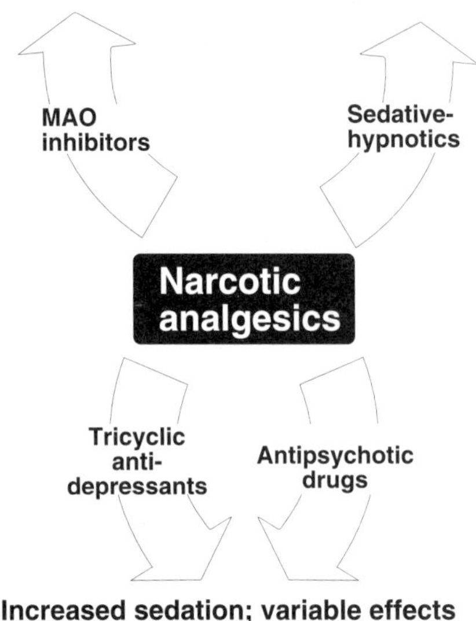
Absolute contra-indication to meperidine and relative contra-indication to other narcotic analgesics because of high incidence of hyperpyrexic coma
Increased CNS depression, particularly respiratory depression
MAO inhibitors
Sedative-hypnotics
Narcotic analgesics
Tricyclic anti-depressants
Antipsychotic drugs
Increased sedation; variable effects on respiratory depression

Figure 14.5
Drugs interacting with narcotic analgesics.

B. Meperidine

Meperidine [me PER i deen] is a synthetic opioid with a structure unrelated to *morphine*. It is used for acute pain.

1. **Mechanism of action:** *Meperidine* binds to opioid receptors, particularly κ receptors.

2. **Actions:** *Meperidine* causes a depression of respiration similar to that of *morphine*, but there is no significant cardiovascular action when the drug is given orally. On intravenous (IV) administration, *meperidine* produces a decrease in peripheral resistance and an increase in peripheral blood flow, and may cause an increase in cardiac rate. As with *morphine*, *meperidine* dilates cerebral vessels, increases cerebrospinal fluid pressure, and contracts smooth muscle (the latter to a lesser extent than does *morphine*). In the gastrointestinal tract, *meperidine* impedes motility, and chronic use results in constipation. *Meperidine* does not cause pinpoint pupils, but rather causes the pupils to dilate because of an *atropine*-like activity.

3. **Therapeutic uses:** *Meperidine* provides analgesia for any type of severe pain. Unlike *morphine*, *meperidine* is not clinically useful in the treatment of diarrhea or cough. *Meperidine* produces less of an increase in urinary retention than does *morphine*.

4. **Pharmacokinetics:** Unlike *morphine*, *meperidine* is well absorbed from the gastrointestinal tract and is useful when an orally-administered, potent analgesic is needed. However, *meperidine* is most often administered intramuscularly. The drug has a duration of action of 2 to 4 hours, which is shorter than that of *morphine* (see Figure 14.6). *Meperidine* is N-demethylated in the liver and is excreted in the urine. [Note: Because of its shorter action and dif-

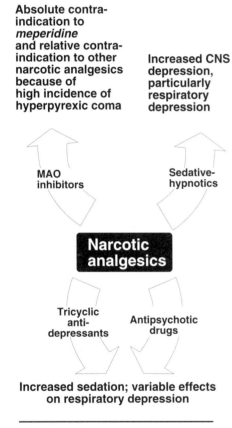

ferent route of metabolism, *meperidine* is preferred for analgesia during labor.]

5. **Adverse effects:** Large doses of *meperidine* cause tremors, muscle twitches, and rarely, convulsions. The drug differs from opioids in that in large doses it dilates the pupil and causes hyperactive reflexes. Severe hypotension can occur when the drug is administered postoperatively. When used with major neuroleptics, depression is greatly enhanced. Administration to patients taking monoamine oxidase inhibitors (see p. 123) can provoke severe reactions such as convulsions and hyperthermia. *Meperidine* can cause dependence, and can substitute for *morphine* or *heroin* in use by addicts. Cross-tolerance with the other opioids occurs.

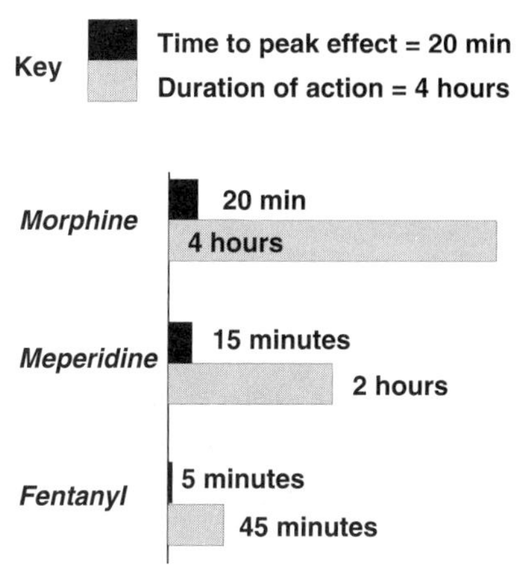

Figure 14.6
Time to peak effect and duration of action of several opioids administered intravenously.

C. Methadone

Methadone [METH a don] is a synthetic, orally effective opioid that is approximately equal in potency to *morphine*, but induces less euphoria and has a longer duration of action.

1. **Mechanism of action:** *Methadone* has its greatest action on μ receptors.

2. **Actions:** The analgesic activity of *methadone* is equivalent to that of *morphine*. *Methadone* exhibits strong analgesic action when administered orally, in contrast to *morphine*, which is only partially absorbed from the gastrointestinal tract. The miotic and respiratory depressant actions of *methadone* have average half-lives of 24 hours. Like *morphine*, *methadone* increases biliary pressure, and is also constipating.

3. **Therapeutic uses:** *Methadone* is used in the controlled withdrawal of addicts from *heroin* and *morphine*. Orally administered, *methadone* is substituted for the injected opioid. The patient is then slowly weaned from *methadone*. *Methadone* causes a milder withdrawal syndrome, which also develops more slowly than that seen during withdrawal from *morphine*.

4. **Pharmacokinetics:** Readily absorbed following oral administration, *methadone* has a longer duration of action than does *morphine*. It accumulates in tissues, where it remains bound to protein from which it is slowly released. The drug is biotransformed in the liver and excreted in the urine, mainly as inactive metabolites.

5. **Adverse effects:** *Methadone* can produce dependence like that of *morphine*. The withdrawal syndrome is much milder but is more protracted (days to weeks) than with opiates.

D. Fentanyl

Fentanyl [FEN ta nil], which is chemically related to *meperidine,* has 80 times the analgesic potency of *morphine*, and is used in anesthesia. It has a rapid onset and short duration of action (15 to 30 minutes). When combined with *droperidol* (see p.117) it produces a dissociative anesthesia. *Sufentanil* [soo FEN ta nil], a related drug, is even more potent than *fentanyl*.

E. Heroin

Heroin [HAIR o in] does not occur naturally but is produced by acetylation of *morphine*, which leads to a three-fold increase in its potency. Its greater lipid solubility allows it to cross the blood-brain barrier more rapidly than *morphine*, causing a more exaggerated euphoria when the drug is taken by injection. *Heroin* is converted to *morphine* in the body, but lasts about half as long. It has no accepted medical use in the United States.

IV. MODERATE AGONISTS

A. Propoxyphene

Propoxyphene [proe POX i feen] is a derivative of *methadone*. The dextro isomer is used as an analgesic to relieve mild to moderate pain. The levo isomer is not analgesic but has antitussive action. *Propoxyphene* is a weaker analgesic than *codeine,* requiring approximately twice the dose to achieve an equianalgesic effect as *codeine*. *Propoxyphene* is often used in combination with *aspirin* (see p. 403) or *acetaminophen* (see p. 412) for a greater analgesia than that obtained with either drug alone. It is well absorbed orally, with peak plasma levels occurring in 1 hour, and it is metabolized in the liver. *Propoxyphene* can produce nausea, anorexia, and constipation. In toxic doses, it can cause respiratory depression, convulsions, hallucinations and confusion. When toxic doses are taken, a very serious problem can arise in some individuals, with resultant cardiotoxicity and pulmonary edema. [Note: When used with alcohol and sedatives, a severe CNS depression is produced and death by respiratory depression and cardiotoxicity can result. The respiratory depression and sedation can be antagonized by *naloxone* (see p. 141), but the cardiotoxicity cannot.]

B. Codeine

Codeine [KOE deen] is a much less potent analgesic than *morphine*, but it has a higher oral efficacy. *Codeine* shows good antitussive activity at doses that do not cause analgesia. The drug has a lower abuse potential than *morphine* and rarely produces dependence. *Codeine* produces less euphoria than *morphine*. *Codeine* is often used in combination with *aspirin* or *acetaminophen*. [Note: In most nonprescription cough preparations, *codeine* has been replaced by newer drugs, such as *dextromethorphan* (see p. 222), a synthetic cough depressant that has no analgesic action and a low potential for abuse.] Figure 14.7 shows some of the actions of *codeine.*

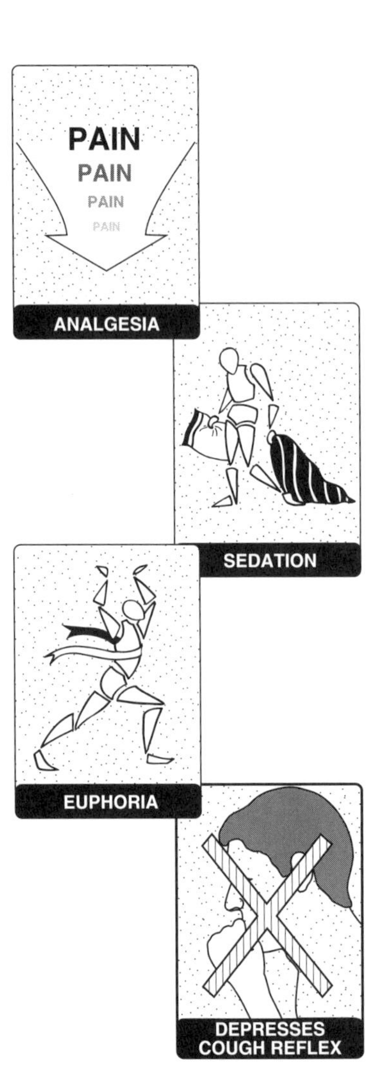

Figure 14.7
Some actions of *codeine.*

V. MIXED AGONIST-ANTAGONISTS

Drugs that stimulate one receptor but block another are termed mixed agonist-antagonists. The effects of these drugs depend on previous exposure to opioids. In individuals who have not recently received opioids, mixed agonist-antagonists show agonist activity and are used to relieve pain. In the patient with opioid dependence, the agonist-antagonist drugs may show primarily blocking effects, that is, produce withdrawal symptoms. Most of the drugs in this group cause dysphoria, rather than euphoria, mediated by activation of σ receptors.

A. Pentazocine

Pentazocine [pen TAZ oh seen] acts as an agonist on κ receptors and is a weak antagonist at μ and δ receptors. It also binds to σ receptors, which may account for its dysphoric properties. *Pentazocine* promotes analgesia by activating receptors in the spinal cord, and is used to relieve moderate pain. It may be administered either orally or parenterally. *Pentazocine* produces less euphoria than does *morphine*. In higher doses, the drug causes respiratory depression and decreases the activity of the gastrointestinal tract. High doses increase blood pressure and can cause hallucinations, nightmares, tachycardia, and dizziness. In angina, *pentazocine* increases the mean aortic pressure and pulmonary arterial pressure and thus increases the work of the heart. The drug decreases renal plasma flow. Despite its antagonist action, *pentazocine* does not antagonize the respiratory depression of *morphine*, but it can precipitate a withdrawal syndrome in a *morphine* abuser. *Pentazocine* should not be used with agonists such as *morphine*, since the antagonist action of *pentazocine* may block the analgesic effects of *morphine*. Tolerance and dependence develop on repeated use.

B. Buprenorphine

Although *buprenorphine* [byou preh NOR feen] is classified as a partial agonist acting at the μ receptor, it behaves like *morphine* in naive patients. However, it can also antagonize *morphine*. *Buprenorphine* is administered parenterally and has a long duration of action because of its tight binding to the receptor. It is metabolized by the liver and excreted in the bile and urine. Adverse effects include respiratory depression, decrease (or, rarely, increase) in blood pressure, nausea and dizziness.

VI. ANTAGONISTS

The opioid antagonists bind with high affinity to opioid receptors but fail to activate the receptor-mediated response. Administration of opioid antagonists produces no profound effects in normal individuals. However, in patients addicted to opioids, antagonists rapidly reverse the effect of agonists, such as *heroin*, and precipitate the symptoms of opiate withdrawal.

A. Naloxone

Naloxone [nal OX own] is used to reverse the coma and respiratory depression of opioid overdose. It rapidly displaces all receptor-

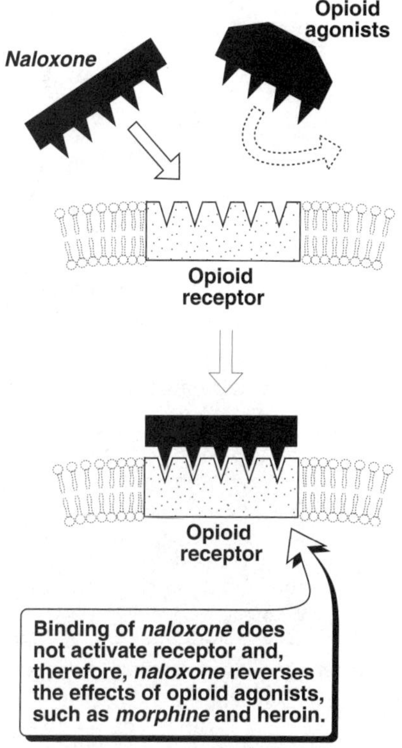

Figure 14.8
Competition of *naloxone* with opioid agonists.

bound opioid molecules and therefore is able to reverse the effect of a *heroin* overdose (Figure 14.8). Within 30 seconds of intravenous injection of *naloxone*, the respiratory depression and coma characteristic of high doses of *heroin* are reversed, causing the patient to be revived and alert. *Naloxone* has a half-life of 60 to 100 minutes. *Naloxone* is a competitive antagonist at μ, κ and δ, receptors, with a 10-fold higher affinity for μ receptors than for κ. This may explain why *naloxone* readily reverses respiratory depression with only minimal reversal of analgesia that results from agonist stimulation of κ receptors in the spinal cord. *Naloxone* produces no pharmacologic effects in normal individuals, but it precipitates withdrawal symptoms in *morphine* or *heroin* abusers.

B. Naltrexone

Naltrexone [nal TREX own] has actions similar to those of *naloxone*. This drug has a longer duration of action than *naloxone*, and a single oral dose of *naltrexone* blocks the effect of injected *heroin* for up to 48 hours. *Naltrexone* is used in opiate-dependence maintenance programs and may also be beneficial in treating chronic alcoholism.

Study Questions

Choose the ONE best answer.

14.1 All of the following statements concerning methadone are correct EXCEPT:

A. It has less potent analgesic activity than that of morphine.

B. It has a longer duration of action than that of morphine.

C. It is effective by oral administration.

D. It causes a milder withdrawal syndrome than morphine.

E. It has its greatest action on μ receptors

> Correct choice = A. Methadone shows an analgesic action similar to that of morphine. Methadone is effective for 15 to 20 hr, whereas morphine acts for 4 to 6 hr. A major advantage of using methadone in the controlled withdrawal of heroin and morphine abusers is that it can be given orally.

14.2 Which of the following statements about pentazocine is INCORRECT?

A. It is a mixed agonist-antagonist.

B. It may be administered orally or parenterally.

C. It produces less euphoria than morphine.

D. It is often combined with morphine for maximal analgesic effects.

E. High doses of pentazocine increase blood pressure.

> Correct choice = D. Pentazocine (a mixed agonist-antagonist) should not be used with agonists such as morphine, because it can block their actions. (Pentazocine acts as an agonist on κ receptors, but is an antagonist at μ and δ receptors.)

14.3 Which of the following statements about morphine is INCORRECT?

A. It is used therapeutically to relieve pain caused by severe head injury.

B. Its withdrawal symptoms can be relieved by methadone.

C. It causes constipation.

D. It is most effective by parenteral administration.

E. It rapidly enters all body tissues, including the fetus of a pregnant woman.

> Correct choice = A. Morphine causes increased cerebrospinal fluid pressure secondary to dilation of cerebral vasculature. Methadone can relieve withdrawal symptoms because opioids show cross sensitivity. It is administered parenterally because absorption from the gastrointestinal tract is unreliable.

Drugs Used to Treat Epilepsy

15

I. OVERVIEW OF EPILEPSY

Epilepsy is widespread among the general population with over two million affected individuals in the United States. Epilepsy is not a single entity; it is a family of different recurrent seizure disorders that have in common the sudden, excessive and disorderly discharge of cerebral neurons. This results in abnormal movements or perceptions that are of short duration but that tend to recur. The site of the electrical discharge determines the symptoms that are produced. For example, epileptic seizures may cause convulsions if the motor cortex is involved. The seizures may include visual, auditory, or olfactory hallucinations if the parietal or occipital cortex plays a role. Drug therapy is the most widely effective mode of treatment for epilepsy. Seizures can be controlled completely in approximately 50% of epileptic patients, and meaningful improvement is achieved in at least one half of the remaining patients. (See Figure 15.1 for a summary of the antiepileptic drugs.)

A. Etiology

The neuronal discharge in epilepsy results from the firing of a small population of neurons in some specific area of the brain, referred to as the primary focus. Anatomically, this focal area may appear perfectly normal. There is usually no identifiable cause for epilepsy, although the focal areas that are functionally abnormal may be triggered into activity by changes in any of a variety of environmental factors, including alteration in blood gases, pH, electrolytes, or glucose availability.

1. **Primary epilepsy:** When no specific anatomic cause for the seizure, such as trauma or neoplasm, is evident the syndrome is called idiopathic or primary epilepsy. These seizures may be produced by an inherited abnormality in the central nervous system (CNS). Patients are treated chronically with antiepileptic drugs, often for life.

2. **Secondary epilepsy:** A number of reversible disturbances, such as tumors, head injury, hypoglycemia, meningeal infection, or rapid withdrawal of alcohol from an alcoholic, can precipitate seizures. Antiepileptic drugs are given until the primary cause of the seizures can be corrected. Seizures secondary to stroke or trauma may cause irreversible CNS damage.

ANTIEPILEPTIC DRUGS

- *Carbamazepine*
- *Clonazepam*
- *Clorazepate*
- *Diazepam*
- *Ethosuximide*
- *Gabapentin*
- *Lamotrigine*
- *Phenobarbital*
- *Phenytoin*
- *Primidone*
- *Tiagabine*[1]
- *Topiramate*[1]
- *Valproic acid*
- *Vigabatrin*[1]

Figure 15.1
Summary of agents used in the treatment of epilepsy.
[1]Described in Pharmacology update, p. 445

Lippincott's Illustrated Reviews: Pharmacology, Second Edition.
by Mary J. Mycek, Richard A. Harvey and Pamela C. Champe.
Lippincott Williams & Wilkins, Philadelphia, PA © 2000.

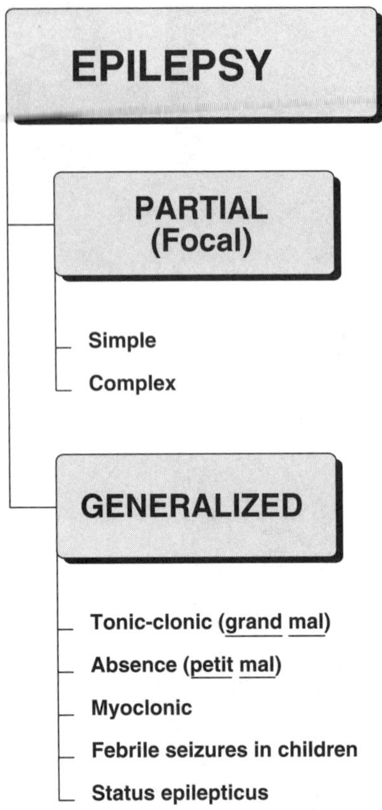

Figure 15.2
Classification of epilepsy.

B. Classification of epilepsy

Seizures have been classified into two broad groups, partial (or focal), and generalized. Choice of drug treatment is based on the classification of the epilepsy being treated (Figure 15.2).

1. **Partial:** The symptoms of each seizure type depend on the site of neuronal discharge and on the extent to which the electrical activity spreads to other neurons in the brain. Partial seizures may progress, becoming generalized tonic-clonic seizures.

   a. **Simple partial:** These seizures are caused by a group of hyperactive neurons exhibiting abnormal electrical activity and are confined to a single locus in the brain; the electrical disorder does not spread. The patient does not lose consciousness and often exhibits abnormal activity of a single limb or muscle group that is controlled by the region of the brain experiencing the disturbance. The patient may also show sensory distortions. Simple partial seizures may occur at any age.

   b. **Complex partial:** These seizures exhibit complex sensory hallucinations, mental distortion, and loss of consciousness. Motor dysfunction may involve chewing movements, diarrhea, urination. Most (80%) of individuals with complex partial epilepsy experience their initial seizures before 20 years of age.

2. **Generalized:** These seizures begin locally, but they rapidly spread, producing abnormal electrical discharge throughout both hemispheres of the brain. Generalized seizures may be convulsive or nonconvulsive; the patient usually has an immediate loss of consciousness.

   a. **Tonic-clonic (grand mal):** This is the most commonly encountered and the most dramatic form of epilepsy. Seizures result in loss of consciousness, followed by tonic, then clonic phases. The seizure is followed by a postictal period of confusion and exhaustion.

   b. **Absence (petit mal):** These seizures involve a brief, abrupt, and self-limiting loss of consciousness. The onset occurs in patients at ages 3 to 5 years and lasts until puberty. The patient stares and exhibits rapid eye-blinking, which lasts for 3 to 5 seconds.

   c. **Myoclonic:** These seizures consist of short episodes of muscle contractions that may reoccur for several minutes. Myoclonic seizures are rare, occur at any age, and are often a result of permanent neurologic damage acquired as a result of hypoxia, uremia, encephalitis, or drug poisoning.

   d. **Febrile seizures:** Young children (3 months to 5 years of age) frequently develop seizures with illness accompanied by high fever. The febrile seizures consist of generalized tonic-clonic convulsions of short duration. Although febrile seizure may be frightening to observers, they are benign and do not cause death, neurologic damage, injury, or learning disorders, and they rarely require medication.

e. **Status epilepticus:** Seizures are rapidly recurrent.

C. Mechanism of action of antiepileptic drugs

Drugs that are effective in seizure reduction can either block the initiation of the electrical discharge from the focal area or, more commonly, prevent the spread of the abnormal electrical discharge to adjacent brain areas.

II. ANTIEPILEPTIC DRUGS

Initial drug treatment to suppress or reduce the incidence of seizures is based on the specific type of seizure (see Figure 15.3). Thus, tonic-clonic (grand mal) seizures are treated differently than absence seizures (petit mal). Several drugs may be equally effective, and the toxicity of the agent is often a major consideration in drug selection. Monotherapy is instituted with a single agent until seizures are controlled or toxic signs occur. When therapy with a single drug is ineffective, a second drug may be added to the therapeutic regimen. Antiepileptic therapy for tonic-clonic seizures should never be terminated abruptly, otherwise seizures may result.

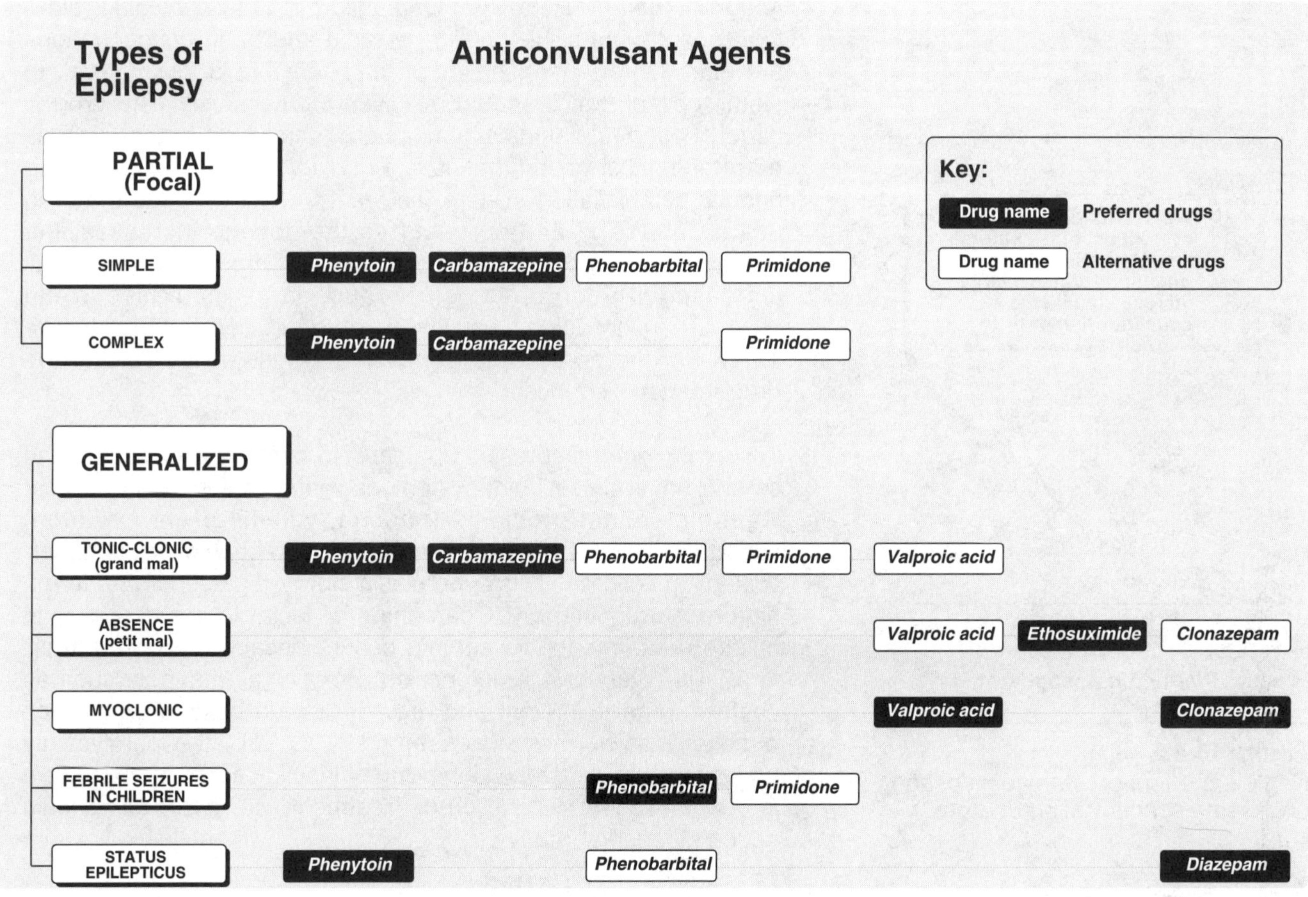

Figure 15.3
Therapeutic indications for anticonvulsant agents.

A. Phenytoin

Phenytoin [FEN i toy in] (formerly called *diphenylhydantoin*) is effective in suppressing tonic-clonic and partial seizures, and is a drug of choice for initial therapy, particularly in treating adults.

1. **Mechanism of action:** *Phenytoin* stabilizes neuronal membranes to depolarization by decreasing the flux of sodium ions in neurons in the resting state or during depolarization. It also reduces the influx of calcium ions during depolarization and suppresses repetitive firing of neurons.

2. **Actions:** *Phenytoin* is not a generalized CNS depressant like the barbiturates, but it does produce some degree of drowsiness and lethargy without progression to hypnosis. *Phenytoin* reduces the propagation of abnormal impulses in the brain.

3. **Therapeutic uses:** *Phenytoin* is highly effective for all partial seizures (simple and complex), for tonic-clonic seizures, and in the treatment of status epilepticus caused by recurrent tonic-clonic seizures (Figure 15.3). *Phenytoin* is not effective for absence seizures, which often may worsen if such a patient is treated with this drug.

4. **Absorption and Metabolism:** Oral absorption of *phenytoin* is slow, but once it occurs, distribution is rapid and brain concentrations are high. Chronic administration of *phenytoin* is always oral; in status epilepticus, it should be given intravenously. The drug is largely bound to plasma albumin. Less than 5% of a given dose is excreted unchanged in the urine. *Phenytoin* is metabolized by the hepatic hydroxylation system (see p. 14). At low doses the drug has a half-life of 24 hours, but as the dosage increases, the hydroxylation system becomes saturated. Thus, relatively small increases in each dose can produce large increases in the plasma concentration, resulting in drug-induced toxicity (Figure 15.4). Furthermore, large genetic variations in the rate of the drug's metabolism occur.

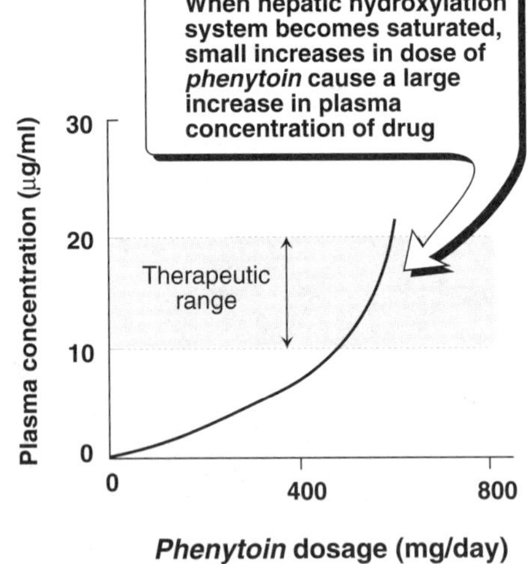
When hepatic hydroxylation system becomes saturated, small increases in dose of *phenytoin* cause a large increase in plasma concentration of drug
Plasma concentration (μg/ml)
30
20
10
0
Therapeutic range
0
400
800
Phenytoin dosage (mg/day)

Figure 15.4
Nonlinear effect of *phenytoin* dosage on plasma concentration of drug.

5. **Adverse effects:** Depression of the CNS occurs particularly in the cerebellum and vestibular system, causing nystagmus and ataxia. Gastrointestinal problems (nausea, vomiting) are common. Gingival hyperplasia may cause the gums to grow over teeth, particularly in children. This hyperplasia slowly regresses after termination of drug therapy. Coarsening of facial features occurs in children. Megaloblastic anemia occurs because the drug interferes with vitamin B_{12} metabolism. Behavioral changes, such as confusion, hallucination, and drowsiness are common. Inhibition of antidiuretic hormone release occurs as well as hyperglycemia and glycosuria caused by inhibition of insulin secretion. *Phenytoin* is also an antiarrhythmic drug. Treatment with *phenytoin* should not be stopped abruptly.

6. **Teratogenic effects:** *Phenytoin* causes teratogenic effects in offspring of mothers given the drug during pregnancy. "Fetal hydantoin syndrome" includes cleft lip, cleft palate, congenital heart

disease, as well as slowed growth and mental deficiency. Almost half of untreated epileptic women have an increased seizure frequency during pregnancy. These seizures can lead to anoxic episodes, which yield a higher incidence of congenital birth defects. Antiepileptic drugs are given at the lowest possible dose to control seizures.

7. **Drug interactions:**

a. **Inhibition of phenytoin metabolism:** Inhibition of microsomal metabolism of *phenytoin* in the liver is caused by *chloramphenicol*, *dicumarol*, *cimetidine*, sulfonamides, and *isoniazid*. When used chronically, these drugs increase the concentration of *phenytoin* in plasma by preventing its metabolism. A decrease in the plasma concentration of *phenytoin* is caused by *carbamazepine*, which enhances *phenytoin* metabolism (Figure 15.5).

b. **Increase in metabolism of other drugs by phenytoin:** *Phenytoin* induces the P-450 system (see p. 14) which leads to an increase in the metabolism of other antiepileptics, anticoagulants, oral contraceptives, *quinidine*, *doxycycline*, *cyclosporine*, *mexiletine*, *methadone*, and *levodopa*.

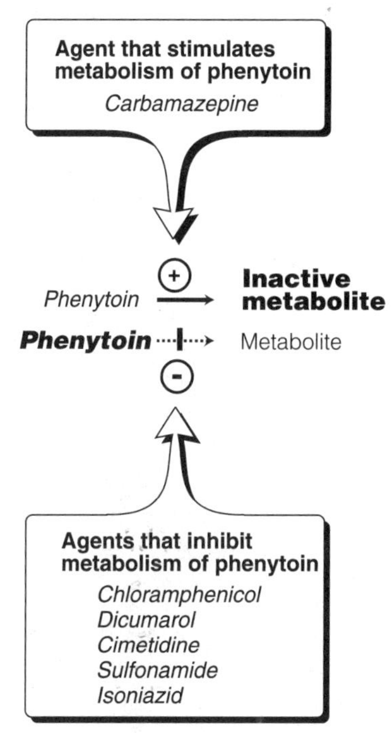

Figure 15.5
Drugs affecting the metabolism of *phenytoin*.

B. Carbamazepine

1. **Actions:** *Carbamazepine* [kar ba MAZ a peen] reduces the propagation of abnormal impulses in the brain by blocking sodium channels, thereby inhibiting the generation of repetitive action potentials in the epileptic focus.

2. **Therapeutic uses:** *Carbamazepine* is highly effective for all partial seizures (simple and complex) and is often the drug of first choice. In addition the drug is highly effective for tonic-clonic seizures and is used to treat trigeminal neuralgia. It has occasionally been used in manic-depressive patients to ameliorate the symptoms.

3. **Absorption and metabolism:** *Carbamazepine* is absorbed slowly following oral administration. It enters the brain rapidly because of its high lipid solubility. *Carbamazepine* induces the drug metabolizing enzymes in the liver, and its half-life therefore decreases with chronic administration. The enhanced hepatic P-450 system activity also increases the metabolism of other antiepileptic drugs.

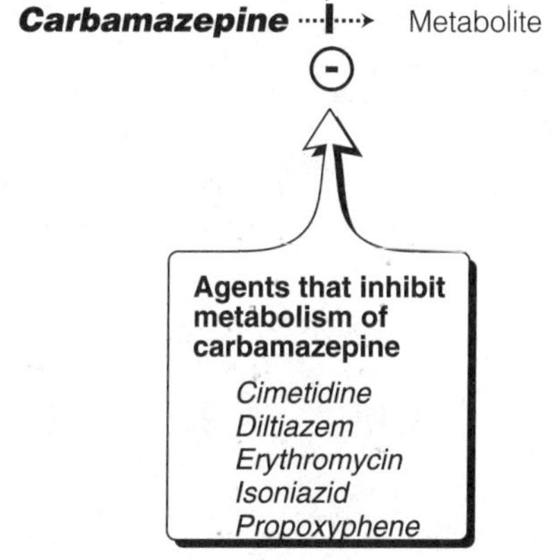

Figure 15.6
Drugs affecting the metabolism of *carbamazepine*.

4. **Adverse effects:** Chronic administration of *carbamazepine* can cause stupor, coma, and respiratory depression, along with drowsiness, vertigo, ataxia, and blurred vision. The drug is irritating to the stomach, and nausea and vomiting may occur. Aplastic anemia, agranulocytosis, and thrombocytopenia have occurred in some patients. This drug has the potential for inducing serious liver toxicity. Therefore, anyone being treated with *carbamazepine* should have frequent liver function tests.

5. **Drug interactions:** The hepatic metabolism of *carbamazepine* is inhibited by several drugs (Figure 15.6). Toxic symptoms may arise if the dose is not adjusted.

C. Phenobarbital

1. **Actions:** *Phenobarbital* (see p. 94) has antiepileptic activity, limiting the spread of seizure discharges in the brain and elevating the seizure threshold. Its mechanism of action is unknown but may involve potentiation of the inhibitory effects of γ-aminobutyric acid (GABA)-mediated neurons. Doses required for antiepileptic action are lower than those that cause pronounced CNS depression.

2. **Therapeutic uses:** *Phenobarbital* provides a 50% favorable response rate for simple partial seizures, but it is not very effective for complex partial seizures. The drug has been regarded as the first choice in treating recurrent seizures in children, including febrile seizures. However, *phenobarbital* can depress cognitive performance in children treated for febrile seizures, and the drug should be used cautiously. *Phenobarbital* is also used to treat recurrent tonic-clonic seizures, especially in patients who do not respond to *diazepam* plus *phenytoin*. *Phenobarbital* is also used as a mild sedative to relieve anxiety, nervous tension and insomnia, although benzodiazepines (see p. 89) are superior.

3. **Absorption and metabolism:** *Phenobarbital* is well absorbed orally. The drug freely penetrates the brain. Approximately 75% of the drug is inactivated by the hepatic microsomal system; the remaining drug is excreted unchanged by the kidney. *Phenobarbital* is a potent inducer of the P-450 system, and when given chronically, it enhances the metabolism of other agents.

4. **Adverse effects:** Sedation, ataxia, nystagmus, vertigo, and acute psychotic reactions may occur with chronic use. Nausea and vomiting are seen as well as a morbilliform rash in sensitive individuals. Agitation and confusion occur at high doses. Rebound seizures can occur on discontinuance of *phenobarbital*.

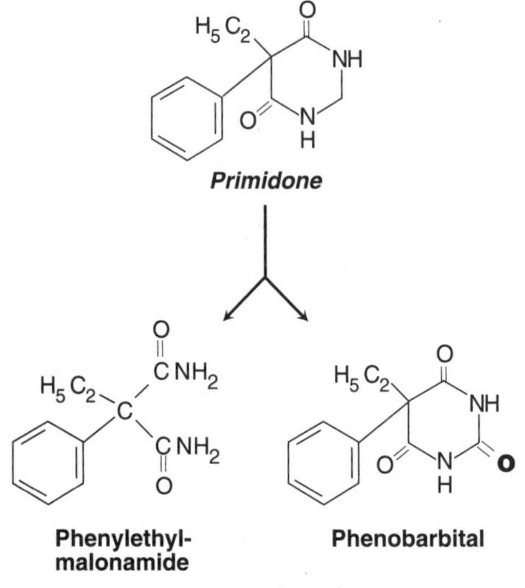

Figure 15.7
Metabolism of *primidone*.

D. Primidone

Primidone [PRI mi done] is structurally related to *phenobarbital*, and resembles *phenobarbital* in its anticonvulsant activity. *Primidone* is an alternate choice in partial seizures and tonic-clonic seizures. Much of *primidone*'s efficacy comes from its metabolites *phenobarbital* and phenylethylmalonamide (see Figure 15.7), which have longer half-lives than the parent drug. *Phenobarbital* is effective against tonic-clonic and simple partial seizures, and phenylethylmalonamide is effective against complex partial seizures. *Primidone* is often used with *carbamazepine* and *phenytoin*, allowing smaller doses of these agents to be used. It is ineffective in absence seizures (Figure 15.3). *Primidone* is well absorbed orally. It exhibits poor protein binding. This drug has the same adverse effects as those seen with *phenobarbital*.

E. Valproic acid

Valproic acid [val PROE ic] reduces the propagation of abnormal electrical discharge in the brain. It may enhance GABA action at inhibitory synapses. *Valproic acid* is the most effective agent available for treatment of myoclonic seizures. The drug diminishes absence seizures but is a second choice because of its hepatotoxic potential. *Valproic acid* also reduces the incidence and severity of tonic-clonic seizures (see Figure 15.3). The drug is effective orally and is rapidly absorbed. About 90% is bound to plasma proteins. Only 3% is excreted unchanged; the rest is converted to active metabolites by the liver. *Valproic acid* is metabolized by the P-450 system, but it does not induce P-450 enzyme synthesis. The glucuronylated metabolites are excreted in the urine. *Valproic acid* can cause nausea and vomiting; sedation, ataxia, and tremor are common (Figure 15.8). Hepatic toxicity may cause a rise in hepatic enzymes in plasma, which should be monitored frequently. In some individuals, a rash and alopecia may occur. Bleeding times may increase because of both thrombocytopenia and an inhibition of platelet aggregation. *Valproic acid* inhibits *phenobarbital* metabolism, thereby increasing circulating levels of that barbiturate.

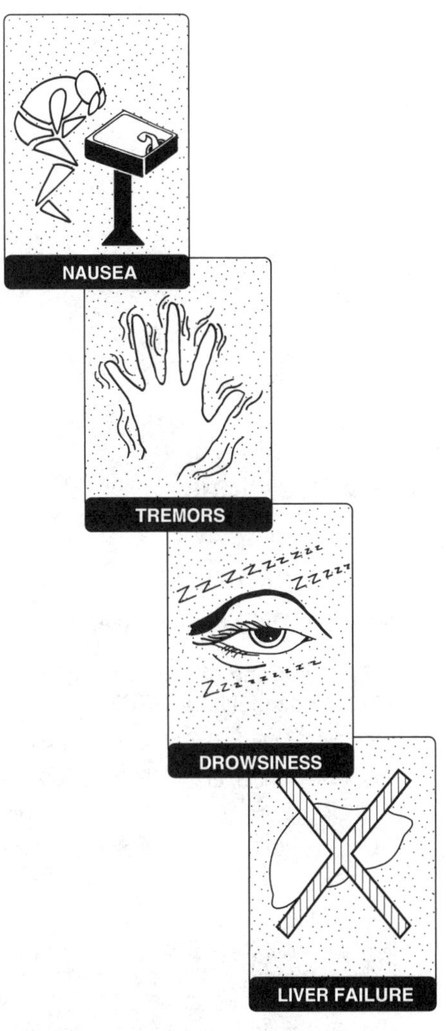

Figure 15.8
Some adverse effects of *valproic acid.*

F. Ethosuximide

Ethosuximide [eth oh SUX i mide] reduces propagation of abnormal electrical activity in the brain, and is the first choice in absence seizures (see Figure 15.3). *Ethosuximide* is well absorbed orally. It is not bound to plasma proteins. About 25% of the drug is excreted unchanged in the urine, and 75% is converted to inactive metabolites in the liver by the microsomal P-450 system. *Ethosuximide* does not induce P-450 enzyme synthesis. The drug is irritating to the stomach, and nausea and vomiting may occur on chronic administration. Drowsiness, lethargy, dizziness, restlessness, agitation, anxiety, and the inability to concentrate are often observed. In sensitive individuals, a Stevens-Johnson syndrome or urticaria may occur, as well as leukopenia, aplastic anemia, and thrombocytopenia.

G. Benzodiazepines

Several of the benzodiazepines show antiepileptic activity. *Clonazepam* and *clorazepate* are used for chronic treatment, whereas *diazepam* is the drug of choice in the acute treatment of status epilepticus (see p. 91). *Clonazepam* suppresses seizure spread from the epileptogenic focus, and is effective in absence and myoclonic seizures (see Figure 15.3), but tolerance develops. *Clorazepate* is effective in partial seizures when used in conjunction with other drugs. Of all the antiepileptics, the benzodiazepines are the safest and most free from severe side effects. All benzodiazepines have sedative properties; thus, drowsiness, somnolence, and fatigue can occur with higher dosage as well as ataxia, dizziness and behavior changes. Respiratory depression and cardiac depression may occur when given intravenously in acute situations.

H. Gabapentin and Lamotrigine

For the first time in many years, new classes of antiepileptic drugs are becoming available. *Gabapentin* [gah ah PEN tin] is an analogue of GABA, but its mechanism is not known. *Lamotrigine* [la MO tri geen] inhibits glutamate and aspartate release, blocks sodium channels, and prevents repetitive firing. Both drugs are approved for the treatment of simple or complex partial seizures and generalized tonic-clonic seizures. *Gabapentin* does not bind to plasma proteins and is excreted unchanged through the kidneys, minimizing the likelihood of drug interactions. *Lamotrigine* is metabolized in the liver. Its $t_{1/2}$ is decreased by enzyme-inducing drugs (*carbamazepine, phenytoin*) and is increased by *valproic acid*. Mild CNS effects occur with both drugs, and development of a rash with *lamotrigine*, have been the most noted adverse reactions.

See pp. 445-446 for a description of the newly approved drugs, *tiagabine*, *topiramate* and *vigabatin*.

Study Questions

Choose the ONE best answer.

15.1 For which one of the following drugs is the therapeutic indication INCORRECT?

A. Ethosuximide: Absence seizures
B. Phenobarbital: Febrile seizures in children
C. Diazepam: Status epilepticus
D. Phenytoin: Absence seizures
E. Carbamazepine: Tonic-clonic seizures

Correct choice = D. Phenytoin is effective in suppressing tonic-clonic and partial seizures, and in the treatment of status epilepticus caused by recurrent tonic-clonic seizures. It is not effective for absence seizures.

15.2 Which of the following statements concerning phenytoin is INCORRECT?

A. Causes less sedation than phenobarbital.
B. Causes gingival hyperplasia.
C. May cause fetal hydantoin syndrome if given during pregnancy.
D. Is excreted unchanged in the urine.
E. The plasma half-life increases as the dose is increased.

Correct choice = D. Less than 5% of phenytoin is excreted unchanged in the urine; it is metabolized by the hepatic hydroxylation system. Saturation of hepatic metabolizing enzymes at high doses of phenytoin leads to an increase in the half-life of the drug.

15.3 All the following drugs are useful in treating complex partial seizures EXCEPT:

A. Ethosuximide
B. Phenobarbital
C. Carbamazepine
D. Phenytoin
E. Gabapentin

Correct choice = A. Ethosuximide is used in the treatment of absence seizures.

15.4 Which of the following drug/toxicity pairs is INCORRECT?

A. Valproic acid: Nausea and vomiting
B. Ethosuximide: Stevens-Johnson syndrome
C. Carbamazepine: Bone marrow suppression
D. Primidone: Hepatotoxicity
E. Phenobarbital: Sedation

Correct choice = D. Primidone does not cause hepatotoxicity. The adverse effects seen with this drug are the same as those seen with phenobarbital.

UNIT IV: Drugs Affecting the Cardiovascular System

16 Treatment of Congestive Heart Failure

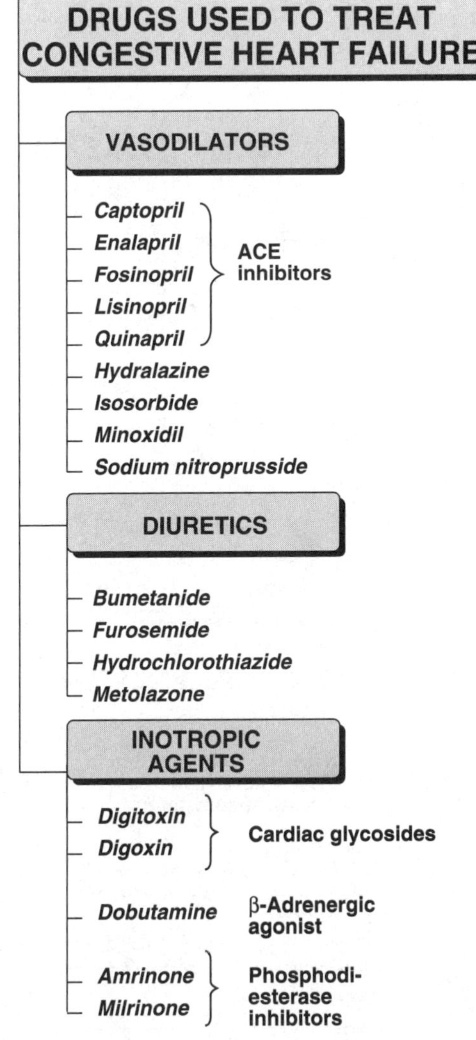

DRUGS USED TO TREAT CONGESTIVE HEART FAILURE
VASODILATORS
Captopril
Enalapril
Fosinopril
Lisinopril
Quinapril
ACE inhibitors
Hydralazine
Isosorbide
Minoxidil
Sodium nitroprusside
DIURETICS
Bumetanide
Furosemide
Hydrochlorothiazide
Metolazone
INOTROPIC AGENTS
Digitoxin
Digoxin
Cardiac glycosides
Dobutamine
β-Adrenergic agonist
Amrinone
Milrinone
Phosphodi-esterase inhibitors

Figure 16.1
Summary of drugs used to treat congestive heart failure.

I. OVERVIEW OF CONGESTIVE HEART FAILURE

Congestive heart failure (CHF) is a condition in which the heart is unable to pump sufficient blood to meet the needs of the body. CHF can be caused by an impaired ability of the cardiac muscle to contract or by an increased workload imposed on the heart. CHF is accompanied by abnormal increases in blood volume and interstitial fluid; the heart, veins, and capillaries are therefore generally dilated with blood. Hence the term "congestive" heart failure, since the symptoms include pulmonary congestion with left heart failure, and peripheral edema with right heart failure. Underlying causes of CHF include arteriosclerotic heart disease, hypertensive heart disease, valvular heart disease, dilated cardiomyopathy, and congenital heart disease. Left systolic dysfunction secondary to coronary artery disease is the most common cause of heart failure. The number of newly diagnosed patients with CHF is increasing because more individuals now survive acute myocardial infarction.

The therapeutic goal for CHF is to increase cardiac output. Three classes of drugs have been shown to be clinically effective in reducing symptoms and prolonging life: 1) vasodilators that reduce the load on the myocardium; 2) diuretic agents that decrease extracellular fluid volume; and 3) inotropic agents that increase the strength of contraction of cardiac muscle (Figure 16.1). [Note: These agents relieve the symptoms of cardiac insufficiency but do not reverse the underlying pathologic condition.] Knowledge of the physiology of cardiac muscle contraction is clearly essential to an understanding of the compensatory responses evoked by the failing heart, as well as the actions of drugs used to treat CHF.

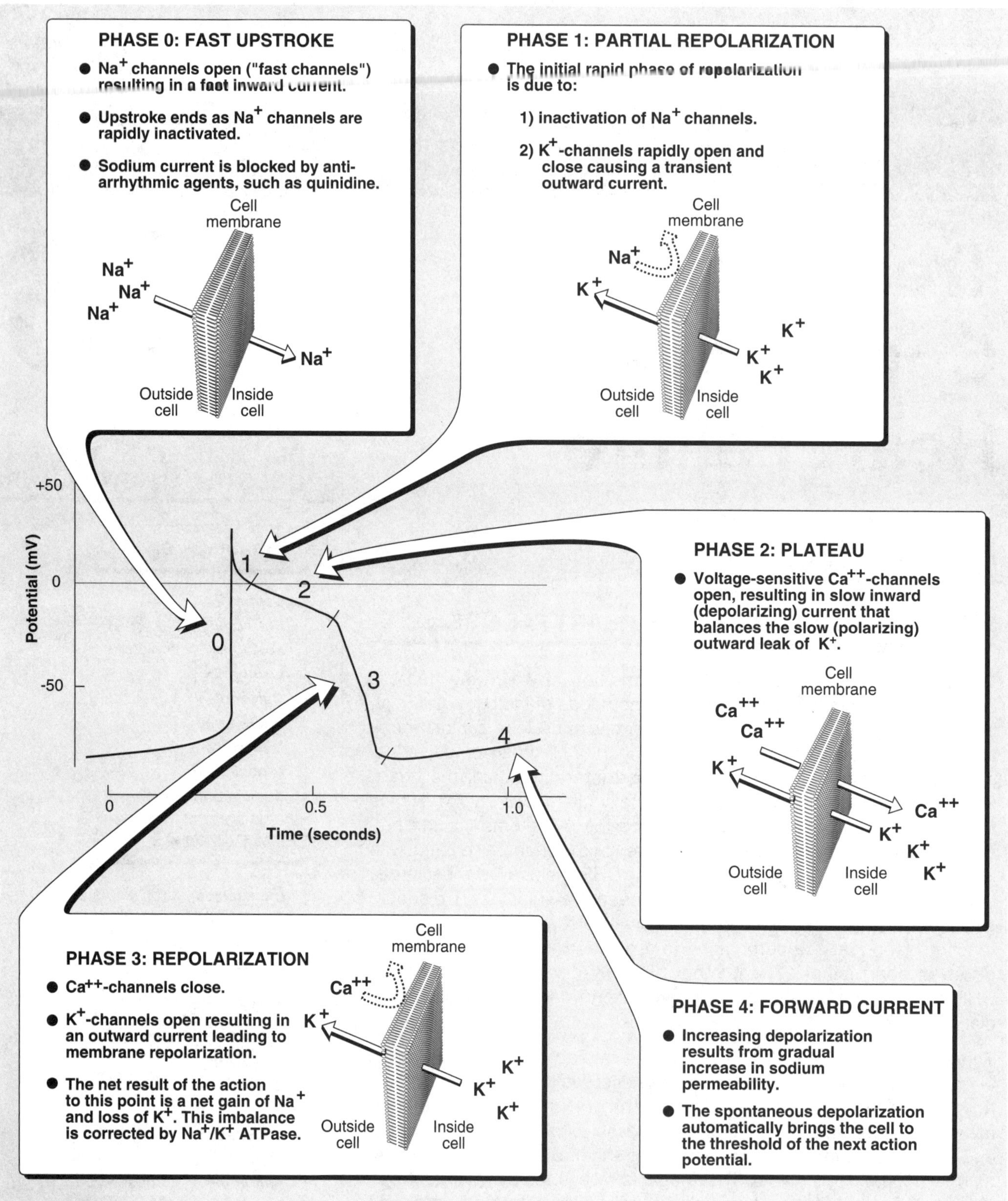
PHASE 0: FAST UPSTROKE
● Na+ channels open ("fast channels") resulting in a fast inward current.
● Upstroke ends as Na+ channels are rapidly inactivated.
● Sodium current is blocked by anti-arrhythmic agents, such as quinidine.
Cell membrane
Na+
Na+
Na+
Na+
Outside cell
Inside cell
PHASE 1: PARTIAL REPOLARIZATION
● The initial rapid phase of repolarization is due to:
1) inactivation of Na+ channels.
2) K+-channels rapidly open and close causing a transient outward current.
Cell membrane
Na+
K+
K+
K+
K+
Outside cell
Inside cell
+50
0
-50
Potential (mV)
1
2
0
3
4
0
0.5
1.0
Time (seconds)
PHASE 2: PLATEAU
● Voltage-sensitive Ca++-channels open, resulting in slow inward (depolarizing) current that balances the slow (polarizing) outward leak of K+.
Cell membrane
Ca++
Ca++
K+
Ca++
K+
K+
K+
Outside cell
Inside cell
PHASE 3: REPOLARIZATION
● Ca++-channels close.
● K+-channels open resulting in an outward current leading to membrane repolarization.
● The net result of the action to this point is a net gain of Na+ and loss of K+. This imbalance is corrected by Na+/K+ ATPase.
Cell membrane
Ca++
K+
K+
K+
K+
Outside cell
Inside cell
PHASE 4: FORWARD CURRENT
● Increasing depolarization results from gradual increase in sodium permeability.
● The spontaneous depolarization automatically brings the cell to the threshold of the next action potential.

Figure 16.2
Action potential of a Purkinje fiber.

II. PHYSIOLOGY OF MUSCLE CONTRACTION

The myocardium, like smooth and skeletal muscle, responds to stimulation by depolarization of the membrane; this is followed by shortening of the contractile proteins and ends with relaxation and return to the resting state (Figure 16.2). However, unlike skeletal muscle, which shows graded contractions depending on the number of muscle cells stimulated, the cardiac muscle cells are interconnected in groups that respond to stimuli as a unit, contracting together whenever a single cell is stimulated.

A. Action potential

Cardiac muscle cells are electrically excitable. However, unlike the cells of other muscles and nerves, the cells of cardiac muscle show a spontaneous, intrinsic rhythm generated by specialized "pacemaker" cells located in the sinoatrial (SA), and atrioventricular (AV) nodes. The cardiac cells also have an unusually long action potential, which can be divided into five phases (0 to 4). Figure 16.2 illustrates the major ions contributing to depolarization and polarization of cardiac cells. These ions pass through channels in the sarcolemmal membrane and thus create a current. The channels open and close at different times during the action potential; some respond primarily to changes in ion concentration, whereas others are either adenosine triphosphate (ATP)- or voltage-sensitive.

B. Cardiac contraction

The contractile machinery of the myocardial cell is essentially the same as in striated muscle. The force of contraction of the cardiac muscle is directly related to the concentration of free (unbound) cytosolic calcium. Therefore agents that increase these calcium levels (or increase the sensitivity of the contractile machinery to calcium) result in an increase in the force of contraction (inotropic effect). [Note: The inotropic agents increase the contractility of the heart by directly or indirectly altering the mechanisms that control the concentration of intracellular calcium.]

1. **Sources of free intracellular calcium:** Calcium comes from two sources. The first is from outside the cell, where opening of voltage-sensitive calcium channels causes an immediate rise in free cytosolic calcium. The second source is the release of calcium from the sarcoplasmic reticulum and mitochondria, which further increases the cytosolic level of calcium (Figure 16.3).

2. **Removal of free cytosolic calcium:** If free cytosolic calcium levels were to remain high, the cardiac muscle would be in a constant state of contraction, rather than showing a periodic contraction. Mechanisms of removal include two alternatives.

   a. **Sodium-calcium exchange:** Calcium is removed by a sodium-calcium exchange reaction that reversibly exchanges calcium ions for sodium ions across the cell membrane (Figure 16.3).

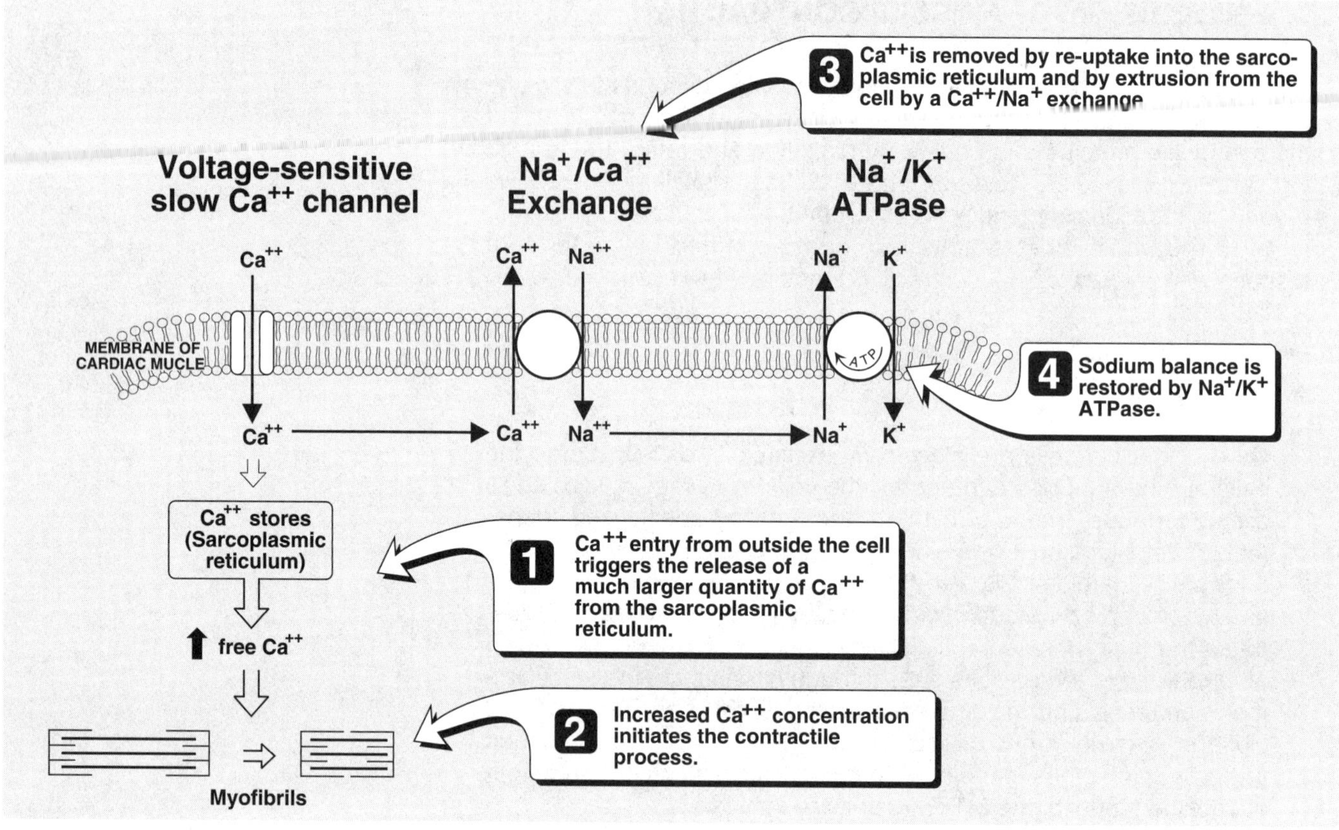

Figure 16.3
Ion movements during the contraction of cardiac muscle.

This interaction between the movement of calcium and sodium ions is significant, since changes in intracellular sodium can affect cellular levels of calcium.

b. **Uptake of calcium by the sarcoplasmic reticulum and mitochondria:** Calcium is also recaptured by the sarcoplasmic reticulum and the mitochondria. More than 99% of the intracellular calcium is located in these organelles, and even a modest shift between these stores and free calcium can lead to large changes in the concentration of free cytosolic calcium.

C. Compensatory physiological responses in CHF

The failing heart evokes three major compensatory mechanisms to enhance cardiac output (Figure 16.4).

1. **Increased sympathetic activity:** Baroreceptors sense a decrease in blood pressure, and trigger activation of β-adrenergic receptors in the heart. This results in an increase in heart rate and a greater force of contraction of the heart muscle (Figure 16.4). In addition, vasoconstriction (α_1-mediated) enhances venous return and increases cardiac preload. These compensatory responses increase the work of the heart and, therefore, can contribute to the further decline in cardiac function.

2. **Fluid retention:** A fall in cardiac output decreases blood flow to the kidney, prompting the release of renin, with a resulting increase in the synthesis of angiotensin II and aldosterone (see p. 181). This results in increased peripheral resistance and retention of sodium and water. Blood volume increases, and more blood is returned to the heart. If the heart is unable to pump this extra volume, venous pressure increases and peripheral edema and pulmonary edema occur (Figure 16.4). These compensatory responses increase the work of the heart and, therefore, can contribute to the further decline in cardiac function.

3. **Myocardial hypertrophy:** The heart increases in size, and the chambers dilate. Initially, stretching of the heart muscle leads to a stronger contraction of the heart. However, excessive elongation of the fibers results in weaker contractions. This type of failure is termed systolic failure and is a result of a ventricle unable to pump effectively. Less commonly, patients with CHF may have diastolic dysfunction—a term applied when the ventricles' ability to relax and accept blood is impaired by structural changes, such as hypertrophy. The thickening of the ventricular wall and subsequent decrease in ventricular volume decreases the ability of heart muscle to relax. In this case, the ventricle does not fill adequately, and the inadequacy of cardiac output is termed diastolic heart failure.

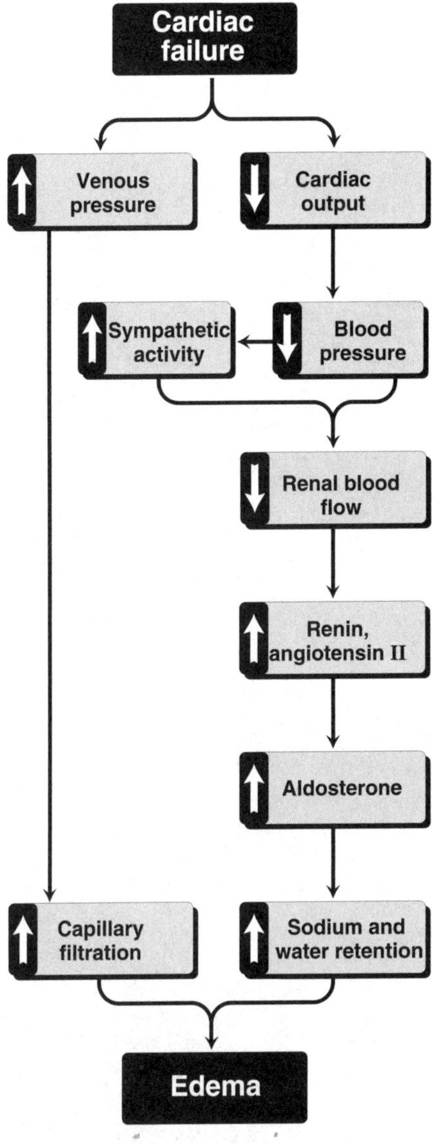

Figure 16.4
Cardiovascular consequences of heart failure.

D. Decompensated heart failure

If the mechanisms listed above adequately restore cardiac output, then the heart failure is said to be compensated. However, these compensations increase the work of the heart and contribute to further decline in cardiac performance. If the adaptive mechanisms fail to maintain cardiac output, the heart failure is termed decompensated.

E. Therapeutic strategies in CHF

Chronic heart failure is typically managed by reduction in physical activity, low dietary intake of sodium (less than 1500 mg sodium per day), and treatment with vasodilators, diuretics and inotropic agents. Drugs that may precipitate or exacerbate CHF—nonsteroidal anti-inflammatory drugs (NSAIDs), alcohol, β-blockers, calcium channel-blockers and some antiarrhythmic drugs—should be avoided if possible. Patients with CHF complain of dyspnea on exertion, orthopnea, paroxysmal nocturnal dyspnea, fatigue, and dependent edema.

III. VASODILATORS

In CHF, the impaired contractile function of the heart is exacerbated by compensatory increases in both preload and afterload. Preload is the volume of blood that fills the ventricle during diastole. Elevated preload causes overfilling of the heart, which increases the workload. Afterload is the pressure that must be overcome for the heart to pump blood into the arterial system. Elevated afterload causes the heart to work harder to pump blood into the arterial system. Vasodilators are useful in reducing excessive preload and afterload. Dilation of venous blood vessels leads to a decrease in cardiac preload by increasing venous capacitance; arterial dilators reduce systemic arteriolar resistance and decrease afterload.

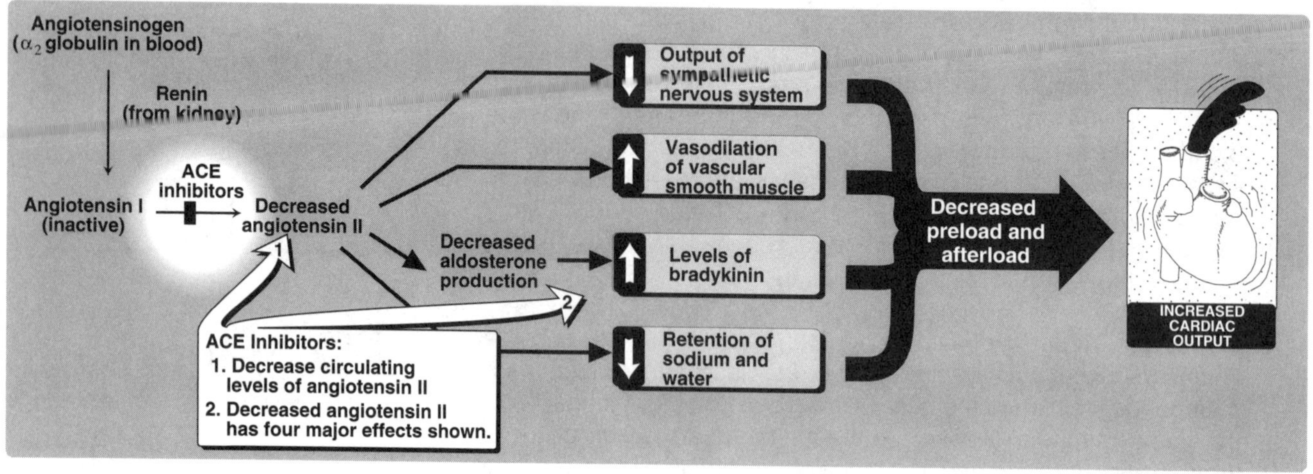

Figure 16.5
Effects of ACE inhibitors.

A. Angiotensin converting enzyme (ACE) inhibitors

ACE inhibitors are the agents of choice in CHF and are superior to other vasodilators.These drugs block the enzyme that cleaves angiotensin I to form the potent vasoconstrictor, angiotensin II (Figure 16.5). These agents also diminish the rate of bradykinin inactivation. [Note: Vasodilation occurs as a result of the combined effects of lower vasoconstriction caused by diminished levels of angiotensin II and the potent vasodilating effect of increased bradykinin.] By reducing circulating angiotensin II levels, ACE inhibitors also decrease the secretion of aldosterone, resulting in decreased sodium and water retention.

1. **Actions on heart:** ACE inhibitors decrease vascular resistance, venous tone, and blood pressure, resulting in an increased cardiac output (Figure 16.5). ACE inhibitors also blunt the usual angiotensin II-mediated increase in epinephrine and aldosterone seen in CHF. ACE inhibitors improve clinical signs and symptoms in patients also receiving a diuretic and/or *digoxin* (see p. 157). The use of ACE inhibitors in the treatment of CHF has significantly decreased both morbidity and mortality. For example, Figure 16.6 shows that the ACE inhibitor *enalapril* [e NAL a pril] decreases the cumulative mortality in patients with congestive heart failure. [Note: Reduction in mortality is due primarily to a decrease in deaths caused by progressive heart failure.] Treatment with *enalapril* also reduced arrhythmic death, myocardial infarction, and strokes. Similar data have been obtained with other ACE inhibitors.

2. **Indications:** ACE inhibitors may be considered for single-agent therapy in patients who present with mild dyspnea on exertion and who do not show signs or symptoms of volume overload. ACE inhibitors are useful in decreasing CHF in asymptomatic patients with ejection fraction less than 35% (left ventricular dysfunction). Patients who have had a recent myocardial infarction also benefit from long-term ACE inhibitor therapy. Patients with the lowest ejection fraction show the greatest benefit. Early use of ACE

inhibitors is indicated in treating patients with all stages of left ventricular failure, with and without symptoms, and therapy should be initiated immediately after myocardial infarction. See p. 186 for the use of ACE inhibitors in the treatment of hypertension.

3. **Adverse effects:** These include postural hypotension, renal insufficiency, hyperkalemia, and a persistent dry cough. The potential of symptomatic hypotension with ACE inhibitor therapy requires careful monitoring. ACE inhibitors should not be used in pregnant women.

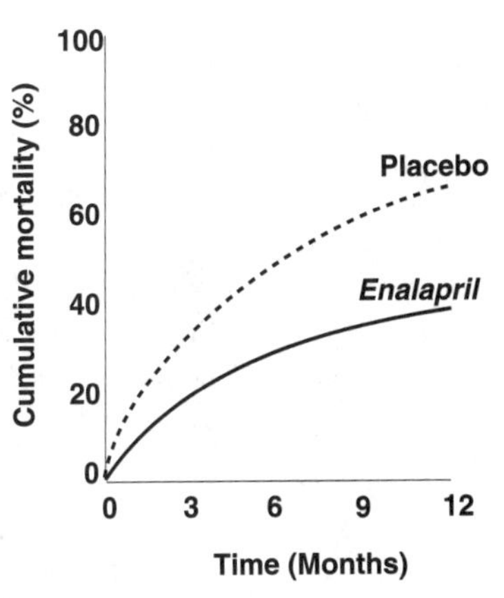

Figure 16.6
Effect of *enalapril* on mortality of patients with congestive heart failure.

B. Direct smooth muscle relaxants

Dilation of venous blood vessels leads to a decrease in cardiac preload by increasing venous capacitance; arterial dilators reduce systemic arteriolar resistance and decrease afterload. Nitrates (see p. 175) are commonly employed venous dilators for patients with congestive heart failure. If the patient is intolerant of ACE inhibitors, the combination of *hydralazine* and *isosorbide dinitrate* is most commonly used. *Amlodipine* and *felodipine* (see p. 188) have less negative inotropic effect than other calcium channel blockers, and seem to decrease sympathetic nervous activity.

IV. DIURETICS

Diuretics relieve pulmonary congestion and peripheral edema. These agents are useful in reducing the symptoms of volume overload, including orthopnea and paroxysmal nocturnal dyspnea. Diuretics decrease plasma volume and subsequently decrease venous return to the heart (preload). This decreases the cardiac workload and oxygen demand. Diuretics also decrease afterload by reducing plasma volume, thus decreasing blood pressure. Thiazide diuretics (see p. 229) are relatively mild diuretics and lose efficacy if patient creatinine clearance is less than 50 ml/min. Loop diuretics (see p. 227) are used in patients with renal insufficiency. [Note: Overdoses of loop diuretics can lead to profound hypovolemia.]

V. INOTROPIC DRUGS

Positive inotropic agents enhance cardiac muscle contractility, and thus increase cardiac output. Although these drugs act by different mechanisms, in each case the inotropic action is the result of an increased cytoplasmic calcium concentration that enhances the contractility of cardiac muscle.

A. Digitalis

The cardiac glycosides are often called digitalis or digitalis glycosides because most of the drugs come from the digitalis (foxglove) plant. They are a group of chemically similar compounds that can increase the contractility of the heart muscle and are therefore widely used in treating heart failure. Like the antiarrhythmic drugs described in Chapter 17, the cardiac glycosides influence the

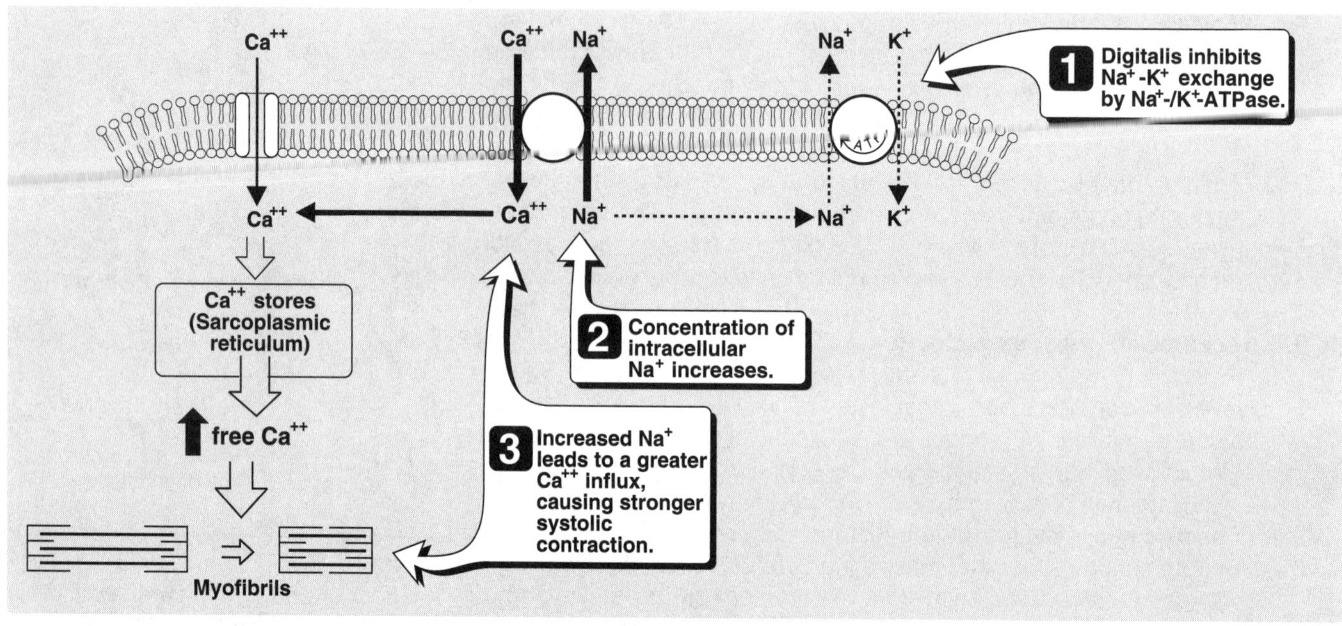

Figure 16.7
Mechanism of action of cardiac glycosides, or digitalis.

sodium and calcium ion flows in the cardiac muscle, thereby increasing contraction of the atrial and ventricular myocardium (positive inotropic action). The digitalis glycosides show only a small difference between a therapeutically effective dose and doses that are toxic or even fatal. Therefore, the drugs have a low therapeutic index (see p. 23). The digitalis glycosides include *digitoxin* [di ji TOX in], and the most widely used agent, *digoxin* [di JOX in].

1. Mode of action:

a. Regulation of cytosolic calcium concentration: Cardiac glycosides combine reversibly with the sodium-potassium ATPase of the cardiac cell membrane (Figure 16.7), resulting in an inhibition of pump activity. This causes an increase in the intracellular sodium concentration, which favors the transport of calcium into the cell via the sodium-calcium exchange mechanism (Figure 16.7). The elevated intracellular calcium levels result in an increase in the systolic force of contraction.

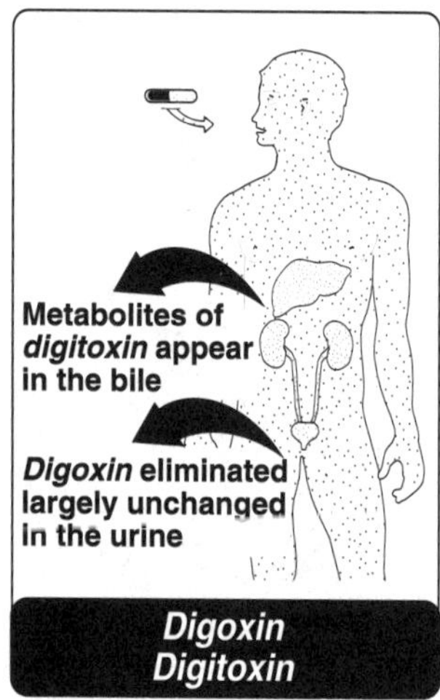

b. Increased contractility of the cardiac muscle: Administration of digitalis glycosides increases the force of cardiac contractility causing the cardiac output to more closely resemble that of the normal heart (Figure 16.8). An increased myocardial contraction leads to a decrease in end diastolic volume, thus increasing the efficiency of contraction (increased ejection fraction). The resulting improved circulation leads to reduced sympathetic activity, which then reduces peripheral resistance. Together, these effects cause a reduction in heart rate. Vagal tone is also enhanced so the heart rate decreases and myocardial oxygen demand is diminished. [Note: In the normal heart, the positive inotropic effect of digitalis is counteracted by compensatory autonomic reflexes.]

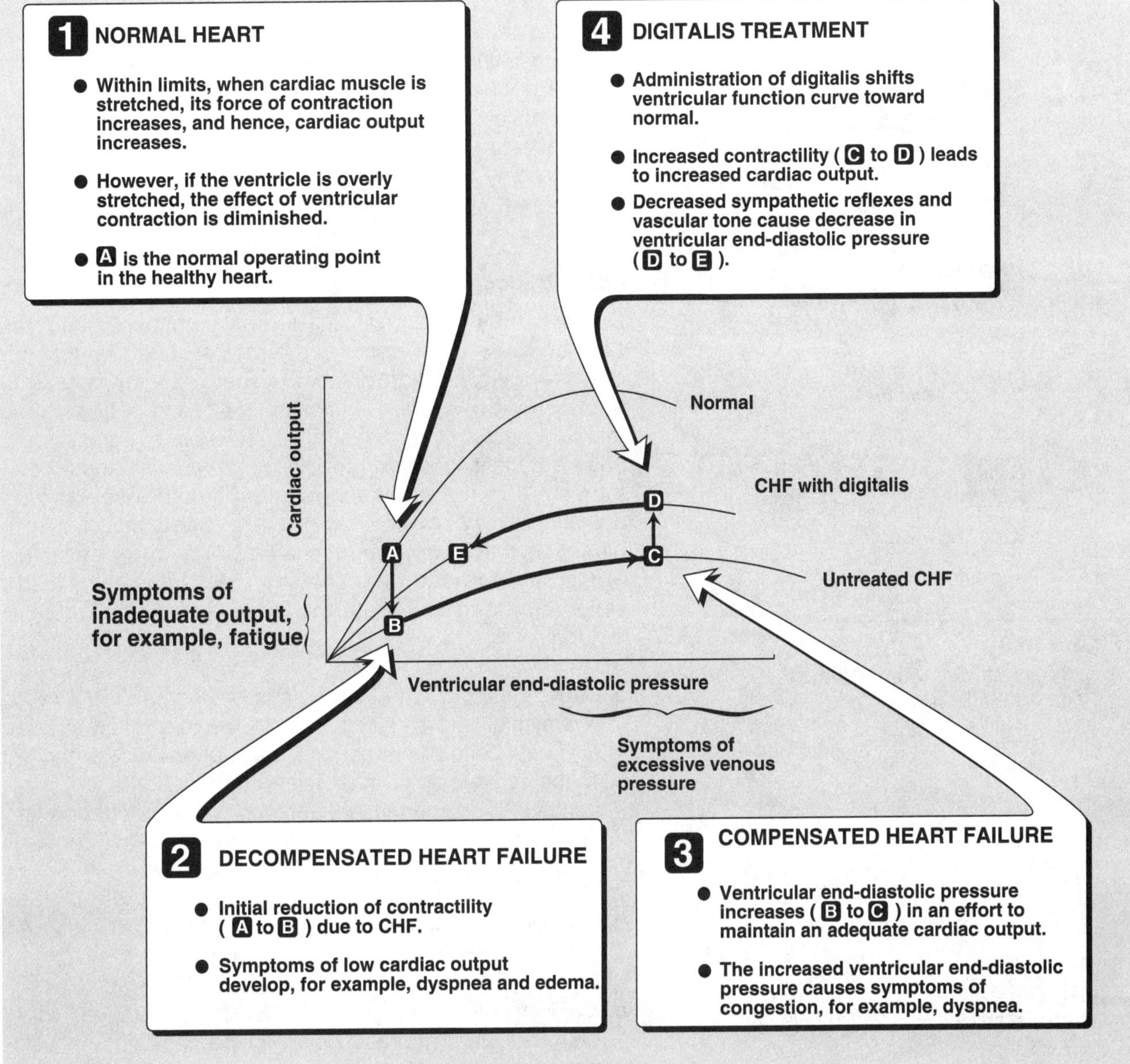

1 NORMAL HEART
Within limits, when cardiac muscle is stretched, its force of contraction increases, and hence, cardiac output increases.
However, if the ventricle is overly stretched, the effect of ventricular contraction is diminished.
A is the normal operating point in the healthy heart.
4 DIGITALIS TREATMENT
Administration of digitalis shifts ventricular function curve toward normal.
Increased contractility (C to D) leads to increased cardiac output.
Decreased sympathetic reflexes and vascular tone cause decrease in ventricular end-diastolic pressure (D to E).
Cardiac output
Normal
CHF with digitalis
Untreated CHF
A
B
C
D
E
Symptoms of inadequate output, for example, fatigue
Ventricular end-diastolic pressure
Symptoms of excessive venous pressure
2 DECOMPENSATED HEART FAILURE
Initial reduction of contractility (A to B) due to CHF.
Symptoms of low cardiac output develop, for example, dyspnea and edema.
3 COMPENSATED HEART FAILURE
Ventricular end-diastolic pressure increases (B to C) in an effort to maintain an adequate cardiac output.
The increased ventricular end-diastolic pressure causes symptoms of congestion, for example, dyspnea.

Figure 16.8
Ventricular function curves in the normal heart, in congestive heart failure (CHF), and in CHF treated with digitalis.

2. **Therapeutic uses:** *Digoxin* therapy is indicated in patients with severe left ventricular systolic dysfunction after initiation of diuretic and vasodilation therapy. *Digoxin* is not indicated in patients with diastolic or right-sided heart failure. *Dobutamine*, another inotropic agent, can be given intravenously in the hospital, but at present no good oral inotropic agents exist other than *digoxin*. Patients with mild to moderate heart failure will often respond to treatment with ACE inhibitors and diuretics and do not require *digoxin*.

3. **Pharmacokinetics:** All digitalis glycosides possess the same pharmacologic actions, but they vary in potency and pharmacokinetics

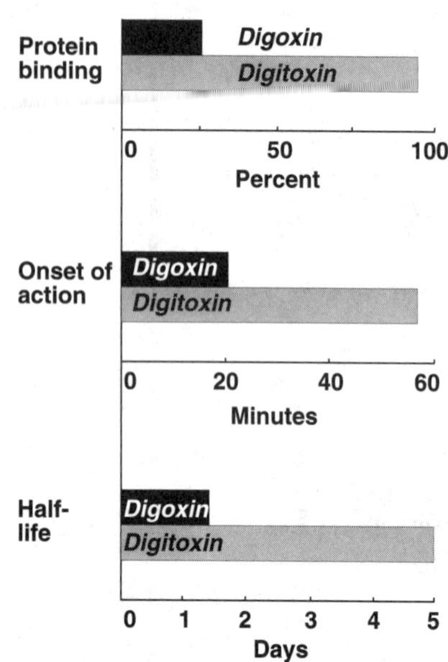

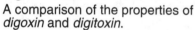

Figure 16.9
A comparison of the properties of *digoxin* and *digitoxin*.

(Figure 16.9). These drugs are absorbed after oral administration. Note that *digitoxin* binds strongly to proteins in the extravascular space, resulting in a large volume of distribution. *Digoxin* has the advantage of a relatively short half-life, which allows better treatment of toxic reactions. *Digoxin* also has a more rapid onset of action, making it useful in emergency situations. *Digoxin* is eliminated largely unchanged in the urine. *Digitoxin* is extensively metabolized by the liver before excretion in the feces, and hepatic disease may require decreased doses.

4. Adverse effects

Digitalis toxicity is one of the most commonly encountered adverse drug reactions. Side effects can often be managed by discontinuing cardiac glycoside therapy, determining serum potassium levels, and if indicated, by giving potassium supplements. In general, decreased serum levels of potassium predispose a patient to *digoxin* toxicity. *Digoxin* levels must be closely monitored in the presence of renal insufficiency and dosage adjustment may be necessary. Severe toxicity resulting in ventricular tachycardia may require administration of antiarrhythmic drugs, and the use of antibodies (FAB fragments) to *digoxin,* which bind and inactivate the drug. Types of adverse effects include:

a. **Cardiac effects:** The major effect is progressively more severe dysrhythmia, moving from decreased or blocked atrioventricular nodal conduction, paroxysmal supraventricular tachycardia, to the conversion of atrial flutter to atrial fibrillation, premature ventricular depolarization, ventricular fibrillation, and finally, to complete heart block. A decrease in intracellular potassium is the primary predisposing factor in these effects.

b. **Gastrointestinal effects:** Anorexia, nausea, and vomiting are commonly encountered adverse effects.

c. **CNS effects:** These include headache, fatigue, confusion, blurred vision, alteration of color perception, and haloes on dark objects.

5. Factors predisposing to digitalis toxicity:

a. **Electrolytic disturbances:** Hypokalemia can precipitate serious arrhythmia. Reduction of serum potassium levels is most frequently observed in patients receiving *thiazide* or loop diuretics, and can usually be prevented by use of a potassium sparing diuretic or supplementation with potassium chloride. Hypercalcemia and hypomagnesemia also predispose to digitalis toxicity.

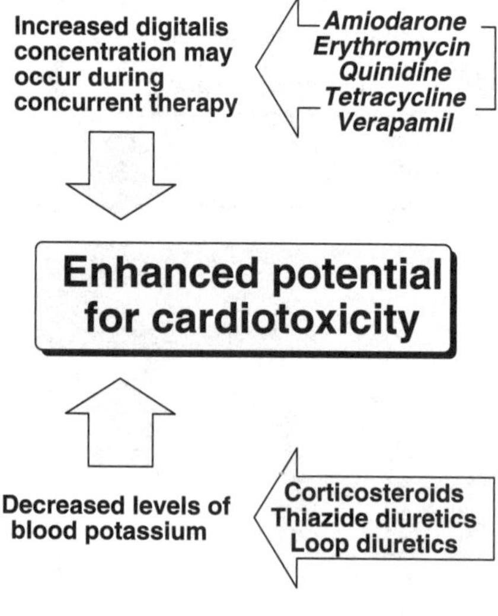

Figure 16.10
Drugs interacting with *digoxin* and other digitalis glycosides.

b. **Drugs:** *Quinidine* can cause *digitalis* intoxication both by displacing *digitalis* from plasma protein binding sites, and by competing with *digitalis* for renal excretion. *Verapamil* also displaces *digitalis* from plasma protein binding sites and can increase *digoxin* levels by 50 to 75%; this may require a reduction in the dose of *digoxin*. Potassium-depleting diuretics, corticosteroids, and a variety of other drugs can also increase digitalis toxicity (Figure 16.10). Hypothyroidism, hypoxia, renal failure, and myocarditis are also predisposing factors to *digitalis* toxicity.

B. β-Adrenergic agonists

β-Adrenergic stimulation improves cardiac performance by positive inotropic effects and vasodilation. *Dobutamine* (see p. 66) is the most commonly used inotropic agent other than digitalis. *Dobutamine* leads to an increase in intracellular cAMP, which results in the activation of protein kinase. Slow calcium channels are one important site of phosphorylation by protein kinase. When phosphorylated, the entry of calcium ion into the myocardial cells increases, thus enhancing contraction (Figure 16.11). *Dobutamine* must be given by intravenous infusion, and is primarily used in the treatment of acute heart failure in a hospital setting.

C. Phosphodiesterase inhibitors

Amrinone [AM ri none] and *milrinone* [MIL ri none] are phosphodiesterase inhibitors that increase the intracellular concentration of cAMP (Figure 16.11). This results in an increase in intracellular calcium, and therefore cardiac contractility, as discussed above for the β-adrenergic agonists. [Note: Recent clinical trials have shown that *amiodarone* did not reduce the incidence of sudden death or prolong survival in patients with CHF (see p. 172). *Milrinone* showed increased mortality and no beneficial effects.]

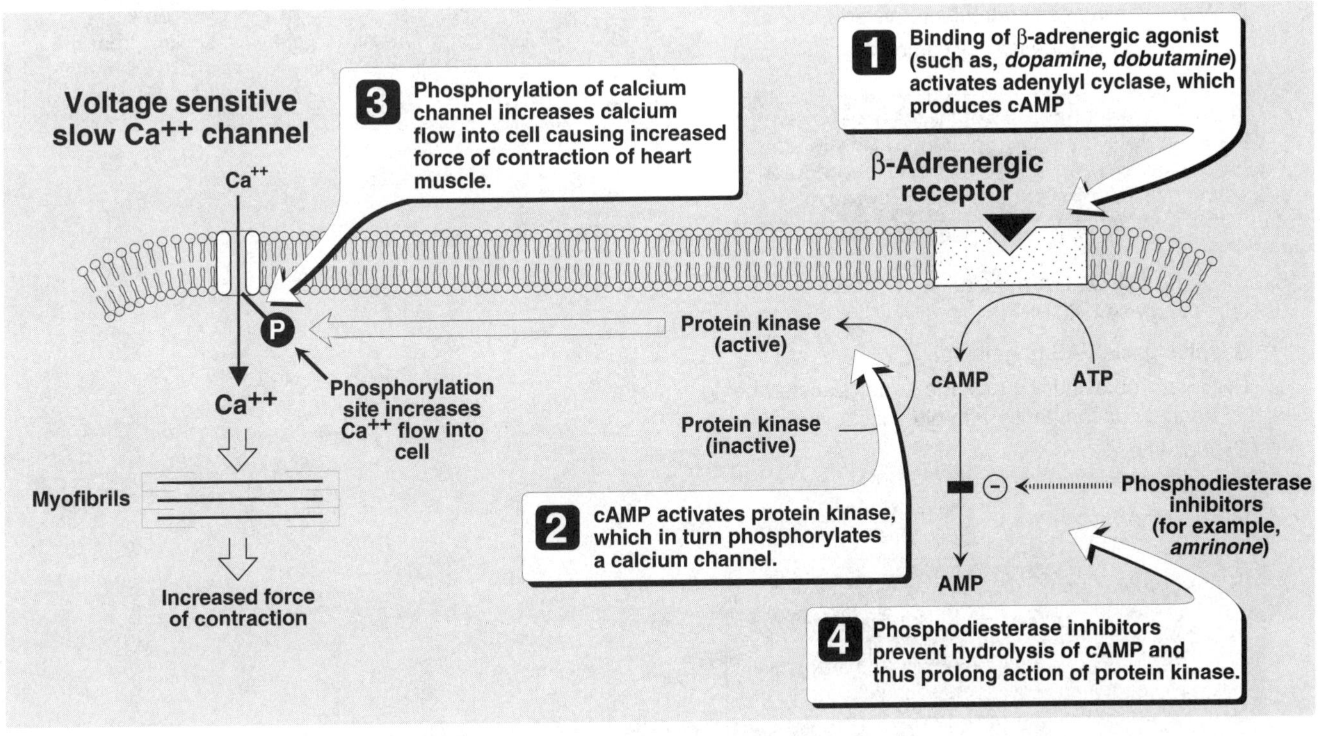

Figure 16.11
Sites of action of β-adrenergic agonists on heart muscle.

Choose the ONE best answer.

16.1 Which of the following most directly describes the mechanism of action of digitalis?

A. Inhibits sodium-potassium ATPase.

B. Decreases intracellular sodium concentration.

C. Increases the intracellular level of ATP.

D. Stimulates production of cAMP.

E. Decreases release of calcium from the sarcoplasmic reticulum.

Correct answer = A. The cardiac glycosides bind to and block the action of the sodium-potassium ATPase. The cardiac glycosides inhibit the extrusion of sodium from the cell, leading to an increase in sodium levels within the cell. The production of ATP is not significantly changed in the treated heart. Stimulation of the production of cAMP is the mechanism of action of the β-adrenergic agonists. By increasing intracellular calcium, digitalis stimulates the SR to release additional calcium.

16.2 Which one of the following drugs would be the most appropriate single drug therapy for mild congestive heart failure?

A. A vasodilator such as hydralazine.

B. A cardiac glycoside such as digoxin.

C. A β-adrenergic agonist such as norepinephrine.

D. A diuretic such as hydrochlorothiazide.

E. An ACE inhibitor, such as captopril.

Correct answer = E. ACE inhibitors may be considered sole therapy in patients who present with mild dyspnea on exertion and who do not show signs or symptoms of volume overload.

16.3 All of the following are useful in the treatment of digitalis overdose EXCEPT:

A. anti-digoxin FAB fragments.

B. dietary potassium supplements for patients being treated concomitantly with diuretics.

C. lidocaine.

D. phenytoin.

E. quinidine.

Correct choice = E. Quinidine may increase digitalis concentration by reducing renal clearance. Purified fragments of antibodies specific for digoxin are used to treat potentially lethal toxicities. Hypokalemia is frequently encountered in individuals taking loop or thiazide diuretics and can predispose the patient to digitalis toxicity. Antiarrhythmic drugs, such as lidocaine and phenytoin, are used for ventricular tachycardia.

16.4 Which one of the following statements concerning congestive heart failure is correct?

A. Digitoxin is more widely used than digoxin because it has a shorter half-life.

B. Serum levels of digoxin can be decreased by quinidine.

C. Loop diuretics are used in patients with renal insufficiency.

D. Digoxin is eliminated primarily in the bile.

E. Congenital heart defects are the most common cause of congestive heart failure.

Correct answer = C.

16.5 Which one of the following aggravates a digitalis-induced arrhythmia?

A. Decreased serum calcium.

B. Decreasing heart rate with propranolol.

C. Decreased serum sodium.

D. Decreased serum potassium.

E. Decreased serum angiotensin II.

Correct answer = D. Low serum potassium further decreases the efflux of sodium from the cardiac cell, leading to an enhanced toxicity. Low levels of circulating calcium diminish the digitalis-stimulated calcium uptake into the cardiac cell. Agents that decrease the heart rate tend to diminish the toxicity of digitalis. Low serum sodium enhances the efflux of sodium from the cardiac cell, leading to a diminished sodium-calcium exchange.

Antiarrhythmic Drugs

17

I. OVERVIEW

In contrast to skeletal muscle, which contracts only when it receives a stimulus, the heart contains specialized cells that exhibit automaticity, that is, they can intrinsically generate rhythmic action potentials in the absence of external stimuli. These "pacemaker" cells differ from other myocardial cells in showing a slow, spontaneous depolarization during diastole (Phase 4) caused by an inward positive current carried by sodium and calcium currents (see p. 152). This depolarization is fastest in the sinoatrial (SA) node (the normal initiation site of the action potential) and decreases throughout the normal conduction pathway through the atrioventricular (AV) node to the bundle of His and the Purkinje system. Dysfunction of impulse generation or conduction at any of a number of sites in the heart can cause an abnormality in cardiac rhythm. Figure 17.1 summarizes the drugs used to treat cardiac arrhythmias.

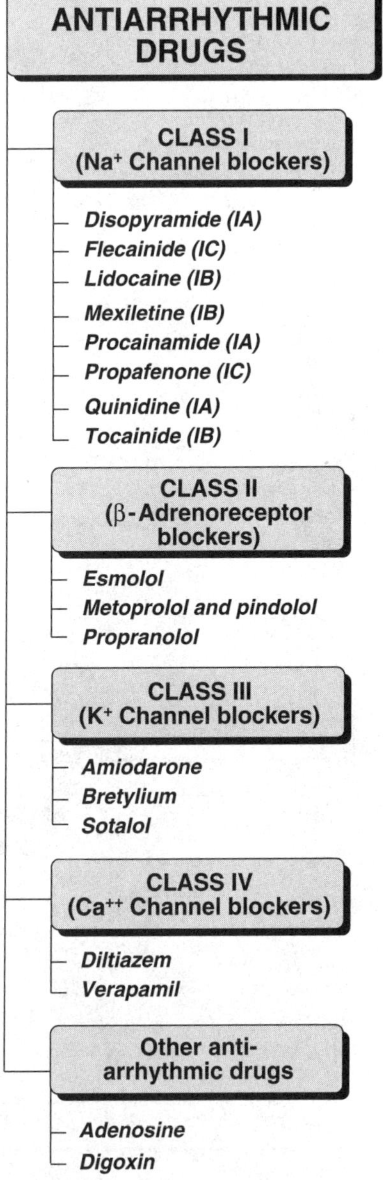

ANTIARRHYTHMIC DRUGS
CLASS I (Na+ Channel blockers)
Disopyramide (IA)
Flecainide (IC)
Lidocaine (IB)
Mexiletine (IB)
Procainamide (IA)
Propafenone (IC)
Quinidine (IA)
Tocainide (IB)
CLASS II (β-Adrenoreceptor blockers)
Esmolol
Metoprolol and pindolol
Propranolol
CLASS III (K+ Channel blockers)
Amiodarone
Bretylium
Sotalol
CLASS IV (Ca++ Channel blockers)
Diltiazem
Verapamil
Other anti-arrhythmic drugs
Adenosine
Digoxin

Figure 17.1
Summary of antiarrhythmic drugs.

II. INTRODUCTION TO THE ARRHYTHMIAS

The arrhythmias are conceptually simple—dysfunctions cause abnormalities in impulse formation and conduction in the myocardium. However, in the clinic, arrhythmias present as a complex family of disorders that show a variety of symptoms. For example, cardiac arrhythmias may cause the heart (1) to beat too slowly (sinus bradycardia); (2) to beat too rapidly (sinus or ventricular tachycardia, atrial or ventricular premature depolarization, atrial flutter); (3) to respond to impulses originating from sites other than the SA node; or (4) to respond to impulses traveling along accessory (extra) pathways that lead to deviant depolarizations (A-V reentry, Wolff-Parkinson White syndrome). In order to make sense of this large group of disorders, it is useful to organize the arrhythmias into groups according to the anatomic site of the the abnormality—the atria, AV node, or the ventricles. Figure 17.2 summarizes several commonly occurring atrial, AV junction or ventricular arrhythmias. Although not shown here, each of these abnormalities can be further divided into subgroups depending on the electrocardiogram (ECG) findings.

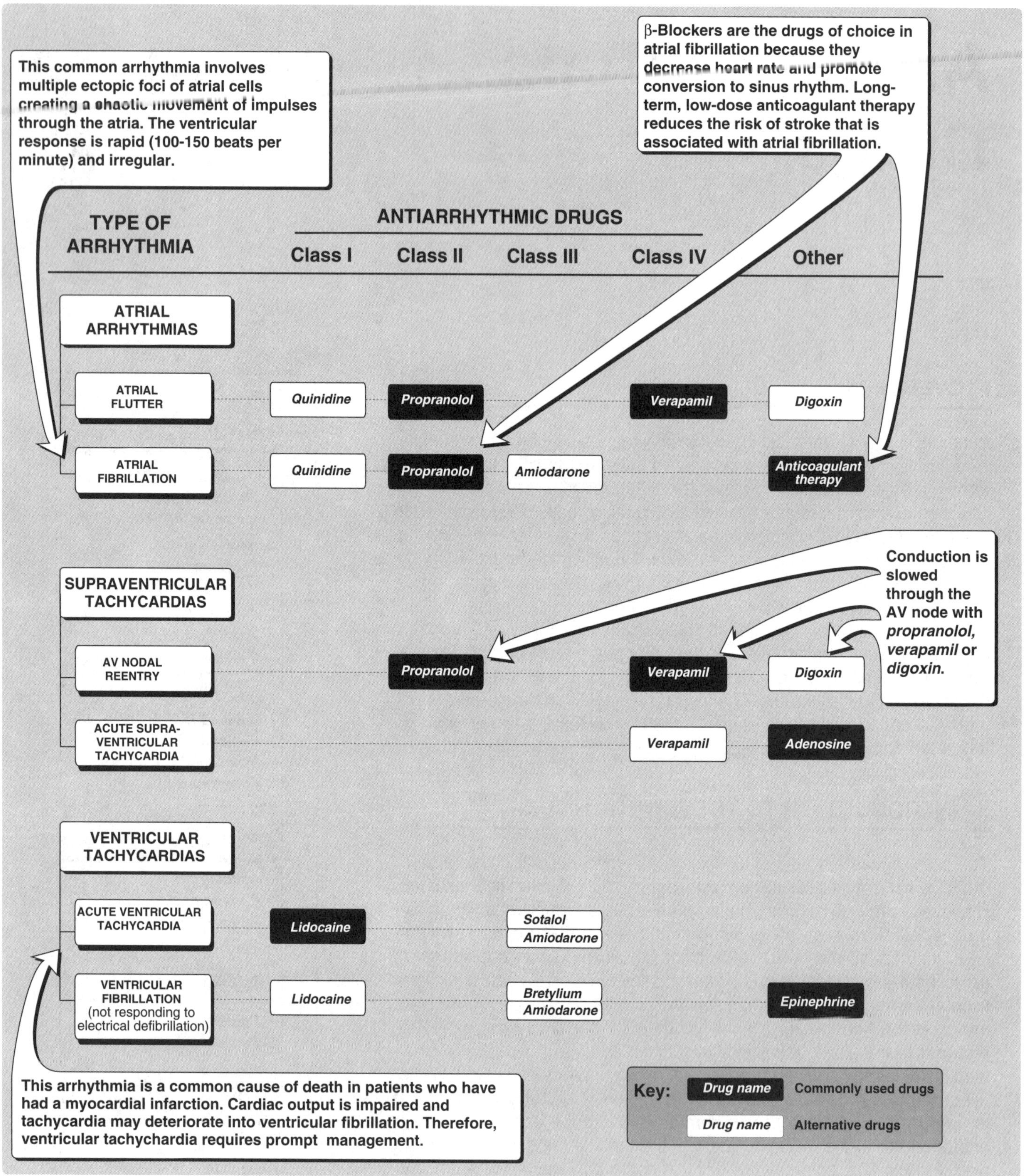

Figure 17.2
Therapeutic indications for some commonly encountered arrhythmias.

A. Causes of arrhythmias

Most arrhythmias arise either from aberrations in impulse generation (abnormal automaticity) or from a defect in impulse conduction.

1. **Abnormal automaticity:** The SA node shows the fastest rate of Phase 4 depolarization and therefore, exhibits a higher rate of discharge than that occurring in other pacemaker cells exhibiting automaticity. The SA node thus normally sets the pace of contraction for the myocardium, and latent pacemakers are depolarized by impulses coming from the SA node. However, if cardiac sites other than the SA node show enhanced automaticity, they may generate competing stimuli, and arrhythmias may arise. Abnormal automaticity may also occur if the myocardial cells are damaged, for example, by hypoxia or potassium imbalance. These cells may remain partially depolarized during diastole and therefore can reach the firing threshold earlier than normal cells. Abnormal automatic discharges may thus be induced.

2. **Effect of drugs on automaticity:** Most of the antiarrhythmic agents suppress automaticity (1) by decreasing the slope of Phase 4 (diastolic) depolarization and/or (2) by raising the threshold of discharge to a less negative voltage. Such drugs cause the frequency of discharge to decrease, an effect that is more pronounced in cells with ectopic pacemaker activity than in normal cells.

3. **Abnormalities in impulse conduction:** Impulses from higher pacemaker centers are normally conducted down pathways that bifurcate to activate the entire ventricular surface (Figure 17.3). A phenomenon called reentry can occur if a unidirectional block caused by myocardial injury or a prolonged refractory period results in an abnormal conduction pathway. Reentry is the most common cause of arrhythmias and can occur at any level of the cardiac conduction system. For example, consider a single Purkinje fiber with two conduction pathways to ventricular muscle. An impulse normally travels down both limbs of the conduction path. However, if myocardial injury results in a unidirectional block, the impulse may only be conducted down pathway #1 (see Figure 17.3). If the block in pathway #2 is in the forward direction only, the impulse may travel in a retrograde fashion through pathway #2 and reenter the point of bifurcation. This short-circuit pathway results in reexcitation of the ventricular muscle, causing premature contraction or sustained ventricular arrhythmia.

4. **Effects of drugs on conduction abnormalities:** Antiarrhythmic agents prevent reentry by slowing conduction and/or increasing the refractory period required to convert a unidirectional block into a bidirectional block.

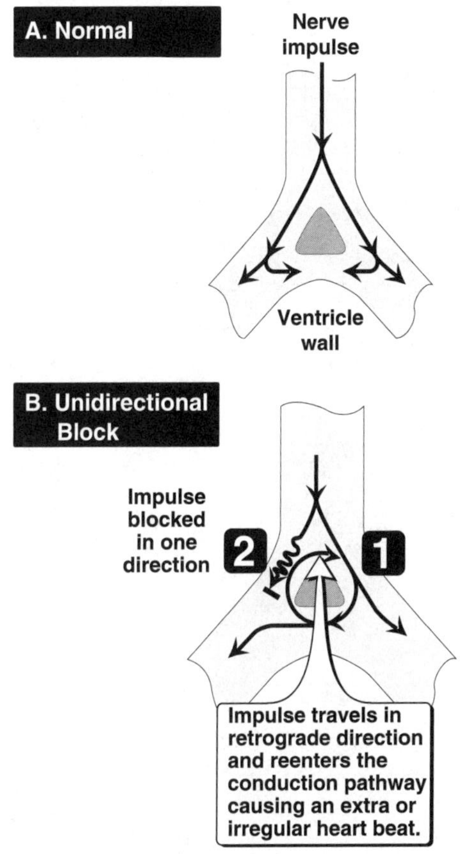

Figure 17.3
Schematic representation of reentry.

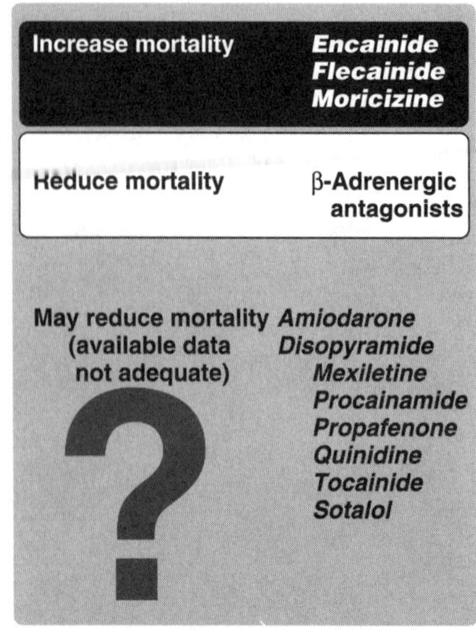

Increase mortality
Encainide
Flecainide
Moricizine
Reduce mortality
β-Adrenergic antagonists
May reduce mortality (available data not adequate)
Amiodarone
Disopyramide
Mexiletine
Procainamide
Propafenone
Quinidine
Tocainide
Sotalol
?

Figure 17.4
Effect of long-term antiarrhythmic therapy on mortality based on placebo-controlled, randomized trials.

B. Antiarrhythmic drugs

As noted above, the antiarrhythmic drugs can modify impulse generation and conduction. More than a dozen such drugs that are potentially useful in treating arrhythmias are currently available. However, only a limited number of these agents are clinically beneficial in the treatment of selected arrhythmias. For example, the acute termination of ventricular tachycardia by *lidocaine* or supraventricular tachycardia by *adenosine* or *verapamil* are examples in which antiarrhythmic therapy results in decreased morbidity. In contrast, many of the antiarrhythmic agents are now known to have lethal proarrhythmic actions, that is, to cause arrhythmias.

1. **Proarrhythmic effects of antiarrhythmic drugs:** In the Cardiac Arrhythmia Suppression Trial (CAST) treatment with *encainide* and *flecainide*, two class IC antiarrhythmic agents, successfully prevented ventricular ectopic beats in patients who had myocardial infarction. However, continued therapy with either drug was associated with a two- to three-fold increase in death due to cardiac arrhythmias. Similar results were reported for *moricizine*. Increased death was probably due to drug-induced fatal arrhythmias triggered by recurrent myocardial ischemia.

2. **The unexpected conclusion:** The results of CAST challenged the assumption that treating postmyocardial arrhythmia—and perhaps arrhythmias in general—was in fact beneficial. CAST accentuated the fact that the efficacy of many antiarrhythmic agents remains unproven in placebo-controlled, random trials (Figure 17.4). This has caused many clinicians to review current drug recommendations, particularly as new data from clinical trials become available.

III. CLASS I ANTIARRHYTHMIC DRUGS

The antiarrhythmic drugs can be classified according to their predominant effects on the action potential. Although this classification is convenient, it is not entirely clear-cut, because many of the drugs have

Classification of Drug	Mechanism of Action	Comment
IA	Na^+ channel blocker	Slows Phase 0 depolarization
IB	Na^+ channel blocker	Shortens Phase 3 repolarization
IC	Na^+ channel blocker	Markedly slows Phase 0 depolarization
II	β Adrenoreceptor blocker	Suppresses Phase 4 depolarization
III	K^+ channel blocker	Prolongs Phase 3 repolarization
IV	Ca^{++} channel blocker	Shortens action potential

Figure 17.5
Actions of antiarrhythmic drugs.

actions relating to more than one class or they may have active metabolites with a different class of action. Class I antiarrhythmic drugs act by blocking voltage-sensitive sodium channels by the same mechanism as local anesthetics (see p. 117). The decreased rate of entry of sodium slows the rate of rise of Phase 0 of the action potential. [Note: At therapeutic doses, these drugs have little effect on the resting, fully polarized membrane.] Class I antiarrhythmic drugs therefore generally cause a decrease in excitability and conduction velocity.

A. Use-dependence

Class I drugs bind more rapidly to open or inactivated sodium channels than to channels that are fully repolarized following recovery from the previous depolarization cycle. Therefore, these drugs show a greater degree of blockade in tissues that are frequently depolarizing (for example, during tachycardia when the sodium channels open often). This property is called use-dependence (or state-dependence) and enables these drugs to block cells that are discharging at an abnormally high frequency without interfering with the normal low-frequency beating of the heart. The Class I drugs have been subdivided into three groups according to their effect on the duration of the action potential. Class IA agents slow the rate of rise of the action potential, thus slowing conduction, and prolong the action potential and increase the ventricular effective refractory period. They have an intermediate speed of association with activated/inactivated sodium channels, and an intermediate rate of dissociation from resting channels. Class IB drugs have little effect on the rate of depolarization, but rather they decrease the duration of the action potential by shortening repolarization. They rapidly interact with sodium channels. Class IC agents markedly depress the rate of rise of the membrane action potential, and therefore they cause marked conduction slowing but have little effect on the duration of the membrane action potential or the ventricular effective refractory period. They bind slowly to sodium channels. [See Figure 17.5 for a summary of the actions of the antiarrhythmic drugs.]

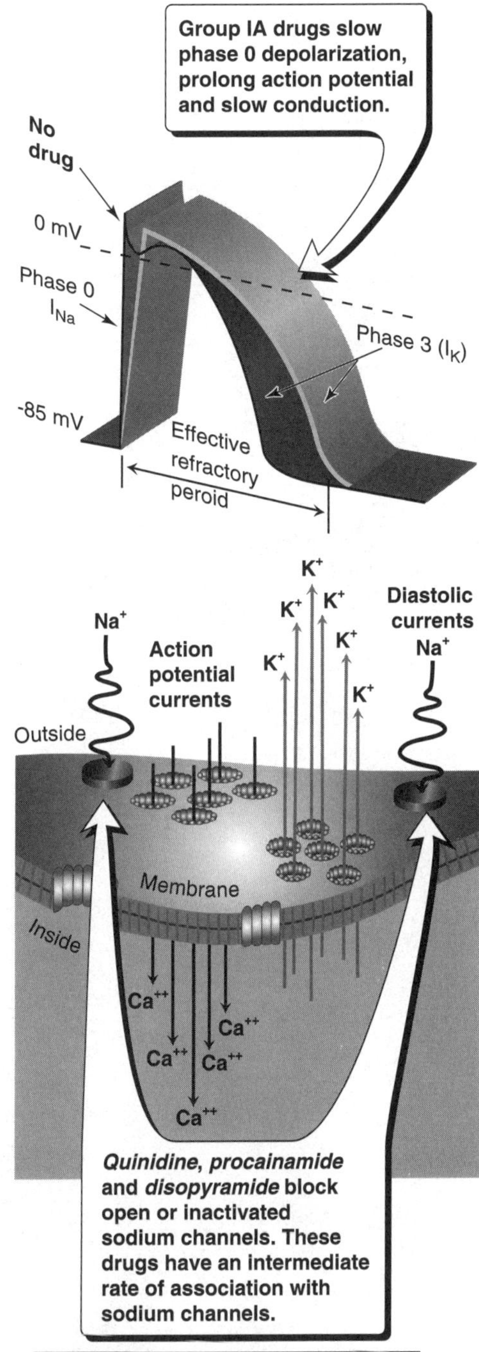

Group IA drugs slow phase 0 depolarization, prolong action potential and slow conduction.
No drug
0 mV
Phase 0
I_{Na}
Phase 3 (I_K)
-85 mV
Effective refractory peroid
K^+
Na^+
Action potential currents
Diastolic currents
Na^+
Outside
Membrane
Inside
Ca^{++}
Quinidine, procainamide and *disopyramide* block open or inactivated sodium channels. These drugs have an intermediate rate of association with sodium channels.

Figure 17.6
Schematic diagram of the effects of Group IA agents.

B. Quinidine

Quinidine [KWIN i deen] is the prototype Class IA drug. At high doses, it can actually precipitate arrhythmias, which can lead to fatal ventricular fibrillation. Because of *quinidine's* toxic potential, calcium antagonists, such as *verapamil*, are increasingly replacing this drug in clinical use.

1. **Mechanism of action:** *Quinidine* binds to open and inactivated sodium channels and prevents sodium influx, thus slowing the rapid upstroke during Phase 0 (Figure 17.6). It also decreases the slope of Phase 4 spontaneous depolarization.

2. **Actions:** *Quinidine* inhibits ectopic arrhythmias and ventricular arrhythmias caused by increased normal automaticity. *Quinidine* also prevents reentry arrhythmias by producing bidirectional block through decreasing membrane responsiveness and pro-

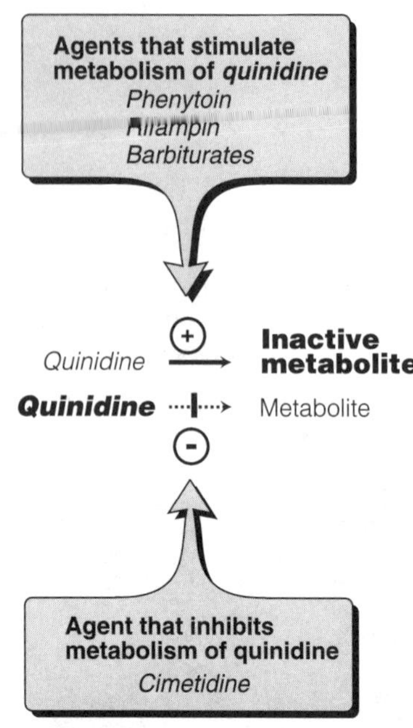

Figure 17.7
Drugs affecting the metabolism of *quinidine*.

longing the effective refractory period. The drug has little effect on normal automaticity. [Note: *Quinidine* can induce a tachycardia in normal individuals because of its atropine-like (anticholinergic) effect.]

3. **Therapeutic uses:** *Quinidine* is used in the treatment of a wide variety of arrhythmias, including atrial, AV junctional, and ventricular tachyarrhythmias. *Quinidine* is used to maintain sinus rhythm after direct current cardioversion of atrial flutter or fibrillation and to prevent frequent ventricular tachycardia.

4. **Pharmacokinetics:** *Quinidine sulfate* is rapidly and almost completely absorbed after oral administration.

5. **Adverse effects:** A potential adverse effect of *quinidine* (or any antiarrhythmic drug) is exacerbation of the arrhythmia. *Quinidine* may cause SA and AV block or asystole. At toxic levels, the drug may induce ventricular tachycardia. Cardiotoxic effects are exacerbated by hyperkalemia. *Quinidine* can increase the steady state concentration of *digoxin* by displacement of *digoxin* from tissue binding sites. Nausea, vomiting, and diarrhea are commonly observed. Large doses may induce the symptoms of cinchonism, for example, blurred vision, tinnitus, headache, disorientation, and psychosis. The drug has a mild α-adrenergic blocking action as well as an *atropine*-like effect. Drugs interacting with *quinidine* are shown in Figure 17.7

C. Procainamide

1. **Actions:** This Class IA drug, a derivative of the local anesthetic *procaine* (see p. 117), shows actions similar to those of *quinidine*.

2. **Pharmacokinetics** *Procainamide* [pro kane A mide] is absorbed following oral administration. [Note: The intravenous route is rarely used because hypotension occurs if the drug is too rapidly infused.] *Procainamide* has a relatively short half-life of 2-3 hours. A portion of the drug is acetylated in the liver to N-acetylprocainamide (NAPA), which has little effect on the maximum polarization of Purkinje fibers but prolongs the duration of the action potential. Thus, NAPA has properties of a Class III drug. NAPA is eliminated via the kidney, and dosages of *procainamide* may need to be adjusted in patients with renal failure.

3. **Adverse effects:** With chronic use, *procainamide* causes a high incidence of side effects, including a reversible lupus erythematosus-like syndrome that develops in 25 to 30% of patients. Toxic concentrations of *procainamide* may cause asystole or induction of ventricular arrhythmias. Central nervious system (CNS) side effects include depression, hallucination and psychosis. With this drug, gastrointestinal intolerance is less frequent than with *quinidine*.

D. Disopyramide

1. **Actions:** This Class IA drug shows actions similar to those of *quinidine*. *Disopyramide* [dye so PEER a mide] produces a negative inotropic effect that is greater than the weak effect exerted by *quinidine* and *procainamide*, and unlike the latter drugs, *disopyramide* causes peripheral vasoconstriction. The drug may produce a clinically important decrease in myocardial contractility in patients with preexisting impairment of left ventricular function. *Disopyramide* is used for treatment of ventricular arrhythmias as an alternative to *procainamide* or *quinidine*.

2. **Pharmacokinetics** Approximately one half of the orally ingested drug is excreted unchanged by the kidneys. About 30% of the drug is converted by the liver to the less active mono-N-dealkylated metabolite.

3. **Adverse effects:** *Disopyramide* shows effects of anticholinergic activity, for example, dry mouth, urinary retention, blurred vision, and constipation.

E. Lidocaine

Lidocaine [LYE doe kane] is a Class IB drug. The IB agents rapidly associate and dissociate from sodium channels. Thus the actions of Class IB agents are manifested when the cardiac cell is depolarized or firing rapidly. Class IB drugs are particularly useful in treating ventricular arrhythmias. *Lidocaine* is the drug of choice for emergency treatment of cardiac arrhythmias.

1. **Actions:** *Lidocaine*, a local anesthetic, shortens phase 3 repolarization and decreases the duration of the action potential (Figure 17.8). Unlike *quinidine*, which suppresses arrhythmias caused by increased normal automaticity, *lidocaine* suppresses arrhythmias caused by abnormal automaticity. *Lidocaine*, like *quinidine*, abolishes ventricular reentry.

2. **Therapeutic uses:** *Lidocaine* is useful in treating ventricular arrhythmias arising during myocardial ischemia, such as that experienced during a myocardial infarction. The drug does not markedly slow conduction and thus has little effect on atrial or AV junction arrhythmias.

3. **Pharmacokinetics:** *Lidocaine* is given intravenously because of extensive first-pass transformation by the liver, which precludes oral administration. The drug is dealkylated and eliminated almost entirely by the liver, consequently dosage adjustment may be necessary in patients with liver dysfunction.

4. **Adverse effects:** *Lidocaine* has a fairly wide toxic-to-therapeutic ratio; it shows little impairment of left ventricular function, and has no negative inotropic effect. The CNS effects include drowsiness, slurred speech, paresthesia, agitation, confusion, and convulsions; cardiac arrhythmias may also occur.

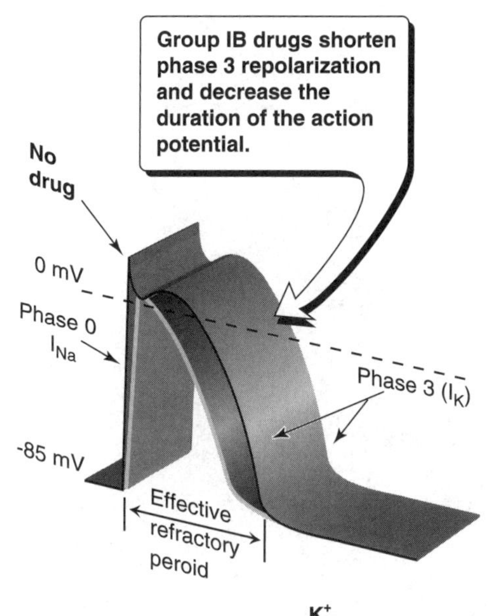

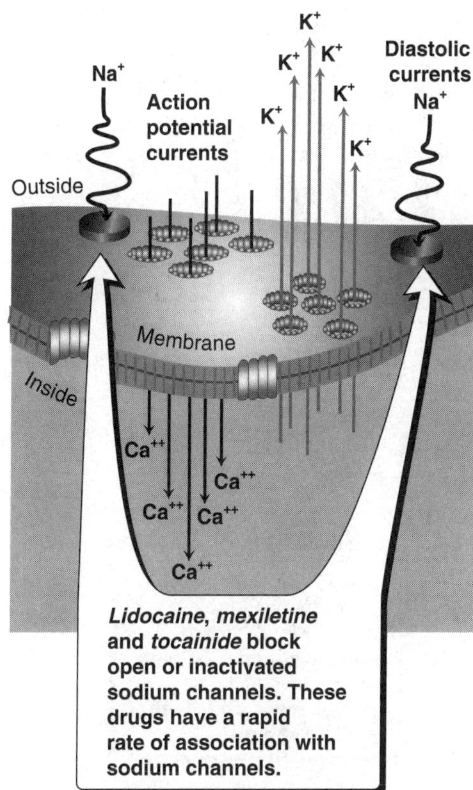

Figure 17.8
Schematic diagram of the effects of Group IB agents.

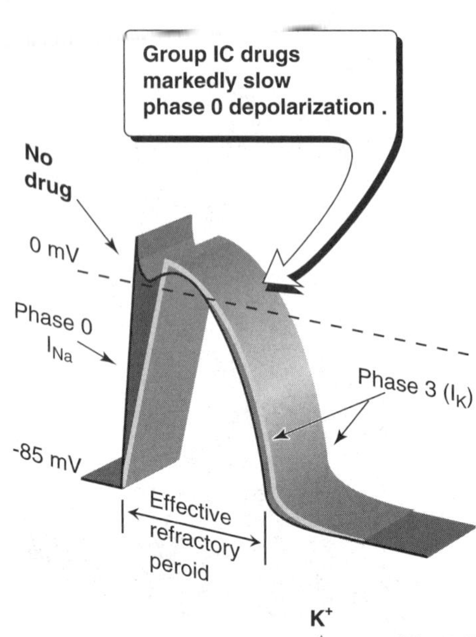

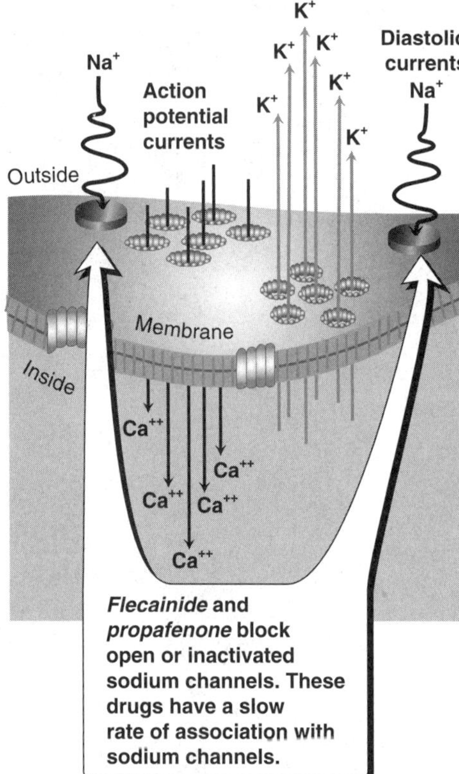

Figure 17.9
Schematic diagram of the effects of Group IC agents.

F. Mexiletine and tocainide

These are Class IB drugs with actions similar to those of *lidocaine*. These agents can be administered orally. *Mexiletine* [mex IL e teen] is used for chronic treatment of ventricular arrhythmias associated with previous myocardial infarction. *Tocainide* [toe KAY nide] is used for treatment of ventricular tachyarrhythmias. *Tocainide* has pulmonary toxicity, which may lead to pulmonary fibrosis.

G. Flecainide

Flecainide [fle KAY nide] is a Class IC drug. These drugs slowly dissociate from resting sodium channels and show prominent effects, even at normal heart rates. These drugs are approved only for refractory ventricular arrhythmias. However, recent data have cast serious doubts on the safety of the Class IC drugs.

1. **Actions:** *Flecainide* suppresses Phase 0 upstroke in Purkinje and myocardial fibers (Figure 17.9). This causes marked slowing of conduction in all cardiac tissue, with a minor effect on the duration of the action potential and refractoriness. Automaticity is reduced by an increase in the threshold potential rather than a decrease in the slope of Phase 4 depolarization.

2. **Therapeutic uses:** *Flecainide* is useful in treating refractory ventricular arrhythmias. It is particularly useful in suppressing premature ventricular contraction. *Flecainide* has a negative inotropic effect and can aggravate congestive heart failure.

3. **Pharmacokinetics:** *Flecainide* is absorbed orally, undergoes minimal biotransformation, and has a half-life of 16 to 20 hours.

4. **Adverse effects:** *Flecainide* can cause dizziness, blurred vision, headache, and nausea. Like other Class IC drugs, *flecainide* can aggravate preexisting arrhythmias or induce life-threatening ventricular tachycardia that is resistant to treatment (see p. 166).

H. Propafenone

This Class IC drug shows actions similar to those of *flecainide*. *Propafenone* [proe POF en one], like *flecainide*, slows conduction in all cardiac tissues and is considered a broad spectrum antiarrhythmic agent.

IV. CLASS II ANTIARRHYTHMIC DRUGS

The Class II agents include the β-adrenergic antagonists (see p. 73). These drugs diminish Phase 4 depolarization, thus depressing automaticity, prolonging AV conduction, and decreasing heart rate and contractility. Class II agents are useful in treating tachyarrhythmias caused by increased sympathetic activity. They are also used for atrial flutter and fibrillation, and for AV nodal reentrant tachycardia.

A. Propranolol

Propranolol reduces the incidence of sudden arrhythmic death after myocardial infarction (the most common cause of death in this group of patients). The mortality rate in the first year after a heart attack is significantly reduced by *propranolol*, partly because of its ability to prevent ventricular arrhythmias. (*Propranolol* is described in detail on p. 74)

B. Metoprolol and pindolol

Propranolol is the β-adrenergic antagonist most widely used in the treatment of cardiac arrhythmias. However, β_1-specific drugs, such as *metoprolol* (see p. 77) reduce the risk of bronchospasm, and drugs with partial agonist activity, such as *pindolol* (see p. 77), may decrease the frequency of cardiac failure.

C. Esmolol

Esmolol [ESS moe lol] is a very short-acting β blocker used for intravenous administration in acute arrhythmias occurring during surgery or emergency situations.

V. CLASS III ANTIARRHYTHMIC DRUGS

Class III agents block potassium channels and thus diminish the outward potassium current during repolarization of cardiac cells. These agents prolong the duration of the action potential without altering Phase 0 of depolarization or the resting membrane potential (Figure 17.10). Instead, they prolong the effective refractory period. All Class III drugs have the potential to induce arrhythmias.

A. Sotalol

Sotalol [SOE ta lol], although a class III antiarrhythmic agent, also has potent β-blocker activity. It is well established that β-blockers reduce mortality associated with acute myocardial infarction.

1. **Actions:** *Sotalol* blocks a rapid outward potassium current, known as the delayed rectifier. This blockade prolongs both repolarization and the duration of the action potential, thus lengthening the effective refractory period.

2. **Therapeutic uses:** β-Blockers are used for long-term therapy to decrease the rate of sudden death following an acute myocardial infarction. β-Blockers have modest ability to suppress ectopic beats and reduce myocardial oxygen demand. They have strong antifibrillary effects, particularly in the ischemic myocardium. *Sotalol* was more effective in preventing arrhythmia recurrence and in decreasing mortality than *imipramine*, *mexiletine*, *procainamide*, *propafenone* and *quinidine* in patients with sustained ventricular tachycardia (Figure 17.11).

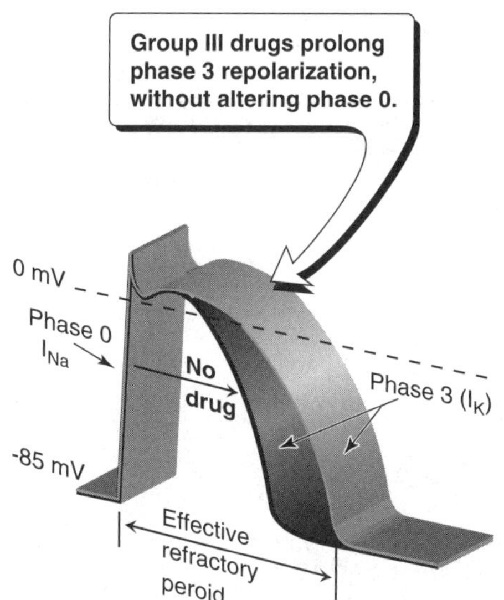

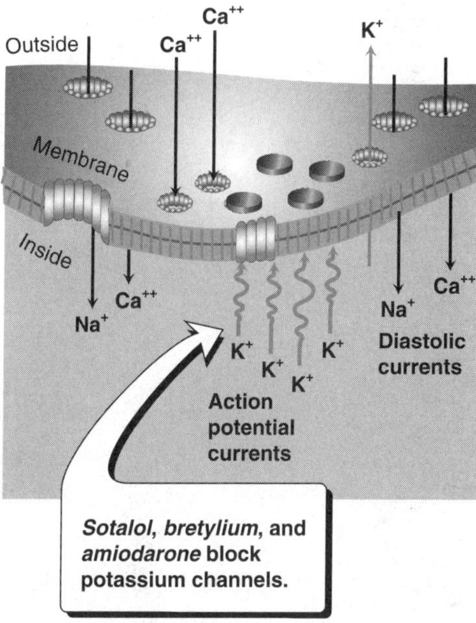

Figure 17.10
Schematic diagram of the effects of Group III agents.

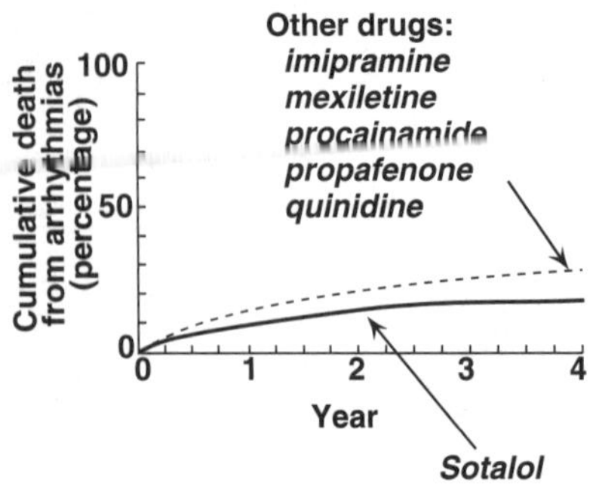

Figure 17.11
Comparison of *sotalol* with six other drugs with respect to deaths due to cardiac arrhythmias.

3. **Adverse effects:** This drug also had the lowest rate of acute or long-term adverse effects. As with all drugs that prolong the QT interval, the syndrome of torsade de pointes is a serious potential adverse effect, typically seen in 3 to 4% of patients.

B. Bretylium

1. **Actions:** *Bretylium* has a number of direct and indirect electrophysiological actions, the most prominent of which are prolongation of the refractory period and raising of the intensity of the electrical current necessary to induce ventricular fibrillation in the His-Purkinje system.

2. **Therapeutic uses:** *Bretylium* is reserved for life-threatening ventricular arrhythmias, especially recurrent ventricular fibrillation or tachycardia.

3. **Pharmacokinetics:** *Bretylium* is poorly absorbed from the gastrointestinal tract and therefore is usually administered parenterally. The drug is excreted unchanged in the urine, and dosage may have to be adjusted in patients with kidney dysfunctions.

4. **Adverse effects:** *Bretylium* can cause severe postural hypotension.

C. Amiodarone

1. **Actions:** *Amiodarone* [a MEE oh da rone] contains iodine and is related structurally to thyroxine. It has complex effects showing Class I, II, III and IV actions. Its dominant effect is prolongation of the action potential duration and the refractory period. *Amiodarone* has antianginal as well as antiarrhythmic activity.

2. **Therapeutic uses:** *Amiodarone* is effective in the treatment of severe refractory supraventricular and ventricular tachyarrhythmia. Its clinical usefulness is limited by its toxicity.

3. **Pharmacokinetics:** *Amiodarone* is incompletely absorbed after oral administration. The drug is unusual in having a prolonged half-life of several weeks. Full clinical effects may not be achieved until 6 weeks after initiation of treatment.

4. **Adverse effects:** *Amiodarone* shows a variety of toxic effects. After long-term use, more than one half of the patients receiving the drug show side effects sufficiently severe to prompt its discontinuation. Some of the more common effects include interstitial pulmonary fibrosis, gastrointestinal tract intolerance, tremor, ataxia, dizziness, hyper- or hypothyroidism, liver toxicity, photosensitivity, neuropathy, muscle weakness, and blue skin discoloration caused by iodine accumulation in the skin. As noted earlier (see p. 166) recent clinical trials have shown that *amiodarone* did not reduce incidence of sudden death or prolong survival in patient with congestive heart failure (CHF).

VI. CLASS IV ANTIARRHYTHMIC DRUGS

The Class IV drugs are calcium channel blockers. They decrease the inward current carried by calcium, resulting in a decrease in the rate of Phase 4 spontaneous depolarization and slowed conduction in tissues dependent on calcium currents, such as the AV node (Figure 17.12). Although voltage-sensitive calcium channels occur in many different tissues, the major effect of calcium-channel blockers is on vascular smooth muscle and the heart.

A. Verapamil and diltiazem

Verapamil [ver AP a mill] shows greater action on the heart than on vascular smooth muscle, whereas *nifedipine*, a calcium channel-blocker used to treat hypertension (see p. 187) exerts a stronger effect on vascular smooth muscle than on the heart. *Diltiazem* [dil TYE a zem] is intermediate in its actions.

1. **Actions:** Calcium enters cells by voltage-sensitive channels and by receptor-operated channels that are controlled by the binding of agonists, such as catecholamines, to membrane receptors. Calcium channel blockers, such as *verapamil* and *diltiazem*, are more effective against the voltage-sensitive channels, causing a decrease in the slow inward current that triggers cardiac contraction (see p. 152). *Verapamil* and *diltiazem* bind only to open, depolarized channels, thus preventing repolarization until the drug dissociates from the channel. These drugs are therefore use-dependent (see p. 166), that is, they block most effectively when the heart is beating rapidly, since in a normally paced heart, the calcium channels have time to repolarize, and the bound drug dissociates from the channel before the next conduction pulse. By decreasing the inward current carried by calcium, *verapamil* and *diltiazem* slow conduction and prolong the effective refractory period in tissues dependent on calcium currents, such as the AV node. These drugs are therefore effective in treating arrhythmias that must traverse calcium-dependent cardiac tissues.

2. **Therapeutic uses:** *Verapamil* and *diltiazem* are more effective against atrial than ventricular dysrhythmias. They are useful in treating reentrant supraventricular tachycardia and reducing ventricular rate in atrial flutter and fibrillation. In addition, these drugs are used to treat hypertension (see p. 187) and angina (see p. 177).

3. **Pharmacokinetics:** *Verapamil* and *diltiazem* are absorbed after oral administration. *Verapamil* is extensively metabolized by the liver; thus, care should be taken in administration of this drug to patients with hepatic dysfunction.

4. **Adverse effects:** *Verapamil* and *diltiazem* have negative inotropic properties and therefore may be contraindicated in patients with preexisting depressed cardiac function. Both drugs can also cause a decrease in blood pressure caused by peripheral vasodilation.

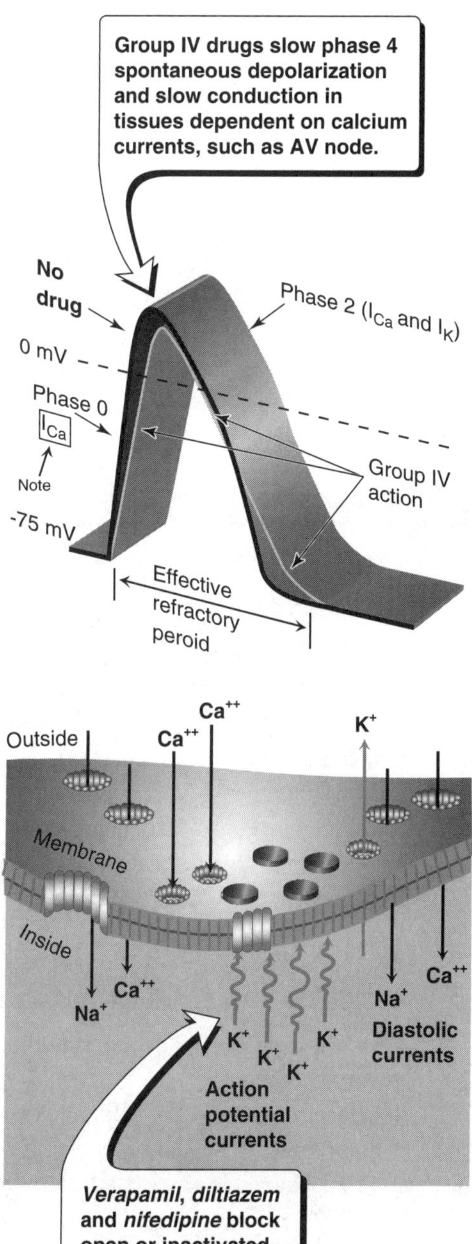

Figure 17.12
Schematic diagram of the effects of Group IV agents.

VII. OTHER ANTIARRHYTHMIC DRUGS

A. Digoxin

Digoxin (see p. 158) shortens the refractory period in atrial and ventricular myocardial cells while prolonging the effective refractory period and diminishing conduction velocity in Purkinje fibers. *Digoxin* is used to control the ventricular response rate in atrial fibrillation and flutter. At toxic concentrations, *digoxin* causes ectopic ventricular beats that may result in ventricular tachycardia and fibrillation. [Note: This arrhythmia is usually treated with *lidocaine* or *phenytoin.*]

B. Adenosine

Adenosine is a naturally occurring nucleoside, but at high doses the drug decreases conduction velocity, prolongs the refractory period, and decreases automaticity in the AV node. Intravenous *adenosine* is the drug of choice for abolishing acute supraventricular tachycardia. It has low toxicity, but causes flushing, chest pain and hypotension. *Adenosine* has an extremely short duration of action (about 15 seconds).

Study Questions

Choose the ONE best answer.

17.1 All of the following mechanisms of action correctly match a drug EXCEPT:

A. Quinidine: Blocks Na^+ channels
B. Bretylium: Blocks K^+ channels
C. Verapamil: Blocks Ca^{++} channels
D. Propranolol: Blocks β adrenoceptors
E. Procainamide: Blocks K^+ channels

> Correct answer = E. Procainamide blocks Na^+ channels.

17.2 Which one of the following statements is INCORRECT?

A. Lidocaine must be given parenterally.
B. Lidocaine is used mainly for atrial arrhythmias.
C. Procainamide is associated with a reversible lupus phenomenon.
D. Quinidine is active orally.
E. All antiarrhythmic drugs can suppress cardiac contractions.

> Correct answer = B. Lidocaine is useful in treating ventricular arrhythmias. Lidocaine is given intravenously because of extensive first-pass transformation by the liver, which precludes oral administration. All of the antiarrhythmic drugs can exert a negative inotropic effect.

17.3 Which one of the following statements is INCORRECT?

A. Quinidine prolongs repolarization and the effective refractory period.
B. Mexiletine shortens repolarization and decreases the effective refractory period.
C. Propranolol increases Phase 4 depolarization.
D. Verapamil shortens the duration of the action potential .
E. Amiodarone prolongs repolarization.

> Correct choice = C. Propranolol decreases Phase 4 depolarization.

17.4 Which one of the following statements about antiarrhythmic drugs is CORRECT?

A. They may act by converting unidirectional block to a bidirectional block.
B. They often cause an increase in cardiac output.
C. As a group they have mild side effects.
D. They all affect Na^+ channels in the cell membrane.
E. They are equally useful in atrial and ventricular arrhythmias.

> Correct answer = A. A bidirectional block can decrease arrhythmias caused by reentry. All antiarrhythmic drugs exert some negative inotropic effect and decrease cardiac output. The side effects of this group of drugs are serious and include arrhythmias that can lead to sudden death. Some antiarrhythmic drugs affect K^+ or Ca^{++} channels, or β adrenoreceptors.

Antianginal Drugs

18

I. OVERVIEW

Angina pectoris is a characteristic chest pain caused by coronary blood flow that is insufficient to meet the oxygen demands of the myocardium. The imbalance between oxygen delivery and utilization may result from a spasm of the vascular smooth muscle or from obstruction of blood vessels caused by atherosclerotic lesions. Angina is characterized by a sudden, severe pressing substernal pain radiating to the left arm. Three classes of drugs are effective, either alone or in combination, in treating patients with stable angina: nitrates, β-blockers, and calcium channel-blockers. Nitrates decrease coronary vasoconstriction or spasm and increase perfusion of the myocardium by relaxing coronary arteries. β-Blockers decrease the oxygen demands of the heart. Variant angina (also called Prinzimetal's angina) caused by spontaneous coronary spasm, either at work or at rest, rather than by increases in myocardial oxygen requirements, is controlled by organic nitrates or calcium channel blockers, but β-blockers are contraindicated. (See Figure 18.1 for a summary of these antianginal agents.)

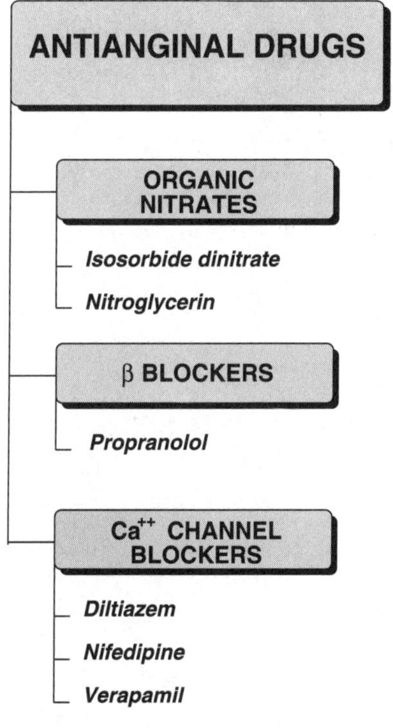

Figure 18.1
Summary of antianginal drugs.

II. ORGANIC NITRATES

Organic nitrates (and nitrites) are simple nitric and nitrous acid esters of alcohols. They differ in their volatility; for example, *isosorbide dinitrate* is solid at room temperature, *nitroglycerin* is only moderately volatile, whereas *amyl nitrate* is extremely volatile. These compounds cause a rapid reduction in myocardial oxygen demand followed by rapid relief of symptoms. They are effective in stable and unstable angina, as well as Prinzmetal's or variant angina pectoris.

A. Nitroglycerin

Nitrates, β-blockers, and calcium channel blockers are equally effective for relief of anginal symptoms. However, for prompt relief of an ongoing attack of angina precipitated by exercise or emotional stress, sublingual (or spray form) *nitroglycerin* is the drug of choice.

Lippincott's Illustrated Reviews: Pharmacology, Second Edition.
by Mary J. Mycek, Richard A. Harvey and Pamela C. Champe.
Lippincott Williams & Wilkins, Philadelphia, PA © 2000.

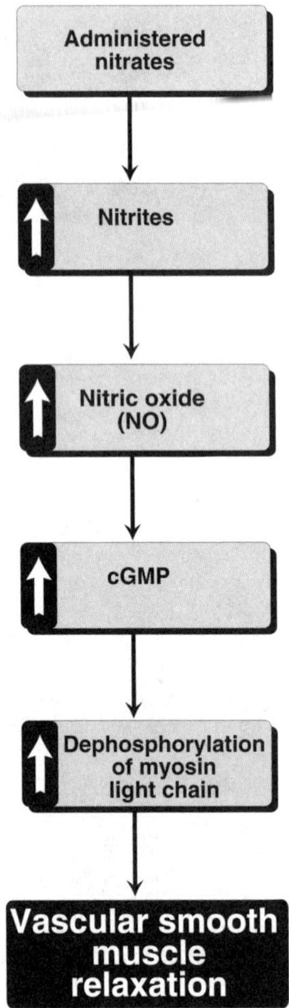

Figure 18.2
Effects of nitrates and nitrites on smooth muscle.

1. **Mechanisms of action:** The organic nitrates, such as *nitroglycerin* [nye troe GLI ser in], are thought to relax vascular smooth muscle by their intracellular conversion to nitrite ions and then to nitric oxide (NO), which in turn activates guanylate cyclase and increases the cells' cyclic GMP. Elevated cGMP ultimately leads to dephosphorylation of the myosin light chain, resulting in vascular smooth muscle relaxation (Figure 18.2).

2. **Effects on cardiovascular system:** At therapeutic doses, *nitroglycerin* has two major effects. First, it causes dilation of the large veins, resulting in pooling of blood in the veins. This diminishes preload (venous return to the heart), and reduces the work of the heart. Second, *nitroglycerin* dilates the coronary vasculature, providing increased blood supply to the heart muscle. *Nitroglycerin* causes a decrease in myocardial oxygen consumption because of decreased cardiac work.

3. **Pharmacokinetics:** The time to onset of action varies from one minute for *nitroglycerin* to more than one hour for *isosorbide mononitrate* (Figure 18.3). Significant first-pass metabolism of *nitroglycerin* occurs in the liver. Therefore, it is common to give the drug either sublingually or via a transdermal patch.

4. **Adverse effects:** The most common adverse effect of *nitroglycerin,* as well as the other nitrates, is headache. Thirty to sixty percent of patients receiving intermittent nitrate therapy with long-acting agents develop headaches. High doses of organic nitrates can also cause postural hypotension, facial flushing, and tachycardia.

5. **Tolerance:** Tolerance to the actions of nitrates develops rapidly. It can be overcome by provision of a daily "nitrate-free interval" to restore sensitivity to the drug. This interval is typically 6 to 8 hours, usually at night because there is decreased demand on the heart at that time. *Nitroglycerin* patches are worn for 12 hours and removed for 12 hours. However, Prinzimetal's or variant angina worsens early in the morning, perhaps due to circadian catecholamine surges. These patients' nitrate-free interval should be late afternoon.

B. Isosorbide dinitrate

Isosorbide dinitrate [eye soe SOR bide] is an orally active nitrate (Figure 18.3). The drug is not readily metabolized by the liver or smooth muscle and has a lower potency than *nitroglycerin* in relaxing vascular smooth muscle.

III. β-ADRENERGIC BLOCKERS

The β-adrenergic blocking agents suppress the activation of the heart by blocking β_1 receptors (see p. 73). They also reduce the work of the heart by decreasing cardiac output and causing a slight decrease in blood pressure. *Propranolol* (see p. 74) is the prototype of this class of compounds, but other β-blockers, such as *metoprolol* and *atenolol* are equally effective. However, agents with intrinsic sympathomimetic activity (for example, *pindolol* and *acebutolol*) are less effective and should be avoided. The β-blockers reduce the frequency and severity of angina attacks. These agents are particularly useful in the treatment of patients with myocardial infarction. The β-blockers can be used with nitrates to increase exercise duration and tolerance. They are, however, contraindicated in patients with diabetes, peripheral vascular disease, or chronic obstructive pulmonary disease.

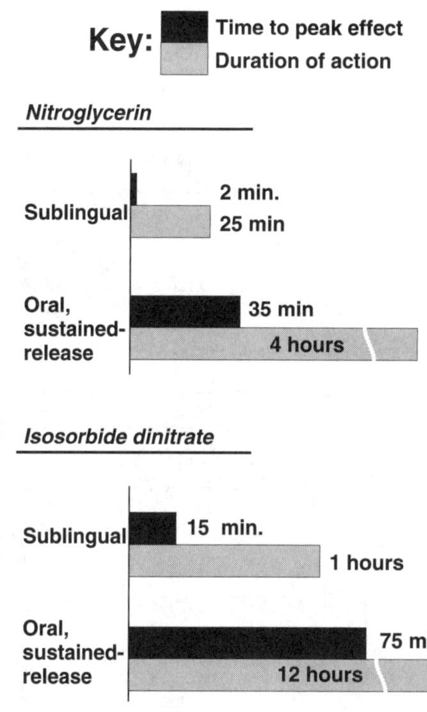

Figure 18.3
Time to peak effect and duration of action for two organic nitrate agents.

IV. CALCIUM CHANNEL BLOCKERS

The calcium channel blockers inhibit the entrance of calcium into cardiac and smooth muscle cells of the coronary and systemic arterial beds. All calcium channel blockers are therefore vasodilators that cause a decrease in smooth muscle tone and vascular resistance. (See p. 187 for a description of the mechanism of action of this group of drugs.) At clinical doses, these agents affect primarily the resistance of vascular smooth muscle and the myocardium. [Note: *Verapamil* mainly affects the myocardium, whereas *nifedipine* exerts a greater effect on smooth muscle in the peripheral vasculature. *Diltiazem* is intermediate in its actions.]

A. Nifedipine:

Nifedipine [nye FED i peen] functions mainly as an arteriolar vasodilator. This drug has minimal effect on cardiac conduction or heart rate. *Nifedipine* is administered orally and has a short half-life (about 4 hours) requiring multiple dosing. The vasodilation effect of *nifedipine* is useful in the treatment of variant angina caused by spontaneous coronary spasm. *Nifedipine* can cause flushing, headache, hypotension, and peripheral edema as side effects of its vasodilation activity. The drug may cause reflex tachycardia if peripheral vasodilation is marked resulting in a substantial decrease in blood pressure.

B. Verapamil

Verapamil [ver AP a mill] slows cardiac conduction directly and thus decreases heart rate and oxygen demand. *Verapamil* causes greater negative inotropic effects than does *nifedipine*, but it is a weaker vasodilator. *Verapamil* is contraindicated in patients with preexisting depressed cardiac function or AV conduction abnormalities. It also causes constipation. *Verapamil* should be used with caution in digitalized patients, since it increases *digoxin* levels (see p. 160).

C. Diltiazem

Diltiazem [dil TYE a zem] has cardiovascular effects that are similar to those of *verapamil*. It reduces the heart rate, although to a lesser extent than *verapamil*, and also decreases blood pressure. In addition, *diltiazem* can relieve coronary artery spasm and is therefore particularly useful in patients with variant angina. The incidence of adverse side effects is low. Figure 18.4 shows treatment of angina in patients with concomitant diseases.

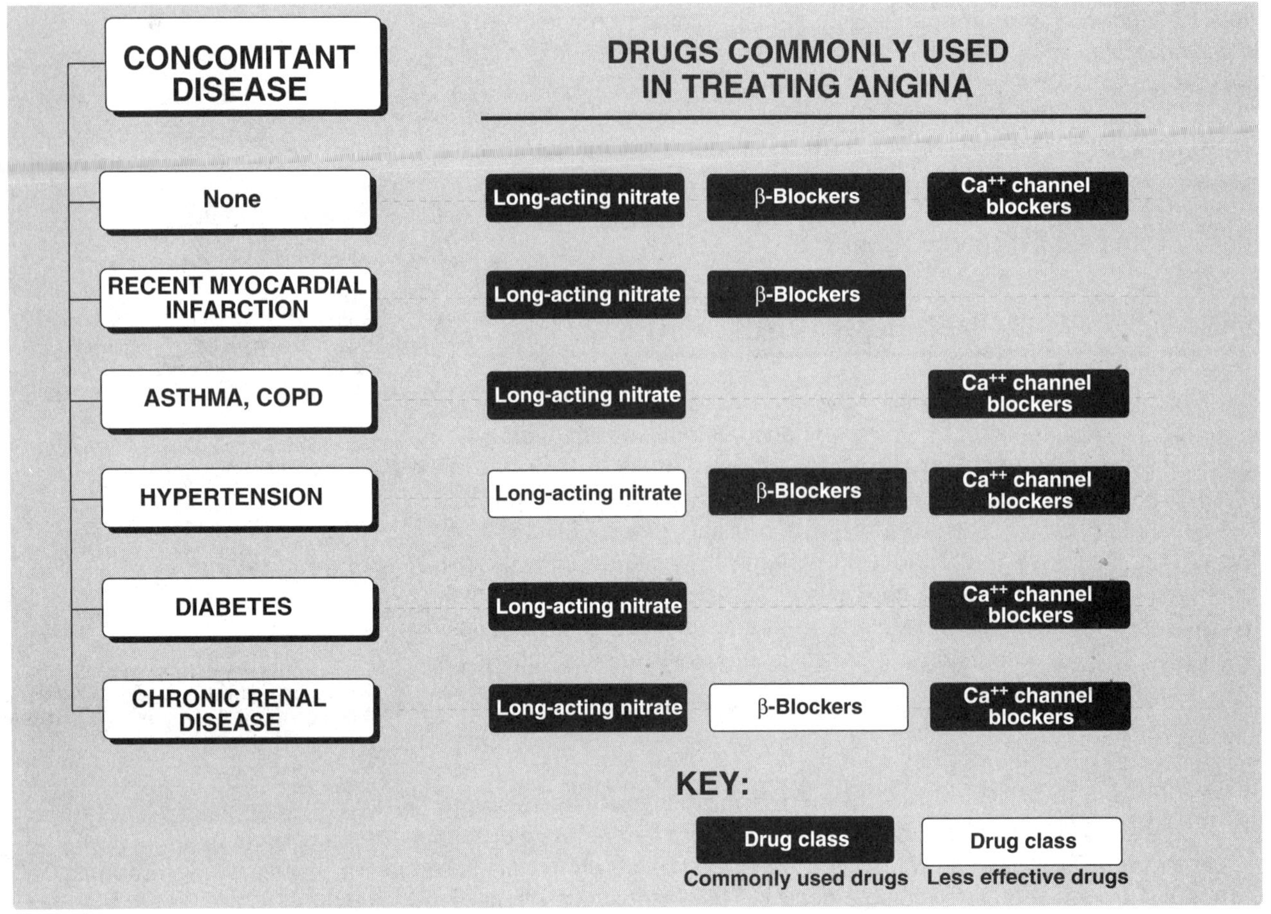

Figure 18.4
Treatment of angina in patients with concomitant diseases. COPD, chronic obstructive pulmonary disease.

Study Questions

Choose the ONE best answer.

18.1 All of the following statements concerning nitroglycerin are correct EXCEPT:

A. It causes an elevation of intracellular cGMP.
B. It undergoes significant first-pass metabolism in the liver.
C. It may cause significant reflex tachycardia.
D. It significantly decreases AV conduction.
E. It can cause postural hypotension.

> Correct choice = D. In contrast to other antianginal drugs, such as calcium channel blockers and β-adrenergic blockers, nitroglycerin does not block impulse conduction in the heart. Nitroglycerin causes increased cGMP, leading to vascular smooth muscle relaxation. The drug is commonly administered sublingually or transdermally to avoid hepatic inactivation. Increased heart rate results from the decrease in peripheral resistance and drop in blood pressure induced by nitroglycerin.

18.2 Which one of the following adverse effects is associated with nitroglycerin?

A. Hypertension
B. Throbbing headache
C. Bradycardia
D. Sexual dysfunction
E. Anemia

> Correct answer = B. Nitroglycerin causes throbbing headache in 30 to 60% of patients taking the drug. The other choices are incorrect. [Note: Nitroglycerin may cause postural hypotension.]

Antihypertensive Drugs

19

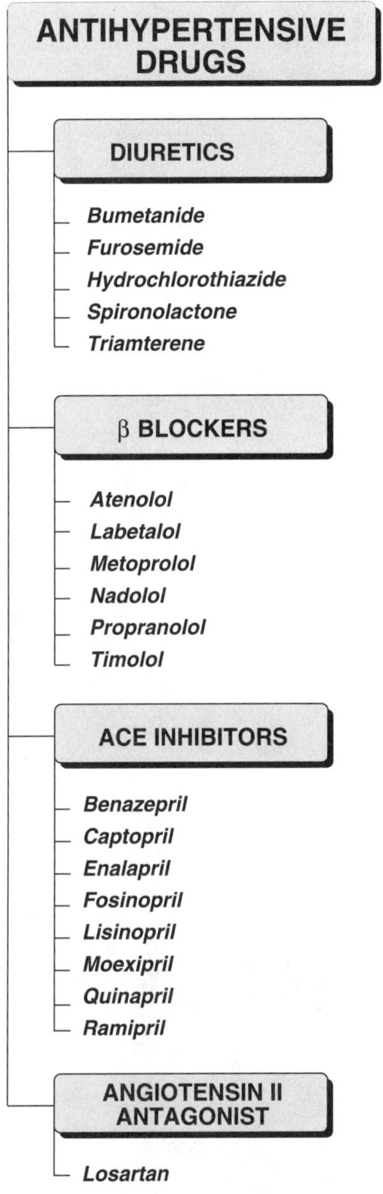

ANTIHYPERTENSIVE DRUGS
DIURETICS
Bumetanide
Furosemide
Hydrochlorothiazide
Spironolactone
Triamterene
β BLOCKERS
Atenolol
Labetalol
Metoprolol
Nadolol
Propranolol
Timolol
ACE INHIBITORS
Benazepril
Captopril
Enalapril
Fosinopril
Lisinopril
Moexipril
Quinapril
Ramipril
ANGIOTENSIN II ANTAGONIST
Losartan

Figure 19.1
Summary of antihypertensive drugs. (Figure continues on next page.)

I. OVERVIEW

Hypertension is defined as a sustained diastolic blood pressure greater than 90 mm Hg accompanied by an elevated systolic blood pressure (>140 mm Hg). Hypertension results from increased peripheral vascular smooth muscle tone, which leads to increased arteriolar resistance and reduced capacitance of the venous system. Elevated blood pressure is an extremely common disorder, affecting approximately 15% of the population of the United States (60 million people). Although many of these individuals have no symptoms, chronic hypertension—either systolic or diastolic—can lead to congestive heart failure, myocardial infarction, renal damage, and cerebrovascular accidents. The incidence of morbidity and mortality significantly decreases when hypertension is diagnosed early and is properly treated.

II. ETIOLOGY OF HYPERTENSION

Although hypertension may occur secondary to other disease processes, more than 90% of patients have essential hypertension, a disorder of unknown origin affecting the blood pressure-regulating mechanism. A family history of hypertension increases the likelihood that an individual will develop hypertensive disease. Essential hypertension occurs four times more frequently among blacks than among whites, and it occurs more often among middle-aged males than among middle-aged females. Environmental factors such as a stressful lifestyle, high dietary intake of sodium, obesity, and smoking all further predispose an individual to the occurrence of hypertension. Figure 19.1 summarizes the drugs used to treat hypertension. [Note: Nonsteroidal anti-inflammatory drugs (NSAID) (see p. 403) interfere with the hypotensive action of many antihypertensives.]

Lippincott's Illustrated Reviews: Pharmacology, Second Edition.
by Mary J. Mycek, Richard A. Harvey and Pamela C. Champe.
Lippincott Williams & Wilkins, Philadelphia, PA © 2000.

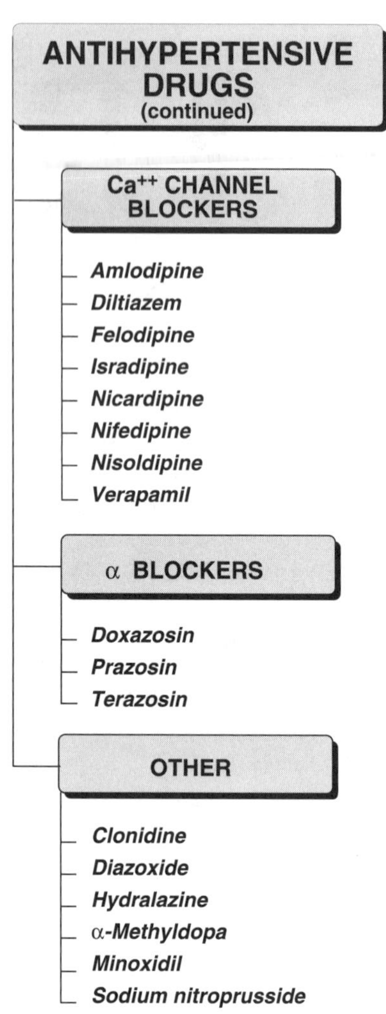

ANTIHYPERTENSIVE DRUGS (continued)
Ca++ CHANNEL BLOCKERS
Amlodipine
Diltiazem
Felodipine
Isradipine
Nicardipine
Nifedipine
Nisoldipine
Verapamil
α BLOCKERS
Doxazosin
Prazosin
Terazosin
OTHER
Clonidine
Diazoxide
Hydralazine
α-Methyldopa
Minoxidil
Sodium nitroprusside

Figure 19.1
Summary of antihypertensive drugs.

III. MECHANISMS FOR CONTROLLING BLOOD PRESSURE

Arterial blood pressure is regulated within a narrow range to provide adequate perfusion of the tissues without causing damage to the vascular system, particularly the arterial intima. Arterial blood pressure is directly proportional to the product of the cardiac output and the peripheral vascular resistance (Figure 19.2). In both normal and hypertensive individuals, cardiac output and peripheral resistance are controlled mainly by two overlapping control mechanisms: the baroreflexes mediated by the sympathetic nervous system, and the renin-angiotensin-aldosterone system (Figure 19.3). Most antihypertensive drugs lower blood pressure by reducing cardiac output and/or decreasing peripheral resistance.

A. Baroreceptors and the sympathetic nervous system

Baroreflexes involving the sympathetic nervous system are responsible for the rapid moment-to-moment regulation of blood pressure. A fall in blood pressure causes pressure-sensitive neurons (baroreceptors in the aortic arch and carotid sinuses) to send fewer impulses to cardiovascular centers in the spinal cord. This prompts a reflex response of increased sympathetic and decreased parasympathetic output to the heart and vasculature, resulting in vasoconstriction and increased cardiac output. These changes result in a compensatory rise in blood pressure (Figure 19.3, and Figure 3.5, see p. 31).

B. Renin-angiotensin-aldosterone system

The kidney provides for the long-term control of blood pressure by altering the blood volume. Baroreceptors in the kidney respond to reduced arterial pressure (and to sympathetic stimulation of β-adrenoceptors) by releasing the enzyme renin (see Figure 19.3). This peptidase converts angiotensinogen to angiotensin I, which is in turn converted to angiotensin II in the presence of angiotensin converting enzyme (ACE, see p. 186). Angiotensin II is the body's most

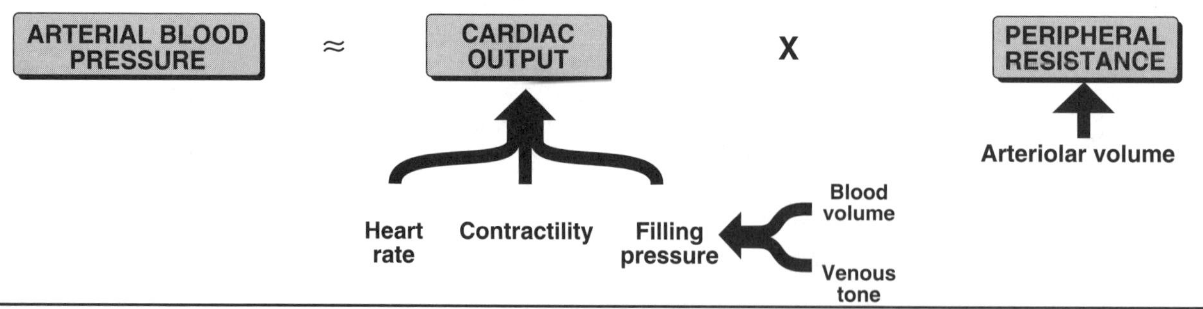

Figure 19.2
Major factors influencing blood pressure.

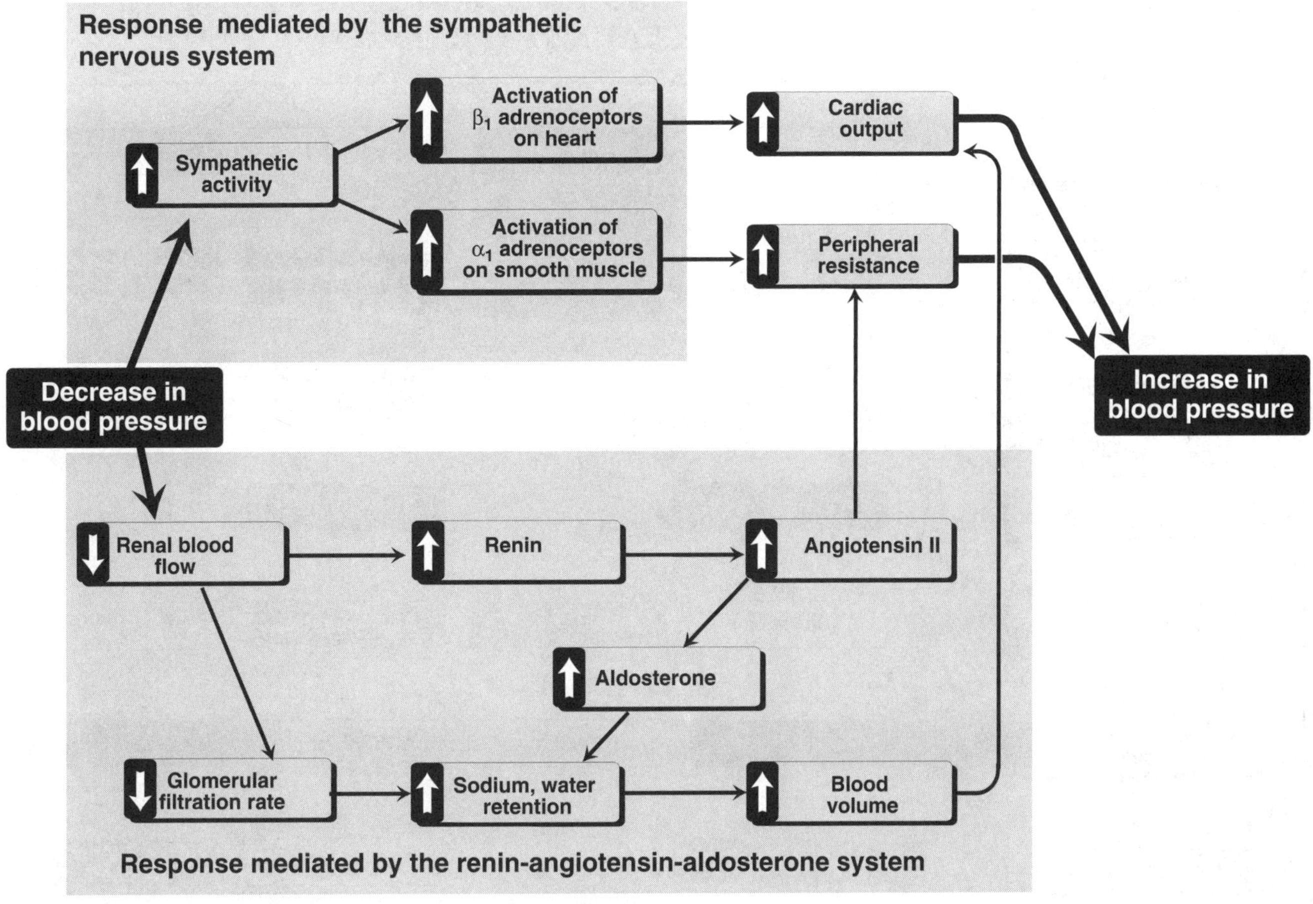

Figure 19.3
Response of the autonomic nervous system and the renin-angiotensin-aldosterone system to a decrease in blood pressure.

potent circulating vasoconstrictor, causing an increase in blood pressure. Furthermore, angiotensin II stimulates aldosterone secretion, leading to increased renal sodium reabsorption and an increase in blood volume, which contribute to a further increase in blood pressure).

IV. TREATMENT STRATEGIES

Mild hypertension can often be controlled with a single drug. More severe hypertension may require treatment with several drugs that are selected to minimize adverse effects of the combined regimen. Treatment is initiated with any of four drugs depending on the individual patient: a diuretic, a β-blocker, an ACE inhibitor, or a calcium channel blocker. If blood pressure is inadequately controlled, a second drug is added. A β-blocker is usually added if the initial drug was a diuretic, or a diuretic is added if the first drug was a β-blocker. A vasodilator can be added as a third step for those patients who still fail to respond.

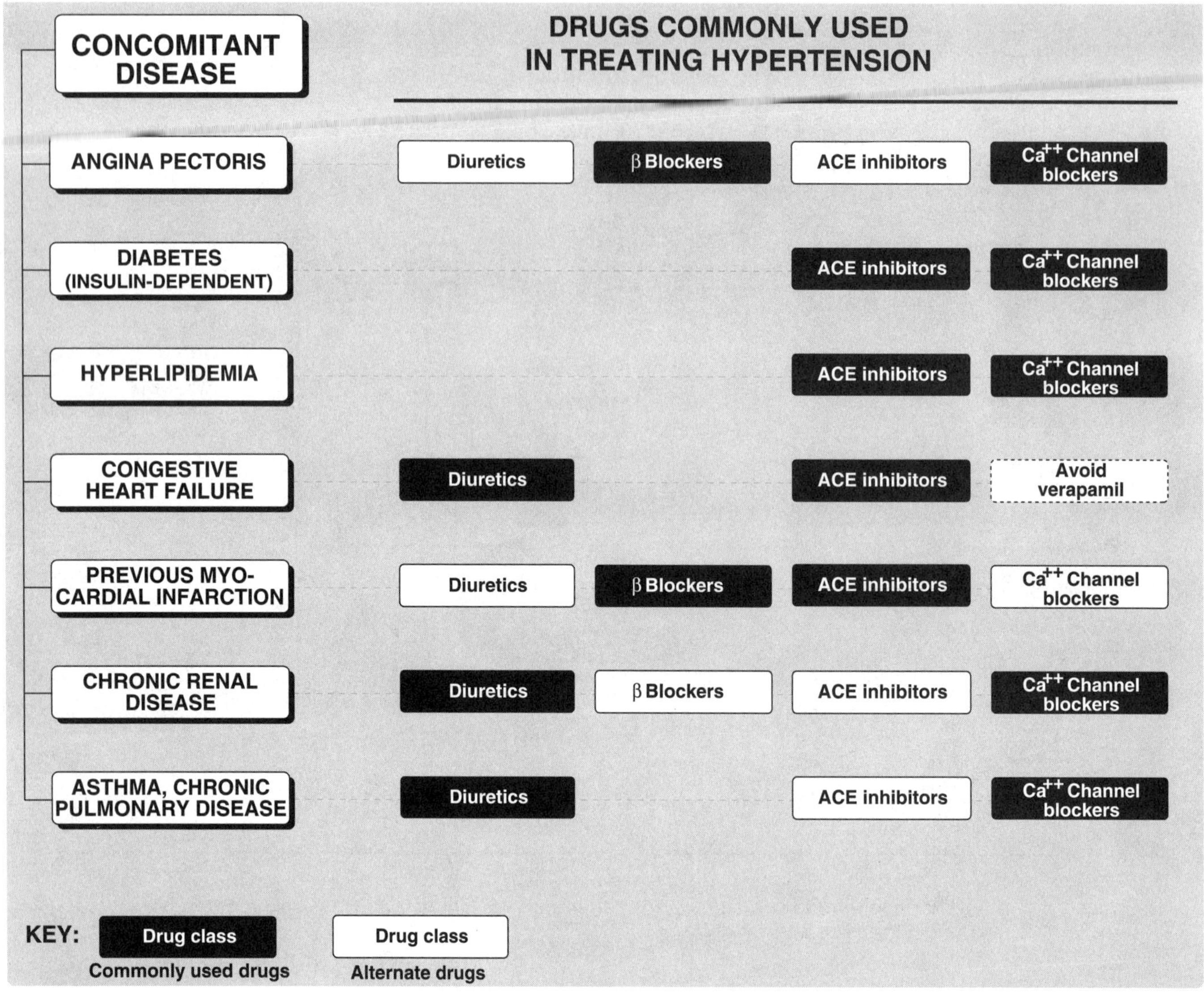

Figure 19.4
Treatment of hypertension in patients with concomitant diseases.

A. Individualized care

Certain subsets of the hypertensive population respond better to one class of drug than another. For example, black patients respond well to diuretics and calcium channel blockers, but therapy with β-blockers or ACE inhibitors is often less effective. Similarly, calcium channel blockers, ACE inhbibitors, and diuretics are favored for treatment of hypertension in the elderly, whereas β-blockers and α-antagonists are less well tolerated. Furthermore, hypertension may coexist with other diseases that can be aggravated by some of the antihypertensive drugs. For example, Figure 19.4 shows the preferred therapy in hypertensive patients with various concomitant diseases. In such cases, it is important to match antihypertensive drugs to the particular patient. Figure 19.5 shows the frequency of concomitant disease in the hypertensive patient population.

B. Patient compliance in antihypertensive therapy

Lack of patient compliance is the most common reason for failure of antihypertensive therapy. The hypertensive patient is usually asymptomatic and is diagnosed by routine screening before the occurrence of overt end-organ damage. Thus, therapy is directed at preventing disease sequelae (that occur in the future), rather than in relieving present discomfort of the patient. The adverse effects associated with the hypertensive therapy may influence the patient more than future benefits. For example, β-blockers can decrease libido and induce impotence in males, particulary middle-aged and elderly men. This drug-induced sexual dysfunction may prompt the patient to discontinue therapy. Thus, it is important to enhance compliance by carefully selecting a drug regimen that both reduces adverse effects and minimizes the number of doses required daily.

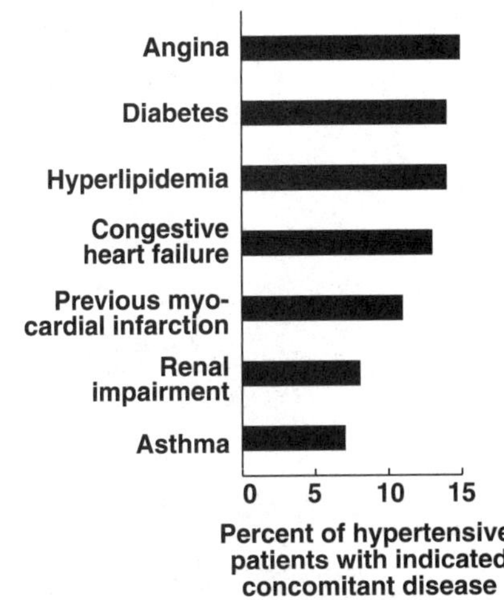

Figure 19.5
Frequency of occurrence of concomitant disease among the hypertensive patient population.

V. DIURETICS

Diuretics and/or β-blockers are currently recommended as the first-line drug therapy for hypertension. Low-dose diuretic therapy is safe and effective in preventing stroke, myocardial infarction, congestive heart failure and total mortality. Recent data suggest that diuretics are superior to β-blockers in older adults.

A. Thiazide diuretics

All oral diuretic drugs are effective in the treatment of hypertension, but the thiazides have found the most widespread use.

1. **Actions:** Thiazide diuretics, such as *hydrochlorothiazide* [hye droe klor oh THYE a zide], lower blood pressure, initially by increasing sodium and water excretion. This causes a decrease in extracellular volume, resulting in a decrease in cardiac output and renal blood flow (Figure 19.6). With long-term treatment, plasma volume approaches a normal value, but peripheral resistance decreases. *Spironolactone* [spye row no LAK tone], a potassium-sparing diuretic, is often used with thiazides. (A complete discussion of diuretics is found on p. 223.)

2. **Therapeutic uses:** Thiazide diuretics decrease blood pressure in both the supine and standing positions; postural hypotension is rarely observed, except in elderly, volume-depleted patients. These agents counteract the sodium and water retention observed with other agents used in the treatment of hypertension (for example, *hydralazine*). Thiazides are therefore useful in combination therapy with a variety of other antihypertensive agents including β-blockers and ACE inhibitors. Thiazide diuretics are particularly useful in the treatment of black or elderly patients, and in those with chronic renal disease. Thiazide diuretics are not effective in patients with inadequate kidney function (creatinine clearance less than 50 mls/min). Loop diuretics may be required in these patients.

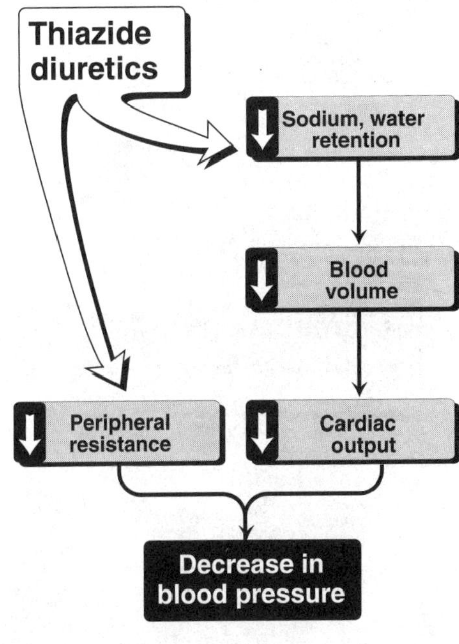

Figure 19.6
Actions of thiazide diuretics.

3. **Pharmacokinetics:** Thiazide diuretics can be administered orally. They induce considerable disturbances in electrolyte balance. For example, blood levels of K^+ and Mg^{++} are reduced, and Ca^{++} is retained by the body (see p. 220).

4. **Adverse effects:** Thiazide diuretics induce hypokalemia and hyperuricemia in 70% of patients, and hyperglycemia in 10% of patients. Serum potassium levels should be monitored closely in patients who are predisposed to cardiac arrhythmias (particularly individuals with left ventricular hypertrophy, ischemic heart disease, or chronic congestive heart failure) and who are concurrently being treated with both thiazide diuretics and *digitalis* glycosides (see p. 160). Diuretics should be avoided in the treatment of hypertensive diabetics or patients with hyperlipidemia.

B. Loop diuretics

The loop diuretics act promptly, even in patients who have poor renal function or who have not responded to thiazides or other diuretics. The loop diuretics cause decreased renal vascular resistance and increased renal blood flow. [Note: Loop diuretics increase the Ca^{++} content of urine (see p. 227), whereas thiazide diuretics decrease the Ca^{++} concentration of the urine.]

VI. β-ADRENOCEPTOR BLOCKING AGENTS

β-Blockers and/or diuretics are currently recommended as first-line drug therapy for hypertension. These drugs are efficacious but have some contraindications.

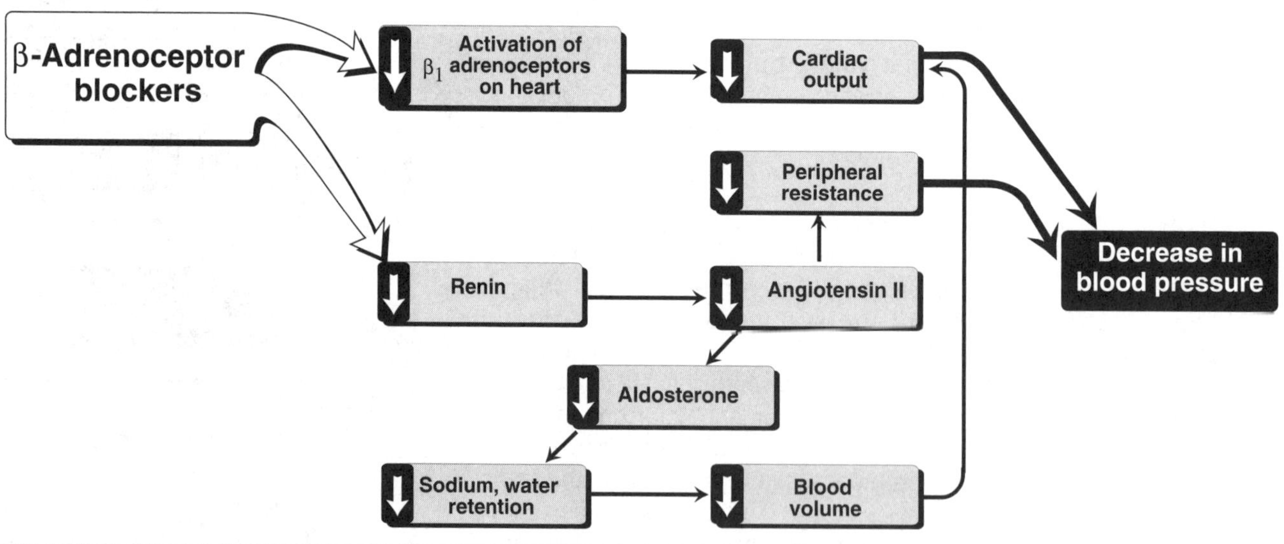

Figure 19.7
Actions of β-adrenoceptor blocking agents.

A. Actions

The β-blockers reduce blood pressure primarily by decreasing cardiac output (Figure 19.7). They may also decrease sympathetic outflow from the CNS and inhibit the release of renin from the kidneys, thus decreasing the formation of angiotensin II and secretion of aldosterone. The prototype β-blocker is *propranolol*, which acts at both β_1 and β_2 receptors. Newer agents, such as *atenolol* and *metoprolol*, are selective for β_1 receptors. These agents are commonly used in disease states such as asthma, in which *propanolol* is contraindicated due to its β_2-mediated bronchoconstriction. (See p. 73 for a complete discussion of β-blockers.)

B. Therapeutic uses

1. **Subsets of the hypertensive population:** The β-blockers are more effective for treating hypertension in white than in black patients, and in young patients compared to the elderly. [Note: Conditions that discourage the use of β-blockers (for example, severe chronic obstructive lung disease, chronic congestive heart failure, severe symptomatic occlusive peripheral vascular disease) are more commonly found in the elderly and in diabetics.]

2. **Hypertensive patients with concomitant diseases:** The β-blockers are useful in treating conditions that may coexist with hypertension, such as supraventricular tachyarrhythmia, previous myocardial infarction, angina pectoris, glaucoma (applied topically), and migraine headache.

C. Pharmacokinetics

The β-blockers are orally active. *Propranolol* undergoes extensive first-pass metabolism. The β-blockers may take several weeks to develop their full effects.

D. Adverse effects

1. **Common effects:** The β-blockers may cause CNS side effects such as fatigue, lethargy, insomnia, and hallucinations; these drugs can also cause hypotension. The β-blockers may decrease libido and cause impotence; drug-induced sexual dysfunction can severely reduce patient compliance (Figure 19.8).

2. **Alterations in serum lipid patterns:** The β-blockers may disturb lipid metabolism, decreasing high-density lipoproteins (HDL) and increasing plasma triacylglycerol.

3. **Drug withdrawal:** Abrupt withdrawal may cause rebound hypertension, probably as a result of up-regulation of β-receptors. Patients should be tapered off of β-blocker therapy in order to avoid precipitation of arrhythmias.The β-blockers should be avoided in treating patients with asthma, congestive heart failure, and peripheral vascular disease.

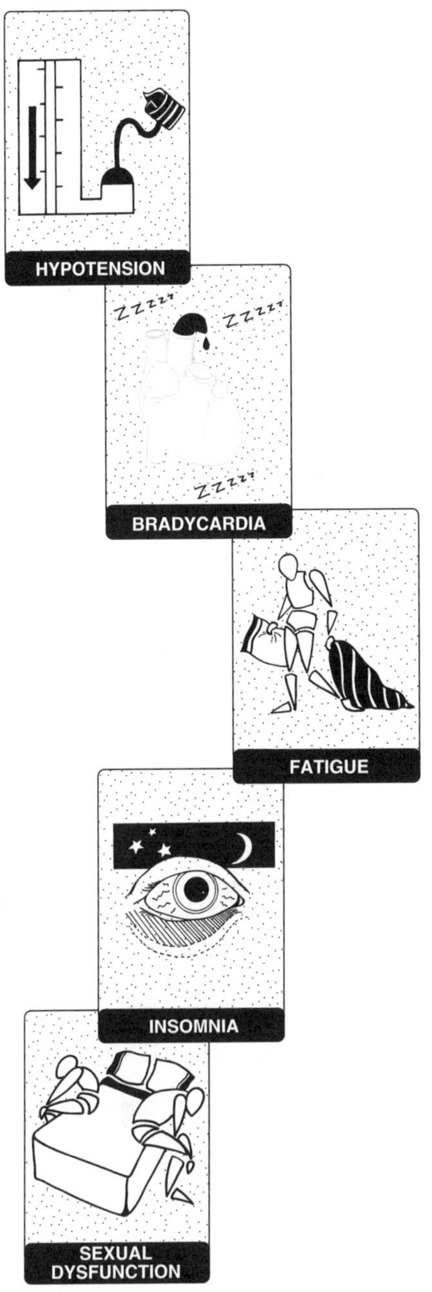

Figure 19.8
Some adverse effects of β blockers.

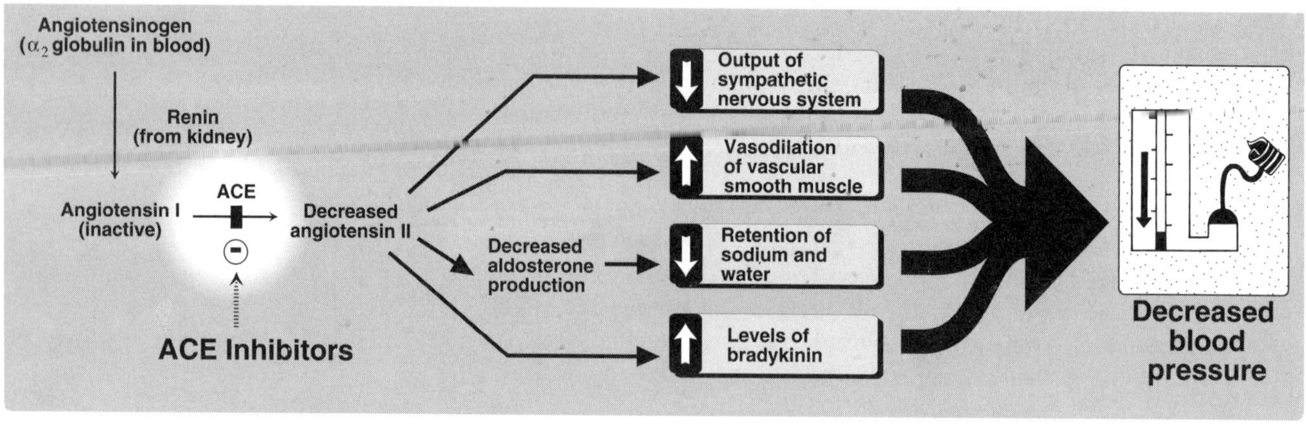

Figure 19.9
Effects of ACE inhibitors.

VII. ACE INHIBITORS

The angiotensin-converting enzyme (ACE) inhibitors are recommended when the preferred first-line agents (diuretics or β-blockers) are contraindicated or ineffective. Despite their wide-spread use, it is not clear if antihypertensive therapy with ACE inhibitors increases the risk of other major diseases.

A. Actions

The ACE inhibitors lower blood pressure by reducing peripheral vascular resistance without reflexly increasing cardiac output, rate, or contractility. These drugs block the angiotensin converting enzyme that cleaves angiotensin I to form the potent vasoconstrictor, angiotensin II (Figure 19.9). These inhibitors also diminish the rate of bradykinin inactivation. Vasodilation occurs as a result of the combined effects of lower vasoconstriction caused by diminished levels of angiotensin II and the potent vasodilating effect of increased bradykinin. By reducing circulating angiotensin II levels, ACE inhibitors also decrease the secretion of aldosterone, resulting in decreased sodium and water retention.

B. Therapeutic uses

Like β-blockers, ACE inhibitors are most effective in hypertensive patients who are white and young. However, when used in combination with a diuretic, the effectiveness of ACE inhibitors is similar in white and black hypertensive patients. Unlike β-blockers, ACE inhibitors are effective in the management of patients with chronic congestive heart failure (see p. 156). ACE inhibitors are now a standard in the care of a patient following a myocardial infarction. Therapy is started 24 hours after the end of the infarction.

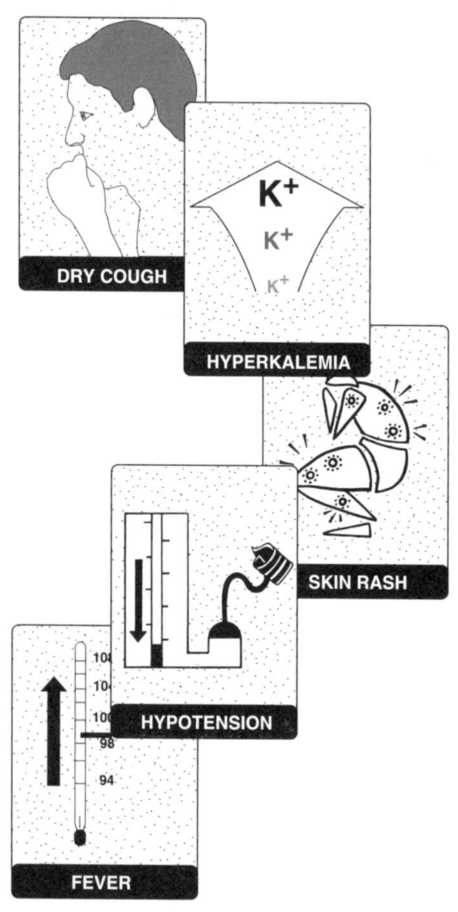

Figure 19.10
Some common adverse effects of the ACE inhibitors.

C. Adverse effects

Common side effects include dry cough, rashes, fever, altered taste, hypotension (in hypovolemic states), and hyperkalemia (Figure 19.10). Potassium levels must be monitored, and potassium supplements or *spironolactone* (see p. 232) are contraindicated. Angioedema is a rare but potentially life-threatening reaction. Because of the risk of angioedema and first dose syncope, ACE inhibitors are first administered in the physician's office with close observation. Reversible renal failure can occur in patients with severe renal artery stenosis. ACE inhibitors are fetotoxic and should not be used in pregnant women.

VIII. ANGIOTENSIN II ANTAGONISTS

The nanopeptide *losartan* [LOW sar tan], a highly selective angiotensin II receptor blocker, has recently been approved for antihypertensive therapy. Its pharmacologic effects are similar to ACE inhibitors in that it produces vasodilation and blocks aldosterone secretion. Its adverse effects profile is improved over the ACE inhibitors, although it is fetotoxic.

IX. CALCIUM CHANNEL BLOCKERS

Calcium channel blockers are recommended when the preferred first-line agents are contraindicated or ineffective. Despite their wide-spread use, it is not clear what effects antihypertensive therapy with these drugs has on major disease. In hypertensive patients, one retrospective study suggests that use of short-acting calcium channel blockers, especially in high doses, is associated with an increased risk of myocardial infarction. If confirmed in more rigorous randomized trials, these findings will reinforce the importance of diuretics and β-blockers as first-line agents unless contraindicated.

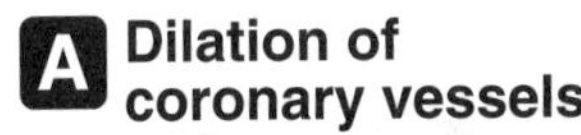

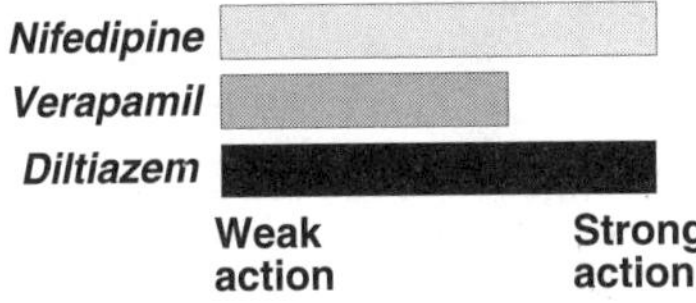

B AV Conduction

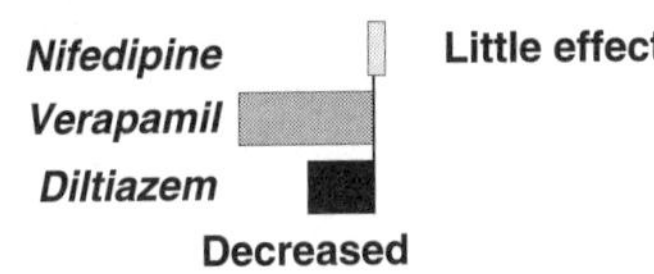

C Frequency of adverse effects

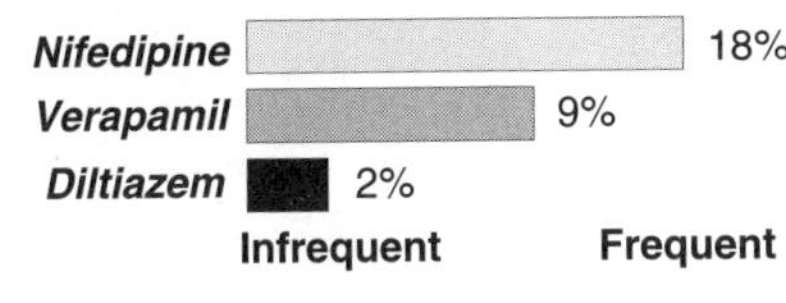

Figure 19.11
Actions of calcium channel blockers.

A. Classes of calcium channel blockers

The calcium channel blockers are divided into three chemical classes, each with different pharmacokinetic properties and clinical indications (Figures 19.11 and 19.12).

1. **Diphenylalkylamines:** *Verapamil* [ver AP a mill] is the only member of this class that is currently approved in the United States. *Verapamil* is the least selective of any calcium channel blocker, and has significant effects on both cardiac and vascular smooth-muscle cells. It is used to treat angina, supraventricular tachyarrhythmias, and migraine headache.

2. **Benzothiazepines:** *Diltiazem* [dil TYE a zem] is the only member of this class that is currently approved in the United States. Like *verapamil, diltiazem* affects both cardiac and vascular smooth-muscle cells; however, it has a less pronounced negative inotropic effect on the heart than does *verapamil. Diltiazem* has a favorable side-effect profile.

3. **Dihydropyridines:** This rapidly expanding class of calcium channel blockers includes the first-generation *nifedipine* [nye FED i peen],

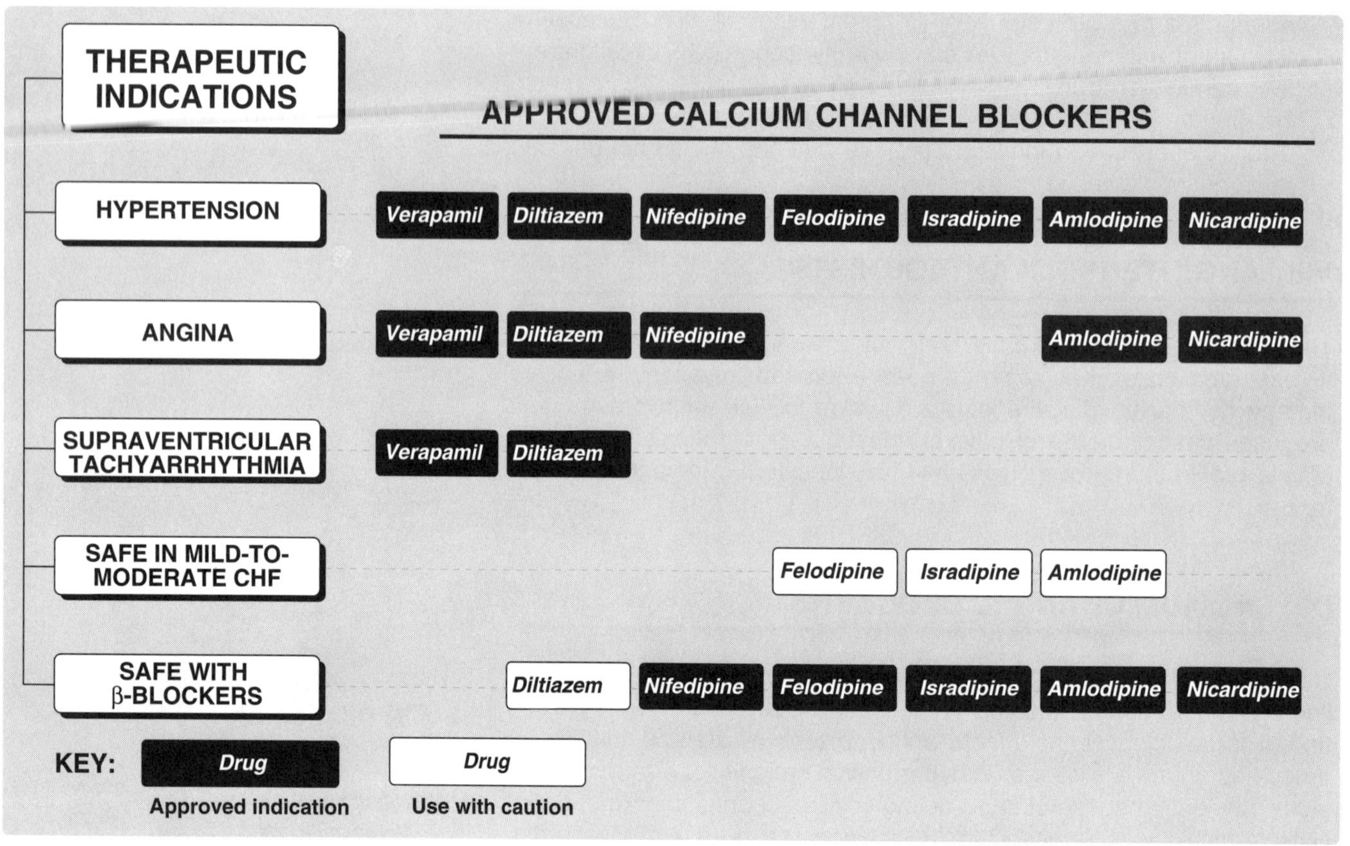

Figure 19.12
Some therapeutic applications of calcium channel blockers. CHF, congestive heart failure.

and five new agents for treating cardiovascular disease: *amlodipine* [am LOE di peen], *felodipine* [fell OH di peen], *isradipine* [eyes RAD i pen], *nicardipine* [nye KAR de peen] and *nisoldipine* [ni SOL de peen]. These second-generation calcium channel blockers differ in pharmacokinetics, approved uses, and drug interactions. All the dihydropyridines have a much greater affinity for vascular calcium channels than for calcium channels in the heart. They are therefore particularly attractive in treating hypertension. Some of the newer agents, such as *amlodipine* and *nicardipine*, have the advantage that they show little interaction with other cardiovascular drugs, such as *digoxin* (see p. 160) or *warfarin* (see p. 199) that are often used concomitantly with calcium channel blocker drugs.

B. Actions

The intracellular concentration of calcium plays an important role in maintaining the tone of smooth-muscle and in the contraction of the myocardium. Calcium enters muscle cells through special voltage-sensitive calcium channels. This triggers release of calcium from the sarcoplasmic reticulum and mitochondria, which further increases the cytosolic level of calcium. Calcium channel antagonists block the inward movement of calcium by binding to L-type calcium channels in the heart and in smooth-muscle of the coronary and peripheral vasculature. This causes vascular smooth muscle to relax, dilating mainly arterioles.

C. Therapeutic uses

Calcium channel blockers have an intrinsic natriuretic effect; therefore, they do not usually require the addition of a diuretic. These agents are useful in the treatment of hypertensive patients who also have asthma, diabetes, angina, and/or peripheral vascular disease.

D. Pharmacokinetics

Most of these agents have short half-lives ($t_{1/2}$ = 3 to 8 hours) following an oral dose. Treatment is required three times a day to maintain good control of hypertension. Sustained release preparations permit less frequent dosing.

E. Adverse effects

Although infrequent, side effects include constipation in 10% of patients, dizziness, headache, and a feeling of fatigue caused by a decrease in blood pressure (Figure 19.13). *Verapamil* should be avoided in treating patients with congestive heart failure due to its negative inotropic effects.

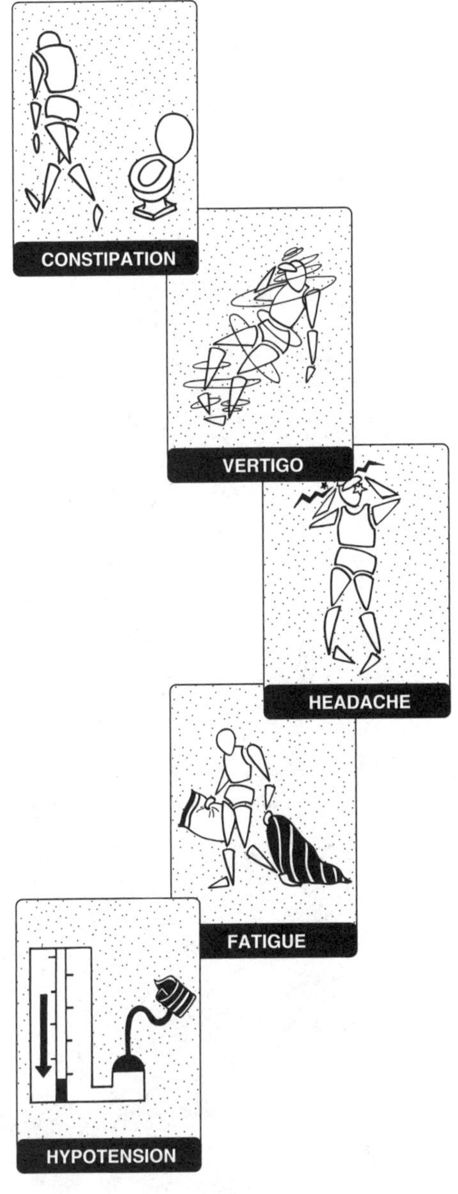

Figure 19.13
Some common adverse effects of the calcium channel blockers.

X. α-ADRENERGIC BLOCKING AGENTS

Prazosin, *oxazosin* and *terazosin* (see p. 73) produce a competitive block of α_1 adrenoceptors. They decrease peripheral vascular resistance and lower arterial blood pressure by causing the relaxation of both arterial and venous smooth muscle. These drugs cause only minimal changes in cardiac output, renal blood flow, and glomerular filtration rate. Therefore, long-term tachycardia and increased renin release do not occur. Postural hypotension may occur in some individuals. *Prazosin* is used to treat mild to moderate hypertension and is prescribed in combination with *propranolol* or a diuretic for additive effects. Reflex tachycardia and first dose syncope are almost universal adverse effects. Concomitant use of a β-blocker may be necessary to blunt the short-term effect of reflex tachycardia.

XI. CENTRALLY-ACTING ADRENERGIC DRUGS

A. Clonidine

This α_2-agonist diminishes central adrenergic outflow. *Clonidine* [KLOE ni deen] (see p. 67) is used primarily for the treatment of mild to moderate hypertension that has not responded adequately to treatment with diuretics alone. *Clonidine* does not decrease renal blood flow or glomerular filtration and therefore is useful in the treatment of hypertension complicated by renal disease. *Clonidine* is absorbed well after oral administration and is excreted by the kidney. Because it causes sodium and water retention, *clonidine* is usually administered in combination with a diuretic. Adverse effects are generally mild, but the drug can produce sedation and drying of nasal mucosa. Rebound hypertension occurs following abrupt withdrawal of *clonidine*. The drug should therefore be withdrawn slowly if the clinician wishes to change agents.

B. α-Methyldopa

This α-adrenergic agonist diminishes the adrenergic outflow from the CNS, leading to reduced total peripheral resistance and a decreased blood pressure. Cardiac output is not decreased and blood flow to vital organs is not diminished. Because blood flow to the kidney is not diminished by its use, *α-methyldopa* [meth ill DOE pa] is especially valuable in treating hypertensive patients with renal insufficiency. The most common side effects of *α-methyldopa* are sedation and drowsiness.

XII. VASODILATORS

The direct-acting smooth muscle relaxants, such as *hydralazine* and *minoxidil*, have traditionally not been used as primary drugs to treat hypertension. Vasodilators act by producing relaxation of vascular smooth muscle, which decreases resistance and therefore decreases blood pressure. These agents produce reflex stimulation of the heart, resulting in the competing symptoms of increased myocardial contractility, heart rate, and oxygen consumption. These actions may prompt angina pectoris, myocardial infarction, or cardiac failure in predisposed individuals. Vasodilators also increase plasma renin concentration, resulting in sodium and water retention. These undesirable side effects can be blocked by concomitant use of a diuretic and a β-blocker.

A. Hydralazine

This drug causes direct vasodilation, acting primarily on arteries and arterioles. This results in a decreased peripheral resistance, which in turn prompts a reflex elevation in heart rate and cardiac output. *Hydralazine* [hye DRAL a zeen] is used to treat moderately severe hypertension. It is almost always administered in combination with a β-blocker such as *propranolol* (to balance the reflex tachycardia) and a diuretic (to decrease sodium retention). Together, the three drugs decrease cardiac output, plasma volume, and peripheral vascular resistance. Adverse effects of hydralazine therapy include headache, nausea, sweating, arrhythmia, and precipitation of angina. A lupus-like syndrome can occur with high dosage, but it is reversible on discontinuation of the drug.

B. Minoxidil

This drug causes dilation of resistance vessels (arterioles) but not of capacitance vessels (venules). *Minoxidil* [mi NOX i dill] is administered orally for treatment of severe to malignant hypertension that is refractory to other drugs. Reflex tachycardia may be severe and may require the concomitant use of a diuretic and a β-blocker. *Minoxidil* causes serious sodium and water retention, leading to volume overload, edema, and congestive heart failure. [Note: *Minoxidil* treatment also causes hypertrichosis (the growth of body hair). This drug is now used topically to treat male pattern baldness.]

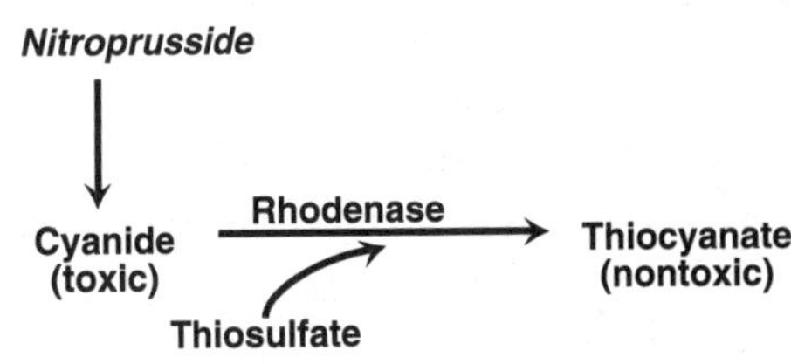

Figure 19.14
Detoxification of cyanide with thiosulfate and rhodenase

XIII. HYPERTENSIVE EMERGENCY

Hypertensive emergency is a rare, but life-threatening situation in which the diastolic blood pressure is either over 150 mm Hg (with systolic blood pressure greater than 210 mm Hg) in an otherwise healthy person, or 130 mm Hg in an individual with preexisting complications, such as encephalopathy, cerebral hemorrhage, left ventricular failure, or aortic stenosis. The therapeutic goal is to rapidly reduce blood pressure.

A. Sodium nitroprusside

Nitroprusside [nye troe PRUSS ide] is administered intravenously, and causes prompt vasodilation, with reflex tachycardia. It is capable of reducing blood pressure in all patients, regardless of the cause of hypertension. The drug has little effect outside the vascular system, acting equally on arterial and venous smooth muscle. [Note: Because *nitroprusside* also acts on the veins, it can reduce cardiac preload.] *Nitroprusside* is metabolized rapidly ($t_{1/2}$ of minutes) and requires continuous infusion to maintain its hypotensive action. *Sodium nitroprusside* exerts few adverse effects except for those of hypotension caused by overdose. *Nitroprusside* metabolism results in cyanide ion production, although cyanide toxicity is rare and can be effectively treated with an infusion of *sodium thiosulfate* to produce thiocyanate, which is less toxic and is eliminated by the kidneys (Figure 19.14). [Note: *Nitroprusside* is poisonous if given orally because of its hydrolysis to cyanide.]

B. Diazoxide

Diazoxide [dye az OX ide] is a direct-acting arteriolar vasodilator. It has vascular effects like those of *hydralazine*. For patients with coronary insufficiency, *diazoxide* is administered intravenously with a β-blocker, which diminishes reflex activation of the heart. *Diazoxide* is useful in the treatment of hypertensive emergencies, hypertensive encephalopathy, and eclampsia. Excessive hypotension is the most serious toxicity.

C. Labetalol

Labetalol (see p. 78) is both an α- and β-blocker that has been successfully used in hypertensive emergencies. *Labetalol* does not cause the reflex tachycardia that may be associated with *diazoxide*. *Labetalol* carries the contraindications of a nonselective β-blocker (see p. 78).

Choose the ONE best answer.

19.1 Which of the following patients is most suited for primary therapy with hydrochlorothiazide?

A. Patients with gout
B. Patients with hyperlipidemia
C. Young hypertensive patients with rapid resting heart rates
D. Black patients and elderly patients
E. Patients with impaired renal function

Correct answer = D. Among black patients, diuretic and calcium channel blockers are more effective than ACE inhibitors or β-blockers. Diuretics are effective among the elderly. Thiazide diuretics cause hyperuricemia and can precipitate a gout attack in susceptible individuals. Thiazide diuretics increase LDL cholesterol and may increase the risk of atherosclerosis in patients with hyperlipidemia. Patients with evidence of elevated catecholamines are best treated with β-blockers. Thiazides cannot promote sodium excretion when renal function is severely impaired. The loop diuretics, such as furosemide, are used in patients with impaired renal function.

19.2 All of the following produce a significant decrease in peripheral resistance except:

A. chronic administration of diuretics.
B. hydralazine.
C. β-blockers.
D. ACE inhibitors.
E. clonidine.

Correct choice = C. β-blockers act primarily by decreasing heart rate and cardiac output.

19.3 Which one of the following drugs acts at central presynaptic α_2 receptors?

A. Minoxidil
B. Verapamil
C. Clonidine
D. Enalapril
E. Hydrochlorothiazide

Correct answer = C. Clonidine reduces sympathetic outflow by stimulating α-adrenergic receptors. Minoxidil is a direct-acting vasodilator. Verapamil causes vasodilation by inhibiting calcium ion flow into smooth muscle. Enalapril blocks the enzyme that converts angiotensin I to angiotensin II. Hydrochlorothiazide acts by decreasing blood volume.

19.4 Which one of the following antihypertensives is most likely to cause reflex tachycardia?

A. Propranolol
D. Nifedipine
C. Prazosin
D. Hydralazine
E. Captopril

Correct answer = D. Hydralazine has a significant hypotensive effect that activates baroreceptors.

19.5 From the list of antihypertensive drugs below select the one most likely to lower blood sugar.

A. Prazosin
B. Propranolol
C. Nifedipine
D. Captopril
E. Hydralazine

Correct answer = B. Propranolol blocks glycogenolysis.

19.6 Which one of the following drugs should not be given to a pregnant, hypertensive woman?

A. Hydrochlorothiazide
B. Propranolol
C. α-Methyldopa
D. Lisinopril
E. Verapamil

Correct answer = D. Lisinopril blocks the formation of angiotensin II, which is essential for normal growth and development of fetal kidney and other organs.

Drugs Affecting Blood

20

I. OVERVIEW

This chapter describes drugs useful in treating three important dysfunctions of blood: thrombosis, bleeding, and anemia. Thrombosis—the formation of an unwanted clot within the blood vessels or heart—is the most common abnormality of hemostasis. Bleeding disorders involving failure of hemostasis are less common than thromboembolic diseases and include hemophilia and vitamin K deficiency. Anemias caused by nutritional deficiencies can be treated with either dietary or pharmaceutical supplementation. Recently, *hydroxyurea* has been found to be beneficial in the treatment of sickle cell anemia. See Figure 20.1 for a summary of drugs affecting blood.

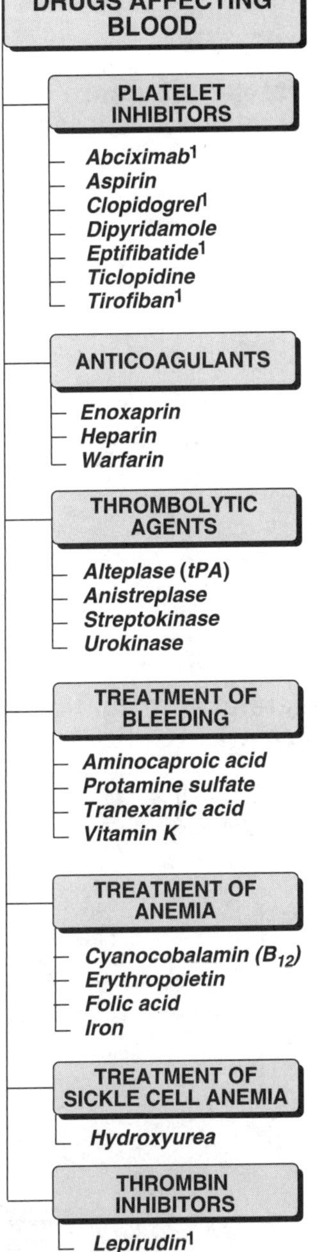

Figure 20.1
Summary of drugs used in treating dysfunctions of blood. [1]Described in Pharmacology update, pp. 446-448

II. NORMAL RESPONSE TO VASCULAR TRAUMA

Physical trauma to the vascular system, such as a puncture or cut, initiates a complex series of interactions between platelets, endothelial cells, and the coagulation cascade. This results in the formation of a platelet-fibrin plug. The creation of an unwanted thrombus involves many of the same steps, except that the triggering stimulus is a pathologic condition in the vascular system rather than physical trauma.

A. Formation of a clot

Clot formation requires platelet activation and aggregation, followed by formation of thrombin. This serum protease catalyzes the production of fibrin which, when cross-linked, stabilizes the clot.

1. **Role of platelets:** Platelets respond to vascular trauma by "activation" processes, which involve three steps: adhesion to the site of injury, release of intracellular granules, and aggregation of the platelets (Figure 20.2). Normally, platelets circulate in the blood in an inactive form, but in response to various stimuli they become activated. Activated platelets undergo modifications that culminate in morphologic changes and in the expression of proteins and cell receptors. For example, after adhering to exposed collagen in the subendothelial layers of injured blood vessels, the platelets release granules containing chemical mediators. These promote platelet aggregation and the formation of a plug, composed of the viscous contents of lysed platelets, neutrophils and monocytes, that rapidly arrests bleeding.

Lippincott's Illustrated Reviews: Pharmacology, Second Edition.
by Mary J. Mycek, Richard A. Harvey and Pamela C. Champe.
Lippincott Williams & Wilkins, Philadelphia, PA © 2000.

1 Damage to vessel exposes collagen of subendothelium

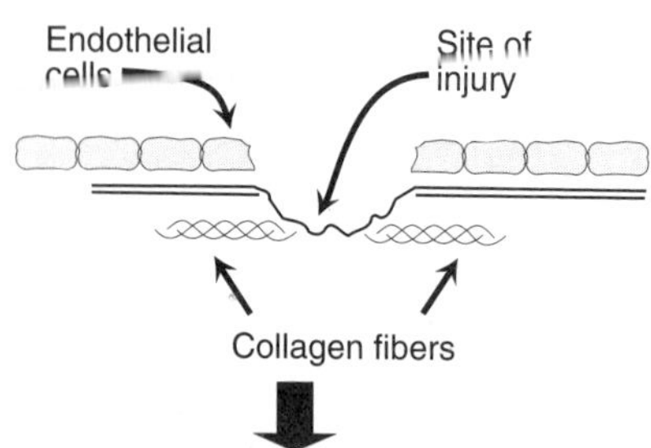

2 Platelet adhesion and release of granules

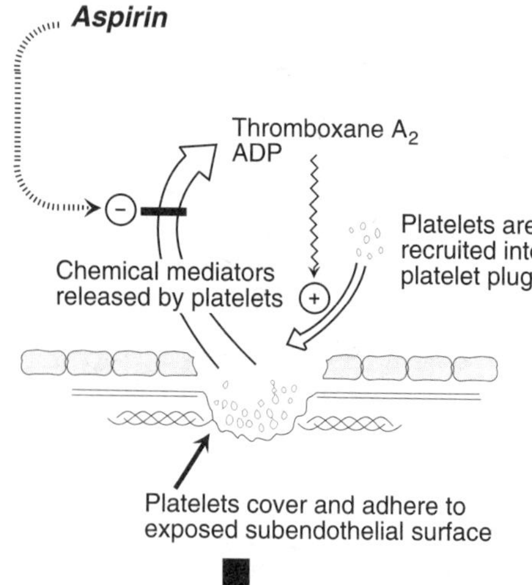

3 Platelet aggregation and formation of fibrin plug

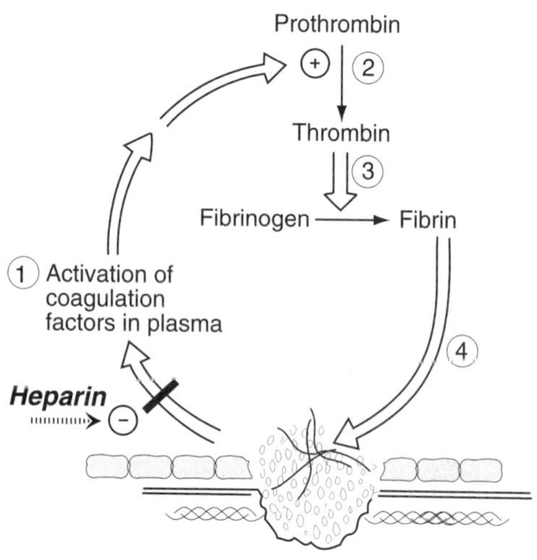

Figure 20.2
Formation of a hemostatic plug.

2. **Role of fibrin:** Local stimulation of the coagulation cascade by factors released from the injured tissue and platelets results in the formation of thrombin (Factor II). In turn, thrombin, a serine protease, catalyzes the conversion of fibrinogen to fibrin, which is incorporated into the plug. Subsequent cross-linking of the fibrin strands stabilizes the clot and forms a hemostatic plug.

3. **Thrombus versus embolus:** A clot that adheres to a vessel wall is called a thrombus, whereas an intravascular clot that floats within the blood is termed an embolus. Thus, a detached thrombus becomes an embolus. Both thrombi and emboli are dangerous, because they may occlude blood vessels and deprive tissues of oxygen and nutrients. Arterial thrombosis most often involves medium-sized vessels rendered thrombogenic by surface lesions of endothelial cells caused by atherosclerosis. In contrast, venous thrombosis is triggered by blood stasis or inappropriate activation of the coagulation cascade, often as a result of a defect in the normal defense hemostatic mechanisms.

B. Fibrinolysis

During platelet plug formation, the fibrinolytic pathway is locally activated. Plasminogen is enzymatically processed to plasmin (fibrinolysin) by plasminogen activators present in the tissue. Plasmin interferes in clot propagation and dissolves the fibrin network as wounds heal. At present, a number of fibrinolytic enzymes are available for treatment of myocardial infarctions or pulmonary emboli (see p. 201).

III. PLATELET ACTIVATION

The outer membrane of platelets contains a variety of receptors that function as sensors capable of responding to physiologic signals present in the plasma (Figure 20.3). These chemical stimuli are classified as platelet-activating if they promote platelet aggregation and the subsequent release of granules stored in the platelet. Conversely, other chemical signals are classified as platelet-inhibiting, if they inhibit platelet activation and the release of platelet granules. Whether platelets remain in a quiescent state or become activated is determined by the balance of activating and inhibiting chemical signals.

A. Chemical signals that oppose platelet activation

1. **Elevated prostacyclin levels:** In a normal, undamaged vessel, platelets circulate freely, since the balance of chemical signals indicates that the vascular system is not damaged. For example, prostacyclin (see p. 403), synthesized by the intact endothelial cells and released into plasma, binds to a specific set of platelet membrane receptors that are coupled to the synthesis of cyclic adenosine monophosphate (cAMP) as an intracellular messenger. Elevated levels of intracellular cAMP inhibit platelet activation, and the subsequent release of platelet aggregation agents (Figure 20.3).

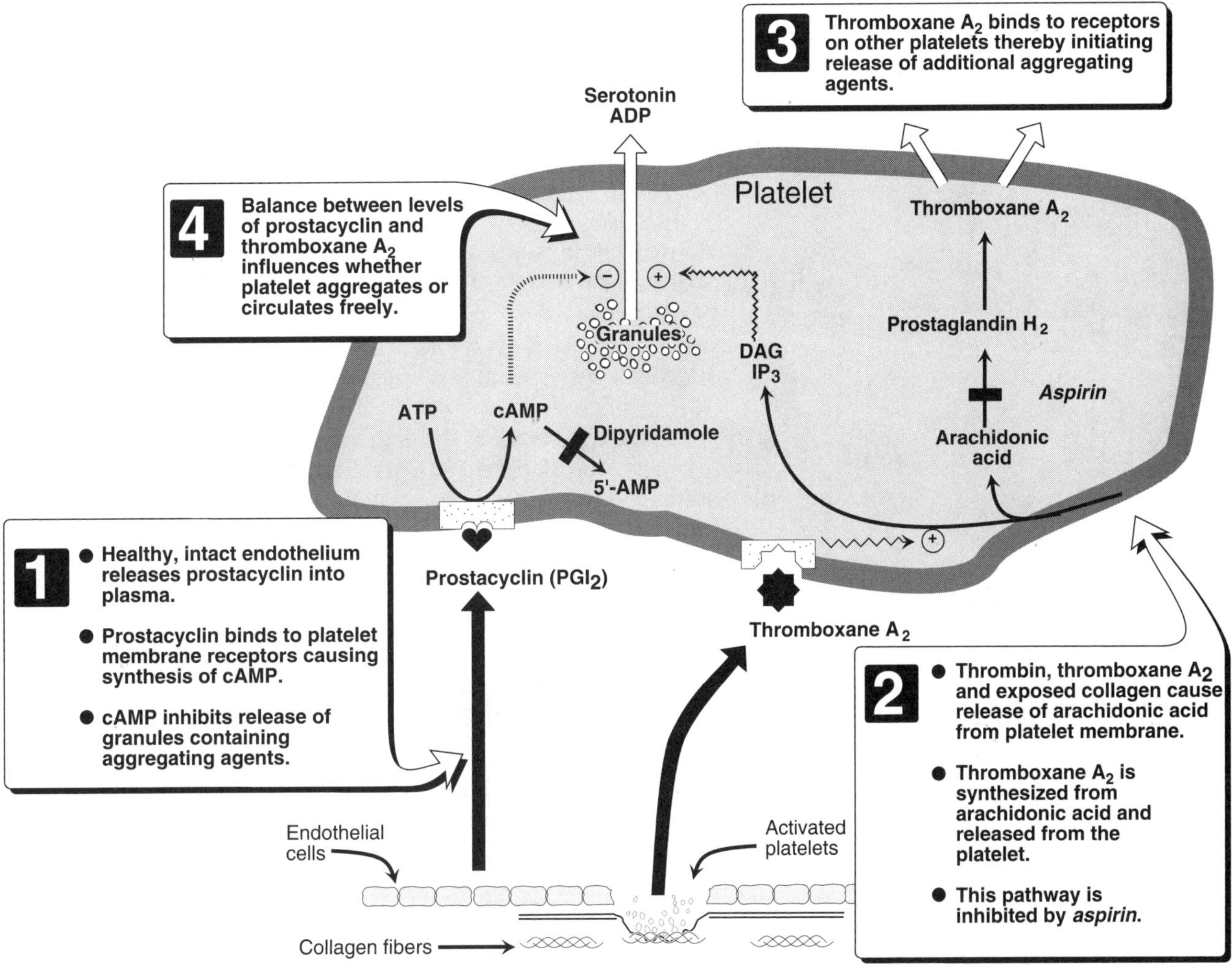

Figure 20.3
Chemical mediators influencing platelet activation and aggregation (relative size of platelets and endothelial cells are not to scale).

2. **Decreased plasma levels of thrombin and thromboxanes:** The platelet membrane also contains receptors that can bind thrombin, thromboxanes, and exposed collagen. When occupied, each of these receptor types triggers a series of reactions leading to the release into the circulation of intracellular granules and ultimately, to platelet aggregation. However, in the intact, normal vessel, circulating levels of thrombin and thromboxanes are low and the intact endothelium covers the collagen present in the subendothelial layers. The corresponding platelet receptors are thus unoccupied, and remain inactive. Consequently, platelet activation and aggregation are not initiated.

B. Chemical signals that promote platelet aggregation

1. **Decreased prostacyclin levels:** Damaged endothelial cells synthesize less prostacyclin, resulting in a localized reduction in

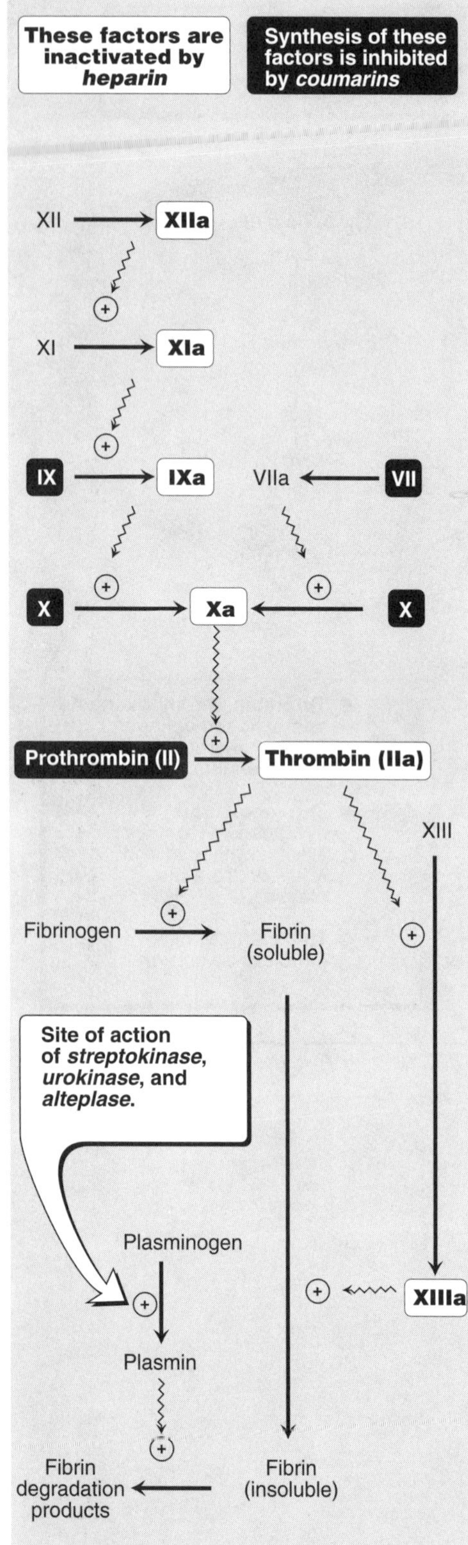

Figure 20.4
Formation of fibrin clot and its ultimate dissolution.

prostacyclin levels. The binding of prostacyclin to platelet receptors is decreased; thus lower levels of intracellular cAMP permit platelet aggregation.

2. **Exposed collagen:** Within seconds of vascular injury, platelets adhere to and virtually cover the exposed collagen of the subendothelium. Receptors on the surface of the platelet are activated by the collagen of this underlying connective tissue, which triggers the release of platelet granules containing adenosine diphosphate (ADP) and serotonin. This process is sometimes referred to as the "platelet release reaction," and the platelet is then said to be activated. Fibrinogen receptors are expressed on the platelet surface and the fibrinogen can then act as a bridge between two platelets.

3. **Increased synthesis of thromboxanes:** Stimulation of platelets by thrombin, collagen, and ADP results in activation of platelet membrane phospholipases, which liberate arachidonic acid from membrane phospholipid. Arachidonic acid is first converted to prostaglandin H_2 by cyclooxygenase, an enzyme that is irreversibly inactivated by *aspirin* (see p. 403). Prostaglandin H_2 is metabolized to thromboxane A_2, which is released into the plasma. Thromboxane A_2 produced by the aggregating platelets further promotes the clumping process that is essential to the rapid formation of a hemostatic plug (see Figure 20.3).

IV. BLOOD COAGULATION

The coagulation process that generates thrombin consists of two interrelated pathways—the extrinsic and the intrinsic systems. The extrinsic system, which is probably the more important in vivo, is initiated by the activation of clotting Factor VII by a tissue factor, thromboplastin—a phospholipid and protein mixture. The intrinsic system is triggered by the activation of clotting Factor XII, following its contact in vitro with glass or highly charged surfaces. Both systems involve a cascade of enzymatic reactions that sequentially transform various plasma factors (proenzymes) to their active (enzymatic) forms, ultimately producing thrombin (Figure 20.4). Thrombin plays a key role in coagulation, since it is responsible for generation of fibrin, a glycoprotein that forms the meshlike matrix of the blood clot. Thrombin also activates clotting Factor XIII (necessary for stabilizing and crosslinking the fibrin molecules into an insoluble clot) as well as activating other blood clotting factors and platelet aggregation. If thrombin is not formed, or its function is impeded, for example, with antithrombin III, coagulation is inhibited.

V. PLATELET AGGREGATION INHIBITORS

Platelet aggregation inhibitors decrease the formation or the action of chemical signals that promote platelet aggregation. These agents have proven beneficial in the prevention and treatment of occlusive cardiovascular diseases, the maintenance of vascular grafts and arterial patency, and as adjuncts to thrombolytic therapy in myocardial infarction.

A. Aspirin

Aspirin [AS pir in] blocks thromboxane A_2 synthesis from arachidonic acid in platelets by irreversible acetylation and inhibition of cyclooxygenase, a key enzyme in prostaglandin and thromboxane A_2 synthesis[1]. (See p. 405 for a discussion of the actions of aspirin on platelets.) The inhibitory effect is rapid, apparently occurring in the portal circulation. The *aspirin*-induced suppression of thromboxane A_2 synthetase and the resulting suppression of platelet aggregation last for the life of the platelet—approximately 7 to 10 days. *Aspirin* is currently employed in the prophylactic treatment of transient cerebral ischemia, to reduce the incidence of recurrent myocardial infarction and to decrease mortality in postmyocardial infarction patients. Currently, a single loading dose of 200 to 300 mg of *aspirin* followed by a daily dose of 75 to 100 mg is recommended. Bleeding time is prolonged, causing complications that include an increased incidence of hemorrhagic stroke as well as gastrointestinal bleeding, especially at higher doses of the drug.

B. Ticlopidine

Ticlopidine [Tye CLO pih deen] also acts as an inhibitor of platelet aggregation but by a mechanism other than that of *aspirin*. The drug inhibits the ADP pathway involved in the binding of platelets to fibrinogen and to each other. *Ticlopidine* has been shown to decrease the incidence of thrombotic stroke. After oral ingestion it is extensively bound to plasma proteins and undergoes hepatic metabolism. The drug can cause prolonged bleeding; its most serious adverse effect is neutropenia. Therefore, it is reserved for patients who cannot tolerate *aspirin*.

C. Dipyridamole

Dipyridamole [dye peer ID a mole], a coronary vasodilator, is employed to prophylactically treat angina pectoris. It is usually given in combination with *aspirin*. *Dipyridamole* increases intracellular levels of cyclic AMP by inhibiting cyclic nucleotide phosphodiesterase[2]. This inhibits thromboxane A_2 synthesis and may potentiate the effect of prostacyclin (PGI_2) to antagonize platelet stickiness and therefore decrease platelet adhesion to thrombogenic surfaces (see Figure 20.2). The meager data available suggest that *dipyridamole* makes only a marginal contribution to the antithrombotic action of *aspirin*. In combination with *warfarin*, however, *dipyridamole* is effective in inhibiting embolization from prosthetic heart valves. See pp. 446-448 for a description of newly approved drugs, *clopidogrel*, *abciximab, eptifibatide* and *tirofiban*.

VI. ANTICOAGULANTS

Two types of drugs are employed in preventing blood coagulation, *heparin* and the *vitamin K* antagonists. Their mechanisms of action differ, as do their clinical uses.

A. Heparin

Heparin [HEP a rin] is an injectable, rapidly-acting anticoagulant that is often used acutely to interfere with the formation of thrombi.

[1,2]See p. 206 for Infolink references to other books in this series.

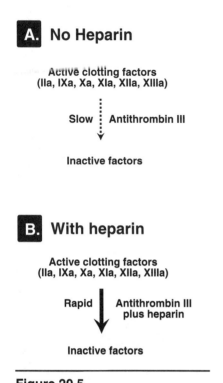

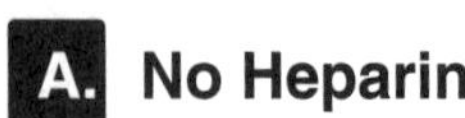
A. No Heparin
Active clotting factors
(IIa, IXa, Xa, XIa, XIIa, XIIIa)
Slow
Antithrombin III
Inactive factors
B. With heparin
Active clotting factors
(IIa, IXa, Xa, XIa, XIIa, XIIIa)
Rapid
Antithrombin III plus heparin
Inactive factors

Figure 20.5
Heparin binds to antithrombin III and enhances its proteolytic activity.

Heparin normally occurs as a macromolecule complexed with histamine in mast cells where its physiologic role is unknown. It is extracted for commercial use from porcine intestine or bovine lung. *Heparin* is a mixture of straight-chain anionic glycosaminoglycans with a mean molecular weight of 15,000. It is strongly acidic because of the presence of sulfate and carboxylic acid groups[3]. The realization that low molecular weight forms of *heparin* also can act as anticoagulants led to the isolation of *enoxaprin* [e NOX a prin], the first low molecular weight *heparin* (<6000) available in the USA.

1. **Mechanism of action:** *Heparin* acts indirectly by binding to antithrombin III to cause a rapid anticoagulant effect. Maximal anticoagulation occurs within minutes after intravenous *heparin* injection (unlike vitamin K antagonist anticoagulants, such as *warfarin*, whose maximum activity requires 8 to 12 hours). Antithrombin III, sometimes referred to as *heparin* cofactor, is an α-globulin that inhibits serine proteases, including several of the clotting factors, for example, thrombin (Factor II, Figure 20.5). In the absence of *heparin*, antithrombin III interacts with thrombin very slowly. The binding of *heparin* to antithrombin III produces a conformational change allowing the antithrombin to rapidly combine with and inhibit thrombin except that already bound to fibrin. [Note: While the *heparin*-antithrombin III complex readily inactivates thrombin, the complex of low molecular weight *heparin* with antithrombin is more specific against Factor Xa.] Chronic or intermittent administration of *heparin* can lead to a reduction in antithrombin III activity thus, increasing the risk of thrombosis. To minimize this risk, low-dose *heparin* therapy is usually employed.

2. **Therapeutic uses:** *Heparin* limits the expansion of thrombi by preventing fibrin formation. *Heparin* is the major antithrombotic drug for the treatment of deep vein thrombosis and pulmonary embolism. It decreases the incidence of recurrent thromboembolic episodes. Clinically, *heparin* is used prophylactically to prevent postoperative venous thrombosis in patients undergoing elective surgery, and in those in the acute phase of myocardial infarction. Coronary artery rethrombosis after thrombolytic treatment is reduced with *heparin.* It is also used in extracorporeal devices (for example, dialysis machines) to prevent thrombosis. It is the anticoagulant of choice for treating pregnant women with prosthetic heart valves or venous thromboembolism, because it does not cross the placenta. *Heparin* has the advantage of speedy onset of action, which is rapidly terminated on suspension of therapy. *Enoxaprin* has been approved for prevention of deep vein thrombosis following hip replacement.

3. **Pharmacokinetics**

   a. **Absorption:** *Heparin* must be given parenterally either in a deep subcutaneous site or intravenously, because the drug does not readily cross membranes. *Enoxaprin* is only given subcutaneously. [Note: Intramuscular administration of either heparin is contraindicated because of hematoma formation.] *Heparin* is often administered intravenously in a bolus to achieve immediate anticoagulation followed by lower doses or

[3]See p. 206 for Infolink references to other books in this series.

continuous infusion. The latter is then maintained for 7 to 10 days, titrating the dose of *heparin* so that the activated partial thromboplastin time (PTT) is 1.5 to 2.5 times the normal control.

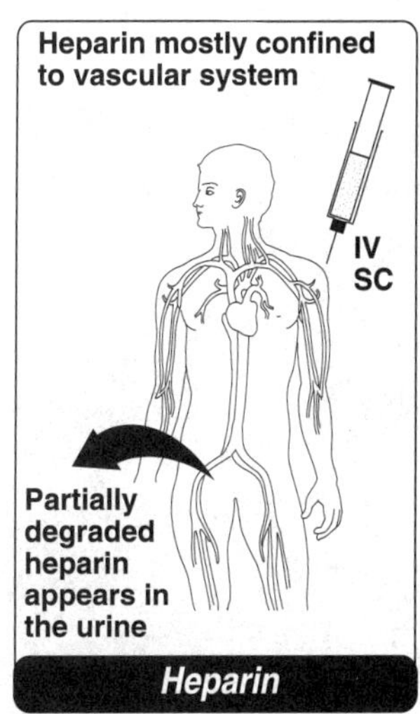
Heparin mostly confined to vascular system
IV
SC
Partially degraded heparin appears in the urine
Heparin

b. Fate: In the blood, *heparin* binds to many proteins that neutralize its activity and can cause resistance to the drug. Although generally restricted to the circulation, *heparin* is taken up by the reticuloendothelial system and undergoes depolymerization to inactive products. *Heparin* therefore has a longer half-life in patients with hepatic cirrhosis. Desulfation occurs in mononuclear phagocytes. The inactive metabolites as well as some of the parent *heparin* are excreted into the urine, therefore renal insufficiency also prolongs the half-life. [Note: *Heparin* does not cross the placental barrier.] The $t_{1/2}$ of *heparin* increases with dose; that of the low molecular weight heparins is about double that of the larger species.

4. Adverse effects: Despite early hopes of fewer side effects with *enoxaprin*, the complications have proven to be similar to those with *heparin*.

a. Bleeding complications: The chief complication of *heparin* therapy is hemorrhage. Careful monitoring of bleeding time is required to minimize this problem. Excessive bleeding may be managed by suspending the drug or treating with *protamine sulfate*. Infused slowly, the latter combines ionically with *heparin* to form a stable, inactive complex.

b. Hypersensitivity reactions: Chills, fever, urticaria, or anaphylactic shock are possible, since the *heparin* preparations are obtained from animal sources and may therefore be antigenic.

c. Thrombocytopenia: A decrease in the number of circulating platelets may occur after about 8 days of therapy. In some patients, *heparin*-induced platelet aggregation is followed by the formation of antiplatelet antibodies. Discontinuance of the drug then becomes necessary. Should *heparin*-induced thromboembolism occur, therapy with a drug that inhibits platelet aggregation or an oral anticoagulant is instituted in place of the *heparin*.

d. Contraindications: *Heparin* is contraindicated for patients who are hypersensitive to it or have bleeding disorders, for alcoholics, and for patients who have had surgery of the brain, eye, or spinal cord.

B. Warfarin

The coumarin anticoagulants, which include *warfarin* [WAR far in] and *dicumarol* [dye KOO ma role] (formerly *bishydroxycoumarin*) owe their action to their ability to antagonize the cofactor functions of *vitamin K*. Initially used as a rodenticide, *warfarin* is now widely employed clinically as an oral anticoagulant. Conflicting opinions exist concerning the usefulness of these agents in clinical situations such as myocardial infarction and hip arthroplasty. The potential morbidity argues for a way to identify those patients who are truly at risk for thrombosis. Even careful monitoring to keep prothrombin time at 1.5 to 2.5 times longer than normal values does not prevent bleeding complications in about 20% of the patients.

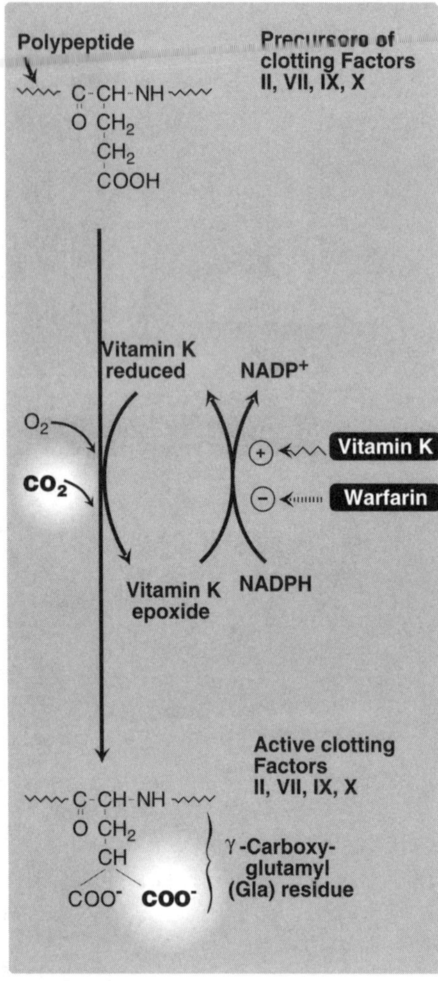

Figure 20.6
Mechanism of action of *warfarin*.

1. **Mechanism of action:** Several of the protein factors (including Factors II, VII, IX, and X; see Figure 20.4) that are involved in the coagulation reactions depend on *vitamin K* as a cofactor in their complete synthesis by the liver. These factors undergo *vitamin K*-dependent posttranslational modification, whereby a number of their glutamic acid residues are carboxylated to form γ-carboxyglutamic acid residues[4] (Figure 20.6). In this reaction, the *vitamin K*-dependent carboxylase fixes CO_2 to form the new COOH group on glutamic acid, and reduced *vitamin K* co-factor is converted to *vitamin K* epoxide. *Vitamin K* is regenerated from the epoxide by vitamin K epoxide reductase. It is this enzyme that is inhibited by *warfarin*. The γ-carboxyglutamyl residues bind calcium ion and are essential for interaction with cell membranes. *Warfarin* or *dicumarol* treatment results in the production of inactive clotting factors, since they lack the γ-carboxyglutamyl side chains. Unlike *heparin*, the anticoagulant effects of *warfarin* are not observed until 8 to 12 hours after drug administration. The anticoagulant effects of *warfarin* can be overcome by the administration of *vitamin K*. However, reversal by *vitamin K* takes approximately 24 hours.

2. **Pharmacokinetics**

   a. **Absorption:** The sodium salt of *warfarin* is rapidly and completely absorbed after oral administration. Though food may delay absorption, it does not affect the extent of absorption of the drug. *Warfarin* is 99% bound to plasma albumin, which prevents its diffusion into the cerebrospinal fluid, urine, and breast milk. However, drugs having a greater affinity for the binding site, such as sulfonamides, can displace the anticoagulant and lead to a transient elevated activity (see p. 12). The drug readily crosses the placental barrier.

   b. **Fate:** The products of *warfarin* metabolism are inactive and, after conjugation to glucuronic acid, are excreted in the urine and stool.

3. **Adverse effects**

   a. **Bleeding disorders:** The principal untoward reaction is hemorrhage. Therefore, it is important to frequently monitor and adjust the anticoagulant effect. Minor bleeding may be treated by withdrawal of the drug and administration of oral *vitamin* K_1; severe bleeding requires greater doses of the vitamin given intravenously. Whole blood, frozen plasma, or plasma concentrates of the blood factors may also be employed to arrest hemorrhaging.

   b. **Drug interactions:** A number of drug interactions that potentiate or attenuate the anticoagulant effects of *warfarin* have been identified. A summary of the most important of these interactions is shown in Figure 20.7.

[4]See p. 206 for Infolink references to other books in this series.

c. **Disease states:** These can also influence the hypoprothrombinemic state of the patient and influence the response to the anticoagulants. For example, a *vitamin K* deficiency, hepatic disease that impairs synthesis of the clotting factors, and hypermetabolic states that increase catabolism of the *vitamin K*-dependent clotting factors, can all augment the response to the oral anticoagulants.

d. **Contraindications:** The drug should never be used in pregnancy because it is teratogenic and can cause abortion.

VII. THROMBOLYTIC DRUGS

Acute thromboembolic disease in selected patients may be treated by the administration of agents that activate the conversion of plasminogen to plasmin, a serine protease that hydrolyzes fibrin and thus dissolves clots (Figure 20.8). The first such agents to be approved, *streptokinase* and *urokinase*, cause a systemic fibrinolytic state that can lead to bleeding problems. *Alteplase*, also known as *tissue-type plasminogen activator (tPA),* acts more locally on the thrombotic fibrin to produce fibrinolysis, and is a potentially important agent in treating thromboembolic disease. (See Figure 20.9 for a comparison of the commonly used thrombolytic agents.) Clinical experience has shown about equal efficacy between *streptokinase* and *tPA*. Unfortunately, thrombolytic therapy is unsuccessful in about 20% of infarcted arteries and about 15% of those opened, reclose.

A. Common characteristics of thrombolytic agents

1. **Actions:** The thrombolytic agents share some common features. All act either directly or indirectly to convert plasminogen to plasmin, which in turn cleaves fibrin, thus lysing thrombi (see Figure 20.8). In each case, clot dissolution and reperfusion occurs with a higher frequency when therapy is initiated early after clot formation, since clots become more resistant to lysis as they age. Unfortunately, increased local thrombin may occur as the clot dissolves, leading to enhanced platelet aggregability and thrombosis. Strategies to prevent this include administration of antiplatelet drugs, such as *aspirin*, or antithrombotics, such as *heparin*.

2. **Administration:** For myocardial infarction, intracoronary delivery of the drugs is the most reliable in terms of achieving recanalization. However, cardiac catheterization may not be possible in the 2 to 6 hour "therapeutic window," beyond which significant myocardial salvage becomes less likely. Thus thrombolytic agents are usually administered intravenously, since this route is rapid, inexpensive, and does not have the risks of catheterization.

3. **Therapeutic uses:** Originally used for the treatment of deep-vein thrombosis and serious pulmonary embolism, thrombolytic drugs are now being used with increasing frequency to treat acute myocardial infarction and peripheral arterial thrombosis and emboli, and for unclotting catheters and shunts.

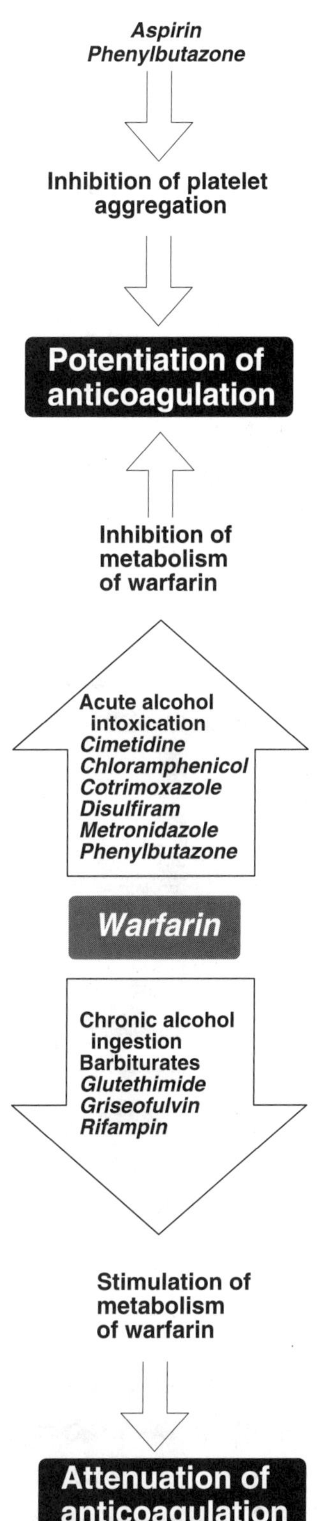

Figure 20.7
Drugs affecting the anticoagulant effect of warfarin.

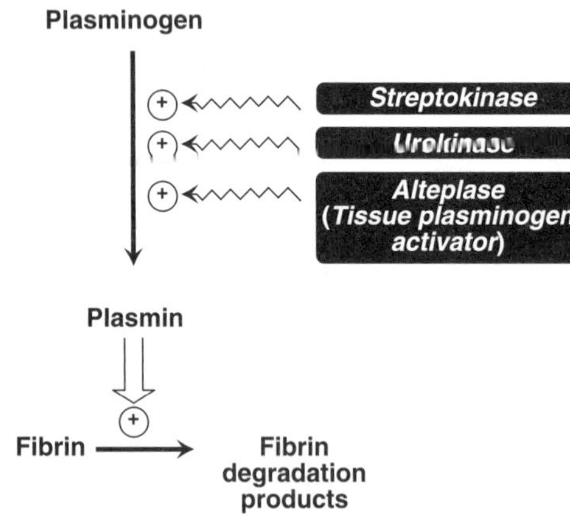

Figure 20.8
Activation of plasminogen by fibrinolytic agents.

4. **Adverse effects:** The thrombolytic agents do not distinguish between the fibrin of an unwanted thrombus and the fibrin of a beneficial hemostatic plug. Thus, hemorrhage is a major side effect. For example, a previously unsuspected lesion, such as a peptic ulcer, may hemorrhage following injection of a thrombolytic agent (Figure 20.10). They are contraindicated in patients with a healing wound, pregnancy, history of cerebrovascular accident, or metastatic cancer. Continued presence of thrombogenic stimuli may cause rethrombosis after lysis of the initial clot.

B. Alteplase (tPA)

Alteplase [AL te place] previously known as *tissue-type plasminogen activator (tPA),* is a serine protease originally derived from cultured human melanoma cells. It is now obtained as a product of recombinant DNA technology.

1. **Mechanism of action:** *Alteplase* has a low affinity for free plasminogen, but it rapidly activates plasminogen bound to fibrin in a thrombus or a hemostatic plug. Thus, *alteplase* is said to be "fibrin selective" and at low doses, has the advantage of lysing only fibrin, without unwanted degradation of other proteins, notably fibrinogen. This contrasts with *urokinase* and *streptokinase*, which act on free plasminogen and induce a thrombolytic state. [Note: At dose levels of *alteplase* currently in use clinically, circulating plasminogen may be activated, resulting in hemorrhage.]

2. **Therapeutic uses:** Currently *alteplase* is approved for the treatment of myocardial infarction, massive pulmonary embolism, and acute ischemic stroke. *Alteplase* seems to be superior to *streptokinase* and *urokinase* in dissolving older clots, and may ultimately be approved for other applications. *Alteplase* administered within 3 hours of the onset of ischemic stroke significantly improves clinical outcome, that is, the patients' ability to perform activites of daily living.

3. **Pharmacokinetics:** The agent has a very short $t_{1/2}$ (about 5 minutes) and therefore is administered as a 100-mg dose with 10 mg injected intravenously as a bolus and the rest over 90 minutes.

4. **Adverse effects:** Bleeding complications, including gastrointestinal and cerebral hemorrhages, may occur.

C. Streptokinase

Streptokinase [strep toe KYE nase] is an extracellular protein purified from culture broths of Group C β-hemolytic streptococci.

1. **Mechanism of action:** *Streptokinase* has no enzymic activity; instead it forms an active 1:1 complex with plasminogen, which then converts uncomplexed plasminogen to the active enzyme plasmin (Figure 20.11). In addition to the hydrolysis of fibrin plugs, the complex also catalyzes the degradation of fibrinogen as well as clotting Factors V and VII.

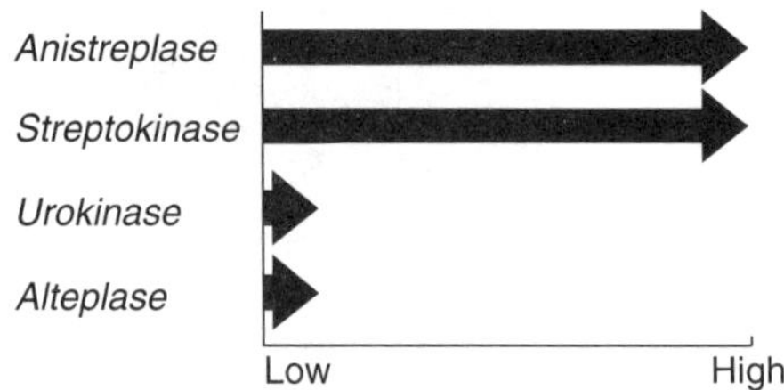

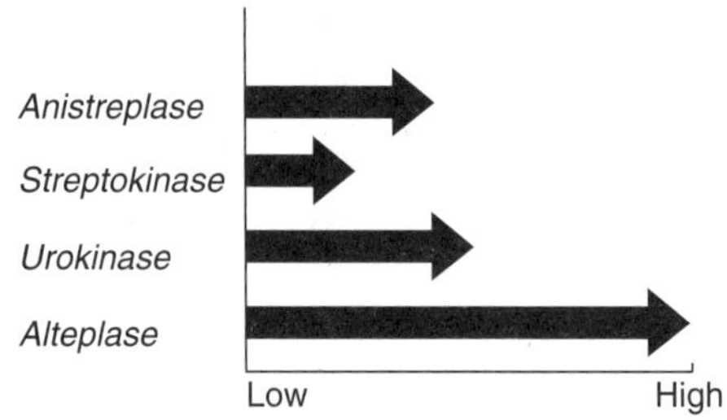

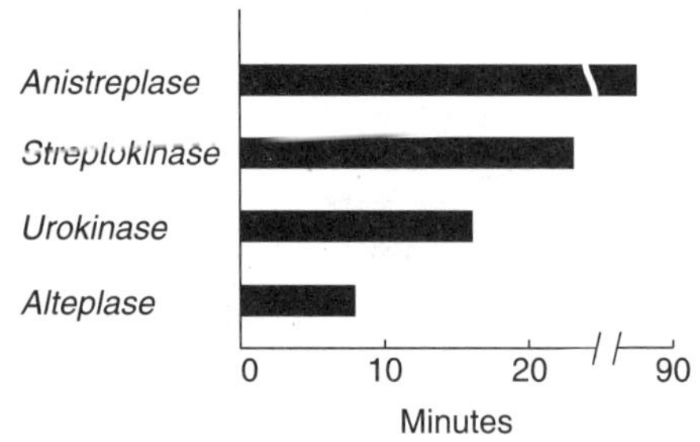

Figure 20.9
A comparison of commonly used thrombolytic agents.

2. **Therapeutic uses:** *Streptokinase* is approved for use in acute pulmonary embolism, deep venous thrombosis, acute myocardial infarction, arterial thrombosis, and occluded access shunts.

3. **Pharmacokinetics:** *Streptokinase* therapy is instituted within 4 hours of a myocardial infarction and is infused for 1 hour. Its $t_{1/2}$ is less than a half-hour. Thromboplastin time is monitored and maintained at two to five times control value. On discontinuation of treatment, either *heparin* or oral anticoagulants may be administered.

4. **Adverse effects**

   a. **Bleeding disorders:** Activation of circulating plasminogen leads to elevated levels of plasmin, which may precipitate bleeding by dissolving hemostatic plugs (Figure 20.12). In the rare instance of life-threatening hemorrhage, *aminocaproic acid* (see p. 204) may be administered.

   b. **Hypersensitivity:** *Streptokinase* is a foreign protein and is antigenic. Rashes, fever, and rarely, anaphylaxis occur. Since most individuals have had a streptococcal infection sometime in their lives, circulating antibodies against *streptokinase* are likely to be present in most patients. These antibodies can combine with *streptokinase* and neutralize its fibrinolytic properties. Therefore, sufficient quantities of *streptokinase* must be administered to overwhelm the antibodies and provide a therapeutic concentration of plasmin. Fever, allergic reactions, and therapeutic failure may be associated with the presence of antistreptococcal antibodies in the patient. The incidence of allergic reactions is approximately 3%.

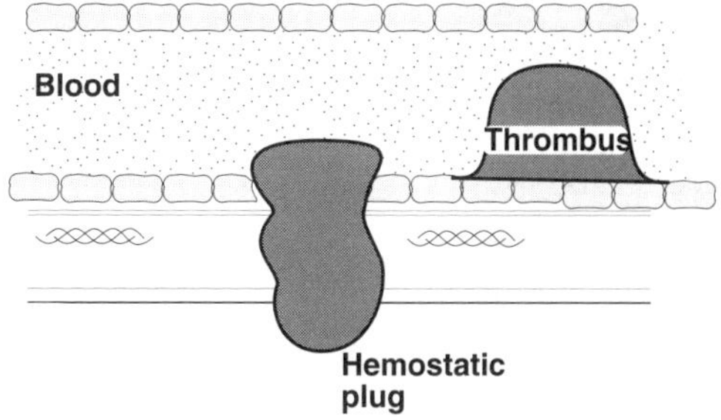

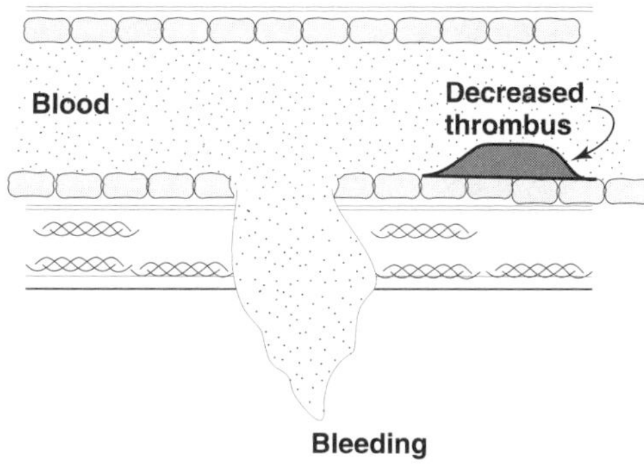

Figure 20.10
Degradation of an unwanted thrombus and a beneficial hemostatic plug by plasminogen activators.

D. Anistreplase

Anistreplase [annie STREP lase] (*anisoylated plasminogen streptokinase activator complex; APSAC*) was synthesized in vitro to improve the kinetics of the *streptokinase-plasminogen* complex. Acylation blocks the lysine at the active site of plasminogen so that the complex is inactive until it binds to fibrin, a property that is retained. On binding, the anisoyl group is removed and fibrinolysis proceeds; thus the complex is semiselective for lysis at the clot site. The plasma half-life of *anistreplase* is long (about 90 minutes) compared to *streptokinase*. It is injected intravenously from 2 to 5 minutes. Reperfusion of the tissue compares favorably with *streptokinase*. Like other thrombolytic agents, bleeding is a complication, as well as are arrhythmias and hypotension.

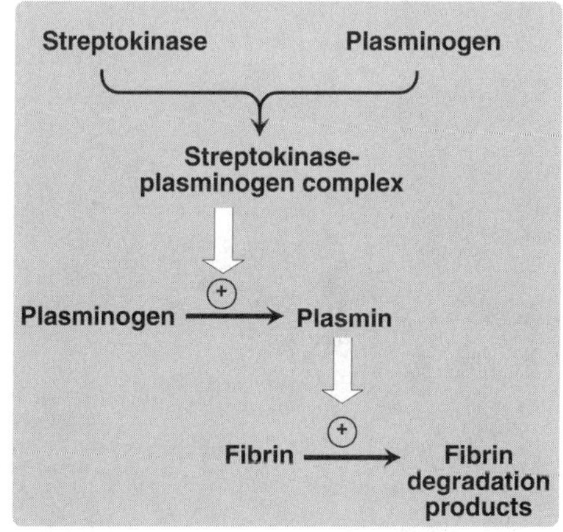

Figure 20.11
Mechanism of action of streptokinase.

E. Urokinase

Urokinase [yoor oh KINE ase] is an enzyme capable of directly degrading both fibrin and fibrinogen (see Figure 20.12). *Urokinase* was originally isolated from human urine, but it is now obtained from cultures of human fetal renal cells. *Urokinase* is more expensive than *streptokinase* and is usually employed in patients who are sensitive to *streptokinase*. [Note: *Urokinase* is not a foreign protein and is therefore nonantigenic.] Like *streptokinase, urokinase* is effective in treating severe pulmonary emboli and deep vein thrombosis. Bleeding complications are the most important side effects of this drug therapy.

VIII. DRUGS USED TO TREAT BLEEDING

Bleeding problems may have their origin in naturally occurring pathologic conditions such as hemophilia, or as a result of fibrinolytic states that may arise after gastrointestinal surgery or prostatectomy. The use of anticoagulants may also give rise to hemorrhaging. Certain natural proteins and *vitamin K* as well as synthetic antagonists are effective in controlling this bleeding. For example, hemophilia is a consequence of a deficiency in plasma coagulation factors, most frequently Factors VIII and IX. Concentrated preparations of these factors are available from human donors. However, they hold the risk of transferring viral infections.

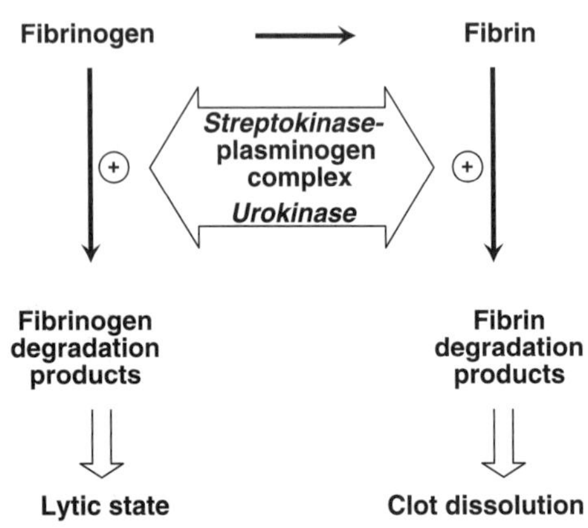

Figure 20.12
Streptokinase and *urokinase* degrade both fibrin and fibrinogen.

A. Aminocaproic acid and tranexamic acid

Fibrinolytic states can be controlled by the administration of *aminocaproic acid* [a mee noe ka PROE ic] or *tranexamic acid* [tran ex AM ic]. Both agents are synthetic and inhibit plasminogen activation. A potential side effect is intravascular thrombosis.

B. Protamine sulfate

Protamine sulfate [PROE ta meen] antagonizes the anticoagulant effects of *heparin*. This protein is derived from fish sperm or testes and is high in arginine content, which explains its basicity. The positively charged protein interacts with the negatively charged *heparin* to form a stable complex without anticoagulant activity. *Protamine sulfate* itself can interfere in coagulation when it is given in the absence of *heparin*, since the basic protein interacts with platelets and fibrinogen. Adverse effects include hypersensitivity, as well as dyspnea, flushing, bradycardia, and hypotension when rapidly injected.

C. Vitamin K

That *vitamin K1* (*phytonadione*) administration can stem bleeding problems due to the oral anticoagulants is not surprising, since those substances act by interfering in the action of the vitamin (see Figure 20.6). The response to *vitamin K* is slow, requiring about 24 hours; thus if immediate hemostasis is required, fresh frozen plasma should be infused. [Note: *Vitamin K* supplementation is required for patients receiving the cephalosporins, *cefamandole*, *cefoperazone*, and *moxalactam* (see p. 306).]

IX. AGENTS USED TO TREAT ANEMIA

Anemia is defined as a below-normal plasma hemoglobin concentration resulting from a decreased number of circulating red blood cells or an abnormally low total hemoglobin content per unit of blood volume. Anemia can be caused by chronic blood loss, bone marrow abnormalities, increased hemolysis, infections, malignancy, endocrine deficiencies, and a number of other disease states. These conditions can be corrected by transfusion of whole blood. A large number of drugs cause toxic effects on blood cells, hemoglobin production, or erythropoietic organs, which in turn may cause anemia. In addition, nutritional anemias are caused by dietary deficiencies of substances [for example, *iron*, *folic acid*, *vitamin B_{12}* (*cyanocobalamin*)] necessary for normal erythropoiesis.

A. Iron

Iron is stored in intestinal mucosal cells as ferritin (an iron/protein complex) until needed by the body. Iron deficiency results from acute or chronic blood loss, from insufficient intake during periods of accelerated growth in children, or in heavily menstruating or pregnant women. Therefore it essentially results from a negative iron balance due to depletion of iron stores and inadequate intake, culminating in hypochromic microcytic anemia. Supplementation with *ferrous sulfate* is required to correct the deficiency. Gastrointestinal disturbances caused by local irritation are the most common adverse effects caused by iron supplements.

B. Folic acid

The primary use of *folic acid* is in treating deficiency states that arise from inadequate levels of the vitamin. *Folate* deficiency may be caused by (1) increased demand (for example, pregnancy and lactation), (2) poor absorption caused by pathology of the small intestine, (3) alcoholism, or (4) treatment with drugs that are dihydrofolate reductase inhibitors (for example, *methotrexate* and *trimethoprim*, see p. 293). A primary result of *folic acid* deficiency is megaloblastic anemia, caused by diminished synthesis of purines and pyrimidines. This leads to an inability of erythropoietic tissue to make DNA and proliferate (Figure 20.13). [Note: It is important to evaluate the basis of the megaloblastic anemia prior to instituting therapy, because *vitamin B_{12}* deficiency indirectly causes symptoms of this disorder (see following paragraph).] *Folic acid* is well absorbed in the jejunum unless pathology is present. If excessive amounts of the vitamin are ingested, they are excreted in the urine and feces. *Folic acid* administered orally has no known toxicity.

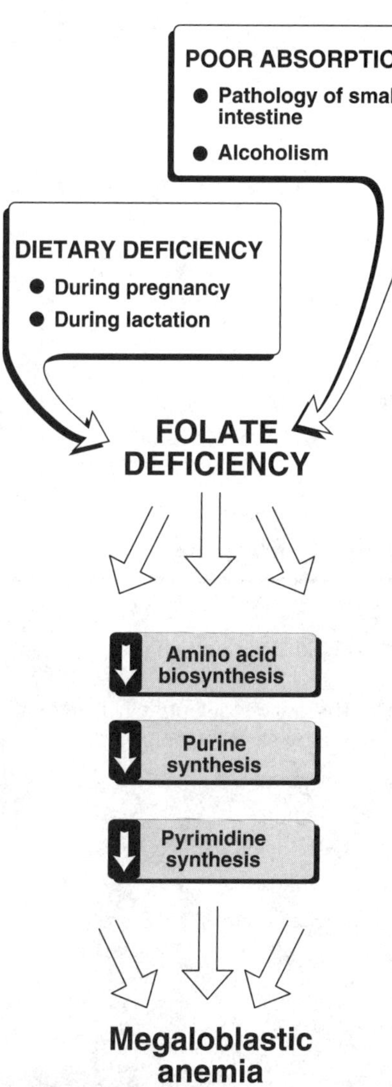

Figure 20.13
Causes and consequences of folic acid depletion.

C. Cyanocobalamin (vitamin B_{12})

Deficiencies of *vitamin B_{12}* can result from either low dietary levels or, more commonly, from poor absorption of the vitamin due to the failure of gastric parietal cells to produce intrinsic factor (as in pernicious anemia) or to a loss of activity of the receptor needed for intestinal uptake of the vitamin.[5] Nonspecific malabsorption syndromes or gastric resection can also cause *vitamin B_{12}* deficiency. The vitamin may be administered orally (for dietary deficiencies), or intramuscularly or deep subcutaneously (for pernicious anemia). [Note: *Folic acid* administration alone reverses the hematologic abnormality and thus masks the *B_{12}* deficiency, which can then proceed to severe neurologic dysfunction and disease. Therefore, megaloblastic anemia should not be treated with *folic acid* alone, but rather with a combination of *folate* and *vitamin B_{12}*.] Therapy must be continued for the remainder of the life of a patient suffering from pernicious anemia. There are no known adverse effects of this vitamin.

[5]See p. 206 for Infolink references to other books in this series.

D. Erythropoietin

Erythropoietin [ery throw PO eetin] is a glycoprotein, normally made by the kidney, that regulates red cell proliferation and differentiation in bone marrow. Human *erythropoietin*, produced by recombinant DNA technology, is effective in the treatment of anemia caused by end-stage renal disease, anemia associated with HIV-infected patients, and anemia in some cancer patients. Supplementation with iron may be required to assure an adequate response. The protein is usually administered intravenously in renal dialysis patients, but in others the subcutaneous route is preferred. Side effects such as iron deficiency and an elevation in blood pressure occur. [Note: The latter may be due to increases in peripheral vascular resistance and/or blood viscosity.]

X. AGENTS USED TO TREAT SICKLE CELL DISEASE

Recent clinical trials have shown that *hydroxyurea* can relieve the painful clinical course of sickle cell disease (anemia). *Hydroxyurea* is currently used to treat chronic myelogenous leukemia and polycythemia vera. In sickle cell disease, the drug apparently increases fetal hemoglobin (HbF) levels, thus diluting the abnormal hemoglobin S (HbS). This process takes several months. Polymerization of HbS is delayed in the treated patients so that painful crises are not caused by sickled cells blocking capillaries and causing tissue anoxia.[6] The optimal dose of *hydroxyurea,* and its safety over the long run remain to be determined.

See p. 448 for a description of the newly approved drug *lepirudin.*

Study Questions

Choose the ONE best answer.

20.1. The anticoagulant activity of warfarin can be potentiated by all of the following EXCEPT:

A. Rifampin.
B. Aspirin.
C. Phenylbutazone.
D. Cimetidine.
E. Disulfiram.

Correct choice = A. Rifampin induces the hepatic mixed function oxidases that metabolize warfarin. Platelet inhibitors, such as aspirin, increase the anticoagulant effect of warfarin. Phenylbutazone can transiently increase the level of free warfarin by displacing it from the plasma albumin binding site. Cimetidine inhibits warfarin metabolism and causes potentiation of the anticoagulant. Disulfiram inhibits warfarin metabolism.

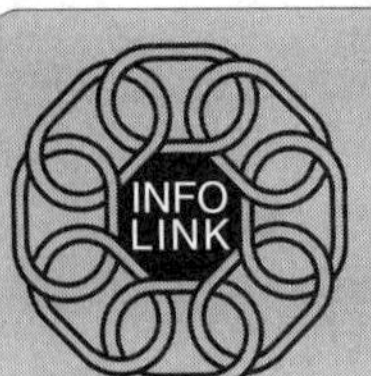

[1]See p. 185 in **Biochemistry** (2nd ed.) for a discussion of prostaglandin synthesis.

[2]See p. 83 in **Biochemistry** (2nd ed.) for a discussion of the hydrolysis of cAMP.

[3]See p. 149 in **Biochemistry** (2nd ed.) for a discussion of the structure of heparin.

[4]See p. 338 in **Biochemistry** (2nd ed.) for a discussion of vitamin K.

[5]See p. 326 in **Biochemistry** (2nd ed.) for a discussion of vitamine B_{12}.

[6]See p. 36 in **Biochemistry** (2nd ed.) for a discussion of sickle cell disease.

Antihyperlipidemic Drugs

21

I. OVERVIEW

Coronary artery disease (CAD) is the cause of about half of all deaths in the United States. CAD has been shown to be correlated with the levels of plasma cholesterol- and/or triacylglycerol-containing lipoprotein particles. These particles, which are key to the development of atherogenesis, are initially synthesized by the intestinal mucosa and the liver, and undergo extensive metabolism in the plasma. They also play an essential role in the transport of lipids between tissues. [Note: Because lipids are insoluble in aqueous solutions, they must be transported in the plasma from tissue to tissue, bound to proteins, hence the name, lipoprotein.] Their levels can be elevated by environmental causes, such as diet, or by inherited genetic defects in the appropriate synthesis or degradation of these compounds. Drugs used in the treatment of elevated serum lipids (hyperlipidemias) generally are targeted to (1) decrease production of a lipoprotein by the tissues, (2) increase catabolism of a lipoprotein in the plasma, or (3) increase removal of cholesterol from the body. Such treatments lead to a decline in the progression of coronary plaque and a possible regression of pre-existing lesions. The antihyperlipidemic drugs are listed in Figure 21.1.

ANTIHYPERLIPIDEMIC DRUGS

- ***Atorvastatin***[1]
- ***Cerivastatin***[1]
- ***Cholestyramine***
- ***Clofibrate***
- ***Colestipol***
- ***Fluvastatin***
- ***Gemfibrozil***
- ***Lovastatin***
- ***Niacin***
- ***Pravastatin***
- ***Probucol***
- ***Simvastatin***

Figure 21.1
Summary of antihyperlipidemic drugs. [1]Described in Pharmacology update, p. 449.

II. HYPERLIPIDEMIAS

The hyperlipidemias are a complex group of diseases that can be designated either primary or secondary, depending on their causes. Primary hyperlipidemias can result from a single inherited gene defect, or more commonly, are caused by a combination of genetic and environmental factors. Secondary hyperlipidemias are the result of a more generalized metabolic disorder, such as diabetes mellitus, excessive alcohol intake, hypothyroidism, or primary biliary cirrhosis. Therapeutic strategies for treating secondary hyperlipidemia caused by one of these disorders include dietary intervention plus a regimen of drugs used to treat the primary cause of the hyperlipidemia. Figure 21.2 illustrates the normal metabolism of serum lipoproteins, and the characteristics of the major genetic hyperlipidemias.

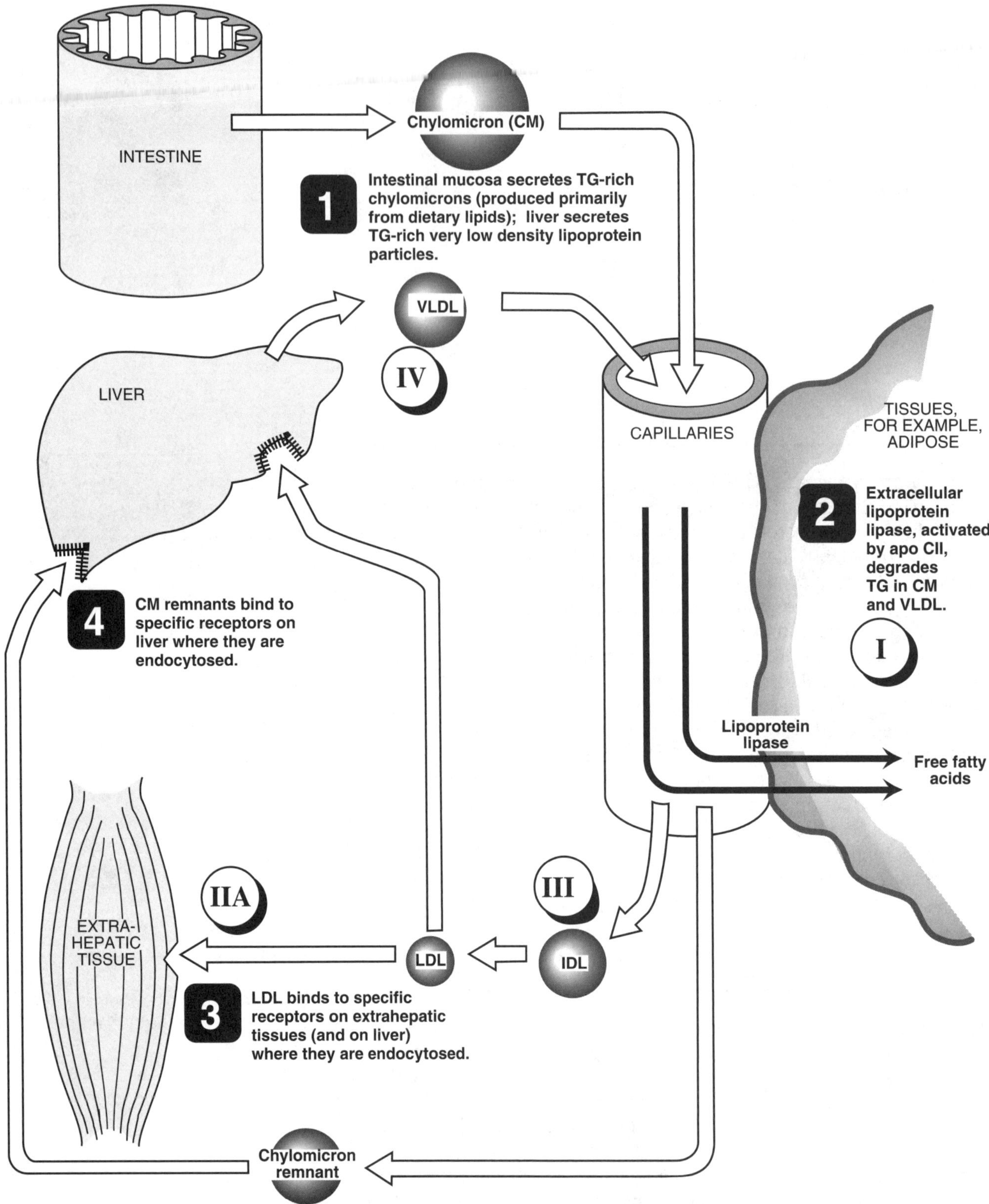

Figure 21.2
Metabolism of plasma lipoproteins and related genetic diseases. CM=chylomicron, TG=triacylglycerol, VLDL=very low density lipoprotein, LDL=low density lipoprotein, IDL=intermediate density lipoprotein, apo CII= apolipoprotein CII found in chylomicrons and VLDL. The Roman numerals in the white circles refer to specific genetic types of hyperlipidemias summarized on the facing page.

Type I [FAMILIAL HYPERCHYLOMICRONEMIA]

- Massive fasting hyperchylomicronemia even following normal dietary fat intake, resulting in greatly elevated serum triacylglycerol.
- Deficiency of lipoprotein lipase or deficiency of normal apolipoprotein CII (rare).
- Type I is not associated with an increase in coronary heart disease.
- Treatment: Low fat diet. No drug therapy is effective for Type I hyperlipidemia.

Type IIA [FAMILIAL HYPERCHOLESTEROLEMIA]

- Elevated LDL with normal VLDL levels due to block in LDL degradation, therefore increased serum cholesterol but normal triacylglycerol.
- Caused by decreased numbers of normal LDL receptors.
- Ischemic heart disease is greatly accelerated.
- Treatment: Low cholesterol and low saturated fat in the diet. Heterozygotes: Cholestyramine or colestipol, and/or lovastatin or mevastatin. Homozygotes: As above, plus niacin.

Type IIB [FAMILIAL COMBINED (MIXED) HYPERLIPIDEMIA]

- Similar to IIA except VLDL are also increased, resulting in elevated serum triacylglycerol as well as cholesterol.
- Caused by overproduction of VLDL by the liver.
- Relatively common.
- Treatment: Dietary restriction of cholesterol and saturated fat and alcohol. Drug therapy similar to IIA except heterozygotes also receive niacin.

Type III [FAMILIAL DYSBETALIPOPROTEINEMIA]

- Serum concentrations of IDL are increased resulting in increased triacylglycerol and cholesterol levels.
- Cause is either overproduction or underutilization of IDL, due to mutant apolipoprotein E.
- Xanthomas and accelerated coronary and peripheral vascular disease develop in patients by middle age.
- Treatment: Weight reduction (if necessary). Dietary restriction of cholesterol and alcohol. Drug therapy includes niacin and clofibrate (or gemfibrozil), or lovastatin (or mevastatin).

Type IV [FAMILIAL HYPERTRIGLYCERIDEMIA]

- VLDL levels are increased, while LDL levels are normal or decreased, resulting in normal to elevated cholesterol, and greatly elevated circulating triacylglycerol levels.
- Cause is overproduction and/or decreased removal of VLDL triacylglycerol in serum.
- This is a relatively common disease. It has few clinical manifestations other than accelerated ischemic heart disease. Patients with this disorder are frequently obese, diabetic, and hyperuricemic. Also seen in individuals undergoing estrogen therapy, or are in their third trimester of pregnancy, or are alcoholic.
- Treatment: Weight reduction (if necessary) is of primary importance. Dietary restriction of controlled carbohydrate, modified fat, low alcohol consumption. If necessary, drug therapy includes niacin and/or gemfibrozil (or clofibrate), or lovastatin (or mevastatin).

Type V [FAMILIAL MIXED HYPERTRIGLYCERIDEMIA]

- Serum VLDL and chylomicrons are elevated. LDL is normal or decreased. This results in elevated cholesterol and greatly elevated triacylglycerol levels.
- Cause is either increased production or decreased clearance of VLDL and chylomicrons. Usually a genetic defect.
- Occurs most commonly in adults who are obese and/or diabetic.
- Treatment: Weight reduction (if necessary) is important. Diet should include protein, low fat and controlled carbohydrate, and no alcohol. If necessary, drug therapy includes niacin, clofibrate and/or gemfibrozil, or lovastatin (or mevastatin).

Figure 21.2 (continued).

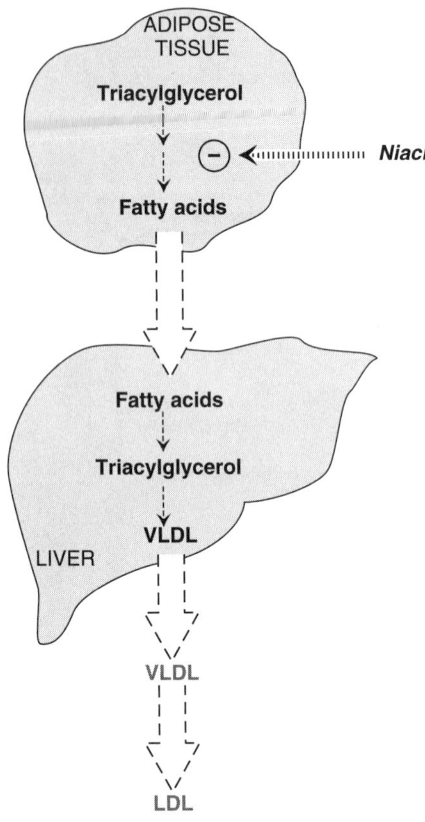

Figure 21.3
Niacin inhibits lipolysis in adipose tissue, resulting in decreased hepatic VLDL and LDL synthesis.

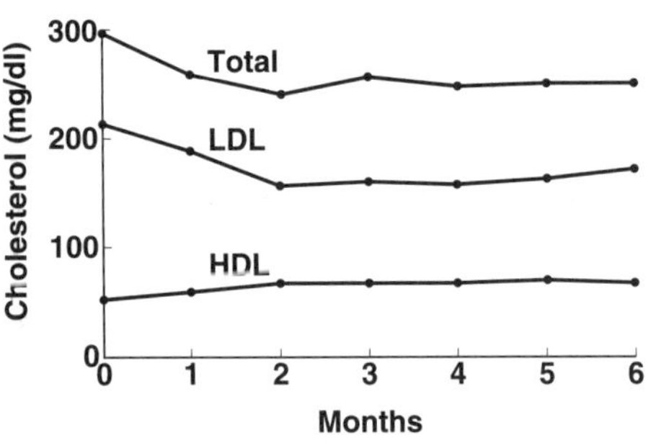

Figure 21.4
Plasma levels of cholesterol in hyperlipidemic patients during treatment with *niacin*.

III. DRUGS THAT LOWER SERUM LIPOPROTEIN CONCENTRATION

Antihyperlipidemic drugs target the problem of elevated serum lipids (in both primary and secondary hyperlipidemias) with complementary strategies; some of these agents decrease production of the lipoprotein carriers of cholesterol and triacylglycerol, whereas others increase lipoprotein degradation. Still others directly increase cholesterol removal from the body. These drugs may be used singly or in combination, but are always accompanied by the requirement that dietary lipid intake be significantly low, especially cholesterol and saturated fats, and the caloric content of the diet must be closely monitored.

A. Niacin (nicotinic acid)

Nicotinic acid has a broad lipid-lowering ability, but its clinical use is limited due to its unpleasant side effects. Derivatives of this drug that are not available in the United States appear to have fewer adverse effects.

1. **Mechanism of Action:** At gram doses, *niacin* [NYE a sin], a water-soluble vitamin[1], strongly inhibits lipolysis in adipose tissue—the primary producer of circulating free fatty acids. The liver normally utilizes these circulating fatty acids as a major precursor for triacylglycerol synthesis. Thus, *niacin* causes a decrease in liver triacylglycerol synthesis, which is required for very low density lipoprotein (VLDL) production (Figure 21.3).[2] Low density lipoprotein (LDL, the cholesterol-rich lipoprotein) is derived from VLDL in the plasma. Therefore a reduction in the VLDL concentration also results in a decreased plasma LDL concentration. Thus, both plasma triacylglycerol (in VLDL) and cholesterol (in VLDL and LDL) are lowered (Figure 21.4). Furthermore, *niacin* treatment increases HDL-cholesterol levels (HDL is the "good" cholesterol carrier). Moreover, by boosting secretion of tissue plasminogen activator and lowering plasma fibrinogen, *niacin* can reverse some of the endothelial cell dysfunction contributing to thrombosis associated with hypercholesterolemia and atherosclerosis.

2. **Therapeutic uses:** *Niacin* lowers plasma levels of both cholesterol and triacylglycerol. Therefore, it is particularly useful in the treatment of Type IIb and IV hyperlipoproteinemia, in which both VLDL and LDL are elevated. *Niacin* is also used to treat other severe hypercholesterolemias, often in combination with other antihyperlipidemic agents (see p. 215). In addition, it is the most potent antihyperlipidemic agent for raising plasma HDL levels.

3. **Pharmacokinetics:** *Niacin* is administered orally. It is converted in the body to nicotinamide, which is incorporated into the cofactor nicotinamide adenine dinucleotide (NAD^+). *Niacin,* its nicotinamide derivative and other metabolites are excreted in the urine. [Note: Nicotinamide alone does not decrease plasma lipid levels.]

4. **Adverse effects:** The most common side effects of *niacin* therapy are an intense cutaneous flush (accompanied by an uncomfort-

[1,2]See p. 216 for Infolink references to other books in this series.

able feeling of warmth) and pruritus. Administration of *aspirin* prior to taking *niacin* decreases the flush, which is prostaglandin-mediated. Some patients also experience nausea and abdominal pain. Nicotinic acid inhibits tubular secretion of uric acid and thus predisposes to hyperuricemia and gout. Impaired glucose tolerance and hepatotoxicity have also been reported.

B. The fibrates—clofibrate and gemfibrozil

These agents are derivatives of fibric acid and both have the same mechanism of action. However, *gemfibrozil* [gem FYE bro zil] has largely replaced *clofibrate* [kloe FYE brate] clinically because of the higher incidence of mortality with the latter agent. The deaths were not associated with cardiovascular causes, but rather with malignancy or complications due to postcholecystectomy and pancreatitis.

1. **Mechanism of action:** Both drugs cause a decrease in plasma triacylglycerol levels by stimulating lipoprotein lipase activity, thereby hydrolyzing triacylglycerols in chylomicrons and VLDL, and thus hastening the removal of these particles from the plasma (Figure 21.5). In contrast, HDL levels rise moderately. Animal studies show that the fibrates can cause a lowering of plasma cholesterol by inhibiting cholesterol synthesis in the liver (mechanism unknown) and by increasing biliary excretion of cholesterol into the feces. The fibrates also appear to lower plasma fibrinogen levels.

2. **Therapeutic uses:** The fibrates are used in the treatment of hypertriglyceridemias, causing a significant decrease in plasma triacylglycerol levels. [Note: They are not indicated for Type I hyperlipidemia in which chylomicron levels are elevated but VLDL levels are normal.] *Clofibrate* and *gemfibrozil* are particularly useful in treating Type III hyperlipidemia (dysbetalipoproteinemia), in which intermediate density lipoproteins (IDL) particles accumulate. Patients with hypertriglyceridemia [Type IV (elevated VLDL) or Type V (elevated VLDL plus chylomicron) disease] who do not respond to diet or other drugs may also benefit from treatment with these agents.

3. **Pharmacokinetics:** Both drugs are completely absorbed after an oral dose. *Clofibrate* is deesterified to the active *clofibric acid*, which binds to albumin and distributes widely in body tissues. Likewise, *gemfibrozil* distributes extensively, bound to albumin. Both drugs undergo extensive biotransformation and are excreted in the urine as their glucuronide conjugates.

4. **Adverse effects**

   a. **GI effects:** The most common adverse effects are mild gastrointestinal disturbances. These lessen as the therapy progresses.

   b. **Lithiasis:** Because these drugs increase biliary cholesterol excretion, there is a predisposition to the formation of gallstones.

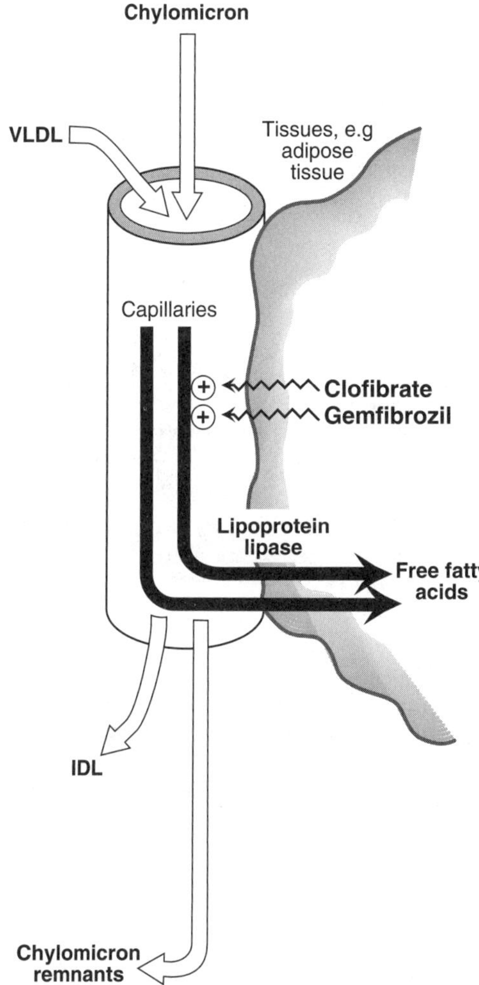

Figure 21.5
Activation of lipoprotein lipase by *clofibrate* and *gemfibrozil*.

c. **Malignancy:** Treatment with *clofibrate* has resulted in a significant number of malignancy–related deaths.

d. **Muscle:** Myositis (inflammation of a voluntary muscle) can occur with both drugs, thus muscle weakness or tenderness should be evaluated. Though rare, patients with renal insufficiency are at risk. Myopathy and rhabdomyolysis have been reported in a few patients taking *gemfibrozil* and *lovastatin* together.

e. **Drug interactions:** Both fibrates compete with the *coumarin* anticoagulants for binding sites on plasma proteins, thus transiently potentiating anticoagulant activity. Prothrombin levels should therefore be monitored when a patient is taking both these drugs. Similarly, these drugs may transiently elevate the levels of sulfonyl ureas.

f. **Contraindications:** The safety of these agents in pregnant or lactating women has not been established. They should not be used in patients with severe hepatic and renal dysfunction or in patients with pre-existing gall bladder disease.

A. Untreated hyperlipidemic patient

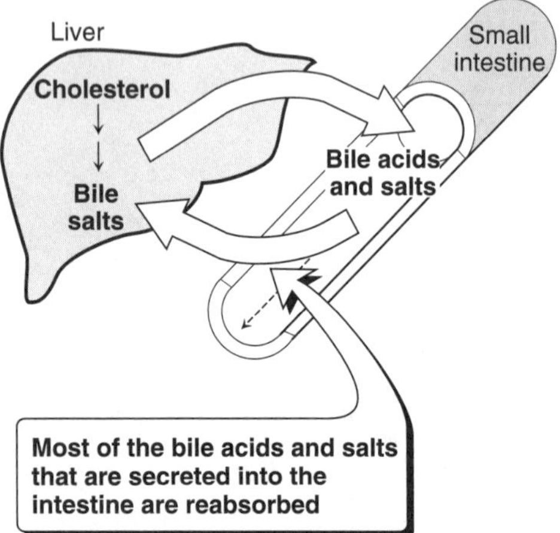
Liver
Small intestine
Cholesterol
Bile salts
Bile acids and salts
Most of the bile acids and salts that are secreted into the intestine are reabsorbed

B. Hyperlipidemic patient treated with bile acid binding resins

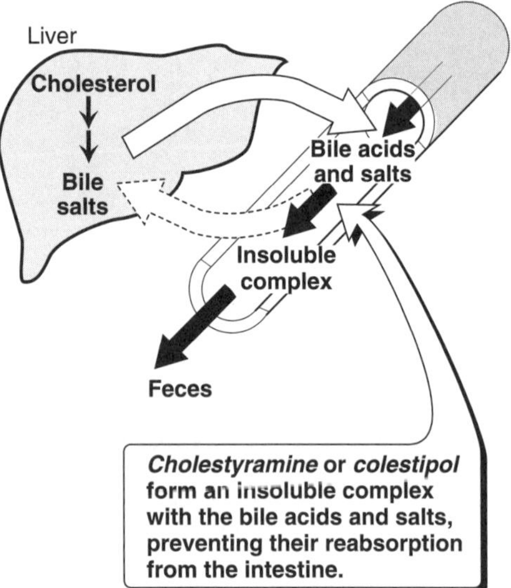
Liver
Cholesterol
Bile salts
Bile acids and salts
Insoluble complex
Feces
Cholestyramine or *colestipol* form an insoluble complex with the bile acids and salts, preventing their reabsorption from the intestine.

Figure 21.6
Mechanism of bile acid binding resins.

C. Bile acid binding resins: cholestyramine and colestipol

1. **Mechanism of action:** *Cholestyramine* [koe less TYE ra meen] and *colestipol* [koe LES tih pole] are anion exchange resins that bind negatively charged bile acids and bile salts in the small intestine (Figure 21.6). The resin/bile acid complex is excreted in the feces, thus preventing the bile acids from returning to the liver by the enterohepatic circulation. Lowering the bile acid concentration causes hepatocytes to increase conversion of cholesterol to bile acids, resulting in a replenished supply of these compounds, which are essential components of the bile. Consequently, the intracellular cholesterol concentration decreases, which activates an increased hepatic uptake of cholesterol-containing LDL particles, leading to a fall in plasma LDL. [Note: This increased uptake is mediated by an upregulation of cell-surface LDL receptors.] In some patients, a modest rise in plasma HDL levels is also observed. The final outcome of this sequence of events is a decreased total plasma cholesterol concentration.

2. **Therapeutic uses:** The bile acid binding resins are the drugs of choice (often in combination with diet or *niacin*) in treating Type IIa and IIb hyperlipidemias. [Note: In those rare individuals who are homozygous for Type IIa, that is, for whom functional LDL receptors are totally lacking, these drugs have little effect on plasma LDL levels.] *Cholestyramine* can also relieve pruritus caused by accumulation of bile acids in patients with biliary obstruction.

3. **Pharmacokinetics**: *Cholestyramine* and *colestipol* are taken orally. Because they are insoluble in water and are very large (molecular weights are greater than 10^6), they are neither absorbed nor metabolically altered by the intestine. Instead, they are totally excreted in the feces.

4. **Adverse effects**

a. **GI effects:** The most common side effects are gastrointestinal disturbances, such as constipation, nausea, and flatulence.

b. **Impaired absorptions:** Absorption of the fat-soluble vitamins, A, D, E, and K can be impaired if high doses of the resin are present. Folic acid and ascorbic acid absorption may also be reduced.

c. **Drug interactions:** *Cholestyramine* and *colestipol* interfere with the intestinal absorption of many drugs, for example, *tetracycline*, *phenobarbital*, *digoxin*, *warfarin, pravastatin, fluvastatin, aspirin,* and *thiazide* diuretics. Therefore, drugs should be taken at least 1 to 2 hours before, or 4 to 6 hours after, the bile acid binding resins.

D. Probucol

Probucol [PROE byoo kole] was introduced in the 1970s, but because it reduced HDL levels to a greater extent than those of LDLs, it fell into disfavor. Newer information indicating that its antioxidant properties may be important in blocking atherosclerosis has resulted in renewed interest.

1. **Mechanism of action:** A number of mechanisms have been proposed to explain how *probucol* lowers serum cholesterol, but its mechanism of action remains uncertain. Recently it has been found that *probucol* inhibits the oxidation of cholesterol, resulting in the ingestion of the oxidized cholesterol-laden LDLs by macrophages (Figure 21.7). Loaded with cholesterol, these macrophages become foam cells that adhere to the vascular endothelium and are the basis for plaque formation. Thus prevention of the cholesterol oxidation reaction might slow the development of atherosclerosis.

2. **Therapeutic uses:** *Probucol* is useful in treating Type IIA and IIB hypercholesterolemia, although less so than the bile acid binding resins. Because a low HDL level is at least as great a risk for atherosclerosis as an elevated LDL level, the usefulness of this drug is limited to instances in which other antihyperlipidemic agents are ineffective. [Note: *Probucol* does not affect plasma triacylglycerol levels.]

3. **Pharmacokinetics:** *Probucol* is very lipophilic, and its absorption is highly variable. Administration with food improves absorption and reduces variability. *Probucol* is carried in the LDL particles and accumulates in adipose tissues where it may persist for months. Excretion is via the bile into the feces.

4. **Adverse effects:** Mild gastrointestinal disturbance is a common adverse effect that generally disappears with continued treatment. A more serious problem is its tendency to prolong the QT interval. Thus *probucol* is contraindicated in those patients who have an abnormally long QT interval. Care should also be taken with patients receiving drugs that prolong this interval, such as

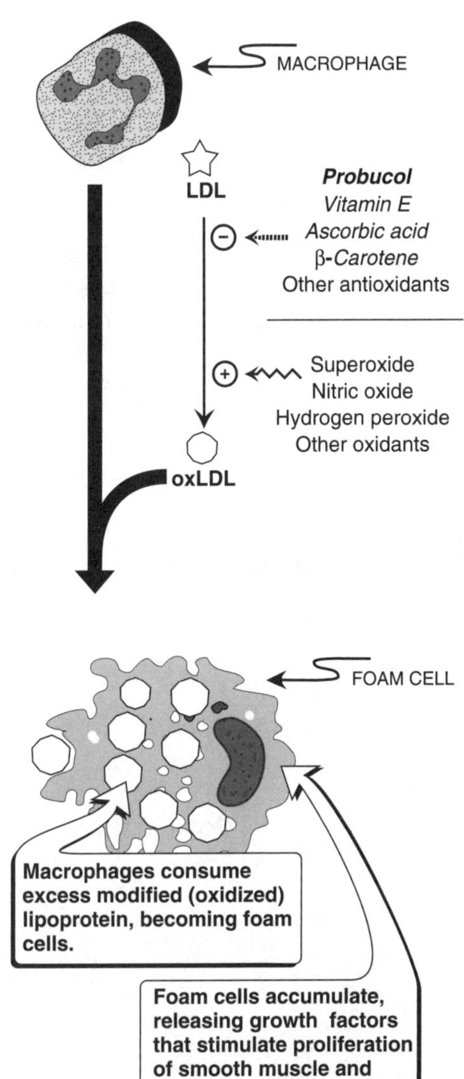

Figure 21.7
Role of *probucol* in preventing oxidation of lipoproteins.

digitalis, *quinidine*, *sotalol*, *astemizole* and *terfenadine*. Because of its long sojourn in the body, a woman should discontinue the drug at least 6 months before attempting pregnancy.

F. HMG-CoA reductase inhibitors: lovastatin, pravastatin, simvastatin and fluvastatin

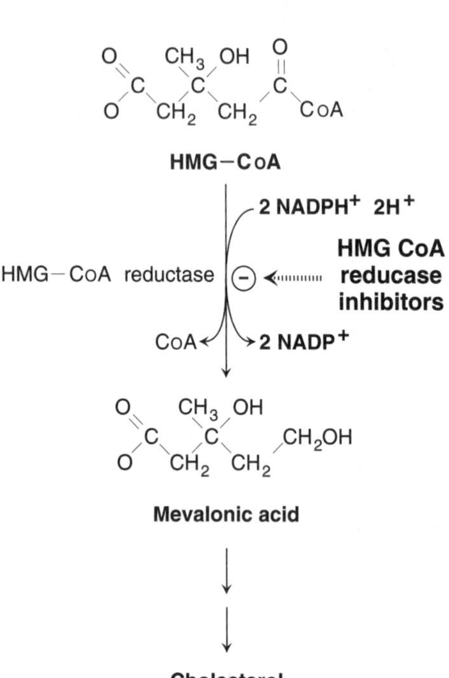

Figure 21.8
Inhibition of HMG-CoA reductase.

This novel group of antihyperlipidemic agents inhibits the first committed enzymatic step of sterol synthesis. As structural analogs of the natural substrate, 3-hydroxy-3-methylglutaric acid (HMG), all members of this group compete to block hydroxymethylglutaryl-Coenzyme A reductase (HMG-CoA reductase).[3] Except for *fluvastatin*, the other HMG reductase inhibitors are chemical modifications of compounds occurring naturally in fungi.

1. Mechanism of action

a. **Inhibition of HMG-CoA reductase:** *Lovastatin* [loe vah STAT in] *simvastatin* [sim vah STAT in], *pravastatin* [prah vah STAT in] and *fluvastatin* [flew vah STAT in] are analogs of 3-hydroxy-3-methylglutarate, the precursor of cholesterol. *Lovastatin* and *simvastatin* are lactones that are hydrolyzed to the active drug. *Pravastatin* and *fluvastatin* are active as such. Because of their strong affinity for the enzyme, all compete effectively to inhibit HMG-CoA reductase, the rate-limiting step in cholesterol synthesis. By inhibiting de novo cholesterol synthesis, they deplete the intracellular supply of cholesterol (Figure 21.8).

b. **Decrease in LDL receptors:** Depletion of intracellular cholesterol causes the cell to increase the number of specific cell-surface LDL receptors that can bind and internalize circulating LDLs. Thus the end result is a reduction in plasma cholesterol both by lowered cholesterol synthesis and by increased catabolism of LDL. [Note: Because these agents undergo a marked first-pass extraction by the liver, their dominant effect is on that organ.] The HMG-CoA reductase inhibitors, like *cholestyramine*, can increase plasma HDL levels in some patients, resulting in an additional lowering of risk for coronary artery disease. Small decreases in triacylglycerol can also occur.

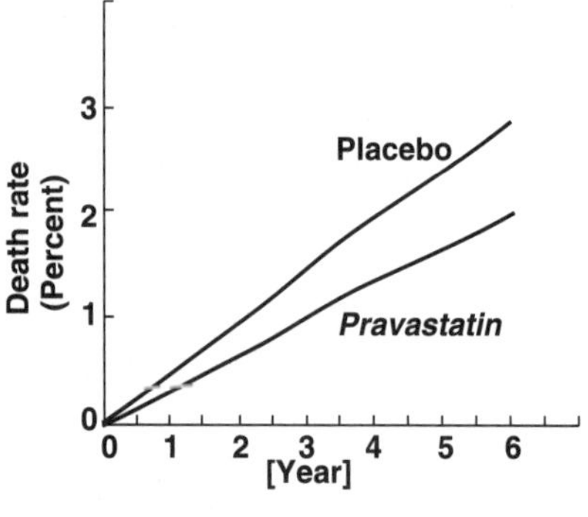

Figure 21.9
Effect of *pravastatin* therapy on deaths from all cardiovascular causes.

2. Therapeutic uses: These drugs are effective in lowering plasma cholesterol levels in all types of hyperlipidemias (Figure 21.9). However, patients who are homozygous for familial hypercholesterolemia lack LDL receptors and therefore benefit much less from treatment with these drugs. [Note: These drugs are often given in combination with other antihyperlipidemic drugs, see later.] It should be noted that in spite of the protection afforded by cholesterol lowering, about one fourth of the patients treated with these drugs still presented with coronary events. Thus, additional strategies such as diet, exercise, or additional agents may be warranted.

[3]See p. 216 for Infolink references to other books in this series.

3. Pharmacokinetics

Pravastatin and *fluvastatin* are almost completely absorbed after oral administration; oral doses of *lovastatin* and *simvastatin* are absorbed from 30 to 50%. Similarly, *pravastatin* and *fluvastatin* are active as such, whereas *lovastatin* and *simvastatin* must be hydrolyzed to the acid. Due to first-pass extraction, the primary action of these drugs is on the liver. All are biotransformed, with some of the products retaining activity. Excretion takes place principally through the bile and feces, but some urinary elimination also occurs. Their half-lives range from 1.5 to 2 hours.

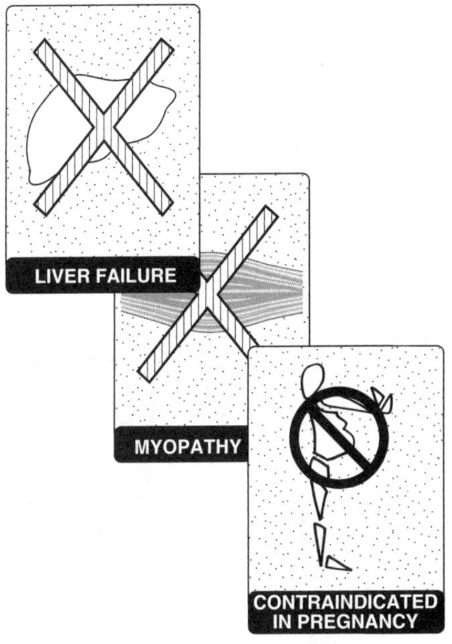

Figure 21.10
Some adverse efffects and precautionsassociated with HMG-CoA reductase inhibitors.

4. **Adverse effects**: It is noteworthy that during the 5-year trials of *simvastatin* and *lovastatin*, only a few adverse effects, related to liver and muscle function, were reported (Figure 21.10).

   a. **Liver:** Biochemical abnormalities in liver function have occurred with the HMG-CoA reductase inhibitors. Therefore it is prudent to evaluate liver function and measure serum transaminase levels periodically. These return to normal on suspension of the drug. [Note: Hepatic insufficiency can cause drug accumulation.]

   b. **Muscle:** Myopathy and rhabdomyolysis (disintegration or dissolution of muscle) have been rarely reported. In most of these cases, patients usually suffered from renal insufficiency or were taking drugs such as *cyclosporine, itraconazole, erythromycin, gemfibrozil,* or *niacin.* Plasma creatine kinase levels should be determined regularly.

   c. **Drug interactions:** The HMG-CoA reductase inhibitors also increase *coumarin* levels. Thus, it is important to evaluate prothrombin times frequently.

   d. **Contraindications:** These drugs are contraindicated in pregnancy and nursing mothers. They should not be used in children or teen-agers.

See p. 449 for a description of the newly approved drug *atorvastatin*.

G. Combination Drug Therapy

It is sometimes necessary to employ two antihyperlipidemia drugs in order to achieve a significant decrease in plasma lipid levels. For example, in Type II hyperlipidemias, patients are commonly treated with a combination of *niacin* plus a bile acid binding agent, such as *cholestyramine*. [Note: Remember that *cholestyramine* causes an increase in LDL receptors that clears the plasma of circulating LDL, whereas *niacin* decreases synthesis of VLDL and therefore also the synthesis of LDL.] The combination of an HMG-CoA reductase inhibitor with a bile acid binding agent has also been shown to be useful in lowering LDL cholesterol (Figure 21.11).

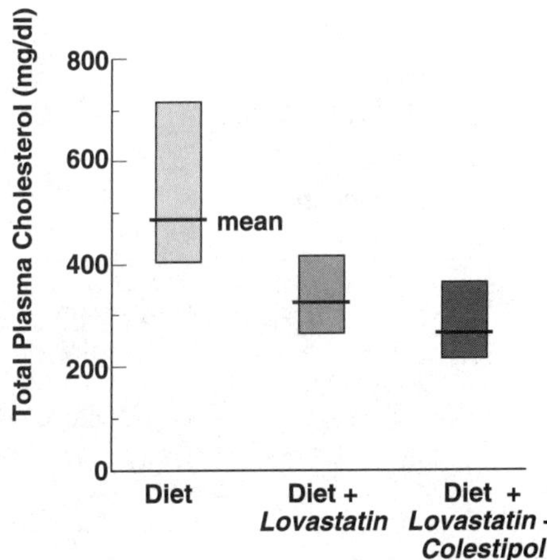

Figure 21.11
Response of total plasma cholesterol in patients with heterozygous familial hypercholesterolemia to diet (low cholesterol, low saturated fat) and hyperlipidemic drugs.

Choose the ONE best answer.

21.1 Which one of the following is the most common side effect of antihyperlipidemic drug therapy?

A. Elevated blood pressure
B. Gastrointestinal disturbance
C. Neurological problems
D. Heart palpitations
E. Migraine headaches

Correct answer = B. Gastrointestinal disturbances frequently occur as a side effect of antihyperlipidemic drug therapy.

21.2 Which one of the following hyperlipidemias is characterized by elevated plasma levels of chylomicrons and has no drug therapy available to lower the plasma lipoprotein levels?

A. Type I
B. Type II
C. Type III
D. Type IV
E. Type V

Correct answer = A. Type I hyperlipidemia (hyperchylomicronemia) is treated with a low fat diet. No drug therapy is effective for this disorder.

21.3 Which one of the following drugs decreases de novo cholesterol synthesis by inhibiting the enzyme 3-hydroxy-3-methylglutaryl CoA reductase?

A. Clofibrate
B. Niacin
C. Cholestyramine
D. Lovastatin
E. Gemfibrozil

Correct answer = D. Clofibrate and gemfibrozil increase the activity of lipoprotein lipase, thereby increasing the removal of VLDL from plasma. Niacin inhibits lipolysis in adipose tissue and thus eliminates the building blocks needed by the liver to produce triacylglycerol and therefore VLDL. Cholestyramine lowers the amount of bile acids returning to the liver via the enterohepatic circulation.

QUESTIONS 21.4 - 21.7

DIRECTIONS: The group of questions below consists of five drugs (A–E) followed by a list of numbered statements. For each numbered statement, select the ONE drug from the list (A–E) that is most closely associated with it. Each drug may be selected once, more than once, or not at all.

Match each drug with the statement that best describes its mode of action:

A. Niacin
B. Clofibrate
C. Cholestyramine
D. Probucol
E. Lovastatin

21.4 Binds bile acids in the intestine, thus preventing their return to the liver via the enterohepatic circulation.

Correct answer = C: Cholestyramine.

21.5 Causes a decrease in plasma triacylglycerol levels by increasing the activity of lipoprotein lipase.

Correct answer = B: Clofibrate.

21.6 Causes a decrease in liver triacylglycerol synthesis by limiting available free fatty acids needed as building blocks for this pathway.

Correct answer = A: Niacin.

21.7 Inhibits 3-hydroxy-3-methylglutaryl CoA reductase, the rate-limiting step in cholesterol synthesis.

Correct answer = E: Lovastatin.

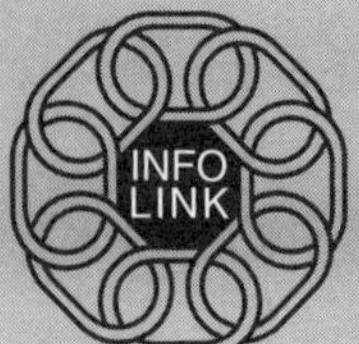

[1]See p. 323 in **Biochemistry** (2nd ed.) for a discussion of niacin as a vitamin.

[3]See p. 206 in **Biochemistry** (2nd ed.) for a discussion of the synthesis of cholesterol.

[2]See p. 213 in **Biochemistry** (2nd ed.) for a discussion of plasma lipoproteins.

UNIT V: Drugs Affecting Other Organ Systems

Drugs Affecting the Respiratory System

22

DRUGS AFFECTING THE RESPIRATORY SYSTEM

DRUGS USED TO TREAT ASTHMA
- β-Adrenergic agonists
- Corticosteroids
- *Cromolyn* and *nedocromil*
- *Ipratropium*
- *Montelukast*[1]
- *Theophylline*
- Zafirlukast[1]
- Zileuton[1]

DRUGS USED TO TREAT RHINITIS
- α-Adrenergic agonists
- Antihistamines
- Corticosteroids
- *Cromolyn*

DRUGS USED TO TREAT CHRONIC OBSTRUCTIVE PULMONARY DISEASES
- β-Adrenergic agonists
- Corticosteroids
- *Ipratropium*

DRUGS USED TO TREAT COUGH
- *Dextromethorphan*
- Opiates

Figure 22.1
Summary of drugs affecting the respiratory system. [1]Described in Pharmacology update, pp. 450-451

I. OVERVIEW

Drugs can be delivered to the lungs by inhalation, oral, or parenteral routes. Inhalation is often preferred because the drug is delivered directly to the target tissue—the airways—and is effective in doses that do not cause significant systemic side effects. Clinically useful drugs act by various mechanisms, for example, by relaxing bronchial smooth muscle, or modulating the inflammatory response. Drugs used to treat asthma, rhinitis, chronic obstructive pulmonary disease, and cough—commonly encountered respiratory disorders—are summarized in Figure 22.1.

II. DRUGS USED TO TREAT ASTHMA

Asthma is a chronic disease that affects 4 to 5% of the U.S. population, or approximately 10 million patients. The disease is characterized by episodes of acute bronchoconstriction causing shortness of breath, cough, chest tightness, wheezing and rapid respirations. These acute symptoms may resolve spontaneously, or more often, require therapy such as a β_2-agonist (see p. 218). A second delayed or late-phase response may occur 4 to 12 hours later, and may require treatment with steroids. Asthma, unlike chronic bronchitis, cystic fibrosis or bronchiectasis, is usually not a progressive disease—it does not inevitably lead to crippling chronic obstructive lung disease. Rather, the clinical course of asthma is characterized by exacerbations and remissions. Deaths due to asthma are infrequent, but morbidity results in significant hospitalization and outpatient costs. The goal of therapy is to relieve symptoms and to prevent recurrence of asthmatic attacks, if possible.

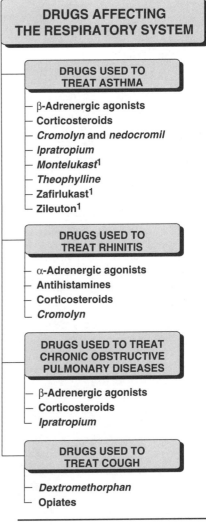

Lippincott's Illustrated Reviews: Pharmacology, Second Edition.
by Mary J. Mycek, Richard A. Harvey and Pamela C. Champe.
Lippincott Williams & Wilkins, Philadelphia, PA © 2000.

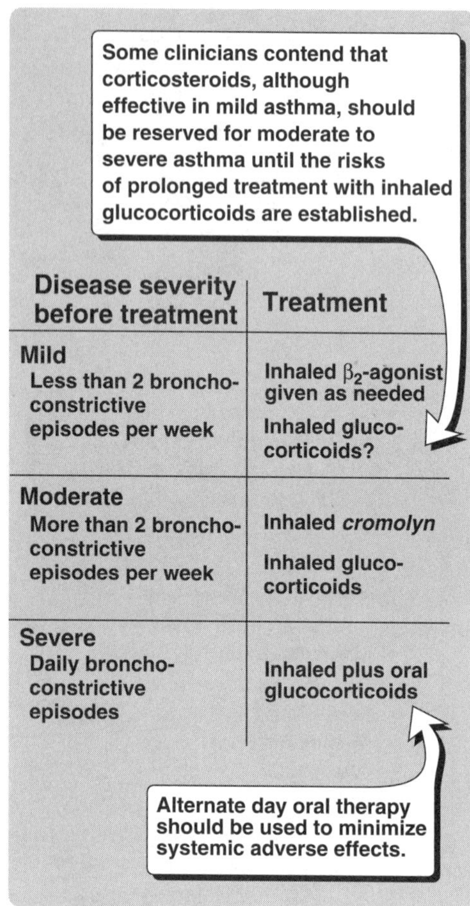

Some clinicians contend that corticosteroids, although effective in mild asthma, should be reserved for moderate to severe asthma until the risks of prolonged treatment with inhaled glucocorticoids are established.
Disease severity before treatment
Treatment
Mild
Less than 2 broncho-constrictive episodes per week
Inhaled β_2-agonist given as needed
Inhaled gluco-corticoids?
Moderate
More than 2 broncho-constrictive episodes per week
Inhaled cromolyn
Inhaled gluco-corticoids
Severe
Daily broncho-constrictive episodes
Inhaled plus oral glucocorticoids
Alternate day oral therapy should be used to minimize systemic adverse effects.

Figure 22.2
Summary of treatments for asthma of varying severity.

A. Role of inflammation in asthma

Airflow obstruction in asthma is due to bronchoconstriction resulting from contraction of bronchial smooth muscle, inflammation of the bronchial wall, and increased mucous secretion. Asthmatic attacks may be related to recent exposure to allergens, inhaled irritants leading to bronchial hyperactivity and inflammation of the airway mucosa. The symptoms of asthma may be effectively treated by several drugs, but none of the agents provide a cure for this obstructive lung disease.

A. Adrenergic agonists

Inhaled adrenergic agonists with β_2 activity are the drugs of choice for mild asthma, that is, in patients showing only occasional, intermittent symptoms (Figure 22.2). β_2-Agonists are potent bronchodilators that relax airway smooth muscle directly .

1. **Short acting drugs:** Most clinically useful β-agonists have a rapid (15 to 30 minutes) onset of action and provide relief for 4 to 6 hours. They are used for symptomatic treatment of bronchospasm and as "rescue agents" to combat acute bronchoconstriction. [Note: *Epinephrine* (see p. 61) is the drug of choice for treatment of acute anaphylaxis.] β_2-Agonists have no anti-inflammatory effects and they should never be used as the sole therapeutic agents for patients with chronic asthma. The β_2-selective agents, such as *pirbuterol*, *terbutaline*, and *albuterol* (see p. 67), offer the advantage of providing maximally attainable bronchodilation with little of the undesired effect of α or β_1 stimulation. (See p. 60 for the receptor-specific actions of adrenergic agonists.) The β_2-agonists are not catecholamines and thus are not destroyed by catechol O-methyltransferase (COMT). Toxic side effects, such as tachycardia, hyperglycemia, hypokalemia and hypomagnesemia, are minimized when the drugs are delivered by inhalation rather than by systemic routes. Though tolerance to the β-agonists' effects on non-airway tissues occurs, it is uncommon with normal dosages.

2. **Long acting drugs:** *Salmeterol xinatoate* [sal MEE ter ol] is a chemical analog of *albuterol*, but differs by having a long lipophilic side chain that increases the affinity of the drug for the β-adrenoceptor. *Salmeterol* has a long duration of action, providing bronchodilation for at least 12 hours. *Salmeterol* has a slow onset of action and should not be used in acute asthmatic attacks; it should only be prescribed for administration at regular intervals and not to relieve symptoms. Like the others in this drug class, it is not a substitute for anti-inflammatory therapy.

B. Corticosteroids

Inhaled glucocorticoids are the drugs of first choice in patients with moderate to severe asthma who require inhalation of β_2-adrenergic agonists more than once daily (see Figure 22.2). Severe asthma may also require systemic glucocorticoids, usually for short term. Inhaled glucocorticoids often reduce (or eliminate) the need for oral glucocorticoids in patients with severe asthma. To be effective in controlling inflammation, glucocorticoids must be taken continuously. (See p. 272 for a summary of the mechanism of action of corticosteroids.)

1. **Actions on lung:** Steroids have no direct effect on the airway smooth muscle. Instead, inhaled glucocorticoids decrease the number and activity of cells involved in airway inflammation—macrophages, eosinophils, and T-lymphocytes. Prolonged (several months) inhalation of steroids reduces the hyperresponsiveness of the airway smooth muscle to a variety of bronchoconstrictor stimuli, such as allergens, irritants, cold air, and exercise. Anti-inflammatory steroids reduce inflammation by reversing mucosal edema, decreasing the permeability of capillaries, and inhibiting the release of leukotrienes. Bronchial reactivity is greatly reduced.

2. **Pharmacokinetics**

   a. **Inhaled drugs:** The development of inhaled steroids has markedly reduced the need for systemic corticosteroid treatment. However, a few precautions are required for successful inhalation therapy. A large fraction (typically 80 to 90%) of inhaled glucocorticoids is deposited in the mouth and pharynx, or is swallowed (Figure 22.3). These glucocorticosteroids are absorbed from the gut and enter the systemic circulation through the liver. However, many of the clinically useful corticosteroids, such as *beclomethasone*, *triamcinolone*, and *flunisolide* [floo NISS oh lide], undergo extensive first-pass metabolism in the liver so that only a small amount of these drugs reaches the systemic circulation. The 10 to 20% of the metered dose of inhaled glucocorticoids that is not swallowed is deposited in the airway.

   b. **Systemic steroids:** Patients with severe exacerbation of asthma (status asthmaticus) may require intravenous administration of *methylprednisolone* or oral *prednisone* (see p. 275). Once the patient has improved, the dose of drug is gradually reduced, leading to discontinuance in 1 to 2 weeks.

   c. **Spacers:** A spacer is a large volume chamber that is attached to the metered-dose inhaler and is used to decrease the deposition of drug in the mouth (Figure 22.4). The chamber serves to reduce the velocity of the injected aerosol before it enters the mouth, and allows large drug particles to be deposited in the device. The smaller, low-velocity drug particles are less likely to be deposited in the mouth and more likely to reach the target airway tissue. Spacers improve delivery of inhaled glucocorticoids and are advised in virtually all patients. [Note: Rinsing the mouth after inhalation can also decrease systemic absorption and the possibility of oropharyngeal candidiasis.]

3. **Adverse effects:** Oral or parenteral glucocorticoids have a variety of potentially serious side effects (see p. 277). However, inhaled glucocorticoids, particularly if used with a spacer, have few systemic effects. Oropharyngeal candidiasis—sometimes called thrush—may be a problem in patients who inhale glucocorticoids,

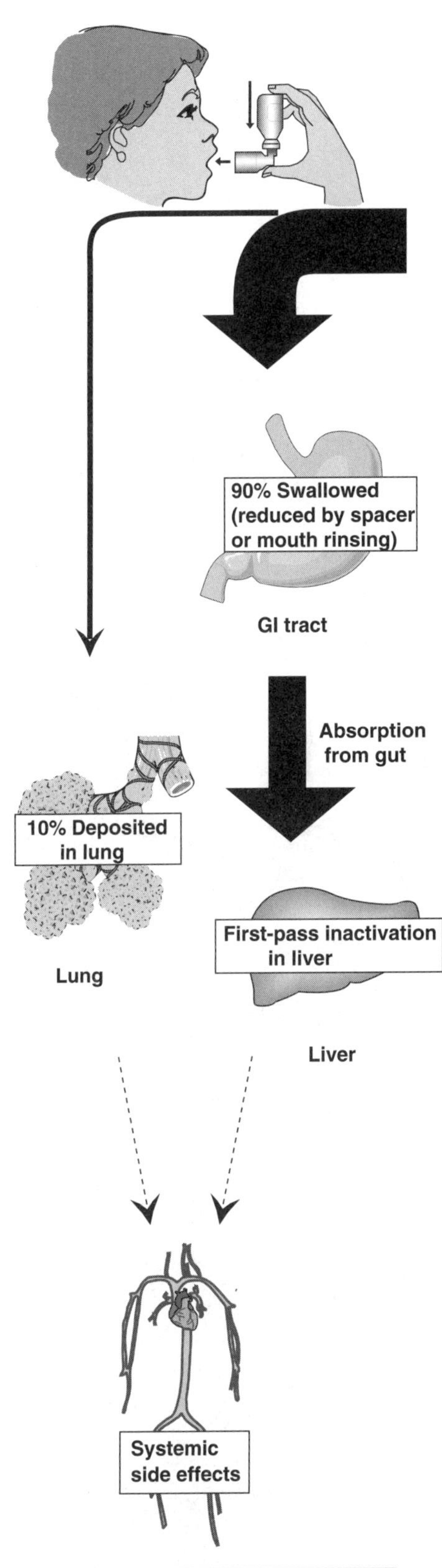

Figure 22.3
Pharmacokinetics of inhaled glucocorticoids.

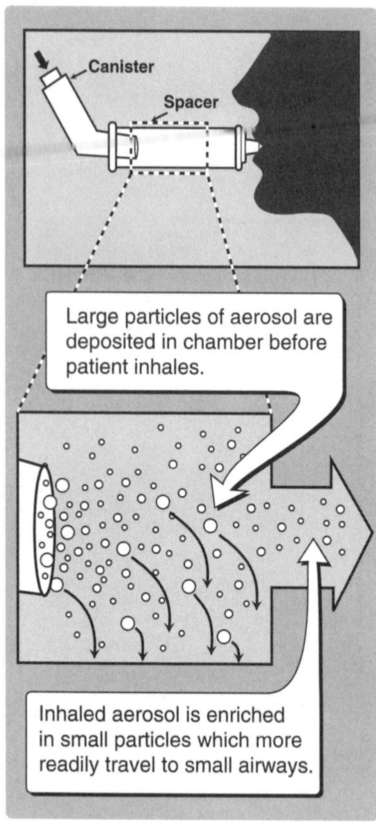

Figure 22.4
Effect of spacer on the delivery of an inhaled aerosol.

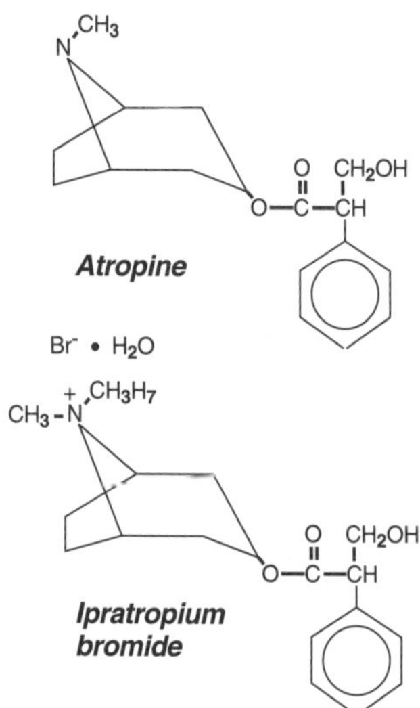

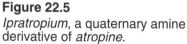

Figure 22.5
Ipratropium, a quaternary amine derivative of *atropine*.

particularly immunosuppressed patients. Spacers minimize the problem of adrenal suppression by reducing the amount of glucocorticoid deposited in the oropharynx.

C. Cromolyn and nedocromil

Cromolyn [KROE moe lin] and *nedocromil* [neh DOC ro mil] are effective prophylactic anti-inflammatory agents, but are not useful in managing an acute asthmatic attack because they are not direct bronchodilators. These agents can block the precipitation of immediate and delayed asthmatic reactions. For use in asthma, *cromolyn* is administered by inhalation of a microfine powder, or as an aerosolized solution. Because it is poorly absorbed, only minor adverse effects are associated with it. Pretreatment with *cromolyn* blocks allergen-induced and exercise-induced bronchoconstriction. *Cromolyn* is also useful in reducing the symptoms of allergic rhinitis (see p. 222). A 4- to 6-week trial is required to determine efficacy. Given its safety, an initial trial of *cromolyn* is often recommended, particularly in children and pregnant women. Toxic reactions are mild; they include a bitter taste and irritation of the pharynx and larynx.

D. Cholinergic antagonists

Anticholinergic agents are generally less effective than β-adrenergic agonists. They block the vagally mediated contraction of airway smooth muscle and mucus secretion. Inhaled *ipratropium* [i pra TROE pee um], a quaternary derivative of *atropine* (Figure 22.5), is useful in patients unable to tolerate adrenergic agonists. *Ipratropium* is slow in onset, and is nearly free of side-effects.

E. Theophylline

Theophylline [the OFF i lin] is a bronchodilator that relieves airflow obstruction in chronic asthma, and decreases the symptoms of the chronic disease. Previously the main-stay of asthma therapy, *theophylline* has been largely replaced with β-agonists and corticosteroids. *Theophylline* is well absorbed by the gastrointestinal tract, and several sustained-release preparations are available. The drug has a narrow therapeutic window, and an overdose of the drug may cause seizures or potentially fatal arrhythmias. Further, *theophylline* interacts adversely with many drugs. See pp. 450-451 for a description of newly approved drugs, *zileuton, zafirlukast,* and *montelukast.*

III. DRUGS USED TO TREAT ALLERGIC RHINITIS

Rhinitis is an inflammation of the mucous membranes of the nose, and is characterized by sneezing, nasal itching, watery rhinorrhea and congestion. An attack may be precipitated by inhalation of allergen (such as dust, pollen, or animal dander), which interacts with mast cells coated with IgE, generated in response to a previous exposure to the allergen (Figure 22.6). The mast cells release mediators, such as histamine, leukotrienes, and chemotactic factors, which promote bronchiolar spasm and mucosal thickening from edema and cellular infiltration. Combinations of oral antihistamines with decongestants are the first-line therapy for allergic rhinitis. However, the systemic effects sometimes associated with these oral preparations (sedation, insomnia, and rarely cardiac arrhythmias) have prompted interest in topical intranasal delivery of drugs for the treatment of allergic rhinitis.

A. Antihistamines (H_1 receptor blockers)

Antihistamines are the most frequently used agents in the treatment of sneezing and watery rhinorrhea associated with allergic rhinitis. H_1-Histamine receptor blockers, such as *diphenhydramine, chlorpheniramine, loratadine, terfenadine* and *astemizole* (see p. 422), are useful in treating the symptoms of allergic rhinitis caused by histamine release. Combinations of antihistamines with decongestants (see below) are effective when congestion is a feature of rhinitis. They differ in their ability to cause sedation, and their duration of action.

B. α-Adrenergic agonists

α-Adrenergic agonists ("nasal decongestants") such as *phenylephrine*, constrict dilated arterioles in the nasal mucosa and reduce airway resistance. Long-acting *oxymetazoline* [ox i met AZ oh leen] is also available. When administered as an aerosol, these drugs have a rapid onset of action and show few systemic effects. Oral administration results in longer duration of action but increased systemic effects. Combinations of these agents with antihistamines are frequently used. However, they should be used no longer than several days because rebound nasal congestion often occurs upon discontinuance of these drugs. Therefore, α-adrenergic agents have no place in the long-term treatment of allergic rhinitis.

C. Corticosteroids

Corticosteroids, such as *beclomethasone, fluticasone, flunisolide* and *triamcinolone* (see p. 275), are effective when administered as nasal sprays. [Note: Systemic absorption is minimal and side effects of intranasal corticosteroid treatment are localized—nasal irritation, nosebleed, sore throat and, rarely candidiasis.] Topical steroids may be more effective than systemic antihistamines in relieving the nasal symptoms of both allergic and nonallergic rhinitis. The effects of long-term usage are unknown, although they are considered to be generally safe. Periodic assessment of the patient is advised. Treatment of chronic rhinitis may not result in improvement until 1 to 2 weeks after starting therapy.

D. Cromolyn

Intranasal *cromolyn* may be useful, particularly when administered before contact with an allergen.

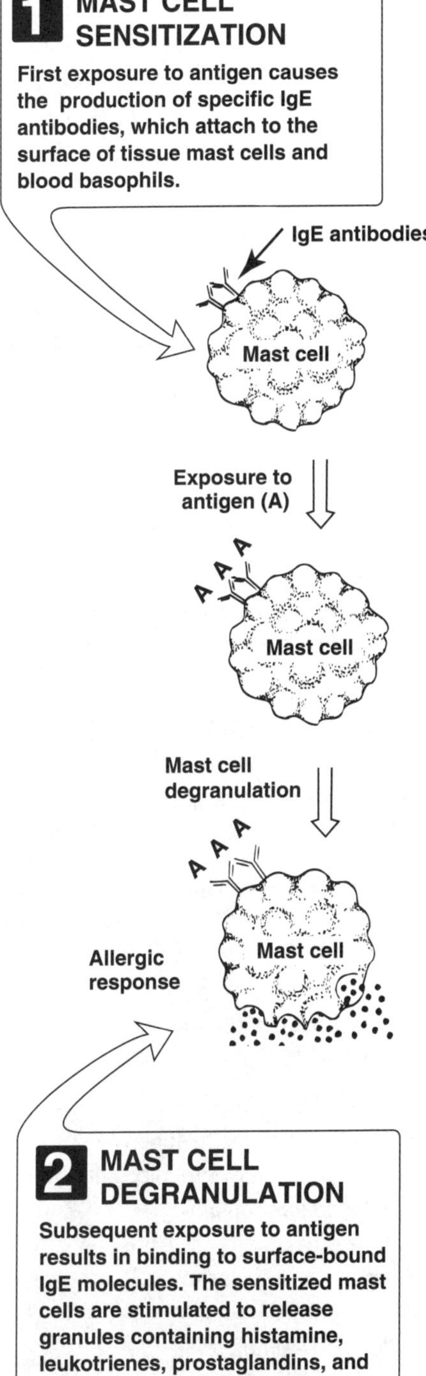

1 MAST CELL SENSITIZATION
First exposure to antigen causes the production of specific IgE antibodies, which attach to the surface of tissue mast cells and blood basophils.
IgE antibodies
Mast cell
Exposure to antigen (A)
Mast cell
Mast cell degranulation
Allergic response
Mast cell
2 MAST CELL DEGRANULATION
Subsequent exposure to antigen results in binding to surface-bound IgE molecules. The sensitized mast cells are stimulated to release granules containing histamine, leukotrienes, prostaglandins, and other potent chemical mediators.

Figure 22.6
Hypersensitivity reactions mediated by IgE molecules can cause rhinitis.

IV. DRUGS USED TO TREAT CHRONIC OBSTRUCTIVE PULMONARY DISEASE

Chronic obstructive pulmonary disease (COPD) affects approximately 30 million people in the U.S., and is the fifth most common cause of death. It is a chronic, irreversible obstruction of air flow. Smoking is the greatest risk factor for COPD. The disease may respond to bronchodilators, such as anticholinergic agents, β-adrenergic agents and *theophylline*. Therapy does not cure the disease or even significantly slow its progress. Treatment consists of a trial of β_2-agonist or *ipratropium* to assess any reversible component of the disease, and is a reasonable first-line initial therapy for all patients. Glucocorticoids may be helpful in the treatment of acute exacerbations in some patients.

V. DRUGS USED TO TREAT COUGH

Codeine, *hydrocodone*, and *hydromorphone* decrease the sensitivity of CNS cough centers to peripheral stimuli, and decrease mucosal secretion. These actions occur at doses lower than required for analgesia (see p. 135 for a more complete discussion of the opiates). *Dextromethorphan* [dex troe meth OR fan], a synthetic derivative of morphine, suppresses the response of the cough center. It has no analgesic or addictive potential, and is less constipating than codeine.

Study Questions

Questions 22.1 to 22.4:

A 12-year-old girl with a childhood history of asthma complained of cough, dyspnia, and wheezing after visiting a riding stable. Her symptoms became so severe that her parent brought her to the emergency room. Physical examination revealed diaphoresis, dyspnea, tachycardia, and tachypnea. Her respiratory rate was 42/min, pulse rate was 110 beats per minute, and blood pressure was 132/65 mm Hg.

For each of the statements below choose the most appropriate drug from the following list:

A. Inhaled cromolyn
B. Inhaled beclomethasone
C. Oral or IV methylprednisolone
D. Inhaled ipratropium
E. Inhaled albuterol
F. Intravenous propranolol
G. Diphenhydramine
H. Inhaled salmeterol
I. Oxymetazoline

22.1 The most appropriate drug to rapidly reverse bronchoconstriction.

> 22.1 Correct answer = E. Inhalation of a rapid acting β_2 agonist, such as albuterol, usually provides immediate bronchodilation.

22.2 The drug most likely to provide sustained resolution of the patient's symptoms.

> 22.2 Correct answer = C. An acute asthmatic crisis often requires IV corticosteroids, often methylprednisolone. Inhaled beclomethasone will not deliver enough steroid to fully combat airway inflammation.

22.3 A drug contraindicated in this patient.

> 22. 3. Correct answer = F. Propranolol is a β-blocker and would aggravate the patient's bronchoconstriction

22.4 A drug likely to be ineffective in this patient.

> 22. 4. Correct answer = A. Cromolyn can be used prophylactically to reduce the inflammatory response, but is ineffective in relieving acute symptoms.

Diuretic Drugs

23

I. OVERVIEW

Drugs inducing a state of increased urine flow are called diuretics. These agents are ion transport inhibitors that decrease the reabsorption of Na^+ at different sites in the nephron. As a result, Na^+ and other ions such as Cl^- enter the urine in greater amounts than normal along with water, which is carried passively to maintain osmotic equilibrium. Diuretics thus increase the volume of the urine and often change its pH as well as the ionic composition of the urine and blood. The efficacy of the different classes of diuretics varies considerably, with the increase in secretion of Na^+ varying from less than 2% for the weak, potassium-sparing diuretics, to over 20% for the potent loop diuretics. Their major clinical uses are in managing disorders involving abnormal fluid retention (edema) or in treating hypertension in which their diuretic action causes a decreased blood volume, leading to a reduction in blood pressure. In this chapter, the diuretic drugs (Figure 23.1) are discussed in the order of their site of action along the nephron (Figure 23.2).

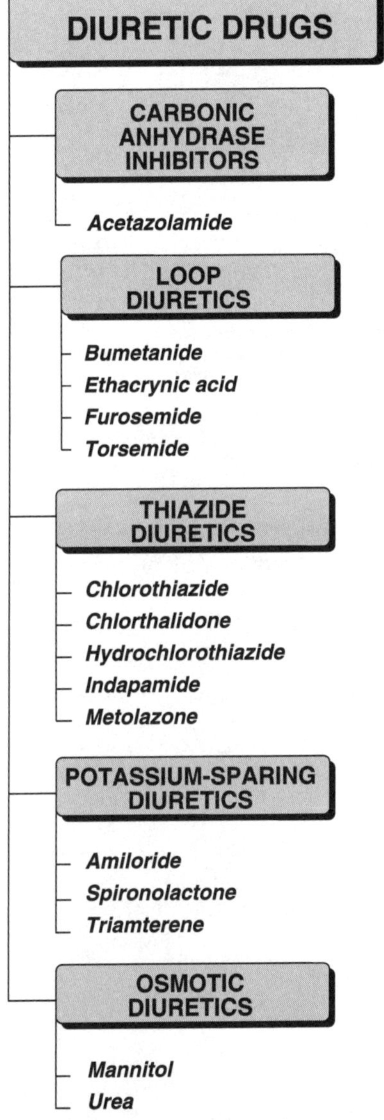

Figure 23.1
Summary of diuretic drugs.

II. NORMAL REGULATION OF FLUID AND ELECTROLYTES BY THE KIDNEYS

Approximately 16–20% of the blood plasma entering the kidneys is filtered from the glomerular capillaries into Bowman's capsule. The filtrate, although normally free of proteins and blood cells, does contain most low molecular weight plasma components in approximately the same concentrations as are found in the plasma. These include glucose, sodium bicarbonate, amino acids, and other organic solutes, plus electrolytes, such as Na^+, K^+, and Cl^-. The kidney regulates the ionic composition and volume of urine by the reabsorption or secretion of ions and/or water at five functional zones along the nephron, namely the proximal convoluted tubule, the descending loop of Henle, the ascending loop of Henle, the distal convoluted tubule, and the collecting duct (Figure 23.2).

A. Proximal convoluted tubule

In the extensively convoluted proximal tubule located in the cortex of the kidney, almost all of the glucose, bicarbonate, amino acids, and other metabolites are reabsorbed. Approximately two thirds of the Na^+ is also reabsorbed in the proximal tubule; chloride and

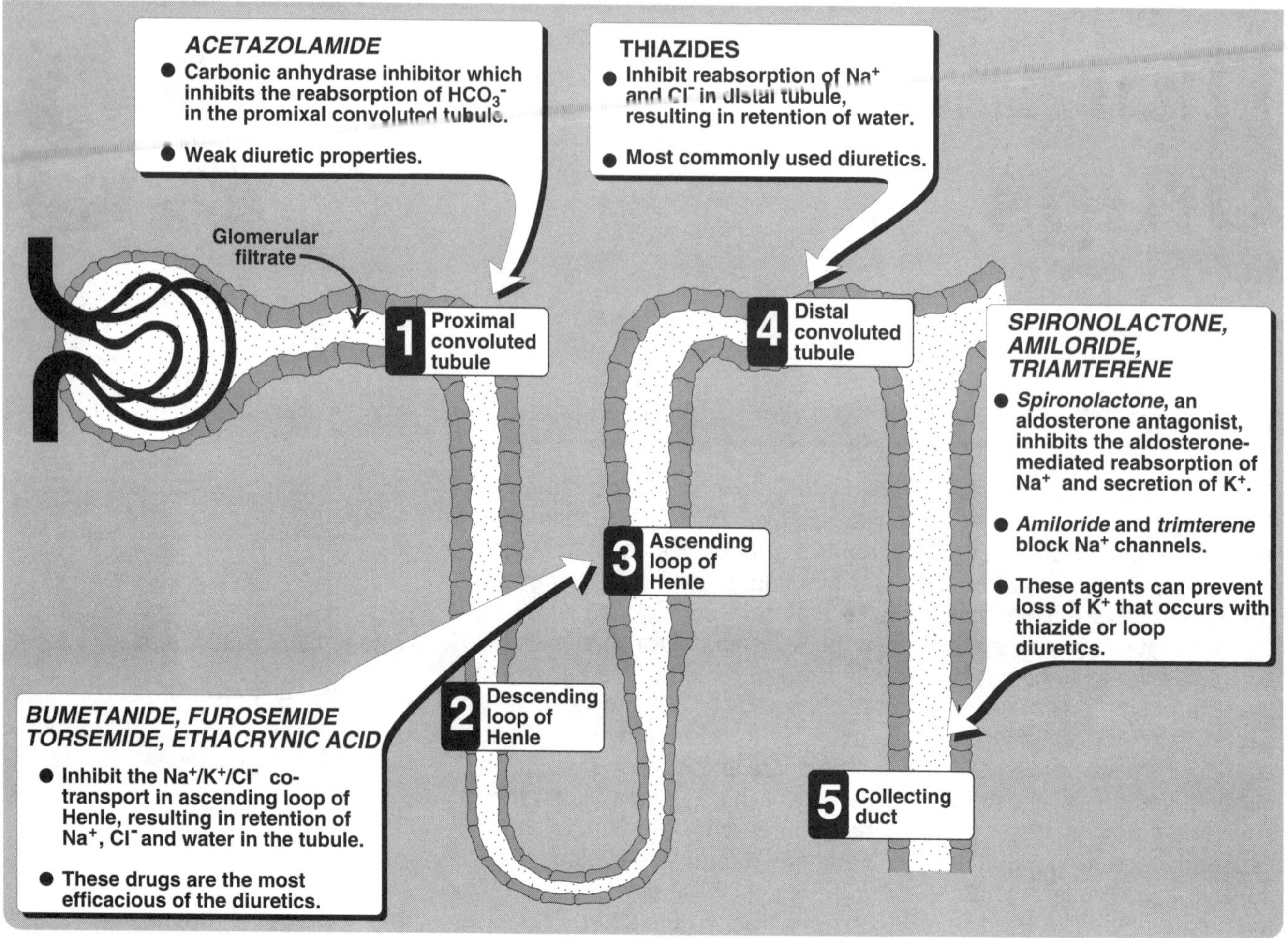

Figure 23.2
Major locations of ion and water exchange in the nephron, showing sites of action of the diuretic drugs.

water follow passively to maintain electrical and osmolar equality. If it were not for the extensive reabsorption of solutes and water in the proximal tubule, the mammalian organism would rapidly become dehydrated and lose its normal osmolarity.

1. **Acid secretory system:** The proximal tubule is the site of the organic acid and base secretory systems (Figure 23.3). The organic acid secretory system secretes a variety of organic acids (such as uric acid, some antibiotics, diuretics) from the blood-stream into the proximal tubule's lumen. Most diuretic drugs are delivered to the tubular fluid via this system. The organic acid secretory system is saturable, and diuretic drugs in the blood-stream compete for transfer with endogenous organic acids, such as uric acid. This explains the hyperuricemia seen with certain of the diuretic drugs, such as *furosemide* or *chlorothiazide*.

B. Descending loop of Henle

The remaining filtrate, which is isotonic, next enters the descending limb of the loop of Henle and passes into the medulla of the kidney.

The osmolarity increases along the descending portion of the loop of Henle because of the countercurrent mechanism. This results in a tubular fluid with a three-fold increase in salt concentration.

C. Ascending loop of Henle

The cells of the ascending tubular epithelium are unique in being impermeable to water. Active reabsorption of Na^+, K^+ and Cl^- is mediated by a $Na^+/K^+/2Cl^-$ cotransporter. Mg^{++} and Ca^{++} enter the interstitial fluid via the paracellular pathway. The ascending loop is thus a diluting region of the nephron. Approximately 25–30% of the tubular sodium chloride returns to the interstitial fluid, thus helping to maintain the fluid's high osmolarity. Since the loop of Henle is a major site for salt reabsorption, drugs affecting this site, such as loop diuretics, are the most efficacious of all the diuretic classes.

D. Distal convoluted tubule

The cells of the distal convoluted tubule are also impermeable to water. About 10% of the filtered sodium chloride is reabsorbed via a Na^+/Cl^- transporter, which is sensitive to thiazide diuretics. Additionally, Ca^{++} excretion is regulated by parathyroid hormone in this portion of the tubule.

E. Collecting tubule and duct

The principal and intercalated cells of the collecting tubule are responsible for Na^+– K^+ exchange and for H^+ secretion and K^+ reabsorption, respectively. Stimulation of aldosterone receptors in the principal cells results in Na^+ reabsorption and K^+ secretion. Antidiuretic hormone (ADH, vasopressin) receptors promote the reabsorption of water from the collecting tubules and ducts (Figure 23.3). This action is mediated by cAMP.

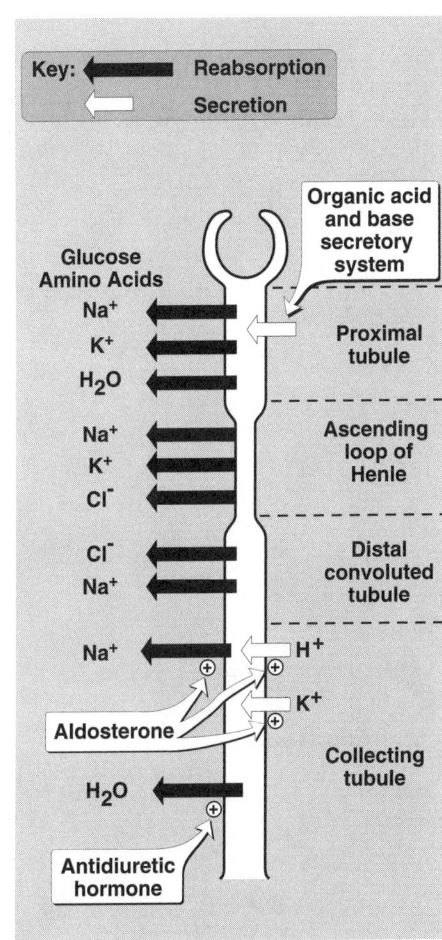

Figure 23.3
Sites of transport of solutes and water along the nephron.

III. KIDNEY FUNCTION IN DISEASE

In many diseases the amount of sodium chloride reabsorbed by the kidney tubules is abnormally high. This leads to the retention of water, an increase in blood volume, and expansion of the extravascular fluid compartment, resulting in edema of the tissues. Several commonly encountered causes of edema include:

A. Congestive heart failure

The decreased ability of the failing heart to sustain adequate cardiac output causes the kidney to respond as if there were a decrease in blood volume. The kidney, as part of the normal compensatory mechanism, retains more salt and water as a means of raising blood volume and increasing the amount of blood that is returned to the heart. However, the diseased heart cannot increase its output, and the increased vascular volume results in edema (see p. 151 for causes and treatment of congestive heart failure).

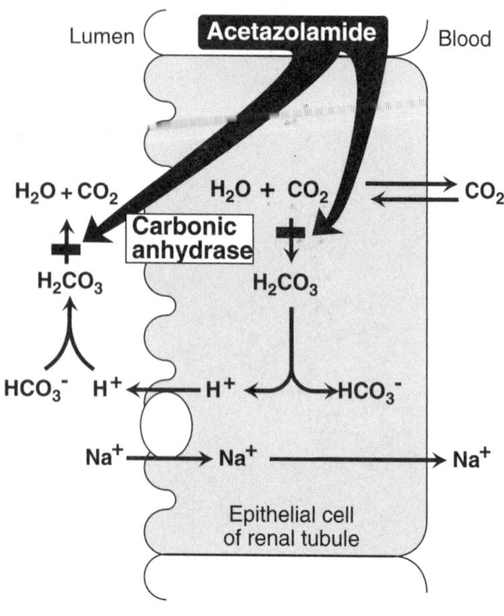

Figure 23.4
Role of carbonic anhydrase in sodium retention by epithelial cells of renal tubule.

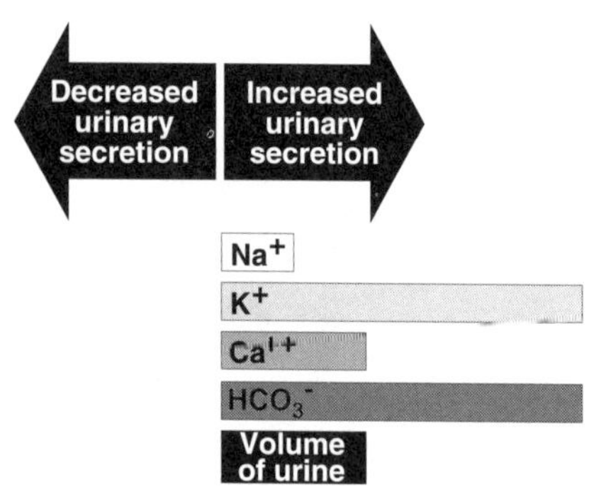

Figure 23.5
Relative changes in the composition of urine induced by *acetazolamide*.

B. Hepatic ascites

Ascites, the accumulation of fluid in the abdominal cavity, is a common complication of cirrhosis of the liver.

1. **Increased portal blood pressure:** Blood flow in the portal system is often obstructed in cirrhosis, resulting in an increased portal blood pressure. Further, colloidal osmotic pressure of the blood is decreased as a result of impaired synthesis of plasma proteins by the diseased liver. Increased portal blood pressure and low osmolarity of the blood cause fluid to escape from the portal vascular system and collect in the abdomen.

2. **Secondary hyperaldosteronism:** Fluid retention is also promoted by elevated levels of circulating aldosterone. This secondary hyperaldosteronism results from the decreased ability of the liver to inactivate the steroid hormone and leads to increased Na^+ and water reabsorption, increased vascular volume, and exacerbation of fluid accumulation (see Figure 23.3).

C. Nephrotic syndrome

When damaged by disease, the glomerular membranes allow plasma proteins to enter the glomerular ultrafiltrate. The loss of protein from the plasma reduces the colloidal osmotic pressure resulting in edema. The low plasma volume stimulates aldosterone secretion through the renin-angiotensin-aldosterone system (see p. 180). This leads to retention of Na^+ and fluid, further aggravating the edema.

D. Premenstrual edema

Edema associated with menstruation is the result of imbalances in hormones such as estrogen excess, which facilitates the loss of fluid into the extracellular space. Diuretics can reduce the edema.

IV. CARBONIC ANHYDRASE INHIBITORS

Acetazolamide [a set a ZOLE a mide] is a sulfonamide without antibacterial activity. Its main action is to inhibit the enzyme carbonic anhydrase in the proximal tubular epithelial cells. However, carbonic anhydrase inhibitors are more often used for their other pharmacologic actions rather than for their diuretic effect, because these agents are much less efficacious than the thiazides or loop diuretics.

A. Acetazolamide

1. **Mechanism of action:** *Acetazolamide* inhibits carbonic anhydrase, located intracellularly and on the apical membrane of the proximal tubular epithelium (Figure 23.4). [Note: Carbonic anhydrase catalyzes the reaction of CO_2 and H_2O leading to H^+ and HCO_3^- (bicarbonate)]. The decreased ability to exchange Na^+ for H^+ in the presence of *acetazolamide* results in a mild diuresis. Additionally, HCO_3^- is retained in the lumen with marked elevation in urinary pH. The loss of HCO_3^- causes a hyperchloremic

metabolic acidosis and decreased diuretic efficacy following several days of therapy. Changes in the composition of urinary electrolytes induced by *acetazolamide* are summarized in Figure 23.5.

2. Therapeutic uses:

a. Treatment of glaucoma: The most common use of *acetazolamide* is to reduce the elevated intraocular pressure of open-angle glaucoma. *Acetazolamide* decreases the production of aqueous humor, probably by blocking carbonic anhydrase in the ciliary body of the eye. It is useful in the chronic treatment of glaucoma but should not be used for an acute attack; *pilocarpine* (see p. 41) is preferred for an acute attack because of its immediate action.

b. Epilepsy: *Acetazolamide* is sometimes used in the treatment of epilepsy—both generalized and partial. It reduces the severity and magnitude of the seizures. Often *acetazolamide* is used chronically in conjunction with antiepileptic medication to enhance the action of these other drugs.

c. Mountain sickness: Less commonly *acetazolamide* can be used in the prophylaxis of acute mountain sickness among healthy, physically active individuals who rapidly ascend above 10,000 feet. *Acetazolamide* given nightly for 5 days before the ascent prevents the weakness, breathlessness, dizziness, nausea, and cerebral and pulmonary edema characteristic of the syndrome.

3. Pharmacokinetics: *Acetazolamide* is given orally once a day.

4. Adverse effects: Metabolic acidosis (mild), potassium depletion, renal stone formation, drowsiness, and paresthesia may occur.

V. LOOP OR HIGH-CEILING DIURETICS

Bumetanide [byoo MET a nide], *furosemide* [fur OH se mide], *torsemide* [TOR se myde] and *ethacrynic acid* [eth a KRIN ik] are four diuretics that have their major action on the ascending limb of the loop of Henle (Figure 23.2). Compared to all other classes of diuretics, these drugs have the highest efficacy in mobilizing Na^+ and Cl^- from the body. *Ethacrynic acid* has a steeper dose-response curve (see p. 21) than *furosemide*; it shows greater side effects than those seen with the other loop diuretics and is not as widely used. *Bumetanide* is much more potent than *furosemide*, and its use is increasing.

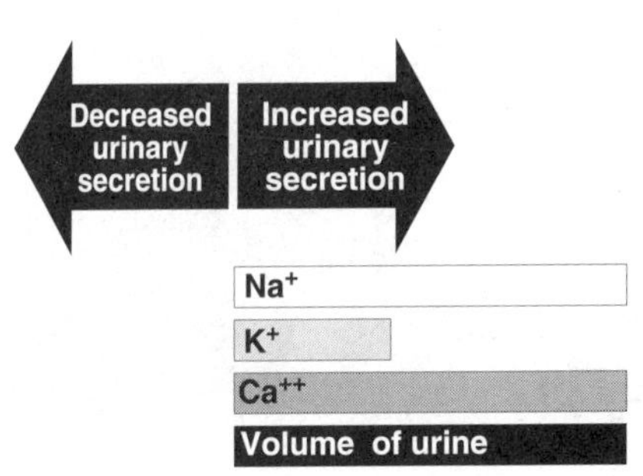

Figure 23.6
Relative changes in the composition of urine induced by loop diuretics.

A. Bumetanide, furosemide, torsemide, ethacrynic acid

1. Mechanism of action: Loop diuretics inhibit the $Na^+/K^+/Cl^-$ cotransport of the luminal membrane in the ascending limb of the loop of Henle. Therefore reabsorption of Na^+, K^+, and Cl^- is decreased (Figure 23.6). The loop diuretics are the most efficacious of the diuretic drugs, because the ascending limb accounts for the reabsorption of 25–30% of filtered NaCl and downstream sites are not able to compensate for this increased Na^+ load.

2. **Actions:** The loop diuretics act promptly, even among patients who have poor renal function or who have not responded to thiazides or other diuretics. Changes in the composition of the urine induced by loop diuretics are shown in Figure 23.6. [Note: Loop diuretics increase the Ca^{++} content of urine, while thiazide diuretics (see p. 229) decrease the Ca^{++} concentration of the urine.] The loop diuretics cause decreased renal vascular resistance and increased renal blood flow.

3. **Therapeutic uses:** The loop diuretics are the drugs of choice for reducing the acute pulmonary edema of congestive heart failure. Because of their rapid onset of action, the drugs are useful in emergency situations, such as acute pulmonary edema, which calls for a rapid, intense diuresis. Loop diuretics (along with hydration) are also useful in treating hypercalcemia because they stimulate tubular Ca^{++} secretion.

4. **Pharmacokinetics:** Loop diuretics are administered orally or parenterally. Their duration of action is relatively brief, 1 to 4 hours.

5. **Adverse effects:**

   a. **Ototoxicity:** Hearing can be affected adversely by the loop diuretics, particularly when used in conjunction with the aminoglycoside antibiotics (see p. 314). Permanent damage may result with continued treatment. Vestibular function is less likely to be disturbed, but it too may be affected by combined treatment.

   b. **Hyperuricemia:** *Furosemide* and *ethacrynic acid* compete with uric acid for the renal and biliary secretory systems, thus blocking its secretion and thereby causing or exacerbating gouty attacks.

   c. **Acute hypovolemia:** Loop diuretics can cause a severe and rapid reduction in blood volume, with the possibility of hypotension, shock, and cardiac arrhythmias.

   d. **Potassium depletion:** The heavy load of Na^+ presented to the collecting tubule results in increased exchange of tubular Na^+ for K^+, with the possibility of inducing hypokalemia. The loss of K^+ from cells in exchange for H^+ leads to hypokalemic alkalosis. Potassium depletion can be averted by use of potassium-sparing diuretics or dietary supplementation with K^+. The adverse effects of the loop diuretic are summarized in Figure 23.7.

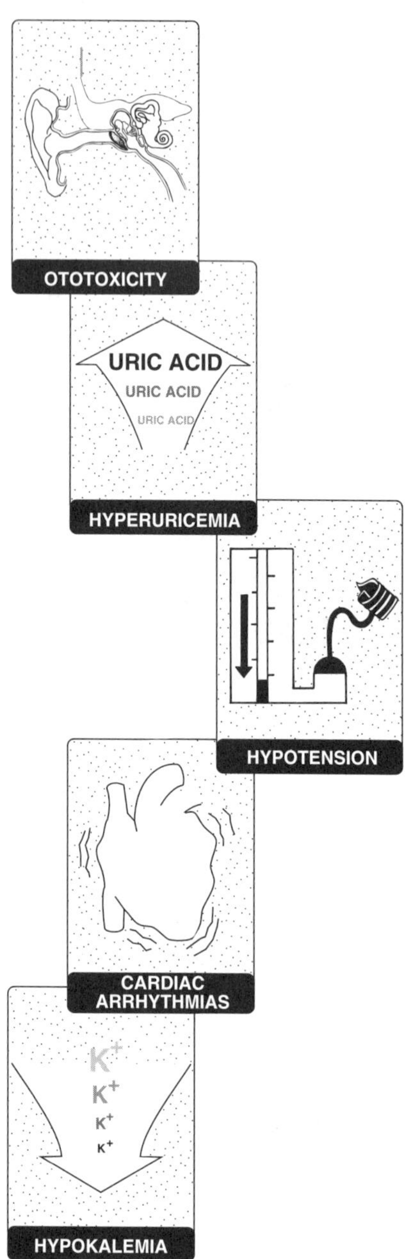

Figure 23.7
Summary of adverse effects commonly observed with loop diuretics.

VI. THIAZIDES AND RELATED AGENTS

The thiazides are the most widely used of the diuretic drugs. They are sulfonamide derivatives and are related in structure to the carbonic anhydrase inhibitors. The thiazides have significantly greater diuretic activity than *acetazolamide*, and they act on the kidney by different mechanisms. All thiazides affect the distal tubule, and all have equal maximum diuretic effect, differing only in potency, expressed on a per - milligram basis.

A. Chlorothiazide

Chlorothiazide [klor oh THYE a zide], the prototype thiazide diuretic, was the first modern diuretic that was active orally and was capable of affecting the severe edema of cirrhosis and congestive heart failure with a minimum of side effects. Its properties are representative of the thiazide group, although newer derivatives such as *hydrochlorothiazide* or *chlorthalidone* are now used more commonly.

1. **Mechanism of action:** The thiazide derivatives act mainly in the distal tubule to decrease the reabsorption of Na^+ by inhibition of a Na^+/Cl^- cotransporter on the luminal membrane (see Figure 23.2). They have a lesser effect in the proximal tubule. As a result, these drugs increase the concentration of Na^+ and Cl^- in the tubular fluid. The acid-base balance is not usually affected. [Note: Because the site of action of the thiazide derivatives is on the luminal membrane, these drugs must be excreted into the tubular lumen to be effective. Therefore, with decreased renal function, thiazide diuretics lose efficacy.]

2. **Actions:**

   a. **Increased excretion of Na^+ and Cl^-:** *Chlorothiazide* causes diuresis with increased Na^+ and Cl^- excretion, which can result in the excretion of a very hyperosmolar urine. This latter effect is unique among the other diuretic classes, which are unlikely to produce a hyperosmolar urine. The diuretic action is not affected by the acid-base status of the body, nor does *chlorothiazide* use change the acid-base status of the blood. The relative changes in the ionic composition of the urine during therapy with thiazide diuretics is given in Figure 23.8.

   b. **Loss of K^+:** Because thiazides increase the Na^+ in the filtrate arriving at the distal tubule, more K^+ is also exchanged for Na^+. Thus, prolonged use of these drugs results in continual loss of K^+ from the body. Therefore, it is imperative to measure serum K^+ once per month (more frequently at the beginning of therapy) to assure that hypokalemia does not develop. Often, K^+ can be supplemented by diet alone, such as by increasing the intake of citrus fruits, bananas, and prunes. In some cases, K^+ salt supplementation may be necessary.

   c. **Decreased urinary calcium excretion:** Thiazide diuretics decrease the Ca^{++} content of urine by promoting the reabsorption of Ca^{++}. This contrasts with the loop diuretics (see p. 227), which increase the Ca^{++} concentration of the urine.

   d. **Reduced peripheral vascular resistance:** An initial reduction in blood pressure results from a decrease in blood volume and therefore a decrease in cardiac output (see p. 180). With continued therapy, volume recovery occurs. However, there are continued hypotensive effects, resulting from reduced peripheral vascular resistance caused by relaxation of arteriolar smooth muscle. This usually occurs prior to the diuretic effect.

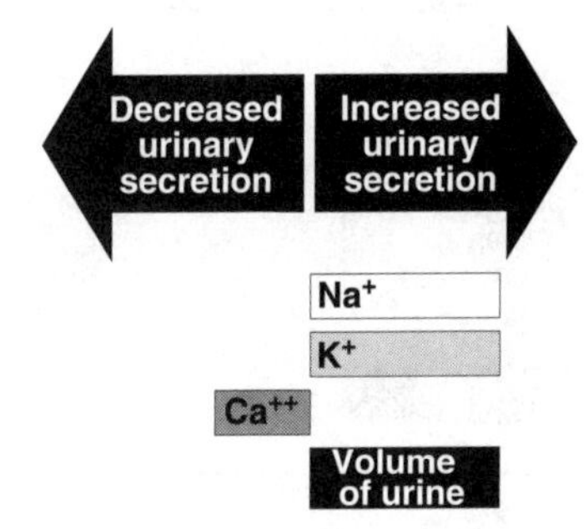

Figure 23.8
Relative changes in the composition of urine induced by thiazide diuretics.

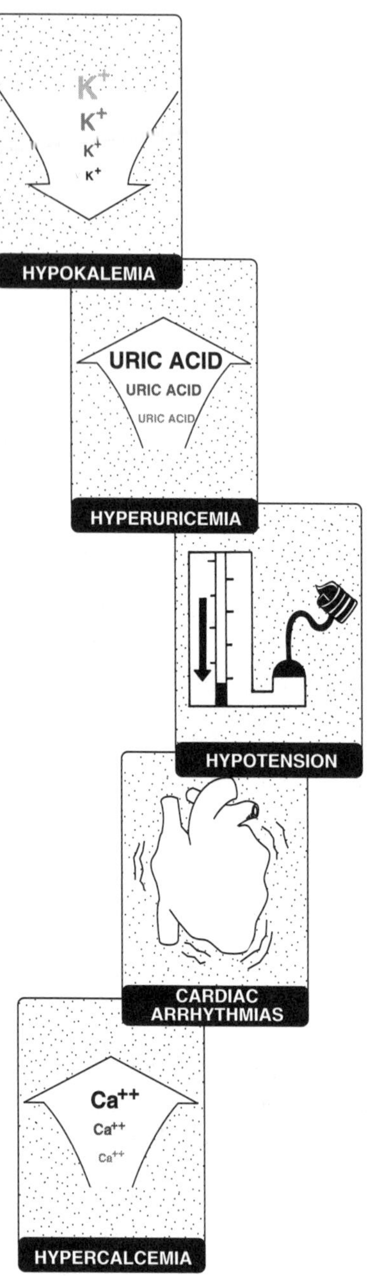

Figure 23.9
Summary of adverse effects commonly observed with thiazide diuretics.

3. Therapeutic uses:

a. **Hypertension:** Clinically, the thiazides have long been the mainstay of antihypertensive medication, since they are inexpensive, convenient to administer, and well tolerated. They are effective in reducing systolic and diastolic blood pressure for extended periods in the majority of patients with mild to moderate essential hypertension (see p. 181 for details on treatment of hypertension). After 3–7 days of treatment, the blood pressure stabilizes at a lower level and can be maintained indefinitely by a daily dosage level of the drug, which causes lower peripheral resistance without having a major diuretic effect. Many patients can be continued for years on the thiazides alone, although a small percentage of patients require additional medication, such as β-adrenergic blockers (see p. 189).

b. **Congestive heart failure:** Thiazides can be the diuretic of choice in reducing extracellular volume in mild to moderate congestive heart failure (see p. 157). If the thiazide fails, loop diuretics may be useful.

c. **Renal impairment:** Patients with nephrotic syndrome accompanied by edema are initially treated with loop diuretics; only if this treatment fails are they given *metolazone* in conjunction with a loop diuretic.

d. **Hypercalciuria:** The thiazides can be useful in treating idiopathic hypercalciuria because they inhibit urinary Ca^{++} excretion. This is particularly beneficial for patients with calcium oxalate stones in the urinary tract.

e. **Diabetes insipidus:** Thiazides have the unique ability to produce a hyperosmolar urine. Thiazides can substitute for the antidiuretic hormone in the treatment of nephrogenic diabetes insipidus. The urine volume of such individuals may drop from 11 L/day to about 3 L/day when treated with the drug.

4. Pharmacokinetics: The drugs are effective orally. Most thiazides take 1 to 3 weeks to produce a stable reduction in blood pressure, and they exhibit a prolonged biological half-life (40 hours). All thiazides are secreted by the organic acid secretory system of the kidney (see p. 224).

5. Adverse effects:

a. **Potassium depletion:** Hypokalemia is the most frequent problem encountered with the thiazide diuretics and can predispose patients on *digitalis* (see p. 160) to ventricular arrhythmias (Figure 23.9). Activation of the renin-angiotensin-aldosterone system by the decrease in intravascular volume contributes significantly to urinary K^+ losses. The K^+ deficiency can be overcome by *spironolactone*, which interferes with aldosterone action, or by administering *triamterene*, which acts to retain K^+ (see p. 223). Low sodium diets blunt the potassium depletion caused by thiazide diuretics.

b. **Hyperuricemia:** Thiazides increase serum uric acid by decreasing the amount of acid excreted by the organic acid secretory system. Being insoluble, the uric acid deposits in the joints, and a full-blown attack of gout may result in individuals predisposed to gouty attacks. It is important, therefore, to perform periodic blood tests for uric acid levels.

c. **Volume depletion:** This can cause orthostatic hypotension or light-headedness.

d. **Hypercalcemia:** The thiazides inhibit the secretion of Ca^{++}, sometimes leading to elevated levels of Ca^{++} in the blood.

e. **Hyperglycemia:** Patients with diabetes mellitus, who are taking thiazides for hypertension, may become hyperglycemic and have difficulty in maintaining appropriate blood sugar levels.

f. **Hypersensitivity:** Bone marrow suppression, dermatitis, necrotizing vasculitis, and interstitial nephritis are very rare.

B. Hydrochlorothiazide

Hydrochlorothiazide is a thiazide derivative that has proven to be more popular than the parent drug. This is because it has far less ability to inhibit carbonic anhydrase as compared to *chlorothiazide*. It is also more potent, so that the required dose is considerably less than that of *chlorothiazide*. On the other hand, the efficacy is exactly the same as that of the parent drug.

C. Chlorthalidone

Chlorthalidone [klor THAL i done] is a thiazide derivative that behaves like *hydrochlorothiazide*. It has a very long duration of action and therefore is often used to treat hypertension. It is given once per day for this indication.

D. Thiazide analogs

1. **Metolazone:** *Metolazone* [me TOLE a zone] is more potent than the thiazides and, unlike the thiazides, causes Na^{+} excretion in advanced renal failure.

2. **Indapamide:** *Indapamide* [in DAP a mide] is a lipid soluble, nonthiazide diuretic that has a long duration of action. At low doses, it shows significant antihypertensive action with minimal diuretic effects. *Indapamide* is often used in advanced real failure to stimulate additional diuresis on top of that achieved by loop diuretics. *Indapamide* is metabolized and excreted by the gastrointestinal tract and the kidneys; it therefore is less likely to accumulate in patients with renal failure and may be useful in their treatment.

VII. POTASSIUM-SPARING DIURETICS

These agents act in the collecting tubule to inhibit Na^+ reabsorption, K^+ secretion, and H^+ secretion (Figure 23.10). Potassium-sparing diuretics are used primarily when aldosterone is present in excess. The major use of potassium-sparing agents is in the treatment of hypertension, most often in combination with a thiazide. It is extremely important that patients treated with any potassium-sparing diuretic be closely monitored for potassium levels. Exogenous potassium supplementation is usually discontinued when potassium-sparing diuretic therapy is instituted.

A. Spironolactone

1. **Mechanism of action:** *Spironolactone* [spye row no LAK tone] is a synthetic aldosterone antagonist that competes with aldosterone for intracellular cytoplasmic receptor sites. The *spironolactone*-receptor complex is inactive, that is, it prevents translocation of the receptor complex into the nucleus of the target cell, and thus does not bind to DNA. This results in a failure to produce proteins that are normally synthesized in response to aldosterone. These mediator proteins normally stimulate the Na^+–K^+ exchange sites of the collecting tubule. Thus, a lack of mediator proteins prevents Na^+ reabsorption and therefore K^+ and H^+ secretion.

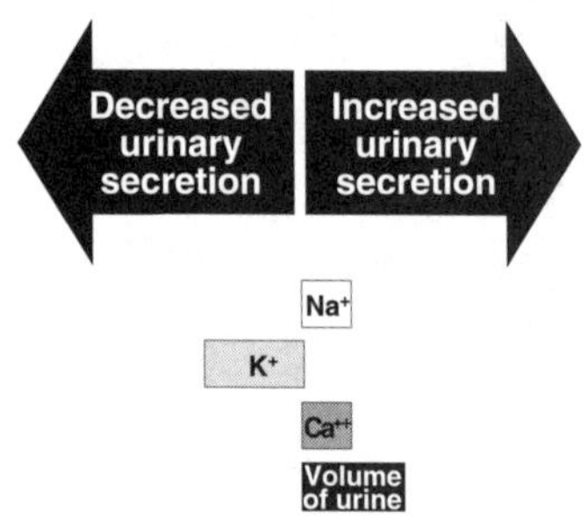

Figure 23.10
Relative changes in the composition of urine induced by potassium-sparing diuretics.

2. **Actions:** In most edematous states, blood levels of aldosterone are high, which is instrumental in retaining Na^+ (see p. 225). When *spironolactone* is given to a patient with elevated circulating levels of aldosterone, the drug antagonizes the activity of the hormone, resulting in retention of K^+ and excretion of Na^+ (Figure 23.10). Where there are no significant circulating levels of aldosterone, such as in Addison's disease (primary adrenal insufficiency), no diuretic effect of the drug occurs.

3. **Therapeutic uses:**

   a. **Diuretic:** Although *spironolactone* has a low efficacy in mobilizing Na^+ from the body in comparison with the other drugs, it has the useful property of causing the retention of K^+ (Figure 23.10). Because of this latter action, *spironolactone* is often given in conjunction with a thiazide or loop diuretic to prevent K^+ excretion that would otherwise occur with these drugs.

   b. **Secondary hyperaldosteronism:** *Spironolactone* is the only potassium-sparing diuretic that is routinely used alone to induce net negative salt balance. It is particularly effective in clinical situations associated with secondary hyperaldosteronism.

4. **Pharmacokinetics**: *Spironolactone* is completely absorbed orally and is strongly bound to proteins. It is rapidly converted to an active metabolite, *canrenone* [KAN ra none]. The action of *spironolactone* is largely due to the effect of *canrenone*, which has mineralocorticoid-blocking activity. *Spironolactone* induces hepatic cytochrome P-450.

5. **Adverse effects:** Because *spironolactone* chemically resembles some of the sex steroids, it does have minimal hormonal activity and may induce gynecomastia in males and menstrual irregularities in females. Because of this, the drug should not be given in high doses on a chronic basis. It is most effectively employed in mild edematous states where it is given for a few days at a time. At low doses, *spironolactone* can be used chronically with few side effects. Hyperkalemia, nausea, lethargy, and mental confusion can occur.

B. Triamterene and amiloride

Triamterene [trye AM ter een] and *amiloride* [a MIL oh ride] block Na^+ transport channels resulting in a decrease in Na^+–K^+ exchange; they have K^+–sparing diuretic actions similar to that of *spironolactone*. However, the ability of these drugs to block the K^+–Na^+ exchange site in the collecting tubule does not depend on the presence of aldosterone. Thus, they have diuretic activity even in individuals with Addison's disease. They, like *spironolactone*, are not very efficacious diuretics. Both *triamterene* and *amiloride* are frequently used in combination with other diuretics, usually for their potassium-sparing properties. For example, much like *spironolactone*, they prevent K^+ loss that occurs with thiazides and *furosemide*. The side effects of *triamterene* are leg cramps and the possibility of increased blood urea nitrogen (BUN) as well as uric acid and K^+ retention.

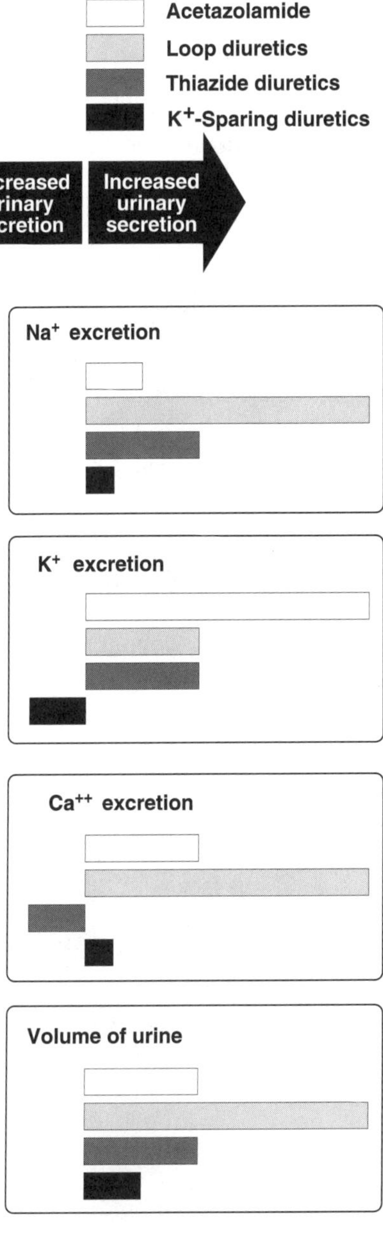

Figure 23.11
Summary of relative changes in urinary composition induced by diuretic drugs.

VIII. OSMOTIC DIURETICS

A number of simple, hydrophilic, chemical substances that are filtered through the glomerulus, such as *mannitol* [MAN i tole] and *urea* [yu REE ah], result in some degree of diuresis. This is due to their ability to carry water with them into the tubular fluid. If the substance that is filtered subsequently undergoes little or no reabsorption, then the filtered substance will cause an increase in urinary output. Only a small amount of additional salt may also be excreted. Because osmotic diuretics are used to effect increased water excretion rather than Na^+ excretion, they are not useful in treating conditions in which Na^+ retention occurs. They are used to maintain urine flow following acute toxic ingestion of substances capable of producing acute renal failure. Osmotic diuretics are a mainstay of treatment for patients with increased intracranial pressure, or acute renal failure due to shock, drug toxicities and trauma. Maintaining urine flow preserves long-term kidney function and may save the patient from dialysis. [Note: *Mannitol* is not absorbed when given orally; the agent can only be given intravenously.]

Figure 23.11 summarizes the relative changes in urinary composition induced by diuretic drugs.

23.1–23.4 From the list of diuretic drugs below choose the agent that is most appropriate for the numbered conditions.

A. Acetazolamide
B. Amiloride
C. Chlorothiazide
D. Furosemide
E. Spironolactone
F. Triamterene

23.1 Acute pulmonary edema

Correct answer = D (Furosemide).

23.2 Acute hypercalcemia

Correct answer = D (Furosemide).

23.3 Essential hypertension

Correct answer = C (Chlorthiazide).

23.4 Glaucoma

Correct answer = A (Acetazolamide).

23.5-23.8 Match the drug from the list below to its appropriate target in the nephron.

A. Amiloride
B. Acetazolamide
C. Chlorthalidone
D. Ethacrynic acid
E. Spironolactone

23.5 $Na^+/K^+/2Cl^-$ cotransporter

Correct answer = D (Ethacrynic acid).

23.6 Carbonic anhydrase

Correct answer = B (Acetazolamide).

23.7 Aldosterone receptors

Correct answer = E (Spironolactone).

23.8 Na^+/Cl^- cotransporter

Correct answer = C (Chlorthalidone).

23.9-23.12 Match the drug from the list below to its most appropriate adverse effect.

A. Ethacrynic acid
B. Chlorthalidone
C. Acetazolamide
D. Furosemide
E. Spironolactone

23.9 Ototoxicity

Correct answer = D (Furosemide).

23.10 Hyperuricemia

Correct answer = B (Furosemide).

23.11 Gynecomastia (development of enlarged breats) in males

Correct answer = E (Spironolactone).

23.12 Metabolic acidosis

Correct answer = C (Acetazolamide).

23.13 Chlorothiazide can produce which one of the following actions?

A. Hyperkalemia
B. Hyperuricemia
C. Increase in blood pressure
D. Hypoglycemia in diabetic patients
E. Hypercalcemia

Correct answer = B. Thiazide decreases the excretion of uric aid by the acid secretory system. Hypokalemia is the most frequently encountered adverse effect of thiazide treatment. Chlorothiazide may induce hyperglycemia and hypotension.

23.14 In an Addisonian patient, all of the following agents would have diuretic actions EXCEPT which one?

A. Amiloride
B. Chlorothiazide
C. Triamterene
D. Spironolactone
E. Torsemide

Correct choice = D. Spironolactone competes with aldosterone, and thus the drug would have no effect in the absence of endogenous hormone.

Gastrointestinal and Antiemetic Drugs

24

I. OVERVIEW

This chapter describes drugs used to treat three common medical conditions involving the gastrointestinal tract: peptic ulcers, control of chemotherapy-induced emesis, and diarrhea and constipation. Many drugs described in other chapters also find application in the treatment of gastrointestinal disorders. For example, the morphine derivative *diphenoxylate* (see p. 244), which decreases peristaltic activity of the gut, is useful in the treatment of severe diarrhea, and the corticosteroid *dexamethasone* (see p. 275) has excellent antiemetic properties. Other drugs, (for example, H_2-receptor antagonists and proton pump inhibitors employed to heal peptic ulcers, and the selective inhibitors of the serotonin receptors, such as *ondansetron* or *granisetron*, which prevent vomiting) are used almost exclusively to treat gastrointestinal tract disorders.

II. DRUGS USED TO TREAT PEPTIC ULCER DISEASE

Although the pathogenesis of peptic ulcer disease is not fully understood, three major factors are recognized: infection with gram-negative Helicobacter pylori, increased hydrochloric acid secretion, and inadequate mucosal defense against gastric acid. Treatment approaches include (1) eradicating H. pylori infection, (2) reducing secretion of gastric acid or neutralizing the acid after it is released, and/or (3) providing agents that protect the gastric mucosa from damage. Figure 24.1 summarizes the agents effective in treating peptic ulcer disease.

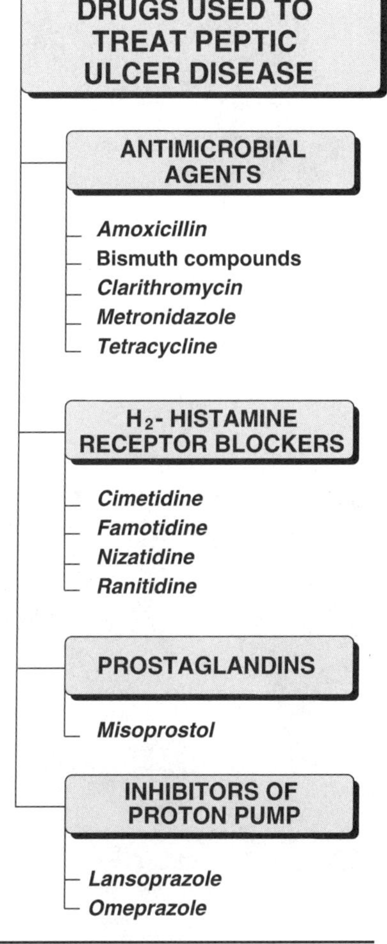

DRUGS USED TO TREAT PEPTIC ULCER DISEASE
ANTIMICROBIAL AGENTS
Amoxicillin
Bismuth compounds
Clarithromycin
Metronidazole
Tetracycline
H2- HISTAMINE RECEPTOR BLOCKERS
Cimetidine
Famotidine
Nizatidine
Ranitidine
PROSTAGLANDINS
Misoprostol
INHIBITORS OF PROTON PUMP
Lansoprazole
Omeprazole

Figure 24.1
Summary of drugs used to treat peptic ulcer disease.
(Figure continues on next page.)

A. Antimicrobial agents

Optimal therapy of patients with peptic ulcer disease (both duodenal and gastric ulcers) who are infected with H. pylori requires antimicrobial treatment. To document infection with H. pylori, endoscopic biopsy of the gastric mucosa or various noninvasive methods are available, including serologic tests and breath tests for urea. Figure 24.2 shows a biopsy sample with H. pylori closely associated with the gastric mucosa. Eradication of H. pylori results in rapid healing

Lippincott's Illustrated Reviews: Pharmacology, Second Edition.
by Mary J. Mycek, Richard A. Harvey and Pamela C. Champe.
Lippincott Williams & Wilkins, Philadelphia, PA © 2000.

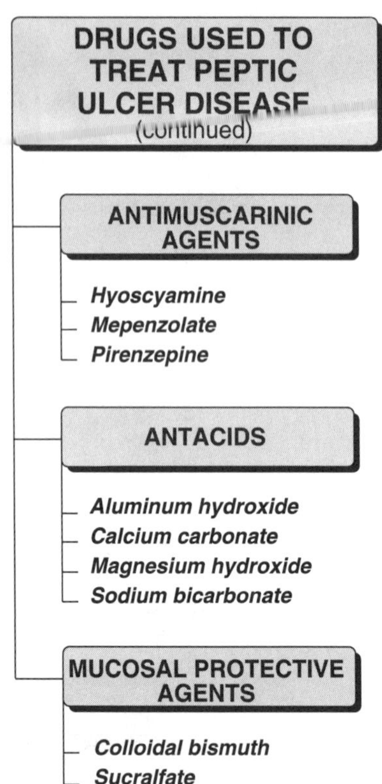

Figure 24.1 (continuted)
Summary of drugs used to treat peptic ulcer disease.

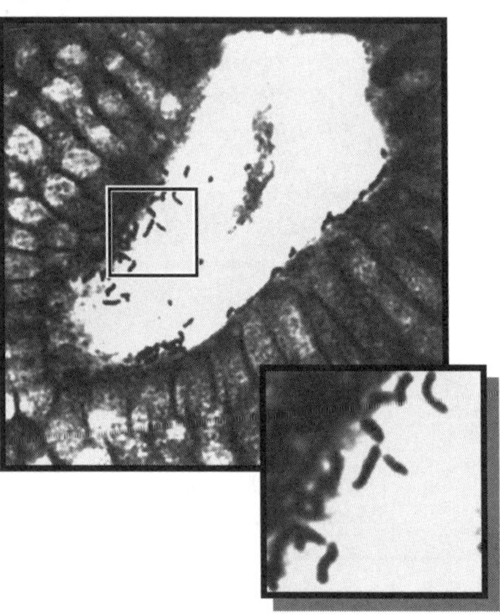

Figure 24.2
Helicobacter pylori in association with gastric mucosa.

of active peptic ulcers and low recurrence rates (less than 15% compared to 60 to 100% per year for patients with initial ulcers healed by traditional antisecretory therapy). Successful eradication of H. pylori (80 to 90%) is possible with various combinations of antimicrobial drugs. For example, a current regimen of choice based on efficacy (about 90% eradication rate) and cost, is a two-week course of triple therapy with *bismuth*, *metronidazole* and *tetracycline*. Often an antisecretory drug is added (see p. 239). Second-line regimens include combinations of two antimicrobial agents (*metronidazole*, *amoxiciliin* or *clarithromycin*) with an antisecretory agent (preferably *omeprazole*). Treatment with a single antimicrobial drug is less effective (20 to 40% eradication rates).

B. Regulation of gastric acid secretion

Gastric acid secretion by parietal cells of the gastric mucosa is controlled by acetylcholine, histamine, prostaglandins E_2 and I_2, and gastrin (Figure 24.3). The receptor-mediated binding of acetylcholine, histamine, or gastrin results in the activation of a H^+/K^+-ATPase proton pump that secretes hydrochloric acid (HCl) into the lumen of the stomach. In contrast, receptor binding of prostaglandins E_2 and I_2 diminishes gastric acid production. [Note: Histamine binding causes activation of adenylyl cyclase (see p. 421), whereas binding of prostaglandin E_2 and I_2 inhibits this enzyme. Gastrin and acetylcholine act by inducing an increase in intracellular calcium levels).]

C. H_2-receptor antagonists

Although antagonists of the histamine H_2-receptor (H_2 antagonists) block the actions of histamine at all H_2 receptors (see p. 421), their chief clinical use is as inhibitors of gastric acid secretion. By competitively blocking the binding of histamine to H_2 receptors, these agents reduce intracellular concentrations of cyclic AMP and thereby, secretion of gastric acid. The four drugs used in the United States, *cimetidine* [sye MET i deen], *ranitidine* [ra NYE ta deen], *famotidine* [fa MOE ti deen] and *nizatidine* [nye ZAT i deen], potently inhibit (>90%) basal, food-stimulated, and nocturnal secretion of gastric acid after a single dose. *Cimetidine* is the prototype histamine H_2-receptor antagonist.

1. **Actions:** The histamine H_2-receptor antagonists—*cimetidine, ranitidine, famotidine*, and *nizatidine*—act on H_2-receptors in the stomach, blood vessels, and other sites. They are competitive antagonists of histamine and are fully reversible. These agents completely inhibit gastric acid secretion induced by histamine, or gastrin. However, they only partially inhibit gastric acid secretion induced by *acetylcholine* or *bethanechol*.

2. **Therapeutic uses:**

   a. **Peptic ulcers:** All four agents are equally effective in promoting healing of duodenal and gastric ulcers. However, recurrence is common after treatment with H_2 antagonists is stopped (60 to

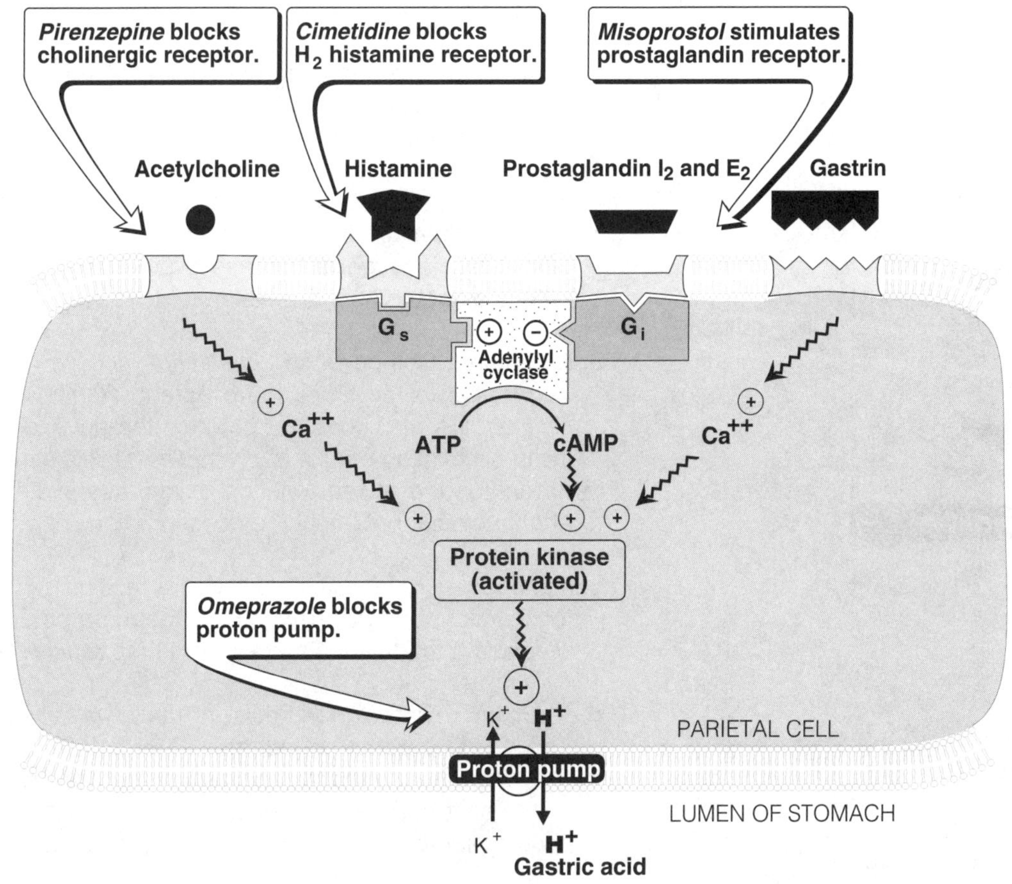

Figure 24.3
Effects of acetylcholine, histamine, prostaglandin I_2, and E_2, and gastrin on gastric acid secretion by the parietal cells of stomach; G_s and G_i are membrane proteins that mediate the stimulatory or inhibitory effect of receptor coupling to adenylyl cyclase.

100% per year). This can be effectively prevented by eradication of H. pylori, and H_2 antagonists continue to be widely used in peptic ulcer therapy in combination with antimicrobial drugs.

b. **Zollinger-Ellison syndrome:** Zollinger-Ellison syndrome is a rare condition in which a gastrin-producing tumor causes hypersecretion of HCl. With H_2 antagonists, the hypersecretion of gastric acid can be kept at safe levels in patients with Zollinger-Ellison syndrome.

c. **Acute stress ulcers:** These drugs are useful in managing acute stress ulcers associated with major physical trauma in high-risk patients in intensive care units.

d. **Gastroesophageal reflux disease (heartburn):** Low doses of H_2 antagonists, recently released for over-the-counter sale, appear to be effective for prevention and treatment of heartburn (gastroesophageal reflux). Because they act by stopping acid secretion, they may not relieve symptoms for at least 45 minutes. Antacids more efficiently neutralize secreted acid already in the stomach.

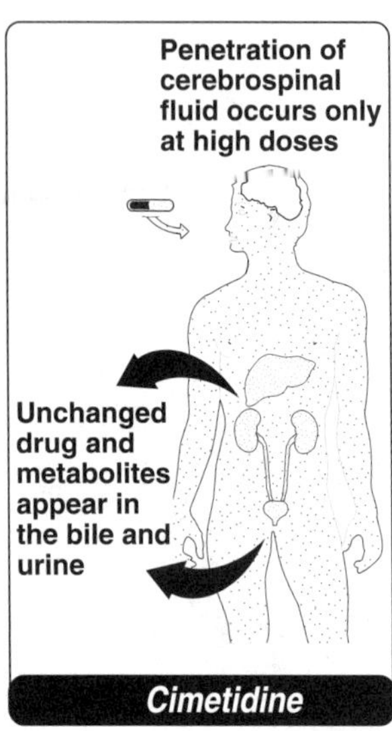

3. **Pharmacokinetics:**

a. **Cimetidine:** *Cimetidine* and the other H_2-antagonists are given orally, distribute widely throughout the body (including in breast milk and across the placenta) and are excreted mainly in the urine. *Cimetidine* normally has a short serum half-life, which is increased in renal failure. Approximately 30% of a dose of *cimetidine* is slowly inactivated by the liver's microsomal mixed function oxygenase system (see p. 14); the other 70% is excreted unchanged in the urine.

b. **Ranitidine:** Compared to *cimetidine*, *ranitidine* is longer acting and is five to ten times more potent. *Ranitidine* has minimal side effects, and does not produce the antiandrogenic or prolactin-stimulating effects of *cimetidine*. Unlike cimetidine, it does not inhibit the mixed function oxygenase system in the liver, and thus does not affect the concentrations of other drugs.

c. **Famotidine:** *Famotidine* is similar to *ranitidine* in its pharmacologic action, but it is 20 to 160 times more potent than *cimetidine* and 3 to 20 times more potent than *ranitidine*.

d. **Nizatidine:** *Nizatidine* is similar to *ranitidine* in its pharmacologic action and potency. In contrast to *cimetidine*, *ranitidine*, and *famotidine* (which are metabolized by the liver), *nizatidine* is eliminated principally by the kidney. Since little first-pass metabolism occurs with *nizatidine*, its bioavailability is nearly 100%.

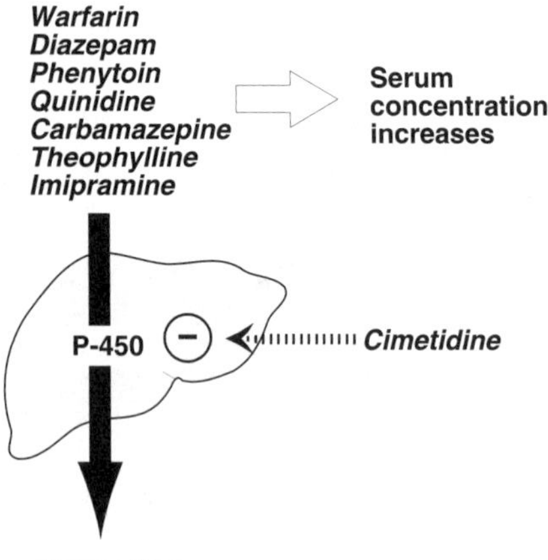

4. **Adverse effects:** The adverse effects of *cimetidine* are usually minor and are associated mainly with the major pharmacologic activity of the drug, namely reduced gastric acid production. Side effects occur only in a small number of patients and generally do not require discontinuation of the drug. The most common side effects are headache, dizziness, diarrhea, and muscular pain. Other central nervous system (CNS) effects (confusion, hallucinations) occur primarily in elderly patients or after prolonged administration. *Cimetidine* can also have endocrine effects, since it acts as a nonsteroidal antiandrogen. These effects include gynecomastia, galactorrhea (continuous release/discharge of milk), and reduced sperm count. *Cimetidine* inhibits cytochrome P-450 and can slow metabolism (and thus potentiate the action) of several drugs (for example, *warfarin*, *diazepam*, *phenytoin*, *quinidine*, *carbamazepine*, *theophylline*, *imipramine*), sometimes resulting in serious adverse clinical effects.

D. Prostaglandins

Prostaglandins E_2 and I_2, produced by the gastric mucosa, inhibit secretion of HCl and stimulate secretion of mucus and bicarbonate (cytoprotective effect). A deficiency of prostaglandins is thought to be involved in the pathogenesis of peptic ulcers. *Misoprostol* [miz o PROS tol], a stable analog of prostaglandin E_1, is currently the only agent approved for prevention of gastric ulcers induced by nonsteroidal anti-inflammatory agents (NSAIDs) (see p. 405). It is less effective than H_2 antagonists for acute treatment of peptic ulcers.

Although *misoprostol* has cytoprotective actions, it is clinically effective only at higher doses that diminish gastric acid secretion. Routine prophylactic use of *misoprostol* may not be justified except in patients taking NSAIDs who are at high risk of NSAID-induced ulcers, such as the elderly or patients with ulcer complications. Like other prostaglandins, *misoprostol* produces uterine contractions and is contraindicated during pregnancy. Dose-related diarrhea and nausea are the most common adverse effects.

E. Inhibitors of the H^+/K^+-ATPase proton pump

Omeprazole [om ME pary zol] is the first of a new class of drugs that binds to the H^+/K^+-ATPase enzyme system (proton pump) of the parietal cell, suppressing secretion of hydrogen ions into the gastric lumen. The membrane-bound proton pump is the final step in the secretion of gastric acid (see Figure 24.3). A second proton pump inhibitor, *lansoprazole* [lan SOP ra zol], is also available.

1. **Actions:** At standard doses, both *omeprazole* and *lansoprazole* inhibit basal and stimulated gastric acid secretion more than 90%. Acid suppression begins within 1 to 2 hr after the first dose of *lansoprazole*, and slightly earlier with *omeprazole*.

2. **Therapeutic uses:** *Omeprazole* and *lansoprazole* are used for short-term treatment of erosive esophagitis and active duodenal ulcer, and for long-term treatment of pathologic hypersecretory conditions (for example, Zollinger-Ellison syndrome). Only *omeprazole* is approved for refractory gastroesophageal reflux disease and maintenance therapy of erosive esophagitis. Clinical studies to date have shown *lansoprazole*, like *omeprazole*, is more effective in the short term than the H_2 antagonist, *ranitidine*. *Omeprazole* is successfully used with antimicrobial regimens to eradicate H. pylori.

3. **Pharmacokinetics:** *Omeprazole* and *lansoprazole* are enteric-coated to protect them from premature activation by gastric acid. After absorption in the duodenum, they are transported to the acid parietal cell canaliculus, where they are converted to active species. Metabolites of these agents are excreted in urine and feces.

4. **Adverse effects:** *Omeprazole* and *lansoprazole* are generally well tolerated, but concerns about long-term safety have been raised. In animal studies, both drugs increase the incidence of gastric carcinoid tumors, possibly related to the effects of prolonged hypochlorhydria and secondary hypergastrinemia. Increased concentration of viable bacteria in the stomach have been reported with continued use of these drugs. *Omeprazole* interferes in the oxidation of *warfarin*, *phenytoin*, *diazepam* and *cyclosporine*; *lansoprazole* does not.

F. Antimuscarinic agents

Muscarinic receptor stimulation increases gastrointestinal motility and secretory activity (see p. 29). Cholinergic antagonists, such as *hyoscyamine*, are used as adjuncts in the management of peptic ulcer disease and Zollinger-Ellison syndrome, particularly in patients refractory to standard therapies. In contrast to the classic anticholinergics, the relatively specific muscarinic M_1-receptor antagonist *pirenzepine* is under investigation for its clinical usefulness as an antisecretory agent (see p. 38). *Pirenzepine* suppresses basal and stimulated gastric acid secretion at doses having a minimal effect on salivary glands, the heart and eye.

G. Antacids

Antacids are weak bases that react with gastric acid to form water and a salt, thereby diminishing gastric acidity. Since pepsin is inactive at pH>4.0, antacids also reduce peptic activity. They may have other actions as well, such as reduction of <u>H. pylori</u> colonization and stimulation of prostaglandin synthesis.

1. **Chemistry of antacids:** Antacid products vary widely in their chemical composition, acid-neutralizing capacity, sodium content, palatability and price. The acid-neutralizing ability of an antacid depends on its capacity to neutralize gastric HCl and on whether the stomach is full or empty (food delays stomach emptying, allowing more time for the antacid to react). Commonly used antacids are salts of aluminum and magnesium, such as *aluminum hydroxide* (usually a mixture of $Al(OH)_3$ and aluminum oxide hydrates) or *magnesium hydroxide* [$Mg(OH)_2$] ("milk of magnesia"), either alone or in combination. Since calcium salts stimulate gastrin release, use of calcium-containing antacids, such as *calcium carbonate* [$CaCO_3$] (*Tums*, *Rolaids*) may be counterproductive. Systemic absorption of *sodium bicarbonate* [$NaHCO_3$] can produce transient metabolic alkalosis; this antacid is not recommended for long-term use.

2. **Therapeutic uses:** Aluminum- and magnesium-containing antacids can promote healing of duodenal ulcers; evidence for efficacy in treatment of acute gastric ulcer is less compelling.

3. **Adverse effects:** *Aluminum hydroxide* may be constipating; *magnesium hydroxide* may produce diarrhea. Preparations that combine these agents aid in normalizing bowel function. In addition to the potential for systemic alkalosis, *NaHCO3* liberates CO_2, causing belching and flatulence. Absorption of cations from antacids (Mg^{++}, Al^{+++}, Ca^{++}) is usually not a problem in patients with normal renal function, but the sodium content of antacids can be an important consideration in patients with hypertension or congestive heart failure.

4. **Drug interactions:** It is usually advisable to avoid concurrent administration of antacids and other drugs. By altering gastric and urinary pH or delaying gastric emptying, antacids can affect rates of dissolution and absorption, bioavailability, and renal elimination of many drugs. By binding to drugs (for example, *tetracycline*), Al^{+++} compounds can form insoluble complexes that are not absorbed. On the other hand, antacids can increase the rate of absorption of some drugs, for example, *levodopa*.

H. Mucosal Protective Agents

These compounds, known as cytoprotective, have several actions that enhance mucosal protection mechanisms, thereby preventing mucosal injury, reducing inflammation, and healing existing ulcers.

1. **Sucralfate:** This complex of aluminum hydroxide and sulfated sucrose, binds to positively charged groups in proteins, glycoproteins, etc, of both normal and necrotic mucosa. By forming complex gels with mucus, *sucralfate* [soo KRAL fate] creates a physical barrier that impairs diffusion of HCl and prevents degradation of mucus by pepsin. It also stimulates prostaglandin release and mucus and bicarbonate output, and inhibits peptic digestion. By these and many other mechanisms, *sucralfate* effectively heals duodenal ulcers and is used in long-term maintenance therapy to prevent their recurrence. Because it requires an acidic pH for activation, *sucralfate* should not be administered with H_2 antagonists or antacids. Little of the drug is absorbed systemically. It is very well tolerated.

2. **Colloidal bismuth:** Preparations of this compound effectively heal peptic ulcers. In addition to their antimicrobial actions (see p. 236), they inhibit the activity of pepsin, increase mucus secretion and interact with proteins in necrotic mucosal tissue to coat and protect the ulcer crater.

III. DRUGS USED TO CONTROL CHEMOTHERAPY-INDUCED EMESIS

Although nausea and vomiting may occur in a variety of conditions (for example motion sickness, pregnancy, hepatitis) and are always unpleasant for the patient, it is the nausea and vomiting produced by many chemotherapeutic agents that demand effective management. Nearly 70 to 80% of all patients given chemotherapy experience nausea or vomiting. Several factors influence the incidence and severity of chemotherapy-induced emesis, including the specific chemotherapeutic drug (see Figure 24.4), dose, route and schedule of administration, and patient variables (for example, 10 to 40% of patients experience nausea or vomiting in anticipation of their chemotherapy [anticipatory vomiting]). Emesis not only affects quality of life, but can lead to rejection of potentially curative antineoplastic treatment. In addition, uncontrolled vomiting can produce dehydration, profound metabolic imbalances and nutrient depletion.

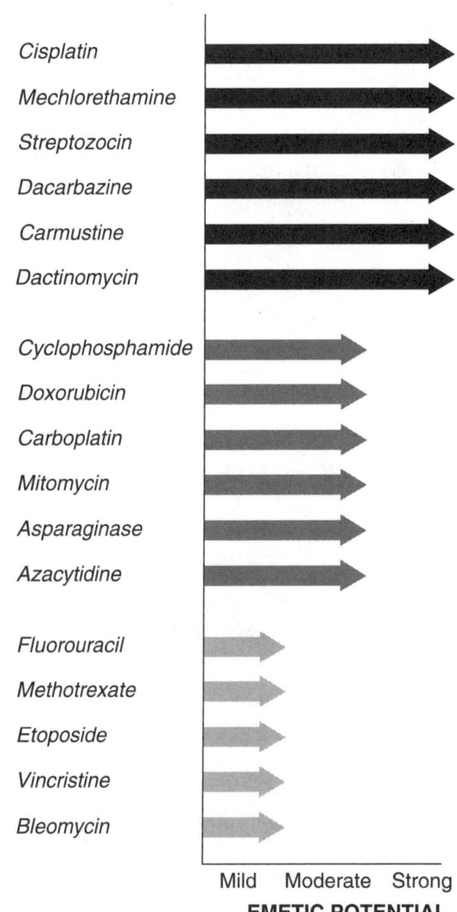

Figure 24.4
Comparison of emetic potential of anticancer drugs.

A. Mechanisms that trigger vomiting

Two brain stem sites have key roles in the vomiting reflex pathway. The chemoreceptor trigger zone, located in the area postrema (a circumventricular structure at the caudal end of the fourth ventricle) is outside the blood-brain barrier. Thus it can respond directly to chemical stimuli in the blood or cerebrospinal fluid. The second important site, the vomiting center, located in the lateral reticular formation of the medulla, coordinates the motor mechanisms of vomiting. The vomiting center also responds to afferent input from the vestibular system, the periphery (pharynx and gastrointestinal tract), and higher brainstem and cortical structures. The vestibular system functions mainly in motion sickness.

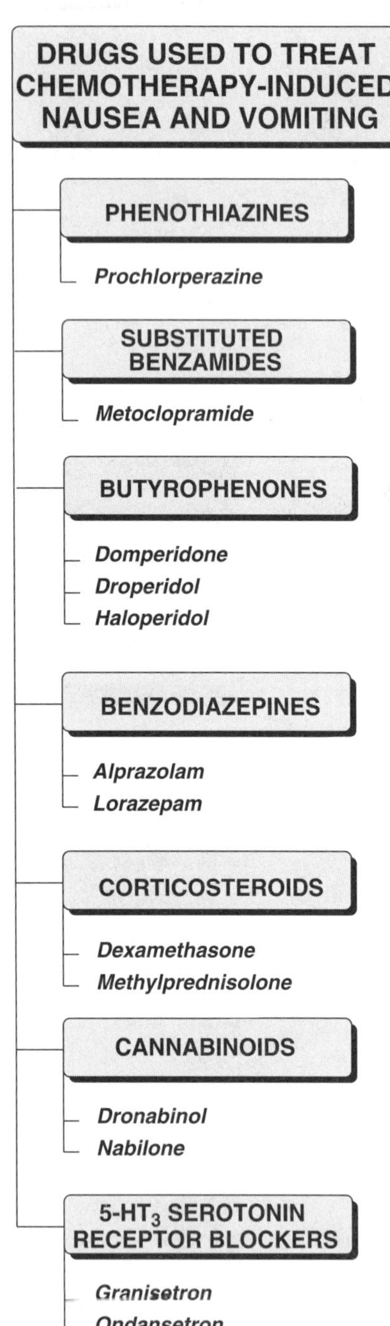

DRUGS USED TO TREAT CHEMOTHERAPY-INDUCED NAUSEA AND VOMITING
PHENOTHIAZINES
Prochlorperazine
SUBSTITUTED BENZAMIDES
Metoclopramide
BUTYROPHENONES
Domperidone
Droperidol
Haloperidol
BENZODIAZEPINES
Alprazolam
Lorazepam
CORTICOSTEROIDS
Dexamethasone
Methylprednisolone
CANNABINOIDS
Dronabinol
Nabilone
5-HT3 SEROTONIN RECEPTOR BLOCKERS
Granisetron
Ondansetron

Figure 24.5
Summary of drugs used to treat chemotherapy-induced nausea and vomiting.

B. Emetic actions of chemotherapeutic agents

Chemotherapeutic agents (or their metabolites) can directly activate the medullary chemoreceptor trigger zone or vomiting center; several neuroreceptors, including dopamine type 2 (DA_2, see p. 128) and serotonin type 3 ($5\text{-}HT_3$), play critical roles. Often, the color or smell of chemotherapeutic drugs (and even stimuli associated with chemotherapy, such as cues in the treatment room or the physician or nurse who administers the therapy) can activate higher brain centers and trigger emesis. Chemotherapeutic drugs can also act peripherally by causing cell damage in the gastrointestinal tract and releasing serotonin from the enterochromaffin cells of the small intestinal mucosa. The released serotonin activates $5\text{-}HT_3$ receptors on vagal and splanchnic afferent fibers, which then carry sensory signals to the medulla, leading to the emetic response.

C. Antiemetic drugs

Considering the complexity of the mechanisms involved in emesis, it is not surprising that antiemetics represent a variety of classes (Figure 24.5) and offer a range of efficacies (Figures 24.6 and 13.4). Anticholinergic drugs, especially the muscarinic receptor antagonist *scopolamine* (see p. 48), and H_1-receptor antagonists, such as *dimenhydrinate*), *meclizine* and *cyclizine* (see p. 422), are very useful in motion sickness, but are ineffective against substances that act directly on the chemoreceptor trigger zone. The major categories of drugs used to control chemotherapy-induced nausea and vomiting include:

1. **Phenothiazines:** The first group of drugs shown to be effective antiemetic agents, phenothiazines, such as *prochlorperazine* [proe klor PER a zeen], act by blocking dopamine receptors (see p. 129). They are effective against low or moderately emetogenic chemotherapeutic agents (for example, *fluorouracil* and *doxorubicin*, see Figure 24.5). Although increasing the dose improves antiemetic activity, side effects, including hypotension and restlessness, are dose-limiting. Other adverse reactions include extrapyramidal symptoms and sedation.

2. **Substituted benzamides:** One of several substituted benzamides with antiemetic activity, *metoclopramide* [met oh kloe PRA mide] is highly effective at high doses against the highly emetogenic *cisplatin*), preventing emesis in 30 to 40% of patients and reducing emesis in the majority. Antidopaminergic side effects, including sedation, diarrhea and extrapyramidal symptoms, limit its high-dose use. These adverse reactions are most common in younger patients.

3. **Butyrophenones:** *Haloperidol*, *droperidol* and *domperidone* act by blocking dopamine receptors. The butyrophenones are moderately effective antiemetics, but high-dose *haloperidol* was found to

be nearly as effective as high-dose *metoclopramide* in preventing *cisplatin*-induced emesis.

4. **Benzodiazepines:** The antiemetic potency of *lorazepam* and *alprazolam* (see p. 89) is low. Their beneficial effects may be due to their sedative, anxiolytic and amnesic properties. These same properties make benzodiazepines useful in treating anticipatory vomiting.

5. **Corticosteroids:** *Dexamethasone* and *methylprednisolone* used alone are effective against mildly to moderately emetogenic chemotherapy. Their antiemetic mechanism is not known, but may involve blockade of prostaglandins. These drugs can cause insomnia and hyperglycemia in patients with diabetes mellitus.

6. **Cannabinoids:** Marijuana derivatives, including *dronabinol* [droe NAB i nol] and *nabilone*, are effective against moderately emetogenic chemotherapy. However, they are seldom first-line antiemetics because of their serious side effects, including dysphoria, hallucinations, sedation, vertigo, and disorientation. In spite of their psychotropic properties (see p. 105), the antiemetic action of cannabinoids may not involve the brain; synthetic cannabinoids having no psychotropic activity, nevertheless are antiemetic.

7. **5-HT3 serotonin receptor blockers:** The specific antagonists of the 5-HT_3 receptor, *ondansetron* [on DAN sah tron] and *granisetron* [gran IZ e tron], selectively block 5-HT_3 receptors in the periphery (visceral afferent fibers) and in the brain (chemoreceptor trigger zone). These drugs can be administered as a single dose prior to chemotherapy (intravenously or orally) and are efficacious against all grades of emetogenic therapy. One trial reported both drugs prevented emesis in 50 to 60% of *cisplatin*-treated patients. *Ondansetron* is approved also for prevention of postoperative nausea and/or vomiting. Headache is a common side effect. These drugs are costly.

8. **Combination regimens:** Antiemetic drugs are often combined to increase antiemetic activity or decrease toxicity (Figure 24.7). Corticosteroids, most commonly *dexamethasone*, increase antiemetic activity when given with high-dose *metoclopramide*, a 5-HT_3 antagonist, *phenothiazine*, *butyrophenone*, a cannabinoid or a benzodiazepine. Antihistamines, like *diphenylhydramine*, are often administered in combination with high-dose *metoclopramide* to reduce extrapyramidal reactions, or corticosteroids, to counter *metoclopramide*-induced diarrhea. Supplementing a cannabinoid regimen with *prochlorperazine* diminishes dysphoria.

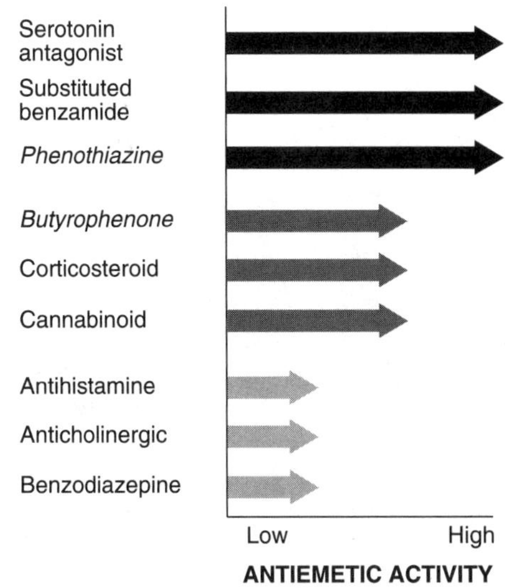

Figure 24.6
Comparison of potency of type of antiemetic drugs.

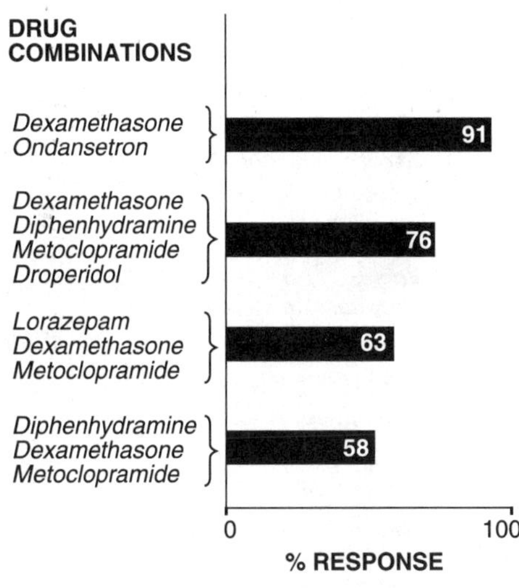

Figure 24.7
Effectiveness of antiemetic activity of some drug combinations against emetic episodes in first 24 hours after *cisplatin* chemotherapy.

IV. ANTIDIARRHEALS

Increased motility of the gastrointestinal tract and decreased absorption of fluid are major factors in diarrhea. Antidiarrheal drugs include antimotility agents, adsorbents, and drugs that modify fluid and electrolyte transport (Figure 24.8).

A. Antimotility agents

Two drugs widely used to control diarrhea are *diphenoxylate* [di PHEN ox a late and *loperamide* [loe PER a mide]. Both are analogues of *meperidine* (see p. 138) and have opioid-like actions on the gut, activating presynaptic opioid receptors in the enteric nervous system to inhibit acetylcholine release and decrease peristalsis. Side effects include drowsiness, abdominal cramps and dizziness. Since these drugs can cause toxic megacolon, they should not be used in young children or patients with severe colitis.

B. Adsorbents

Adsorbent agents such as *kaolin*, *pectin*, *methylcellulose* and *activated attapulgite*, magnesium aluminum silicate, are widely used to control diarrhea, although their efficacy has not been documented by controlled clinical trials. Presumably these agents act by adsorbing intestinal toxins or microorganisms, or by coating or protecting the intestinal mucosa. They are much less effective than antimotility agents and can interfere with absorption of other drugs.

C. Agents that modify fluid and electrolyte transport

Experimental and clinical observations indicate that non-steroidal anti-inflammatory agents (NSAIDs, see p. 403) such as *aspirin* and *indomethacin* are effective in controlling diarrhea. This antidiarrheal action is probably due to inhibition of prostaglandin synthesis. *Bismuth subsalicylate* (PEPTO-BISMOL), used for traveler's diarrhea, decreases fluid secretion in the bowel; its action may be due to its *salicylate* component.

DRUGS USED TO TREAT DIARRHEA AND CONSTIPATION

ANTIDIARRHEALS

- ***Diphenoxylate***
- ***Loperamide***
- ***Kaolin***
- ***Pectin***
- ***Methylcellulose***
- ***Activated attapulgite***
- ***Aspirin***
- ***Indomethacin***
- ***Bismuth subsalicylate***

LAXATIVES

- ***Castor oil***
- ***Senna***
- ***Aloe***
- ***Phenolphthalein***
- ***Bisacodyl***
- ***Hydrophilic colloids***
- ***Methylcellulose***
- ***Psyllium seeds***
- ***Bran***
- ***Magnesium sulfate***
- ***Magnesium hydroxide***
- ***Polyethylene glycol***
- ***Lactulose***
- ***Docusate sodium***
- ***Mineral oil***
- ***Glycerine suppositories***

Figure 24.8
Summary of drugs used to treat diarrhea and constipation.

V. LAXATIVES

Laxatives are commonly used to accelerate the movement of food through the gastrointestinal tract. These drugs can be classified on the basis of their mechanism of action as irritants or stimulants of the gut, bulking agents, and stool softeners.

A. Irritants and stimulants

Castor oil is broken down in the small intestine to ricinoleic acid, which is very irritating to the gut and promptly increases peristalsis. *Cascara*, *senna*, and *aloe* contain *emodin* which stimulates colonic activity. Onset of activity is delayed 6 to 8 hr because *emodin* is excreted into the colon after these agents are absorbed. *Emodin* may pass into breast milk. *Phenolphthalein* and *bisacodyl* are also potent stimulants of the colon. Adverse effects include abdominal cramps and the potential for atonic colon with prolonged use.

B. Bulking agents

The bulk laxatives include *hydrophilic colloids* (from indigestible parts of fruits and vegetables). They form gels in the large intestine, causing water retention and intestinal distension, thereby increasing peristaltic activity. Similar actions are produced by *agar*, *methylcellulose*, *psyllium seeds*, and *bran*. Saline cathartics such as *magnesium sulfate* and *magnesium hydroxide* are nonabsorbable salts that hold water in the intestine by osmosis, and distend the bowel, increasing intestinal activity and producing defecation in about one hour. Isosmotic electrolyte solutions containing *polyethylene glycol* are used as colonic lavage solutions to prepare the gut for radiologic or endoscopic procedures. *Lactulose* is a semisynthetic disaccharide (fructose and galactose) that also acts as an osmotic laxative.

C. Stool Softeners

Surface-active agents that become emulsified with the stool produce softer feces and ease passage. These include *docusate sodium*, *mineral oil* and *glycerin suppositories*.

Study Questions

Choose the ONE best answer

24.1 Which of the following is the most important approach in healing peptic ulcers?

A. Coating the ulcer crater
B. Eradicating infection with H. pylori
C. Inhibiting secretion of gastric acid at the proton pump
D. Blocking receptor activation of gastric acid secretion
E. Neutralizing secreted gastric acid

Correct answer = B. Eradication of H. pylori results in rapid healing of active peptic ulcers and low recurrence rates (less than 15% compared to 60 to 100% per year for patients with initial ulcers healed by traditional antisecretory thrapy).

Questions 24.2–24.7

For each numbered description below, select the most appropriate drug from the following list:

A. Granisetron
B. Ondansetron
C. Dexamethasone
D. Meclizine
E. Lorazepam
F. Metoclopramide

24.2 Given in combination regimens to enhance antiemetic potency

Correct answer = C (Dexamethasone)

24.3 Highly effective against cisplatin-induced emesis

Correct answer = A (Granisetron)

24.4 Can cause extrapyramidal side effects

Correct answer = F (Metoclopramide)

24.5 Approved for managing postoperative nausea and/or vomiting

Correct answer = B (Ondansetron)

24.6 Useful in managing nausea and vomiting due to motion sickness

Correct answer = D (Meclizine)

24.7 Low antiemetic potency

Correct answer = E (Lorazepam)

Questions 24.8–24.13

For each numbered description below, select the most appropriate drug from the following list:

A. Bismuth subsalicylate
B. Phenolphthalein
C. Docusate sodium
D. Loperamide
E. Magnesium sulfate
F. Activated attapulgite

24.8 Softens the stool

Correct answer = C (Docusate sodium)

24.9 May adsorb intestinal toxins

Correct answer = F (Activated attapulgite)

24.10 Diminishes fluid secretion in the bowel

Correct answer = A (Bismuth subsalicylate)

24.11 Irritates the gut and causes increased peristalsis

Correct answer = B (Phenolphthalein)

24.12 Retains water and produces intestinal distension

Correct answer = E (Magnesium sulfate)

24.13 Inhibits peristalsis

Correct answer = D (Loperamide)

Questions 24.14–24.17

For each numbered description below, select the most appropriate drug from the following list:

A. Lansoprazole
B. Misoprostol
C. Prostaglandin E_2
D. Sucralfate
E. Al^{+++}-containing antacids
F. Metronidazole

24.14 Approved for prevention of NSAID-induced gastric ulcers

Correct answer = B (Misoprostol)

24.15 Diminishes gastric acid production by inhibiting adenylyl cyclase

Correct answer = C (Prostaglandin E_2)

24.16 Can alter absorption of other drugs

Correct answer = E (Al^{+++}-containing antacids)

24.17 Binds to mucosa forming physical barrier to HCl and pepsin

Correct answer = D (Sucralfate)

Questions 24.18–24.22

For each numbered description below, select the most appropriate drug from the following list:

A. Sodium bicarbonate
B. Cimetidine
C. Bismuth compounds
D. Diphenoxylate
E. Dronabinol
F. Prochlorperazine

24.18 Gynecomastia

Correct answer = B (Cimetidine)

24.19 Metabolic alkalosis

Correct answer = A (Sodium bicarbonate)

24.20 Extrapyramidal symptoms

Correct answer = F (Prochlorperazine)

24.21 Dysphoria

Correct answer = E (Dronabinol)

24.22 Toxic megacolon

Correct answer = D (Diphenoxylate)

Hormones of the Pituitary and Thyroid

25

I. OVERVIEW

The neuroendocrine system, which is controlled by the pituitary and hypothalamus, coordinates body functions by transmitting messages between individual cells and tissues. The nervous system communicates locally by electrical impulses and neurotransmitters directed through neurons to other neurons or to specific target organs, such as muscle or glands. Nerve impulses generally act within milliseconds. In contrast, the endocrine system releases hormones into the blood stream, which carries these chemical messengers to target cells throughout the body. Hormones have a much broader range of response times than do nerve impulses, requiring from seconds to days or longer to cause a response that may last for weeks or months. The two regulatory systems are closely interrelated. For example, in several instances, the release of hormones is stimulated or inhibited by the nervous system, and some hormones can stimulate or inhibit nerve impulses. Chapters 25–27 in this text focus on drugs that affect the synthesis and/or secretion of specific hormones. In this chapter, the central role of the hypothalamic and pituitary hormones in regulating body functions is briefly presented. In addition, drugs affecting thyroid hormone synthesis and/or secretion are discussed (Figure 25.1).

II. HYPOTHALAMIC AND ANTERIOR PITUITARY HORMONES

The hormones secreted by the hypothalamus and the pituitary are all peptides or low molecular weight proteins that act by binding to specific receptor sites on their target tissues. The hormones of the anterior pituitary are regulated by neuropeptides, called either releasing or inhibiting factors or hormones, which are produced in cell bodies in the hypothalamus and reach the cells of the pituitary by the hypophysial portal system (Figure 25.2). The interaction of the releasing hormones with their receptors results in synthesis and release of the hormones by the pituitary into the circulation. Each hypothalamic regulatory hormone controls the release of a specific hormone from

HYPOTHALAMIC AND ANTERIOR PITUITARY HORMONES

- *Corticotropin (ACTH)*
- *Gonadotropin-releasing hormone (GnRH)*
- *Growth hormone releasing hormone (GHRH), sermorelin*
- *Luteinizing hormone-releasing hormone (LHRH), leuprolide, goserelin, nafarelin, histrelin*
- *Somatostatin, octreotide*
- *Somatotropin (GHIH), somatrem*

HORMONES OF THE POSTERIOR PITUITARY

- *Desmopressin*
- *Oxytocin*
- *Vasopressin (ADH)*

DRUGS AFFECTING THE THYROID

- *Iodide*
- *Levothyronine*
- *Methimazole*
- *Propylthiouracil*
- *Thyroxine*
- *Triiodothyronine*

Figure 25.1
Some of the hormones and drugs affecting the hypothalamus, pituitary and thyroid.

Lippincott's Illustrated Reviews: Pharmacology, Second Edition.
by Mary J. Mycek, Richard A. Harvey and Pamela C. Champe.
Lippincott Williams & Wilkins, Philadelphia, PA © 2000.

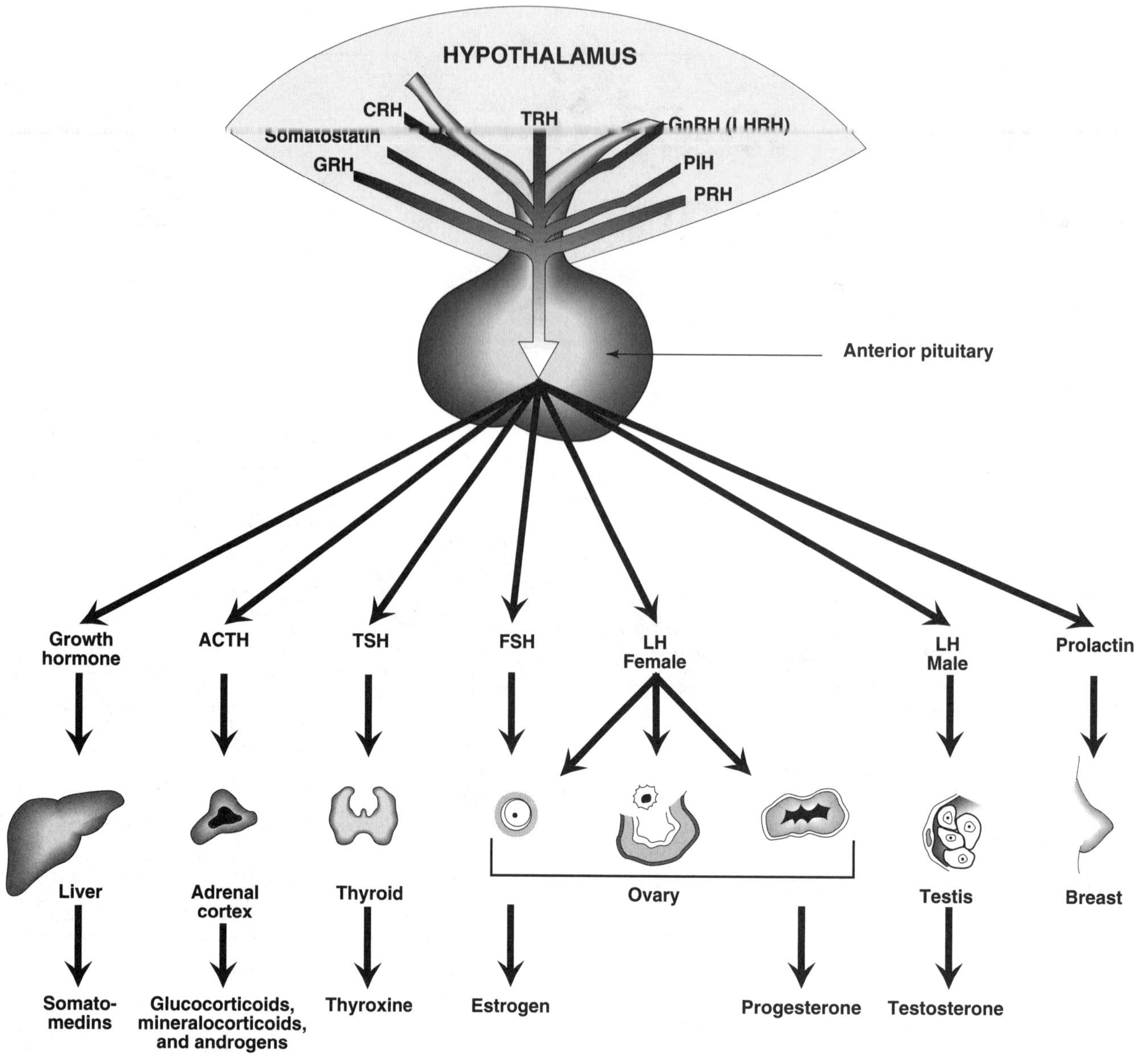

Figure 25.2
Hypothalamic-releasing hormones and actions of anterior pituitary hormones. GRH= growth hormone-releasing hormone; TRH= thyrotropin-releasing hormone; CRH= corticotropin-releasing hormone; GnRH (LHRH)=gonadotropi releasing hormone (luteinizing hormone-releasing hormone); PIH= prolactin-inhibiting hormone (dopamine); and PRH= prolactin-releasing hormone; ACTH= adrenocorticotropic hormone; TSH= thyrotropin-stimulating hormone; FSH= follicle-stimulating hormone; LH= luteinizing hormone

the anterior pituitary. The hypothalamic releasing hormones are primarily used for diagnostic purposes (that is, to determine pituitary insufficiency). [Note: The hypothalamus also synthesizes the hormones vasopressin and oxytocin, which are transported to the posterior pituitary where they are stored until released.] Although a number of pituitary hormone preparations are currently used therapeutically for specific hormonal deficiencies (examples of which follow), most of these agents have limited therapeutic applications. Hormones of the anterior and posterior pituitary are administered either intramuscularly (IM), subcutaneously (SC) or intranasally but not orally, because their peptidic nature makes them susceptible to destruction by the proteolytic enzymes of the digestive tract.

A. Adrenocorticotropic hormone (ACTH or corticotropin)

ACTH is a product of the posttranslational processing of the larger precursor polypeptide, pro-opiomelanocortin. Its target organ is the adrenal cortex where corticotropin [kor ti koe TROE pin] binds to specific receptors on the cell surfaces. The occupied receptors activate G protein-coupled processes to increase cAMP, which in turn stimulates the rate-limiting step in the adrenocorticosteroid synthetic pathway (cholesterol → pregnenolone), concluding with the synthesis and release of the adrenocorticosteroids, and the adrenal androgens (Figure 25.3). The availability of synthetic adrenocorticosteroids with specific properties (see p. 275) has limited the use of corticotropin to serving as a diagnostic tool for differentiating between primary adrenal insufficiency (Addison's disease, associated with adrenal atrophy) and secondary adrenal insufficiency (caused by inadequate secretion of ACTH by the pituitary). Therapeutic corticotropin preparations are extracts from the anterior pituitaries of domestic animals, or synthetic human ACTH. The latter, *cosyntropin* [ko sin TROE pin], is preferred for diagnosis of adrenal insufficiency. Toxicities are similar to those of glucocorticoids. Antibodies can form to ACTH derived from animal sources. [Note: The anterior pituitary is stimulated to synthesize corticotropin by corticotropin-releasing hormone (CRH), produced by the hypothalamus (see Figure 25.3). CRH is used diagnostically to differentiate between Cushing's syndrome and ectopic ACTH-producing cells.]

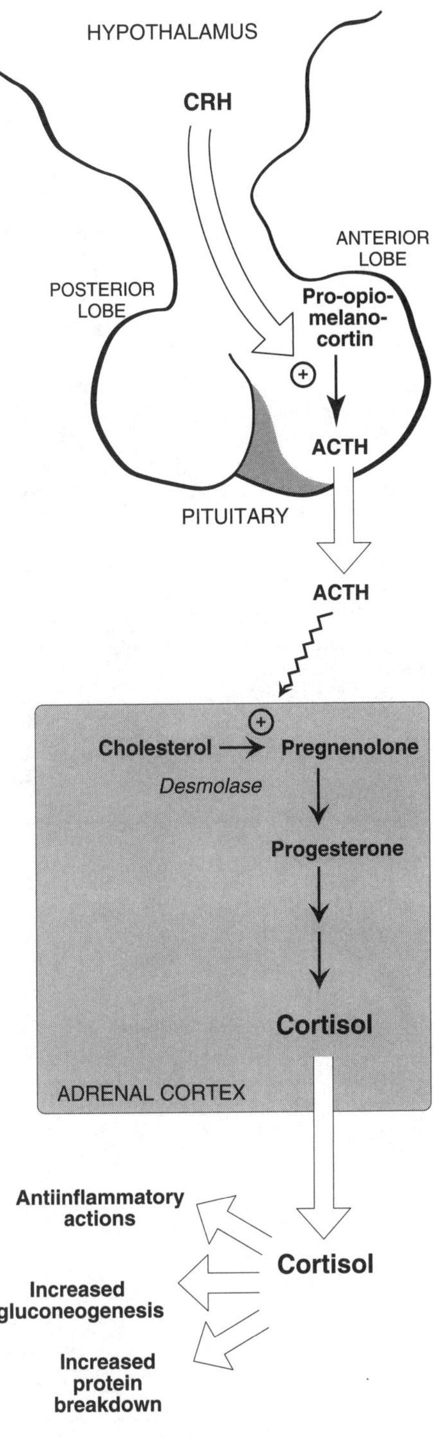

Figure 25.3
Secretion and actions of adrenocorticotropic hormone (ACTH). CRH, corticotropin-releasing hormone.

B. Growth hormone (somatotropin)

Somatotropin [soe ma tee TROE pin] is a large polypeptide, released by the anterior pituitary in response to growth hormone-releasing hormone (GHRH) produced by the hypothalamus. It is produced synthetically by recombinant DNA technology. Growth-hormone (GH) from animal sources is ineffective in humans. *Somatotropin* influences a wide variety of biochemical processes, for example, through stimulation of protein synthetic processes, cell proliferation and bone growth are promoted. Increased formation of hydroxyproline from proline also boosts cartilage synthesis Therefore, *somatotropin* is used in the treatment of growth-hormone (GH) deficiency in children. [Note: It is important to establish whether the deficit in GH is actually due to hypopituitarism, since normal thyroid status is essential to successful somatotropin therapy.] A therapeutically equivalent drug, *somatrem* [soe ma TREM], contains an extra terminal methionyl group not found in *somatotropin.* Though the half-lives of these drugs are short, about 25 minutes, they induce the release from the liver of somatomedin, the insulin-like growth factor-I (IGF-I) that is responsible for subsequent growth hormone-like actions. *Somatotropin* and *somatrem* should not be used in individuals with closed epiphyses or with an enlarging intracranial mass. [Note: Infusion of GHRH, known as *sermorelin* [ser moe REH lyn], can be used to assess the status of GH deficiency.]

C. Growth hormone-inhibiting hormone (somatostatin)

Originally isolated from the hypothalamus, *somatostatin* is a small polypeptide that is also found in neurons throughout the body, as well as in the intestine and pancreas. *Somatostatin* therefore predictably has a number of actions. *Octreotide* [awk TREE oh tide] is a synthetic octapeptide analog of *somatostatin*. It has a much longer half-life than the natural compound and has found use in the treatment of acromegaly caused by hormone-secreting tumors, and secretory diarrhea associated with tumors producing the vasoactive intestinal peptide (VIP). Adverse effects of *octreotide* treatment are flatulence, nausea, and steatorrhea.

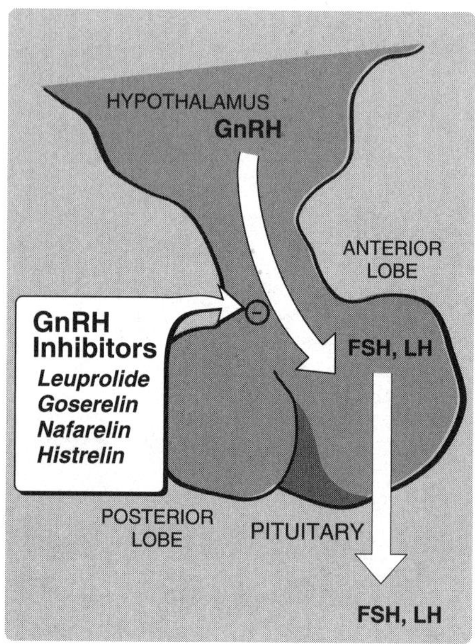

Figure 25.4
Secretion of follicle-stimulating hormone (FSH) and lutenizing hormone (LH).

D. Gonadotropin-releasing hormone (GnRH)/luteinizing hormone-releasing hormone (LHRH)

GnRH, a decapeptide obtained from the hypothalamus, controls the release of follicle-stimulating hormone (FSH) and luteinizing hormone (LH) from the pituitary. GnRH is employed to stimulate gonadal hormone production in hypogonadism. A number of synthetic analogs, such as *leuprolide* [loo PROE lide], *goserelin* [gah SER e lin], *nafarelin* [Neh FAR e lin] *and histrelin* [HIS TRE lin], act as inhibitors of *GnRH* (Figure 25.4). These are effective in suppressing production of the gonadal hormones, and thus are effective in the treatment of prostatic cancer (see p. 395), endometriosis, and precocious puberty.

E. Gonadotropins: human menopausal gonadotropin (hMG), FSH (urofolitropin), human chorionic gonadoptropin (hCG)

The gonadotropins find use in the treatment of infertility in men and women. *Meotropin* (hMG) is partially broken down *FSH* and LH and is obtained from the urine of menopausal women. The *chorionic gonadotropin* (h*CG*) is a placental hormone and an LH agonist. It is also excreted in the urine. Both these hormones are injected intramuscularly. Injection of *hMG* or *FSH* over a period of 5-12 days causes ovarian follicular growth and maturation, and with subsequent injection of *hCG*, ovulation occurs. In men who are lacking gonadoptropins, treatment with *hCG* causes external sexual maturation, and with the subsequent injection hMG spermatogenesis occurs. Adverse effects include ovarian enlargement, and possible hypovolemia. Multiple births are not uncommon. Men may develop gynecomastia.

III. HORMONES OF THE POSTERIOR PITUITARY

In contrast to the hormones of the anterior lobe of the pituitary, those of the posterior lobe, *vasopressin* and *oxytocin*, are not regulated by releasing hormones. Instead, they are synthesized in the hypothalamus, transported to the posterior pituitary and released in response to specific physiologic signals, such as high plasma osmolarity or parturition, respectively. Both are nonapeptides with a circular structure due to a disulfide bridge (Figure 25.5). Reduction of the disulfide inactivates the hormones. They are susceptible to proteolytic cleavage and thus are given parenterally. Both have very short half-lives.

A. Oxytocin

Oxytocin [ox ee TOE sin], originally extracted from animal posterior pituitaries, is now chemically synthesized. Its only use is in obstetrics, where it is employed to stimulate uterine contraction to induce or reinforce labor or to promote breast milk ejection. [Note: The sensitivity of the uterus to *oxytocin* increases with the duration of pregnancy when it is under estrogenic dominance.] To induce labor, the drug is administered intravenously. However, when used to induce "milk let-down", it is given as a nasal spray. *Oxytocin* causes milk ejection by contracting the myoepithelial cells around the mammary alveoli. Although toxicities are uncommon when the drug is used properly, hypertensive crises, uterine rupture, water retention and fetal death have been reported. Its antidiuretic and pressor activities are very much lower than those of *vasopressin*. [Note: *Oxytocin* is contraindicated in abnormal fetal presentation, fetal distress and premature births.]

B. Vasopressin

Vasopressin [vay soe PRESS in] (*antidiuretic hormone*, *ADH*), is structurally related to *oxytocin* (Figure 25.5). The chemically-synthesized nonapeptide has replaced that extracted from animal posterior pituitaries. *Vasopressin* has both antidiuretic and vasopressor effects. In the kidney it binds to the V_2 receptor to increase water permeability and resorption in the collecting tubules. Thus the major use of *vasopressin* is to treat diabetes insipidus. It also finds use in controlling bleeding due to esophageal varices or colonic diverticula. Other effects of *vasopressin* are mediated by the V_1 receptor, found in vascular smooth muscle, liver and other tissues. As might be expected the major toxicity is water intoxication and hyponatremia. Headache, bronchoconstriction and tremor also can occur. Caution must be used in treating patients with coronary artery disease, epilepsy and asthma.

C. Desmopressin

Because of the pressor properties of *vasopressin*, this compound has been modified to *desmopressin* [dez moe PRESS in] (1-desamino-8-D-arginine vasopressin). This analog is now preferred for diabetes insipidus and nocturnal enuresis because it is largely free of pressor effects and is longer-acting than *vasopressin*. *Desmopressin* is conveniently administered intranasally. However, local irritation may occur.

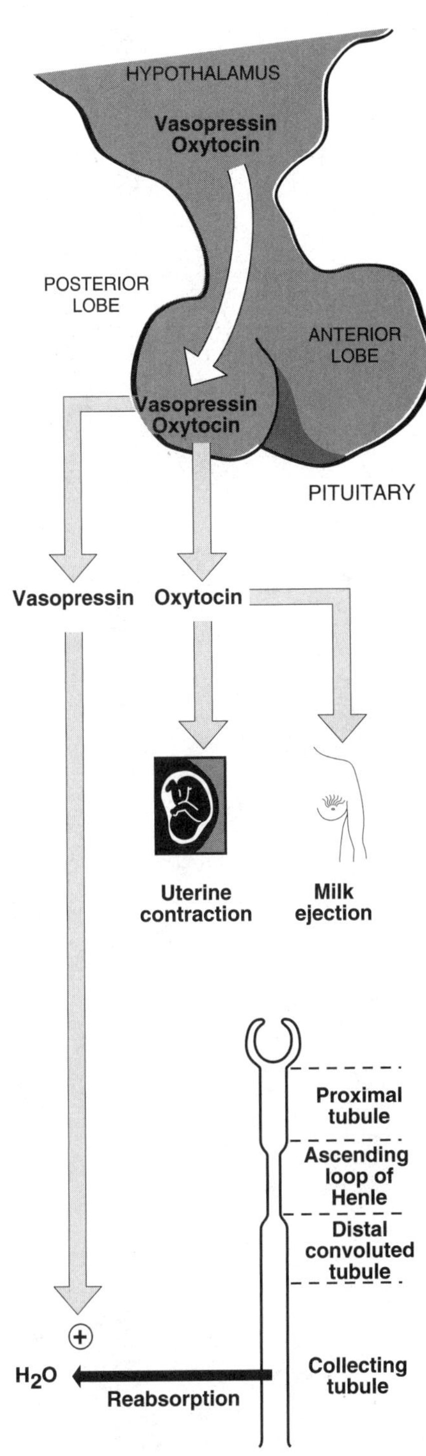

Figure 25.5
Actions of oxytocin and vasopressin.

IV. THYROID HORMONES

The thyroid gland facilitates normal growth and maturation by maintaining the level of metabolism in the tissues that is optimal for their normal function. The two major thyroid hormones are T_3 (triiodothyronine, the most active form), and T_4 (thyroxine). Although the thyroid gland is not essential for life, inadequate secretion of thyroid hormone (hypothyroidism) results in bradycardia, poor resistance to cold, and mental and physical slowing (in children this can cause mental retardation and dwarfism). If, however, an excess of thyroid hormones is

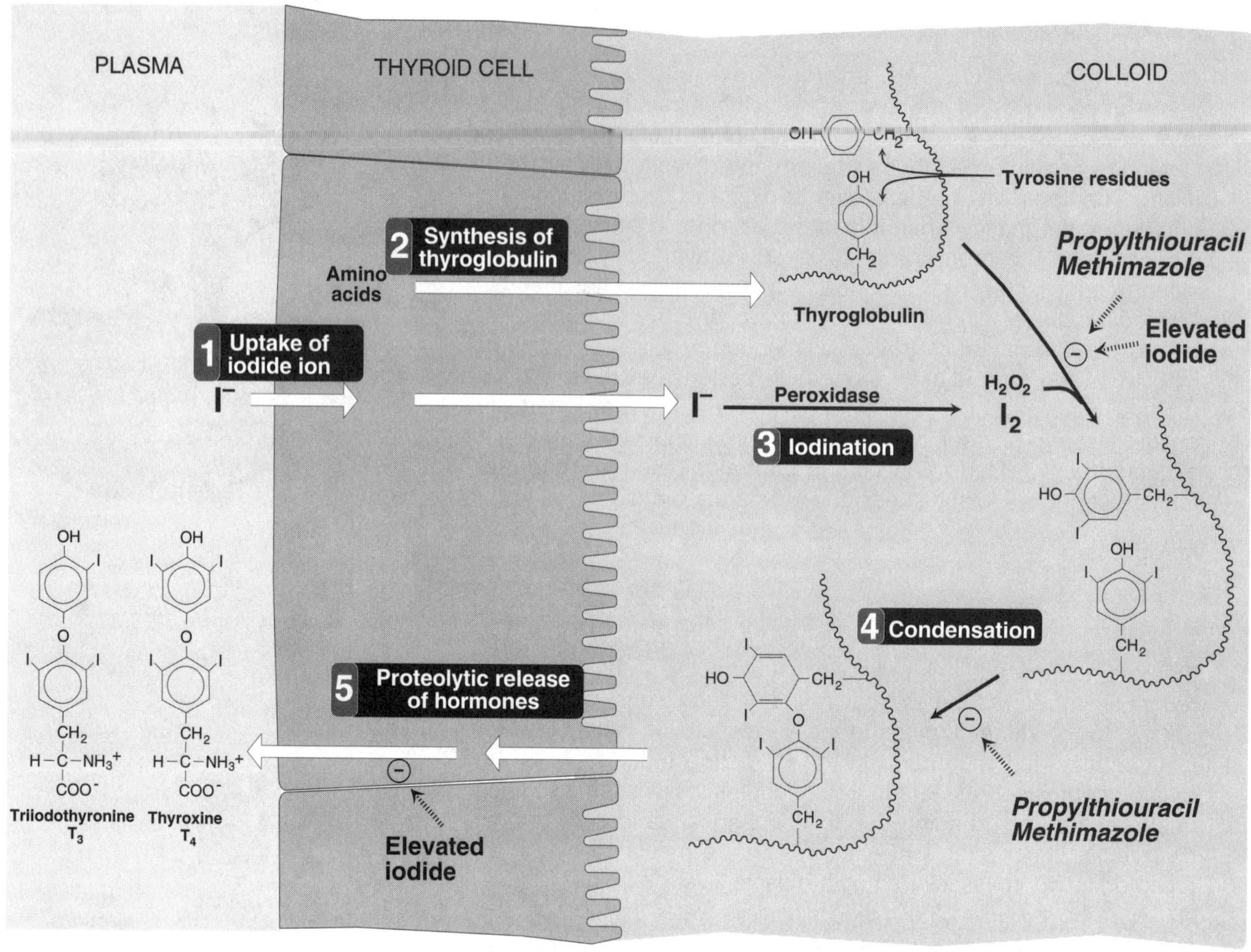

Figure 25.6
Biosynthesis of thyroid hormones.

secreted (hyperthyroidism), tachycardia and cardiac arrhythmias, body wasting, nervousness, tremor, and excess heat production can occur. In mammals, the thyroid gland also secretes the hormone calcitonin, a serum calcium-lowering hormone.

A. Thyroid hormone synthesis and secretion

The thyroid gland is made up of multiple follicles that consist of a single layer of epithelial cells surrounding a lumen filled with colloid (thyroglobulin), the storage form of thyroid hormone. A diagram of the steps in thyroid hormone synthesis and secretion is shown in Figure 25.6.

1. **Regulation of synthesis:** Thyroid function is controlled by a tropic hormone, thyrotropin-stimulating hormone (TSH, thyrotropin), a glycoprotein synthesized by the anterior pituitary (see Figure 25.2). TSH generation is governed by the hypothalamic thy-

rotropin-releasing hormone (TRH). TSH action is mediated by cAMP and leads to stimulation of iodide (I^-) uptake. Oxidation to iodine (I_2) by a peroxidase is followed by iodination of tyrosines on thyroglobulin. Condensation of two diiodotyrosine residues gives rise to T_4 or T_3 still bound to the protein. The hormones are released following proteolytic cleavage of the thyroglobulin.

2. **Regulation of secretion:** Secretion of TSH by the anterior pituitary is stimulated by the hypothalamic TRH. Feedback inhibition of both TRH and TSH secretion occurs with high levels of circulating thyroid hormone or iodide. Most of the hormone (T_3 and T_4) is bound to thyroxine-binding globulin in the plasma.

3. **Pharmacokinetics:** Both T_4 and T_3 are absorbed after oral administration. T_4 is converted to T_3 by one of two distinct deiodinases, depending on the tissue. T_3 combines with a receptor to stimulate subsequent protein synthesis necessary for normal metabolism. The hormones are metabolized through the microsomal P-450 system. Drugs such as *phenytoin*, *rifampin*, *phenobarbital*, etc. that induce the P-450 enzymes accelerate metabolism of the thyroid hormones.

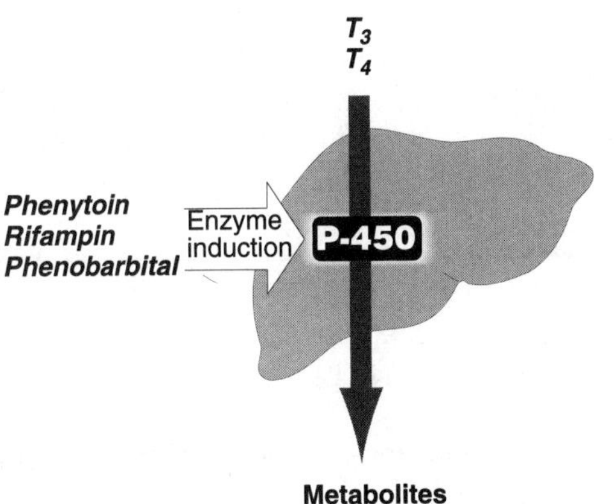

B. Treatment of hypothyroidism

Hypothyroidism is treated with *levothyroxine* (T_4). The drug is given once daily because of its long half-life. Steady state is achieved at 6-8 weeks. Toxicity is directly related to thyroxine levels and manifests itself as nervousness, heart palpitations and tachycardia, intolerance to heat and unexplained weight loss.

C. Treatment of hyperthyroidism (thyrotoxicosis)

Excessive amounts of thyroid hormones in the circulation are associated with a number of disease states, including Graves' disease, toxic adenoma, goiter, and thyroiditis, among others. The goal of therapy is to decrease synthesis and/or release of additional hormone. This can be accomplished by removing part or all of the thyroid gland, by inhibiting synthesis of the hormones, or by blocking release of the hormones from the follicle.

1. **Removal of part or all of the thyroid:** This can be accomplished either surgically or by destruction of the gland by beta particles emitted by radioactive iodine (^{131}I), which is selectively taken up by the thyroid follicular cells.

2. **Inhibition of thyroid hormone synthesis:** The thioamides, *propylthiouracil* [proe pill thye oh YOOR a sil] (*PTU*) and *methimazole* [meth IM a zole], are concentrated in the thyroid where they inhibit both the oxidative processes required for iodination of tyrosyl groups and the coupling of iodotyrosines to form T_3 and T_4 (see Figure 25.6). *PTU* can also block the conversion of T_4 to T_3. [Note: These drugs have no effect on the thyroglobulin already stored in the gland; therefore observation of any clinical effect of these drugs may be delayed until thyroglobulin stores are depleted.] The thioamides are well absorbed from the gas-

trointestinal tract, but they have short half-lives. Several doses of *PTU* are required per day, whereas a single dose of *methimazole* suffices due to the duration of its antithyroid effect. The effects of these drugs are slow in onset and thus they are not effective in the treatment of thyroid storm. Relatively rare adverse effects include agranulocytosis, rash, and edema.

3. **Propranolol:** β-Blockers are effective in blunting the widespread sympathetic stimulation that occurs in hyperthyroidism (see p. 75).

4. **Blockade of hormone release:** A pharmacologic dose of *iodide* inhibits the iodination of tyrosines, thus decreasing the supply of stored thyroglobulin. *Iodide* also inhibits thyroid hormone release by mechanisms not yet understood. Today, *iodide* is rarely used as sole therapy. However, it is employed to treat potentially fatal thyrotoxic crisis (thyroid storm), or prior to surgery, since it decreases the vascularity of the thyroid gland. *Iodide* is not useful for long-term therapy, because the thyroid ceases to respond to the drug after a few weeks. *Iodide* is administered orally. Adverse effects are relatively minor and include sore mouth and throat, rashes, ulcerations of mucous membranes, and a metallic taste in the mouth.

Study Questions

Choose the ONE best answer.

25.1 Symptoms of hyperthyroidism include all of following EXCEPT:

A. tachycardia.
B. nervousness.
C. poor resistance to cold.
D. body wasting.
E. tremor.

Correct choice = C. An individual with hyperthyroidism often experiences excess heat production.

25.2 Which of the following best describes the effect of propylthiouracil on thyroid hormone production?

A. It blocks the release of thyrotropin-releasing hormone.
B. It inhibits uptake of iodide by thyroid cells.
C. It prevents the release of thyroid hormone from thyroglobulin.
D. It blocks iodination and coupling of tyrosines in thyroglobulin to form thyroid hormones.
E. It blocks the release of hormones from the thyroid gland.

Correct answer = D. Propylthiouracil blocks the synthesis of the thyroid hormones, but does not affect the uptake of iodide, proteolytic cleavage of thyroglobulin, or the release of hormones from the thyroid gland. The thyroid hormones inhibit the secretion of thyroid-stimulating hormone from the anterior pituitary.

25.3 Hyperthyroidism can be treated by all but which one of the following?

A. Triiodothyronine
B. Surgical removal of the thyroid gland
C. Iodide
D. Propylthiouracil
E. Methimazole

Correct answer = A. Triiodothyronine is a thyroid hormone that is overproduced in hyperthyroidism.

Insulin and Oral Hypoglycemic Drugs

26

I. OVERVIEW

The pancreas is both an endocrine gland that produces the peptide hormones *insulin*, glucagon and somatostatin, and an exocrine gland that produces digestive enzymes. The peptide hormones are secreted from cells located in the islets of Langerhans (β- or B-cells produce *insulin*, α_2- or A-cells produce glucagon, and α_1- or D-cells produce somatostatin). These hormones play an important role in regulating the metabolic activities of the body, and in doing so, help maintain the homeostasis of blood glucose.[1] Hyperinsulinemia (due, for example, to an insulinoma) can cause severe hypoglycemia. More commonly, a relative or absolute lack of *insulin* (such as in diabetes mellitus) can cause serious hyperglycemia. Administration of *insulin* preparations or hypoglycemic agents (Figure 26.1) can prevent morbidity and reduce mortality associated with diabetes.

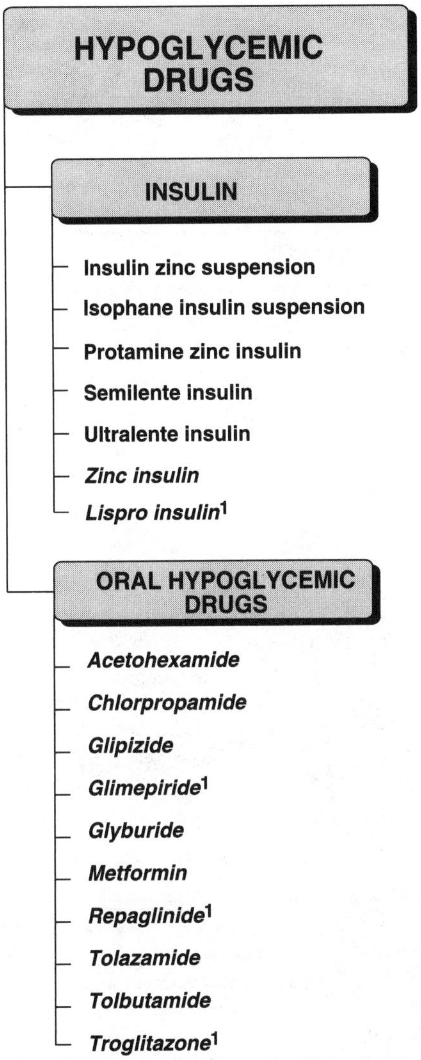

II. DIABETES MELLITUS

Diabetes is not a single disease. Instead, it is a heterogeneous group of syndromes all characterized by an elevation of blood glucose caused by a relative or absolute deficiency of *insulin*. Frequently the inadequate release of *insulin* is aggravated by an excess of glucagon. Diabetes afflicts about 10 million individuals or about 5% of the population of the United States, and is the eighth leading cause of death in this country. Diabetics can be divided into two groups based on their requirements for *insulin: insulin*-dependent diabetes mellitus (IDDM or Type I) and non-*insulin*-dependent diabetes mellitus (NIDDM or Type II).[2] About one to two million patients have IDDM; the remaining 80 to 90% of diabetic patients have NIDDM. Figure 26.2 summarizes the characteristics of Types I and II diabetes.

HYPOGLYCEMIC DRUGS

INSULIN

- **Insulin zinc suspension**
- **Isophane insulin suspension**
- **Protamine zinc insulin**
- **Semilente insulin**
- **Ultralente insulin**
- ***Zinc insulin***
- ***Lispro insulin***[1]

ORAL HYPOGLYCEMIC DRUGS

- ***Acetohexamide***
- ***Chlorpropamide***
- ***Glipizide***
- ***Glimepiride***[1]
- ***Glyburide***
- ***Metformin***
- ***Repaglinide***[1]
- ***Tolazamide***
- ***Tolbutamide***
- ***Troglitazone***[1]

Figure 26.1
Summary of hypoglycemic agents.
[1]Described in Pharmacology update, pp. 452-454

[1,2]See p. 262 for Infolink references to other books in this series.

Lippincott's Illustrated Reviews: Pharmacology, Second Edition.
by Mary J. Mycek, Richard A. Harvey and Pamela C. Champe.
Lippincott Williams & Wilkins, Philadelphia, PA © 2000.

	Insulin-dependent diabetes	Non-insulin-dependent diabetes
Age of onset	Usually during childhood or puberty	Frequently over age 35
Nutritional status at time of onset of disease	Frequently undernourished	Obesity usually present
Prevalence	10-20% of diagnosed diabetics	80-90% of diagnosed diabetics
Genetic predisposition	Moderate	Very strong
Defect or deficiency	β cells destroyed eliminating production of insulin	Inability of β-cells to produce appropriate quantities of insulin; insulin resistance; other unknown defects

Figure 26.2
Comparison of insulin-dependent diabetes and non-insulin-dependent diabetes.

A. Type I diabetes (insulin-dependent diabetes mellitus, IDDM)

Insulin-dependent diabetes most commonly afflicts juveniles, but IDDM can also occur among adults (Figure 26.2). The disease is characterized by an absolute deficiency of *insulin* caused by massive β-cell lesions or necrosis. Loss of β-cell function may be due to invasion by viruses, the action of chemical toxins, or usually, through the actions of autoimmune antibodies directed against the β-cell. As a result of the destruction of β-cells, the pancreas fails to respond to ingestion of glucose, and the Type I diabetic shows classic symptoms of *insulin* deficiency (polydipsia, polyphagia and polyuria). Type I diabetics require exogenous *insulin* to avoid hyperglycemia and life-threatening ketoacidosis.

1. **Cause of Type I diabetes:** A burst of *insulin* secretion normally occurs after ingestion of a meal in response to transient increases in the levels of circulating glucose and amino acids. In the postabsorptive period, low, basal levels of circulating *insulin* are maintained through β-cell secretion. However, the Type I diabetic has virtually no functional β-cells, and can neither respond to variations in circulating fuels nor maintain even a basal secretion level of *insulin* (Figure 26.3). The development and progression of neuropathy, nephropathy and retinopathy are directly related to the extent of glycemic control (most often measured as blood levels of hemoglobin A_{1C}).[3]

2. **Treatment of Type I diabetes:** A Type I diabetic must rely on exogenous (injected) *insulin* in order to control hyperglycemia, maintain acceptable levels of glycosylated hemoglobin (HbA_{1c}), and avoid ketoacidosis. [Note: The rate of formation of HbA_{1C} is proportional to the average blood glucose concentration over the previous several months; thus, HbA_{1C} provides a measure of how well treatment has normalized blood glucose in diabetics.] The goal in administering *insulin* to Type I diabetics is to maintain blood glucose concentrations as close to normal as possible and to avoid wide swings in blood glucose levels that may contribute to long-term complications. The use of portable blood glucose analyzers facilitates close self-monitoring and treatment.

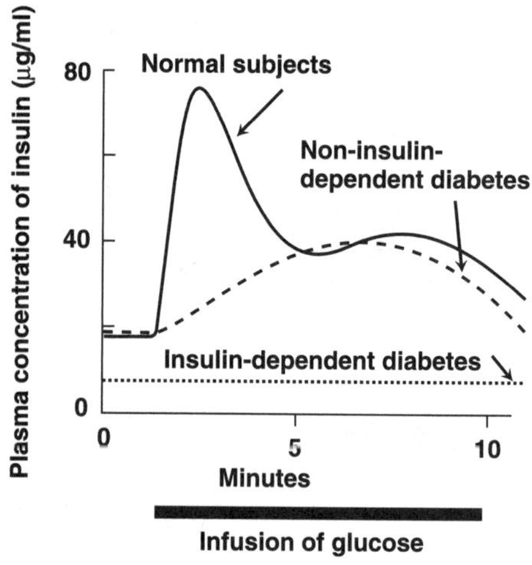

Figure 26.3
Release of insulin that occurs in response to constant infusion of glucose in normal subjects and in diabetic patients.

B. Type II diabetes (non-insulin-dependent diabetes mellitus, NIDDM)

Most diabetics are in this category. Genetic factors rather than viruses or autoimmune antibodies are apparently causal. The metabolic alterations observed are milder than those described for IDDM (for example, NIDDM patients typically are not ketotic), but the long-term clinical consequences can be just as devastating (for example, vascular complications and subsequent infection can lead to amputation of the lower limbs).

1. **Cause of Type II diabetes:** In NIDDM, the pancreas retains some β-cell function, resulting in variable *insulin* levels that are insufficient to maintain glucose homeostasis (see Figure 26.3).

[3]See p. 262 for Infolink references to other books in this series.

Patients with Type II diabetes are often obese. Type II diabetes is frequently accompanied by target organ *insulin* resistance that limits responsiveness to both endogenous and exogenous *insulin*. In some cases, *insulin* resistance is due to a decreased number or mutations of *insulin* receptors. However, an as yet undefined defect in the events that occur after *insulin* binds to its receptor is believed to account for resistance in most patients.

2. **Treatment of Type II diabetes:** The goal in treating Type II diabetes is to maintain blood glucose concentrations within normal limits and to prevent the development of long-term complications of the disease. Weight reduction, exercise and dietary modification decrease *insulin* resistance and correct the hyperglycemia of Type II diabetes in some patients. However, most are dependent on pharmacologic intervention with oral hypoglycemic agents (Figure 26.4). *Insulin* therapy may be required to achieve satisfactory serum glucose levels. [Note: See Figure 26.2 for a summary comparison of Type I and Type II diabetes mellitus.]

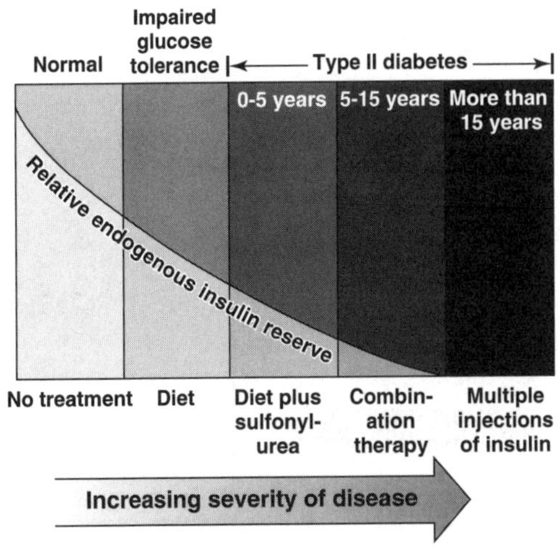

Figure 26.4
Duration of non-insulin-dependent (type II) diabetes mellitus, sufficiency of endogenous insulin, and recommended sequence of therapy.

III. INSULIN

Insulin [IN suh lin] is a small protein consisting of two polypeptide chains that are connected by disulfide bonds. It is synthesized as a precursor protein (pro-*insulin*) that undergoes proteolytic cleavage to form *insulin* and peptide C, both of which are secreted by the β-cells of the pancreas.[4] [Note: Normal individuals secrete less pro-*insulin* than *insulin*, whereas NIDDM patients secrete high levels of the prohormone. Since radioimmunoassays do not distinguish between the two *insulin* types, NIDDM patients may have lower levels of the active hormone than the assay indicates. Thus measurement of circulating C peptide provides a better index of *insulin* levels.]

A. Insulin secretion

Insulin secretion is regulated not only by blood glucose levels but also by other hormones and autonomic mediators. Secretion is most commonly triggered by high blood glucose which is taken up and phosphorylated in the β-cells of the pancreas. Adenosine triphosphate (ATP) levels rise and block K^+ channels, leading to membrane depolarization and an influx of Ca^{++}, which causes pulsatile *insulin* exocytosis. [Note: Glucose given by injection has a lower effect on *insulin* secretion than does glucose taken orally, because orally taken glucose stimulates production of digestive hormones by the gut, which in turn stimulate *insulin* secretion by the pancreas.]

B. Sources of insulin

Insulin is isolated from beef and pork pancreas. However, *human insulin* is replacing the animal hormone for therapy. *Human insulin* is produced by a special strain of Escherichia coli that has been genetically altered to contain the gene for *human insulin*. *Pork insulin* is closest in structure to *human insulin*, differing by only one amino acid.

[4]See p. 262 for Infolink references to other books in this series.

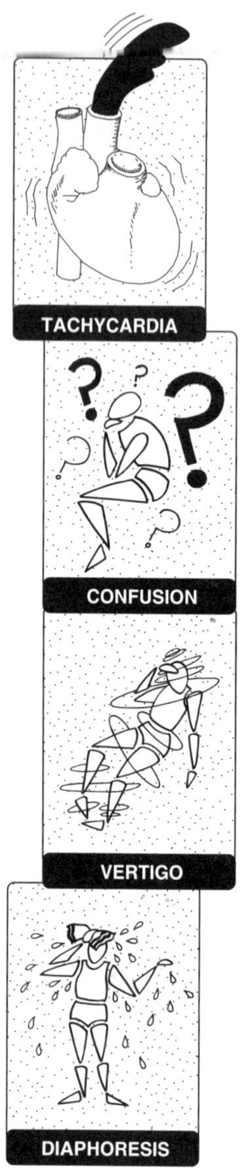

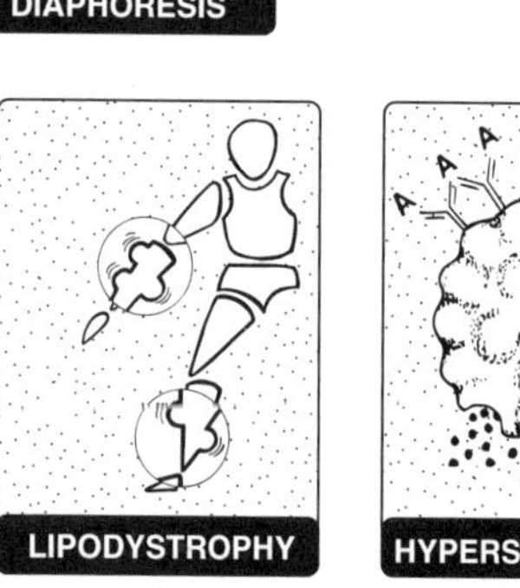

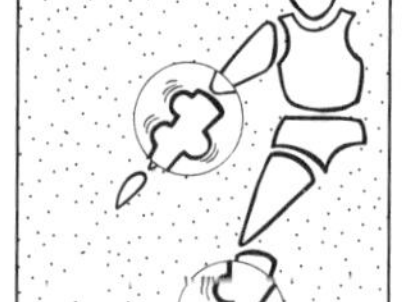

Figure 26.5
Adverse effects observed with *insulin*; Note: lipodystrophy is a local atrophy or hypertrophy of subcutaneous fatty tissue at the site of injections.

C. Insulin administration

Because *insulin* is a protein, it is degraded in the gastrointestinal tract if taken orally. It is therefore generally administered by subcutaneous injection. [Note: In a hyperglycemic emergency, regular *insulin* is injected intravenously.] *Insulin* is inactivated by the reducing enzyme, *insulin*ase, found mainly in the liver and kidney. *Insulin* preparations vary primarily in their times of onset of activity and duration of activity. This is due in large part to the size and composition of the *insulin* crystals in the preparations. [Note: The less soluble an *insulin* preparation is, the longer it acts.] Dose, site of injection, blood supply, temperature and physical activity can affect the duration of action of the various preparations. *Human insulin* is absorbed more quickly from its site of injection than are the beef or pork hormones. Thus, the duration of action of *human insulin* is shorter, and doses must be adjusted accordingly.

D. Adverse reactions to insulin

The symptoms of hypoglycemia are the most serious and common adverse reactions to an overdose of *insulin* (Figure 26.5). Long-term diabetics often do not produce adequate amounts of the counterregulatory hormones (glucagon, epinephrine, cortisol, and growth hormone) that normally provide an effective defense against hypoglycemia. Other adverse reactions include lipodystrophy and allergic reactions. [Note: β-Blockers (p. 74) cause hypoglycemia. Because they inhibit the adrenergic physiologic symptoms of hypoglycemia, except for sweating, these drugs can mask the onset of *insulin* coma.]

IV. INSULIN PREPARATIONS

Most of the *insulin*s derived from beef and pork have been largely replaced by the human form synthesized utilizing recombinant DNA technology.

A. Rapid action insulin preparations

Regular *insulin* is a short-acting soluble crystalline zinc *insulin*. It is usually given subcutaneously (or intravenously in emergencies) and lowers blood sugar within minutes (Figure 26.6). It is the only *insulin* preparation suitable for intravenous administration. The buffered form is used in external *insulin* pumps. Both human recombinant and animal source *insulin* are availble in this form. A new type of insulin, which contains a modification in the amino acid sequence of naturally occuring insulin, has recently been approved. This insulin acts faster than regular insulin.

B. Intermediate action insulin preparations

1. **Semilente insulin suspension:** This *insulin* is an amorphous precipitate of *insulin* with zinc ion in acetate buffer that is not suitable for intravenous administration. Its onset of actions and peak effect are rapid, but somewhat slower than for regular *insulin*.

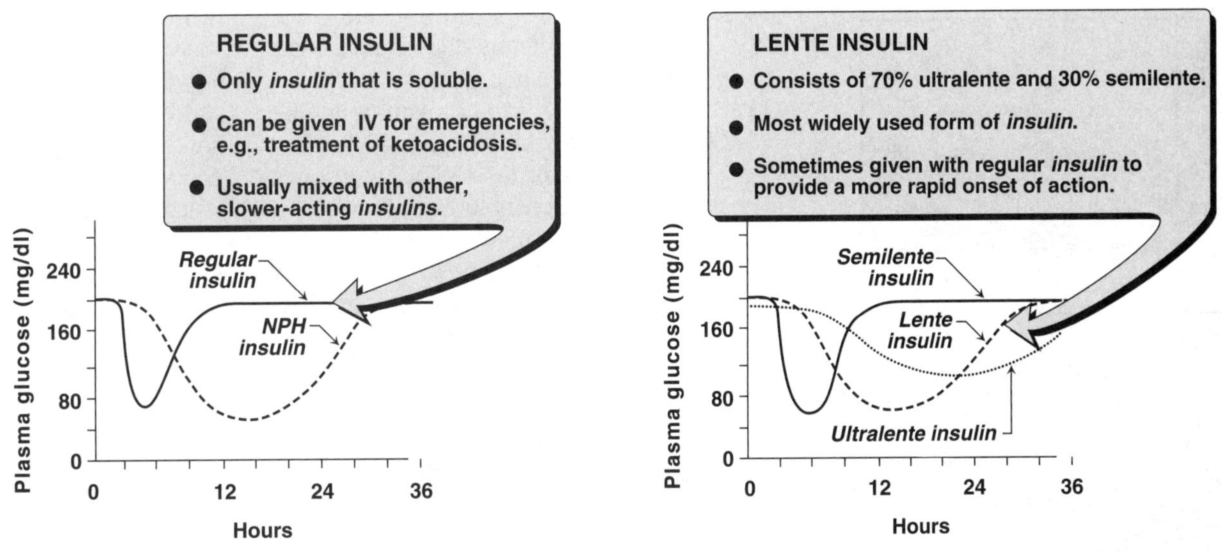

Figure 26.6
Extent and duration of action of various types of *insulin* (in a fasting diabetic). NPH= neutral protamine Hagedorn.

2. **Isophane insulin suspension:** This *insulin*, sometimes called neutral protamine Hagedorn, *NPH*, is a suspension of *crystalline zinc insulin* combined at neutral pH with the positively charged polypeptide, protamine. Its duration of action is intermediate. This is due to delayed absorption of the *insulin* because of conjugation of the *insulin* with protamine to form a less soluble complex. The *NPH* should only be given subcutaneously (never IV), and is useful in treating all forms of diabetes except diabetic ketoacidosis or emergency hyperglycemia.

3. **Lente insulin:** This *insulin* is a mixture of 30% semilente *insulin* (prompt acting) and 70% ultralente *insulin* (prolonged acting). This combination provides a relatively rapid absorption, with a sustained action making lente *insulin* the most widely used of the lente series of *insulins.* It is given only subcutaneously.

4. **Insulin combinations:** Combinations of human *insulin*s such as 70% isophane + 30% regular, or 50% of each of these are also available.

C. Prolonged action insulin preparations

Ultralente *insulin* is a suspension zinc *insulin* (porcine or human) crystals in acetate buffer that is composed of large particles which are slow to dissolve, producing a slow onset of action and a long-lasting hypoglycemic effect.

D. Standard treatment vs. intensive treatment:

Standard treatment of patients with diabetes mellitus involves injection of *insulin* twice daily resulting in mean blood glucose levels in the range of 225 to 275 mg/dL, with HbA_{1C} of 8 to 9% of total hemoglobin. In contrast, intensive treatment seeks to normal-

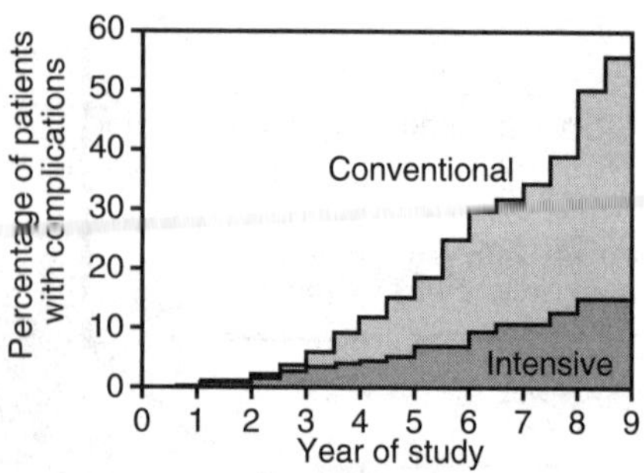

Figure 26.7
Effect of standard and intensive care on the long-term complications of diabetes.

ize blood glucose through more frequent injections of *insulin* (three or more times daily in response to monitoring blood glucose levels). Mean blood glucose levels of 150 mg/dL can be achieved, with an HbA_{1C} of approximately 7% of total hemoglobin. [Note: Normal mean blood glucose is approximately 110 mg/dL, and HbA_{1C} is 6% or less.] Thus, total normalization of blood glucose levels is not achieved even in intensively treated diabetic patients. Nonetheless, patients on intensive therapy show a 60% reduction in the long-term complications of diabetes—retinopathy, nephropathy, and neuropathy—compared to patients receiving standard care (Figure 26.7). However, the frequency of hypoglycemic episodes, coma, and seizures due to excessive *insulin* is particularly high with intensive treatment regimens .

See p. 452 for a description of the newly approved drug, *lispro insulin.*

V. ORAL HYPOGLYCEMIC AGENTS

These agents are useful in the treatment of patients who have non-*insulin*-dependent diabetes (NIDDM) but cannot be managed by diet alone. The patient most likely to respond well to oral hypoglycemic agents is one who develops diabetes after age 40 and has had diabetes less than 5 years. Patients with long-standing disease may require a combination of a hypoglycemic drug and *insulin* to control their hyperglycemia. Oral hypoglycemic agents should not be given to patients with Type I diabetes. Figure 26.8 summarizes some of the interactions of oral hypoglycemic agents with other drugs.

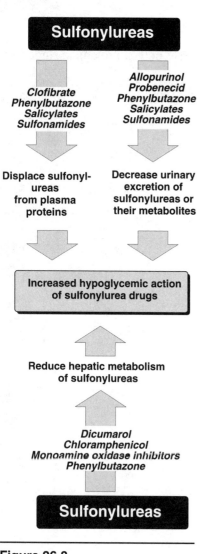

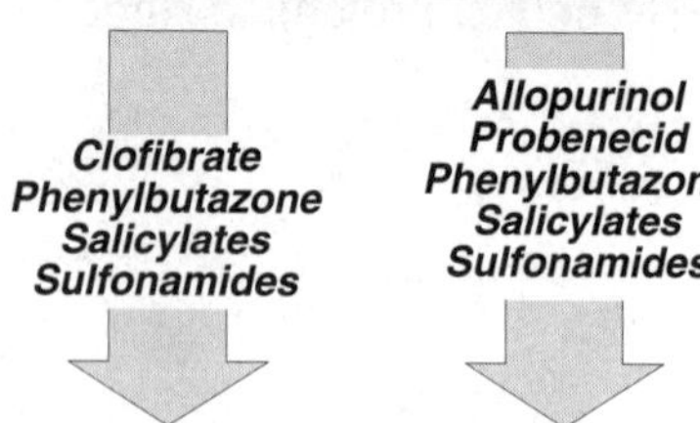

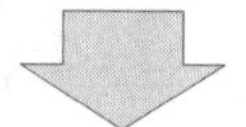

Increased hypoglycemic action of sulfonylurea drugs

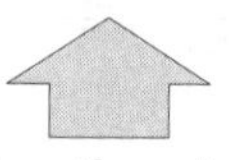

Reduce hepatic metabolism of sulfonylureas

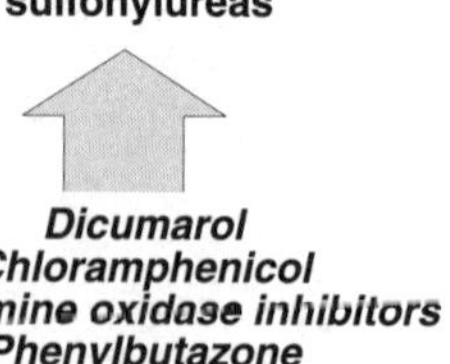

Figure 26.8
Drugs interacting with sulfonylurea drugs.

A. Sulfonylureas

The mechanisms of action of the sulfonylureas include: (1) stimulation of *insulin* release from the β-cells of the pancreas, (2) reduction of serum glucagon levels, and (3) increased binding of *insulin* to target tissues and receptors. The primary drugs used today are *tolbutamide* [tole BYOO ta mide], and the second generation derivatives, *glyburide* [GLYE byoor ide] and *glipizide* [GLIP i zide]. Given orally, they bind to serum proteins, are metabolized by the liver, and are excreted by the liver or kidney. These drugs are contraindicated in patients with hepatic or renal insufficiency, because delayed excretion of the drug, resulting in its accumulation, may cause hypoglycemia. Renal impairment is a particular problem in the case of those agents that are metabolized to active compounds. The sulfonylureas traverse the placenta and can deplete *insulin* from the fetal pancreas; therefore the NIDDM pregnant women should be treated with *insulin*. [Note: *Acetohexamide* [a seat oh HEX a mide], and *tolazamide* [tole AZ a mide] are rarely used today. *Chlorpropamide* [klor PROE pa mide] should be avoided in the elderly. Its effects are very long lasting and it has the highest incidence of side effects in this drug group, causing hyponatremia, hypoglycemia, and if taken with alcohol, a disulfiram reaction (see p. 96) and hypotension.] Figure 26.9 summarizes some properties of the hypoglycemic drugs and Figure 26.10 illustrates some of the common adverse effects of these agents.

B. Biguanides

Metformin [MET for min] is now available in the United States. A biguanide, it differs from the sulfonylureas in not stimulating *insulin* secretion. The risk of hypoglycemia is less than with sulfonylurea agents. *Metformin* may be used alone or in combination with the sulfonylureas. *Metformin* acts primarily by decreasing hepatic glucose output, largely by inhibiting gluconeogenesis. A very important property is its ability to reduce hyperlipidemia (LDL and VLDL cholesterol concentrations fall and HDL cholesterol rises). The patient often loses weight. *Metformin* is considered by some experts as the drug of choice in newly diagnosed Type II diabetics. *Metformin* is well absorbed orally, is not bound to serum proteins and is not metabolized. Excretion is via the urine. Adverse effects are largely gastrointestinal. Rarely, potentially fatal lactic acidosis has occurred. [Note: *Phenformin*, a previous biguanide hypoglycemic agent, was withdrawn for this reason.] Long term use may interfere with B_{12} absorption. The drug is contraindicated in renal and hepatic insufficiency.

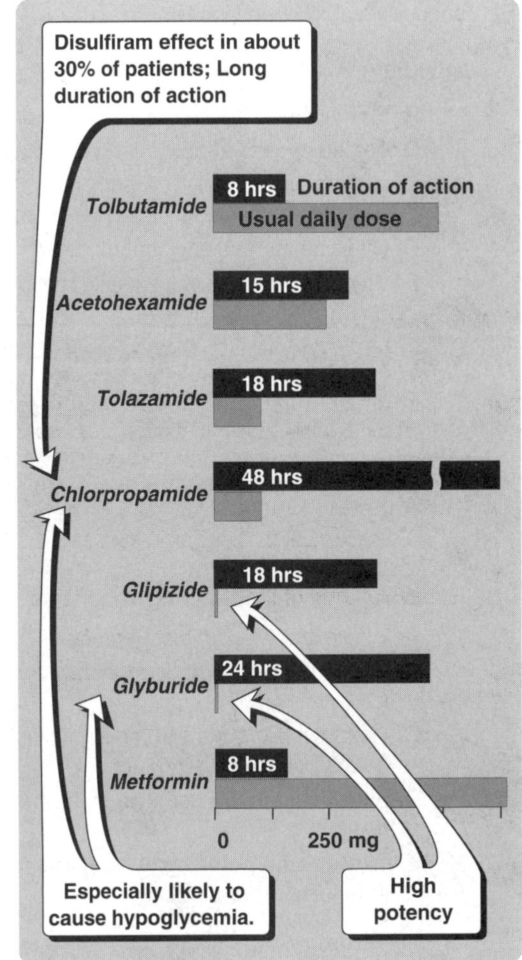

Figure 26.9
Summary of the properties of oral hypoglycemic agents.

C. α-Glucosidase inhibitor

Recently, *acarbose* [ay KAR bose] has been approved as an orally active drug for the treatment of patients with NIDDM and as a possible adjunct to *insulin* for those with IDDM. *Acarbose* inhibits α-glucosidase in the intestinal brush border and thus decreases the absorption of starch and disaccharides. Consequently the postprandial rise of blood glucose is blunted. Unlike the other oral hypoglycemic agents, *acarbose* does not stimulate *insulin* release from the pancreas nor does it increase *insulin* action in peripheral tissues. Thus *acarbose* does not cause hypoglycemia. The drug can be used as monotherapy in those patients being controlled by diet or in combination with oral hypoglycemic agents, or with *insulin*. It is poorly absorbed and its major side effects are flatulence, diarrhea, and abdominal cramping.

See pp. 452-453 for a description of the newly approved hypoglycemic drugs, *glimepiride*, *repaglinide* and *troglitazone*.

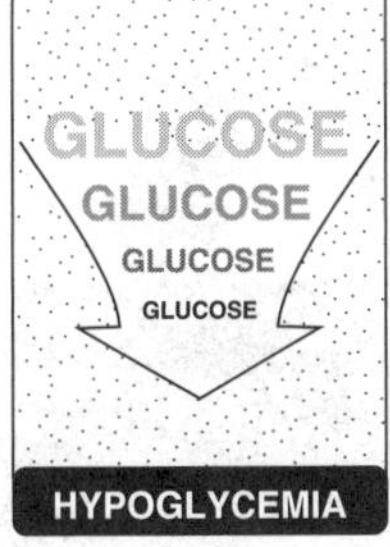

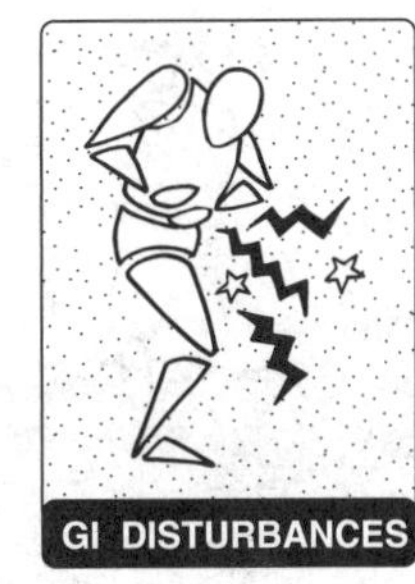

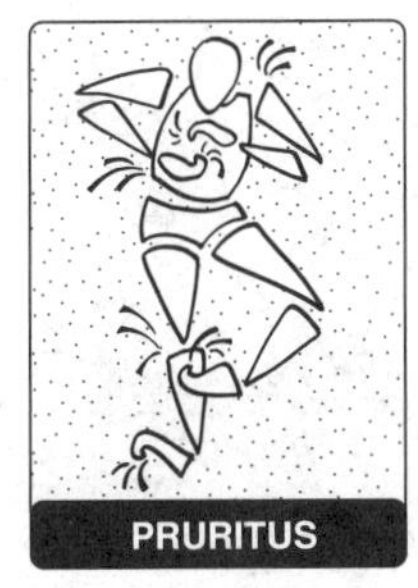

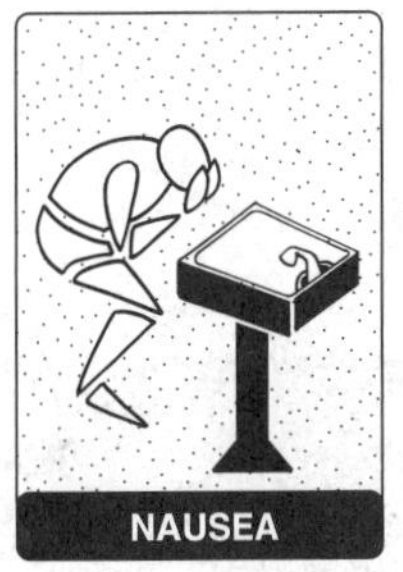

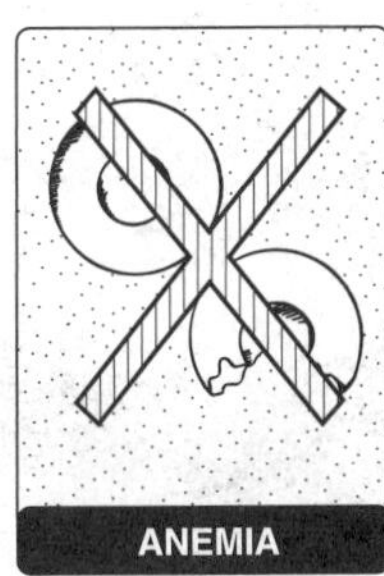

Figure 26.10
Summary of the adverse effects observed with oral hypoglycemic agents.

Choose the ONE best answer.

26.1 Which one of the following statements is correct?

A. Sulfonylureas decrease the secretion of insulin.
B. Tolbutamide is effective in Type I diabetics.
C. Sulfonylureas increase both the release of insulin and the insulin-sensitivity of target tissue.
D. Glipizide increases glucagon secretion.
E. Chlorpropamide blocks insulin receptors.

Correct answer = C. Sulfonylureas increase both insulin release and target tissue sensitivity. Sulfonylureas cannot act to increase insulin secretion in Type I diabetics because these individuals have no β-cell function. Oral hypoglycemic agents often cause a decrease in glucagon release.

26.2 Which one of the following statements is correct?

A. Insulin can be administered orally.
B. Insulin is always required therapy in Type II diabetics.
C. Protamine is added to insulin to decrease the rate of absorption of the hormone.
D. Sulfonylureas are useful in the treatment of ketoacidosis.
E. Insulin acts by binding to receptors in the nucleus of target tissue.

Correct answer = C. Protamine complexes with insulin to form an insoluble complex that is slowly absorbed. Insulin is not administered orally because it is destroyed by proteases in the GI tract. Diet therapy and/or sulfonylureas are often effective without additional insulin in the therapy of Type II diabetics. Ketoacidosis is the most life-threatening consequence of Type I diabetics and requires adequate treatment with insulin, not sulfonylureas. Insulin acts by binding to specific receptors in the cell membrane, not in the nucleus.

26.3 All of the following are correct EXCEPT:

A. One of the most common side effects of oral hypoglycemic agents is gastrointestinal disturbance.
B. The most serious consequence of insulin overdose is hypoglycemia.
C. Weight reduction is often of therapeutic help in obese Type II diabetics.
D. Sulfonylureas are contraindicated in patients with hepatic insufficiency.
E. Insulin and glucagon have similar effects on metabolism.

Correct choice = E. Insulin and glucagon have opposite effects on metabolism. The other statements are correct.

26.4 A female patient with non-insulin-dependent diabetes has been maintained on an oral sulfonylurea hypoglycemic agent. She becomes pregnant. The doctor switches her to insulin. This is necessary for all of the following reasons EXCEPT:

A. Sulfonylureas can traverse the placenta and act on the islet cells of the pancreas of the fetus to deplete them of insulin.
B. Sulfonylureas may provoke pregnancy-induced hypertension.
C. Insulin does not pass through the placenta.
D. There is a greater demand for insulin in pregnancy than can be provided by sulfonylureas.

The correct answer= B In pregnancy, not only is the mother being treated with a drug but so is the fetus. In this case, it is important that the islet cells of the fetal pancreas not be affected by the sulfonylurea, otherwise the infant is born hypoglycemic. Sulfonylureas have no effect on blood pressure. The fact that insulin does not pass through the placenta allows the fetus to develop normally. With the growth of the fetus, there are greater demands on all body processes and thus an increased demand on insulin.

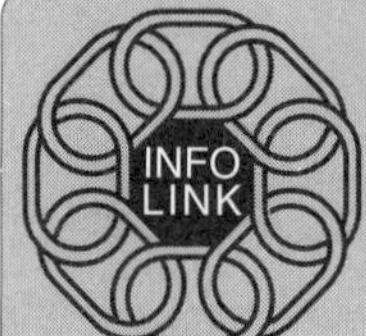

[1]See p. 269 in **Biochemistry** (2nd ed.) for a discussion of hormonal regulation of metabolism.

[2]See p. 295 in **Biochemistry** (2nd ed.) for a discussion of Type I and Type II diabetes.

[3]See p. 34 in **Biochemistry** (2nd ed.) for a discussion of hemoglobin A_{1c}.

[4]See p. 270 in **Biochemistry** (2nd ed.) for a discussion of biosynthesis of insulin.

Steroid Hormones

27

I. OVERVIEW

Steroid hormones include the sex hormones (androgens, progestins and estrogens), and the hormones of the adrenal cortex. Sex hormones produced by the gonads and adrenals are necessary for conception, embryonic maturation, and development of primary and secondary sexual characteristics at puberty. The gonadal hormones are used therapeutically in replacement therapy and, in the case of estrogen, for contraception and osteoporosis. The adrenal cortex produces two major classes of steroid hormones: the adrenocorticosteroids (glucocorticoids and mineralocorticoids) and the adrenal androgens. Their synthesis is stimulated by corticotropin (previously called adrenocorticotropic hormone, ACTH, see p. 247). Hormones of the adrenal cortex are used in replacement therapy, in the treatment and management of inflammatory diseases such as rheumatoid arthritis, in the treatment of severe allergic reactions, and in the treatment of some cancers (see p. 393). Inhibitors of adrenal cortical steroids are used to treat hormonal dysfunctions in which these compounds are produced in excess. Figure 27.1 lists the steroid hormones referred to in this chapter.

II. ESTROGENS

Estradiol [ess tra DYE ole] is the most potent estrogen produced by women; the other major estrogens, *estrone* [ESS trone] and *estriol* [essTRI ole], have about one tenth the potency of estradiol. These naturally occurring steroids are subject to a large first-pass hepatic metabolism and when admistered orally show low bioavailability. PREMARIN—a preparation of conjugated estrogens (contains sulfate esters of *estrone* and *equilin*) obtained from pregnant mare's urine—is a widely used oral preparation. Synthetic estrogens, for example, *ethinyl estradiol* [ETH eye nil ess tra DYE ole], undergo less first-pass metabolism and thus are effective when administered orally at lower doses. Synthetic nonsteroidal compounds with estrogenic activity, for example, *diethylstilbestrol* [dye eth il stil BESS trol] [*DES*], *quinestrol* [kwin ESS trole], *chlorotrianisene* [klor oh trye AN i seen] and others, are used clinically.

STEROID HORMONES

ESTROGENS
- *Chlorotrianisene*
- *Diethylstilbestrol*
- *Estradiol*
- *Estriol*
- *Estrone*
- *Ethinyl estradiol*
- *Mestranol*
- *Quinestrol*

SELECTIVE ESTROGEN MODULATORS
- *Raloxifene*[1]

ANTIESTROGENS
- *Clomiphene*
- *Tamoxifen*

PROGESTINS
- *Hydroxyprogesterone*
- *Medroxyprogesterone*
- *Norethindrone*
- *Norgestrel*

ANTIPROGESTIN
- *Mifepristone*

ANDROGENS
- *Danazol*
- *Fluoxymesterone*
- *Nandrolone*
- *Stanozolol*
- *Testosterone cypionate*

Figure 27.1
Summary of steroid hormones. (figure continues on next page.)
[1]Described in Pharmacology update, pp. 454-455.

Lippincott's Illustrated Reviews: Pharmacology, Second Edition.
by Mary J. Mycek, Richard A. Harvey and Pamela C. Champe.

STEROID HORMONES (continued)

ANTIANDROGENS

- *Cyproterone acetate*
- *Finasteride*
- *Flutamide*

CORTICOSTEROIDS

- *Beclomethasone*
- *Betamethasone*
- *Cortisone*
- *Desoxycorticosterone*
- *Dexamethasone*
- *Fludrocortisone*
- *Hydrocortisone*
- *Methylprednisolone*
- *Paramethasone*
- *Prednisolone*
- *Prednisone*
- *Triamcinolone*

INHIBITORS OF ADRENOCORTICOID BIOSYNTHESIS

- *Aminoglutethimide*
- *Ketoconazole*
- *Metyrapone*
- *Mifepristone*
- *Spironolactone*

Figure 27.1 (continued)
Summary of steroid hormones.

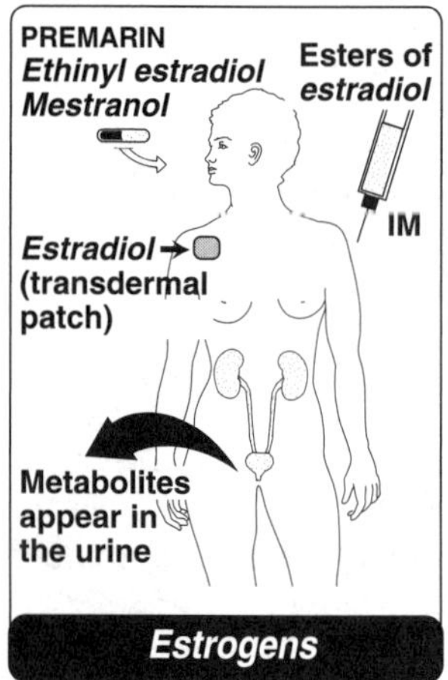

A. Mechanism of action

Steroid hormones diffuse across the cell membrane and bind with high affinity to specific nuclear receptor proteins (see p. 393). Affinity for the receptor varies with the particular estrogen. [Note: The estrogen receptor is a member of a superfamily of receptors that include those for thyroid hormones and vitamin D, as well as ligands not yet identified. The attachment of two estrogen-linked receptors to the genome is required for a response.] The activated steroid-receptor complex interacts with nuclear chromatin to initiate hormone-specific RNA synthesis, resulting in the synthesis of specific proteins that mediate a number of physiologic functions. [Note: The steroid hormones may elicit the synthesis of different RNA species in diverse target tissues and are therefore both receptor- and tissue-specific.]

B. Therapeutic uses of estrogens

The most frequent uses of estrogens are for contraception (see p. 268), for postmenopausal hormone therapy and for osteoporosis. Estrogens are also used extensively for replacement therapy in patients deficient in this hormone. Such a deficiency can be due to lack of development of the ovaries, menopause, or castration.

1. **Postmenopausal hormone therapy:** In the past, estrogen therapy was reserved for postmenopausal women experiencing “hot flashes”, atrophic vaginitis and urethral changes, and women wishing to reduce the risk of osteoporosis. Today, evidence is accumulating that all (except for those with specific contraindications, such as a history of estrogen-dependent cancer) may experience multiple benefits from estrogen replacement therapy (Figure 27.2). For women who have not undergone a hysterectomy, a progestin is usually included with the estrogen therapy, since the combination reduces the risk of endometrial carcinoma associated with estrogen treatment alone. For women whose uterus has been surgically removed, unopposed estrogen therapy is recommended, since progestins may unfavorably alter the high density/low density lipoprotein (HDL/LDL) ratio[1]. [Note: The amounts of estrogen used in replacement therapy are substantially less than the doses used in oral contraception described on p. 268. Thus the adverse effects of estrogen replacement therapy tend to be less severe than side effects seen in women taking estrogen for contraceptive purposes.] Delivery of *estradiol* by transdermal patch is also effective in treating postmenopausal symptoms. Replacement therapy is not universally beneficial; the risk of breast and endometrial cancer is slightly increased and gallbladder disease is more common in women receiving estrogen. However, if these adverse affects are balanced against the favorable actions—particularly the cardioprotective effect—the cumulative effect of estrogen therapy is strongly beneficial. Figure 27.3 summarizes some of the agents useful in the treatment of osteoporosis.

2. **Primary hypogonadism:** Estrogen therapy mimicking the natural cyclic pattern, and usually in combination with progestins is instituted to stimulate development of secondary sex characteristics in young women (11 to 13 years of age) with hypogonadism.

[1]See p. 278 for Infolink references to other books in this series.

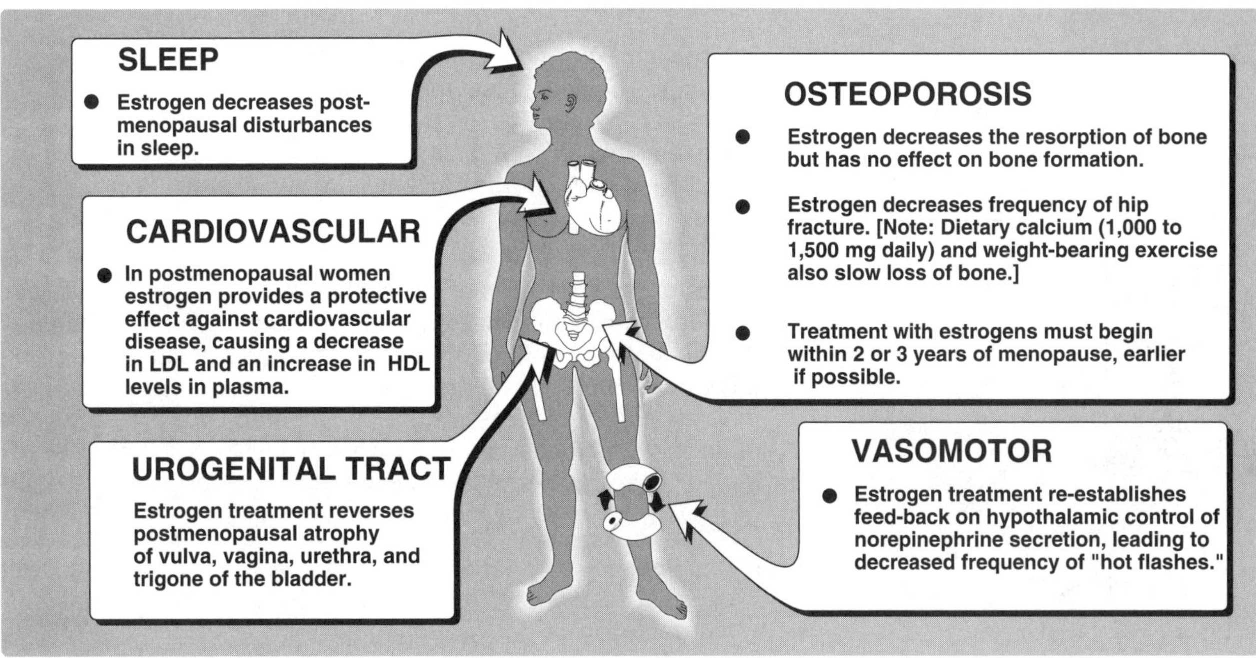

Figure 27.2
Benefits associated with postmenopausal estrogen replacement.

C. Pharmacokinetics

1. **Naturally occurring estrogens:** These agents and their esterified or conjugated derivatives are readily absorbed through the gastrointestinal tract, skin, and mucous membranes. Estrogen is also quickly absorbed when administered intramuscularly. Administered orally, *estradiol* is rapidly metabolized (and partially inactivated) by the microsomal enzymes of the liver.

2. **The synthetic estrogen analogs:** These compounds, for example, *ethinyl estradiol* and *mestranol* [MES tra nole]), are well absorbed after oral administration, and through the skin or mucous membranes. *Mestranol* is quickly oxidized to *ethinyl estradiol,* which is metabolized more slowly than the naturally occurring estrogens by the liver and peripheral tissues. Being fat soluble, they are stored in adipose tissue from which they are slowly released. Therefore, the synthetic estrogen analogs have a prolonged action and higher potency as compared to natural estrogens.

3. **Metabolism:** Estrogens are transported in the blood bound to serum albumin and sex hormone-binding globulin. They are hydroxylated in the liver to derivatives that are subsequently glucuronidated or sulfated. These inactive products are excreted in the urine. [Note: In individuals with liver damage, serum estrogen levels may increase due to reduced metabolism, causing feminization in males or signs of estrogen excess in females.]

Alendronate

- Decreases bone turnover.
- Inhibits osteoclast activity.
- Long term safety remains to be established.

***Cacitonin* nasal spray**

- Interferes with osteoclasts and inhibits bone resorption.
- Generally considered safe, but effectiveness is limited.

***Calcium carbonate* supplements**

- Total dietary calcium should be approximately 1,200 mg/day.
- Minimizes loss of calcium from bones.
- Must be accompanied by adequate intake of vitamin D .

Estrogens

- A progestin is usually included, since the combination reduces the risk of endometrial carcinoma associated with estrogen treatment alone.
- Decreases the incidence of spine fractures by 70% and hip fractures by 50%.

Figure 27.3
Drugs and dietary supplements used in the treatment of osteoporosis.

D. Adverse effects

Nausea and vomiting are the most common adverse effects of estrogen therapy. Other effects of estrogen are shown in Figure 27.4. *Diethylstilbestrol* has been implicated as the possible cause of a rare, clear cell cervical or vaginal adenocarcinoma observed among the daughters of women who took the drug during early pregnancy.

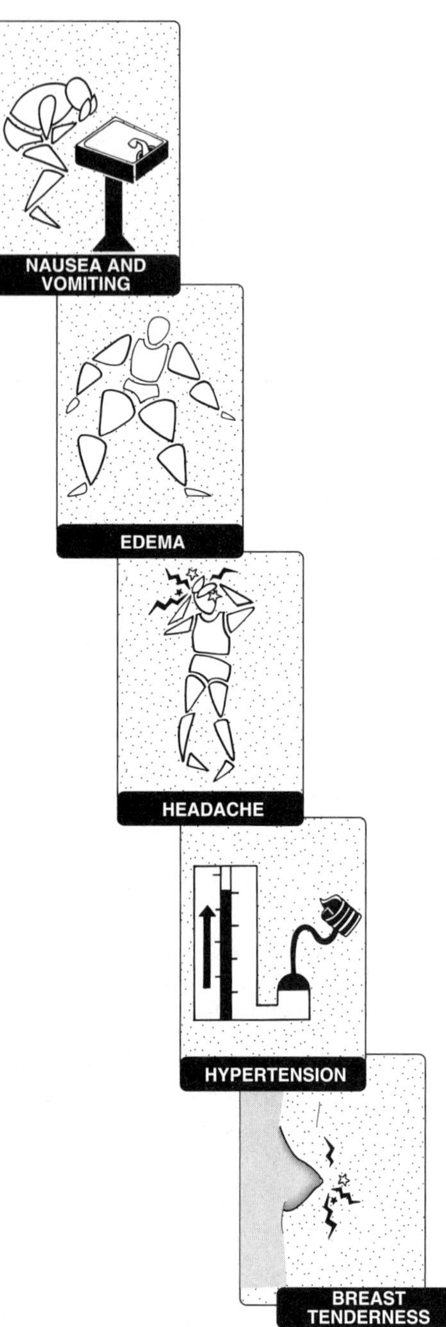

Figure 27.4
Some adverse effects associated with estrogen therapy.

E. Antiestrogens

Antiestrogens, which modify or oppose the action of estrogens, include the nonsteroidal antiestrogenic compounds *clomiphene* [KLOE mi feen] and its structurally related analog, *tamoxifen* [ta MOX i fen]. Both inhibit the action of estrogens by interfering with their access to receptor sites. They act as competitive antagonists or, in a low estrogen milieu, as weak agonists of the natural estrogens. These nonsteroidal antiestrogenic compounds are equally effective when given by mouth or by injection.

1. **Clomiphene:** By interfering with the negative feedback of estrogens on the hypothalamus and pituitary, *clomiphene* increases the secretion of gonadotropin-releasing hormone (Gn-RH) and gonadotropins, leading to a stimulation of ovulation. The drug has been used successfully to treat infertility associated with anovulatory cycles, but it is not effective in women whose ovulatory dysfunction is due to pituitary or ovarian failure. Adverse effects are dose-related and include ovarian enlargement, vasomotor flushes, and visual disturbances.

2. **Tamoxifen:** This drug competes for binding to the estrogen receptor and is currently used in the palliative treatment of advanced breast cancer in postmenopausal women (see p. 394). [Note: Normal breast growth is stimulated by estrogens. It is therefore not surprising that some breast tumors regress following treatment with antiestrogens.] *Tamoxifen's* most frequent adverse effects are hot flashes, nausea and vomiting. Menstrual irregularities and vaginal bleeding can also occur.

See pp. 454-455 for a description of the newly approved selective estrogen modulator drug, *raloxifene*.

III. PROGESTINS

Progesterone, the natural progestin, is produced in response to luteinizing hormone (LH) by both females [secreted by the corpus luteum, primarily during the second half of the menstrual cycle (Figure 27.5), and by the placenta] and by males (secreted by the testes). It is also synthesized by the adrenal cortex in both sexes. In females, progesterone promotes the development of a secretory endometrium that can accommodate implantation of a newly forming embryo. The high levels of progesterone released during the second half of the menstrual cycle (the luteal phase) inhibit the production of gonadotropin, and therefore, further ovulation. If conception takes place, progesterone continues to be secreted, maintaining the endometrium in a favorable state for the continuation of the pregnancy and reducing uterine contractions. If conception does not take place, the release of progesterone from the corpus luteum ceases abruptly. This decline stimulates the onset of menstruation. (See Figure 27.5 for a summary of the hormones produced during the menstrual cycle.)

A. Therapeutic uses of progestins

The major clinical use of progestins is in contraception, in which they are generally used with estrogens, either in combination or in a sequential manner. *Progesterone* by itself is not used widely therapeutically because of its rapid metabolism, resulting in its low bioavailability. Synthetic progestins used in contraception are more stable to first-pass metabolism, allowing for lower doses when administered orally. These agents include *medroxyprogesterone acetate* [meh DROX ee proe JESS ter one], *hydroxyprogesterone acetate* [hye DROX ee proe JESS ter one], *norethindrone* [nor eth IN drone], and *norgestrel* [nor JESS trel]. [Note: *Norethindrone* and *norgestrel* are sometimes called the nortestosterone progestins because of their structural similarity to the androgen. They also possess some androgenic activity.] Other clinical uses of the progestins are in the control of dysfunctional uterine bleeding, the treatment of dysmenorrhea, suppression of postpartum lactation, and the management of endometriosis. They are also used to treat endometrial carcinomas.

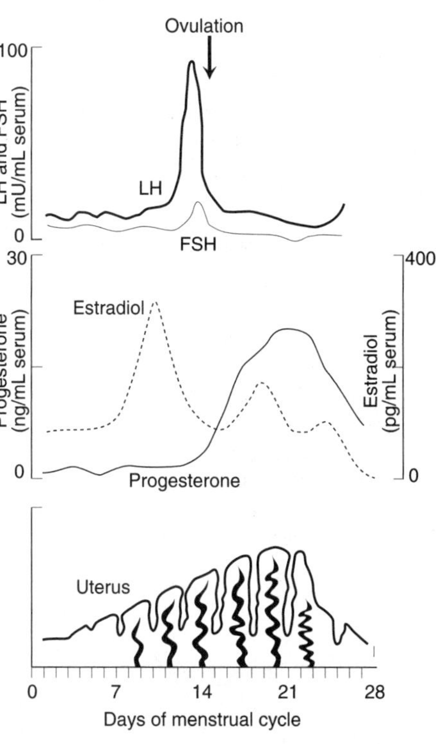

Figure 27.5
Menstrual cycle showing plasma levels of pituitary and ovarian hormones, and a schematic representation of changes in the morphology of the uterine lining. FSH, follicle-stimulating hormone; LH, luteinizing hormone.

B. Pharmacokinetics

Progesterone is rapidly absorbed after its administration by any route. It has a short half-life in the plasma, since it is almost completely metabolized in one passage through the liver. The glucuronidated metabolite (pregnanediol glucuronide) is excreted by the kidney. Synthetic progestins are less rapidly metabolized.

C. Adverse effects

The major adverse effects associated with the use of progestins are edema and depression. The androgen-like progestins can increase the ratio of LDL to HDL cholesterol, cause thrombophlebitis and pulmonary embolism, as well as acne, hirsutism and weight gain.

D. Antiprogestin

Mifepristone (also designated RU 486) is a progestin antagonist with partial agonist activity. [Note: *Mifepristone* is also a potent antiglucocorticoid (see p. 277).] Administration of this drug to females early in pregnancy results in most cases (85%) in abortion of the fetus due to the interference with progesterone and the decline in human chorionic gonadotropin (hCG). The major adverse effects are significant uterine bleeding and the possibility of an incomplete abortion. However, administration of *prostaglandin E_1* intravaginally, or *misoprostol* [miss oh PROH stol] orally, after a single oral dose of *mifepristone*, effectively terminates gestation. *Mifepristone* can also be used as a contraceptive, given once a month during the midluteal phase of the cycle when progesterone is normally high (Figure 27.5).

IV. ORAL AND IMPLANTABLE CONTRACEPTIVES

Drugs have been identified that decrease fertility by a number of different mechanisms, for example, preventing ovulation, impairing gametogenesis or gamete maturation, or interfering with gestation. Currently, interference with ovulation is the most common pharmacologic intervention for preventing pregnancy (Figure 27.6).

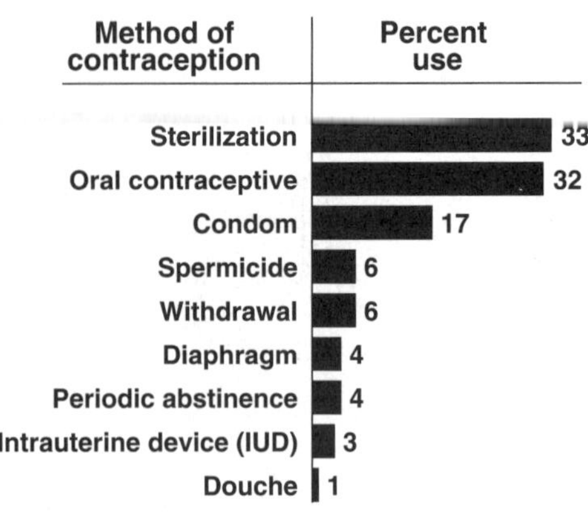

Figure 27.6
Comparison of contraceptive use among U.S. women ages 15 to 44 years.

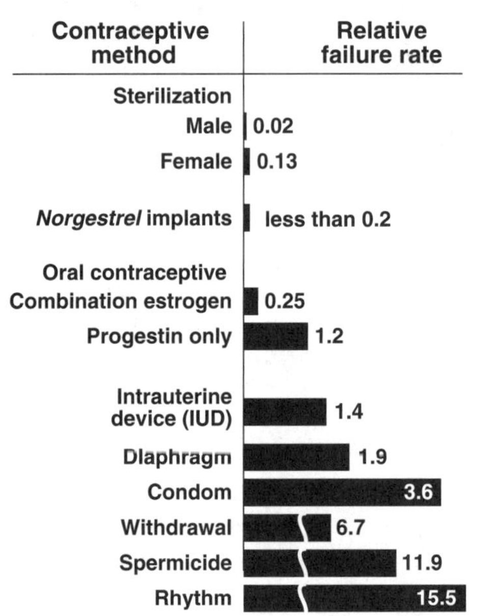

Figure 27.7
Comparison of failure rate for various methods of contraception. Longer bars indicate a higher failure rate, that is, more pregnancies.

A. Major classes of oral contraceptives

1. **Combination pills:** Products containing a combination of estrogen and a progestin are the most common type of oral contraceptives. The estrogen component suppresses ovulation while the progestin prevents implantation in the endometrium and makes the cervical mucus impenetrable to sperm. Combination pills contain a constant low dose of estrogen given over 21 days plus a concurrent low but increasing dose of progestin given over 3 successive 7-day periods (called the "triphasic regimen"). The pills are taken for 21 days followed by a 7-day withdrawal period to induce menses. [Note: Estrogens that are commonly present in the combination pills are *ethinyl estradiol* and *mestranol.*] These preparations are highly effective in achieving contraception (Figure 27.7).

2. **Progestin pills:** Products containing a progestin only, usually *norethindrone* or *norgestrel* (called a "mini-pill"), are taken daily on a continuous schedule. Progestin-only pills deliver a low, continuous dosage of drug. These preparations are less effective than the combination pill (Figure 27.7) and may produce irregular menstrual cycles more frequently than the combination product. The progestin-only pill has limited patient acceptance because of anxiety over the increased possibility of pregnancy and the frequent occurrence of menstrual irregularities.

3. **Progestin implants:** Subdermal capsules containing *levonorgestrel* offer long-term contraception. Six capsules, each the size of a match stick, are placed subcutaneously in the upper arm. The progestin is slowly released from the capsules providing contraceptive protection for approximately 5 years. The implant is cheaper than oral contraceptives, nearly as reliable as sterilization, and totally reversible if the implants are surgically removed. Once the progestin-containing capsules are implanted, this method of contraception does not rely on patient compliance. This may, in part, explain the low failure rate for the method of contraception. For example, Figure 27.8 shows that this use of *levonorgestrel* (NORPLANT) implants by adolescent mothers results in significantly lower rates of new pregnancies when compared to women using oral contraceptives. Principal side effects of the implants are irregular menstrual bleeding and headaches.

4. **Postcoital contraception:** A fourth type of contraceptive strategy uses high-dose estrogen (for example, *ethinyl estradiol* or *diethylstilbestrol*) administered within 72 hours of coitus and continued twice daily for 5 days (the "morning-after" pill). Alternatively, two doses of *ethinyl estradiol* plus *norgestrel* are given within 72 hours of coitus, followed by another two doses 12 hours later. A single dose of *mifepristone* has also been used.

B. Mechanism of action

The mechanism of action of these contraceptives is not completely understood. It is likely that the combination of estrogen and progestin administered over approximately a 3-week period inhibits ovulation.

[Note: The estrogen provides a negative feedback on the release of LH and FSH by the pituitary gland, thus preventing ovulation. The progestin stimulates normal bleeding at the end of the menstrual cycle.] Thickening of cervical mucus prevents access by the sperm.

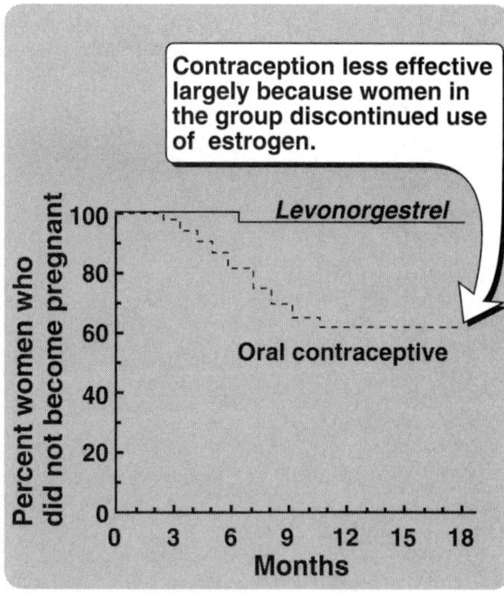

Figure 27.8
Superiority of *levonorgestrel* in preventing pregnancy in adolescent mothers.

C. Adverse effects

Most adverse effects are believed to be due to the estrogen component, but cardiovascular effects reflect the action of both estrogen and progestin. The incidence of side effects with oral contraceptives is relatively low and is determined by the specific compounds and combinations used.

1. **Major adverse effects:** The major side effects are breast fullness, depression, dizziness, edema, headache, nausea, and vomiting.

2. **Cardiovascular:** The most serious side effect of oral contraceptives is cardiovascular disease, including thromboembolism, thrombophlebitis, hypertension, and increased incidences of myocardial infarction and cerebral and coronary thrombosis. These adverse effects are most common among women who smoke and who are over 35 years of age, although they may affect women of any age.

3. **Carcinogenicity:** Oral contraceptives have been shown to decrease the incidence of endometrial and ovarian cancer. Their ability to induce other neoplasms is controversial. The production of benign tumors of the liver that may rupture and hemorrhage is rare.

4. **Metabolic:** Decreased dietary carbohydrate absorption by the intestine is sometimes associated with oral contraceptives, along with an increased incidence of abnormal glucose tolerance tests (similar to the changes seen in pregnancy).

5. **Serum lipids:** The combination pill causes a change in the serum lipoprotein profile: estrogen causes an increase in HDL and a decrease in LDL—a desirable occurrence—whereas progestins have the opposite effect. [Note: The potent progestin, *norgestrel*, causes the greatest increase in the LDL/HDL ratio. Therefore, estrogen-dominant preparations are best for individuals with elevated serum cholesterol.] Cholestatic jaundice, cholecystitis and cholangitis are also encountered.

6. **Contraindications:** Oral contraceptives are contraindicated in the presence of cerebrovascular and thromboembolic disease, estrogen-dependent neoplasms, liver disease, and migraine headache.

V. ANDROGENS

The androgens are a group of steroids that have anabolic and/or masculinizing effects in both males and females. *Testosterone* [tess TOSS ter one], the most important androgen in humans, is synthesized by Leydig cells in the testes, and, in smaller amounts, by cells in the ovary of the female and in the adrenal gland. In adult males, *testosterone* secretion by Leydig cells is controlled by hormonal signals from the hypothalamus (Gn-RH), by way of the pituitary gland secretion of FSH and LH (which was originally known as interstitial cell-stimulating hormone, (ICSH) in males). [Note: LH stimulates steroidogenesis in the Leydig cells, whereas FSH is necessary for the initiation of spermatogenesis.] *Testosterone* or its metabolite *5 α dihydrotestosterone* (DHT, see later) inhibits production of these specific trophic hormones and thus regulates *testosterone* production (Figure 27.9). Synthetic modifications of the androgen structure are designed to (1) modify solubility and susceptibility to enzymatic breakdown (thus prolonging the half-life of the hormone), and (2) separate anabolic and androgenic effects.

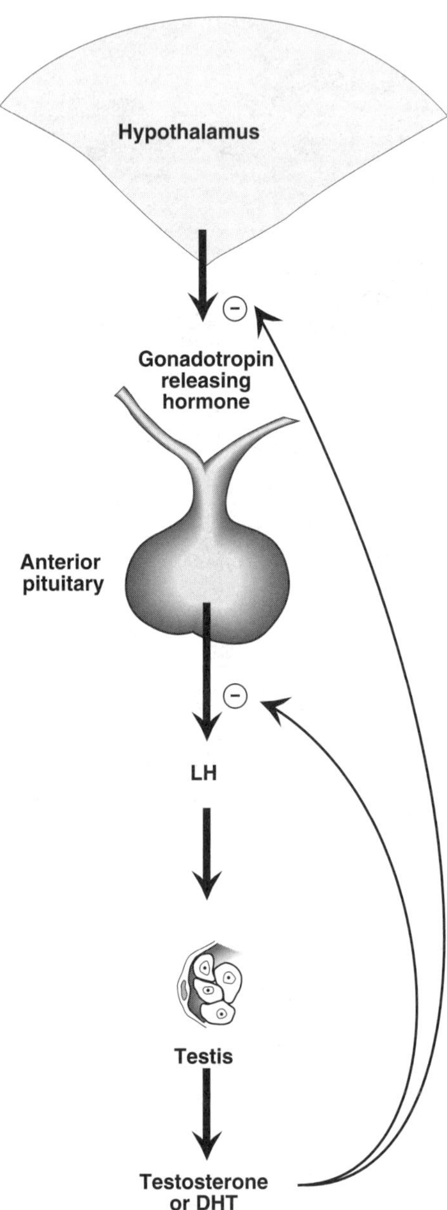

Figure 27.9
Regulation of secretion of testosterone.

A. Mechanism of action

Like the estrogens and progestins, androgens bind to a specific nuclear receptor in a target cell. Although *testosterone* itself is the active ligand in muscle and liver, in other tissues it must be metabolized to derivatives such as DHT. For example, after diffusing into the cells of the prostate, seminal vesicles, epididymis and skin, *testosterone* is converted by 5-α-reductase to DHT, which binds to the receptor. In the brain *testosterone* is biotransformed to *estradiol.* The hormone/receptor complex binds to DNA and stimulates the synthesis of specific RNAs and proteins.[2] [Note: *Testosterone* analogs that cannot be converted to DHT have less effect on the reproductive system than they do on the skeletal musculature.]

B. Therapeutic uses

1. **Androgenic effects:** Androgenic steroids are used in males with inadequate androgen secretion. [Note: Hypogonadism can be due to Leydig cell dysfunction or, secondarily, to failure of the hypothalamic-pituitary unit. In each instance, androgen is indicated.]

2. **Anabolic effects:** Anabolic steroids can be used to treat senile osteoporosis and severe burns, to speed recovery from surgery or from chronic debilitating diseases, and to counteract the catabolic effects of externally administered adrenal cortical hormones.

3. **Growth:** Androgens are used in conjunction with other hormones to promote skeletal growth in prepubertal boys with pituitary dwarfism.

4. **Endometriosis:** *Danazol* [DA na zole], a mild androgen, is used in the treatment of endometriosis (ectopic growth of the endometrium).

5. **Unapproved use:** Androgenic steroids are used to increase lean body mass, muscle strength and aggressiveness in athletes and body builders (see "Adverse Effects").

[2]See p. 278 for Infolink references to other books in this series.

C. Pharmacokinetics

1. **Testosterone:** This agent is ineffective orally because of inactivation by first-pass metabolism. As with the other sex steroids, *testosterone* is rapidly absorbed by the liver and other tissues, and is metabolized to relatively or completely inactive compounds that are excreted primarily in the urine but also in the feces. *Testosterone* and its C-17-esters (for example, *testosterone cypionate* or *enanthate*) are administered intramuscularly. [Note: The addition of the esterified lipid makes the hormone more lipid-soluble, thereby increasing its duration of action.] *Testosterone* and its esters demonstrate a 1:1 relative ratio of androgenic to anabolic activity.

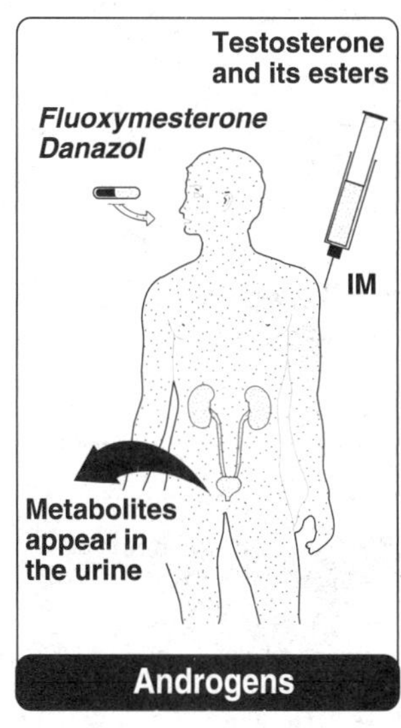

2. **Testosterone derivatives:** Agents such as *fluoxymesterone* [floo ox ee MESS te rone] and *danazol* also have a longer half-life in the body than does the naturally occurring androgen. *Fluoxymesterone* is effective when given orally, and it has a 1:2 androgenic to anabolic ratio. Because it is not readily converted to DHT, it is less active than *testosterone* in the reproductive system and does not induce puberty. It has a longer half-life than does *testosterone*.

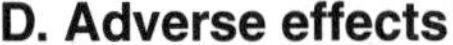

D. Adverse effects

1. **In females:** Androgens can cause masculinization with acne, growth of facial hair, deepening of the voice, male pattern baldness, and excessive muscle development. Menstrual irregularities may also occur. *Testosterone* should not be used by pregnant women, because of the possible virilization of the female fetus.

2. **In males:** Excess androgens can cause priapism, impotence, decreased spermatogenesis, and gynecomastia.

3. **In children:** Androgens can cause growth disturbances resulting from premature closing of the epiphyseal plates and abnormal sexual maturation.

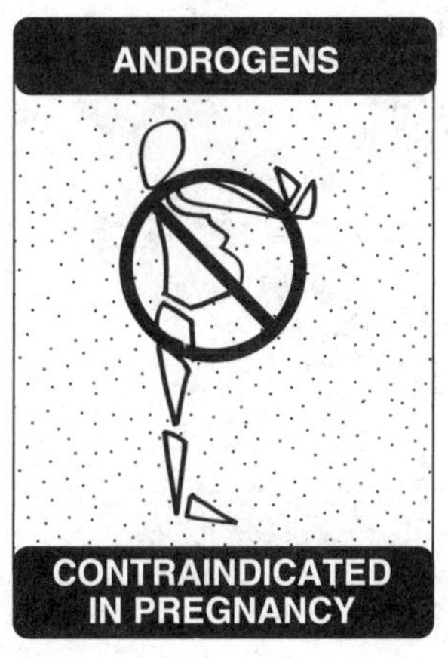

4. **General effects:** Androgens increase serum LDL and lower serum HDL levels; therefore they increase the LDL/HDL ratio and potentially increase the risk for premature coronary heart disease. Androgens can also cause fluid retention leading to edema.

5. **In athletes:** Use of anabolic steroids, (for example, *nandrolone* [nan DRO lone] or *stanozolol* [sta NO zo lol], by athletes can cause premature closing of the epiphysis of the long bones, which interrupts development. The high doses taken by these young athletes may result in hepatic abnormalities, increased aggression ("roid rage"), and psychotic episodes, as well as the other adverse effects described above.

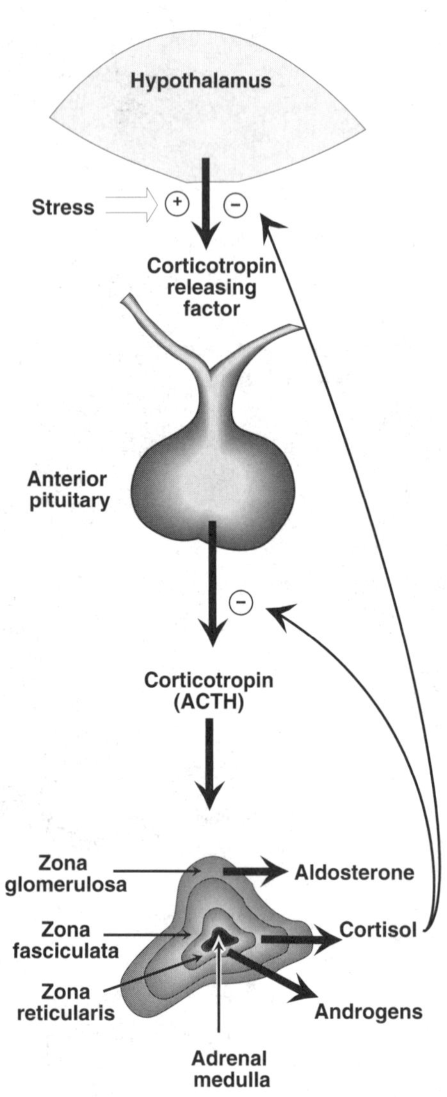

Figure 27.10
Regulation of corticosteroid secretion.

E. Antiandrogens

Antiandrogens counter male hormonal action by interfering with the synthesis of androgens or by blocking their receptors. For example, at high doses, the antifungal *ketoconazole* (see p. 340) inhibits several of the cytochrome P-450 enzymes involved in steroid synthesis. *Finasteride* [fin AS ter eyed], the steroid-like drug recently approved for the treatment of benign prostatic hypertrophy (BPH), inhibits 5-α-reductase; the resulting decrease in formation of DHT by the prostate leads to a reduction in prostate size. Antiandrogens, such as *cyproterone acetate* [sih PROE ter one] and *flutamide* [FLOO ta mide] (see p. 395), act as competitive inhibitors of androgens. They inhibit the action of the androgens at the target cell. *cyproterone acetate* has been used to treat hirsutism in females; wherease *flutamide* is used in the treatment of prostatic carcinoma in males.

VI. ADRENAL CORTICOSTEROIDS

The adrenal cortex is divided into three zones that synthesize various steroids from cholesterol and secrete them (Figure 27.10). The outer zona glomerulosa produces mineralocorticoids (for example, aldosterone), which are responsible for regulating salt and water metabolism. Production of aldosterone is regulated primarily by the renin-angiotensin system (see p. 180). The middle zona fasciculata synthesizes glucocorticoids (for example, cortisol [KOR ti sol]), which are concerned with normal metabolism and resistance to stress. The inner zona reticularis secretes adrenal androgens, such as dehydroepiandrosterone. Secretion by the two inner zones, and to some extent, the outer zone, is controlled by pituitary corticotropin, which is released in response to the hypothalamic corticotropin-releasing hormone (CRH, see p.247). Glucocorticoids serve as feedback inhibitors of corticotropin and corticotropin-releasing factor (CRF) secretion (Figure 27.10).

A. Mechanism of action

The adrenocorticoids bind to specific intracellular cytoplasmic receptors in target tissues. The receptor-hormone complex then translocates into the nucleus where it acts as a transcription factor to turn genes on or off, depending on the tissue. This mechanism requires time to produce an effect. There are other glucocorticoid effects, such as their requirement for catecholamine-mediated dilation of vascular and bronchial musculature or lipolysis, whose effects are immediate. The bases for these actions are unknown.

B. Actions

Some normal actions and some selected mechanisms of adrenocorticoids are described in this section. Understanding these actions aids the reader in better comprehending the results of adrenal insufficiency and the uses of adrenocorticoids as therapeutic agents in a variety of disorders.

1. Glucocorticoids

a. **Promote normal intermediary metabolism:** Glucocorticoids favor gluconeogenesis by both increasing amino acid uptake by the liver and kidney and elevating activities of gluconeogenic enzymes. They stimulate protein catabolism (except in the liver) and lipolysis, thereby providing the building blocks and energy needed for glucose synthesis. [Note: Glucocorticoid insufficiency may result in hypoglycemia, for example, during stressful periods or fasting.]

b. **Increase resistance to stress:** By raising plasma glucose levels, glucocorticoids provide the body with the energy it requires to combat stress caused, for example, by trauma, fright, infection, bleeding, or debilitating disease. Glucocorticoids can cause a modest rise in blood pressure, apparently by enhancing the vasoconstrictor action of adrenergic stimuli on small vessels. [Note: Individuals with adrenal insufficiency may respond to severe stress by becoming hypotensive.]

c. **Alter blood cell levels in plasma:** Glucocorticoids cause a decrease in eosinophils, basophils, monocytes, and lymphocytes by redistributing them to lymphoid tissue from the circulation. In contrast, they increase the blood levels of hemoglobin, erythrocytes, platelets and polymorphonuclear leukocytes. [Note: The decrease in circulating lymphocytes and macrophages compromises the body's ability to fight infections. However, this property is important in the treatment of leukemia (see p. 393).]

d. **Anti-inflammatory action:** The most important therapeutic property of the glucocorticoids is their ability to dramatically reduce the inflammatory response and to suppress immunity. The exact mechanism is complex and incompletely understood. However, it is known that the lowering and inhibition of peripheral lymphocytes and macrophages play a role. Also involved is the indirect inhibition of phospholipase A_2 (due to the steroid mediated elevation of lipocortin), which blocks the release of arachidonic acid, the precursor of the prostaglandins and leukotrienes, from membrane-bound phospholipid (see p. 403).

e. **Affect other components of the endocrine system:** Feedback inhibition of corticotropin production by elevated glucocorticoids causes inhibition of further glucocorticoid synthesis as well as thyroid stimulating hormone production, whereas growth hormone production is increased.

f. **Effects on other systems:** These are mostly associated with the adverse effects of the hormones. High doses of glucocorticoids stimulate gastric acid and pepsin production and may exacerbate ulcers. Effects on the central nervous system that influence mental status have been identified. Chronic glucocorticoid therapy can cause severe bone loss. Myopathy leads patients to complain of weakness.

2. Mineralocorticoids

Mineralocorticoids help control the body's water volume and concentration of electrolytes, especially sodium and potassium. Aldosterone acts on kidney tubule cells, causing a reabsorption of sodium, bicarbonate, and water. Conversely, aldosterone decreases reabsorption of potassium, which is then lost in the urine. [Note: Elevated aldosterone levels may cause alkalosis and hypokalemia, whereas retention of sodium and water leads to an increase in blood volume and blood pressure (see p. 180). Hyperaldosteronism is treated with *spironolactone* (see p. 232).]

C. Therapeutic uses of the adrenal corticosteroids

Several semisynthetic derivatives of the glucocorticoids have been developed that vary in their anti-inflammatory potency, the degree to which they cause sodium retention, and their duration of action. These are summarized in Figure 27.11.

1. **Replacement therapy for primary adrenocortical insufficiency (Addison's disease):** This disease is caused by adrenal cortex dysfunction (as diagnosed by the lack of patient response to corticotropin administration). *Hydrocortisone* [hye droe KOR ti sone], which is identical to the natural *cortisol*, is given to correct the deficiency. Failure to do so results in death. The dosage of *hydrocortisone* is divided so that two thirds of the normal daily dose is given in the morning and one third in the afternoon. [Note: The goal of this regimen is to approximate the daily hormone levels resulting from the circadian rhythm exhibited by cortisol, which causes plasma levels to be maximal around 8 A.M. and then to decrease throughout the day to their lowest level around 1 A.M.] Administration of *fludrocortisone* [floo droe KOR ti sone], a synthetic mineralocorticoid with some glucocorticoid activity, may also be necessary to raise the mineralocorticoid activity to normal levels.

2. **Replacement therapy for secondary or tertiary adrenocortical insufficiency:** These deficiencies are caused by a defect either in CRF production by the hypothalamus or corticotropin production by the pituitary (see p. 247). [Note: Under these conditions, the adrenal cortex synthesis of mineralocorticoids is less impaired than that of glucocorticoids.] The adrenal cortex responds to corticotropin administration by synthesizing and releasing the adrenal corticosteroids. *Hydrocortisone* is also used for these deficiencies.

3. **Diagnosis of Cushing's syndrome:** Cushing's syndrome is caused by a hypersecretion of glucocorticoids that is due to either excessive release of corticotropin by the anterior pituitary or to an adrenal tumor. The *dexamethasone* suppression test is used to diagnose the cause of an individual's case of Cushing's syndrome. This synthetic glucocorticoid suppresses cortisol release in individuals with pituitary-dependent Cushing's syndrome, but it does not suppress glucocorticoid release from adrenal tumors.

4. **Replacement therapy for congenital adrenal hyperplasia (CAH):** This is a group of diseases resulting from an enzyme defect in the

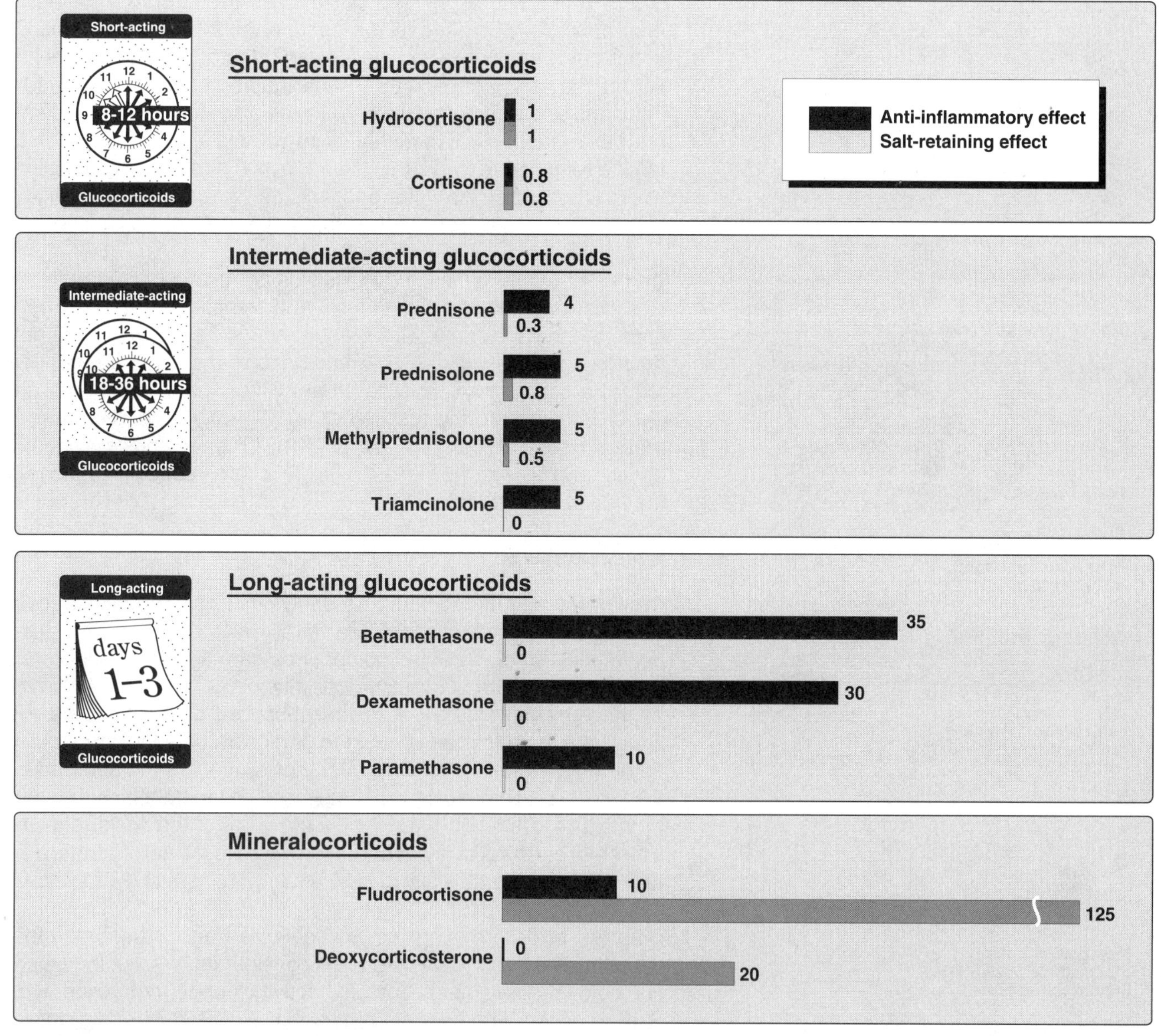

Figure 27.11
Pharmacologic properties of some commonly used natural and synthetic corticosteroids; activities are all relative to hydrocortisone =1. Time refers to duration of action.

synthesis of one or more adrenal steroid hormones. Treatment of this condition requires administration of sufficient corticosteroids to normalize the patient's hormone levels. Choice of replacement hormone depends on the site of the lesion.

5. **Relief of inflammatory symptoms:** Glucocorticoids dramatically reduce the manifestations of inflammations (for example, rheumatoid and osteoarthritic inflammations, inflammatory conditions of the skin), including the redness, swelling, heat, and tenderness that are commonly present at the inflammatory site. The effect of glucocorticoids on the inflammatory process is the result of their effects on the distribution, concentration, and function of leuko-

cytes. These effects include an increase in the concentration of neutrophils; a decrease in the concentration of lymphocytes (T and B cells), basophils, eosinophils and monocytes; and an inhibition of the ability of leukocytes and macrophages to respond to mitogens and antigens. Glucocorticoids also influence the inflammatory response by their ability to reduce the amount of histamine released from basophils and to inhibit the activity of kinins. [Note: The ability of glucocorticoids to inhibit the immune response is also a result of the other actions described above.]

6. **Treatment of allergies:** Glucocorticoids are useful in the treatment of the symptoms of drug, serum, and transfusion allergic reactions, bronchial asthma, and allergic rhinitis. These drugs are not, however, curative. [Note: *Beclomethasone dipropionate* [be kloe METH a sone], *triamcinolone* [tri am SIN o lone] and others are applied topically to the respiratory tract through inhalation from a metered dose dispenser (see p. 219). This minimizes systemic effects and allows the patient to significantly reduce or eliminate the use of oral steroids.]

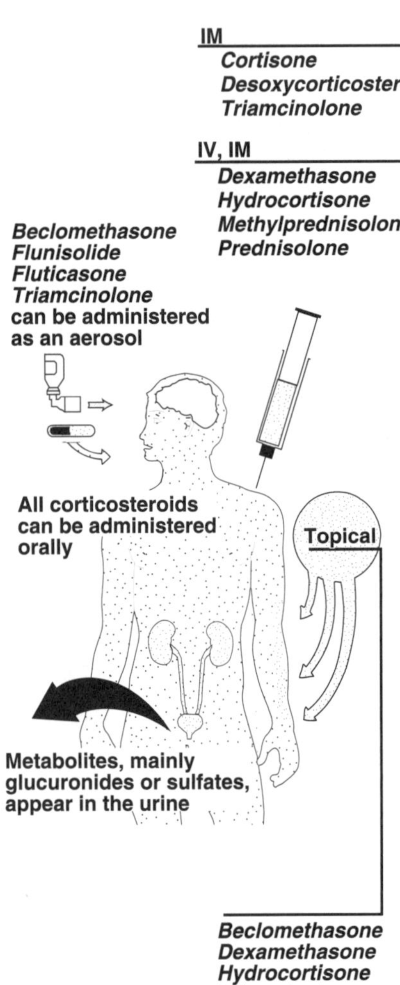

Figure 27.12
Routes of administration and elimination of corticosteriods.

D. Pharmacokinetics

1. **Absorption and metabolism:** Naturally occurring adrenal corticosteroids and their derivatives are readily absorbed from the gastrointestinal tract. Selected compounds can also be administered intravenously, intramuscularly, topically, or as an aerosol (Figure 27.12). Greater than 90% of the absorbed glucocorticoids are bound to plasma proteins: most to corticosteroid-binding globulin, and the remainder to albumin. Corticosteroids are metabolized by the liver microsomal oxidizing enzymes. The metabolites are conjugated to glucuronic acid or sulfate, and the products are excreted by the kidney. [Note: The half-life of adrenal steroids may increase dramatically in individuals with hepatic dysfunction.]

2. **Dosage:** In determining the dosage of adrenocortical steroids, many factors need to be taken into consideration, including glucocorticoid versus mineralocorticoid activity, duration of action, type of preparation, and the time of day that a steroid is administered. For example, when large doses of the hormone are required over an extended period of time (more than 2 weeks), suppression of the hypothalamic-pituitary-adrenal (HPA) axis occurs. To prevent this adverse effect, a regimen of alternate-day administration of the adrenocortical steroid may be useful. This schedule allows the HPA axis to recover/function on the days the hormone is not taken.

E. Adverse effects

The common side effects of long-term corticosteroid therapy are summarized in Figure 27.13. [Note: Increased appetite is not necessarily an adverse effect, since it is one of the reasons for the use of *prednisone* in cancer chemotherapy.] The classic Cushing-like syndrome—redistribution of body fat, puffy face, increased body hair growth, acne, insomnia and increased appetite—are observed when excess corticosteroids are present. Increased frequency of cataracts also occurs with long-term corticosteroid therapy. Withdrawal from the drugs can be a serious problem, because if the patient has experienced hypothalamic-pituitary-adrenal suppression, abrupt removal of the corticosteroids causes an acute adrenal insufficiency syndrome that can be lethal. This fact, coupled with the possibility of psychological dependence on the drug and the fact that withdrawal might cause an exacerbation of the disease, means that the individual schedule for withdrawal may be based on trial and error. The patient must be carefully monitored.

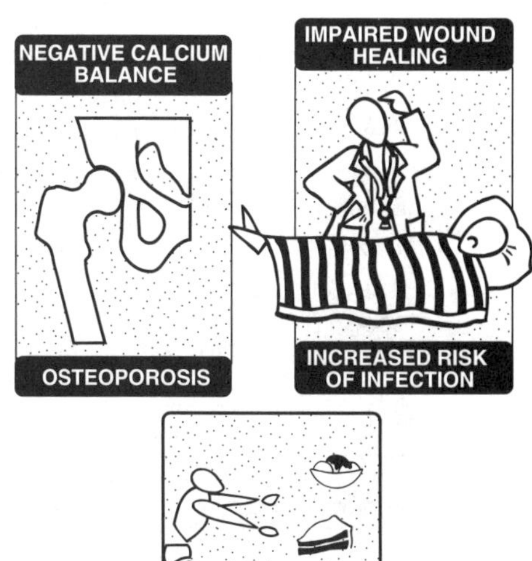

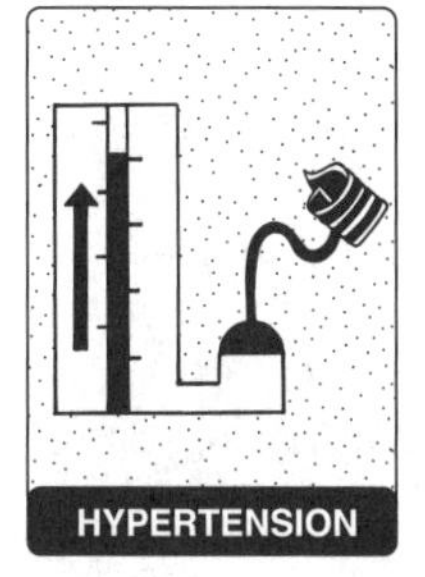

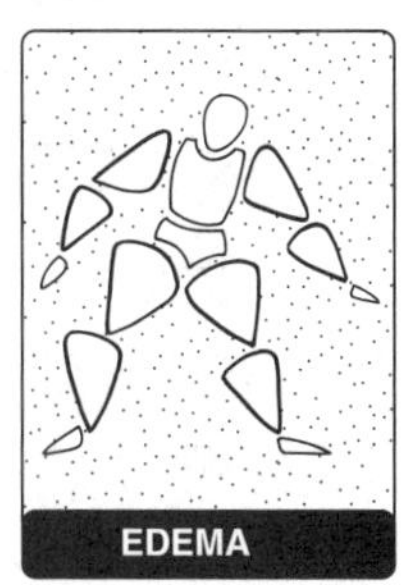

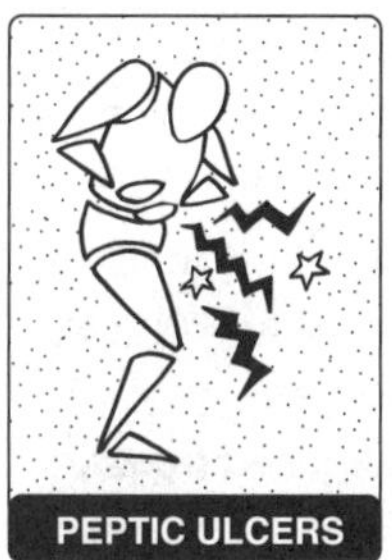

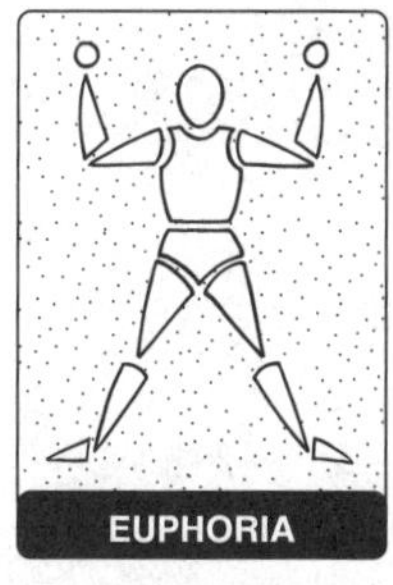

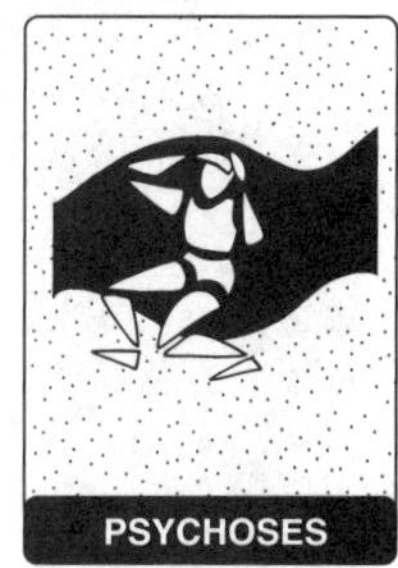

INCREASED APPETITE

Figure 27.13
Some commonly observed effects of long-term corticosteroid therapy.

F. Inhibitors of adrenocorticoid biosynthesis

Several substances have proven to be useful as inhibitors of the synthesis of adrenal steroids: *metyrapone* [me TEER a pone], *aminoglutethimide* [a mee noe glu TETH i mide], *ketoconazole* [kee toe KON a zole], and *spironolactone*. *Mifepristone* competes with glucocorticoids for the receptor.

1. **Metyrapone** is used for the treatment of Cushing's syndrome and can be used for tests of adrenal function. [Note: *Dexamethasone* suppression is now used more commonly for diagnosis.] *Metyrapone* interferes with corticosteroid synthesis by blocking the final step (11-hydroxylation) in glucocorticoid synthesis, leading to an increase in 11-deoxycortisol as well as adrenal androgens and the potent mineralocorticoid, 11-deoxycorticosterone. The adverse effects encountered with *metyrapone* include salt and water retention, hirsutism, transient dizziness, and gastrointestinal disturbances.

2. **Aminoglutethimide** acts by inhibiting the conversion of cholesterol to pregnenolone. As a result, the synthesis of all hormonally active steroids is reduced. *Aminoglutethimide* has been used therapeutically in the treatment of breast cancer to reduce or eliminate androgen and estrogen production. In these cases it is used in conjunction with *dexamethasone*. *Aminoglutethimide* may also be useful in the treatment of malignancies of the adrenal cortex to reduce the secretion of steroids.

3. **Ketoconazole** (an antifungal agent, see p. 340) strongly inhibits all gonadal and adrenal steroid hormone synthesis. It is used in the treatment of patients with Cushing's syndrome.

4. **Mifepristone** is a potent glucocorticoid antagonist as well as an antiprogestin (see p. 267). It forms a complex with the glucocorticoid receptor, but the rapid dissociation of the drug from the receptor leads to a faulty translocation into the nucleus. Its potential use in the treatment of Cushing's syndrome is being explored.

5. **Spironolactone** competes for the mineralocorticoid receptor and thus inhibits sodium reabsorption in the kidney (see p. 232). It can also antagonize aldosterone and testosterone synthesis. It is effective against hyperaldosteronism. The drug is also useful in the treatment of hirsutism in women, probably due to interference at the androgen receptor of the hair follicle.

Choose the ONE best answer.

27.1 All of the following statements about glucocorticoids are correct EXCEPT:

A. They may produce peptic ulcers.
B. They are useful in the treatment of refractory asthma.
C. They are contraindicated in glaucoma.
D. They are used in the treatment of Addison's disease.
E. They exert their effect by binding to receptors in the cell membrane.

Correct answer = E. All steroid hormones bind to receptors in the nucleus or the cytosol.

27.2 Which one of the following statements is true?

A. Diethylstibestrol enhances fertility by blocking the inhibitory effect of estrogen on the pituitary.
B. Tamoxifen is an estrogen antagonist.
C. Dexamethasone has weak anti-inflammatory properties. .
D. Estrogens are mainly excreted unchanged in the urine.
E. Tamoxifen is used to treat infertility.

Correct answer = B. Diethylstibestrol is a synthetic estrogen that acts directly on target tissues. Estrogens are secreted as sulfated or glucuronidated metabolites. Tamoxifen is used in the treatment of advanced breast cancer.

27.3 All of the following are adverse effects associated with the use of oral contraceptive agents EXCEPT:

A. Edema.
B. Breast tenderness.
C. Nausea.
D. Increased frequency of migraine headache.
E. Increased risk of ovarian cancer.

Correct choice = E. Oral contraceptive agents decrease the incidence of ovarian and endometrial cancers.

27.4 Estrogen replacement therapy in menopausal women

A. restores bone loss accompanying osteoporosis.
B. may induce "hot flashes".
C. may cause atrophic vaginitis.
D. is most effective if instituted at the first signs of menopause.
E. requires higher doses of estrogen than are required with oral contraceptive therapy.

Correct answer = D. Estrogens decrease but do not restore the age-related loss of bone. Vasomotor symptoms of menopause, such as hot flashes, are decreased with estrogen replacement therapy. Symptoms of menopause, such as atrophic vaginitis, are decreased with estrogen replacement therapy. Oral contraceptives contain higher doses of estrogen than those used with estrogen replacement therapy.

27.5 Progestins

A. are not produced in males.
B. increase HDL and decrease LDL.
C. attenuate the increased risk of endometrial cancer associated with estrogen-only oral contraceptive agents.
D. such as progesterone are widely used in oral contraceptives.
E. commonly induce weight loss.

The correct answer = C. Progesterone is synthesized by the testes in males. Progestins decrease HDL and increase LDL. When orally administered, progesterone is largely inactivated by hepatic first-pass metabolism. Weight gain is one of the side effects of progestins.

27.6 Which one of the following is a synthetic estrogen used in oral contraceptives?

A. Mestranol.
B. Norgestrel.
C. Clomiphene.
D. Estradiol.
E. Norethindrone.

Correct answer = A. Norgestrel and norethindrone are progestins, and clomiphene is an antiestrogen. Estradiol is largely inactivated by first-pass metabolism when administered orally.

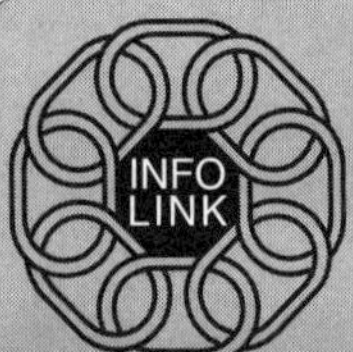

[1]See p. 213 in **Biochemistry** (2nd ed.) for a discussion of plasma lipoproteins.

[2]See p. 383 in **Biochemistry** (2nd ed.) for a discussion of the transcription of eukaryotic genes.

UNIT VI: Chemotherapeutic Drugs

Principles of Antimicrobial Therapy

28

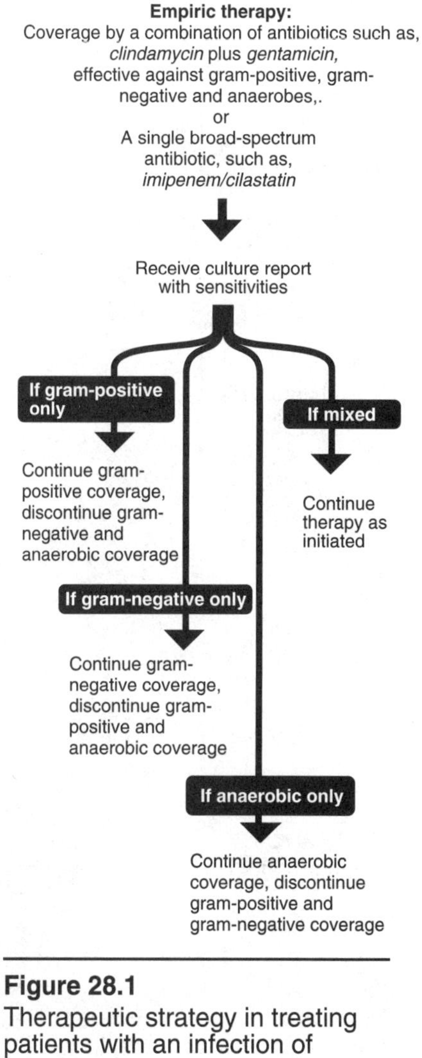

I. OVERVIEW

Antimicrobial drugs are effective in the treatment of infections because of their selective toxicity—the ability to kill an invading microorganism without harming the cells of the host. In most instances, the selective toxicity is relative, rather than absolute, requiring that the concentration of the drug be carefully controlled to attack the microorganism while still being tolerated by the host. Selective antimicrobial therapy takes advantage of the biochemical differences that exist between microorganisms and human beings.

II. SELECTION OF ANTIMICROBIAL AGENTS

Selection of the most appropriate antimicrobial agent requires knowledge of (A) the organism's identity and its sensitivity to a particular agent, (B) the site of the infection, (C) the safety of the agent, (D) patient factors and (E) the cost of therapy. However, some critically ill patients require empiric therapy, that is, immediate administration of drug(s) covering infections by both gram-positive and gram-negative microorganisms (Figure 28.1).

A. Empiric therapy prior to organism identification

Ideally, the antimicrobial agent used to treat an infection is selected after the organism has been identified and its drug sensitivity established. However, in the critically ill patient, such a delay could prove fatal and immediate empiric therapy is indicated.

1. **The acutely ill patient:** Acutely ill patients with infections of unknown origin for example, a neutropenic patient (one who has a reduction in neutrophil count, possibly indicating bacterial

Empiric therapy:
Coverage by a combination of antibiotics such as, *clindamycin* plus *gentamicin,* effective against gram-positive, gram-negative and anaerobes,.
or
A single broad-spectrum antibiotic, such as, *imipenem/cilastatin*
Receive culture report with sensitivities
If gram-positive only
Continue gram-positive coverage, discontinue gram-negative and anaerobic coverage
If mixed
Continue therapy as initiated
If gram-negative only
Continue gram-negative coverage, discontinue gram-positive and anaerobic coverage
If anaerobic only
Continue anaerobic coverage, discontinue gram-positive and gram-negative coverage

Figure 28.1
Therapeutic strategy in treating patients with an infection of unknown origin.

Lippincott's Illustrated Reviews: Pharmacology, Second Edition.
by Mary J. Mycek, Richard A. Harvey and Pamela C. Champe.
Lippincott Williams & Wilkins, Philadelphia, PA © 2000.

infection), or a patient with severe headache, a rigid neck, and sensitivity to bright lights (symptoms characteristic of meningitis) require immediate treatment. Therapy is initiated after specimens for laboratory analysis have been obtained but before the results of the culture are available.

2. **Selecting a drug:** The choice of drug in the absence of sensitivity data is influenced by site of infection and patient history, for example, whether the infection was hospital- or community-acquired, whether the patient is immunocompromised, as well as the patient's travel record and age. Empiric therapy with a combination of antibiotics or a single drug covering infections by both gram-positive and gram-negative microorganisms may be started initially. Figure 28.1 summarizes a typical therapeutic strategy for a patient with a suspected bacterial infection of unknown origin.

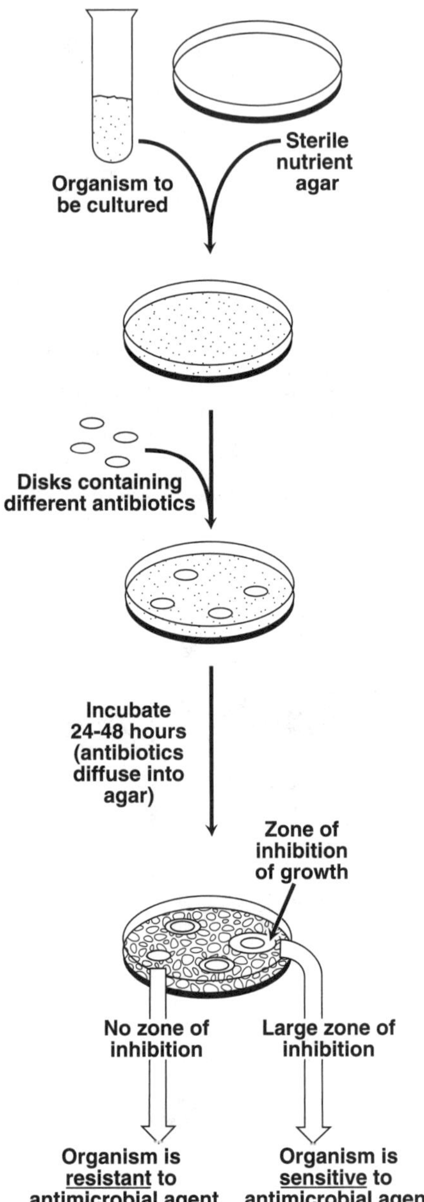

Figure 28.2
Disk diffusion method for determining the sensitivity of bacteria to antimicrobial agents.

B. Identification and sensitivity of the organism

Characterization of the organism is central to the selection of the proper drug. A rapid assessment of the nature of the organism can sometimes be made on the basis of differential stains, such as the Gram stain, but it is generally necessary to culture the infective organism in order to arrive at a conclusive diagnosis and to determine the sensitivity of the bacteria to antimicrobial agents. Thus, it is essential to obtain a sample culture of the organism prior to initiating treatment if possible. Newer methods that use molecular biological techniques to identify microorganisms are making a public health impact in identification of the source of an outbreak of infectious diseases.

C. Laboratory methods of identification

The most commonly used method to test susceptibility to antibiotics has been disk diffusion, in which disks containing antibiotics are placed on culture dishes inoculated with the microorganism to be tested, and the organism's growth (resistance to the drug), or lack of growth (sensitivity to the drug) is then monitored (Figure 28.2). Although this method is still employed in some clinical laboratories, it is being replaced by miniaturized automated procedures that are much faster and more cost effective. In these procedures, plates, called panels, consist of wells containing reactants that permit assessment of unique characteristics of the organism (for example, fermentation of glucose). Other wells may hold various concentrations of clinically useful antibiotics. Results are obtained and printed automatically, identifying the organism and the minimal inhibitory concentration of the antibiotics to which it is susceptible.

D. The effect of the site of infection on therapy

Adequate levels of an antibiotic must reach the site of infection in order for the invading microorganism to be effectively eradicated. Natural barriers such as those described below may cause inadequate penetration of the drug into certain tissues such as the brain, prostate, and bone, although inflammation can influence the response to drug therapy in these tissues.

1. **Blood-brain barrier:** Treatment of central nervous system infections, such as meningitis, depends on the ability of a drug to penetrate into the cerebrospinal fluid (CSF). The blood-brain barrier (see p. 8) ordinarily excludes many antibiotics. However, inflammation facilitates penetration and allows sufficient levels of many (but not all) antibiotics to enter the CSF. [Note: For cure of meningitis, it is important that a bactericidal rather than a bacteriostatic effect is achieved in the CSF. Yet, this is not without its problems, since rapid bacteriolysis in the infected CSF will liberate high concentrations of bacterial cell walls and lipopolysaccharide that can exacerbate the inflammation. This has led to the use of adjunctive (simultaneous administration of) corticosteroids, which diminish the inflammatory process and neurologic sequelae.]

2. **Prostate:** Bacterial prostatitis is difficult to cure, probably because of the failure of many antibiotics to cross the prostatic epithelium, and, therefore, not entering the prostatic fluid and tissue. Furthermore, the pH of prostatic fluid is relatively acidic (pH 6.4) compared to the plasma (pH 7.4). *Trimethoprim*, a basic antimicrobic with a pK_a of 7.3 is effective in bacterial prostatitis. About 50% non-ionized in the plasma, and with good lipid solubility, the drug diffuses into the prostate and concentrates due to ion trapping in the relatively more acidic prostatic fluid (Figure 28.3). In contrast, acidic antibiotics tend to be predominantly ionized at plasma pH in the plasma and do not cross into the prostatic fluid. For example, consider *penicillin G,* which is poorly lipid soluble and has a pK_a of 2.7. The calculated ratio of charged to uncharged drug in the plasma is about 100,000, so it is not surprising that it is ineffective in the treatment of prostatitis even in susceptible organisms (see ion trapping, p. 24).

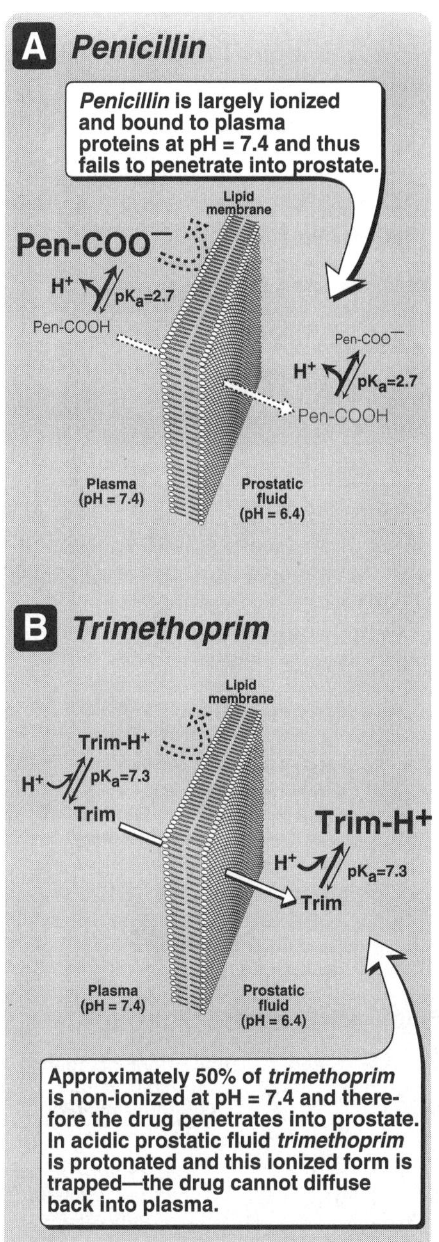

Figure 28.3
A. Diffusion of non-ionized form of a *penicillin* through prostatic membrane; B. Diffusion of non-ionized form of *trimethoprim* through prostatic membrane.

E. Status of the patient

In selecting an antibiotic, attention must be paid to the condition of the patient. For example, the status of the patient's immune system, kidneys, and liver must be considered. In women, pregnancy or breastfeeding an infant also affect the selection of the antimicrobial agent.

1. **Immune system:** Elimination of infecting organisms from the body depends on an intact immune system. Antibacterial drugs decrease the microbial population (bactericidal), or inhibit further bacterial growth (bacteriostatic, p. 283), but the host defense system must ultimately eliminate the invading organisms. Alcoholism, diabetes, infection with the human immunodeficiency virus (HIV), malnutrition, or advanced age can affect a patient's immunocompetency, as can therapy with immunosuppressive drugs. Higher than usual doses of bactericidal agents or longer treatment are required to eliminate the infective organisms in these individuals.

2. **Renal dysfunction:** Poor kidney function (10% or less of normal) causes accumulation of antibiotics that are ordinarily eliminated by this route. This may lead to serious adverse effects unless controlled by adjusting the dose or the dosage schedule of the antibiotic. Although serum creatinine levels are sometimes used as an index of renal function for adjustment of drug regimens, direct monitoring of serum levels of some antibiotics is preferred

to identify maximum and minimum values. Rising minimum values alert the physician to potential toxicity. [Note: The number of functioning nephrons decreases with age. Thus elderly patients are particularly vulnerable to accumulation of drugs eliminated by the kidneys. Antibiotics that undergo extensive metabolism or are excreted via the biliary route are favored in such patients.]

3. **Hepatic dysfunction:** Antibiotics that are concentrated or eliminated by the liver (for example, *erythromycin*, *tetracycline*) are contraindicated in treating patients with liver disease.

4. **Poor Perfusion:** Decreased circulation to an anatomic area, as in the lower limbs of the diabetic, reduces the amount of antibiotic that reaches the extremities and makes infections notoriously difficult to treat.

5. **Pregnancy:** All antibiotics cross the placenta. Adverse effects to the fetus are rare, except for tooth dysplasia and inhibition of bone growth encountered with the tetracyclines. However, some anthelmintics are embryotoxic and teratogenic (p. 359). Aminoglycosides should be avoided in pregnancy because of their ototoxic effect in the fetus.

6. **Lactation:** Drugs administered to a lactating mother may enter the nursing infant via the breast milk. Even though the concentration of an antibiotic in breast milk is usually low, the total dose to the infant may be enough to cause problems.

7. **Age:** Renal or hepatic elimination processes are often poorly developed in newborns, making neonates particularly vulnerable to the toxic effects of *chloramphenicol* (see p. 320) and sulfonamides (see p. 289). Young children should not be treated with tetracyclines (see p. 311) which affect bone growth, or fluoroquinolones (see p. 323), which interfere with cartilage growth.

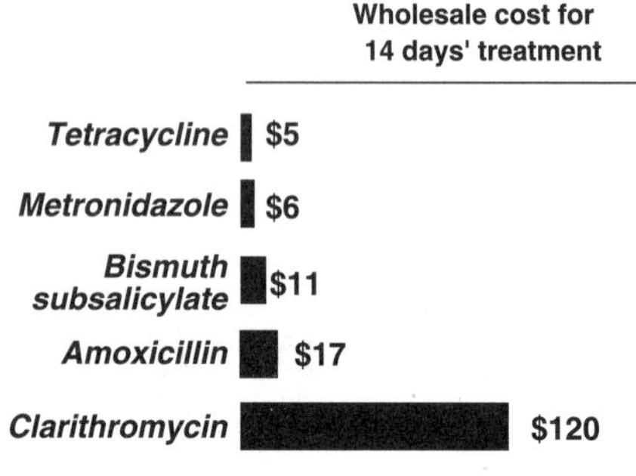

Figure 28.4
Cost of some drugs for treatment of peptic ulcers caused by Helicobacter pylori.

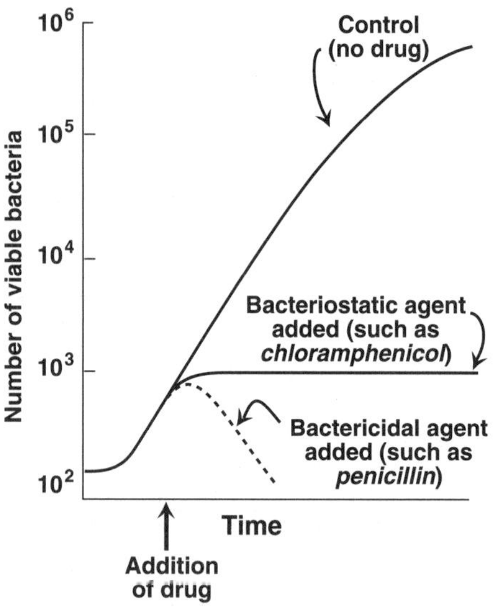

Figure 28.5
Effects of bactericidal and bacteriostatic drugs on the growth of bacteria in vitro.

F. Safety of the agent

Many of the antibiotics, such as the penicillins, are among the least toxic of all drugs because they interfere with a site unique to the growth of microorganisms. Other antimicrobial agents (for example, *chloramphenicol*) are less specific and are reserved for life-threatening infections because of the drug's potential for serious toxicity. [Note: Safety is related not only to the inherent nature of the drug but also to patient factors that can predispose to toxicity (see Section E).]

G. Cost of therapy

Often, several drugs may show similar efficacy in treating an infection, but vary widely in cost. Figure 28.4 illustrates the cost of some antibacterial agents showing similar efficacy in eradicating the gram-negative bacillus Helicobacter pylori from the gastric mucosa. None of these agents shows a clear therapeutic superiority and thus a combination of *metronidazole* with *bismuth subsalicylate* plus one other antibiotic is usually employed. Selecting *clarithromycin* would have a considerable cost impact.

III. BACTERIOSTATIC VERSUS BACTERICIDAL DRUGS

Antimicrobial drugs are classified as either bacteriostatic or bactericidal. Bacteriostatic drugs arrest the growth and replication of bacteria at serum levels achievable in the patient, thus limiting the spread of infection while the body's immune system attacks, immobilizes, and eliminates the pathogens. If the drug is removed before the immune system has scavenged the organisms, enough viable organisms may remain to begin a second cycle of infection. For example, Figure 28.5 shows a laboratory experiment in which the growth of bacteria is arrested by the addition of a bacteriostatic agent. Note that viable organisms remain, even in the presence of the bacteriostatic drug. By contrast, addition of a bactericidal agent kills bacteria and the total number of viable organisms decreases. Though practical, this classification may be too simplistic because it is possible for an antibiotic to be bacteriostatic for one organism and cidal for another, (for example, *chloramphenicol* is static against gram negative rods and cidal against Pneumococci).

IV. CHEMOTHERAPEUTIC SPECTRA

The chemotherapeutic spectrum of a particular drug refers to the species of organisms affected by that drug. In this book, bacteria that are commonly encountered as infectious agents are presented in pie charts in which each segment represents a general class of microorganisms, for example, gram-positive cocci (Figure 28.6A). In each section of the text covering a particular antibiotic, the microbial classes that are generally treated with that agent are highlighted (Figure 28.6B). [Note: One section of the pie chart is labeled "Other" and represents any of several microorganisms specifically covered in different chapters.]

A. Narrow spectrum

Chemotherapeutic agents acting only on a single or a limited group of microorganisms are said to have a narrow spectrum. For example, *isoniazid* is active only against Mycobacteria (Figure 28.6B).

B. Extended spectrum

Extended spectrum is the term applied to antibiotics that are effective against gram-positive organisms and also against a significant number of gram-negative bacteria. For example, *ampicillin* is considered to have an extended spectrum because it acts against gram-positive and some gram-negative bacteria.

C. Broad spectrum

Drugs such as *tetracycline* and *chloramphenicol* affect a wide variety of microbial species and are referred to as broad spectrum antibiotics (Figure 28.6C). Administration of broad spectrum antibiotics can drastically alter the nature of the normal bacterial flora and can precipitate a superinfection of an organism, such as candida whose growth is normally kept in check by the presence of other microorganisms.

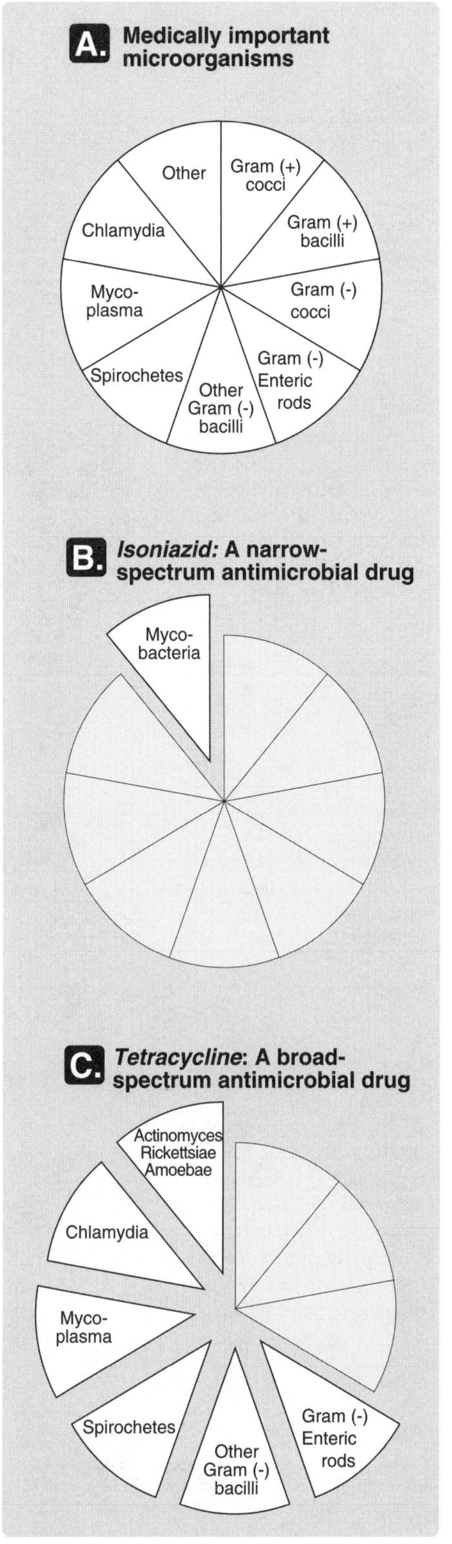

Figure 28.6
A. Medically important bacterial species. B. *Isoniazid*, a narrow-spectrum antimicrobial agent. C. *Tetracycline*, a broad-spectrum antimicrobial agent.

V. COMBINATIONS OF ANTIMICROBIAL DRUGS

It is therapeutically advisable to treat with the single agent that is most specific for the infecting organism. This strategy reduces the possibility of superinfection, decreases the emergence of resistant organisms (see section VI), and minimizes toxicity.. However, situations in which combinations of drugs are employed do exist, for example, the treatment of tuberculosis benefits from drug combinations (p. 331).

A. Advantages of drug combinations

Certain combinations of antibiotics,such as β-lactams and aminoglycosides, show synergism, that is, the combination is more effective than either of the drugs used separately. Because such synergism among antimicrobial agents is rare, they should only be used in special situations summarized in Figure 28.7)

B. Disadvantages of drug combinations

A number of antibiotics act only when organisms are growing. Thus, concomitant administration of a second agent that results in bacteriostasis may interfere with the action of the first drug that is bactericidal.

When mixed infections are present.

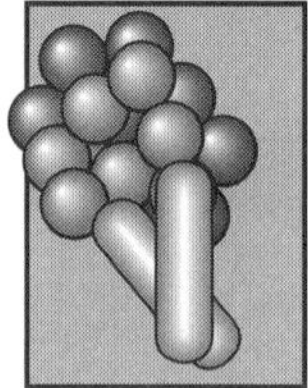

2 **In the treatment of enterococcal endocarditis with *penicillin* and *streptomycin* or cryptococcal meningitis infections with *amphotericin B* in combination with *flucytosine*.**

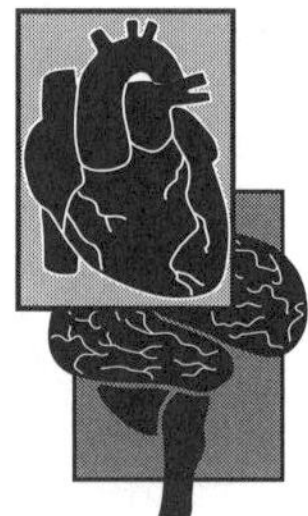

3 **When there is a risk of developing resistant organisms, for example, *isoniazid* plus *pyrazinamide* and *rifampin* in the treatment of tuberculosis.**

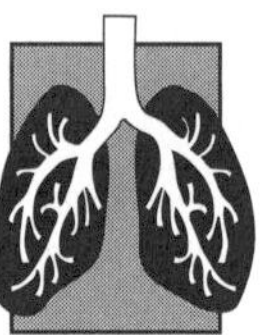

4 **When the greatest antimicrobial coverage is desirable (for example, sepsis, meningitis) or in infections of unknown origin.**

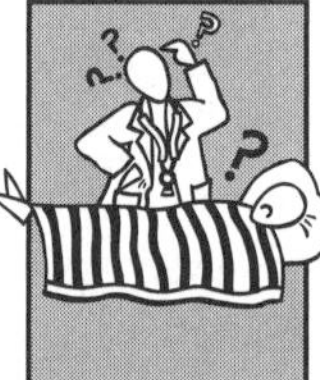

Figure 28.7
Some clinical situations in which combinations of antimicrobial drugs are indicated.

VI. DRUG RESISTANCE

Bacteria are said to be resistant if their growth is not halted by the maximal level of an antibiotic that is tolerated by the host. Some organisms are inherently resistant to an antibiotic. For example, gram-negative organisms are resistant to *vancomycin*. However, microbial species normally responsive to a particular drug may develop resistant strains. Many organisms have adapted, through spontaneous mutation or acquired resistance and selection, and developed more virulent strains many of which are resistant to multiple antibiotics. The emergence of these resistant strains has been ascribed to the imprudent and inappropriate use of antibiotics in conditions that might resolve without treatment or which are not amenable to antibiotic therapy, for example, the common cold. Health professionals are obligated to use antibiotic agents with thoughtful restraint.

A. Genetic alterations leading to drug resistance

Resistance develops due to the ability of DNA to: 1) undergo spontaneous mutation, or 2) move from one organism to another. In the first instance, chromosomal alteration may occur by insertion, deletion or substitution of one or more nucleotides within the genome[1].

1. **Spontaneous mutations of DNA:** The resulting mutation may persist, be corrected, or be lethal to the cell. However, if the cell survives, it may replicate and transmit properties to daughter cells, thus producing resistant strains that may proliferate under certain

[1]See p. 288 for Infolink references to other books in this series.

selective pressures. An example is the emergence of *rifampin*-resistant Mycobacterium tuberculosis when *rifampin* is used as a single drug (see p. 334) .

2. **DNA transfer of drug resistance:** Of particular clinical concern is resistance acquired due to DNA transfer from one organism to another. Resistance properties are usually encoded in extrachromosomal R factors (plasmids). These may enter cells by processes such as transduction (phage-mediated), transformation or, most importantly, bacterial conjugation.

B. Altered expression of proteins in drug-resistant organisms

Drug resistance may be mediated by a variety of mechanisms, such as lack of or an alteration in a target site, lowered penetrability of the drug due to decreased permeability, or increased efflux or presence of antibiotic-inactivating enzymes (Table 28.1).

1. **Modification of target sites:** Alteration of the target site through mutation can confer resistance as occurs with the penicillin binding proteins in *methicillin*-resistant S. aureus, or the enzyme dihydrofolate reductase, which is less sensitive to inhibition in organisms resistant to *trimethoprim.*

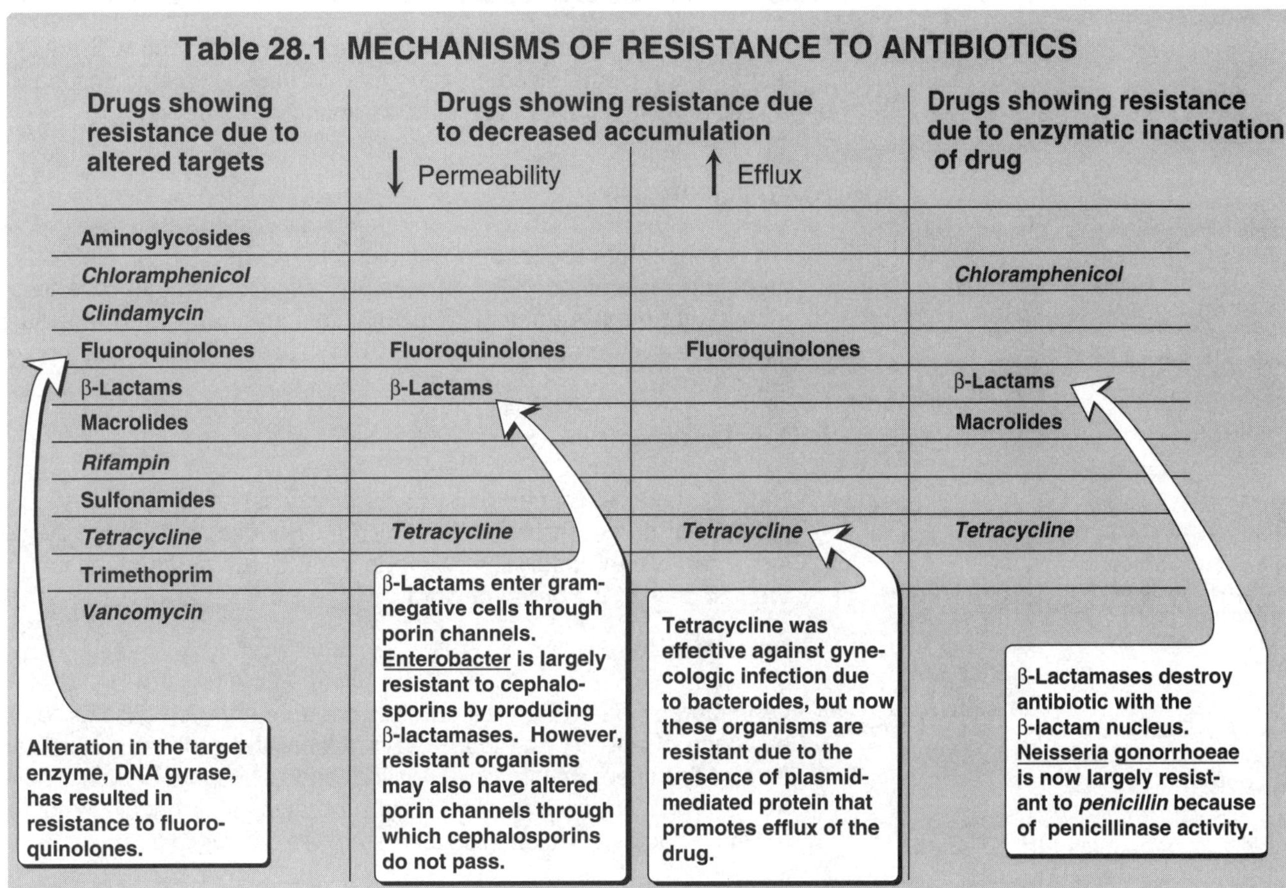

Table 28.1 MECHANISMS OF RESISTANCE TO ANTIBIOTICS

Drugs showing resistance due to altered targets	Drugs showing resistance due to decreased accumulation: ↓ Permeability	Drugs showing resistance due to decreased accumulation: ↑ Efflux	Drugs showing resistance due to enzymatic inactivation of drug
Aminoglycosides			
Chloramphenicol			*Chloramphenicol*
Clindamycin			
Fluoroquinolones	Fluoroquinolones	Fluoroquinolones	
β-Lactams	β-Lactams		β-Lactams
Macrolides			Macrolides
Rifampin			
Sulfonamides			
Tetracycline	*Tetracycline*	*Tetracycline*	*Tetracycline*
Trimethoprim			
Vancomycin			

Alteration in the target enzyme, DNA gyrase, has resulted in resistance to fluoroquinolones.
β-Lactams enter gram-negative cells through porin channels. Enterobacter is largely resistant to cephalosporins by producing β-lactamases. However, resistant organisms may also have altered porin channels through which cephalosporins do not pass.
Tetracycline was effective against gynecologic infection due to bacteroides, but now these organisms are resistant due to the presence of plasmid-mediated protein that promotes efflux of the drug.
β-Lactamases destroy antibiotic with the β-lactam nucleus. Neisseria gonorrhoeae is now largely resistant to *penicillin* because of penicillinase activity.

2. **Decreased accumulation:** Decreased penetrability of an agent can protect organisms against that antibiotic because it is unable to gain access to the site of action due to the presence of either a lipopolysaccharide layer (gram-negative bacteria) or of an efflux system that pumps out the drug (*tetracyclines*, *primaquine*).

3. **Enzymic inactivation:** The ability to destroy or inactivate the antimicrobial agent also can confer resistance on microorganisms. For example, β-lactamases destroy many penicillins and cephalosporins and an acetyltransferase can convert *chloramphenicol* to an inactive compound.

VII. PROPHYLACTIC ANTIBIOTICS

Certain clinical situations (Figure 28.8) require the use of antibiotics for the prevention rather than the treatment of infections. Since the indiscriminate use of antimicrobial agents can result in bacterial resistance and superinfection, prophylactic use is restricted to clinical situations in which benefits outweigh the potential risks. The duration of prophylaxis is dictated by the duration of the risk of infection.

VIII. COMPLICATIONS OF ANTIBIOTIC THERAPY

Selective toxicity to the invading organism does not insure the host against adverse effects, since the drug may produce an allergic response or be toxic in ways unrelated to the drug's antimicrobial activity.

A. Hypersensitivity

Hypersensitivity reactions to antimicrobial drugs or their metabolic products frequently occur. For example, the penicillins, despite their almost absolute selective microbial toxicity, can cause serious hypersensitivity problems, ranging from urticaria (hives) to anaphylactic shock.

B. Direct toxicity

High serum levels of certain antibiotics may cause toxicity by affecting cellular processes in the host directly. For example, aminoglycosides can cause ototoxicity by interfering with membrane function in the hair cells of the organ of Corti.

C. Superinfections

Drug therapy, particularly with broad spectrum antimicrobials or combinations of agents, can lead to alterations of the normal microbial flora of the upper respiratory, intestinal and genitourinary tracts, permitting the overgrowth of opportunistic organisms, especially fungi or resistant bacteria. These infections are often difficult to treat.

Prevention of streptococcal infections in patients with a history of rheumatic heart disease. Patients may require 20 years of treatment.

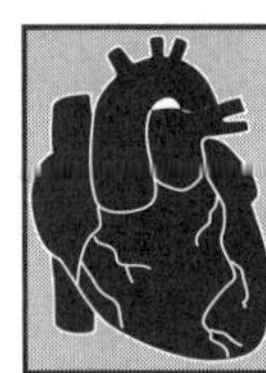

2

Pretreatment of patients undergoing dental extractions who have implanted prosthetic devices, such as artificial heart valves, to prevent seeding of prosthesis.

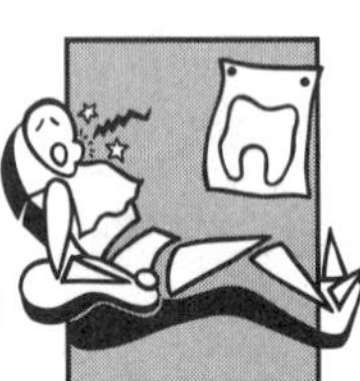

3

Prevention of tuberculosis or meningitis among individuals who are in close contact with infected patients.

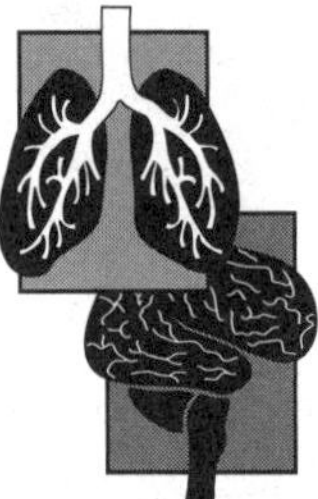

4

Treatment prior to certain surgical produres (such as bowel surgery, joint replacement and some gynecologic interventions) to prevent infection.

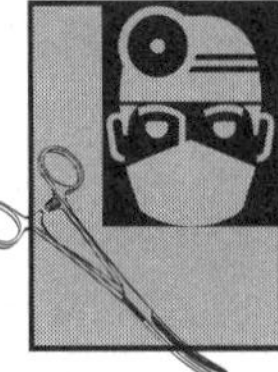

5

Treatment of the mother with *zidovudine* to protect the fetus in the case of an HIV-infected pregnant woman.

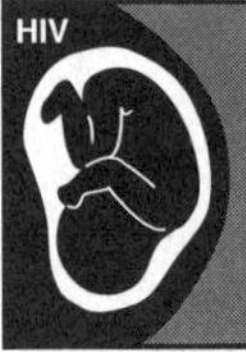

Figure 28.8
Some clinical situations where prophylactic antibiotics are indicated.

IX. CLASSIFICATION OF ANTIMICROBIAL AGENTS

Antimicrobial drugs can be classified in a number of ways, for example, according to their chemical structure (β-lactams, aminoglycosides), mechanism of action (cell wall synthesis inhibitors), or activity against particular types of organisms (bacteria, fungi, viruses). The following chapters will be organized by the mechanisms of action of the drug (Figure 28.9) or according to the type of organisms affected by the drug.

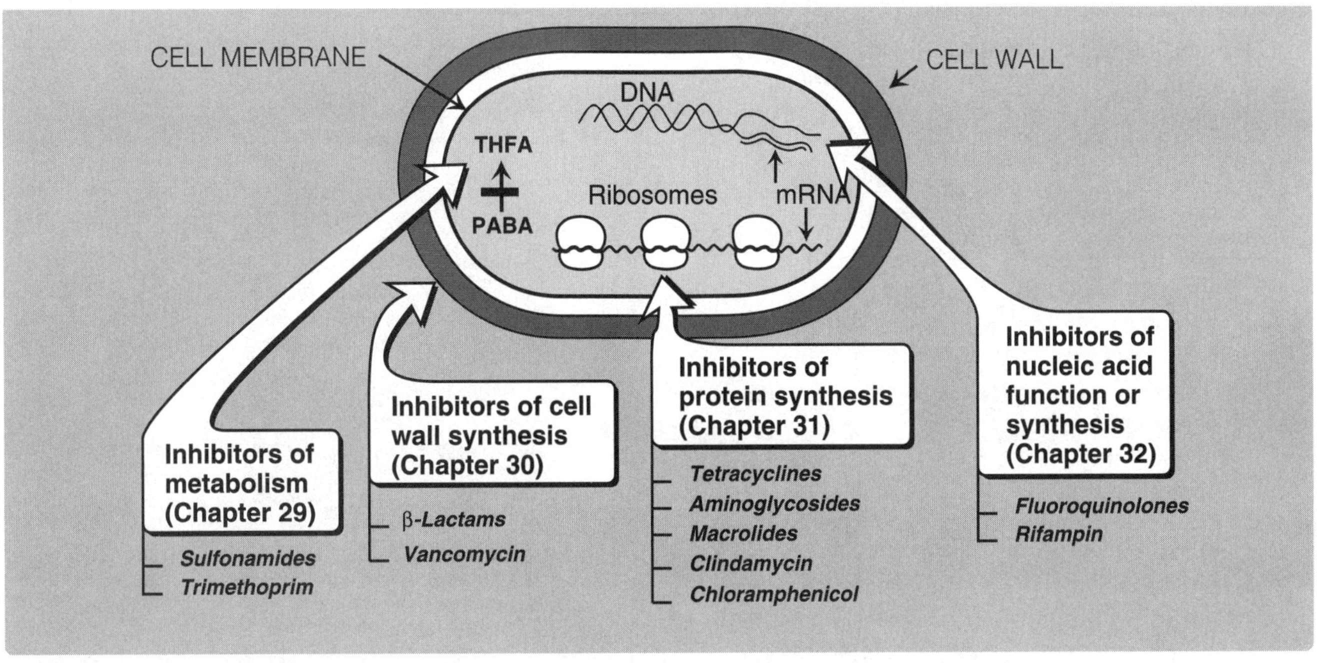

Figure 28.9
Classification of some antimicrobial agents by their sites of action.

Study Questions

Choose the ONE best answer.

28.1 All of the following clinical indications may require a combination of antibiotics (rather than a single agent) EXCEPT:

A. treatment of mixed infections.
B. treatment of enterococcal endocarditis.
C. treatment of tuberculosis.
D. treatment of cryptococcal meningitis.
E. treatment of gonorrhea.

Correct answer = E. Combinations of antibiotics are not indicated in the treatment of gonorrhea. Most Neisseria gonorrhoeae, the causative organism, respond to a single agent—for example, ceftriaxone, a third generation cephalosporin. Combinations of antibiotics are indicated in the treatment of mixed infections, enterococcal endocarditis (with penicillin and streptomycin) and cryptococcal meningitis infection (amphotericin B in combination with flucytosine. Drug combinations are also indicated when there is a risk of developing resistant organisms (for example, isoniazid plus pyrazinamide and rifampin in the treatment of tuberculosis, and when the greatest antimicrobial coverage is desirable (for example, sepsis, meningitis) or in infections of unknown origin.

28.2 Which one of the following patients is least likely to require antimicrobial treatment tailored to the individual's condition?

A. Patient undergoing cancer chemotherapy.
B. Patient with kidney disease.
C. Elderly patient.
D. Patient with hypertension.
E. Patient with liver disease.

Correct answer = D. Elevated blood pressure would not be expected to markedly influence the type of antimicrobial treatment employed. Anticancer drugs often suppress the immune function, and these patients require additional antibiotics to eradicate infections. Impaired renal function may lead to accumulation of toxic levels of antimicrobial drugs. Renal and hepatic function are often decreased among the elderly. Impaired liver function may lead to the accumulation of toxic levels of antimicrobial drugs.

28.3 In which one of the following clinical situations is the prophylactic use of antibiotics NOT warranted?

A. Prevention of meningitis among individuals in close contact with infected patients.
B. Patient with a heart prosthesis having a tooth removed.
C. Presurgical treatment for implantation of a hip prosthesis.
D. Patient who complains of frequent respiratory illness.
E. Presurgical treatment in gastrointestinal procedures.

Correct answer = D. Respiratory illness may be of viral origin; further, consequence of chronic disorder may not warrant prophylactic use of antibiotics. Meningitis is a sufficiently contagious and serious disease to warrant prophylactic use of antibiotics. Following a tooth extraction bacteria of the oral cavity can readily enter the circulation and colonize on a prosthesis, causing a serious and often fatal infection. Infection following implantation of a hip prosthesis is such a serious complication that prophylactic antibiotics are warranted. Infection is such a serious complication of gastrointestinal surgery that prophylactic antibiotics are warranted.

28.4 A 60-year old woman who had undergone chemotherapy for lymphoma the week previously is brought to the emergency room. She has a fever of 101°F and is confused. Respiration is rapid and blood pressure is 78/40. She is neutropenic. Gram stains of the urine and sputum are negative. Which one of the following actions is most likely to be beneficial to this patient?

A. Send a clinical sample to the laboratory for identification and then administer an appropriate antibiotic.
B. Administer a broad spectrum antibiotic like tetracycline.
C. Administer a combination such as clindamycin and an aminoglycoside
D. Administer clindamycin
E. Administer aztreonam.

Correct answer = C. This patient is seriously ill and to wait for identification and sensitivity of the organism would no doubt lead to a worsened condition. Tetracycline is not indicated because it is bacteriostatic and the patient is neutropenic. Its spectrum of activity also does not cover infections due to Pseudomonas aeruginosa, a frequent cause of infection in these patients. Therefore, empiric therapy is required that would employ an antibiotic or a combination of antibiotics to: (1) cover both gram positive and gram negative organisms as well as anaerobes; (2) be bactericidal; (3) cover Pseudomonas aeruginosa; and (4) have good penetrability into tissues. Neither clindamycin or aztreonam by themselves meet these criteria, whereas clindamycin plus an aminoglycoside is appropriate.

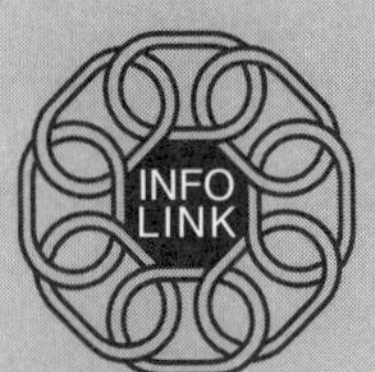

[1]See p. 390 in **Biochemistry** (2nd ed.) for a discussion of mutations in DNA.

Folate Antagonists

29

I. OVERVIEW

Folic acid coenzymes are required for the synthesis of purines and pyrimidines (precursors of RNA and DNA) and other compounds required for cellular growth and replication. In the absence of folic acid, cells cannot grow or divide. The sulfa drugs are inhibitors of folic acid synthesis. They originated from the dye prontosil, which was shown in the early 1930's to be effective against hemolytic streptococcal infections because the body converted it to *sulfanilamide* [sul fa NIL a mide]. Many congeners of the latter compound were synthesized and found to be effective in the treatment of infectious diseases. Today, particularly in developing countries, the sulfas are still employed because of their low cost and efficacy in certain bacterial infections such as those of the urinary tract, and trachoma. However, due to the emergence of resistant bacterial strains, development of patient allergies, and the advent of the penicillins, the sulfas were less frequently prescribed for a time, until their synergistic effect with *trimethoprim* was recognized. With the introduction in the mid-1970s of the synergistic combination of *sulfamethoxazole* [sul fa meth OX a zole] with *trimethoprim* [try METH oh prim] (generic name, *co-trimoxazole* [co try MOX a zole]), there has been a renewed interest in the sulfonamides. *Co-trimoxazole* is effective in treating conditions such as Pneumocystis carinii pneumonia, or *ampicillin-* or *chloramphenicol*-resistant systemic salmonella infections. [Note: Inhibitors of the reduction of folate to its active cofactor form, such as *methotrexate*, are also used in the treatment of certain rapidly growing cancers (see p. 378).]

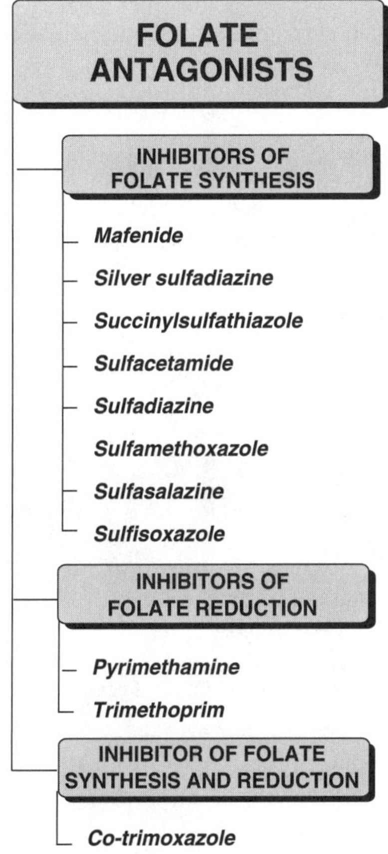

FOLATE ANTAGONISTS
INHIBITORS OF FOLATE SYNTHESIS
Mafenide
Silver sulfadiazine
Succinylsulfathiazole
Sulfacetamide
Sulfadiazine
Sulfamethoxazole
Sulfasalazine
Sulfisoxazole
INHIBITORS OF FOLATE REDUCTION
Pyrimethamine
Trimethoprim
INHIBITOR OF FOLATE SYNTHESIS AND REDUCTION
Co-trimoxazole

Figure 29.1
Summary of folate antagonists.

II. SULFONAMIDES

All sulfonamides in clinical use are synthetic structural analogs of p-aminobenzoic acid (PABA). They differ from each other not only in their chemical and physical properties but also in their pharmacokinetics.

A. Mechanism of action

Being impermeable to folic acid, many bacteria must rely on their ability to synthesize folate from PABA, pteridine, and glutamate. In contrast, human beings cannot synthesize folic acid and must obtain preformed folate as a vitamin in their diet. Because of their structural similarity to PABA, the sulfonamides compete with this substrate for the enzyme dihydropteroate synthetase, thus preventing the synthe-

H_2N–C₆H₄–COOH

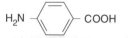

p-Aminobenzoic acid (PABA)

Pteridine precursor

Dihydro-pteroate synthetase

H_2N–C₆H₄–SO_2–NHR

Sulfanilamide (and other sulfonamides)

Folic acid

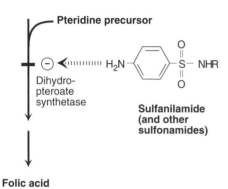

Figure 29.2
Competitive inhibition of folic acid synthesis by sulfonamides.

sis of bacterial folic acid and formation of its one-carbon carrying cofactors.[1] This deprives the cell of essential cofactors for purine, pyrimidine, and amino acid synthesis (Figure 29.2, see also Figure 29.5).

B. Antibacterial spectrum

The sulfas, including *co-trimoxazole* (*sulfamethoxazole* plus *trimethoprim*, see p. 293), are bacteriostatic. These drugs are active against selected enterobacteria, chlamydia, Pneumocystis, and nocardia. Typical clinical applications are shown in Figure 29.3. In addition, *sulfadiazine* [sul fa DYE a zeen] in combination with the dihydrofolate reductase inhibitor *pyrimethamine* [py ri METH a meen] is the only effective form of chemotherapy for toxoplasmosis (p. 353).

C. Resistance

Only organisms that synthesize their own folate are sensitive to the sulfonamides. Bacterial resistance to the sulfas can arise from plasmid transfers or random mutations. The resistance is generally irreversible and may be due to any of the following three possibilities. [Note: Organisms resistant to one member of this drug family are resistant to all, but they may be susceptible to *co-trimoxazole*.]

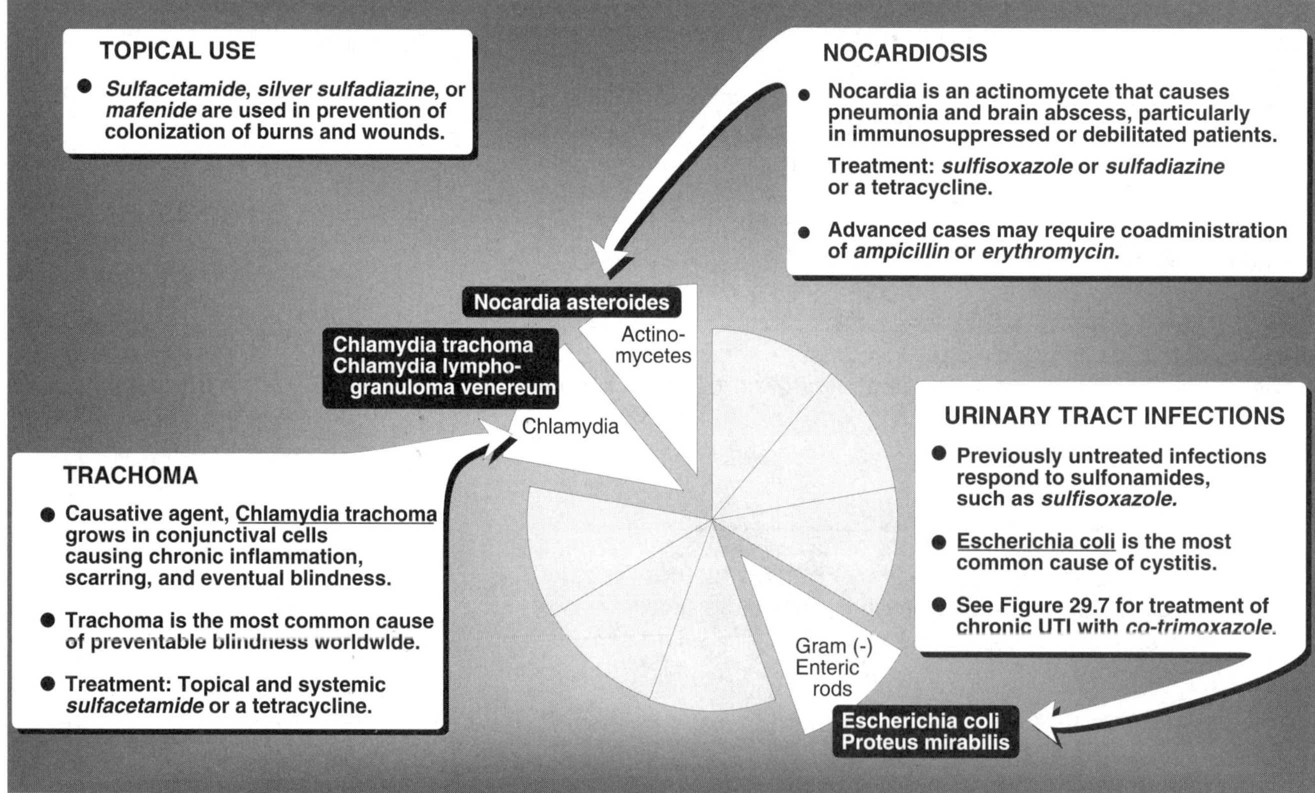

Figure 29.3
Typical therapeutic applications of sulfonamides. UTI= urinary tract infection.

[1]See p. 296 for Infolink references to other books in this series.

1. **Altered enzyme:** Bacterial dihydropteroate synthetase can undergo mutation or be transferred via a plasmid to result in a decreased affinity for the sulfas. The drugs therefore become less effective competitors of PABA.

2. **Decreased uptake:** Permeability to sulfas may be reduced in some resistant strains.

3. **Increased PABA synthesis:** Enhanced production of the natural substrate, PABA, by the microorganism through selection or mutation can overcome the inhibition of the dihydropteroate synthetase by the sulfas.

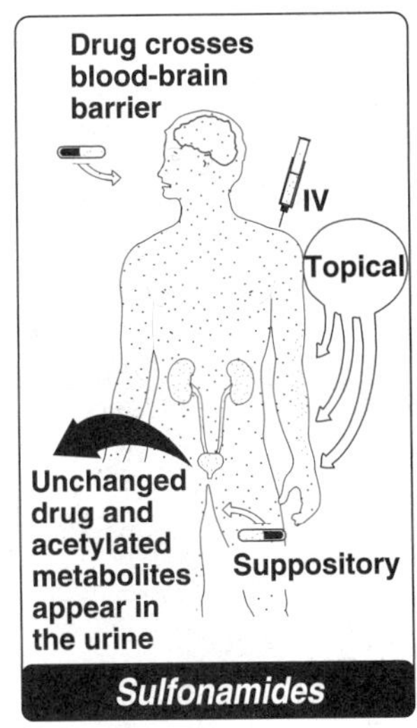

D. Pharmacokinetics

1. **Administration:** Most sulfa drugs are well absorbed after oral administration. *Sulfasalazine* [sul fa SAL a zeen], when administered orally or as a suppository, is reserved for treatment of chronic inflammatory bowel disease (for example, Crohn's disease or ulcerative colitis), because it is not absorbed. Similarly, *succinylsulfathiazole* [suks in ill sul fa THI a zole] is used for the treatment of salmonella and shigella carriers. Intravenous sulfonamides are generally reserved for patients who are unable to take oral preparations. Because of the risk of sensitization, sulfas are not usually applied topically. In burn units, creams of *mafenide acetate* (*p-aminomethylbenzensulfonamide*) or *silver sulfadiazine* have been effective in reducing burn sepsis. However, superinfections with resistant bacteria or fungi may occur.

2. **Distribution:** Sulfa drugs are distributed throughout body water and penetrate well into cerebrospinal fluid, even in the absence of inflammation. They can also pass the placental barrier and into breast milk. Sulfa drugs are bound to serum albumin in the circulation; the extent of binding depends on the particular agent.

3. **Metabolism:** The sulfas are acetylated at N4, primarily in the liver. The product is devoid of antimicrobial activity, but it retains the toxic potential to precipitate at neutral or acidic pH, causing crystalluria ("stone formation") and therefore potential damage to the kidney (Figure 29.4). *Sulfasalazine* is effective in the treatment of inflammatory bowel disease because local intestinal flora split the drug into *sulfapyridine* and *5-aminosalicylate.* The latter exerts the antiinflammatory effect. Absorption of *sulfapyridine* can lead to toxicity in patients who are slow acetylators.

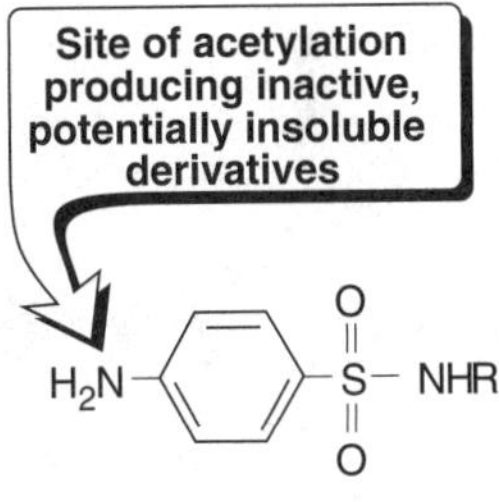

Figure 29.4
Inactivation of sulfonamides.

4. **Excretion:** Elimination of sulfas is by glomerular filtration. Therefore, depressed kidney function causes accumulation of both the parent compounds and their metabolites.

E. Adverse effects

1. **Crystalluria:** Nephrotoxicity develops as a result of crystalluria. Adequate hydration and alkalinization of urine prevent the problem by reducing the concentration of drug and promoting its ion-

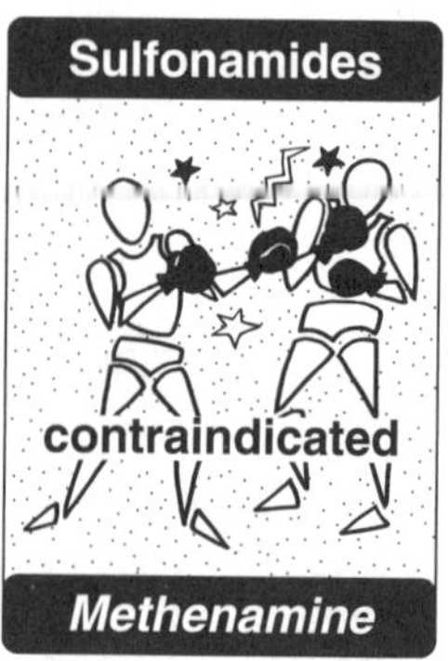

ization. Newer agents, such as *sulfisoxazole* [sul fi SOX a zole] and *sulfamethoxazole* are more soluble at urinary pH than are the older sulfonamides (for example, *sulfadiazine*) and are less liable to cause crystalluria.

2. **Hypersensitivity:** Hypersensitivity reactions, such as rashes, angioedema, and Stevens-Johnson syndrome, are fairly common. The latter occurs more frequently with the longer acting agents. [Note: Many drugs are derived from the sulfas and cross allergenicity has been reported for the diuretics, *acetazolamide*, *thiazides*, *furosemide*, *bumetanide*, *diazoxide* (see p. 226) and the sulfonylurea hypoglycemic drugs (see p. 260).]

3. **Hemopoietic disturbances:** Hemolytic anemia is encountered in patients with glucose 6-phosphate dehydrogenase deficiency[2] (p. 351). Granulocytopenia and thrombocytopenia can also occur.

4. **Kernicterus:** This disorder may occur in newborns because sulfas displace bilirubin from binding sites on serum albumin. The bilirubin is then free to pass into the central nervous system.

5. **Drug potentiation:** Transient potentiation of the hypoglycemic effect of *tolbutamide* (see p. 260) or the anticoagulant effect of *warfarin* or of *bishydroxycoumarin* (see p. 199) results from their displacement from binding sites on serum albumin. Free *methotrexate* (see p. 378) levels may also rise through displacement.

6. **Contraindications:** Sulfas should be avoided in newborns and infants less than 2 months old as well as pregnant women at term, due to the danger of kernicterus. Because sulfonamides condense with formaldehyde, they should not be given to patients receiving *methenamine* (see p. 327) for urinary tract infections.

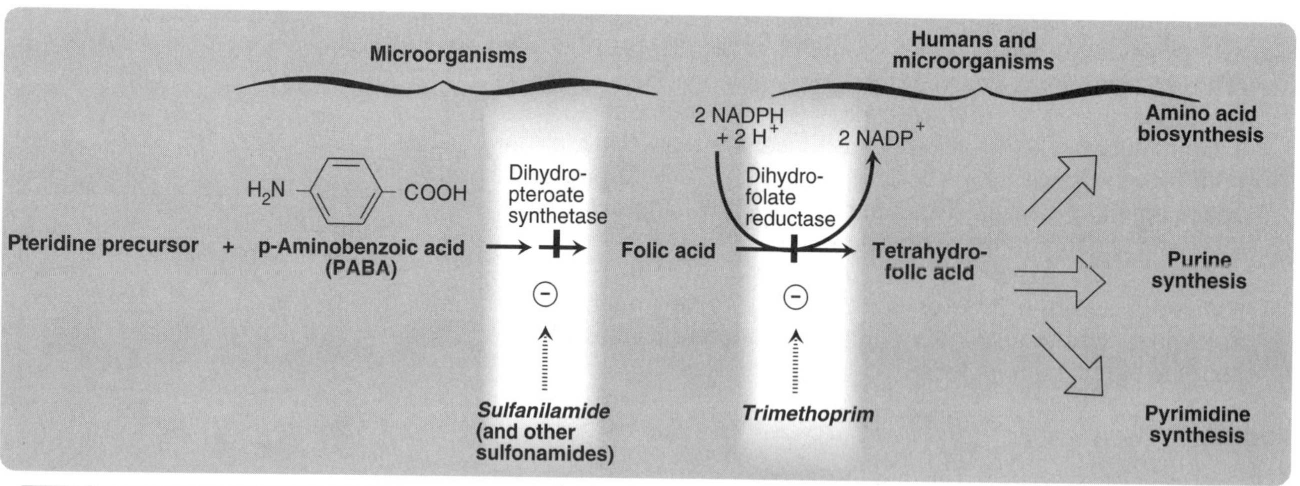

Figure 29.5
Inhibition of tetrahydrofolate synthesis by sulfonamides and *trimethoprim*.

[2]See p. 296 for Infolink references to other books in this series.

III. TRIMETHOPRIM

Trimethoprim [trye METH oh prim], a potent inhibitor of bacterial dihydrofolate reductase[3], exhibits an antibacterial spectrum similar to the sulfonamides. However, *trimethoprim* is most often compounded with *sulfamethoxazole*.

A. Mechanism of action

The active form of folate is the tetrahydro-derivative that is formed through reduction by dihydrofolate reductase. This enzymatic reaction (Figure 29.5) is inhibited by *trimethoprim*, leading to a decrease in the folate coenzymes for purine, pyrimidine, and amino acid synthesis. Bacterial reductase has a much stronger affinity for *trimethoprim* than does the mammalian enzyme, which accounts for the drug's selective toxicity. [Note: Examples of other folate reductase inhibitors include *pyrimethamine*, which is used with sulfonamides in parasitic infections (see p. 353), and *methotrexate*, which is used in cancer chemotherapy (see p. 378).]

B. Antibacterial spectrum

The antibacterial spectrum of *trimethoprim* is similar to that of *sulfamethoxazole* (see p. 290); however, *trimethoprim* is 20 to 50 times more potent than the sulfonamide. *Trimethoprim* may be used alone in acute urinary tract infections and in the treatment of bacterial prostatitis (though fluoroquinolones are preferred).

C. Resistance

Resistance in gram-negative bacteria is due to the presence of an altered dihydrofolate reductase that has a lower affinity for the drug.

D. Pharmacokinetics

The pharmacokinetic characteristics of *trimethoprim* are similar to *sulfamethoxazole*, but higher concentrations are achieved in the relatively acidic prostatic and vaginal fluids since it is a weak base. *Trimethoprim* undergoes O-demethylation.

E. Adverse effects

Trimethoprim can produce the effects of folate deficiency, that is, megaloblastic anemia, leukopenia, and granulocytopenia. These reactions can be reversed by the simultaneous administration of *folinic acid*, which does not enter bacteria (see p. 379).

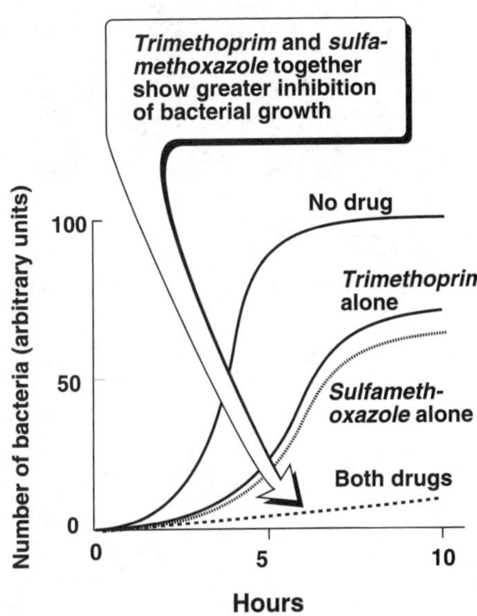

Figure 29.6
Synergism between *trimethoprim* and *sulfamethoxazole* on the inhibition of growth of Escherichia coli

IV. CO-TRIMOXAZOLE

Trimethoprim is most often compounded with the sulfa drug, *sulfamethoxazole*. The resulting combination, called *co-trimoxazole*, shows greater antimicrobial activity than equivalent quantities of either drug used alone (Figure 29.6). The combination was selected because of the similarity in the pharmacokinetics of the two drugs.

[3]See p. 296 for Infolink references to other books in this series.

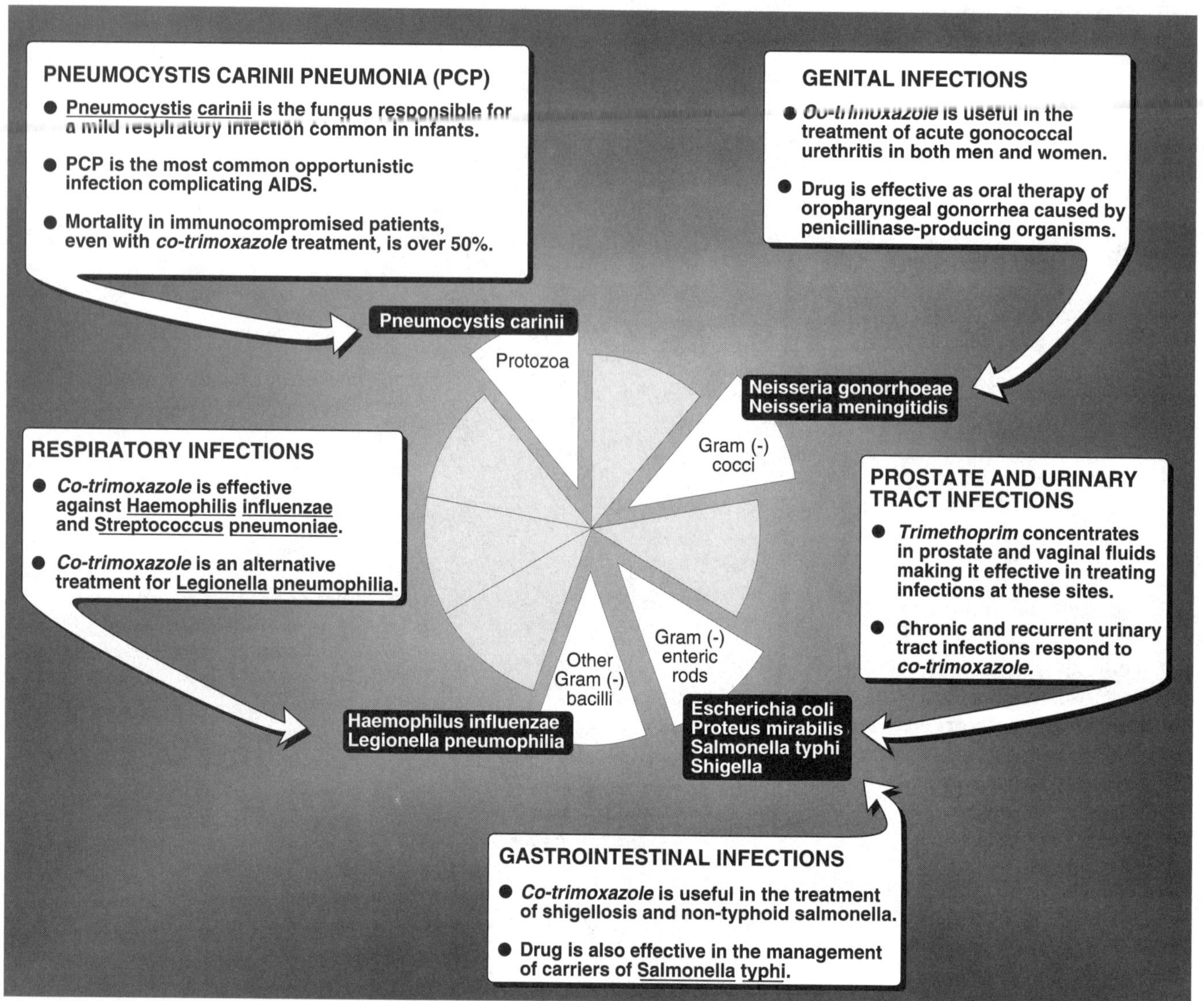

Figure 29.7
Typical therapeutic applications of *co-trimoxazole* (*sulfamethoxazole* plus *trimethoprim*).

A. Mechanism of action

The synergistic antimicrobial activity of *co-trimoxazole* results from its inhibition of two sequential steps in the synthesis of tetrahydrofolic acid: *sulfamethoxazole* inhibits the incorporation of PABA into folic acid, and *trimethoprim* prevents reduction of dihydrofolate to tetrahydrofolate (see Figure 29.5). *Co-trimoxazole* exhibits more potent antimicrobial activity than *sulfamethoxazole* or *trimethoprim* alone (seed Figure 29.6).

B. Antibacterial spectrum

The combination of *trimethoprim-sulfamethoxazole* has a broader spectrum of action than the sulfas (Figure 29.7).

C. Resistance

Resistance to the *trimethoprim-sulfamethoxazole* combination is less frequently encountered than resistance to either of the drugs alone because it requires simultaneous resistance to both drugs.

D. Pharmacokinetics

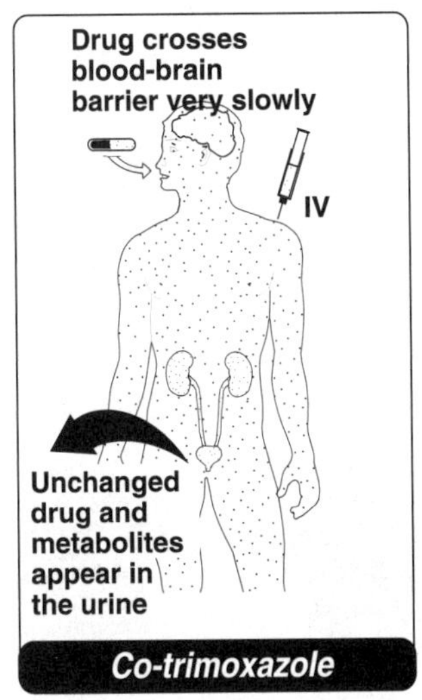
Drug crosses blood-brain barrier very slowly
IV
Unchanged drug and metabolites appear in the urine
Co-trimoxazole

1. **Administration and metabolism:** *Trimethoprim* is more lipid-soluble than *sulfamethoxazole* and has a greater volume of distribution. Administration of 1 part of *trimethoprim* to 5 parts of the sulfa drug produces a ratio of the drugs in the plasma of 20 parts of *sulfamethoxazole* to 1 part *trimethoprim*. This ratio is optimal for the antibiotic effect. *Co-trimoxazole* is generally administered orally. An exception involves intravenous administration to patients with severe pneumonia caused by <u>Pneumocystis</u> <u>carinii</u>, or to patients who cannot take the drug by mouth.

2. **Fate:** Both agents distribute throughout the body. *Trimethoprim* concentrates in the relatively acidic milieu of prostatic and vaginal fluids and accounts for the use of the *trimethoprim-sulfamethoxazole* combination in infections at these sites. Both parent drugs and their metabolites are excreted in the urine.

E. Adverse effects

1. **Dermatologic:** Reactions involving the skin are very common and may be severe in the elderly.

2. **Gastrointestinal:** Nausea, vomiting as well as glossitis, and stomatitis are not unusual.

3. **Hematologic:** Megaloblastic anemia, leukopenia, and thrombocytopenia may occur; all of these effects may be reversed by the concurrent administration of *folinic acid* (see p. 379), which protects the patient and does not enter the microorganism. Hemolytic anemia may occur in patients with glucose-6-phosphate deficiency due to the *sulfamethoxazole* (see p. 351).

4. **HIV patients:** These immunocompromised patients with <u>Pneumocystis</u> pneumonia frequently show drug-induced fever, rashes, diarrhea and/or pancytopenia.

5. **Drug Interactions:** Prolonged prothrombin times in patients receiving *warfarin* have been reported. Plasma half-life of *phenytoin* (see p. 147) may be increased due to an inhibition of its metabolism. *Methotrexate* (see p. 378) levels may rise due to displacement from albumin binding sites by the *sulfamethoxazole*.

Choose the ONE best answer.

29.1 Sulfonamides are useful in the treatment of which one of the following?

A. Influenza.
B. Gonorrhea.
C. Most streptococcal infections.
D. Urinary tract infections.
E. Meningococcal infections.

Correct answer = D. Sulfonamides at one time were the mainstay of the treatment of uncomplicated infections of the urinary tract.

29.2 Trimethoprim:

A. is less potent than sulfamethoxazole.
B. inhibits the enzyme dihydropteroate synthetase.
C. lowers the ratio of tetrahydrofolate to folate in the organism
D. resistance has not been observed in microorganisms.
E. stimulates purine synthesis.

Correct answer = C. Trimethoprim is 20 to 50 times more potent than sulfamethoxazole. It inhibits the enzyme dihydrofolate reductase, thus preventing both purine and pyrimidine synthesis. Trimethoprim resistance has been observed in gram-negative bacteria caused by the presence of a plasmid that codes for an altered dihydrofolate reductase with a lower affinity for the drug.

29.3 All of the following statements concerning sulfonamides are correct EXCEPT:

A. They require actively growing cultures for maximum antimicrobial activity.
B. Allergic reactions are frequent adverse effects.
C. Treatment of patients with severe renal insufficiency may lead to crystalluria.
D. They diminish activity of warfarin.
E. They compete with p-aminobenzoic acid for the enzyme dihydropteroate synthetase.

Correct choice = D. Transient potentiation of the anticoagulant effect of vitamin K antagonists, such as warfarin or bis-hydroxycoumarin, results from their displacement from binding sites on serum albumin. Sulfonamides are bacteriostatic and are most effective against growing microorganisms, where they are competitive inhibitors of dihydropteroate synthetase. Allergic reactions and crystalluria are the two most common adverse effects associated with sulfonamide treatment. The sulfonamides tend to have low solubilities and to form crystals in the kidney or bladder, particularly if urinary output is low.

29.4 Sulfonamides increase the risk of neonatal kernicterus because they

A. diminish the production of plasma albumin.
B. increase the turnover of red blood cells.
C. inhibit the metabolism of bilirubin.
D. compete for bilirubin binding sites on plasma albumin.
E. depress the bone marrow.

Correct answer = D. Increased release of albumin-bound bilirubin increases the plasma concentration of free bilirubin, which can penetrate the CNS.

Questions 29.5 - 29.7: For each phrase, select the ONE drug (A-E) that is most closely associated with it. Each drug (A-E) may be selected once, more than once, or not at all.

A. Sulfasalazine
B. Sulfacetamide
C. Trimethoprim-sulfamethoxazole
D. Mafenide acetate
E. Sulfisoxazole

29.5 It is used to prevent infections among burn patients.

Correct answer = D. Creams containing mafenide acetate are used in burn units where they are used prophylactically to protect against infection with a variety of gram-negative and gram-positive microorganisms.

29.6 It is used in the treatment of ulcerative colitis.

Correct answer = A. Sulfasalazine is reserved for treatment of ulcerative colitis because the drug is not absorbed from the gut and acts locally.

29.7 It is effective in the treatment of pneumonia caused by Pneumocystis carinii.

Correct answer = C. Co-trimoxazole is currently the drug of choice, although high doses are required.

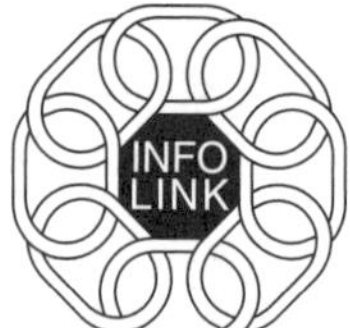

[1]See p. 250 in **Biochemistry** (2nd ed.) for a discussion of synthesis of folic acid and formation of its one-carbon carrying cofactors.

[3]See p. 325 in **Biochemistry** (2nd ed.) for a discussion of a role of dihydrofolate reductase in metabolism.

[2]See p. 115 in **Biochemistry** (2nd ed.) for a discussion of the causes of hemolytic anemia encountered in patients with glucose 6-phosphate dehydrogenase deficiency.

Inhibitors of Cell Wall Synthesis

30

I. OVERVIEW

Some antimicrobial drugs selectively interfere with the synthesis of the bacterial cell wall. Unique to bacteria, this structure is not found in mammalian cells. It is a polymer of glycan units joined to each other by peptide cross-links, hence, the designation of peptidoglycan cell wall. To be maximally effective, these agents require actively proliferating microorganisms; they have little or no effect on bacteria that are not growing. The most important members of the group are the β-lactam antibiotics, named after the β-lactam ring, which is essential to their activity (Figure 30.1).

II. PENICILLINS

The penicillins [pen i SILL in] are the most widely effective antibiotics and are among the least toxic drugs known; the major adverse reaction to penicillins is hypersensitivity. The members of this family differ from one another in the R substituent attached to the 6-aminopenicillanic acid residue. The nature of this side chain affects their antimicrobial spectrum, stability to stomach acid, and susceptibility to bacterial degradative enzymes (β-lactamases). Figure 30.1 shows the main structural features of the penicillins. Figure 30.2 shows the classification of agents affecting cell wall synthesis.

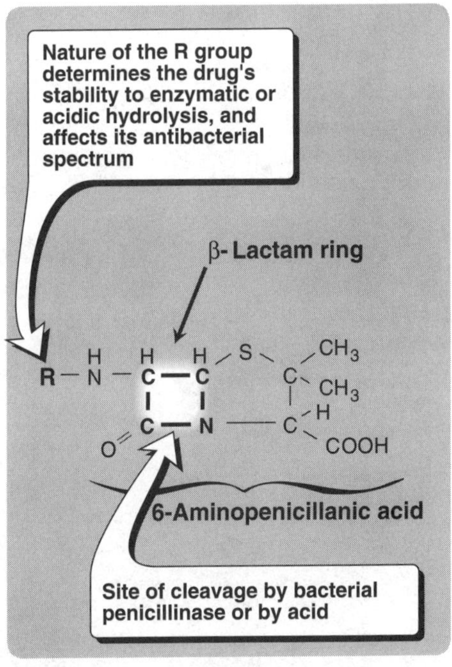

Figure 30.1
Structural features of β-lactam antibiotics.

A. Mechanism of action

The penicillins interfere with the last step of bacterial cell wall synthesis (transpeptidation or cross-linkage), thus exposing the osmotically less stable membrane. Cell lysis can then occur, and these drugs are therefore bactericidal. The success of a penicillin antibiotic in causing cell death is related to its size, charge, and hydrophobicity (see p. 300). Penicillins are, of course, only effective against rapidly growing organisms that synthesize a peptidoglycan cell wall. Consequently, they are inactive against organisms devoid of this structure, such as mycobacteria, protozoa, fungi, and viruses.

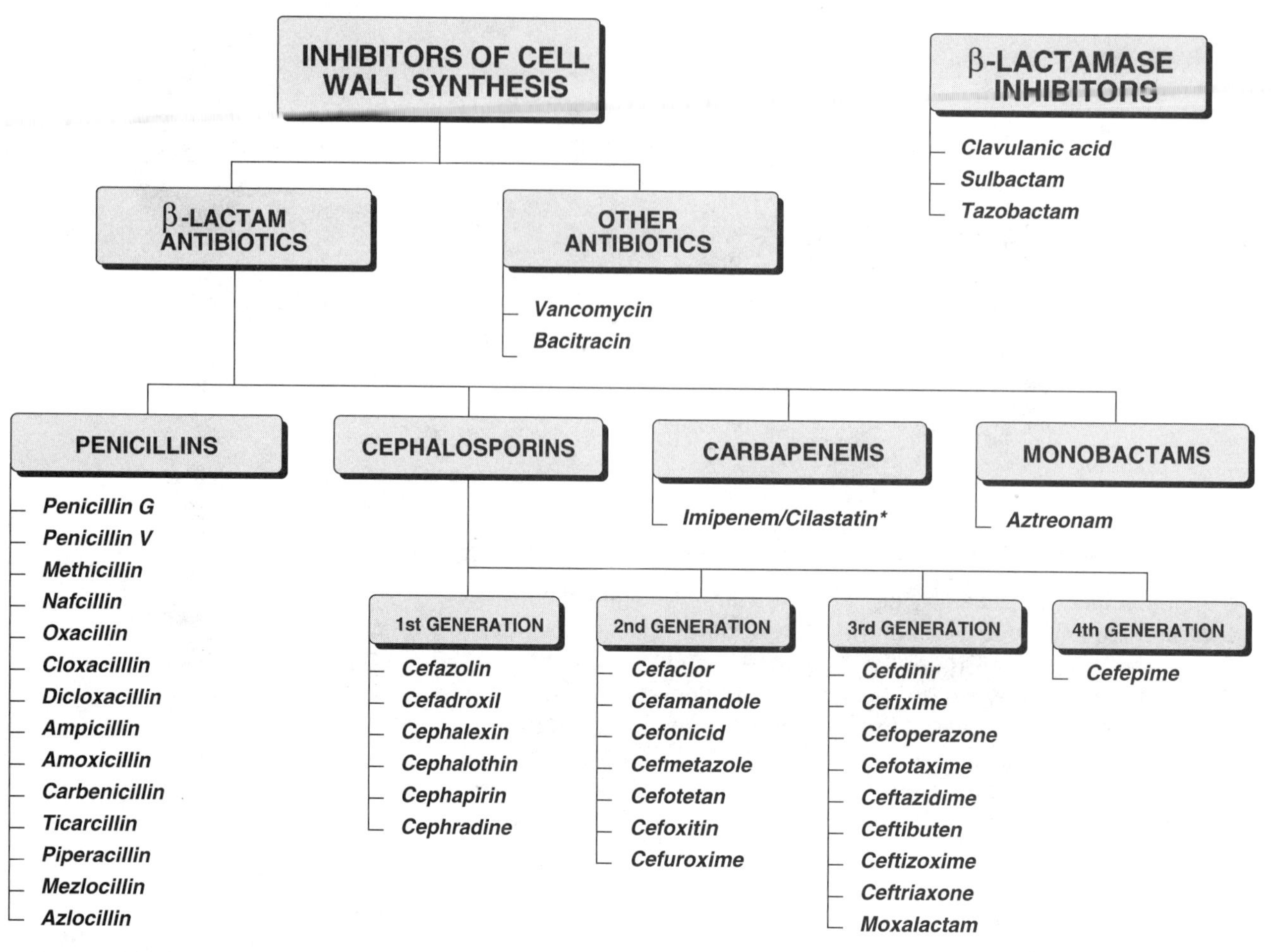

Figure 30.2
Summary of antimicrobial agents affecting cell wall synthesis *[Note: Cilastatin is not an antibiotic but a peptidase inhibitor that protects *imipenem* from degradation.]

1. **Penicillin binding proteins:** Penicillins inactivate proteins present on the bacterial cell membrane. These penicillin binding proteins (PBPs) are bacterial enzymes involved in the synthesis of the cell wall, and in the maintenance of the morphologic features of the bacterium. Exposure to these antibiotics can therefore not only prevent cell wall synthesis but also lead to morphologic changes or lysis of susceptible bacteria. The number of PBPs vary with the type of organism. Alterations in some of these target molecules confer resistance on the organism. [Note: *Methicillin*-resistant Staphylococcus aureus, MRSA, apparently arose because of such an alteration.]

2. **Inhibition of transpeptidase:** Some PBPs catalyze formation of the cross-linkages between peptidoglycan chains. Penicillins inhibit this transpeptidase-catalyzed reaction, thus hindering the formation of crosslinks essential for cell wall integrity. As a result of this blockade of cell wall synthesis, the "Park peptide", UDP-acetylmuramyl-L-Ala-D-Gln-L-Lys-D-Ala-D-Ala, accumulates.

3. **Autolysins:** Many bacteria, particularly the gram-positive cocci, produce degradative enzymes (autolysins) that participate in the normal remodeling of the bacterial cell wall. In the presence of *penicillin*, the degradative action of the autolysins proceeds in the absence of cell wall synthesis. The exact autolytic mechanism is unknown but may be due to a disinhibition of the autolysins. Thus, the antibacterial effect of *penicillin* is the result of both inhibition of cell wall synthesis and destruction of existing cell wall by autolysins.

B. Antibacterial spectrum

The antibacterial spectrum of the various penicillins is determined, in part, by their ability to cross the bacterial peptidoglycan cell wall and to reach the penicillin-binding proteins that are located in the periplasmic space. In general, gram-positive microorganisms have cell walls that are easily traversed by penicillins and therefore (in the absence of resistance) are susceptible to these drugs. Gram-negative microorganisms have an outer lipopolysaccharide membrane surrounding the cell wall that presents a barrier to the water-soluble penicillins. [Note: For this reason, penicillins have little use in the treatment of intracellular pathogens.] Gram-negative bacteria have

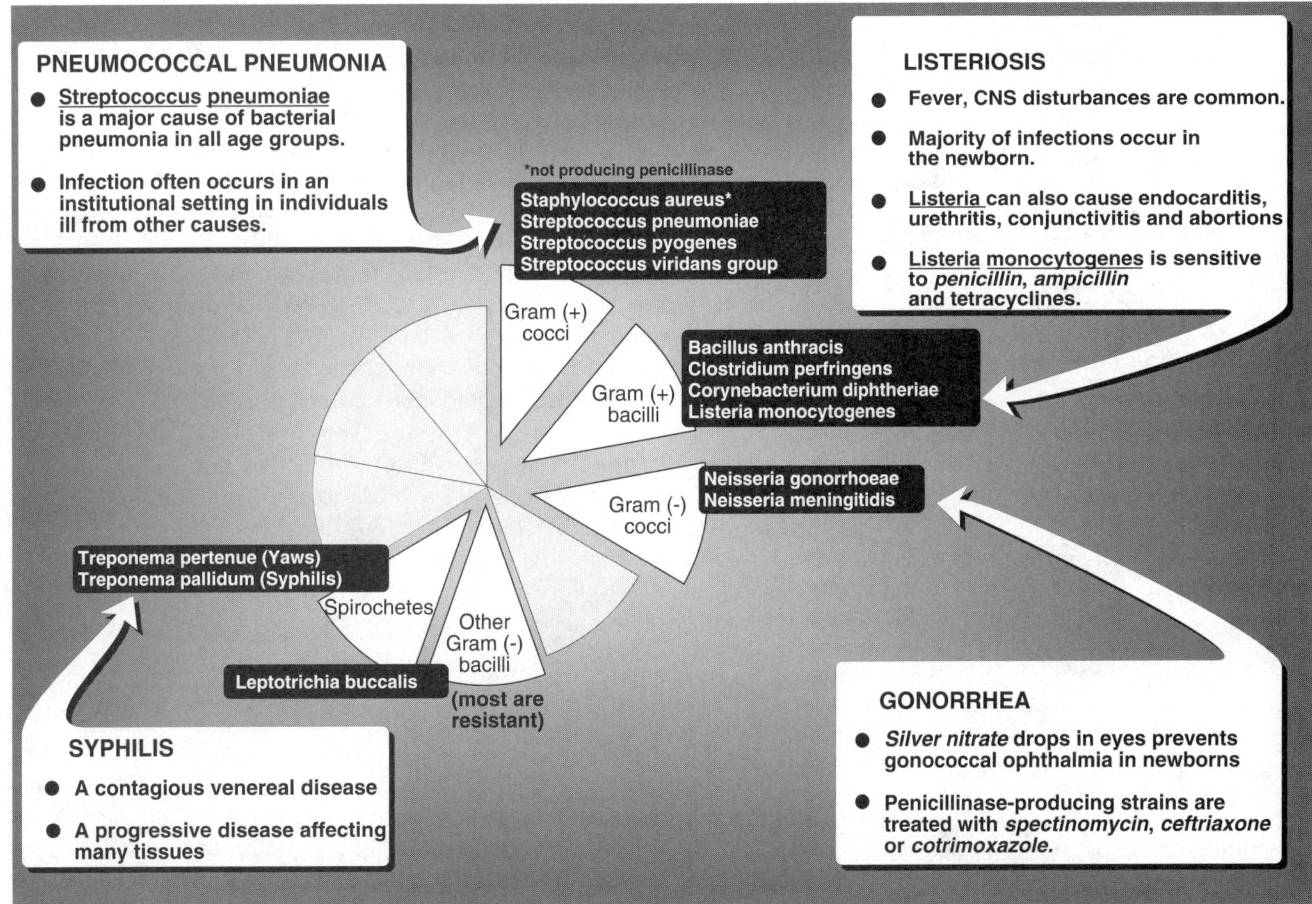

Figure 30.3
Typical therapeutic applications of penicillin G.

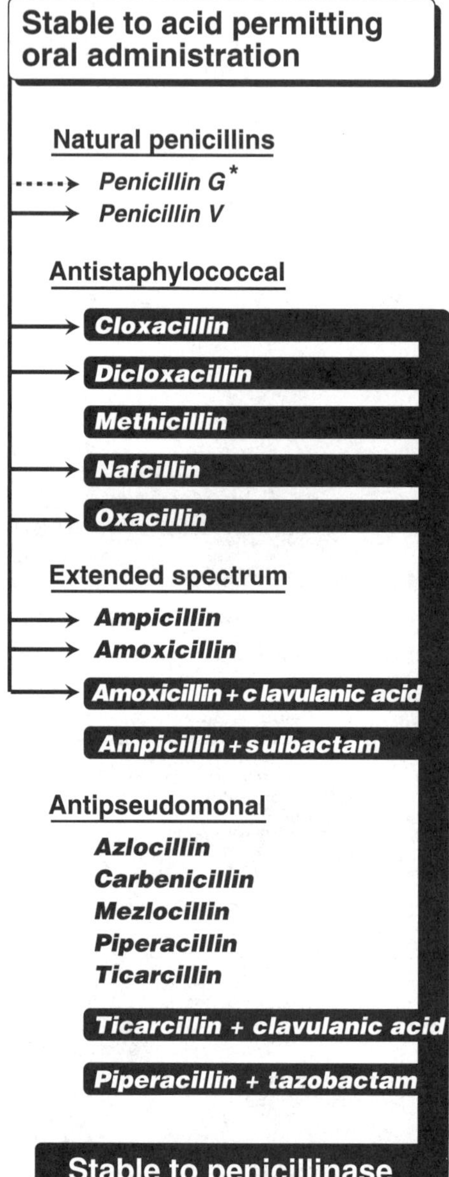

Figure 30.4
Stability of the penicillins to acid or the action of penicillinase
*[Note: *Penicillin G* is largely inactived by stomach acid, but doses can be adjusted so that adequate serum levels are achieved.]

proteins inserted in the lipopolysaccharide layer that act as water-filled channels (also called porins) and permit transmembrane entry. Factors that determine their susceptibility to these antibiotics include the size, charge and hydrophobicity of the particular β-lactam.

1. Natural penicillins

These penicillins, which include those listed as antistaphylococcal, are obtained from fermentations of the mold Penicillium chrysogenum. Other penicillins are called semi-synthetic because the different R groups are attached chemically to the 6-aminopenicillanic acid nucleus obtained from fermentation broths of the mold.

a. **Penicillin G** (*benzylpenicillin*) is the cornerstone of therapy for infections caused by a number of gram-positive and gram-negative cocci, gram-positive bacilli, and spirochetes (Figure 30.3). *Penicillin G* is susceptible to inactivation by β-lactamases (penicillinases, Figure 30.4).

b. **Penicillin V** has a spectrum similar to *penicillin G*, but it is not used for treatment of bacteremia because of its higher minimum lethal concentration (MLC, the minimum amount of the drug needed to eliminate the infection). *Penicillin V* is more acid-stable than *penicillin G*. It is often employed in the treatment of oral infections where it is effective against some anaerobic organisms.

2. Antistaphylococcal penicillins: *Methicillin* [meth i SILL in], *nafcillin* [naf SILL in], *oxacillin* [ox a SILL in], *cloxacillin* [klox a SILL in], and *dicloxacillin* [dye klox a SILL in] are penicillinase-resistant penicillins. Their use is restricted to the treatment of infections caused by penicillinase-producing staphylococci. Because of its toxicity, *methicillin* is rarely used. *Methicillin*-resistant strains of Staphylococcus aureus (MRSA), currently a serious source of nosocomial (hospital-acquired) infections, are usually susceptible to *vancomycin*, and rarely to *ciprofloxacin* or *rifampin*.

3. Extended spectrum penicillins: *Ampicillin* [am pi SIL in] and *amoxicillin* [a mox i SIL in] have an antibacterial spectrum similar to that of *penicillin G*, but are more effective against gram-negative bacilli. They are therefore referred to as extended spectrum penicillins (Figure 30.5). *Ampicillin* is the drug of choice for the gram-positive bacillus, Listeria monocytogenes. These agents are also widely used in the treatment of respiratory infections, and *amoxicillin* is employed prophylactically by dentists for patients with abnormal heart valves who are to undergo extensive oral surgery. Resistance to these antibiotics is now a major clinical problem because of inactivation by plasmid-mediated penicillinase. [Note: Escherichia coli and Haemophilus influenzae are frequently resistant.] Formulation with a β-lactamase inhibitor, such as *clavulanic acid* or *sulbactam*, protects *amoxicillin* or *ampicillin*, respectively, from enzymatic hydrolysis, and extends their antimicrobial spectrum. (See p. 307 for a discussion of these inhibitors.)

4. **Antipseudomonal penicillins:** *Carbenicillin* [kar ben i SILL in], *ticarcillin* [tye kar SILL in], and *piperacillin* [pip er a SILL in] are called antipseudomonal penicillins because of their activity against Pseudomonas aeruginosa. *Piperacillin* is the most potent. These antibiotics are effective against many gram-negative bacilli but not against Klebsiella, because of its constitutive penicillinase (Figure 30.5B). Formulation of *ticarcillin* or *piperacillin* with *clavulanic acid* or *tazobactam*, respectively (see p. 307) extends the antimicrobial spectrum of these antibiotics to include penicillinase-producing organisms. *Mezlocillin* [mez loe SILL in] and *azlocillin* [az loe SILL in] (sometimes referred to as *acylureido penicillins*) are also effective against Pseudomonas aeruginosa, and a large number of gram-negative organisms. They are susceptible to β-lactamase breakdown. (see Figure 30.4).

6. **Penicillins and aminoglycosides:** The antibacterial effects of all the β-lactam antibiotics are synergistic with the aminoglycosides. The ability of penicillins (and other agents that inhibit cell wall synthesis) to alter permeability of the bacterial cell can facilitate entry of antibiotics that might not ordinarily gain access to target sites, thus resulting in enhanced antimicrobial activity. Although the combination is employed clinically, these drug types should never be placed in the same infusion fluid, because on prolonged contact, the positively charged aminoglycosides form an inactive complex with the negatively charged penicillins .

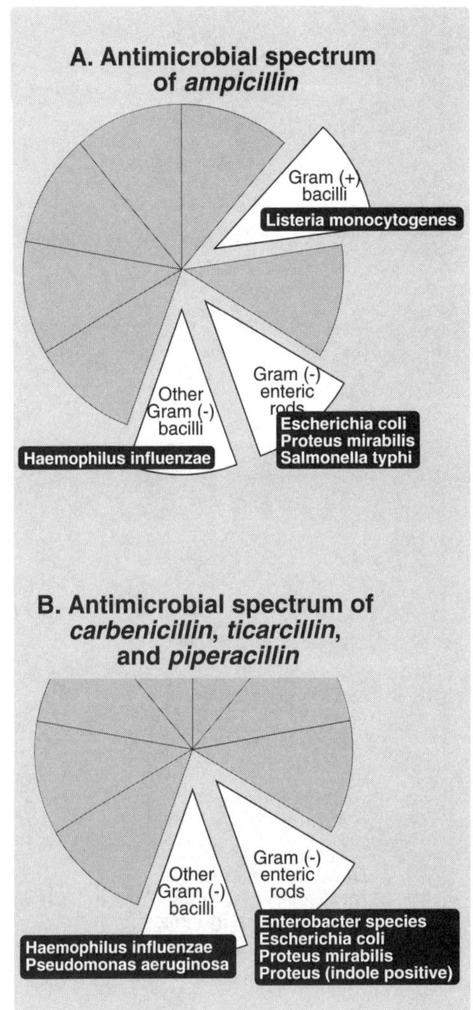

Figure 30.5
Typical therapeutic applications of *ampicillin* (A) and the antipseudomonal penicillins (B).

C. Resistance

Natural resistance to the penicillins occurs in organisms that either lack a peptidoglycan cell wall (for example, Mycoplasma) or that have cell walls that are impermeable to the drugs. **Acquired resistance** to the penicillins by plasmid transfer has become a significant clinical problem, since an organism may become resistant to several antibiotics due to acquisition of a plasmid that encodes resistance for multiple agents. Multiplication of such an organism will lead to increased dissemination of the resistance genes. By obtaining a resistance plasmid, bacteria may acquire one or both of the following properties, thus allowing it to withstand β-lactam antibiotics.

1. **β-lactamase activity:** This family of enzymes hydrolyzes the cyclic amide bond of the β-lactam ring, which results in loss of bactericidal activity (see Figure 30.1). β-Lactamases are either constitutive or, more commonly, are acquired by the transfer of plasmids. Some of the β-lactam antibiotics are poor substrates for β-lactamases and resist cleavage; thus they retain their activity against β-lactamase-producing organisms. [Note: Certain organisms may have chromosome-associated β-lactamases that are inducible by β-lactam antibiotics (for example, *cefoxitin*).]

2. **Decreased permeability to drug**: Decreased penetration of the antibiotic through the outer cell membrane prevents the drug from reaching the target penicillin-binding proteins (PBPs).

3. **Altered penicillin binding proteins:** Modified PBPs have a lower affinity for β-lactam antibiotics, requiring clinically unattainable concentrations of the drug to effect binding and inhibition of bacterial growth. This mechanism may explain *methicillin*-resistant staphylococci, although it does not explain its resistance to non-lactam antibiotics like *erythromycin* to which they are also refractory.

D. Pharmacokinetics

1. **Administration:** The route of administration is determined by the stability of the drug to gastric acid and by the severity of the infection.

   a. **Routes of administration:** *Methicillin*, *ticarcillin*, *carbenicillin*, *mezlocillin*, *piperacillin*, *azlocillin*, and the combinations of *ampicillin* with *sulbactam*, *ticarcillin* with *clavulanic acid*, and *piperacillin* with *tazobactam* must be administered intravenously (IV) or intramuscularly (IM). *Penicillin* V, *amoxicillin*, and *amoxicillin* combined with *clavulanic acid* are only available as oral preparations. Others are effective by the oral, IV, or IM routes (see Figure 30.4).

   b. **Depot forms:** *Procaine penicillin G* and *benzathine penicillin G* are administered intramuscularly and serve as depot forms. They are slowly absorbed into the circulation over a long time period.

2. **Absorption:** Most of the penicillins are incompletely absorbed after oral administration and reach the intestine in sufficient amounts to affect the composition of the intestinal flora. However, *amoxicillin* is almost completely absorbed. Consequently, it is not appropriate therapy for the treatment of shigella- or salmonella-derived enteritis, since therapeutically effective levels do not reach the organisms in the intestinal crypts. Absorption of *penicillin G* and all the penicillinase-resistant penicillins is decreased by food in the stomach since gastric emptying time is reduced and the drugs are destroyed in the acidic environment. Therefore, they must be administered 30-60 minutes before meals or 2-3 hours postprandially. Other penicillins are less affected by food.

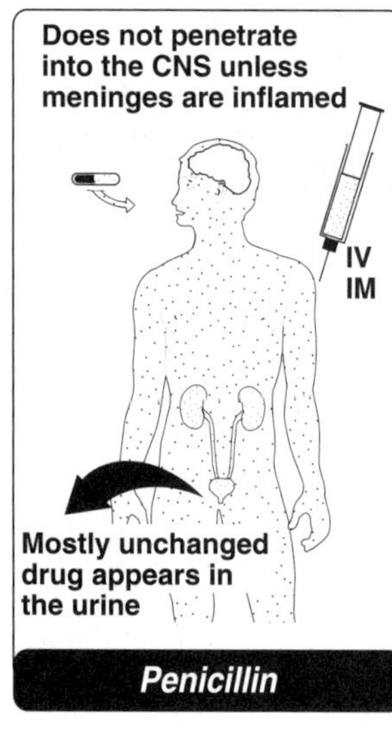
Does not penetrate into the CNS unless meninges are inflamed
IV
IM
Mostly unchanged drug appears in the urine
Penicillin

3. **Distribution:** Distribution of the free drug throughout the body is good. All the penicillins cross the placental barrier, but none have been shown to be teratogenic. However, penetration into certain sites such as bone or cerebrospinal fluid is insufficient for therapy, unless these sites are inflamed (Figure 30.6). During the acute phase (first day), the inflamed meninges are more permeable to penicillins, resulting in an increased ratio in the amount of drug in the central nervous system compared to the amount in the serum. As the infection abates, inflammation subsides, and permeability barriers are reestablished.

4. **Metabolism:** Metabolism of these drugs by the host is usually insignificant, but some metabolism of *penicillin* G has been shown to occur in patients with impaired renal function.

5. **Excretion:** The primary route of excretion is through the organic acid (tubular) secretory system of the kidney (see p. 224), as well as by glomerular filtration. Patients with impaired renal function must have dosage regimens adjusted. Thus the $t_{1/2}$ of *penicillin G* can increase from a normal of $^1/_2$ -1 hour to 10 hours in individuals with renal failure. *Probenecid* inhibits the secretion of penicillins. *Nafcillin* is primarily eliminated through the biliary route. [Note: This is also the preferential route for the *acylureido penicillins* in cases of renal failure.]

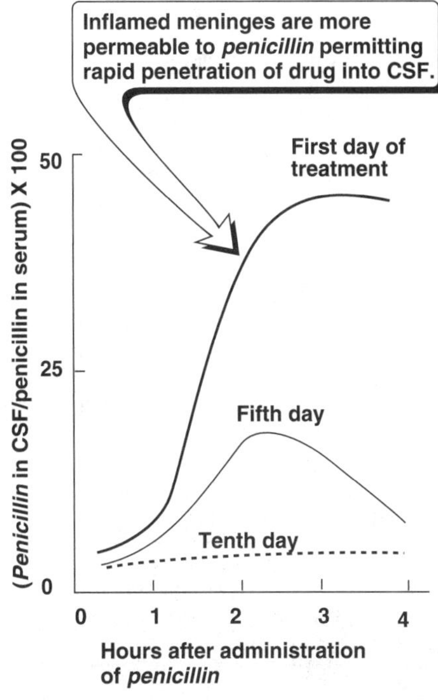

Figure 30.6
Enhanced penetration of *penicillin* into the cerebral spinal fluid (CSF) during inflammation.

E. Adverse reactions

Penicillins are among the safest drugs, and blood levels are not monitored, although adverse reactions do occur.

1. **Hypersensitivity:** This is the most important adverse effect of the penicillins. The major antigenic determinant of penicillin hypersensitivity is its metabolite, penicilloic acid, which reacts with proteins and serves as a hapten to cause an immune reaction. Approximately 5% of patients have some kind of reaction, ranging from maculopapular rash to angioedema (marked swelling of lips, tongue, periorbital area) and anaphylaxis. Cross-allergic reactions do occur among the β-lactam antibiotics. Although rashes can develop with all the penicillins, maculopapular rashes are most common with *ampicillin*. Among patients with mononucleosis who are treated with *ampicillin*, the incidence of maculopapular rash approaches 100%.

2. **Diarrhea:** This effect, which is caused by a disruption of the normal balance of intestinal microorganisms, is a common problem. It occurs to a greater extent with those agents that are incompletely absorbed and have an extended antibacterial spectrum.

3. **Nephritis:** All penicillins, but particularly *methicillin*, have the potential to cause acute interstitial nephritis.

4. **Neurotoxicity**: The penicillins are irritating to neuronal tissue and can provoke seizures if injected intrathecally or if very high blood levels are reached. Epileptic patients are especially at risk.

5. **Platelet dysfunction**: This side effect, which involves decreased agglutination, is observed with the antipseudomonal penicillins (*carbenicillin* and *ticarcillin*) and, to some extent, with *penicillin G*. It is generally a concern when treating patients predisposed to hemorrhage or those receiving anticoagulants.

6. **Cation toxicity:** Penicillins are generally administered as the sodium or potassium salt. Toxicities may be caused by the large quantities of sodium or potassium that accompany the penicillin. Sodium excess may result in hypokalemia. This can be avoided by using the most potent antibiotic, which permits lower doses of drug and accompanying cations.

III. CEPHALOSPORINS

The cephalosporins are β-lactam antibiotics that are closely related both structurally (Figure 30.7) and functionally to the penicillins. Most cephalosporins are produced semi-synthetically by the chemical attachment of side chains to 7-aminocephalosporanic acid. Cephalosporins and cephamycins have the same mode of action as the penicillins and are affected by the same resistance mechanisms, but they tend to be more resistant than the penicillins to β-lactamases.

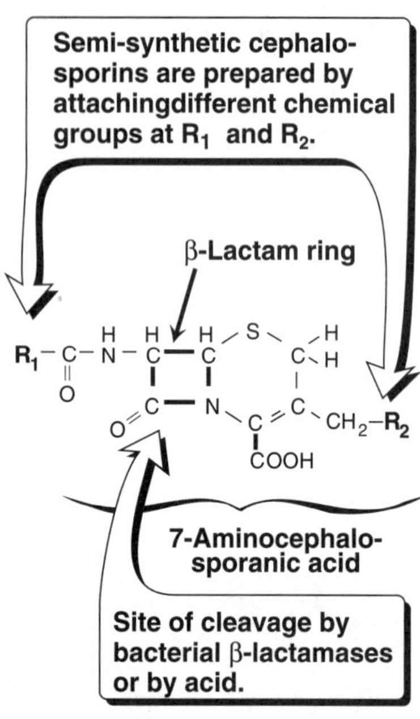

Figure 30.7
Structural features of cephalosporins.

A. Antibacterial spectrum

Cephalosporins have been classified as first, second or third generation, largely on the basis of bacterial susceptibility patterns and resistance to β-lactamases (Figure 30.8). [Note: They are ineffective against *methicillin*-resistant Staphylococcus aureus (MRSA), Listeria monocytogenes, Clostridium difficile and the enterococci.]

1. **First generation:** Cephalosporins designated first generation (Figure 30.8) act as *penicillin G* substitutes that are resistant to the staphylococcal penicillinase. They also have activity against **P**roteus mirabilis, **E**scherichia **c**oli, and **K**lebsiella pneumoniae (the acronym **PEcK** has been suggested).

2. **Second generation:** The second generation cephalosporins display greater activity against three additional gram-negative organisms, **H**aemophilus influenzae, some **E**nterobacter aerogenes and some **N**eisseria species (**HENPEcK**), whereas activity against gram-positive organisms is weaker. [Note: The cephamycins are effective against Bacteroides fragilis; *cefoxitin* is the most potent.]

3. **Third generation:** These cephalosporins have assumed an important role in the treatment of infectious disease. Though greatly inferior to first generation cephalosporins in regard to their activity against gram-positive cocci, the third generation cephalosporins have enhanced activity against gram-negative bacilli, including those mentioned above plus most other enteric organisms and Serratia marcescens. *Ceftriaxone* (sef tree AKS own) or *cefotaxime* [sef oh TAKS eem] have become agents of choice in the treatment of meningitis. *Ceftazidime* (sef TAZ id eem) has activity against Pseudomonas aeruginosa.

4. **Fourth Generation:** *Cefepime* [SEF eh peem] is the most clinically useful fourth generation cephalosporin and must be administered parenterally. *Cefepime* has a wide antibacterial spectrum being active vs. Streptococci and Staphylococci (only those that are *methicillin* susceptible). It is also effective against aerobic Gram negative organisms such as Enterobacter, Escherichia coli, Klebsiella pneumoniae, Proteus mirabilis and Pseudomonas aeruginosa.

B. Resistance

Mechanisms of bacterial resistance to the cephalosporins are essentially the same as those described for the penicillins (see p. 301).

C. Pharmacokinetics

1. **Administration:** All the cephalosporins (except for those highlighted in Figure 30.8) must be administered intravenously because of their poor oral absorption.

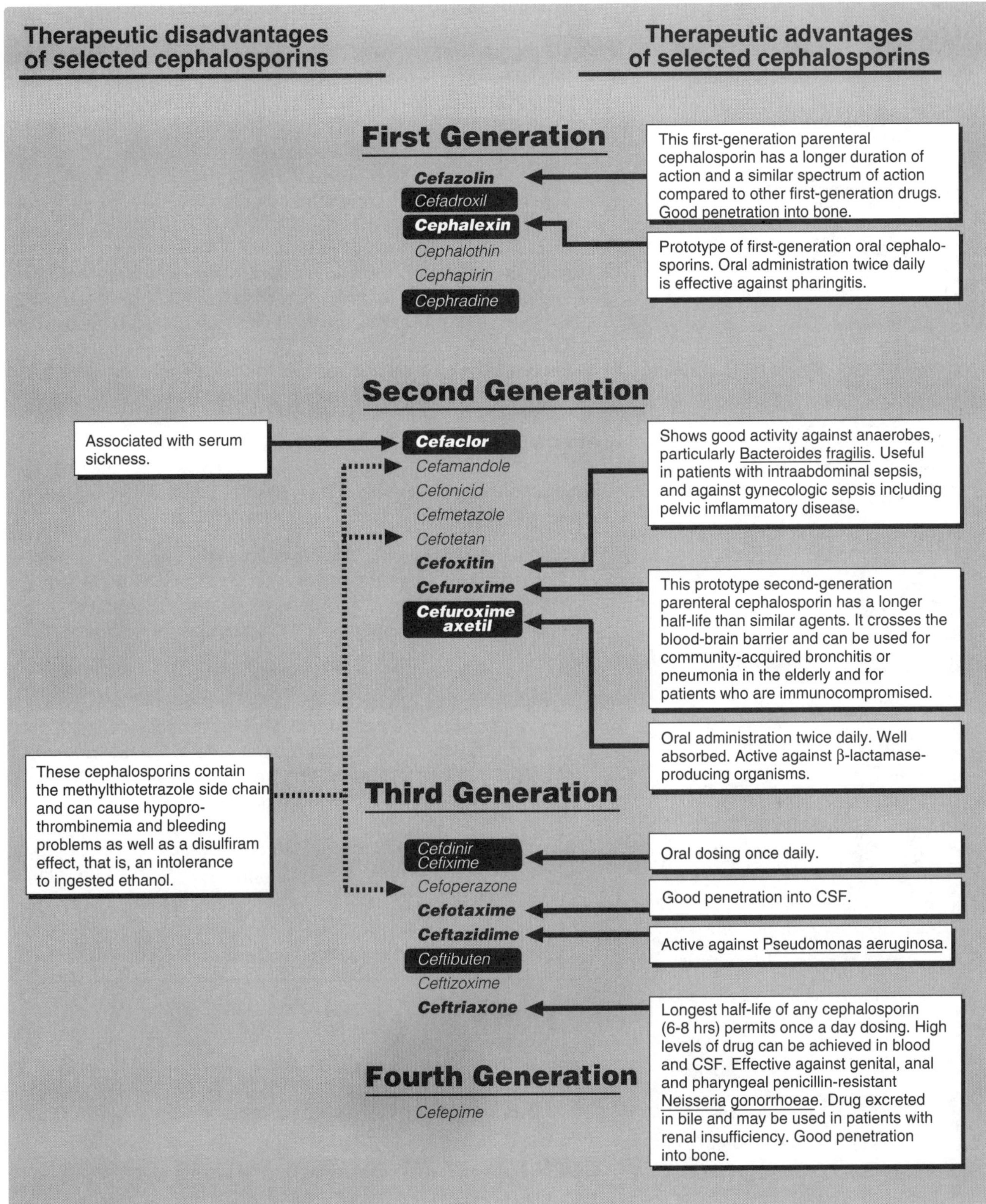

Figure 30.8
Characteristic of some clinically useful cephalosporins. Note: Drugs that can be administered orally are shown in reverse type. More useful drugs shown in **bold**.

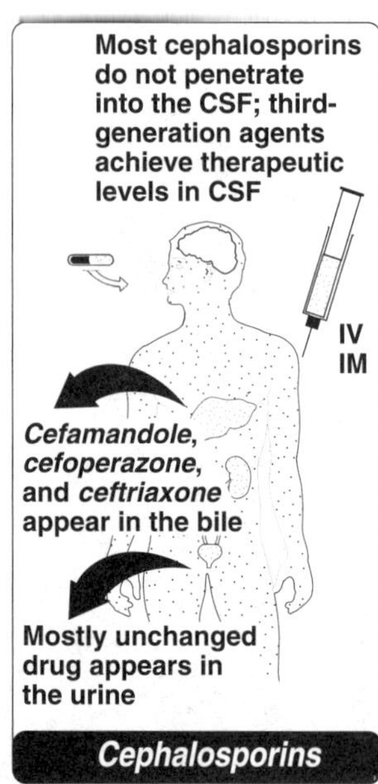

Most cephalosporins do not penetrate into the CSF; third-generation agents achieve therapeutic levels in CSF
IV
IM
Cefamandole, cefoperazone, and ceftriaxone appear in the bile
Mostly unchanged drug appears in the urine
Cephalosporins

2. **Distribution:** All of these antibiotics distribute very well into body fluids. However, adequate therapeutic levels in the cerebrospinal fluid (CSF), regardless of inflammation, are achieved only with the third generation cephalosporins (for example, *ceftriaxone* or *cefotaxime* are effective in the treatment of neonatal and childhood meningitis caused by Haemophilus influenzae). *Cefazolin* (se FA zo lin) finds application in orthopedic surgery because of its activity against penicillinase-producing Staphylococcus aureus, its half-life and its ability to penetrate bone.

3. **Fate:** Biotransformation of cephalosporins by the host is not clinically important. Elimination occurs through tubular secretion and/or glomerular filtration; thus doses must be adjusted in the case of severe renal failure to guard against accumulation and toxicity. *Cefoperazone* (sef oh PER az own) and *ceftriaxone* are excreted through the bile into the feces and are frequently employed in patients with renal insufficiency.

D. Adverse effects

The cephalosporins produce a number of adverse affects, some of which are unique to particular members of the group.

1. **Allergic manifestations**: The cephalosporins should be avoided or used with caution in individuals allergic to penicillins (about 5 to 15% show cross-sensitivity). In contrast, the incidence of allergic reactions to cephalosporins is 1-2% in patients without a history of allergy to penicillins.

2. **A disulfiram-like effect:** When *cefamandole* [se FAM an dol] or *cefoperazone* is ingested with alcohol or alcohol-containing medications, a disulfiram-like effect is seen (see p. 96), because these cephalosporins block the second step in alcohol oxidation, which results in the accumulation of acetaldehyde[1].

3. **Bleeding:** Bleeding can occur with *cefamandole* or *cefoperazone*, because of anti-vitamin K effects; administration of the vitamin corrects the problem.

IV. OTHER β-LACTAM ANTIBIOTICS

A. Carbapenems

Carbapenems are synthetic β-lactam antibiotics that differ from the penicillins in that the sulfur atom of the thiazolidine ring (Figure 30.9) has been externalized and replaced by a carbon atom. *Imipenem* [i mi PEN em] is the only drug of this group currently available.

1. **Antibacterial spectrum:** *Imipenem/cilastatin* is the broadest spectrum β-lactam antibiotic preparation currently available. *Imipenem* resists hydrolysis by most β-lactamases. The drug plays a role in empiric therapy since it is active against penicillinase-producing gram-positive and gram-negative organisms, anaerobes, and

[1]See p. 310 for Infolink references to other books in this series.

Pseudomonas aeruginosa, although other pseudomonas strains are resistant. [Note: Resistant strains of Pseudomonas aeruginosa have been reported to arise during therapy.]

2. **Pharmacokinetics:** *Imipenem* is administered intravenously and penetrates well into body tissues and fluids including cerebral spinal fluid when the meninges are inflamed. It is excreted by glomerular filtration and undergoes cleavage by a dehydropeptidase found in the brush border of the proximal renal tubule to form an inactive metabolite that is potentially nephrotoxic. Compounding the *imipenem* with *cilastatin*, a dehydropeptidase inhibitor, protects the parent drug from cleavage and thus prevents the formation of a toxic metabolite. This allows the drug to be active in the treatment of urinary tract infections. [Note: The dose must be adjusted in patients with renal insufficiency.]

3. **Adverse effects:** *Imipenem/cilastatin* can cause nausea, vomiting, and diarrhea. Eosinophilia and neutropenia are less common. High levels of this agent may provoke seizures.

B. Monobactams

The monobactams, of which *aztreonam* [az TREE oh nam] is the only commercially available example, are unique because the β-lactam ring is not fused to another ring (Figure 30.9). Monobactams also disrupt cell wall synthesis. The drug's narrow antimicrobial spectrum precludes its use alone in empiric therapy (p. 279). *Aztreonam* is resistant to the action of β-lactamases.

1. **Antibacterial spectrum:** The antibacterial activity of *aztreonam* is primarily directed against the enterobacteria. *Aztreonam* is useful because of its action against aerobic gram-negative rods. It lacks activity against gram-positive organisms and anaerobes.

2. **Pharmacokinetics:** *Aztreonam* is administered via IV or IM routes. It is excreted in the urine and can accumulate in patients with renal failure.

3. **Adverse effects:** *Aztreonam* is relatively nontoxic, but it may cause phlebitis, skin rash, and occasionally, abnormal liver function tests. *Aztreonam* has a low immunogenic potential and shows little cross-reactivity with antibodies induced by other β-lactams. Thus *aztreonam* may offer a safe alternative for treating patients allergic to penicillins and/or cephalosporins.

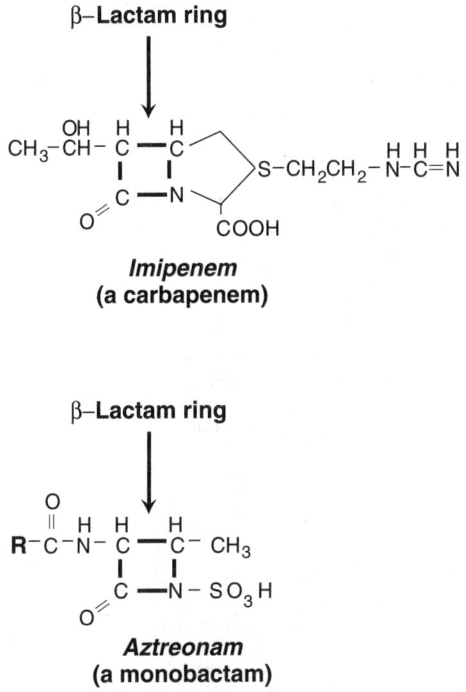

β–Lactam ring

CH_3–CH(OH)–CH–CH–(ring)–S–CH_2CH_2–NH–CH=NH; C=O, N, COOH

Imipenem
(a carbapenem)

β–Lactam ring

R–C(=O)–NH–CH–CH–CH_3; C(=O)–N–SO_3H

Aztreonam
(a monobactam)

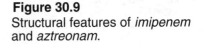

Figure 30.9
Structural features of *imipenem* and *aztreonam*.

V. β-LACTAMASE INHIBITORS

Hydrolysis of the β-lactam ring, either by enzymatic cleavage via a β-lactamase or by acid, destroys antimicrobial activity. β-Lactamase inhibitors, such as *clavulanic acid* [cla vue LA nick], *sulbactam* [sul BACK tam] and *tazobactam* [ta zoh BACK tam], contain a β-lactam ring, but they do not have significant antibacterial activity. Instead, they bind to and inactivate β-lactamases, thereby protecting the antibiotics that are normally substrates for these enzymes. The β-lactamase inhibitors are formulated with the penicillin derivatives to protect the latter from enzy-

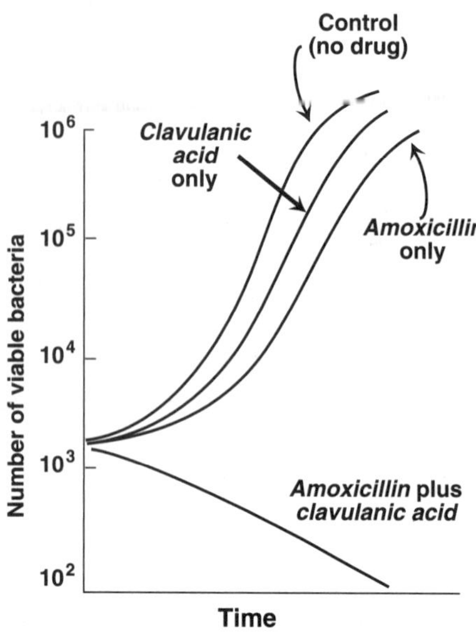

Figure 30.10
The growth of Escherichia coli in the presence of *amoxicillin*, with and without *clavulanic acid*.

matic inactivation. Figure 30.10 shows the effect of *clavulanic acid* and *amoxicillin* on the growth of β-lactamase-producing Escherichia coli. Note that *clavulanic acid* alone is nearly devoid of antibacterial activity.

VI. OTHER AGENTS AFFECTING THE CELL WALL

A. Vancomycin

Vancomycin [van koe MYE sin] is a tricyclic glycopeptide that has become increasingly important because of its effectiveness against multiple drug resistant organisms such as *methicillin*-resistant staphylococci. The medical community is presently concerned about reports of emergence of *vancomycin* resistance in these strains as well as the enterococci.

1. **Mode of action:** *Vancomycin* inhibits synthesis of bacterial cell wall phospholipids as well as peptidoglycan polymerization at a site earlier than that inhibited by the β-lactam antibiotics.

2. **Antibacterial spectrum:** In order to curtail the increase in *vancomycin*-resistant bacteria (for example, the Entercococcus faecium and Entercococcus faecalis), it is important to restrict its use to the treatment of serious infections caused by β-lactam-resistant gram-positive microorganisms, or for patients with gram-positive infections who have a serious allergy to the β-lactams. It is also used for potentially life-threatening antibiotic-associated colitis due to Clostridium difficile or staphylococci. It is used prophylactically in dental patients. *Vancomycin* is used in individuals with prosthetic heart valves or in patients being implanted with prosthetic devices. The latter is of particular concern in those hospitals where there is a problem with *methicillin*-resistant Staphylococcus aureus (MRSA) or Staphylococcus epidermidis (MRSE). *Vancomycin* acts synergistically with the aminoglycosides and this combination can be used in the treatment of enterococcal endocarditis.

3. **Resistance:** Occurring rarely, *vancomycin* resistance is due to plasmid-mediated changes in permeability to the drug and is also due to decreased binding of *vancomycin* to receptor molecules.

4. **Pharmacokinetics:** Slow intravenous infusion is employed for treatment of systemic infections or for prophylaxis. Because *vancomycin* is not absorbed after oral administration, this route is only employed for the treatment of antibiotic-induced colitis due to C. difficile. Inflammation allows penetration into the meninges. Metabolism is minimal; 90-100 % is excreted by glomerular filtration. [Note: Dosage must be adjusted in renal failure since the drug will accumulate. Normal half-life is 6-10 hours compared to over 200 hours in end-stage renal disease.]

5. **Adverse effects:** Side effects are a serious problem with *vancomycin* and include fever, chills, and/or phlebitis at the infusion site. Shock has occurred as a result of rapid administration.

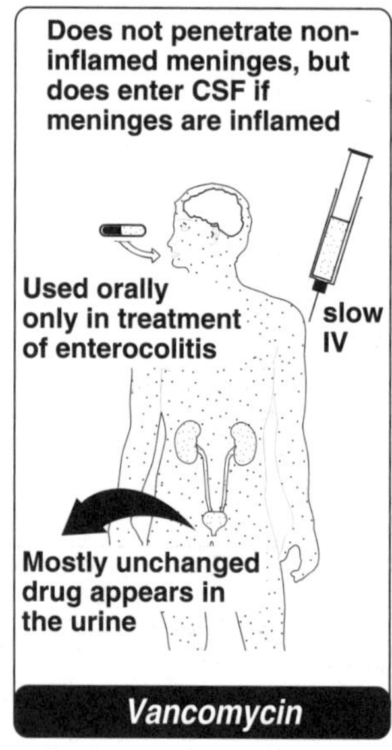

Flushing ("red man syndrome") and shock result due to histamine release caused by rapid infusion. Dose-related hearing loss has occurred in patients with renal failure who accumulate the drug.

B. Bacitracin

Bacitracin [bass i TRAY sin] is a mixture of polypeptides that inhibits bacterial cell wall synthesis. It is active against a wide variety of gram-positive organisms. Its use is restricted to topical application because of its potential for nephrotoxicity.

Study Questions

Choose the ONE best answer.

30.1 Which one of the following drugs is both penicillinase-resistant and effective by oral administration?

A. Methicillin.
B. Carbenicillin.
C. Penicillin V.
D. Amoxicillin plus clavulanic acid.
E. Piperacillin.

Correct answer = D. Amoxicillin plus clavulanic acid is an extended spectrum formulation that is penicillinase resistant because of the presence of a β-lactamase inhibitor, and is stable in acid. Methicillin, an antistaphylococcal penicillin, is penicillinase resistant but is not stable in acid. Carbenicillin and piperacillin, antipseudomonal penicillins, are neither penicillinase resistant nor stable in acid. Penicillin V is a narrow spectrum antibiotic that is not penicillinase resistant but is stable in acid.

30.2 Which one of the following antibiotics is INCORRECTLY matched with an appropriate clinical indication?

A. Penicillin G: Pneumonia caused by Klebsiella pneumoniae
B. Carbenicillin: Urinary tract infection caused by Pseudomonas aeruginosa (β-lactamase negative)
C. Ampicillin: Bacterial meningitis caused by Haemophilus influenzae (β-lactamase negative)
D. Penicillin G: Syphilis caused by Treponema pallidum
E. Cefazolin: Staphyloccocal osteomyelitis

Correct choice = A. Cephalosporins, not penicillins, are effective against Klebsiella.

30.3 A 70 year old alcoholic male with poor dental hygiene is to have his remaining teeth extracted for subsequent dentures. He has mitral valve stenosis with mild cardiac insufficiency and is being treated with captopril, digoxin and furosemide. The dentist decides that his medical history warrants prophylactic antibiotic therapy prior to the procedure and prescribes:

A. Vancomycin
B. Amoxicillin
C. Tetracycline
D. Co-trimoxazole
E. Imipenem

Answer: B (Amoxicillin). The multiple extractions can lead to bacteremia while the mitral valve stenosis and cardiac insufficiency place him at risk for developing endocarditis. The present American Heart Association guidelines indicate amoxicillin (3 gm 1 hour prior to procedure and 1.5 gm 6 hours after original dose.) Vancomycin would only be appropriate if the patient was allergic to penicillins. Tetracycline and cotrimoxazole are bacteriostatic and not effective against the viridans group of Streptococci, the usual causative organism. Imipenem is also inappropriate since its spectrum is too broad.

30.4 All of the following statements about penicillin G are correct EXCEPT:

A. It is excreted from the body primarily via the hepatobiliary route.
B. Administered orally, it is variably absorbed because of its degradation by stomach acid.
C. It is more effective in killing growing bacteria than microorganisms in the stationary phase.
D. It can act synergistically with aminoglycosides.
E. Levels in the blood can be increased by administration of probenecid.

Correct choice = A. The primary route of excretion of penicillin G is via the kidney. Oral administration of penicillin G is unreliable, in part because the β-lactam ring is cleaved in acid. Penicillin G is bactericidal to growing microorganisms when they are actively making new cell wall material, and it facilitates the entry of the aminoglycosides into the cell, leading to synergistic antimicrobial effects. Administration of probenecid interferes with the secretion of penicillins and results in higher blood levels of penicillin and a prolonged half-life of the antibiotic.

30.5 Which one of the following statements about inhibitors of cell wall synthesis is INCORRECT?

A. The concentration of penicillin in the cerebrospinal fluid is higher when administered to patients with meningococcal meningitis than it is when given to normal patients.

B. First generation cephalosporins are more effective against staphylococcal infections than are third generation cephalosporins.

C. Cefoxitin is less likely to cause an allergic reaction in a patient that is hypersensitive to penicillin G than is penicillin V.

D. The half-life of procaine penicillin administered intramuscularly is greater than the half-life of penicillin G administered orally.

E. Third-generation cephalosporins are susceptible to β-lactamase activity.

Correct choice = E. Unlike the penicillins, cephalosporins are less sensitive to β-lactamase activity. Inflammation does increase penetration of penicillin into the CSF. All penicillin derivatives, including penicillin V, can potentially trigger an allergic reaction in patients sensitive to penicillin G. Cefoxitin can often be used in these patients. However, caution should be exercised, since there is about 5 to 15% cross-reactivity.

30.6 A 25-year-old male returns home from a holiday in the Far East and complains of three days of dysuria and a purulent urethral discharge. You diagnose this to be a case of gonorrhea. Which of the following is appropriate treatment?

A. Ceftriaxone IM

B. Penicillin G IM

C. Gentamicin IM

D. Piperacillin/tazobactam IV

E. Vancomycin IV

Correct answer = A. Most gonoccocal infections are now resistant to penicillin, the previous drug of choice. The other antibiotics are inappropriate.

30.7 An eight-month pregnant medical student complains of lower abdominal pain and a 48-hour history of dysuria. She does not have any fever; an analysis of her urine shows protein, but no blood or glucose. A culture is taken. Which of the following is useful for treating this urinary tract infection orally without causing risks to the fetus?

A. Cefadroxil (first generation cephalosporin)

B. Cotrimoxazole (TMP/SM)

C. Penicillin V

D. Ceftriaxone (third generation cephalosporin)

E. Tetracycline

Correct answer = A. Most urinary tract infections are due to E. coli and can usually be treated with cotrimoxazole. However, this patient is near term and the sulfa in the cotrimoxazole might put the infant at risk due to kernicterus. Thus, the first generation cephalosporin, cefadroxil, is appropriate since it would be effective orally against penicillinase producing E. coli. Ceftriaxone, while it would be effective, would have to be administered parenterally. Penicillin V is not effective against E. coli. Tetracycline deposits in teeth and skeleton of the fetus and is contraindicated.

30.8 A patient with degenerative joint disease is to undergo insertion of a hip prosthesis. In order to avoid complications due to post-operative infection, the surgeon will pretreat this patient with an antibiotic. This hospital has a significant problem with methicillin-resistant Staphylococcus aureus. Which of the following antibiotics should the surgeon select?

A. Ampicillin

B. Imipenem/cilastatin

C. Gentamicin/piperacillin

D. Vancomycin

E. Cefazolin

Correct answer = D. The only antibiotic which is effective against methicillin-resistant Staphylococcus aureus is vancomycin.

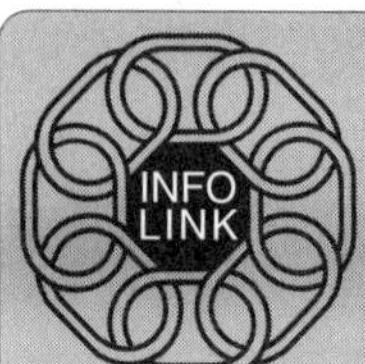

[1]See p. 279 in **Biochemistry** (2nd ed.) for a discussion of ethanol metabolism.

Protein Synthesis Inhibitors

31

I. OVERVIEW

A number of antibiotics exert their antimicrobial effects by targeting the bacterial ribosome, which has components that differ structurally from those of the mammalian cytoplasmic ribosome. The bacterial ribosome is smaller (70S) than the mammalian ribosome (80S) and is composed of 50S and 30S subunits as compared to 60S and 40S subunits[1]. The mammalian mitochondrial ribosome, however, more closely resembles the bacterial ribosome. Thus, although drugs that interact with the bacterial site usually spare the host cells, high levels of drugs like *chloramphenicol* or the tetracyclines may cause toxic effects as a result of interaction with the mitochondrial ribosomes. Figure 31.1 lists the drugs discussed in this chapter

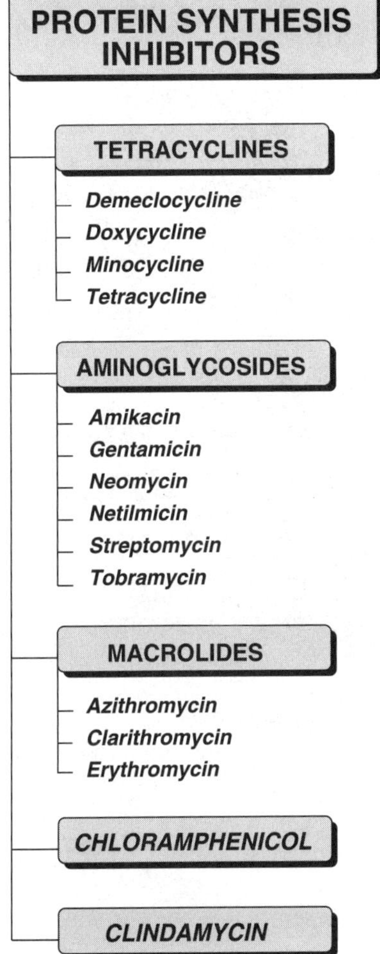

Figure 31.1
Summary of protein synthesis inhibitors.

II. TETRACYCLINES

Tetracyclines [tet ra SYE kleen] are a group of closely related compounds that, as the name implies, consist of 4 fused rings with a system of conjugated double bonds. Their small differences in clinical efficacy reflect a variation in their individual pharmacokinetics due to substitutions on these rings.

A. Mode of action

Entry of these agents into susceptible organisms is mediated by transport proteins unique to the bacterial inner cytoplasmic membrane. Binding of the drug to the 30S subunit of the bacterial ribosome is believed to block access of the amino acyl-tRNA to the mRNA-ribosome complex at the acceptor site, thus inhibiting bacterial protein synthesis.[2]

B. Antibacterial spectrum

As broad spectrum antibiotics, the tetracyclines are also effective against organisms other than bacteria. Tetracyclines are generally bacteriostatic and are the drugs of choice for infections shown in Figure 31.2.

[1,2]See p. 322 for Infolink references to other books in this series.

Lippincott's Illustrated Reviews: Pharmacology, Second Edition.
by Mary J. Mycek, Richard A. Harvey and Pamela C. Champe.

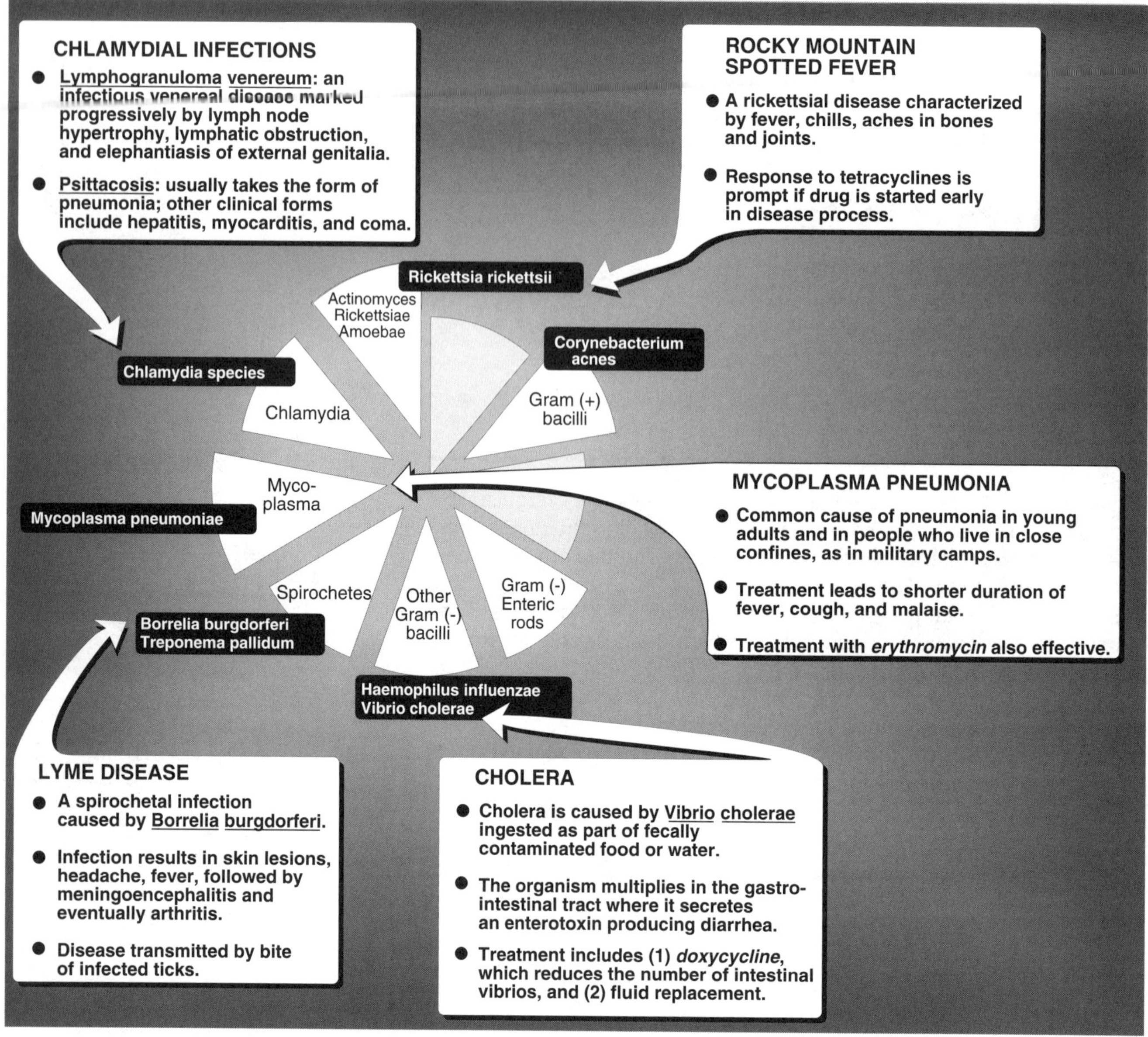

Figure 31.2
Typical therapeutic applications of tetracyclines.

C. Resistance

Widespread resistance to tetracyclines limits their clinical use. The most commonly encountered naturally occurring R factor confers an inability of the organism to accumulate the drug, thus producing resistance. This is accomplished by a Mg^{++}-dependent active efflux of the drug mediated by the resistance protein TetA. Other mechanisms such as possible modification of the tetracycline binding site have also been reported. Any organism resistant to one tetracycline is resistant to all. The majority of penicillinase-producing staphylococci are now also insensitive to tetracyclines.

D. Pharmacokinetics

1. **Absorption:** All tetracyclines are adequately but incompletely absorbed after oral ingestion. However, taking these drugs con-concomitantly with dairy foods in the diet decreases absorption because of the formation of nonabsorbable chelates of the tetracyclines with calcium ions. This is less of a problem with *doxycycline* [dox i SYE kleen]. Nonabsorbable chelates are also formed with other divalent and trivalent cations (for example, those found in magnesium and aluminum antacids, and in iron preparations). [Note: This presents a problem if the patient self-treats the epigastric upsets caused by tetracycline ingestion with antacids (Figure 31.3).]

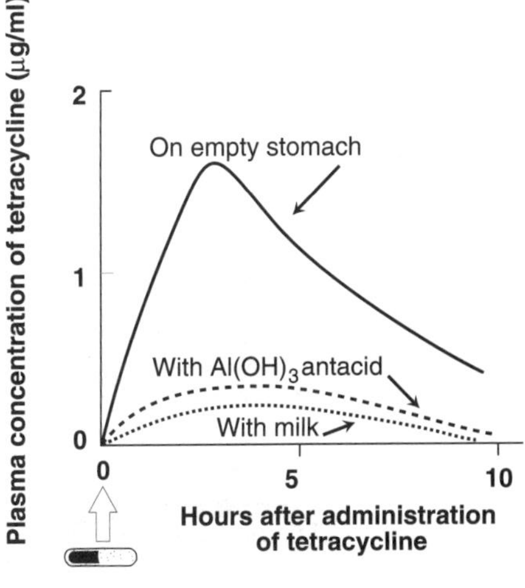

Figure 31.3
Effect of antacids and milk on the absorption of tetracyclines.

2. **Distribution:** The tetracyclines concentrate in the liver, kidney, spleen, and skin and bind to tissues undergoing calcification (for example, teeth and bones), or to tumors that have a high calcium content (for example, gastric carcinoma). Penetration into most body fluids is adequate. Although all tetracyclines enter the cerebrospinal fluid, levels are insufficient for therapeutic efficacy, except for *minocycline* [mi noe SYE kleen]. *Minocycline* enters the brain in the absence of inflammation, and also appears in tears and saliva. Though useful in eradicating the meningococcal carrier state, *minocycline* is not effective for central nervous system (CNS) infections. All tetracyclines cross the placental barrier and concentrate in fetal bones and dentition.

3. **Fate:** All the tetracyclines concentrate in the liver, where they are, in part, metabolized and conjugated to form soluble glucuronides. The parent drug and/or its metabolites are secreted into the bile; most tetracyclines are reabsorbed in the intestine and enter the urine by glomerular filtration. *Doxycycline* is an exception, since its metabolite is preferentially excreted via the bile into the feces. Thus, unlike other tetracyclines, *doxycycline* can be employed in treating infections in renally compromised patients.

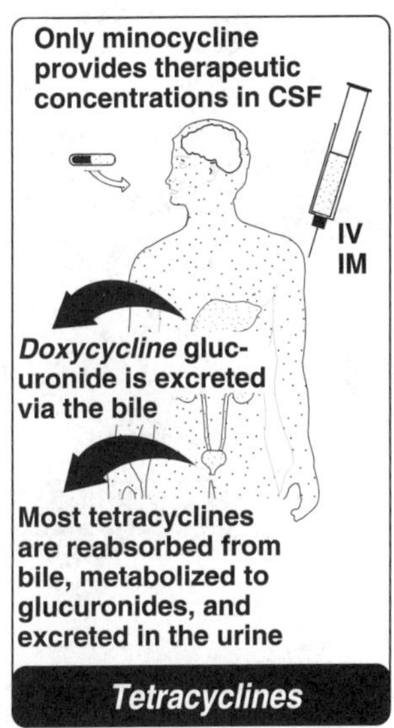

Only minocycline provides therapeutic concentrations in CSF
IV
IM
Doxycycline glucuronide is excreted via the bile
Most tetracyclines are reabsorbed from bile, metabolized to glucuronides, and excreted in the urine
Tetracyclines

E. Adverse effects

1. **Gastric discomfort:** Epigastric distress commonly results from irritation of the gastric mucosa (Figure 31.4) and is often responsible for non-compliance in patients treated with these drugs. The discomfort can be controlled if the drug is taken with foods other than dairy products.

2. **Effects on calcified tissues:** Deposition in the bone and primary dentition occurs during calcification in growing children; this causes discoloration and hypoplasia of the teeth and a temporary stunting of growth.

3. **Fatal hepatotoxicity:** This side effect has been known to occur in pregnant women who received high doses of tetracyclines, especially if they are experiencing pyelonephritis.

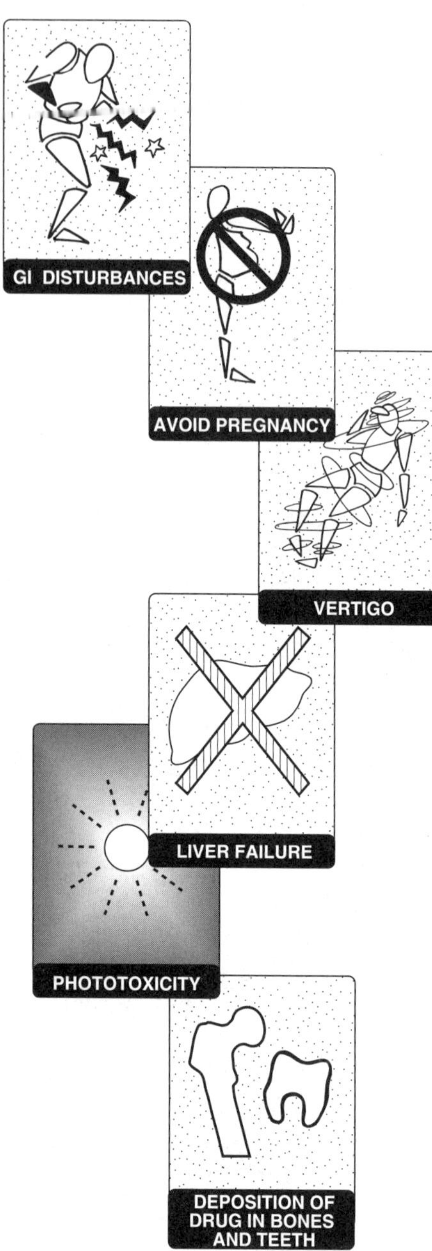

Figure 31.4
Some adverse effects of tetracycline.

4. **Phototoxicity:** Phototoxicity, for example, severe sunburn, occurs when the patient receiving a tetracycline is exposed to sun or ultraviolet rays. This toxicity is encountered most frequently with *tetracycline*, *doxycycline*, and *demeclocycline* [dem e kloe SYE kleen].

5. **Vestibular problems:** These side effects (for example, dizziness, nausea, vomiting) occur with *minocycline*, which concentrates in the endolymph of the ear and affects function.

6. **Pseudotumor cerebri:** Benign intracranial hypertension characterized by headache and blurred vision may occur in adults. Though discontinuation of the drug reverses the condition, it is not clear whether permanent sequelae may occur.

7. **Superinfections:** Overgrowths of Candida (for example in the vagina) or of resistant staphylococci (in the intestine) may occur.

8. **Contraindications:** Renally-impaired patients should not be treated with any of the tetracyclines except *doxycycline*. Accumulation of tetracyclines may aggravate pre-existing azotemia by interfering with protein synthesis, thus promoting amino acid degradation The tetracyclines should not be employed in pregnant or breast-feeding women, or in children under 8 years of age.

III. AMINOGLYCOSIDES

Aminoglycoside antibiotics had been the mainstays of treatment of serious infections due to aerobic gram-negative bacilli. However, since their use was limited by serious toxicities, they have been replaced to some extent by safer antibiotics such as the third generation cephalosporins (see p. 304), the fluoroquinolones (see p. 323), and *imipenem/cilastatin* (see p. 306). Aminoglycosides that are derived from Streptomyces have "mycin" suffixes, whereas those from Micromonospora end in "micin." The terms "aminoglycoside" and "aminocyclitol" stem from their structure — two amino sugars joined in glycosidic linkage to a central hexose (aminocyclitol) nucleus.

A. Mode of action

All members of this family are believed to inhibit bacterial protein synthesis by the mechanism determined for *streptomycin* [strep toe MYE sin]. Susceptible organisms have an oxygen-dependent system that transports the antibiotic across the cell membrane. The antibiotic then binds to the separated 30S ribosomal subunit, interfering with assembly of the functional ribosomal apparatus, or causing the 30S subunit of the complete ribosome to misread the genetic code. Polysomes become depleted because the aminoglycosides interrupt the process of polysome disaggregation and assembly. [Note: The aminoglycosides synergize with β-lactam antibiotics because of the latters' action on cell wall synthesis, which enhances diffusion of the aminoglycosides into the bacterium (see p. 301).]

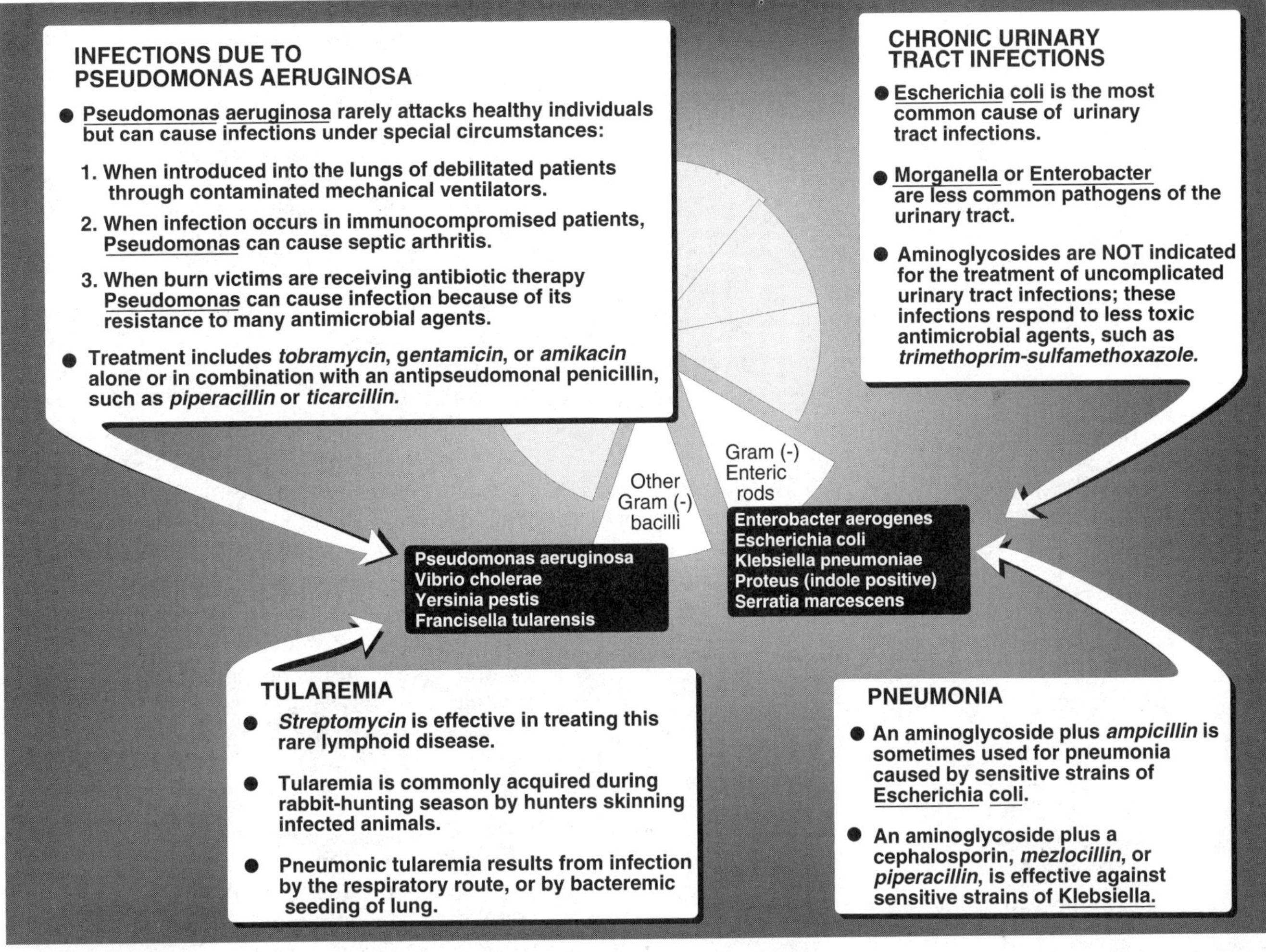

INFECTIONS DUE TO PSEUDOMONAS AERUGINOSA
Pseudomonas aeruginosa rarely attacks healthy individuals but can cause infections under special circumstances:
1. When introduced into the lungs of debilitated patients through contaminated mechanical ventilators.
2. When infection occurs in immunocompromised patients, Pseudomonas can cause septic arthritis.
3. When burn victims are receiving antibiotic therapy Pseudomonas can cause infection because of its resistance to many antimicrobial agents.
Treatment includes tobramycin, gentamicin, or amikacin alone or in combination with an antipseudomonal penicillin, such as piperacillin or ticarcillin.
CHRONIC URINARY TRACT INFECTIONS
Escherichia coli is the most common cause of urinary tract infections.
Morganella or Enterobacter are less common pathogens of the urinary tract.
Aminoglycosides are NOT indicated for the treatment of uncomplicated urinary tract infections; these infections respond to less toxic antimicrobial agents, such as trimethoprim-sulfamethoxazole.
Other Gram (-) bacilli
Gram (-) Enteric rods
Pseudomonas aeruginosa
Vibrio cholerae
Yersinia pestis
Francisella tularensis
Enterobacter aerogenes
Escherichia coli
Klebsiella pneumoniae
Proteus (indole positive)
Serratia marcescens
TULAREMIA
Streptomycin is effective in treating this rare lymphoid disease.
Tularemia is commonly acquired during rabbit-hunting season by hunters skinning infected animals.
Pneumonic tularemia results from infection by the respiratory route, or by bacteremic seeding of lung.
PNEUMONIA
An aminoglycoside plus ampicillin is sometimes used for pneumonia caused by sensitive strains of Escherichia coli.
An aminoglycoside plus a cephalosporin, mezlocillin, or piperacillin, is effective against sensitive strains of Klebsiella.

Figure 31.5
Typical therapeutic applications of *gentamicin*, *tobramycin*, *streptomycin* and *amikacin*.

B. Antibacterial spectrum

All aminoglycosides are bactericidal. They are effective only against aerobic organisms, since anaerobes lack the oxygen-requiring transport system. *Streptomycin* is used to treat tuberculosis, plague, tularemia, and in combination with *penicillin*, endocarditis caused by viridans group streptococci. Some therapeutic applications of four commonly used aminoglycosides, *amikacin* [am i KAY sin], *gentamicin* [jen ta MYE sin], *tobramycin* [toe bra MYE sin] and *streptomycin* are shown in Figure 31.5.

C. Resistance

Resistance can be caused by 1) decreased uptake of drug when the oxygen-dependent transport system for aminoglycosides is absent; an altered receptor where the 30S ribosomal subunit binding site has a lowered affinity for aminoglycosides; plasmid-associated synthesis of enzymes (for example, acetyltransferases, nucleotidyltransferases, and phosphotransferases) that modify and inactivate aminoglycoside antibiotics. Each type of enzyme has its own specificity as to substrate antibiotic; therefore, cross-resistance is not an invariable rule. *Netilmicin* [ne TIL mye sin] and *amikacin* are less vulnerable to these enzymes than are the other antibiotics of this group.

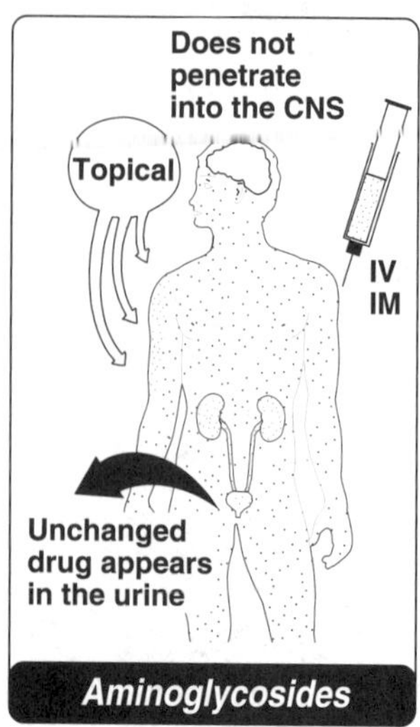

D. Pharmacokinetics

1. **Administration:** The highly polar, polycationic structure of the aminoglycosides prevents adequate absorption after oral administration. Therefore, all aminoglycosides (except *neomycin* [nee oh MYE sin]) must be given parenterally to achieve adequate serum levels. [Note: The severe nephrotoxicity associated with *neomycin* precludes parenteral administration, and its current use is limited to topical application or oral treatment in hepatic coma to reduce the intestinal bacterial population.]

2. **Distribution:** All of the aminoglycosides have similar pharmacokinetic properties. Levels achieved in most tissues are low, and penetration into most body fluids is variable. Concentrations in cerebrospinal fluid are inadequate even when the meninges are inflamed. Except for *neomycin*, the aminoglycosides may be administered intrathecally. High concentrations accumulate in the renal cortex and in the endolymph and perilymph of the inner ear, which may account for their nephrotoxic and ototoxic potential. All cross the placental barrier and may accumulate in fetal plasma and amniotic fluid.

3. **Fate:** Metabolism of the aminoglycosides does not occur in the host. All are rapidly excreted into the urine, predominantly by glomerular filtration. Accumulation occurs in patients with renal failure, and requires dose modification (Figure 31.6).

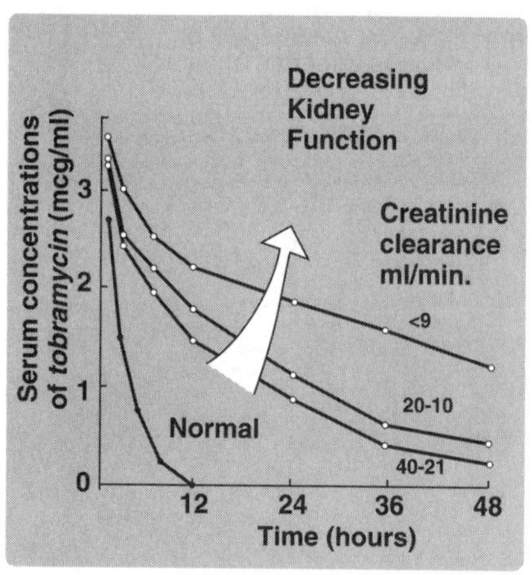

Figure 31.6
Serum concentrations of *tobramycin* following administration of the same dose of drug to normal and azotemic patients.

E. Adverse effects

It is important to monitor peak and trough plasma levels (see p. 20) of *gentamicin*, *tobramycin*, *netilmicin*, and *amikacin* to avoid concentrations that cause dose-related toxicities (Figure 31.7). [Note: Peak levels are defined as those obtained $\frac{1}{2}$ to 1 hour after infusion. Trough levels are obtained immediately before the next dose.] Patient factors, such as old age, previous exposure to aminoglycosides, gender, and liver disease, tend to predispose patients to adverse reactions. The elderly are particularly susceptible to nephrotoxicity and ototoxicity.

1. **Ototoxicity:** Ototoxicity (vestibular and cochlear) is directly related to high peak plasma levels and duration of treatment. Deafness may be irreversible and has been known to affect fetuses in utero. Patients simultaneously receiving another ototoxic drug such as the loop diuretics *furosemide*, *bumetanide*, *ethacrynic acid* (see p. 227) or *cisplatin* (see p. 396), are particulary at risk. Vertigo and loss of balance may also occur because these drugs affect the vestibular apparatus.

2. **Nephrotoxicity:** Retention of the aminoglycosides by the proximal tubular cells disrupts calcium-mediated transport processes and results in kidney damage ranging from mild renal impairment to severe acute tubular necrosis which can be irreversible.

3. **Neuromuscular paralysis:** This side effect most often results after direct intraperitoneal or intrapleural application of large doses of aminoglycosides. The mechanism responsible is a decrease in both the release of acetylcholine from prejunctional nerve endings and the sensitivity of the postsynaptic site. Patients with myasthenia gravis are particularly at risk. Prompt administration of *calcium gluconate* or *neostigmine* can reverse the block.

4. **Allergic reactions:** Contact dermatitis is a common reaction to topically-applied *neomycin.*

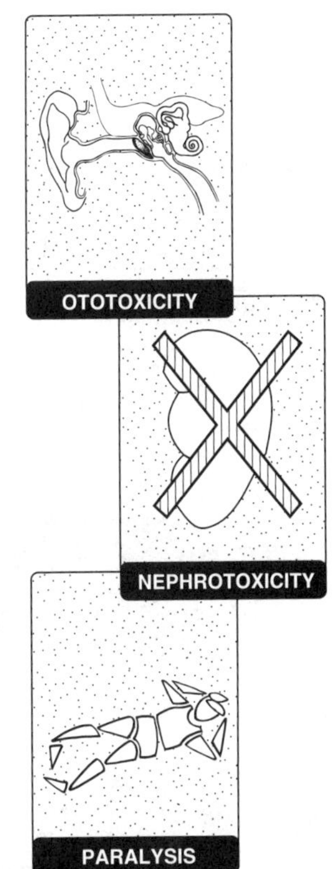

Figure 31.7
Some adverse effects of aminoglycosides.

IV. MACROLIDES

The macrolides are a group of antibiotics with a macrocyclic lactone structure. *Erythromycin* [er ith roe MYE sin] was the first of these to find clinical application both as the drug of first choice, and as an alternative to *penicillin* in individuals who are allergic to β-lactam antibiotics. The new members of this family, *clarithromycin* (a methylated form of *erythromycin*) and *azithromycin* (having a larger lactone ring) have some features in common with and others that improve on, *erythromycin.* Recently, *dirithromycin* [di rith roe MYE sin], a macrolide similar to erythromycin in antibacterial spectrum, but with the advantage of one-daily dosage, has been approved.

A. Mode of action

The macrolides bind irreversibly to a site on the 50S subunit of the bacterial ribosome, thus inhibiting the translocation steps of protein synthesis. Generally considered to be bacteriostatic, they may be cidal at higher doses. The binding site is either identical to or in close proximity to that for *lincomycin*, *clindamycin*, and *chloramphenicol.*

B. Antibacterial spectrum

1. **Erythromycin** is effective against the same organisms as *penicillin G*; therefore, it is used in patients allergic to the penicillins. In addition, it is the drug of choice for the treatment of the infections shown in Figure 31.8.

2. **Clarithromycin** has a spectrum of antibacterial activity similar to that of *erythromycin*, but is also effective against Haemophilus influenzae. Its activity against intracellular pathogens such as Chlamydia, Legionella and Ureaplasma is higher than that of *erythromycin* (Figure 31.9).

CHLAMYDIAL INFECTIONS

- *Erythromycin* is an alternative to *tetracycline* in treating uncomplicated urethral, endocervical, rectal, or epididymal infections due to Chlamydia.
- *Erythromycin* is the drug of choice for urogenital infections due to Chlamydia occuring during pregnancy.

UREAPLASMA

- Causes urethritis in males; genital tract infections in females.
- Major cause of fetal death, miscarriage and low birth weight.

MYCOPLASMAL PNEUMONIA

- Called "atypical" pneumonia because causative mycoplasma escape isolation by standard bacteriological techniques.
- *Tetracyclines* are also effective.

Gram (+) cocci

Gram (+) bacilli

Chlamydia

Myco-plasma

Spirochetes

Other Gram (-) bacilli

Corynebacterium diphtheriae

Mycoplasma pneumoniae

Ureaplasma urealyticum

Treponema pallidum (Syphilis)

Legionella pneumophila

CORYNEBACTERIUM DIPHTHERIAE

- *Erythromycin* or *penicillin* used to eliminate the carrier state.

LEGIONNAIRES' DISEASE (LEGIONELLOSIS)

- Legionellosis represents 0.5-2.0% of all pneumonia in the United States.
- Undiagnosed or asymptomatic infections are common.

SYPHILIS

- *Erythromycin* is used to treat syphilis in patients who are allergic to *penicillin G.*

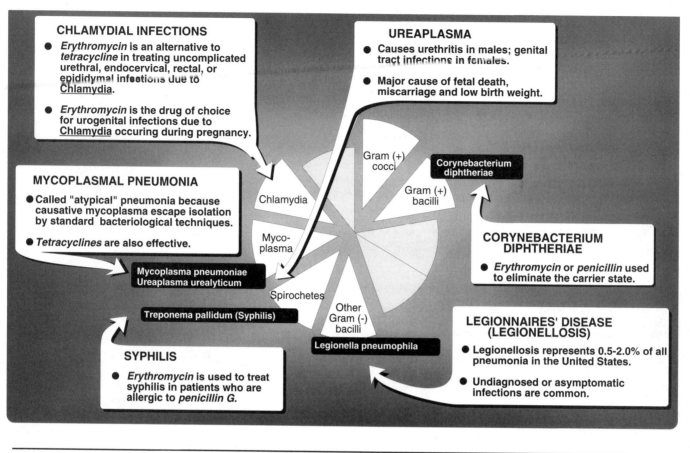

Figure 31.8
Typical therapeutic applications of *erythromycin*.

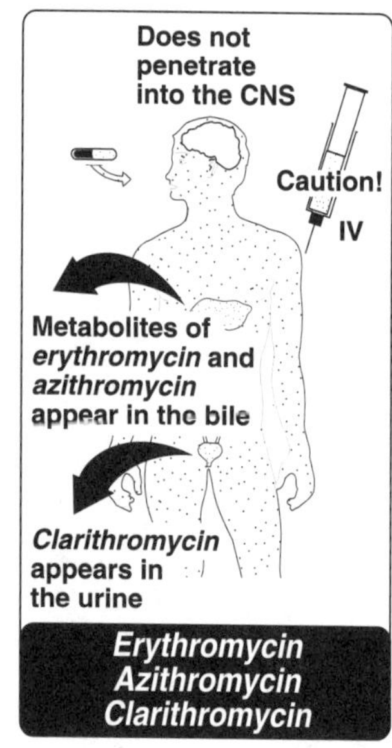

3. **Azithromycin,** though less active against streptococci and staphylococci than *erythromycin*, is far more active against respiratory infections due to Haemophilus influenzae and Moraxella catarrhalis. Except for its cost, it is now the preferred therapy for urethritis caused by Chlamydia trachomatis. Its activity against Mycobacterium avium intracellulare complex has not proven to be clinically important, except in AIDS patients with disseminated infections.

C. Resistance

Resistance to *erythromycin* is becoming a serious clinical problem. For example, most strains of staphylococci in hospital isolates are resistant to this drug. Several mechanisms have been identified: (1) the inability of the organism to take up the antibiotic; (2) a decreased affinity of the 50S ribosomal subunit for the antibiotic resulting from the methylation of an adenine of the 23S bacterial ribosomal RNA; and (3) presence of a plasmid-associated *erythromycin* esterase. Both *clarithromycin* and *azithromycin* show cross-resistance with *erythromycin*.

D. Pharmacokinetics

1. **Administration:** The *erythromycin* base is destroyed by gastric acid; thus either enteric coated tablets or esterified forms are administered. All are adequately absorbed on oral administration. *Clarithromycin* and *azithromycin* are stable to stomach acid and are readily absorbed. Food interferes with the absorption of *erythromycin* and *azithromycin* but can increase that of *clarithromycin*. Intravenous administration of *erythromycin* is associated with a high incidence of thrombophlebitis.

2. **Distribution:** *Erythromycin* distributes well to all body fluids except the cerebrospinal fluid (CSF). It is one of the few antibiotics that diffuses into prostatic fluid and has the unique characteristic of accumulating in macrophages. It concentrates in the liver. Inflammation allows for greater tissue penetration. Similarly, *clarithromycin* and *azithromycin* are widely distributed in tissues. Serum levels of *azithromycin* are low; the drug is concentrated in neutrophils, macrophages, and fibroblasts.

3. **Metabolism:** *Erythromycin* is extensively metabolized and is known to inhibit the oxidation of a number of drugs through its interaction with the cytochrome P-450 system (see p. 14). *Clarithromycin* is oxidized to the 14-hydroxy derivative, which retains antibiotic activity; interference with the metabolism of drugs such as *theophylline* and *carbamazepine* has been reported. *Azithromycin* does not undergo metabolism.

4. **Excretion:** *Erythromycin* and *azithromycin* are primarily concentrated and excreted in an active form in the bile. Partial reabsorption occurs through the enterohepatic circulation. In contrast, *clarithromycin* and its metabolites are eliminated by the kidney as well as the liver and it is recommended that dosage be adjusted in patients with compromised renal function.

E. Adverse effects

1. **Epigastric distress:** This side effect is common and can lead to poor patient compliance for *erythromycin*. The new macrolides seem to be better tolerated by the patient; gastrointestinal problems are their most common side effects.

2. **Cholestatic jaundice:** This side effect occurs, especially with the estolate form of *erythromycin*, presumably as the result of a hypersensitivity reaction to the estolate form (the lauryl salt of the propionyl ester of *erythromycin*). It has also been reported for other forms of the drug.

3. **Ototoxicity:** Transient deafness has been associated with *erythromycin*, especially at high dosages.

4. **Contraindications:** Patients with hepatic dysfunction should not be treated with *erythromycin*, since the drug accumulates in the liver.

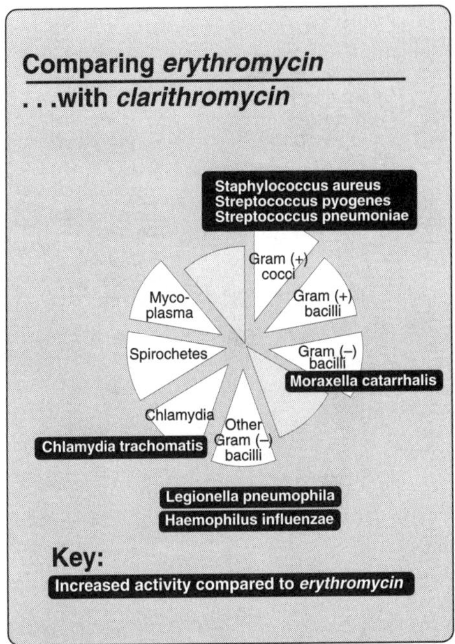

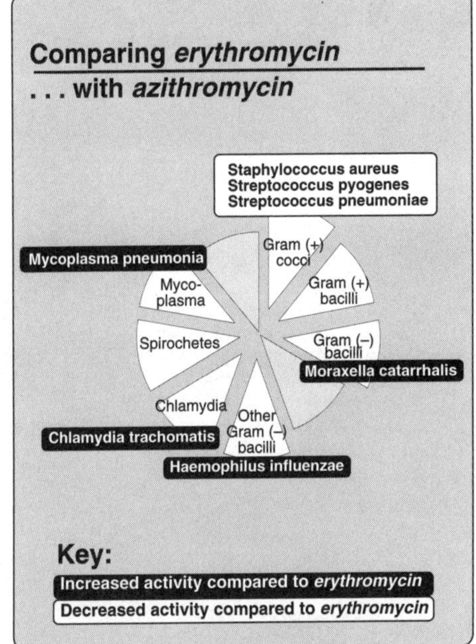

Figure 31.9
Antimicrobial activity of two new macrolides compared with that of *erythromycin*.

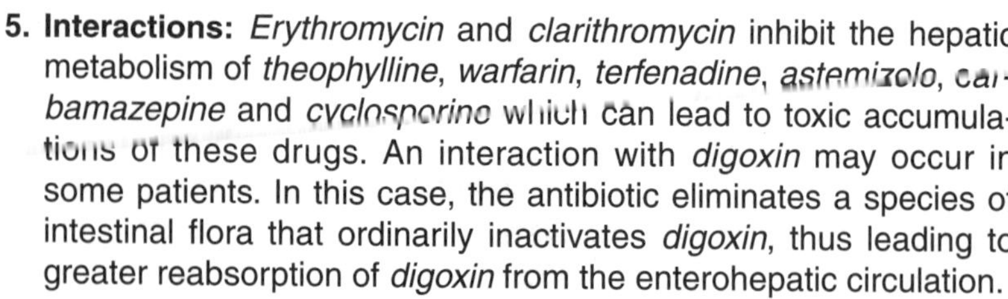

5. **Interactions:** *Erythromycin* and *clarithromycin* inhibit the hepatic metabolism of *theophylline*, *warfarin*, *terfenadine*, *astemizole*, *carbamazepine* and *cyclosporine* which can lead to toxic accumulations of these drugs. An interaction with *digoxin* may occur in some patients. In this case, the antibiotic eliminates a species of intestinal flora that ordinarily inactivates *digoxin*, thus leading to greater reabsorption of *digoxin* from the enterohepatic circulation.

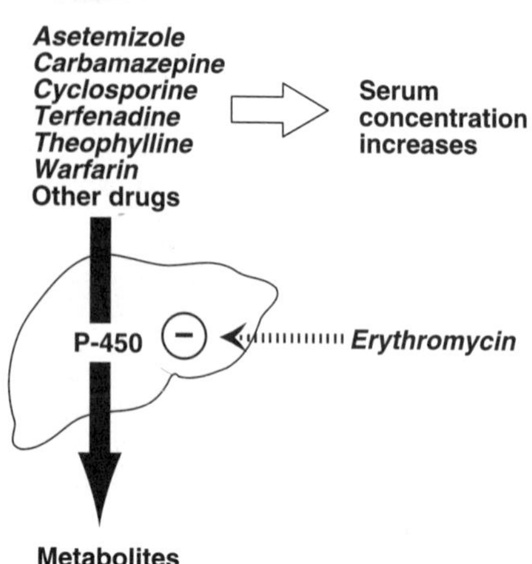

V. CHLORAMPHENICOL

Chloramphenicol [klor am FEN i kole] is active against a wide range of gram-positive and gram-negative organisms, but because of its toxicity, its use is restricted to life-threatening infections in which there are no alternatives.

A. Mode of action

The drug binds to the bacterial 50S ribosomal subunit and inhibits protein synthesis at the peptidyl transferase reaction. Because of the similarity of mammalian mitochondrial ribosomes to those of bacteria, protein synthesis in these organelles may be inhibited at high circulating *chloramphenicol* levels, producing bone marrow toxicity.

B. Antimicrobial spectrum

Chloramphenicol, a broad spectrum antibiotic, is active not only against bacteria but also against other microorganisms, such as rickettsiae. *Chloramphenicol* has excellent activity against anaerobes. The drug is either bactericidal or (more commonly) bacteriostatic, depending on the organism.

C. Resistance

Resistance is conferred by the presence of an R factor, which codes for an acetyl coenzyme A transferase that inactivates *chloramphenicol*. Another mechanism for resistance is associated with an inability of the antibiotic to penetrate the organism. This change in permeability may be the basis of multidrug resistance.

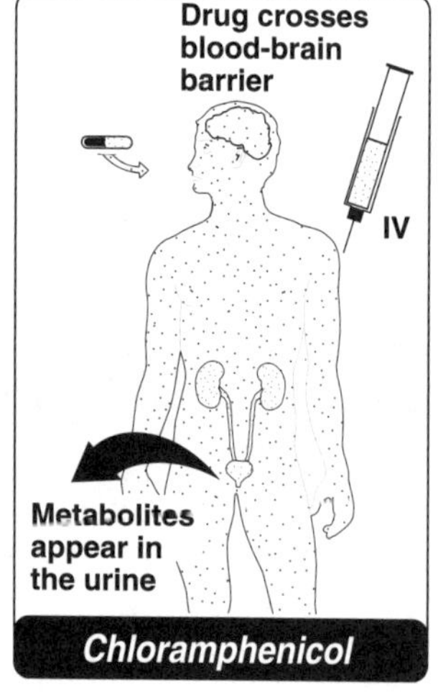

D. Pharmacokinetics

Chloramphenicol may be administered either intravenously or orally. It is completely absorbed via the oral route because of its lipophilic nature and is widely distributed throughout the body. It readily enters the normal CSF. The drug inhibits the hepatic mixed function oxidases. Excretion of the drug depends on its conversion in the liver to a glucuronide that is then secreted by the renal tubule. Only about 10% of the parent compound is excreted by glomerular filtration.

E. Adverse effects

The clinical use of *chloramphenicol* is limited because of the serious adverse effects associated with its administration. In addition to gastrointestinal upsets, overgrowth of Candida may appear on the mucuous membranes.

1. **Anemias:** Hemolytic anemia occurs in patients with low levels of glucose 6-phosphate dehydrogenase[3] (see p. 351). Other types of anemia occurring as a side effect of *chloramphenicol* include reversible anemia, which is apparently dose-related and occurs concomitantly with therapy, and aplastic anemia, which is idiosyncratic and usually fatal. [Note: Aplastic anemia is independent of dose and may occur after therapy has ceased.]

2. **Gray baby syndrome:** This adverse effect occurs in neonates if the dosage regimen of *chloramphenicol* is not properly adjusted. Neonates have a low capacity to glucuronidate the antibiotic and they have underdeveloped renal function. They therefore have a decreased ability to excrete the drug, which accumulates to levels that interfere with the function of mitochondrial ribosomes. This leads to poor feeding, depressed breathing, cardiovascular collapse, cyanosis (hence the term "gray baby") and death.

3. **Interactions:** *Chloramphenicol* is able to inhibit some of the hepatic mixed function oxidases and thus can block the metabolism of such drugs as *warfarin*, *phenytoin*, *tolbutamide* and *chlorpropamide*, thus elevating their concentrations and potentiating their effects.

VI. CLINDAMYCIN

Clindamycin's [klin da MYE sin] mode of action is the same as that of *erythromycin* (see p. 317). *Clindamycin* is employed primarily in the treatment of infections caused by anaerobic bacteria, such as Bacteroides fragilis, which often causes abdominal infections associated with trauma. However, it is also significantly active against non-enterococcal gram-positive cocci. Resistance mechanisms are the same as those for *erythromycin*, but cross-resistance is not a problem. [Note: Clostridium difficile is always resistant to *clindamycin*.] *Clindamycin* is well absorbed by the oral route. It distributes well into all body fluids except the CSF. Adequate levels of *clindamycin* are not achieved in the brain, even when meninges are inflamed. Penetration into bone occurs even in the absence of inflammation. *Clindamycin* undergoes extensive oxidative metabolism to inactive products. The drug is excreted into the bile or urine by glomerular filtration, but therapeutically effective levels of the parent drug are not achieved in the urine. Accumulation has been reported in patients with either severely compromised renal function or hepatic failure. In addition to skin rashes, the most serious adverse effect is potentially fatal pseudomembranous colitis caused by overgrowth of Clostridium difficile, which elaborates necrotizing toxins. Oral administration of either *metronidazole* (see p. 347) or *vancomycin* (see p. 308) is usually effective in controlling this serious problem. Impaired liver function has also been reported.

[3]See p. 322 for Infolink references to other books in this series.

Choose the ONE best answer.

31.1 Which one of the following diseases is NOT treated with a tetracycline?

A. Cholera.
B. Lyme disease.
C. Rocky Mountain spotted fever.
D. Mycoplasma pneumonia.
E. Streptococcal infection.

Correct choice = E. Most strains of streptococci are resistant to tetracycline.

31.2 Which one of the following statements about tetracycline is INCORRECT?

A. Its use is rarely contraindicated because of resistant strains.
B. It is contraindicated in pregnancy.
C. It is effective in treating infections caused by Chlamydiae.
D. It can form poorly absorbable complexes with calcium ions.
E. It can lead to discoloration of teeth if given to children.

Correct choice = A. Widespread resistance to tetracycline limits the clinical uses of this drug. Deposition of tetracycline in calcifying tissues of the fetus and growing children can occur. The drug has the potential for causing hepatic toxicity in the mother. Dairy foods in the diet decrease absorption because of the formation of nonabsorbable chelates of tetracycline with calcium ions.

31.3 Which one of the following statements about tetracyclines is INCORRECT?

A. Accumulation of tetracyclines by susceptible organisms is mediated by transport proteins located in the bacterial membrane.
B. Tetracyclines, even at high concentrations, do not affect mammalian cell metabolism.
C. Tetracyclines bind to the 30S subunit of the bacterial ribosome and block protein synthesis.
D. Phototoxicity is encountered most frequently with demeclocycline and doxycycline.
E. Doxycycline is the only tetracycline that may be used in treating patients with renal failure.

Correct choice = B. At high concentrations, tetracycline enters mammalian cells by diffusion and interacts with mitochondrial ribosomes, blocking access of the amino acyl-tRNA to the mRNA-ribosome complex at the acceptor site. Severe photosensitive dermatitis occurs when the patient receiving tetracycline is exposed to sun or ultraviolet rays.

31.4 All of the following properties are exhibited by aminoglycosides EXCEPT:

A. They are poorly absorbed from gastrointestinal tract.
B. They have bactericidal properties.
C. They can achieve adequate serum levels after oral administration.
D. They bind to the 30S ribosomal subunit.
E. They are not accumulated by anaerobic microorganisms.

Correct choice = C. All aminoglycosides are poorly absorbed from the gastrointestinal tract. All aminoglycosides are given parenterally and are rapidly bactericidal. They interfere with assembly of the functional ribosomal apparatus or cause the 30S subunit of the complete ribosome to misread the genetic code. Anaerobes lack the oxygen-dependent system that is responsible for transporting the antibiotics across the cytoplasmic membrane, therefore, strictly anaerobic organisms are resistant to aminoglycosides.

31.5. A patient being treated for springtime allergies with terfenadine develops an upper respiratory problem. He receives an antibiotic and develops a cardiac arrhythmia. What was the likely antibiotic?

A. Ampicillin
B. Cefaclor
C. Erythromycin
D. Doxycycline
E. Cotrimoxazole

The correct answer is C. Erythromycin and clarithromycin inhibit the metabolism of terfenadine giving rise to cardiac arrhythmias (torsade de pointe). None of the other antibiotics have this effect.

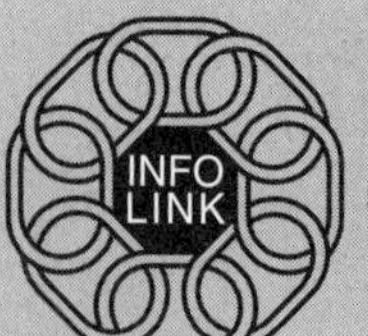

[1]See p. 393 in **Biochemistry** (2nd ed.) for a discussion of structure of ribosomes.

[2]See p. 396 in **Biochemistry** (2nd ed.) for a discussion of drug binding to ribosomes.

[3]See p. 115 in **Biochemistry** (2nd ed.) for a discussion of hemolytic anemia that occurs in patients with low levels of glucose 6-phosphate dehydrogenase.

Quinolones and Urinary Tract Antiseptics

32

I. OVERVIEW

Introduction of the first fluorinated quinolone, *norfloxacin* [nor FLOX a sin], has been rapidly followed by new members of this class. These agents are totally synthetic and are closely related structurally to an earlier quinolone, *nalidixic acid* [nal i DIX ik]. The principal member of this group is *ciprofloxacin* [sip ro FLOX a sin], which has the widest clinical application. Other antibiotics in this group available in the United States are primarily employed to treat urinary infections (Figure 32.1). It seems likely that the size of this class of antibiotics will increase due to its wide antibacterial spectrum, favorable pharmacokinetic properties and relative lack of adverse reactions. Unfortunately, their overuse has already led to the emergence of resistant strains resulting in limitations to their clinical usefulness.

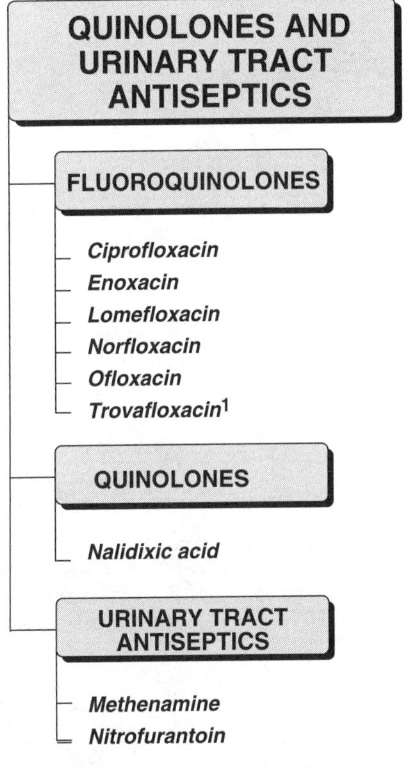

QUINOLONES AND URINARY TRACT ANTISEPTICS
FLUOROQUINOLONES
Ciprofloxacin
Enoxacin
Lomefloxacin
Norfloxacin
Ofloxacin
Trovafloxacin1
QUINOLONES
Nalidixic acid
URINARY TRACT ANTISEPTICS
Methenamine
Nitrofurantoin

Figure 32.1
Summary of drugs described in this chapter. [1]Described in Pharmacology update, p. 456

II. FLUOROQUINOLONES

The older drug, *nalidixic acid*, is a nonfluorinated quinolone, and is not effective against systemic infections. Its use in the treatment of urinary tract infections (UTIs) is limited due to the rapid emergence of resistant strains. It will be considered in a separate section below. Unless care is taken to employ these drugs in appropriate infective states, it is possible that their value will be lost.

A. Mechanism of action

The fluoroquinolones enter the cell by passive diffusion through water-filled protein channels (porins) in the outer membrane. Intracellularly, they uniquely inhibit the replication of bacterial DNA by interfering with the action of DNA gyrase (topoisomerase II) during bacterial growth and reproduction. [Note: Topoisomerases are enzymes that change the configuration or topology of DNA by a nicking, pass-through and re-sealing mechanism without changing its primary structure (Figure 32.2).][1] Binding of the quinolone to both the enzyme and the DNA to form a ternary complex inhibits the rejoining

[1]See p. 330 for Infolink references to other books in this series.

Lippincott's Illustrated Reviews: Pharmacology, Second Edition.
by Mary J. Mycek, Richard A. Harvey and Pamela C. Champe.
Lippincott Williams & Wilkins, Philadelphia, PA © 2000.

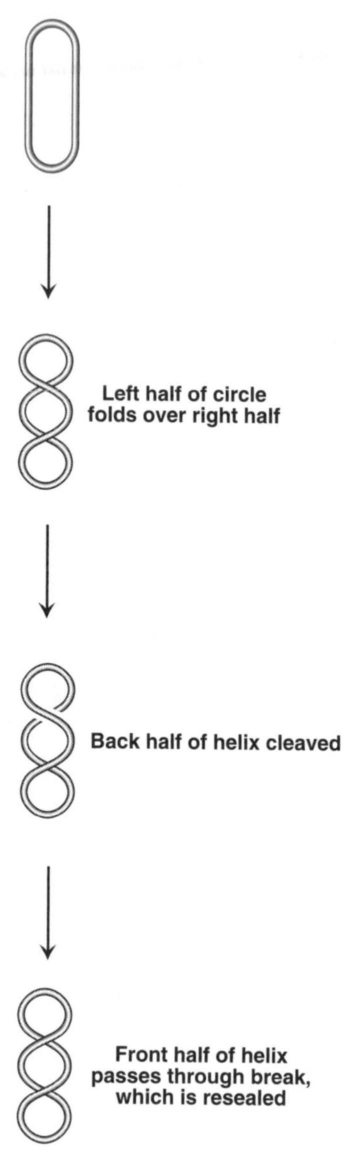
Left half of circle folds over right half
Back half of helix cleaved
Front half of helix passes through break, which is resealed

Figure 32.2
Action of type II DNA topoisomerase.

step and can cause cell death by inducing cleavage of the DNA. Since DNA gyrase is a distinct target for antimicrobial therapy, cross-resistance with other more commonly used antimicrobial drugs is rare but increasing in the case of multi-drug resistant organisms.

B. Antimicrobial spectrum

All of the fluoroquinolones are bactericidal. In general, they are effective against gram-negative organisms such as the enterobacteria, pseudomonas organisms, Haemophilus influenzae, Moraxella catarrhalis, Legionella, Chlamydia and mycobacteria except for M. avium intracellulare complex. They are effective in the treatment of gonorrhea but not syphilis. Though active against some gram-positive organisms, they should be avoided in the treatment of pneumoccal or enterococcal infections. Their activity against anaerobes is poor. If used prophylactically before transurethral surgery, they lower the incidence of postsurgical UTIs.

1. **Ciprofloxacin:** This is the most potent of the fluoroquinolones and has an antibacterial spectrum similar to that of *norfloxacin* (Figure 32.3). *Ciprofloxacin* finds use in the treatment of pseudomonas infections associated with cystic fibrosis. The serum levels achieved are effective against many systemic infections with the exception of serious infections caused by *methicillin*-resistant Staphylococcus aureus (MRSA), the enterococci and pneumococci. *Ciprofloxacin* is particularly useful in treating infections caused by many Enterobacteraceae and other gram-negative bacilli. *Ciprofloxacin* is an alternative to more toxic drugs, such as the aminoglycosides (p. 314). It may act synergistically with β-lactams (p. 297).

2. **Norfloxacin:** This agent is effective against both gram-negative (including Pseudomonas aeruginosa) and gram-positive organisms in treating complicated and uncomplicated UTIs and prostatitis, but not in systemic infections.

3. **Ofloxacin:** Like *norfloxacin, ofloxacin* [oh FLOX a sin] is primarily used in the treatment of prostatitis due to E. coli and of sexually transmitted diseases (STDs) with the exception of syphilis. It may be used as alternative therapy in patients with gonorrhea. It has some benefit in the treatment of skin and lower respiratory tract infections.

4. **Lomefloxacin:** *Lomefloxacin* [loh me FLOX a sin] and *enoxacin* [ee NOX a sin] are useful in the treatment of UTIs and bronchitis caused by Haemophilus influenzae or Moraxella catarrhalis. *Lomefloxacin* is not effective against pseudomonal bacteremia.

See p. 456 for a description of newly approved drug, *trovafloxacin.*

C. Resistance

When the fluoroquinolones were first introduced, there was optimism that resistance would not develop. Although no plasmid-mediated resistance has been reported, resistance of MRSA, pseudomonas, coagulase-negative staphylococci and enterococci has unfortunately emerged due to chromosomal mutations. Cross-resistance exists among the quinolones. The mechanisms responsible for this resistance include:

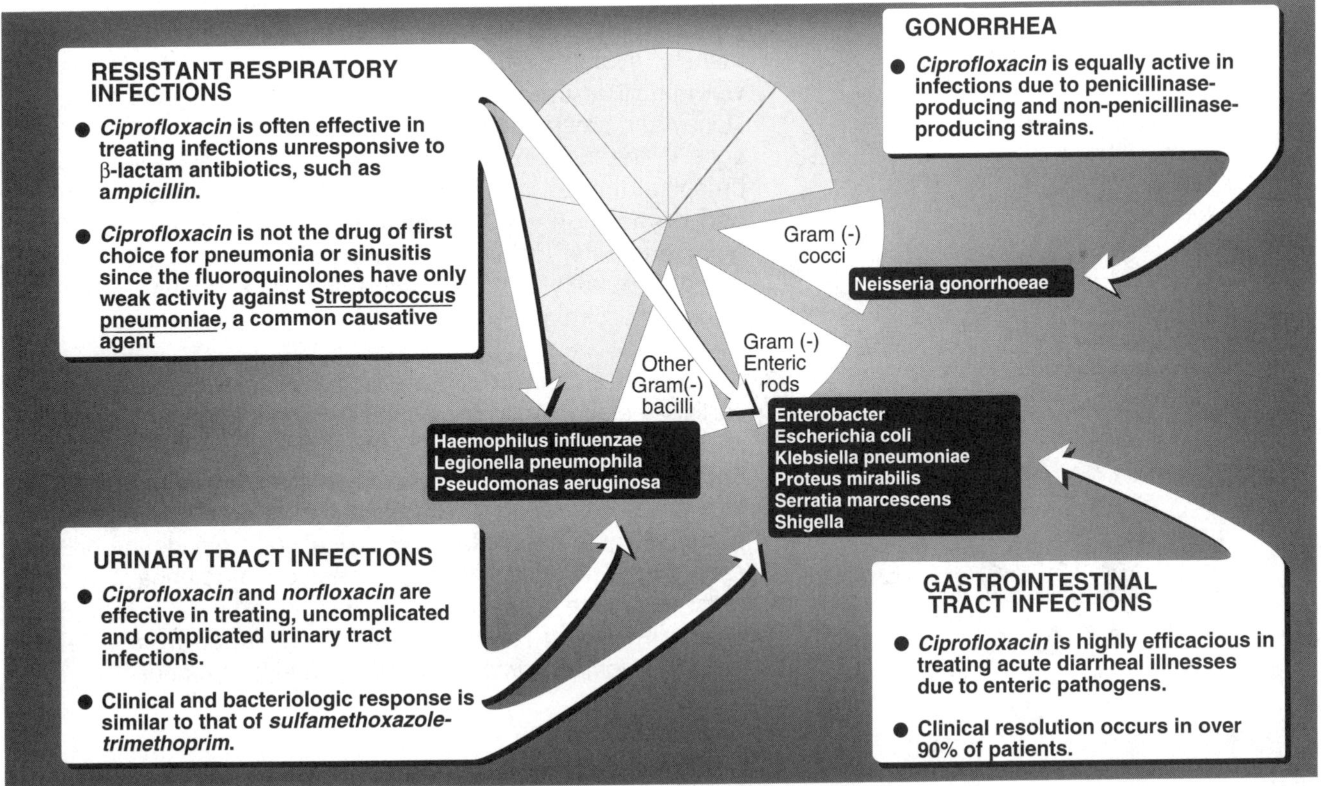

Figure 32.3
Typical therapeutic applications of *ciprofloxacin.*

1. **Altered target:** Modifications in the bacterial DNA gyrase, especially in amino acids at the N-terminus of the A subunit, have been associated with a decreased affinity for the fluoroquinolone. The B subunit of the gyrase is rarely mutated.

2. **Decreased accumulation:** Reduced intracellular concentration of the drugs in the bacterial cell is linked to two mechanisms. One involves a decreased number of porin proteins in the outer membrane of the resistant cell, thereby impairing access of the drugs to the intracellular gyrase. The other mechanism is associated with an energy-dependent efflux system in the cytoplasmic membrane.

D. Pharmacokinetics

1. **Absorption:** Only 35-70% of oral *norfloxacin* is absorbed. However, 70-90% of the other fluoroquinolones are absorbed after oral administration. Bioavailability is greatest for *ofloxacin* and *lomefloxacin.* Intravenous preparations of *ciprofloxacin* and *ofloxacin* are available. Ingestion of the fluoroquinolones with sucralfate, antacids containing aluminum or magnesium, or dietary supplements containing iron or zinc can interfere with the absorption of these antibacterial agents.

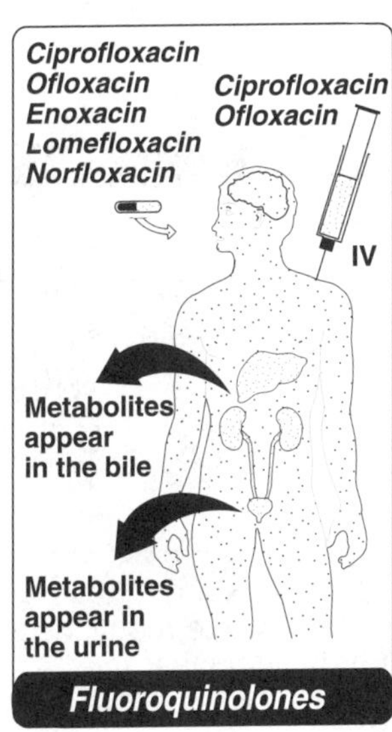

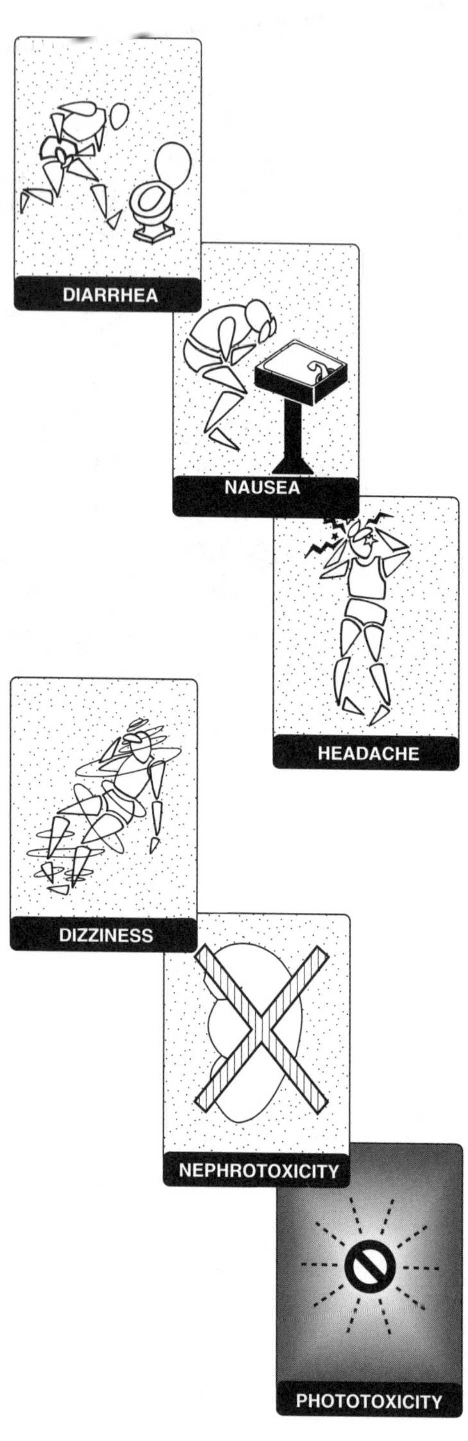

Figure 32.4
Some adverse reactions to fluoroquinolones.

2. **Distribution:** Binding to plasma proteins ranges from 10 to 40%. [Note: Plasma levels of free *norfloxacin* are insufficient for treatment of systemic infections.] All the fluoroquinolones distribute well into all tissues and body fluids. Levels are high in bone, urine, kidney and prostatic tissue (but not prostatic fluid), and concentrations in the lung exceed those in serum. Penetration into cerebrospinal fluid is low except for *ofloxacin* where concentrations can be as high as 90% of those in the serum. The fluoroquinolones also accumulate in macrophages and polymorphonuclear leukocytes, thus being effective against intracellular organisms such as Legionella.

3. **Metabolism:** Except for *ofloxacin* and *lomefloxacin*, these agents are partially metabolized to compounds with less antimicrobial activity.

4. **Excretion:** The parent drugs and their metabolites are excreted into the urine where high levels can occur. This is the major excretory route for *ofloxacin*. Renal failure prolongs the half-life of each drug. The other fluoroquinolones undergo hepatic as well as renal clearance; this route assumes importance in renal failure. The half-lives of the fluoroquinolones range from 3-5 hours, except for *lomefloxacin* which has a half-life of 8 hours.

E. Adverse reactions

Toxicities similar to those for *nalidixic acid* (p. 327) have been reported for the fluoroquinolones (Figure 32.4). Besides diarrhea, the following adverse reactions may be encountered.

1. **CNS problems:** The most prominent side effects are nausea, headache, and dizziness or lightheadedness. Thus, patients with CNS disorders, such as epilepsy, should be treated cautiously with these drugs.

2. **Nephrotoxicity**: Crystalluria has been reported in patients receiving excessive doses (3-4 times normal).

3. **Phototoxicity:** Patients are advised to avoid excessive sunlight and to use sunscreen. However, even sunscreens or sunblocks may not protect against the phototoxicity and the drug should be discontinued at the first sign of this toxicity.

4. **Contraindications:** Fluoroquinolones should be avoided in pregnancy, in nursing mothers and in children under 18 years of age, since articular cartilage erosion (arthropathy) occurs in immature experimental animals.

5. **Drug interactions:** The effect of antacids and cations on the absorption of these agents was considered above. *Ciprofloxacin*, *ofloxacin* and *enoxacin* can increase the serum levels of *theophylline* by inhibiting its metabolism. They also may raise levels of *warfarin*, *caffeine* and *cyclosporine*. *Cimetidine* interferes with the

elimination of the fluoroquinolones. *Enoxacin* when administered concurrently with anti-inflammatory *fenoprofen* has been reported to cause seizures.

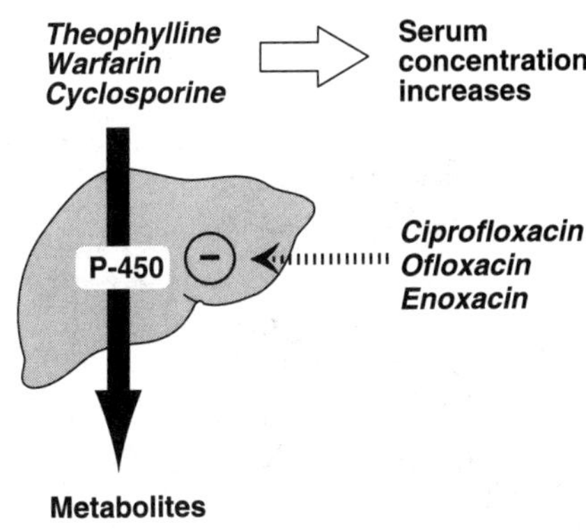

III. QUINOLONES

Nalidixic acid is a nonfluorinated quinolone with the same mechanism of action as that of the fluoroquinolones. It is effective against most of the gram-negative bacteria that commonly cause UTIs but gram-positive organisms are resistant. Its clinical usefulness is limited by the rapid emergence of resistant strains. Well-absorbed, most (>90%) of the drug is protein bound and levels of free drug are therefore inadequate for treatment of systemic infections. Hydroxylation leads to the more potent bactericidal compound, 7-hydroxynalidixic acid, which is excreted in the urine along with the parent drug. Among the adverse effects are nausea, vomiting and abdominal pain. Photosensitivity, urticaria and fever can occur. CNS problems ranging from headache and malaise to visual disturbances are rare. Therapy lasting longer than 2 weeks can adversely affect liver function.

IV. URINARY TRACT ANTISEPTICS

Urinary tract infections (UTI, most commonly uncomplicated acute cystitis and pyleonephritis) in women of child bearing age, and in the elderly, are one of the most common problems seen by primary care physicians. Escherichia coli is the most common pathogen causing about 80% of uncomplicated upper and lower UTI. Staphylococcus saprophyticus is the second most common bacterial pathogen causing UTI; other common causes include Klebsiella pneumoniae and Proteus mirabilis infections. In addition, UTI may be treated with any one of a group of agents called urinary tract antiseptics, including *methenamine* and *nitrofurantoin*. These drugs do not achieve antibacterial levels in the circulation, but because they are concentrated in the urine, microorganisms at that site can be effectively eradicated.

A. Methenamine

1. **Mechanism of action:** In order to act, *methenamine* [meth EN a meen] must decompose at an acidic pH of 5.5 or less in the urine, thus producing formaldehyde, which is toxic to most bacteria (Figure 32.5). The reaction is slow, requiring 3 hours to reach 90% decomposition. *Methenamine* should not be used in patients with indwelling catheters. Bacterial resistance to formaldehyde does not develop. [Note: *Methenamine* is frequently formulated with a weak acid such as mandelic acid, which lowers the pH of the urine thus aiding decomposition of the drug.]

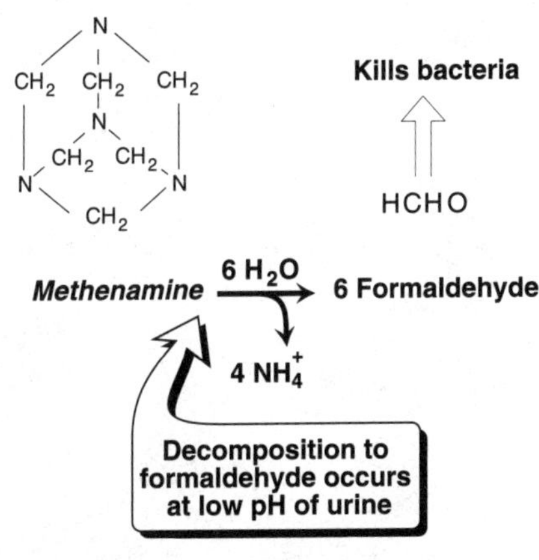

Figure 32.5
Formation of formaldehyde from *methenamine* at acid pH.

2. **Antibacterial spectrum:** *Methenamine* is primarily used for chronic suppressive therapy. Urea-splitting bacteria that alkalinize the urine, such as Proteus, are usually resistant to the action of *methenamine*. *Methenamine* is used to treat UTI, but is not effective in upper UTI.

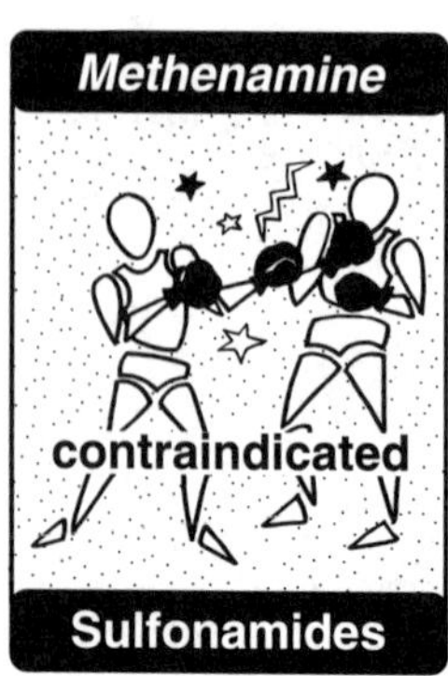

3. **Pharmacokinetics:** *Methenamine* is orally administered. In addition to formaldehyde, ammonium ion is produced in the bladder. Because the liver rapidly metabolizes ammonia to form urea, *methenamine* is contraindicated in patients with hepatic insufficiency, in which elevated levels of circulating ammonium ions would be toxic to the CNS. *Methenamine* is distributed throughout the body fluids, but no decomposition of the drug occurs at pH 7.4; thus, systemic toxicity does not occur. The drug is eliminated in the urine.

4. **Adverse effects:** The side effects include gastrointestinal distress. At higher doses, albuminuria, hematuria and rashes may develop. *Methenamine mandelate* is contraindicated in treating patients with renal insufficiency, because mandelic acid may precipitate. Sulfonamides react with formaldehyde and must not be used concomitantly with *methenamine*.

C. Nitrofurantoin

Nitrofurantoin [nye troe FYOOR an toyn] is less commonly employed for treating UTIs because of its narrow antimicrobial spectrum and its toxicity.

1. **Mechanism of action**: Sensitive bacteria reduce the drug to an active agent that inhibits various enzymes and damages DNA. Activity is greater in acidic urine.

2. **Antimicrobial Spectrum:** The drug is bacteriostatic. It is useful against Escherichia coli, but other common urinary tract gram-negative bacteria may be resistant. Gram-positive cocci are susceptible.

3. **Resistance:** Resistance is constitutive. It is associated with an inability to reduce the nitrogen group in the presence of oxygen. Resistance does not develop during therapy.

4. **Pharmacokinetics:** Absorption is complete after oral administration. The drug is rapidly excreted by glomerular filtration. The presence of the drug turns the urine brown, a surprise for unsuspecting patients.

5. **Adverse effects:**

   a. **Gastrointestinal disturbances:** These side effects include nausea, vomiting, and diarrhea. The macrocrystalline form is better tolerated. Ingestion with food or milk ameliorates these symptoms.

   b. **Acute pneumonitis**: This is a serious complication. Other pul-

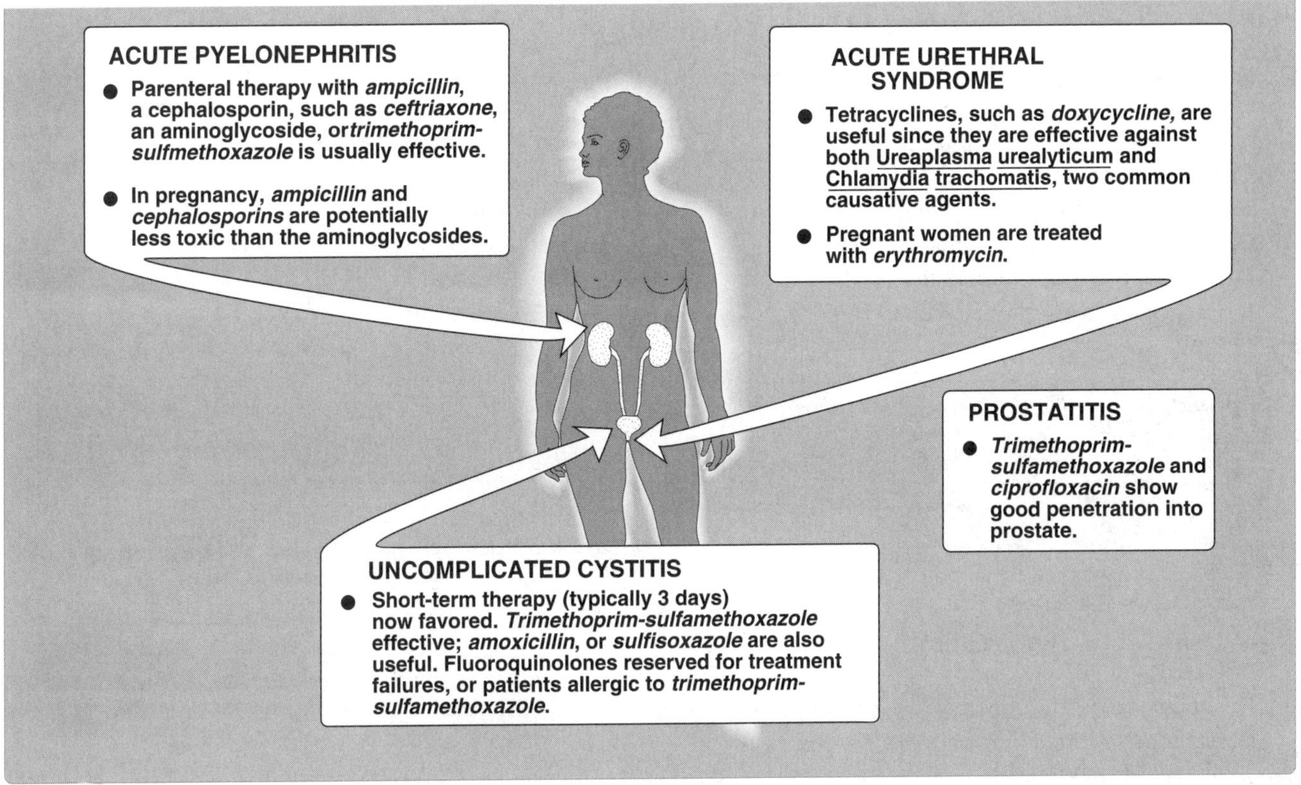

ACUTE PYELONEPHRITIS
Parenteral therapy with ampicillin, a cephalosporin, such as ceftriaxone, an aminoglycoside, ortrimethoprim-sulfmethoxazole is usually effective.
In pregnancy, ampicillin and cephalosporins are potentially less toxic than the aminoglycosides.
ACUTE URETHRAL SYNDROME
Tetracyclines, such as doxycycline, are useful since they are effective against both Ureaplasma urealyticum and Chlamydia trachomatis, two common causative agents.
Pregnant women are treated with erythromycin.
PROSTATITIS
Trimethoprim-sulfamethoxazole and ciprofloxacin show good penetration into prostate.
UNCOMPLICATED CYSTITIS
Short-term therapy (typically 3 days) now favored. Trimethoprim-sulfamethoxazole effective; amoxicillin, or sulfisoxazole are also useful. Fluoroquinolones reserved for treatment failures, or patients allergic to trimethoprim-sulfamethoxazole.

Figure 32.6
Antimicrobial drugs commonly used in treating urinary tract infections.

monary effects, such as interstitial pulmonary fibrosis, can occur in patients being chronically treated.

c. **Neurological problems:** Neurological side effects such as headache, nystagmus, and polyneuropathies with demyelination (sometime leading to footdrop) may develop.

d. **Hemolytic anemia:** The drug is contraindicated in patients with glucose-6-phosphate dehydrogenase deficiency, neonates, and pregnant women.

Agents commonly used in uncomplicated UTI are summarized in Figure 32.6).

Choose the ONE best answer:

32.1 All of the following statements about methenamine are true EXCEPT:

A. It is used in chronic suppressive therapy of urinary tract infections.
B. It has its major antibacterial effect at alkaline pH.
C. It is contraindicated in renal insufficiency.
D. It may cause gastric disturbances.
E. Its antimicrobial activity is confined to the urinary tract.

Correct choice = B. Methenamine has its maximum effect at acidic pH—this is the reason that the drug is often formulated with a weak acid such as mandelic acid

32.2. In which one of the following infections are the fluoroquinolones ineffective?

A. UTIs due to a β-lactamase-producing strain of Klebsiella.
B. Pneumonia due to Streptococcus pneumoniae.
C. Exacerbation of chronic bronchitis due to Moraxella catarrhalis.
D. Urinary tract infection due to E. coli.
E. UTIs due to Pseudomonas aeruginosa.

Correct answer = B. The fluoroquinolones do not have sufficient activity against S. pneumoniae to be effective. Since they are not β-lactams, the fluoroquinolones are effective in treating UTIs caused by β–lactamase-producing organisms. Fluoroquinolones are also indicated for treatment of the other infections listed.

32.3 A 26-year-old young man presents with the symptoms of gonorrhea. Since this condition is often associated with an infection due to Chlamydia trachomatis, which of the following quinolones would be the best choice in treating him?

A. Ciprofloxacin
B. Nalidixic acid
C. Norfloxacin
D. Ofloxacin
E. Lomefloxacin

Correct answer = D. Ofloxacin has the best activity of all the quinolones against both gonorrheal and chlamydial infections. Nalidixic acid is without activity in these conditions.

32.4 Ciprofloxacin and tetracycline have all of the following properties in common EXCEPT:

A. Resistant organisms have an increased ability to pump out the drugs.
B. Absorption can be decreased by concurrent administration with aluminum or magnesium containing antacids.
C. Both can cause severe phototoxicity.
D. Both accumulate with decreased renal function.
E. Both are deposited in developing bones and teeth.

Correct choice = E. Only tetracycline is deposited in bone and thus is contraindicated in children under age 8. Ciprofloxacin damages developing articular cartilage in young experimental animals, which is why it is contraindicated in children under 18 years of age. All the other statements pertain to both antibiotics.

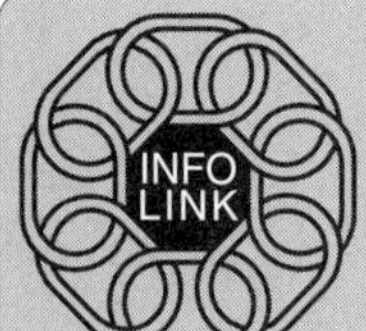

[1]See p. 365 in **Biochemistry** (2nd ed.) for a discussion of topoisomerases and the topology of DNA.

Antimycobacterial Drugs

33

,I. OVERVIEW

The modern era of tuberculosis therapy began with the introduction of *streptomycin*, *isoniazid*, and *p-aminosalicylic acid* and today multidrug therapy includes drugs listed in Figure 33.1. The number of cases of tuberculosis waned and there was hope of complete eradication. Indeed, predictions were made that tuberculosis would be almost nonexistent in the United States by the year 2002. However, in the past decade, tuberculosis cases have significantly increased, chiefly among AIDS patients and the homeless (Figure 33.2). Today tuberculosis is still the leading cause of death by infectious disease throughout the world.

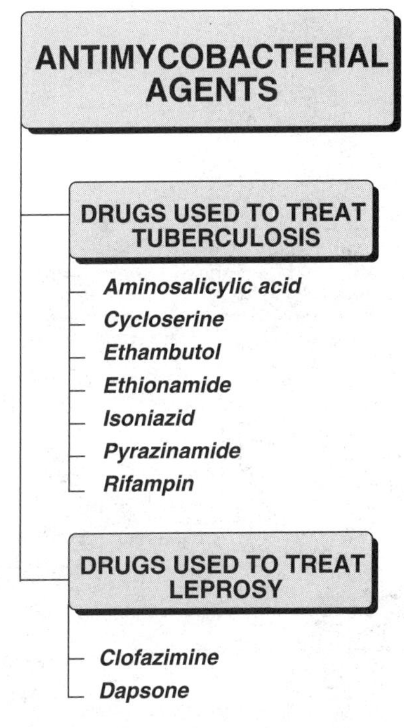

Figure 33.1
Summary of drugs used to treat mycobacterial infections.

II. CHEMOTHERAPY OF TUBERCULOSIS

Mycobacterium tuberculosis, one of a number of mycobacteria, can lead to serious infections of the lungs, the genitourinary tract, skeleton, and meninges. The mycobacteria are classified on the basis of their staining properties. [Note: Though difficult to stain because of the presence of an outer coat of mycolic acid, once stained they hold the stain even in the presence of destaining agents such as acid. Thus they are referred to as "acid-fast".] Treating tuberculosis as well as other mycobacterial infections presents therapeutic problems. The organism grows slowly, and thus the disease may have to be treated for up to 2 years, especially if it is caused by a resistant organism.

A. Strategies for addressing drug resistance

Because strains of the organism resistant to a particular agent emerge during treatment, multiple drug therapy is employed to delay or prevent their emergence. *Isoniazid*, *rifampin*, *ethambutol*, *streptomycin*, and *pyrazinamide* are the principal or so-called "first line" drugs because of their efficacy and acceptable degree of toxicity. However today, because of poor patient compliance and other factors, the number of multidrug-resistant organisms has risen. Some bacteria have been identified that are resistant to as many as seven antitubercular agents. Therefore, although treatment regimens vary

Lippincott's Illustrated Reviews: Pharmacology, Second Edition.
by Mary J. Mycek, Richard A. Harvey and Pamela C. Champe.
Lippincott Williams & Wilkins, Philadelphia, PA © 2000.

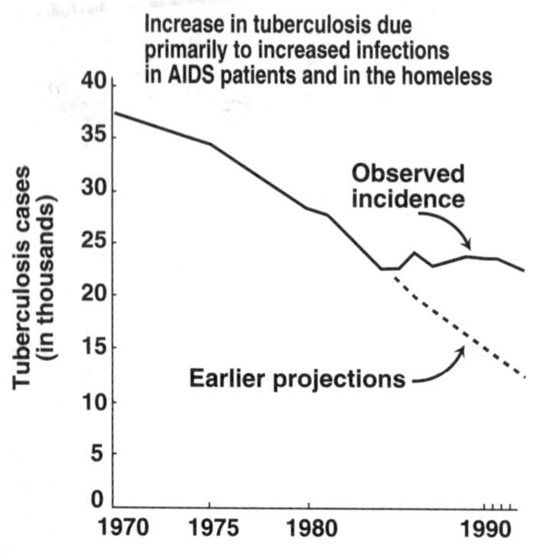

Figure 33.2
Incidence of new cases of tuberculosis.

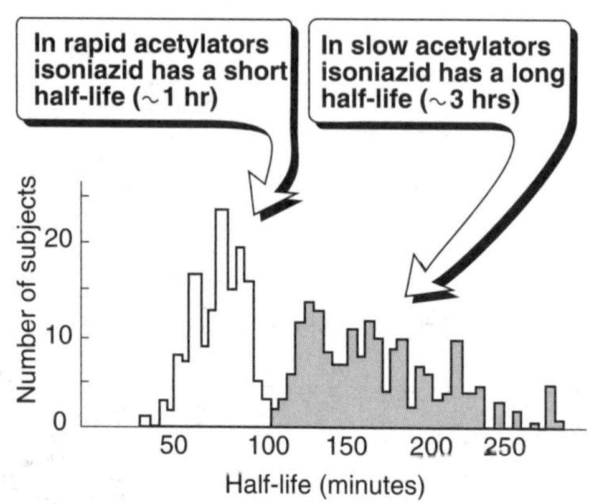

Figure 33.3
Bimodal distribution of *isoniazid* half-lives caused by rapid and slow acetylation of drug.

in duration and in agents employed, they always include a minimum of two drugs, preferably both cidal (see p. 283). Together they should prevent the emergence of resistant strains. The regimen is continued well beyond the disappearance of clinical disease so as to eradicate any persistent organisms. For example, the short course chemotherapy for tuberculosis includes *isoniazid*, *rifampin* and *pyrazinamide* for 2 months, and *isoniazid* and *rifampin* for the next 4 months. *Ethambutol* may also be added to this regimen.

B. Isoniazid

Isoniazid [eye soe NYE a zid], the hydrazide of isonicotinic acid, is a synthetic analog of pyridoxine. It is the most potent of the anti-tubercular drugs, but is never given as a single agent in the treatment of active tuberculosis. Its introduction revolutionized the treatment of tuberculosis.

1. **Mechanism of action:** *Isoniazid*, often referred to as INH, is believed to target the enzyme responsible for assembly of mycolic acids into the outer layer of the mycobacteria, a structure unique to these organisms. Mycolic acids account for the acid-fastness of the mycobacteria; this property is lost after exposure to *isoniazid*.

2. **Antibacterial spectrum:** For bacilli in the stationary phase, the drug is bacteriostatic, but for rapidly dividing organisms, it is bactericidal. It is effective against intracellular bacteria. *Isoniazid* is specific for treatment of M. tuberculosis, although Mycobacterium kansasii may be susceptible at higher drug levels. When it is used alone, resistant organisms rapidly emerge.

3. **Resistance** is associated with the constitutive inability of the organism to accumulate the drug. There is also suggestive evidence that the target enzyme may be altered so as not to bind the *isoniazid,* or that excessive amounts of the enzyme may be produced so that the drug is overwhelmed. No cross-resistance exists between *isoniazid* and other anti-tubercular drugs.

4. **Pharmacokinetics:** The drug is readily absorbed orally. Absorption is impaired if taken with food, particularly carbohydrates, or with aluminum-containing antacids. *Isoniazid* diffuses into all body fluids, cells, and caseous material (necrotic tissue resembling cheese); levels in the cerebrospinal fluid (CSF) are about the same as those in the serum. Infected tissue tends to retain the drug longer. The drug readily penetrates host cells and is effective against bacilli growing intracellularly. *Isoniazid* undergoes N-acetylation and hydrolysis, resulting in inactive products. Acetylation is genetically regulated; the fast acetylator trait is autosomally dominant. A bimodal distribution of fast and slow acetylators exists (Figure 33.3). Chronic liver disease will decrease metabolism, and doses must be reduced. Excretion is through glomerular filtration, predominantly as metabolites. Slow acetylators excrete more of the parent compound. Severely depressed renal function results in accumulation of the drug, primarily in slow acetylators. The drug is also excreted into the saliva, sputum, and milk.

5. **Adverse effects:** The incidence of adverse effects is fairly low. Except for hypersensitivity, they are related to the dosage and duration of administration.

a. **Peripheral neuritis:** Peripheral neuritis (manifest as paresthesia) is the most common adverse effect, which appears to be due to a relative pyridoxine deficiency. This has been attributed to a competition of *isoniazid* with pyridoxal phosphate for the enzyme apotryptophanase. Most of the toxic reactions are corrected by pyridoxine (vitamin B_6) supplementation. [Note: *Isoniazid* can achieve levels in breast milk that are high enough to cause a pyridoxine deficiency in the infant unless the mother is supplemented with the vitamin.]

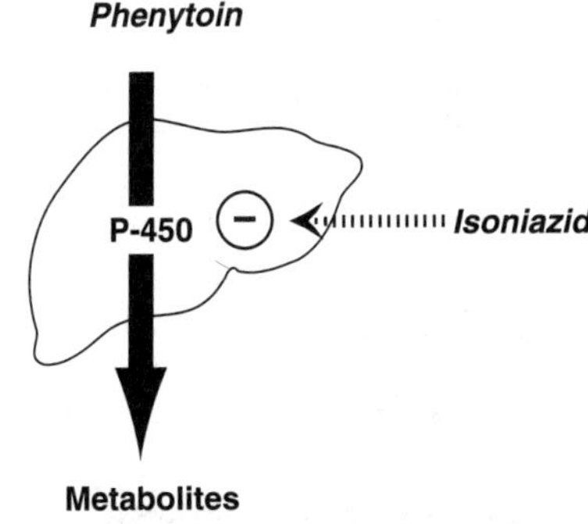

Figure 33.4
Isoniazid potentiates adverse effects of *phenytoin*.

b. **Hepatitis and Idiosyncratic hepatotoxicity:** Potentially fatal hepatitis is the most severe side effect associated with *isoniazid*. It has been suggested that it is caused by a toxic metabolite of monoacetylhydrazine formed during the metabolism of *isoniazid*. Its incidence increases among patients with increasing age, among patients who also take *rifampin*, or among those who imbibe alcohol daily.

c. **Drug interactions:** *Isoniazid* can potentiate the adverse effects of *phenytoin* (for example, nystagmus, ataxia, see p. 146) because the *isoniazid* inhibits metabolism of *phenytoin* (Figure 33.4). Slow acetylators are particularly at risk .

d. **Other adverse effects:** Mental abnormalities, convulsions in patients prone to seizures, and optic neuritis have been observed. Hypersensitivity reactions include rashes and fever.

C. Rifampin

Rifampin [RIF am pin], derived from the soil mold Streptomyces, has a broader antimicrobial activity than *isoniazid* and has found application in the treatment of other bacterial infections. Because resistant strains rapidly emerge during therapy, it is never given as a single agent in the treatment of active tuberculosis.

1. **Mechanism of action:** *Rifampin* blocks transcription by interacting with the β-subunit of bacterial DNA-dependent RNA polymerase[1], thus inhibiting RNA synthesis by suppressing the initiation step. The drug is specific for prokaryotes.

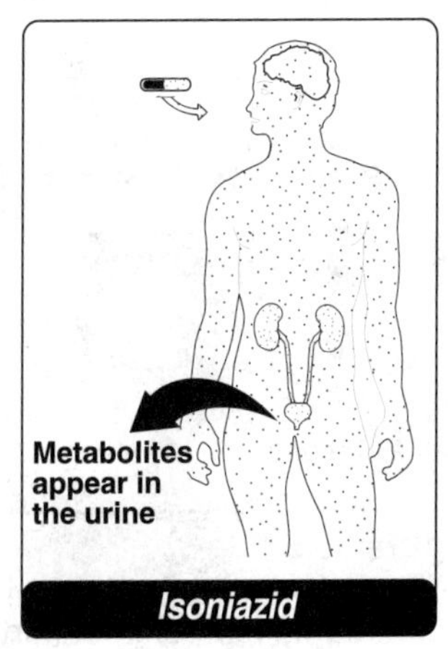

2. **Antimicrobial spectrum:** *Rifampin* is bactericidal for both intracellular and extracellular mycobacteria, including M. tuberculosis, atypical mycobacteria, and Mycobacterium leprae. It is effective against many gram (+) and gram (-) organisms and is frequently used prophylactically for household members exposed to meningitis caused by meningococci or Haemophilus influenzae. *Rifampin* is the most active antileprosy drug at present, but to delay emergence of resistant strains it is usually given in combination with other drugs. *Rifabutin*, an analog of *rifampin*, has some activity against Mycobacterium avium intracellulare complex, but is less active against tuberculosis.

[1]See p. 336 for Infolink references to other books in this series.

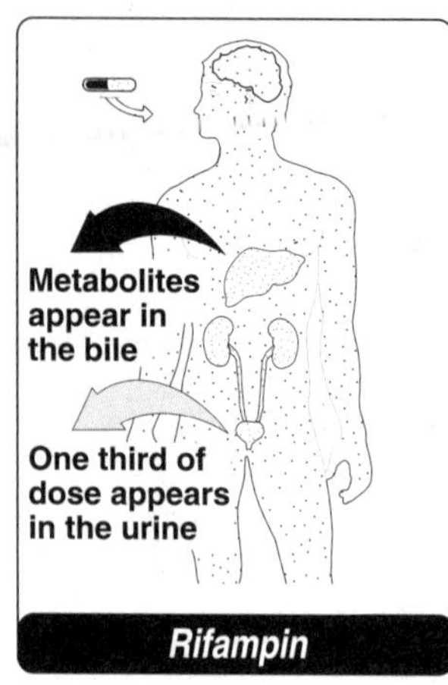

3. **Resistance:** Resistance may be caused by a change in the affinity of the DNA-dependent RNA polymerase for the drug, or by decreased permeability.

4. **Pharmacokinetics:** Absorption is adequate after oral administration. Distribution of *rifampin* occurs to all body fluids and organs. Adequate levels are attained in the CSF even in the absence of inflammation. The drug is taken up by the liver and undergoes enterohepatic cycling. *Rifampin* itself can induce the hepatic mixed function oxidases (see p. 14), leading to a shortened half-life. Elimination is via the bile into the feces and the urine as metabolites and parent drug. Urine and feces as well as other secretions have an orange-red color; patients should be forewarned. [Note: Tears may permantly stain contact lenses orange-red.]

5. **Adverse effects:** Adverse effects are a minor problem with *rifampin*. but can include nausea and vomiting, rash, and fever. The drug should be used judiciously in patients with hepatic failure because of the jaundice that occurs in patients with chronic liver disease, alcoholics, or in the elderly.

6. **Drug interactions:** Because *rifampin* can induce the cytochrome P-450 enzymes (see p. 14), it can decrease the half-lives of other drugs that are coadministered and metabolized by this system (Figure 33.5) This may lead to higher dosage requirements for these agents.

C. Pyrazinamide

Pyrazinamide [peer a ZIN a mide] is a synthetic orally effective bactericidal anti-tubercular agent used along with *isoniazid* and *rifampin*. It is bactericidal to actively dividing organisms. *Pyrazinamide* must be enzymatically hydrolyzed to pyrazinoic acid which is the active form of the drug. Some resistant strains lack the pyrazinamidase. However, the mechanism of its action is unknown. It is active against tubercle bacilli in the acid environment of lysosomes as well as in macrophages. *Pyrazinamide* distributes throughout the body penetrating the CSF; it also undergoes extensive metabolism. About 1-5% of patients taking *isoniazid*, *rifampin*, and *pyrazinamide* may experience liver dysfunction. Urate retention can also occur and may precipitate a gouty attack (Figure 33.6).

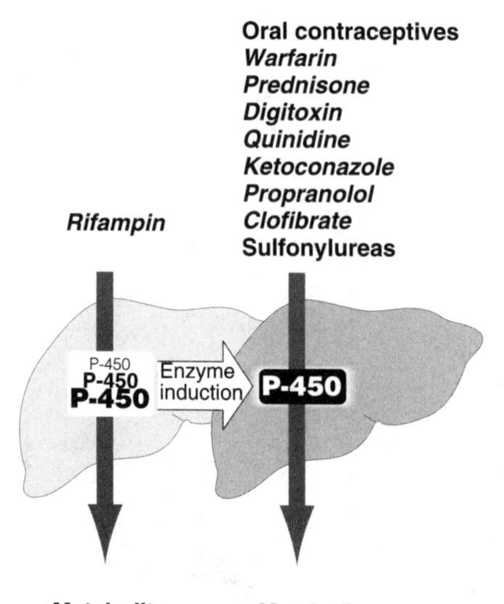

Figure 33.5
Rifampin induces P-450, which can decrease half-life of coadministered drugs that are metabolized by this system.

D. Ethambutol

Ethambutol [e THAM byoo tole] is bacteriostatic and specific for most strains of M. tuberculosis and M. kansasii. Resistance is not a serious problem if the drug is employed with other antituberculous agents. *Ethambutol* can be used in combination with *pyrazinamide*, *isoniazid*, and *rifampin* to treat tuberculosis. Absorbed on oral administration, *ethambutol* is well distributed throughout the body. Penetration into the central nervous system (CNS) is therapeutically adequate in tuberculous meningitis. Both parent drug and metabolites are excreted by glomerular filtration and tubular secretion. The most important adverse effect is optic neuritis, which results in diminished visual acuity and loss of ability to discriminate between red and green. Visual acuity should be periodically examined. Discontinuation of the drug results in reversal of the toxic symptoms. In addition, urate excretion is decreased by the drug, thus gout may be exacerbated (Figure 33.6).

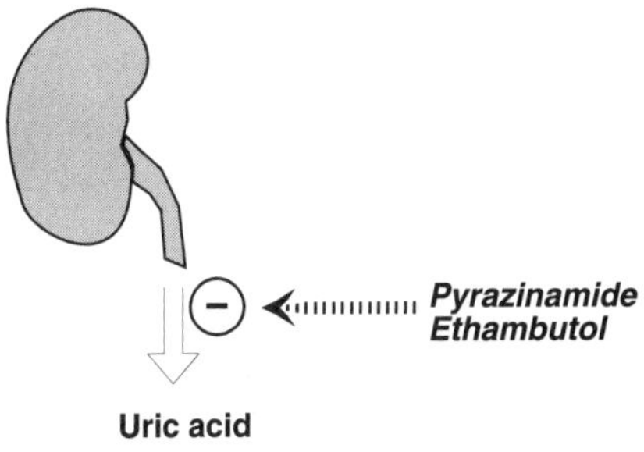

Pyrazinamide
Ethambutol
Uric acid

Figure 33.6
Pyrazinamide and *ethambutol* may cause urate retention and gouty attacks.

E. Alternate second-line drugs

A number of drugs—*aminosalicylic acid* [a mee noe sal i SIL ik], *ethionamide* [e thye on AM ide], *cycloserine* [sye kloe SER een]—are considered second-line drugs because they are no more effective than the first-line agents and their toxicities are often more serious. *Streptomycin*, the first antibiotic effective in the treatment of tuberculosis, has been discussed wth the aminoglycosides (see p. 314). Its action is directed against extracellular organisms.

1. **Aminosalicylic acid:** Because it is poorly tolerated, *aminosalicylic acid* [a mee noe sal i SIL ik] is infrequently used today. It is a bacteriostatic agent that acts as a competitive inhibitor for p-aminobenzoic acid (PABA) in folate biosynthesis[2].

2. **Ethionamide:** This structural analog of *isoniazid* is believed not to act by the same mechanism. It is effective after oral administration, and is widely distributed throughout the body, including the CSF. Metabolism is extensive. *Ethionamide* [e thye on AM ide] can inhibit acetylation of *isoniazid* (Figure 33.7). The urine is the main route of excretion. Adverse effects that limit its use include gastric irritation, hepatotoxicity, peripheral neuropathies, and optic neuritis.

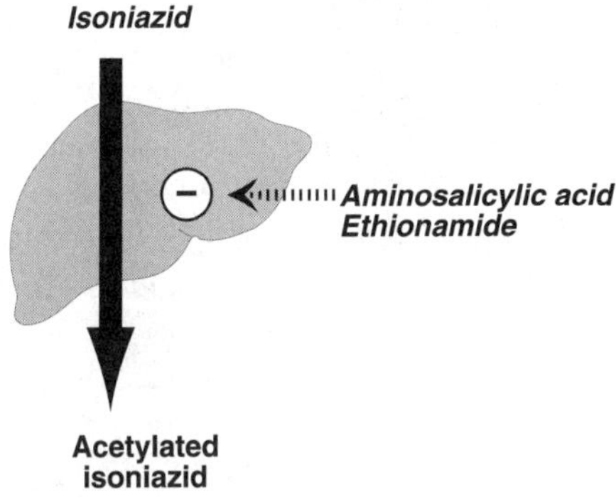

Figure 33.7
Aminosalicylic acid and *ethionamide* can inhibit the acetylation of *isoniazid.*

3. **Cycloserine:** This orally effective tuberculostatic agent appears to antagonize the steps in bacterial cell wall synthesis involving D-alanine. It distributes well throughout body fluids, including the CSF. *Cycloserine* [sye kloe SER een] is metabolized, and both parent and metabolite are excreted in urine. Accumulation occurs with renal insufficiency. Adverse effects involve CNS disturbances; epileptic seizure activity may be exacerbated. Peripheral neuropathies are also a problem.

III. CHEMOTHERAPY OF LEPROSY

Leprosy (Hansen's disease) is caused by M. leprae. Bacilli from skin lesions or nasal discharges of infected patients enter susceptible individuals via the skin or respiratory tract. The World Health Organization recommends the triple drug regimen, *dapsone*, *clofazimine*, and *rifampin* (see p. 333) for 6 to 24 months.

A. Dapsone

Dapsone [DAP sone] is structurally related to the sulfonamides. It is bacteriostatic for M. leprae, but resistant strains are encountered. *Dapsone* is also employed in the treatment of Pneumocystis pneumonia in human immunodeficiency virus (HIV) patients. It acts as a

[2]See p. 336 for Infolink references to other books in this series.

PABA antagonist to inhibit folate biosynthesis. The drug is well absorbed from the gastrointestinal tract and is distributed throughout the body. The parent drug enters the enterohepatic circulation and undergoes heptic acetylation. Both parent drug and metabolites are eliminated through the urine. Adverse reactions include hemolysis, especially in patients with glucose-6-phosphate dehydrogenase deficiency[3], methemoglobinemia, peripheral neuropathy, and the possibility of developing erythema nodosum leprosum. [Note: The latter is treated with corticosteroids (see p. 272) or *thalidomide.*]

B. Clofazimine

Clofazimine [kloe FA zi meen] is a phenazine dye that binds to DNA and inhibits template function. Its redox properties may lead to the generation of cytotoxic oxygen radicals that are also toxic to the bacteria. *Clofazimine* is bactericidal to M. leprae and has some activity against M. avium intracellulare complex. On oral absorption, it accumulates in tissues, allowing for intermittent therapy, but it does not enter the CNS. Patients may develop a red-brown discoloration of the skin. Eosinophilic enteritis has been reported as an untoward effect. The drug also has some anti-inflammatory activity, thus erythema nodosum leprosum does not develop.

Study Questions

Choose the ONE best answer.

33.1 All of the following statements about rifampin are correct EXCEPT:

A. It is frequently used prophylactically for household members exposed to meningitis caused by meningococci or Haemophilus influenzae.
B. It colors body secretions orange-red.
C. It disrupts bacterial lipid metabolism as its major mechanism of action.
D. Although rare, it can cause serious hepatotoxicity.
E. When used alone, there is a high risk of the emergence of resistant strains of mycobacteria.

Correct choice = C. Rifampin interacts with the β-subunit of bacterial DNA-dependent RNA polymerase and thereby inhibits RNA synthesis. Because of the rapid emergence of resistant strains, rifampin is never given as a single agent.

33.2 All of the following statements about isoniazid are correct EXCEPT:

A. It produces age-dependent hepatotoxicity.
B. It readily penetrates into infected cells.
C. It inhibits mycolic acid synthesis in susceptible mycobacteria.
D. It may induce the symptoms of cyanocobalamin (vitamin B_{12}) deficiency.
E. It potentiates the adverse effects of phenytoin when the patient receives both medications concurrently.

Correct choice = D. Isoniazid reacts with pyridoxine (vitamin B_6), which can cause a deficiency of this vitamin. Isoniazid readily penetrates into infected cells and therefore is effective against bacilli growing intracellularly. Isoniazid inhibits the metabolism of phenytoin.

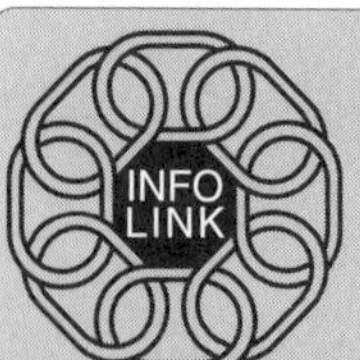

[1]See p. 379 in **Biochemistry** (2nd ed.) for a discussion of DNA-dependent RNA polymerase.

[3]See p. 115 in **Biochemistry** (2nd ed.) for a discussion of glucose-6-P dehydrogenase deficiency.

[2]See p. 325 in **Biochemistry** (2nd ed.) for a discussion of the role of p-aminobenzoic acid in folate biosynthesis.

Antifungal Drugs

34

I. OVERVIEW

Infectious diseases caused by fungi are called mycoses and are often chronic in nature. Many common mycotic infections are superficial and only involve the skin, but fungi may also penetrate the skin, causing subcutaneous infections. The fungal infections that are most difficult to treat are the systemic mycoses, which are often life-threatening. Unlike bacteria, fungi are eukaryotic. They have rigid cell walls containing chitin as well as polysaccharides, and a cell membrane composed of ergosterol. Thus, fungal infections are generally resistant to antibiotics used in the treatment of bacterial infections. Conversely, bacteria are resistant to the antifungal agents. The incidence of fungal infections has escalated as the number of immunosuppressed individuals (e.g. cancer, transplant patients) as well as those debilitated by AIDS, has risen. These patients often suffer from so-called opportunistic fungal infections such as cryptococcal meningitis or aspergillosis. Endemic mycoses, such as blastomycosis, coccidioidomycosis and histoplasmosis, have always been a problem in some geographic locations. The availability of the azole antifungal drugs has been a major advance in the treatment of systemic infections since they are less toxic than *amphotericin B*. Figure 34.1 shows the clinically useful antifungal agents.

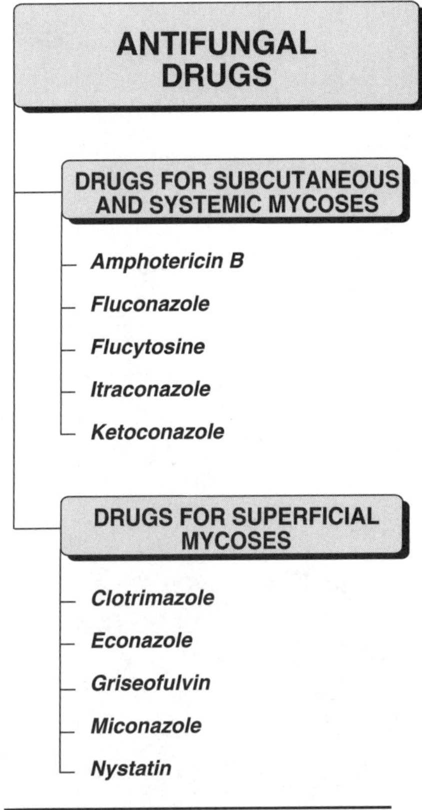

ANTIFUNGAL DRUGS
DRUGS FOR SUBCUTANEOUS AND SYSTEMIC MYCOSES
Amphotericin B
Fluconazole
Flucytosine
Itraconazole
Ketoconazole
DRUGS FOR SUPERFICIAL MYCOSES
Clotrimazole
Econazole
Griseofulvin
Miconazole
Nystatin

Figure 34.1
Summary of antifungal drugs.

II. DRUGS FOR SUBCUTANEOUS AND SYSTEMIC MYCOTIC INFECTIONS

The drugs used in the treatment of subcutaneous and systemic mycoses are *amphotericin B*, *flucytosine*, and the new group of azoles, *ketoconazole*, *fluconazole* and *itraconazole*.

A. Amphotericin B

Amphotericin B [am foe TER i sin] is a naturally occurring polyene macrolide antibiotic, produced by Streptomyces nodosus. In spite of its toxic potential, *amphotericin B* is the drug of choice used in the treatment of the systemic mycoses. It is sometimes used in combination with *flucytosine* so that lower (less toxic) levels of *amphotericin* are possible.

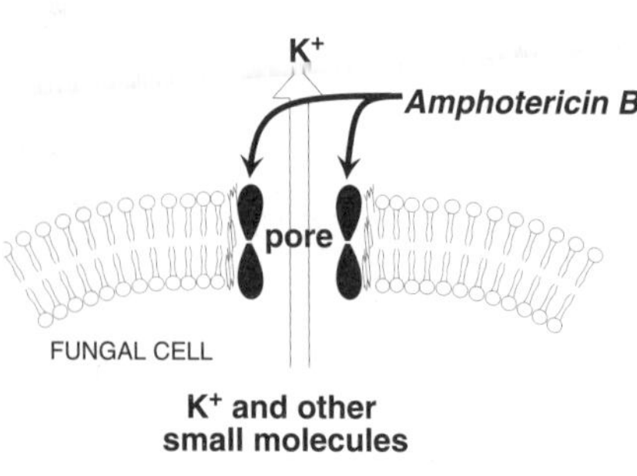

Figure 34.2
Model of pore formed by *amphotericin* in lipid bilayer membrane.

1. **Mode of action:** Several polyene molecules bind to ergosterol present in cell membranes of sensitive fungal cells to form pores or channels that involve hydrophobic bonds between the lipophilic segment of the polyene antibiotic and the sterol (Figure 34.2). This disrupts membrane function, allowing electrolytes (particularly potassium) and small molecules to leak from the cell, resulting in cell death. Since the polyene antibiotics bind preferentially to ergosterol rather than cholesterol, the sterol found in mammalian membranes, a relative (but not absolute) specificity is conferred.

2. **Antifungal spectrum:** *Amphotericin B* is either fungicidal or fungistatic, depending on the organism and the concentration of the drug. It is effective against a wide range of fungi, such as Candida albicans, Histoplasma capsulatum, Cryptococcus neoformans, Coccidioides immitis, many strains of aspergillus, and Blastomyces dermatitidis.

3. **Resistance:** Fungal resistance, though infrequent, is associated with decreased ergosterol content of the fungal membrane.

4. **Pharmacokinetics:** *Amphotericin B* is administered by intravenous infusion. The intrathecal route is sometimes chosen for the treatment of meningitis caused by fungi that are sensitive to *amphotericin B*. *Amphotericin B* is extensively bound to plasma proteins, and is distributed throughout the body becoming highly tissue-bound. Inflammation favors penetration into various body fluids, but little is found in the cerebrospinal fluid, vitreous humor, or amniotic fluid. However, *amphotericin B* does cross the placenta. Low levels of the drug, mostly metabolites, appear in the urine over a long period of time; some is also eliminated via the bile. Adjustment of dose is not required in patients with compromised renal or hepatic function. Liposomal preparations of *amphotericin B* are available and have shown therapeutic efficacy.

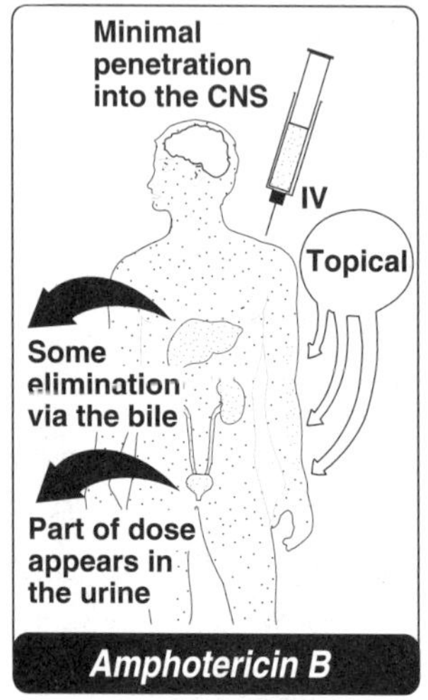

5. **Adverse effects:** *Amphotericin B* has a low therapeutic index. A total daily dose should not exceed 1.5 mg/kg. Small test doses are usually administered to assess the degree of a patient's negative response, for example, anaphylaxis or convulsions. Other toxic manifestations include the following:

   a. **Fever and chills:** These appear with intravenous administration but usually subside with repeated administration of the drug. Premedication with a steroid or an anitpyretic helps prevent this problem. *Meperidine* (see p. 138) can abort fever and chills that have already started.

   b. **Renal impairment:** Despite the low levels of the drug excreted in the urine, patients may exhibit impaired renal function (decrease in glomerular filtration rate and tubular function). Creatinine clearance drops and potassium is lost. The nephrotoxicity may be potentiated by sodium depletion. Normal renal function usually returns on suspension of the drug, but residual damage is likely at high doses. Azotemia is exacerbated by other nephrotoxic drugs such as *aminoglycosides* (see 314), *cyclosporine*, or *pentamidine* (see p. 353), although adequate hydration can decrease its severity.

c. **Hypotension:** A shock-like fall in blood pressure accompanied by hypokalemia may occur, requiring potassium supplementation. Care must be exercised in patients taking *digitalis*.

d. **Anemia:** Normochromic, normocytic anemia caused by a reversible suppression of erythrocyte production may occur. This may be exacerbated in patients with human immunodeficiency virus (HIV) who are taking *zidovudine*.

e. **Neurological effects:** Intrathecal administration can cause a variety of neurologic problems.

f. **Thrombophlebitis:** Adding *heparin* to the infusion can alleviate this problem.

B. Flucytosine

Flucytosine [floo SYE toe seen] (*5-FC*) is a synthetic pyrimidine antimetabolite used only in combination with *amphotericin* for the treatment of systemic mycoses and meningitis caused by Cryptococcus neoformans and Candida.

1. **Mode of action:** The drug enters fungal cells via a cytosine-specific permease, an enzyme not found in mammalian cells. *5-FC* is then converted by a series of steps to 5-fluorodeoxyuridylic acid (5-FdUMP); this false nucleotide inhibits thymidylate synthetase, thus depriving the organism of thymidylic acid, an essential DNA component (Figure 34.3). The unnatural pyrimidine is also metabolized to the nucleotide (5-FUTP) and incorporated into fungal RNA, to disrupt nucleic acid and protein synthesis. The combination of *flucytosine* and *amphotericin B* is synergistic. [Note: The *amphotericin B* affects cell permeability, allowing more of the *flucytosine* to penetrate the cell.]

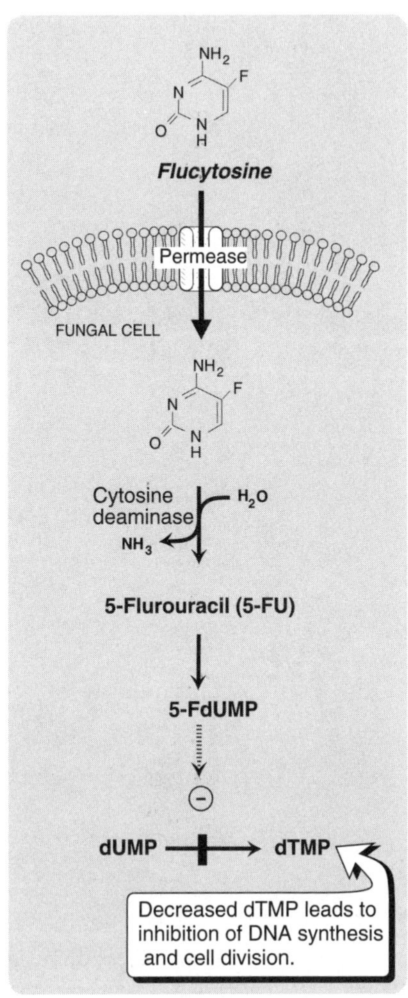

Figure 34.3
Mode of action of *flucytosine*.

2. **Antifungal spectrum:** *Flucytosine* is fungistatic and effective in treating chromoblastomycosis and in combination for candidiasis, and cryptococcosis.

3. **Resistance:** Resistance can develop during therapy and is the reason that *flucytosine* is not used as a single antimycotic drug except for chromoblastomycosis. The rate of emergence of resistant fungal cells is lower with the combination of *amphotericin B* and *flucytosine* than it is with *flucytosine* alone. Decreased levels of any of the enzymes in the conversion of *5-FC* to 5-FU and beyond, or increased synthesis of cytosine, can confer resistance.

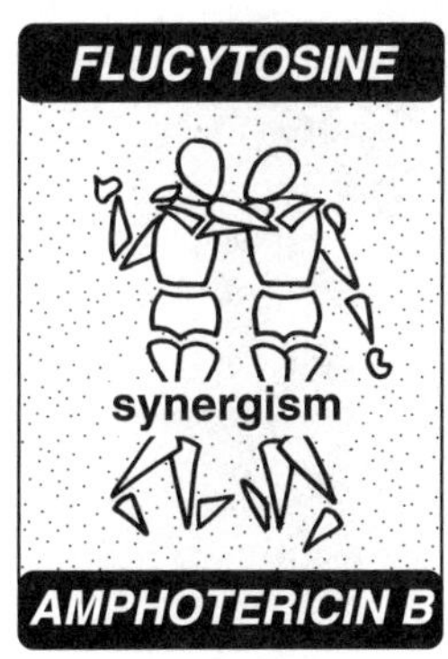

4. **Pharmacokinetics:** *Flucytosine* is well absorbed by the oral route, distributes throughout the body water, and penetrates well into cerebrospinal fluid (CSF). 5-Fluorouracil is detectable in patients and probably is due to metabolism of *5-FC* by intestinal bacteria. Excretion of both the parent drug and its metabolites is by glomerular filtration, and the dose must be adjusted in patients with compromised renal function.

5. **Adverse effects:** Some of these adverse effects may be related to 5-FU formed by intestinal organisms from *5-FC.*

a. **Hematologic toxicity:** *Flucytosine* causes reversible neutropenia, thrombocytopenia, and occasional bone marrow depression. Caution must be exercised in patients undergoing radiation or chemotherapy with drugs that depress bone marrow.

b. **Hepatic dysfunction:** Reversible hepatic dysfunction with elevation of serum transaminases and alkaline phosphatase may occur.

c. **Gastrointestinal disturbances:** Nausea, vomiting, and diarrhea are common, and severe enterocolitis may occur.

C. Ketoconazole

Ketoconazole [kee toe KON a zole], a substituted imidazole, is one of a family of azoles useful in treating systemic mycoses. In addition to its antifungal activity, *ketoconazole* also inhibits gonadal and adrenal steroid synthesis in humans by blocking C17-20 lyase, 11β-hydroxylase, and cholesterol side-chain cleavage; thus, it suppresses *testosterone* and *cortisol* synthesis.

1. **Mode of action:** *Ketoconazole* interacts with C-14 α-demethylase (a cytochrome P-450 enzyme) to block demethylation of lanosterol to ergosterol, the principal sterol of fungal membranes Figure 34.4). This inhibition disrupts membrane function and increases permeability. *Ketoconazole* acts in an additive manner with *flucytosine* against Candida, but antagonizes *amphotericin B*'s antifungal activity.

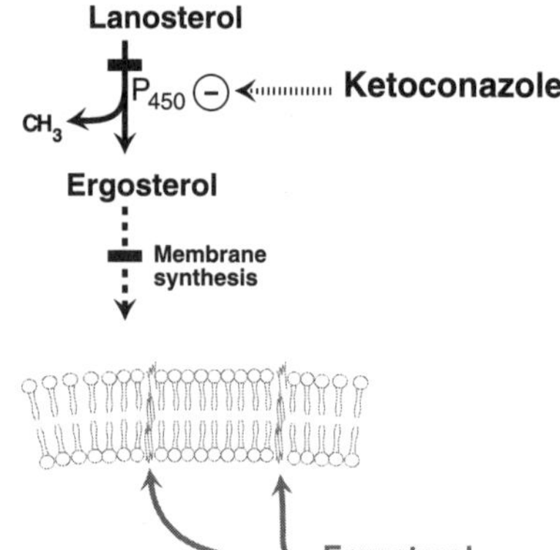

Figure 34.4
Mode of action of *ketoconazole.*

2. **Antifungal spectrum:** *Ketoconazole* is either fungistatic or fungicidal, depending on the dose. Although active against the same fungi as *amphotericin B*, it is most useful in the treatment of histoplasmosis. *Ketoconazole* is also effective against nonmeningeal coccidiomycosis and blastomycosis. Candida, and various dermatophytic infections, including those resistant to *griseofulvin* are also susceptible.

3. **Resistance:** No resistance has been observed.

4. **Pharmacokinetics:** *Ketoconazole* is only administered orally. It dissolves in the acidic gastric contents and is absorbed through the gastric mucosa. Food, antacids, *cimetidine*, and *rifampin* impair absorption. Coca-Cola being acidic has been shown to improve absorption of *ketoconazole*. The drug is highly bound to plasma proteins. Although penetration into tissues is limited, it is effective in the treatment of histoplasmosis in lung, bone, skin, and soft tissues. It does not enter the CSF. Extensive metabolism occurs in the liver. Induction of the cytochrome P-450 system enzymes (see p. 14) in the liver shortens the half-life of *ketoconazole,* but the drug can also inhibit certain cytochromes P-450 to potentiate the effects of some drugs (see p. 341). Excretion is primarily through the bile. Levels of parent drug in the urine are too low to be effective against urinary tract mycotic infections.

5. **Adverse effects:** These effects are primarily gastrointestinal. In addition to allergies, other toxicities include the following effects:

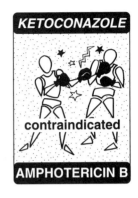

a. **Gastrointestinal distress** is a common side effect.

b. **Endocrine effects:** These result from the blocking of androgen and adrenal steroid synthesis by *ketoconazole*. Among the effects are gynecomastia, decreased libido, impotence, and menstrual irregularities.

c. **Hepatic dysfunction:** Although the incidence is low, hepatic dysfunction, with elevation of serum transaminase levels, is a serious toxic manifestation. *Ketoconazole* may accumulate in patients with hepatic dysfunction. Plasma concentrations of the drug should be monitored in these individuals.

d. **Contraindications:** *Ketoconazole* and *amphotericin B* should not be used together.

e. **Drug interactions:** By inhibiting cytochrome P-450, *ketoconazole* can potentiate the toxicities of *cyclosporine*, *phenytoin*, and the H_1-histamine antagonists, *terfenadine* and *astemizole*. It can also increase the levels of *sucralfate, tolbutamide* and *warfarin*. *Rifampin*, an inducer of the cytochrome P-450 system, can shorten the duration of *ketoconazole* and the other azoles (see Figure 33.5, p. 334). Drugs that decrease gastric acidity such as H_2-receptor blockers and antacids also can decrease absorption of *ketoconazole*.

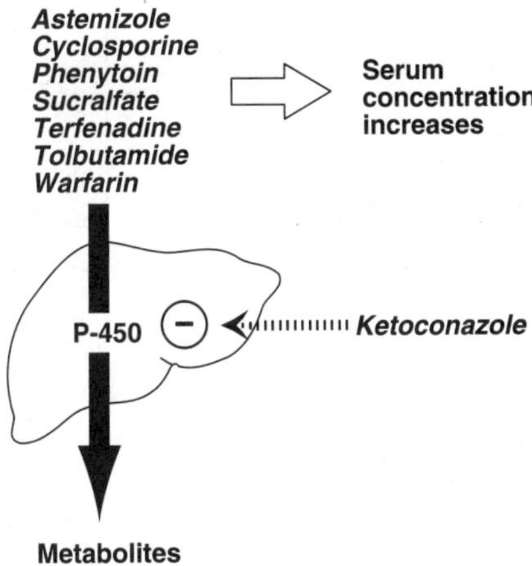

D. Fluconazole

Fluconazole [floo KON a zole] is clinically important because of its lack of the endocrine side effects of *ketoconazole,* and its excellent penetrability into the CSF. *Fluconazole* is employed prophylactically, with some success, for reducing fungal infections in recipients of bone marrow transplants.

1. **Mode of action:** It inhibits the synthesis of fungal membrane ergosterol in the same manner as *ketoconazole.*

2. **Antifungal spectrum:** It is the drug of choice for Cryptococcus neoformans, for candidemia, and for coccidioidomycosis. *Fluconazole* has also been shown to be useful in the treatment of blastomycosis, candidiasis, and histoplasmosis. These infections are characterized by a high rate of relapse, and *fluconazole* has proved effective in chronic ambulatory treatment.

3. **Resistance:** Treatment failures have been reported in some HIV-infected patients.

4. **Pharmacokinetics:** *Fluconazole* is administered orally or intravenously. Its absorption is excellent and, unlike *ketoconazole*, is not dependent on gastric acidity. Binding to plasma proteins is minimal. Its importance lies in its ability to penetrate the CSF of

normal and inflamed meninges. Unlike *ketoconazole*, *fluconazole* is poorly metabolized. The drug is excreted via the kidney, and doses must be reduced in patients with compromised renal function.

5. **Adverse effects:** Its adverse effects are less of a problem than with *ketoconazole*. *Fluconazole* has no endocrinologic effects because it does not inhibit the cytochrome P-450 responsible for the synthesis of androgens. However, it can inhibit the cytochromes P-450 that metabolize the other drugs listed on p. 341 under *ketoconazole*. Besides nausea and vomiting, rashes are a problem. Hepatitis is rare. Recent reports indicate that *fluconazole* is a potent teratogen and suggest that other of the azoles may also be teratogenic.

E. Itraconazole

Itraconazole [it ra KON a zole] is a recent addition to the azole family of antifungal agents. Like fluconazole it is a synthetic triazole, and it also lacks the endocrinologic side effects of *ketoconazole*. Its mode of action is the same as that of the other azoles. *Itraconazole* is now the drug of choice for the treatment of blastomycosis. Unlike *ketoconazole*, it is effective in AIDS-associated histoplasmosis. However, current studies show that it may also be effective in the treatment of aspergillosis, candidemia, coccidioidomycosis, and cryptococcosis. Thus it has a broad antifungal spectrum.

1. **Pharmacokinetics:** *Itraconazole* is well-absorbed orally and food increases its bioavailability. It is extensively bound to plasma proteins and distributes well throughout most tissues, including bone, sputum and adipose tissues. However, therapeutic concentrations are not attained in the CSF. Like *ketoconazole* it is extensively metabolized in the liver but does not inhibit androgen synthesis. Little of the parent drug appears in the urine and thus doses do not have to be reduced in renal failure.

2. **Adverse effects**: Adverse effects include nausea and vomiting, rash (especially in immunocompromised patients), hypokalemia, hypertension, edema, and headache. Drug interactions listed above are also possible with *itraconazole*. Figure 34.5 summarizes the azole antifungal agents.

	Ketoconazole	*Fluconazole*	*Itraconazole*
Spectrum	Narrow	Expanded	Expanded
Route(s) of administration	Oral	Oral, IV	Oral
$t_{1/2}$ (hours)	6-9	30	30-40
CSF penetration	No	Yes	No
Renal excretion	No	Yes	No
Interaction with other drugs	Frequent	Occasional	Occasional
Inhibition of mammalian sterol synthesis	Dose-dependent inhibitory effect	No inhibition	No inhibition

Figure 34.5
Summary of azole fungistatic drugs.

III. DRUGS FOR SUPERFICIAL MYCOTIC INFECTIONS

Fungi that cause superficial skin infections are called dermatophytes. Common dermatomycoses, such as tinea infections, are often referred to as ringworm, which is a misnomer, since fungi rather than worms cause the disease.

A. Griseofulvin

1. **Mode of action:** *Griseofulvin* [gri see oh FUL vin] enters susceptible fungal cells by an energy-dependent process. It is believed to

interact with the microtubules within the fungus to disrupt the mitotic spindle and inhibit mitosis (Figure 34.6). It accumulates in the infected, newly synthesized, keratin-containing tissues, making them unsuitable for the growth of the fungi. Therapy must be continued until normal tissue replaces infected tissue. This usually requires weeks to months of therapy.

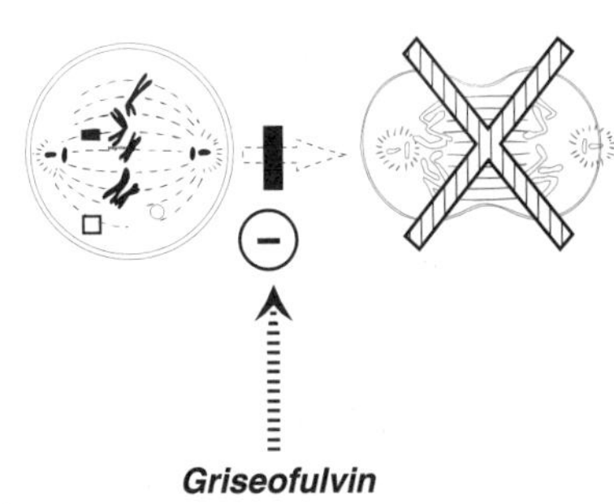

Figure 34.6
Inhibition of mitosis by *griseofulvin.*

2. **Antifungal spectrum:** The drug is principally fungistatic. It is effective only against the dermatophytes—Trichophyton, Microsporum, and Epidermophyton. It is used in the treatment of severe tinea infections that do not respond to other antifungal agents.

3. **Resistance:** Resistance is due to the lack of the energy-dependent uptake system.

4. **Pharmacokinetics:** Ultra-fine crystalline preparations are absorbed adequately from the gastrointestinal tract. Absorption is promoted if ingested with a high fat diet. *Phenobarbital* can interfere with the absorption of *griseofulvin.* The drug is ineffective topically. *Griseofulvin* distributes chiefly to infected keratinized tissue where it becomes bound; therefore, it is uniquely suited for the treatment of dermatophytic infections. Concentrations in other tissues and body fluids are much lower. *Griseofulvin* is extensively metabolized to the demethylated and glucuronidated forms. *Griseofulvin* induces hepatic cytochrome P-450 activity, and can increase the rate of metabolism of a number of drugs including oral anticoagulants (see p. 199). Excretion of the drug occurs via the kidney, primarily as metabolites.

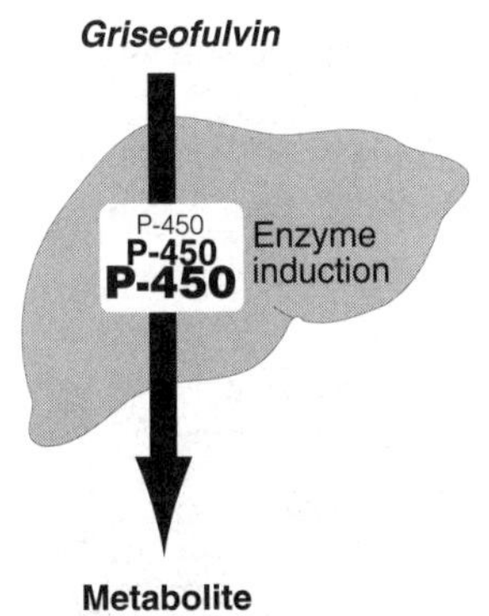

Figure 34.7
Induction of hepatic cytochrome P-450 activity by *griseofluvin.*

5. **Adverse effects:** Toxicity is not generally a clinical problem although allergic reactions and a number of adverse effects (e.g., headache, nausea) have been reported. *Griseofulvin* may cause hepatotoxicity and is contraindicated in patients with acute intermittent porphyria. The drug potentiates the intoxicating effects of alcohol. *Griseofulvin* is teratogenic in laboratory animals.

B. Nystatin

Nystatin [nye STAT in] is a polyene antibiotic; its structure, chemistry, mode of action, and resistance resemble those of *amphotericin B.* Its use is restricted to topical treatment of Candida infections because of its systemic toxicity. The drug is negligibly absorbed from the gastrointestinal tract, and it is never used parenterally. It is administered as an oral agent ("swish and swallow") for the treatment of oral candidiasis. Excretion in the feces is nearly quantitative. Adverse effects are rare because of its lack of absorption, but occasionally nausea and vomiting occur.

C. Miconazole and other topical agents

Miconazole [my KON a zole], *clotrimazole* [kloe TRIM a zole], and *econazole* [e KON a zole] are topically active drugs and are only rarely administered parenterally because of their severe toxicity. Their mechanism of action, antifungal spectrum, distribution, and type of metabolism are the same as *ketoconazole.*

Choose the ONE best answer.

Questions 34.1 - 34.3: For each numbered phrase, select the ONE drug (A-E) that is most closely associated with it. Each drug may be selected once, more than once, or not at all.

A. Flucytosine
B. Griseofulvin
C. Penicillin G
D. Amphotericin-B
E. Ketoconazole

34.1 Binds to ergosterol present in cell membranes of sensitive fungal cells, thereby disrupting membrane function.

The correct answer = D. (Amphotericin B).

34.2 Blocks lanosterol demethylation to ergosterol, thus disrupting fungal membrane integrity.

The correct answer = E. (Ketoconazole).

34.3 Is metabolized to a product that inhibits thymidylate synthetase and thus prevents fungal DNA synthesis.

The correct answer = A. (Flucytosine).

Choose the ONE best answer:

34.4 Which one of the following drugs is not used for the treatment of systemic fungal infections?

A. Amphotericin B.
B. Flucytosine.
C. Ketoconazole.
D. Griseofulvin.
E. Fluconazole.

Correct answer = D. Griseofulvin use is restricted to the treatment of superficial mycotic infections.

34.5 All of the following statements correctly describe ketoconazole EXCEPT:

A. It inhibits the conversion of lanosterol to ergosterol.
B. It may produce gastrointestinal upsets.
C. It can cause gynecomastia in males.
D. It penetrates into the cerebrospinal fluid.
E. It should not be combined with amphotericin B.

Correct answer = D. Ketoconazole does not enter the CSF.

34.6 All of the following statements concerning griseofulvin are correct EXCEPT:

A. It is only effective against dermatophytic infections.
B. It exacerbates acute intermittent porphyria.
C. It induces the hepatic cytochrome P-450 system.
D. It enhances CNS depressant effects of ethanol.
E. Its use in therapy for superficial mycotic infections is usually short term (several days).

Correct answer = E. Griseofulvin accumulates in the infected, newly synthesized keratin containing tissues making them unsuitable for the growth of the fungi. Therapy must be continued until normal tissue replaces infected tissue. This usually requires long-term therapy.

34.7 A 25-year-old male AIDS patient has a fever of 102°F and complains of severe headaches during the past week. Staining of his cerebrospinal fluid with India ink reveals Cryptococcus neoformans. The patient is admitted to the hospital and is treated with:

A. Intravenous amphotericin B plus flucytosine.
B. Oral ketoconazole.
C. Intrathecal amphotericin B.
D. Oral fluconazole.
E. Intravenous amphotericin B plus ketoconazole.

The correct answer = C. Intrathecal administration of amphotericin B is indicated as the most effective way to treat cryptococcal meningitis. Although intravenous amphotericin B may be useful, the addition of flucytosine with its potential for bone marrow toxicity would not be appropriate therapy. Oral ketoconazole is also wrong because of its inability to cross into the CSF. Although fluconazole is very effective against Cryptococcus neoformans and does enter the CSF, the oral route is only used for chronic suppressive therapy and not meningitis. The combination of amphotericin B and ketoconazole is a poor one since ketoconazole disrupts fungal membrane function and thus interferes with the action of amphotericin B.

34. 8 A 30-year-old male has had a heart transplant and is being maintained on the immunosuppressant, cyclosporine. He develops a Candida infection and is treated with ketoconazole. Why is this poor therapy?

A. Ketoconazole is not effective against Candida.
B. Ketoconazole reacts with cyclosporine to inactivate it.
C. Ketoconazole has a potential for cardiotoxicity.
D. Ketoconazole inhibits cytochrome P-450 enzymes that inactivate cyclosporine.
E. Ketoconazole causes gynecomastia and decreased libido in the male.

The correct answer = D. Ketoconazole is effective against Candida, but it does not react with cyclosporine nor is it cardiotoxic. Ketoconazole inhibits the hepatic cytochrome P-450 enzymes that inactivate cyclosporine. Thus in this instance the patient would be in danger of increased cyclosporine toxicity. Though ketoconazole does cause gynecomastia and decreased libido, this would not be of primary concern.

Antiprotozoal Drugs

35

I. OVERVIEW

Protozoal infections are common among people in underdeveloped tropical and subtropical countries where sanitary conditions, hygienic practices, and control of the vectors of transmission are inadequate. However, with increased world travel, protozoal diseases such as malaria, amebiasis, leishmaniasis, trypanosomiasis, trichomoniasis, and giardiasis are no longer confined to specific geographic locales. Because they are eukaryotes, the unicelluar protozoal cells have metabolic processes closer to those of the human host than to prokaryotic bacterial pathogens. Protozoal diseases are thus less easily treated than bacterial infections, and many of the antiprotozoal drugs cause serious toxic effects in the host, particularly on cells showing high metabolic activity—neuronal, renal tubular, intestinal and bone marrow stem cells. Most antiprotozoal agents have not proved safe for pregnant patients. Drugs used to treat protozoan infections are summarized in Figure 35.1.

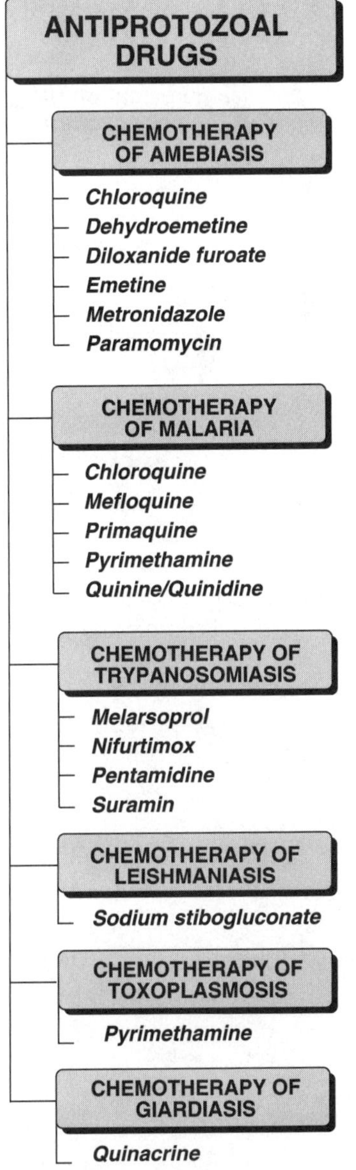

Figure 35.1
Summary of antiprotozoal agents

II. CHEMOTHERAPY OF AMEBIASIS

Amebiasis (also called amebic dysentery) is an infection of the intestinal tract caused by Entamoeba histolytica. The disease can be acute or chronic with patients showing varying degrees of illness, from no symptoms to mild diarrhea to fulminating dysentery. Diagnosis is made by isolating E. histolytica in fresh feces. Therapy is aimed not only at the acutely ill patient but also at those who are asymptomatic carriers since dormant E. histolytica may cause future infections in the carrier and may be a potential source of infection of others.

A. Life cycle of E. histolytica

E. histolytica exists in two forms: cysts that can survive outside the body, and labile but invasive trophozoites that do not persist outside the body. Cysts, ingested through feces-contaminated food or water, pass into the intestine where trophozoites are liberated. The trophozoites multiply, and either invade and ulcerate the mucosa of the large intestine, or simply feed on intestinal bacteria. [Note: One strategy for treating luminal amebiasis is to add antibiotics, such as *tetra-*

Lippincott's Illustrated Reviews: Pharmacology, Second Edition.
by Mary J. Mycek, Richard A. Harvey and Pamela C. Champe.
Lippincott Williams & Wilkins, Philadelphia, PA © 2000.

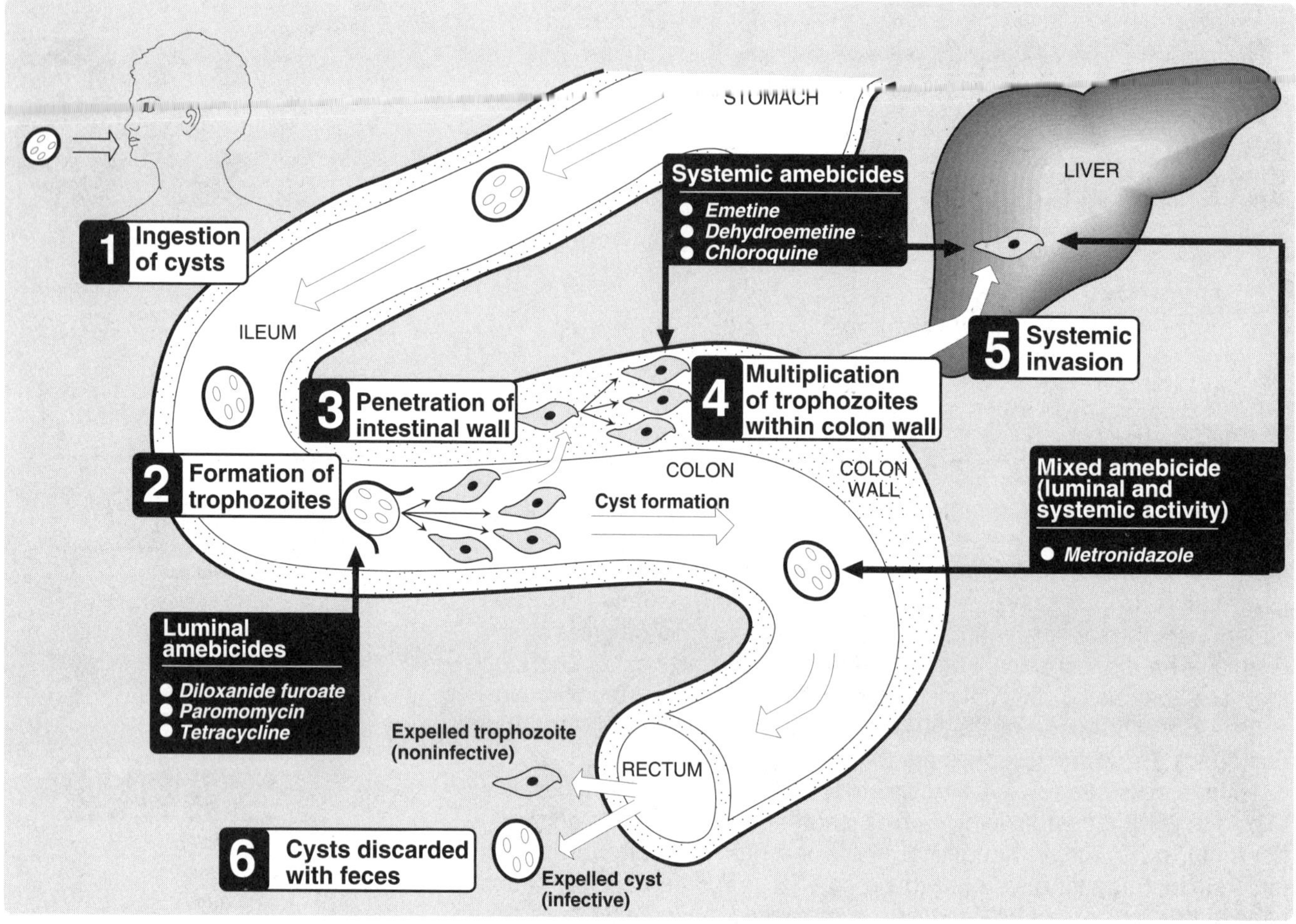

Figure 35.2
Life cycle of Entamoeba histolytica showing sites of action of amebicidic drugs.

cycline, to the treatment regimen resulting in a reduction in intestinal flora, the amebae's major food source.] Large numbers of trophozoites within the colon wall can lead to systemic invasion. The trophozoites within the intestine are slowly carried toward the rectum where they return to the cyst form and are excreted in feces. A summary of the life cycle of this organism is presented in Figure 35.2.

B. Classification of antiprotozal drugs

Therapeutic agents are classified as mixed, luminal, or systemic amebicides according to the site where the drug is effective (see Figure 35.2). For example, mixed amebicides are effective against both the luminal and systemic forms of the disease, though luminal concentrations are too low for single drug treatment. Luminal amebicides act on the parasite in the lumen of the bowel, whereas systemic agents are effective against amebae in the intestine wall and the liver.

C. Mixed amebicide: metronidazole

Amebiasis is generally treated with a combination of *metronidazole* [me troe NYE da zole] plus a luminal amebicidal drug, such as *diloxanide furoate*. This combination provides cure rates of greater than 90%. *Metronidazol* also has important antibacterial activity.

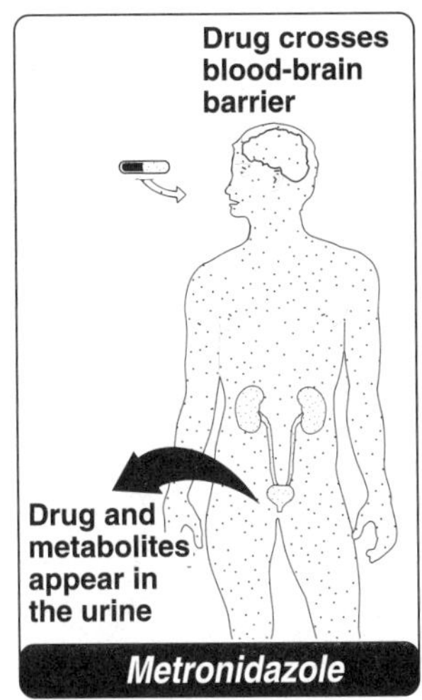
Drug crosses blood-brain barrier
Drug and metabolites appear in the urine
Metronidazole

1. **Mode of action:** *Metronidazole* is selectively toxic not only for amebae but also for anaerobic organisms (including bacteria), and for anoxic or hypoxic cells. Some anaerobic protozoan parasites (including amebae) possess ferrodoxin-like, low-redox potential, electron transport proteins that participate in metabolic electron removal reactions. The nitro group of *metronidazole* is able to serve as an electron acceptor, forming reduced cytotoxic compounds that bind to proteins and DNA to result in cell death.

2. **Antimicrobial spectrum:** *Metronidazole* is the agent of choice for treating infections caused by E. histolytica in which it kills the E. histolytica trophozoites, Giardia lamblia, and Trichomonas vaginalis in both males and females. *Metronidazole* also finds extensive use in the treatment of infections caused by anaerobic cocci and anaerobic gram-negative bacilli (for example, bacteroides species). Anaerobic gram-positive bacilli, such as Clostridia, which cause pseudomembranous colitis, are also sensitive. The drug is effective in the treatment of brain abscesses caused by these organisms.

3. **Resistance:** Resistance is not a therapeutic problem, although strains of trichomonads resistant to *metronidazole* have been reported.

4. **Pharmacokinetics**

   a. **Administration and distribution:** *Metronidazole* is completely and rapidly absorbed after oral administration and for the treatment of amebiasis, is usually administered with a luminal amebicide, such as *diloxanide furoate*. It distributes well throughout body tissues and fluids. Therapeutic levels can be found in vaginal and seminal fluids, saliva, breast milk and cerebrospinal fluid (CSF).

   b. **Fate:** Metabolism depends on hepatic oxidation of the *metronidazole* side-chain by mixed function oxidase, followed by glucuronidation (see p. 14). Therefore, concomitant treatment with inducers of this enzymatic system, such as *phenobarbital* (see p. 94), enhances the rate of metabolism. Conversely, those that inhibit this system, such as *cimetidine* (see p. 236), prolong the plasma half-life ($t_{1/2}$). The drug accumulates in patients with severe hepatic disease. The parent drug and metabolites are excreted in the urine.

5. **Adverse effects:** The most common adverse effects are those associated with the gastrointestinal tract—nausea, vomiting, epigastric distress, and abdominal cramps. An unpleasant metallic taste is often experienced. Other effects include oral moniliasis

(yeast infection of the mouth) and rarely, neurotoxicologic problems, such as dizziness, vertigo, and numbness or paresthesias in the peripheral nervous system. [Note: The latter are reasons for discontinuing the drug.] If taken with alcohol, a *disulfiram*-like effect occurs (see p. 96).

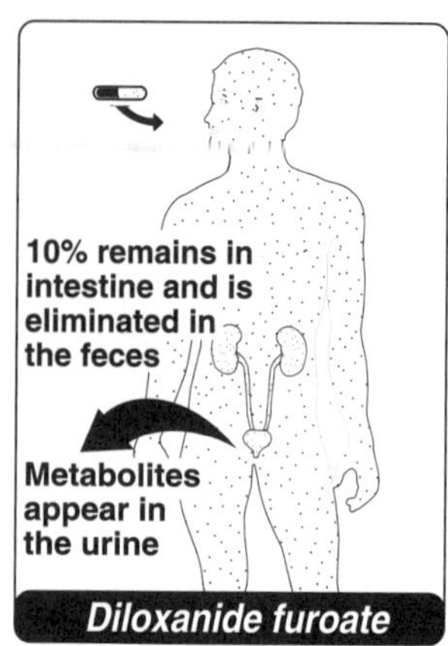
10% remains in intestine and is eliminated in the feces
Metabolites appear in the urine
Diloxanide furoate

D. Luminal amebicide: Diloxanide furoate

Diloxanide furoate [dye LOX a nide] is useful in the treatment of asymptomatic passers of cysts. Its only indication is in the treatment of intestinal amebiasis. After oral administration, *diloxanide furoate* is hydrolyzed in the intestinal mucosa, and the diloxanide is about 90% absorbed. However, the unabsorbed drug is the active amebicide. Adverse effects are mild. They include flatulence, dryness of the mouth, pruritus, and urticaria. The drug is contraindicated in pregnant women and children under 2 years of age.

E. Luminal amebicide: Paromomycin

Paromomycin [par oh moe MYE sin], an aminoglycoside antibiotic, is only effective against the intestinal (luminal) forms of E. histolytica and tapeworm, since it is not significantly absorbed from the gastrointestinal tract. It is an alternative agent for cryptosporidiosis. Although directly amebicidal, *paromomycin* also exerts its antiamebic actions by reducing the population of the intestinal flora. Its direct amebicidal action is probably due to the effects it has on cell membranes to cause leakage. Very little of the drug is absorbed on oral ingestion; that which is, is excreted in the urine. Gastrointestinal distress and diarrhea are the principal adverse effects.

F. Systemic amebicide: Chloroquine

Chloroquine [KLOR oh kwin] is used in conjunction with *metronidazole* and *diloxanide furoate* to treat and prevent amebic liver abscesses. It eliminates trophozoites in liver abscesses, but it is not useful in treating luminal amebiasis. *Chloroquine* is also effective in the treatment of malaria and is more fully described in the malaria section (see p. 349).

G. Systemic amebicides: Emetine and dehydroemetine

Emetine [EM e teen] and *dehydroemetine* [de hye dro EM e teen] are alternate agents for the treatment of amebiasis. They inhibit protein synthesis by blocking chain elongation[1]. Intramuscular injection is the preferred route. *Emetine* is concentrated in the liver where it persists for a month after a single dose. It is slowly metabolized and excreted and can accumulate. Its $t_{1/2}$ is 5 days. The use of these ipecac alkaloids is limited by their toxicities. *Dehydroemetine* is probably less toxic than *emetine*. Close clinical observation is necessary when these drugs are used. Among the untoward effects are pain at the site of injection, transient nausea, cardiotoxicity (e.g., arrhythmias, congestive heart failure), neuromuscular weakness, dizziness, and rashes.

[1]See p. 358 for Infolink references to other books in this series.

III. CHEMOTHERAPY OF MALARIA

Malaria is an acute infectious disease caused by four species of the protozoal genus plasmodium. The parasite is transmitted to humans through the bite of female anopheles mosquito, which thrives in humid, swampy areas. Plasmodium falciparum is the most dangerous species, causing an acute, rapidly fulminating disease characterized by persistent high fever, orthostatic hypotension and massive erythrocytosis (swollen and reddish condition of the limbs). Plasmodium falciparum infection can lead to capillary obstruction and death if treatment is not instituted promptly. Plasmodium vivax causes a milder form of the disease. P. malariae is common to many tropical regions but Plasmodium ovale is rarely encountered. Resistance acquired by the mosquito to insecticides, and by the parasite to drugs, has led to new therapeutic challenges, particularly in the treatment of P. falciparum.

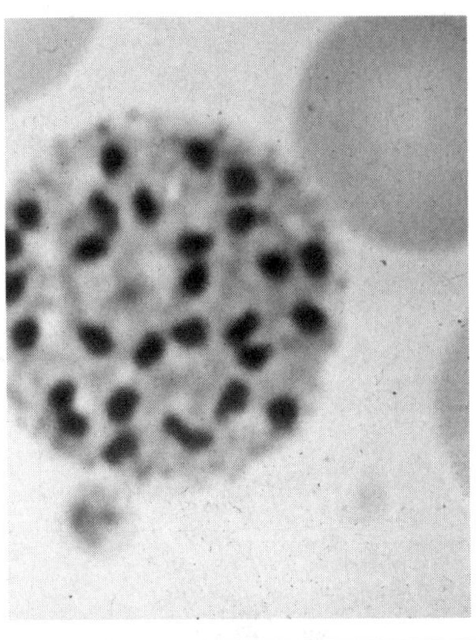

Figure 35.3
Red blood cells containing Plasmodium vivax.

A. Life cycle of the malaria parasite

When an infected mosquito bites, it injects Plasmodium sporozoites into the blood stream. The sporozoites migrate through the blood to the liver where they form cyst-like structures containing thousands of merozoites. [Note: Diagnosis depends on laboratory identification of the parasites in red blood cells of peripheral blood smears (Figure 35.3).] Upon release, each merozoite invades red blood cells, using hemoglobin as a nutrient. Eventually the infected cell ruptures, releasing heme and merozoites that can enter other erythrocytes. The effectiveness of a drug treatment is related to the particular species of infecting plasmodium and the stage of its life cycle. A summary of the life cycle of the parasite and the sites of therapeutic interventions are presented in Figure 35.4.

B. Tissue schizonticide: Primaquine

Primaquine [PRIM a kwin] is an 8-aminoquinoline that eradicates primary exoerythrocytic forms of P. falciparum and P. vivax and the secondary exoerythrocytic forms of recurring malarias (P. vivax and P. ovale). In addition, the sexual (gametocytic) forms of all four plasmodia are destroyed in the blood or are prevented from maturing later in the mosquito. Because of its lack of activity against the erythrocytic schizonts, *primaquine* is often used in conjunction with a schizonticide.

1. **Mode of action:** This is not completely understood. Intermediates are believed to act as oxidants that are responsible for the schizonticidal action as well as for hemolysis and methemoglobinemia encountered as toxicities.

2. **Antimicrobial spectrum:** In spite of structural similarity to the 4-aminoquinolines (for example, *chloroquine*), the 8-aminoquinolines are effective only against the exoerythrocytic (tissue) stages and not the erythrocytic stage of malaria. It is the only agent that can lead to radical cures of the P. vivax and P. ovale malarias, which may remain in the liver after the erythrocytic form of the disease is

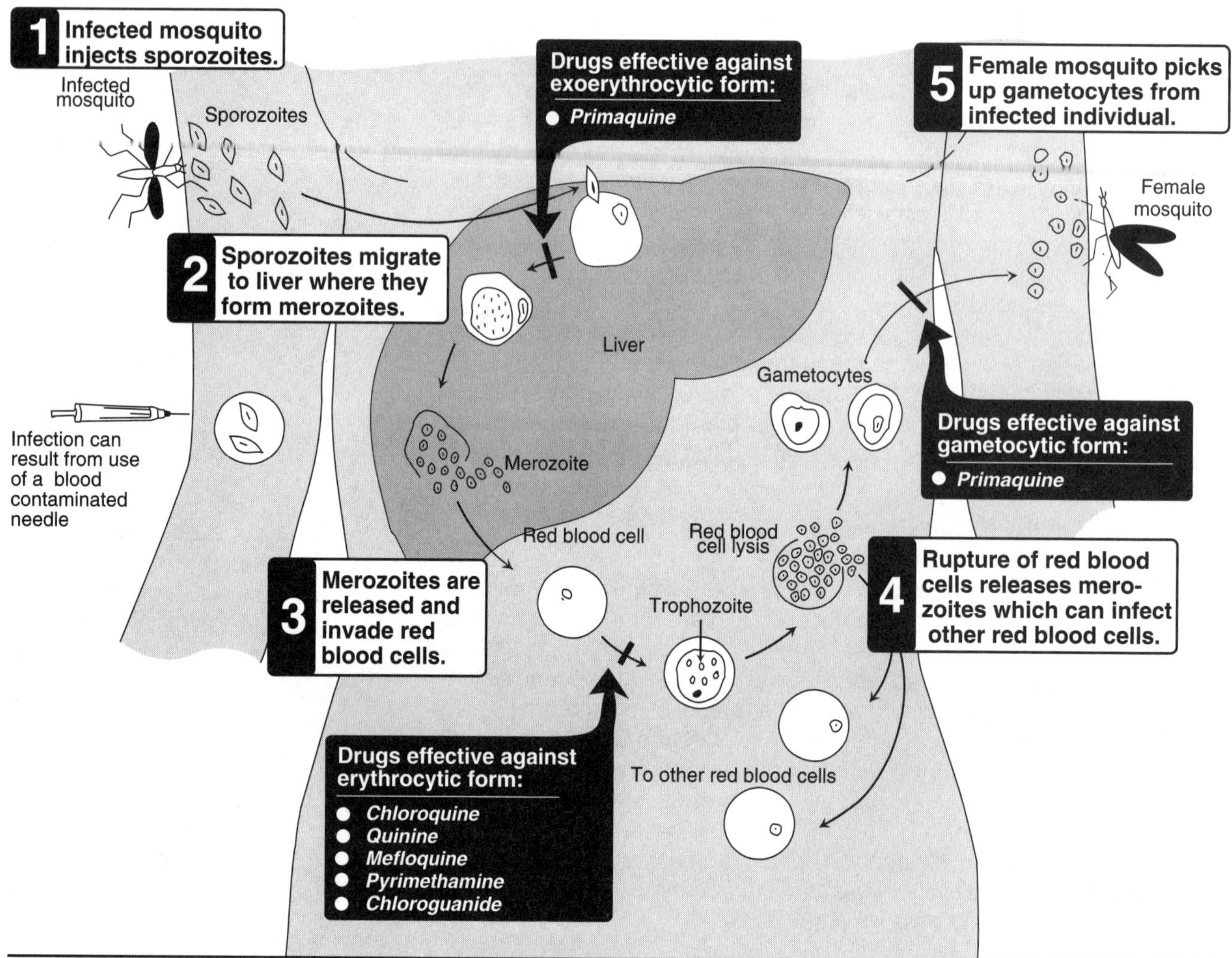

Figure 35.4
Life cycle of the malarial parasite showing the sites of action of antimalarial drugs.

eliminated. Because *primaquine* is also gametocidal for all four plasmodia species, transmission of the disease can be interrupted.

3. **Pharmacokinetics:** *Primaquine* is well absorbed on oral administration and is not concentrated in tissues. It is rapidly oxidized to many compounds, the major one being the deaminated drug. It has not been established which compound possesses the schizonticidal activity. Metabolites appear in urine.

4. **Adverse effects:** *Primaquine* has a low incidence of adverse effects except for drug-induced hemolytic anemia in patients with genetically low levels of glucose-6-phosphate dehydrogenase (Figure 35.5).[2] Other toxic manifestations observed after large doses of the drug include abdominal discomfort, especially in combination with *chloroquine*, (which may affect patient compliance), and occasional methemoglobinemia; granulocytopenia and agranulocytosis are rarely seen except in patients with lupus or arthritis, in whom the drug aggravates both these conditions.

[2]See p. 358 for Infolink references to other books in this series.

C. Blood schizonticide: Chloroquine

Chloroquine [KLOR oh kwin] is a synthetic 4-aminoquinoline that has been the mainstay of antimalarial therapy until the recent appearance of drug resistant strains of P. falciparum.

1. **Mode of action:** Several mechanisms have been identified by which *chloroquine* kills the organism after accumulating in the organism.

   a. **Damage mediated by accumulated heme:** *Chloroquine* enters the red blood cells and interferes with a unique enzyme that is essential to the survival of the parasites in the red blood cells. The parasites digest the host cell's hemoglobin to get essential amino acids and iron. However, this process also releases large amounts of soluble heme that is toxic to the parasites. To protect itself, the parasite ordinarily polymerizes the heme to hemozoin (a pigment) that is sequestered in the parasite's food vacuole. *Chloroquine* inhibits the polymerase and thus soluble heme kills the organism by inhibiting proteinases in the food vacuole. *Chloroquine* also binds to ferriprotoporphyrin IX, which is formed from the breakdown of hemoglobin in infected erythrocytes. The resulting complex damages the membranes and leads to lysis of both the parasite and the red blood cell.

   b. **Alkalinization of food vacuole:** *Chloroquine* is taken up into the parasite's food vacuole by an active transport system. Inside the acidic vacuole the drug, which is very basic, combines with a proton and is trapped, resulting in alkalinization of this organelle. This causes an inability of the parasite to carry out hemoglobin digestion.

   c. **Decreased DNA synthesis:** The drug can also decrease DNA synthesis in the parasite by disrupting the tertiary structure of the nucleic acid.

2. **Resistance:** Resistance of plasmodia to available drugs has become a serious medical problem throughout Asia and some areas of Central and South America. *Chloroquine*-resistant P. falciparum contain membrane-associated P-glycoprotein (see p. 377) that extrudes the drug from the organism.

3. **Antimicrobial spectrum:** *Chloroquine* is the drug of choice in the treatment of erythrocytic falciparum malaria, except in resistant strains. *Chloroquine* is less effective against vivax malaria. It is highly specific for the asexual form of P. vivax and P. falciparum. It is also effective in the treatment of extraintestinal amebiasis (see p. 346). The anti-inflammatory action of *chloroquine* explains its occasional use in rheumatoid arthritis and discoid lupus erythematosus.

4. **Pharmacokinetics**

   a. **Administration and distribution:** *Chloroquine* is rapidly and completely absorbed following oral administration. Usually 4

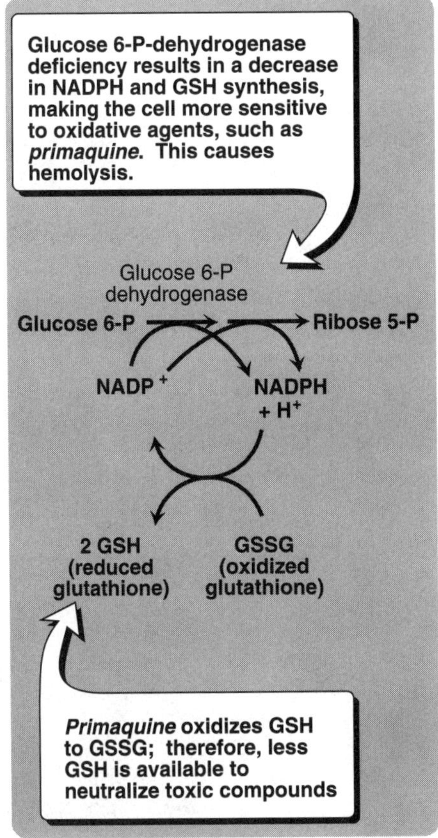

Glucose 6-P-dehydrogenase deficiency results in a decrease in NADPH and GSH synthesis, making the cell more sensitive to oxidative agents, such as *primaquine*. This causes hemolysis.
Glucose 6-P dehydrogenase
Glucose 6-P
Ribose 5-P
NADP$^+$
NADPH + H$^+$
2 GSH (reduced glutathione)
GSSG (oxidized glutathione)
Primaquine oxidizes GSH to GSSG; therefore, less GSH is available to neutralize toxic compounds

Figure 35.5
Mechanism of *primaquine*-induced hemolytic anemia. GSH, reduced glutathione; GSSG, oxidized glutathione; NADPH, reduced nicotinamide adenine dinucleotide phosphate.

days of therapy suffice to cure the disease. The drug concentrates in erythrocytes, liver, spleen, kidney, lung, and melanin-containing tissues as well as leukocytes. Thus it has a very large volume of distribution. It persists in erythrocytes (see mode of action above). The drug also penetrates into the central nervous system and traverses the placenta.

b. **Fate:** *Chloroquine* is dealkylated by the hepatic mixed function oxidases (see p. 14), but some metabolic products retain antimalarial activity. Both parent drug and metabolites are excreted predominantly in the urine. Excretion rate is enhanced as urine is acidified.

5. **Adverse effects:** Side effects are minimal at low doses used in the chemosuppression of malaria. At higher doses, many more toxic effects occur, such as gastrointestinal upset, pruritus, headaches (Figure 35.6), and visual disturbances (an ophthalmological examination should be routinely performed). Discoloration of the nail beds and mucous membranes may be seen on chronic administration. *Chloroquine* should be used cautiously in patients with hepatic dysfunction or severe gastrointestinal problems, or in patients with neurologic or blood disorders. *Chloroquine* can cause electrocardiographic changes, since it has a *quinidine*-like effect (see p. 167). It may also exacerbate dermatitis produced by *gold* (see p. 414) or *phenylbutazone* (see p. 411) therapy. [Note: Patients with psoriasis or porphyria should not be treated with *chloroquine* because an acute attack may be provoked.]

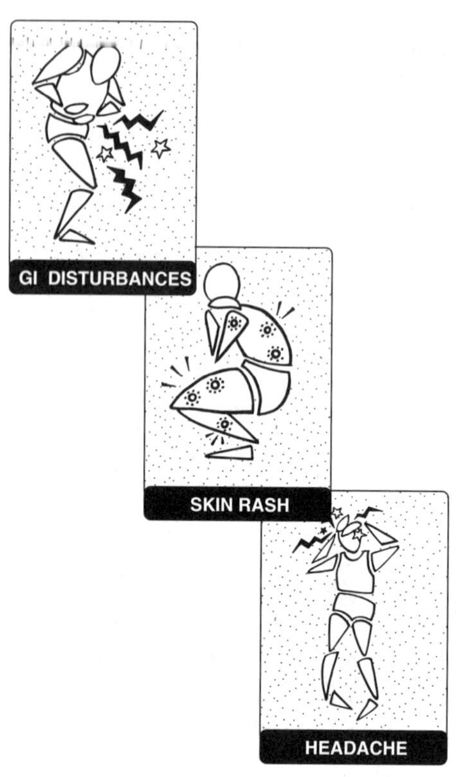

Figure 35. 6
Some adverse effects commonly associated with *chloroquine*.

D. Blood schizonticide: Quinine

Quinine [KWYE nine] is now reserved for malarial strains resistant to other agents. The drug can affect DNA synthesis.

1. **Pharmacokinetics:** When a *chloroquine*-resistant organism is encountered, therapy usually consists of a combination of *quinine*, *pyrimethamine*, and a *sulfonamide*. All are administered orally. [Note: FANSIDAR, a combination of *pyrimethamine* and *sulfadoxime* is used.] Taken orally, *quinine* is well distributed throughout the body and can reach the fetus across the placenta. Alkalinization of the urine decreases its excretion.

2. **Adverse effects:** The major adverse effect of *quinine* is cinchonism, a syndrome causing nausea, vomiting, tinnitus, and vertigo. These effects are reversible and are not considered reason to suspend therapy. However, *quinine* should be suspended if a positive result to a Coombs' test for hemolytic anemia occurs. Among the drug interactions are 1) retardation of absorption when *quinine* is taken with aluminum-containing antacids, 2) potentiation of neuromuscular blocking agents, and 3) elevation of *digoxin* (see p. 158) levels if taken concurrently with *quinine*. *Quinine* is fetotoxic.

E. Blood schizonticide: Mefloquine:

Mefloquine [MEF lo kween] appears promising as an effective single agent for suppressing and curing multidrug-resistant forms of P. -

falciparum. Its exact mechanism of action remains to be determined, but it apparently can damage the parasite's membrane like *quinine* does. Resistant strains have been identified. *Mefloquine* is absorbed well after oral administration and concentrates in the liver and lung. It has a long half-life (17 days) because of concentration in various tissues and because of its continuous circulation through the enterohepatic and enterogastric systems. The drug undergoes extensive metabolism. Its major excretory route is the feces. Adverse reactions at high doses range from nausea, vomiting, and dizziness to disorientation, hallucinations, and depression. Electrocardiographic abnormalities and cardiac arrest are possible if *mefloquine* is taken concurrently with *quinine*, or *quinidine* or β-blockers.

F. Blood schizonticide and sporontocide: Pyrimethamine

The antifolate agent, *pyrimethamine*, is frequently employed as a blood schizonticide to effect a radical cure. It also acts as a strong sporonticide in the mosquito's gut when the mosquito ingests it with the blood of the human host. *Pyrimethamine* inhibits plasmodial dihydrofolate reductase[3] at much lower concentrations than those that inhibit the mammalian enzyme. The inhibition deprives the protozoan of tetrahydrofolate, a cofactor required in the de novo biosynthesis of purines and pyrimidines, and interconversions of certain amino acids. *Pyrimethamine* alone is effective against P. falciparum. In combination with a sulfonamide, it is also used against P. malariae and Toxoplasma gondii. If megaloblastic anemia occurs, it may be reversed with *leucovorin* (see p. 379)

IV. CHEMOTHERAPY OF TRYPANOSOMIASIS

Trypanosomiasis refers to two chronic and eventually fatal diseases caused by species of Trypanosoma: African sleeping sickness and American sleeping sickness (Figure 35.7). In African sleeping sickness, the causative organisms, Trypanosoma brucei gambiense and Trypanosoma brucei rhodiense, initially live and grow in the blood. The parasite invades the CNS, causing an inflammation of the brain and spinal cord that produces the characteristic lethargy and eventually continuous sleep. Chagas' disease (American sleeping sickness) caused by Trypanosoma cruzi occurs in South America.

TRYPANOSOMIASIS
AMERICAN caused by Trypanosoma cruzi (also called Chagas' disease)
Causes cardio-myopathy
Treated with *nifurtimox*
AFRICAN caused by Trypanosoma brucei
Trypanosoma brucei gambiense
Slow to enter CNS
Causes "sleeping sickness"
Trypanosoma brucei rhodesiense
Early invasion of CNS
Usually fatal if not treated
Suramin and *pentamidine* are used only in the early stage of disease. *Melarsoprol* used when there is CNS involvement.

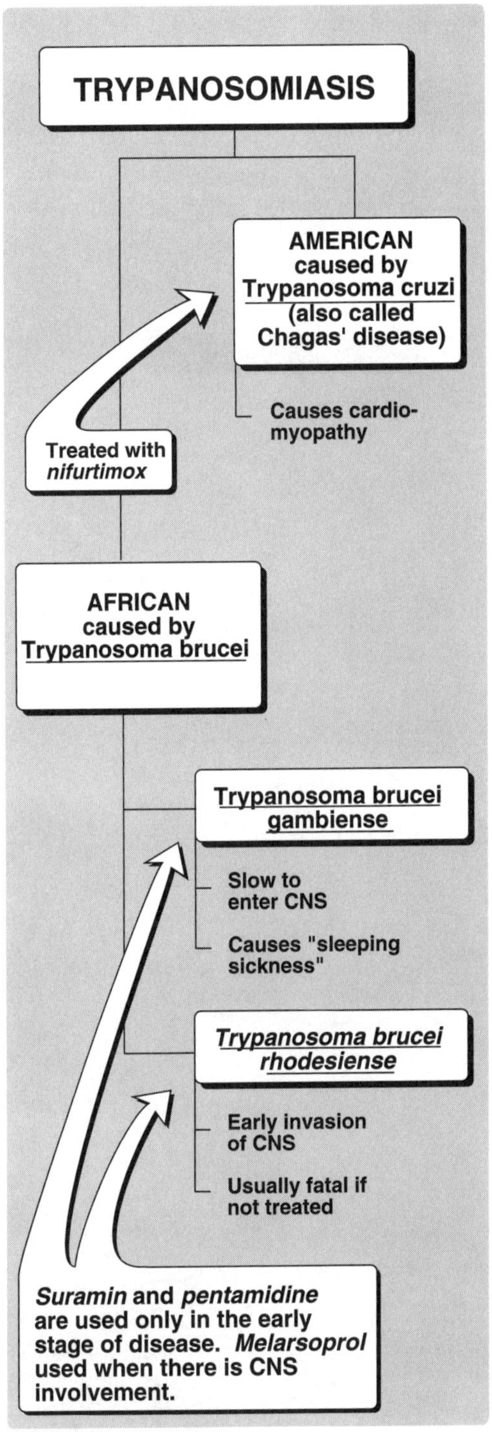

Figure 35.7
Summary of trypanosomiasis.

A. Melarsoprol

Melarsoprol [me LAR soe prole] is a derivative of *mersalyl oxide*, a trivalent arsenical.

1. **Mode of action:** The drug reacts with sulfhydryl groups of various substances including enzymes in both the organism and host. Parasitic enzymes may be more sensitive than are those of the host. There is evidence that mammalian cells may be less permeable to the drug and thus protected from its toxic effects.

2. **Antimicrobial spectrum:** *Melarsoprol* is limited to the treatment of trypanosomal infections, usually in the late stage with CNS involvement, and is lethal for these parasites.

[3]See p. 358 for Infolink references to other books in this series.

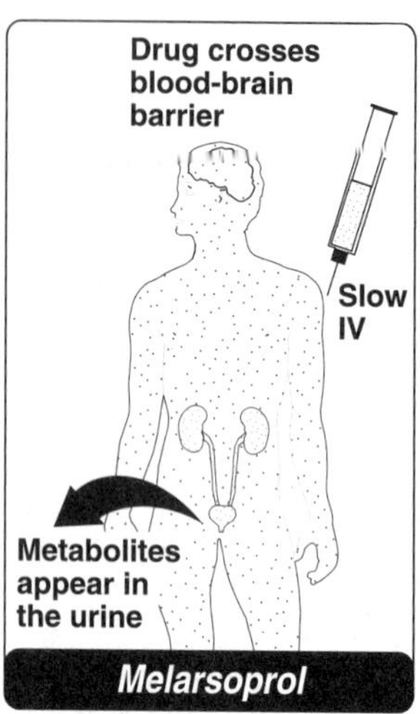
Drug crosses blood-brain barrier
Slow IV
Metabolites appear in the urine
Melarsoprol

3. **Resistance:** may be due to decreased permeability to the drug.

4. **Pharmacokinetics:**

   a. **Administration and distribution:** *Melarsoprol* is usually slowly administered intravenously through a fine needle, even though it is absorbed from the gastrointestinal tract. Because it is very irritating, care should be taken not to infiltrate surrounding tissue. Adequate trypanocidal concentrations appear in the cerebrospinal fluid, which contrasts with *pentamidine* (see p. 355), which does not enter the cerebrospinal fluid. *Melarsoprol* is therefore the agent of choice in the treatment of T. brucei rhodesiense, which rapidly invades the CNS, as well as for meningoencephalitis caused by T.brucei gambiense.

   b. **Fate:** The host readily oxidizes the drug to the relatively nontoxic pentavalent arsenic compound. The drug has a very short half-life and is rapidly excreted into the urine.

5. **Adverse effects**

   a. **Central nervous system toxicities:** These side effects are the most serious. Encephalopathy may appear soon after the first course of treatment but usually subsides. It may, however, be fatal.

   b. **Hypersensitivity reactions:** Such reactions may also occur. Fever may follow injection.

   c. **Gastrointestinal disturbance:** Severe vomiting and abdominal pain can be minimized if the patient is in the fasting state during drug administration and for several hours thereafter.

   d. **Contraindications:** *Melarsoprol* is contraindicated in patients with influenza. Hemolytic anemia has been seen in patients with glucose 6-phosphate dehydrogenase deficiency.

B. Pentamidine isethionate

Pentamidine [pen TAM i deen] is active against protozoal infections, as well as those caused by Pneumocystis carinii. [Note: P. carinii is now considered to be a fungus, but it is not susceptible to antifungal drugs.] Because of the increased incidence of pneumonia caused by this organism in immunocompromised patients such as those infected with human immunodeficiency virus (HIV), *pentamidine* has assumed an important place in chemotherapy. *Pentamidine* is one of the drugs for the prevention and treatment of the hematologic stage of T. brucei gambiense.

1. **Mode of action:** T. brucei concentrates the drug by an energy-dependent, high-affinity uptake system. Although its mode of action has not been defined, evidence exists that the drug binds to the parasite's DNA, and interferes in the synthesis of RNA, DNA, phospholipid and protein of the parasite.

2. **Antimicrobial spectrum:** *Pentamidine* is not effective against all trypanosomes, for example, T. cruzi is resistant. However, it is effective in the treatment of systemic blastomycosis. *Pentamidine* is also effective against P. carinii, but *trimethoprim-sulfamethoxazole* (see p. 293) is preferred. *Pentamidine* is the drug of choice in treating patients with pneumonia caused by P. carinii who have failed to respond to *trimethoprim-sulfamethoxazole*, or in treating individuals who are allergic to sulfonamides. It is an alternative drug to *stibogluconate* in the treatment of leishmaniasis.

3. **Resistance:** Resistance is associated with an inability of the trypanosome to concentrate the drug.

4. **Pharmacokinetics**

   a. **Administration and distribution:** Fresh solutions are administered intramuscularly or as an aerosol. [Note: The intravenous route is avoided because of severe adverse reactions such as a sharp fall in blood pressure and tachycardia.] The drug is concentrated and stored in the liver and kidney for a long period of time. Because it does not enter the CSF, it is ineffective against the meningoencephalitic stage of trypanosomiasis.

   b. **Fate:** The drug is not metabolized and is excreted very slowly into the urine. Its $t_{1/2}$ is about 5 days.

5. **Adverse effects:** Serious renal dysfunction may occur, which reverses on discontinuation of the drug. Other adverse reactions are hypotension, dizziness, rash and toxicity to β-cells of pancreas.

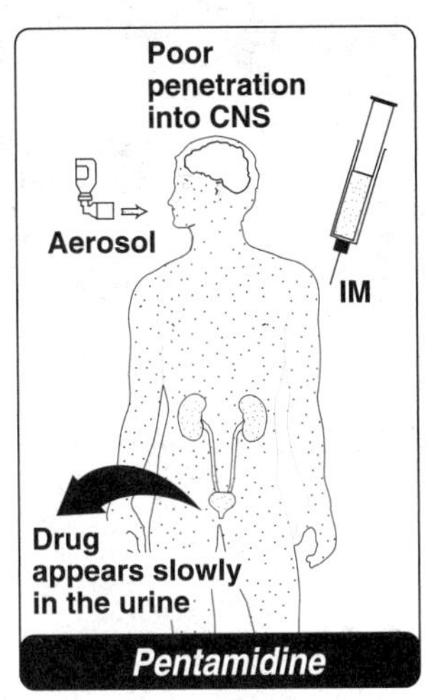

C. Nifurtimox

Nifurtimox [nye FOOR ti mox] has found use only in the treatment of acute T. cruzi infections (Chagas' disease) although treatment of the chronic stage of such infections has led to variable results. [Note: *Nifurtimox* is suppressive not curative.] Being a nitroaromatic compound, *nifurtimox* undergoes reduction and eventually generates intracellular oxygen radicals, such as superoxide radicals and hydrogen peroxide, in both the amastigote and trypomastigote of T. cruzi. These highly reactive radicals are toxic to the organism, which lacks catalase[4]. Mammalian cells are partially protected from such substances by the presence of enzymes such as catalase, glutathione peroxidase, and superoxide dismutase. The drug is administered orally and is rapidly absorbed and metabolized to unidentified products, which are excreted in the urine. Adverse effects are common following chronic administration, particularly among the elderly. Major toxicities include immediate hypersensitivity reactions, such as anaphylaxis; delayed hypersensitivity reactions, for example dermatitis and icterus; and gastrointestinal problems that may be so severe as to cause weight loss. Peripheral neuropathy is relatively common, and disturbances in the CNS may also occur. In addition, cell-mediated immune reactions may be suppressed.

[4]See p. 358 for Infolink references to other books in this series.

D. Suramin

Suramin [SOO ra min] is used primarily in the early treatment and especially in the prophylaxis of African trypanosomiasis. It is very reactive and inhibits many enzymes, among them, those involved in energy metabolism (e.g., glycerol phosphate dehydrogenase) which appears to be the mechanism most closely correlated with trypanocidal activity. *Suramin* is also the drug of choice in treatment of patients with the adult forms of the filarial parasite, Onchocerca volvulus. The drug must be injected intravenously. It binds to plasma proteins and remains in the plasma for a long time, accumulating in the liver and in the proximal tubular cells of the kidney. The severity of the adverse reactions demands that the patient be carefully followed, especially if debilitated. Although infrequent, these reactions include nausea and vomiting (which causes further debilitation of the patient), shock and loss of consciousness, acute urticaria, and neurologic problems that include paresthesia, photophobia, palpebral edema, and hyperesthesia of the hands and feet. Albuminuria tends to be common, but when cylindruria (the presence of renal casts in the urine) and hematuria occur, treatment should cease.

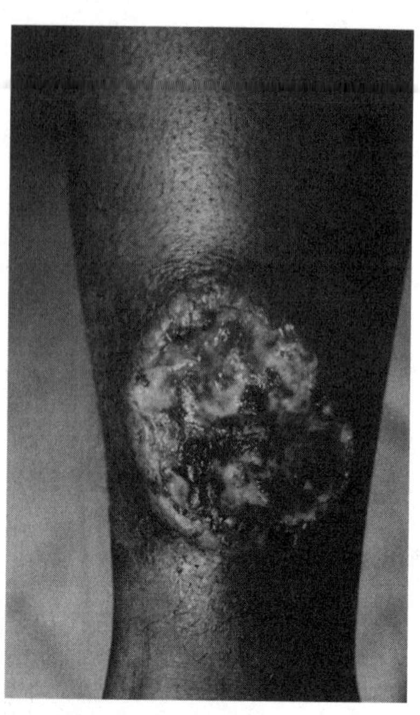

Figure 35.8
Mucocutaneous leishmaniasis.

V. CHEMOTHERAPY OF LEISHMANIASIS

There are three types of leishmaniasis: the cutaneous, mucocutaneous (Figure 35.8), and visceral. [Note: In the visceral type (liver and spleen), the parasite is in the bloodstream and can cause very serious problems.] Leishmaniasis is transmitted from animal to humans (and between humans) by the bite of infected sandflies. The treatments of leishmaniasis and trypanosomiasis (see p. 337), are difficult, because the effective drugs are limited by their toxicities and failure rates. Pentavalent antimonials, such as *sodium stibogluconate*, are the conventional therapy used in the treatment of leishmaniasis, with *pentamidine* (see p. 354) and *amphotericin B* (see p. 357) as back-up agents. *Allopurinol* (see p. 417) has also been reported to be effective. The drug is converted to a toxic metabolite by the amastigote form. The diagnosis is made by demonstrating the organism in biopsy material and skin lesions.

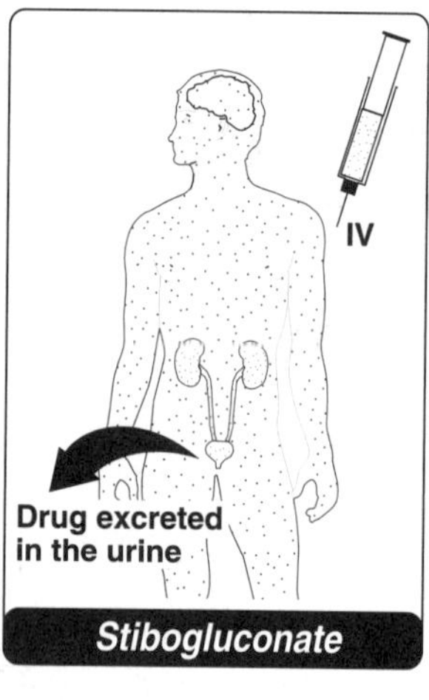

A. Life cycle of the causative organism, Leishmania

The sandfly transfers the flagellated promastigote form of the protozoa, which is rapidly phagocytized by macrophages. In the macrophage, the promastigotes rapidly change to nonflagellated amastigotes and multiply, killing the cell. The newly released amastigotes are again phagocytized, and the cycle continues.

B. Sodium stibogluconate

Stibogluconate [stib o GLOO koe nate] is not effective in vitro; therefore it has been proposed that reduction to the trivalent antimony compound is essential for activity. The exact mechanism of action has not been determined. Evidence for inhibition of glycolysis in the parasite at the phosphofructokinase reaction[5] has been found.

[5]See p. 358 for Infolink references to other books in this series.

Because it is not absorbed on oral administration, *sodium stibogluconate* must be administered parenterally. It is distributed in the extravascular compartment. Metabolism is minimal and the drug is excreted into the urine. Adverse effects include pain at the injection site, gastrointestinal upsets, and cardiac arrhythmias. Renal and hepatic function should be periodically monitored.

VI. CHEMOTHERAPY OF TOXOPLASMOSIS

One of the most common infections in man is caused by the protozoan, Toxoplasma gondii, which is transmitted to humans when they consume raw or inadequately cooked, infected meat. Infected pregnant women can transmit the organism to the fetus. Cats are the only animals that shed oocysts that can infect other animals as well as man. The treatment of choice for this condition is the antifolate drug, *pyrimethamine* [peer i METH a meen] (see p. 353). A combination of *sulfadiazine* (see p. 289) and *pyrimethamine* is also efficacious. *Leucovorin* is often administered to protect against folate deficiency. Other inhibitors of folate biosynthesis, such as *trimethoprim* (see p. 293) and *sulfamethoxazole* (see p. 289) are without therapeutic efficacy in toxoplasmosis. [Note: At the first appearance of a rash, *pyrimethamine* should be discontinued since hypersensitivity to this drug can be severe.]

VII. CHEMOTHERAPY OF GIARDIASIS

Giardia lamblia is the most commonly diagnosed intestinal parasite in the United States. It has only two life-cycle stages: the binucleate trophozoite with 4 flagellae, and the drug-resistant 4-nucleate cyst. Ingestion, usually from contaminated drinking water, leads to infection. The trophozoites exist in the small intestine and divide by binary fission. Occasionally, cysts are formed that pass out in the stool. Though some infections are asymptomatic, severe diarrhea can occur which can be very serious in immune-suppressed patients. The treatment is usually either *quinacrine* or *metronidazole* (see p. 347).

A. Quinacrine

Quinacrine is an acridine derivative that is primarily used in the treatment of giardiasis, but is also effective against tapeworm and malaria, and topically, against leishmaniasis. It binds to membrane phospholipids, blocking phospholipase A_2 activity. *Quinacrine* also binds to the acetylcholine receptor. Given orally, *quinacrine* concentrates in the liver. Because it crosses the placenta, it should be avoided in pregnant women. Adverse effects range from the more common dizziness, headaches, and vomiting to more serious psychosis, urticaria, exfoliative dermatitis and pigmentation of the skin. *Quinacrine* and *primaquine* should not be given together because of increased toxicity.

Questions 35.1 - 35.3: For each numbered phrase, select the ONE drug (A-E) that is most closely associated with it. Each drug (A-E) may be selected once, more than once, or not at all.

A. Sodium stibogluconate
B. Diloxanide furoate
C. Pyrimethamine
D. Emetine
E. Metronidazole

35.1 A systemic amebicide.

Correct answer = D (emetine).

35.2 Used in the treatment of toxoplasmosis.

Correct answer = C (pyrimethamine).

35.3 Used in the treatment of leishmaniasis.

Correct answer = A (sodium stibogluconate).

Choose the ONE best answer.

35.4 All of the following statements about chloroquine are true EXCEPT:

A. It blocks protozoal DNA and RNA synthesis.
B. Infected cells can concentrate the drug to a greater extent than can uninfected cells.
C. It is the drug of choice for the treatment of an acute attack of falciparum or vivax malaria.
D. Chronic administration may cause discoloration of nail beds and mucous membranes.
E. Only exoerythrocytic forms of plasmodium are susceptible.

Correct choice = E. Only the erythrocytic form of the parasite is susceptible to chloroquine.

35.5 All of the following statements about metronidazole are true EXCEPT:

A. It is administered intravenously because it is poorly absorbed after oral administration.
B. It is effective against a wide variety of anaerobic bacteria.
C. It produces a disulfiram-like effect on the ingestion of alcohol.
D. Dosage should be reduced in patients with hepatic dysfunction.
E. Therapeutic levels can be found in the cerebral spinal fluid.

Correct choice = A. Metronidazole is rapidly and nearly completely absorbed after oral administration.

35.6 All of the following statements about melarsoprol are true EXCEPT:

A. It reacts with sulfhydryl groups of various cellular substances, including enzymes.
B. It is equally effective against African and American trypanosomiasis.
C. Adequate trypanocidal concentrations of the drug appear in the cerebral spinal fluid.
D. It can cause serious encephalopathy.
E. It has a very short half-life in the body.

Correct choice = B. American trypanosomiasis, which is caused by T. cruzi, is not successfully treated with melarsoprol.

35.7 Which one of the following statements about primaquine is correct?

A. It is effective against erythrocytic forms of malaria.
B. It is ineffective in treating relapsing vivax malaria.
C. High (toxic) doses may produce corneal opacities.
D. Glucose 6-phosphate dehydrogenase deficient individuals are at risk for hemolytic anemia.
E. It is administered only by intravenous route.

Correct choice = D. See mechanism on p. 351 (Figure 35.5)

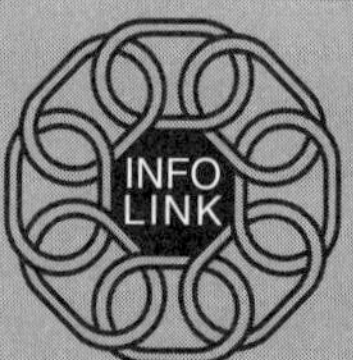

[1]See p. 398 in **Biochemistry** (2nd ed.) for a discussion of inhibitors of protein elongation.

[2]See p. 115 in **Biochemistry** (2nd ed.) for a discussion of glucose 6-phosphate dehydrogenase deficiency.

[3]See p. 250 in **Biochemistry** (2nd ed.) for a discussion of metabolic roles of tetrahydrofolate.

[4]See p. 114 in **Biochemistry** (2nd ed.) for a discussion of catalase and reactive oxygen intermediates.

[5]See p. 90 in **Biochemistry** (2nd ed.) for a discussion of phosphofructokinase reaction

Anthelmintic Drugs

36

I. OVERVIEW

Three major groups of helminths (or worms), the nematodes, trematodes and cestodes, infect humans. As in all antibiotic regimens, the anthelminthic drugs (Figure 36.1) are aimed at metabolic targets that are present in the parasite but are either absent from or have different characteristics than those of the host. Figure 36.2 illustrates the high incidence of helminthic infections.

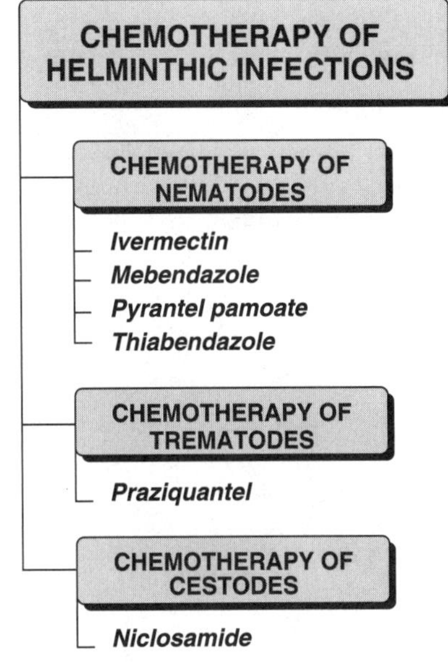

Figure 36.1
Summary of anthelminthic agents.

II. DRUGS FOR THE TREATMENT OF NEMATODES

Nematodes are elongated roundworms that possess a complete digestive system, including both a mouth and an anus (Figure 36.3). They cause infections of the intestine as well as the blood and tissues. Figure 36.4 summarizes the infections caused by nematodes, and the common therapies used for these infections.

A. Mebendazole

Mebendazole [me BEN da zole] a synthetic benzimidazole compound, is effective against a wide spectrum of nematodes. It is a drug of choice in the treatment of infections by whipworm (Trichuris trichiura), pinworm (Enterobius vermicularis), hookworm (Necator americanus and Ancylostoma duodenale), and roundworm (Ascariasis lumbricoides, Figure 36.5). *Mebendazole* acts by binding to and interfering with the synthesis of the parasite's microtubules and also by decreasing glucose uptake. Affected parasites are expelled with the feces. *Mebendazole* is nearly insoluble in aqueous solution, and little of an oral dose (which is chewed) is absorbed by the body unless taken with a high fat meal. Therefore, this drug is relatively free of toxic effects, although patients may complain of abdominal pain and diarrhea. However, it is contraindicated in pregnant women, because it has been shown to be embryotoxic and teratogenic in experimental animals.

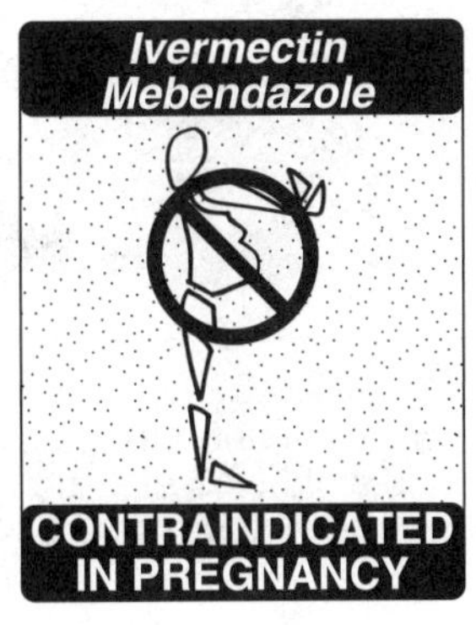

B. Pyrantel pamoate

Pyrantel pamoate [pi RAN tel] along with *mebendazole* is effective in the treatment of infections caused by roundworms, pinworms (see Figure 36.4), and hookworms. *Pyrantel pamoate* is poorly absorbed orally and exerts its effects in the intestinal tract. It acts as a depolarizing neuromuscular blocking agent, causing persistent

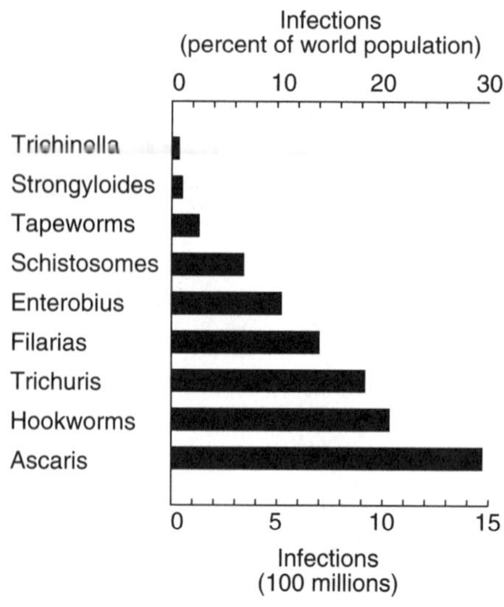

Figure 36.2
Relative incidence of helminth infections worldwide.

activation of the parasite's nicotinic receptors. The paralyzed worm is then expelled from the host's intestinal tract. Adverse effects are mild, and include nausea, vomiting, and diarrhea.

C. Thiabendazole

Thiabendazole [thye a BEN da zole], another synthetic benzimidazole, is effective against strongyloidiasis due to Strongyloides stercoralis (threadworm), cutaneous larva migrans (or creeping eruption) and early stages of trichinosis (caused by Trichinella spiralis). It, too, affects microtubular aggregation. Though nearly insoluble in water, the drug is readily absorbed on oral administration. The drug is hydroxylated in the liver and excreted in the urine. The adverse effects most often encountered are dizziness, anorexia, nausea, and vomiting. There have been reports of central nervous system (CNS) symptomatology. Among the cases of erythema multiforme and Stevens-Johnson syndrome reportedly caused by *thiabendazole*, there have been a number of fatalities.

D. Ivermectin

Ivermectin [eye ver MEK tin] is the drug of choice for the treatment of onchocerciasis (river blindness) caused by Onchocerca volvulus and has been shown to be effective against scabies. *Ivermectin* targets the parasite's γ-aminobutyric acid (GABA) receptors. Chloride efflux is enhanced and hyperpolarization occurs, resulting in paralysis of the worm. The drug is given orally. It does not cross the blood-brain barrier and has no pharmacologic effects. However, it is contraindicated in patients with meningitis, since their blood-brain barrier is more permeable, and CNS effects might be expected. *Ivermectin* is also contraindicated in pregnancy. It should be avoided in patients who are taking benzodiazepines or barbiturates—drugs that act at the GABA receptor. The killing of the microfilaria can result in a Mazotti-like reaction (fever, headache, dizziness, somnolence, hypotension, etc.).

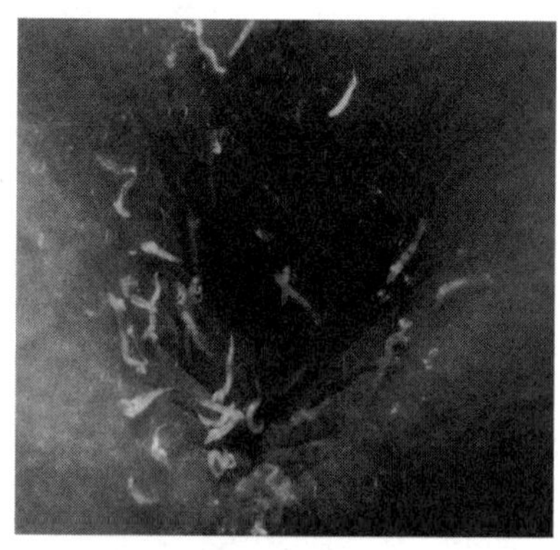

Figure 36.3
Pinworms leaving the anus of a five-year-old child who presented with crying, restlessness and abdominal pain.

III. DRUGS FOR THE TREATMENT OF TREMATODES

The trematodes (flukes) are leaf-shaped flatworms that are generally characterized by the tissues they infect. For example, they may be categorized as liver, lung, intestinal, or blood flukes.

A. Praziquantel

Trematode infections are generally treated with *praziquantel* [pray zi KWON tel]. This drug is an agent of choice for the treatment of all forms of schistosomiasis and for cestode infections like cysticercosis. Permeability of the cell membrane to calcium is increased, causing contracture and paralysis of the parasite. *Praziquantel* is rapidly absorbed after oral administration and distributes into the cerebrospinal fluid. High levels occur in the bile. The drug is extensively metabolized oxidatively, resulting in a short half-life. The metabolites are inactive and are excreted through the urine and bile.

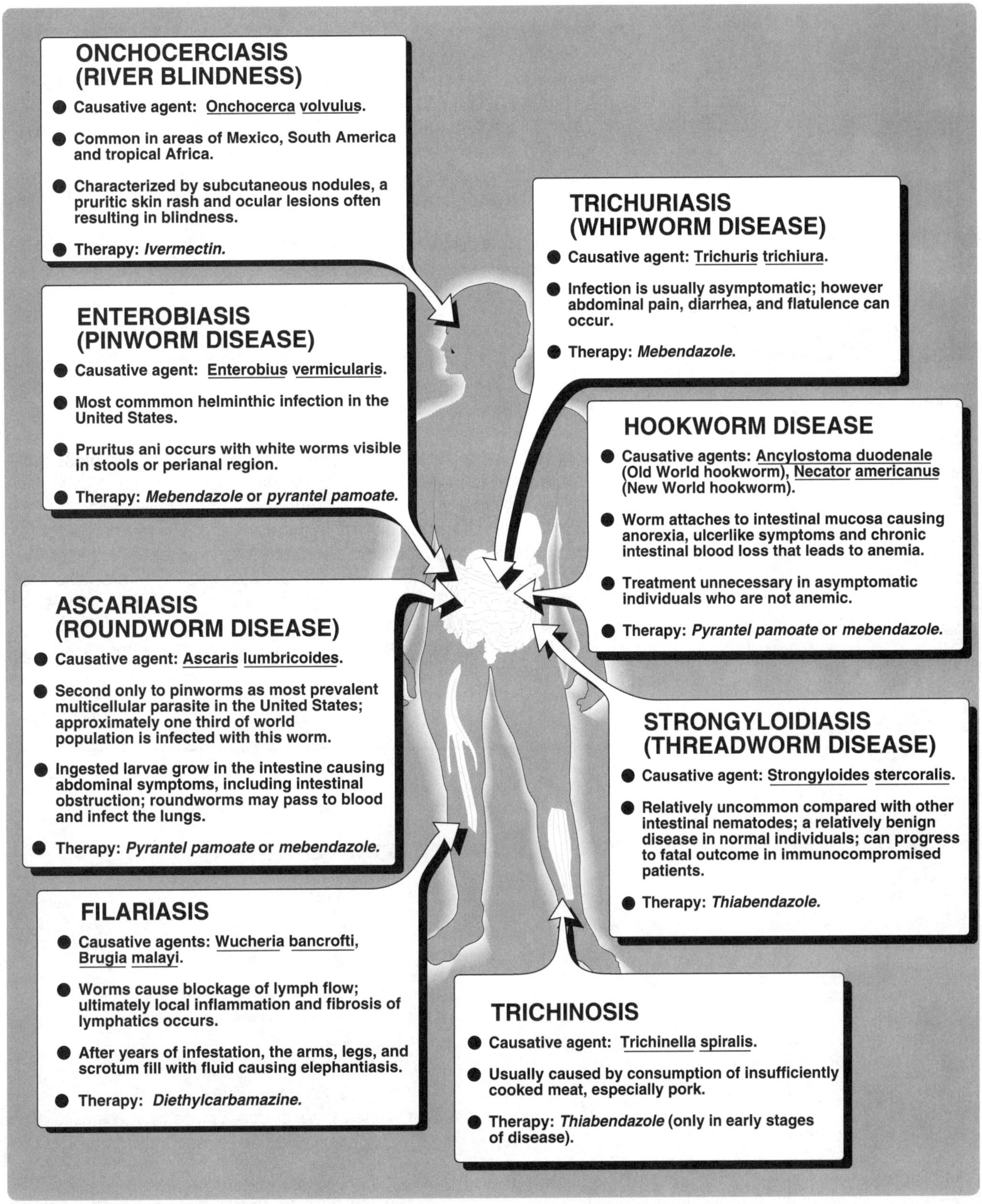

ONCHOCERCIASIS (RIVER BLINDNESS)

- Causative agent: Onchocerca volvulus.
- Common in areas of Mexico, South America and tropical Africa.
- Characterized by subcutaneous nodules, a pruritic skin rash and ocular lesions often resulting in blindness.
- Therapy: *Ivermectin.*

ENTEROBIASIS (PINWORM DISEASE)

- Causative agent: Enterobius vermicularis.
- Most commmon helminthic infection in the United States.
- Pruritus ani occurs with white worms visible in stools or perianal region.
- Therapy: *Mebendazole* or *pyrantel pamoate.*

ASCARIASIS (ROUNDWORM DISEASE)

- Causative agent: Ascaris lumbricoides.
- Second only to pinworms as most prevalent multicellular parasite in the United States; approximately one third of world population is infected with this worm.
- Ingested larvae grow in the intestine causing abdominal symptoms, including intestinal obstruction; roundworms may pass to blood and infect the lungs.
- Therapy: *Pyrantel pamoate* or *mebendazole.*

FILARIASIS

- Causative agents: Wucheria bancrofti, Brugia malayi.
- Worms cause blockage of lymph flow; ultimately local inflammation and fibrosis of lymphatics occurs.
- After years of infestation, the arms, legs, and scrotum fill with fluid causing elephantiasis.
- Therapy: *Diethylcarbamazine.*

TRICHURIASIS (WHIPWORM DISEASE)

- Causative agent: Trichuris trichiura.
- Infection is usually asymptomatic; however abdominal pain, diarrhea, and flatulence can occur.
- Therapy: *Mebendazole.*

HOOKWORM DISEASE

- Causative agents: Ancylostoma duodenale (Old World hookworm), Necator americanus (New World hookworm).
- Worm attaches to intestinal mucosa causing anorexia, ulcerlike symptoms and chronic intestinal blood loss that leads to anemia.
- Treatment unnecessary in asymptomatic individuals who are not anemic.
- Therapy: *Pyrantel pamoate* or *mebendazole.*

STRONGYLOIDIASIS (THREADWORM DISEASE)

- Causative agent: Strongyloides stercoralis.
- Relatively uncommon compared with other intestinal nematodes; a relatively benign disease in normal individuals; can progress to fatal outcome in immunocompromised patients.
- Therapy: *Thiabendazole.*

TRICHINOSIS

- Causative agent: Trichinella spiralis.
- Usually caused by consumption of insufficiently cooked meat, especially pork.
- Therapy: *Thiabendazole* (only in early stages of disease).

Figure 36.4
Characteristics and therapy for commonly encountered nematode infections.

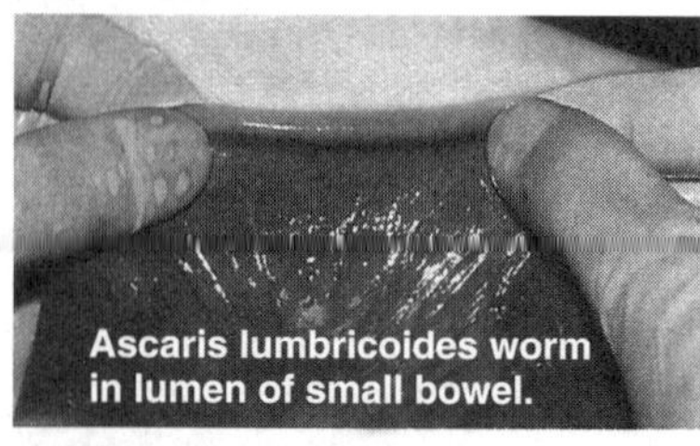
Ascaris lumbricoides worm in lumen of small bowel.

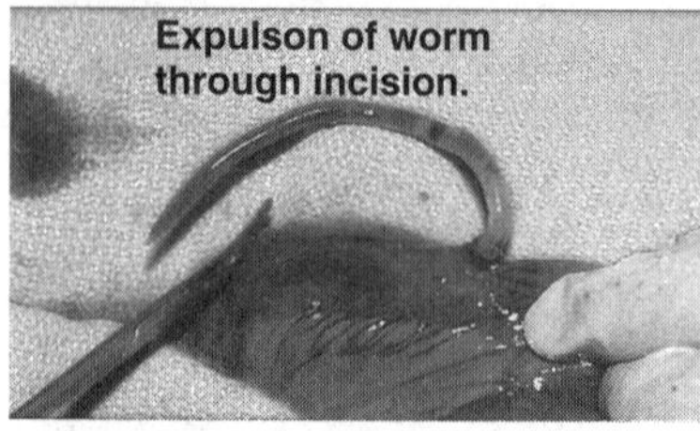
Expulson of worm through incision.

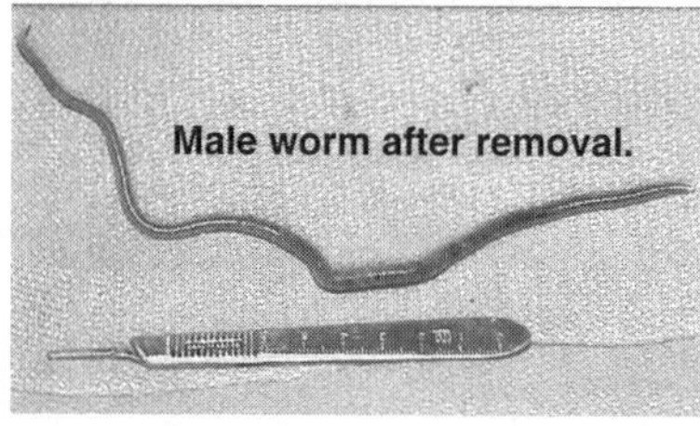
Male worm after removal.

Figure 36.5
Ascaris lumbricoides worm in lumen of small bowel of 52-year-old woman from Africa.

Common adverse effects include drowsiness, dizziness, malaise, and anorexia, as well as gastrointestinal upsets. The drug is not recommended for pregnant women or nursing mothers. Drug interactions due to increased metabolism have been reported with *dexamethasone*, *phenytoin*, and *carbamazepine*. *Cimetidine*, known to inhibit cytochrome P-450 isozymes, causes increased *praziquantel* levels. *Praziquantel* is contraindicated for the treatment of ocular cysticercosis since destruction of the organism in the eye may damage the organ.

IV. DRUGS FOR THE TREATMENT OF CESTODES

The cestodes, or "true tapeworms," typically have a flat, segmented body and attach to the host's intestine. Like the trematodes, the tapeworms lack a mouth and a digestive tract throughout their life cycle.

A. Niclosamide

Niclosamide [ni KLOE sa mide] is the drug of choice for most cestode (tapeworm) infections. Its action has been ascribed to inhibition of the parasite's mitochondrial anaerobic phosphorylation of ADP which produces usable energy in the form of ATP. The drug is lethal for the cestode's scolex and segments of cestodes but not for the ova. A laxative is administered prior to oral administration of *niclosamide*. This is done to purge the bowel of all dead segments in order to preclude digestion and liberation of the ova, which may lead to cysticercosis. Alcohol should be avoided within 1 day of *niclosamide*.

Study Questions

Questions 35.1 - 35.4: For each numbered phrase, select the ONE drug (A-E) that is most closely associated with it. Each drug (A-E) may be selected once, more than once, or not at all.

A. Mebendazole
B. Praziquantel
C. Niclosamide
D. Pyrantel pamoate
E. Thiabendazole

35.1 A drug which affects microtubular function in roundworm, pinworm, and hookworm.

Correct answer = A (mebendazole)

35.2 Acts as a depolarizing neuromuscular blocking agent.

Correct answer = D (pyrantel pamoate)

35.3 A drug of choice for the treatment of all forms of schistosomiasis.

Correct answer = B (praziquantel)

35.4 Drug of choice for the treatment of most tapeworm infections.

Correct answer = C (niclosamide)

Choose the ONE best answer.

35.5 All of the following statements about mebendazole are correct EXCEPT:

A. It is contraindicated in pregnant women.
B. It is the drug of choice in the treatment of whipworm infections.
C. It is effective by oral administration.
D. It is active against cestodes.
E. It interferes with glucose uptake by the parasite.

Correct answer = D. Mebendazole is effective against nematodes, in part by decreasing glucose uptake, and thus causing the parasite to starve. Mebendazole has been shown to be embryotoxic and teratogenic in experimental animals

Antiviral Drugs

37

I. OVERVIEW

Viruses are obligate intracellular parasites. They lack both a cell wall and a cell membrane and do not carry out metabolic processes. Viral reproduction uses much of the host's metabolic machinery, and few drugs are selective enough to prevent viral replication without injury to the host. For example, viruses are not affected by antimicrobial agents. Nevertheless, some drugs sufficiently discriminate between cellular and viral reactions to be effective and yet relatively nontoxic. Unfortunately, only a few virus groups, including those that cause the viral infections discussed in this chapter, respond to these drugs (Figure 37.1).

ANTIVIRAL DRUGS

FOR RESPIRATORY VIRUS INFECTIONS
- *Amantadine*
- *Ribavirin*
- *Rimantadine*

FOR HERPES AND CYTOMEGALOVIRUS INFECTIONS
- *Acyclovir*
- *Cidofovir*[1]
- *Famciclovir*
- *Foscarnet*
- *Ganciclovir*
- *Penciclovir*[1]
- *Trifluridine*
- *Vidarabine*

FOR HUMAN IMMUNODEFICIENCY VIRUS (HIV) INFECTIONS
- *Abacavir*[1]
- *Adefovir*[1]
- *Amprenavir*[1]
- *Delavirdine*[1]
- *Didanosine (ddI)*
- *Efavirenz*[1]
- *Indinavir*[1]
- *Nelfinavir*[1]
- *Nevirapine*[1]
- *Ritonavir*[1]
- *Saquinavir*[1]
- *Stavudine (d4T)*
- *Zalcitabine (ddC)*
- *Zidovudine (AZT)*

FOR HEPATITIS, LEUKEMIA AND KAPOSI'S SARCOMA
- *Interferon*

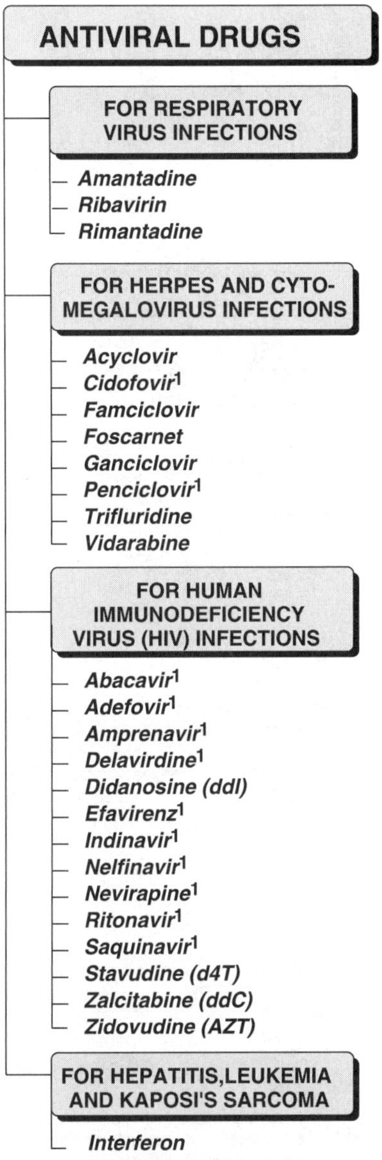

Figure 37.1
Summary of antiviral drugs.
[1]Described in Pharmacology update, p. 457.

II. TREATMENT OF VIRAL RESPIRATORY INFECTIONS

Viral respiratory tract infections for which treatments exist include those of influenza types A and B, and respiratory syncytial virus (RSV). [Note: Immunization against influenza A is the preferred approach. However, antiviral agents are employed when patients are allergic to the vaccine or when the outbreak is due to an immunologic variant of the virus not covered by vaccines, or when outbreaks occur among unvaccinated individuals at risk who are in closed settings, for example, in a nursing home.]

A. Amantadine and rimantadine

In many viral infections the clinical symptoms appear late in the course of the disease at a time when most of the virus particles have replicated. [Note: This contrasts with bacterial diseases in which the clinical symptoms are usually coincident with bacterial proliferation.] At this late, symptomatic stage of the viral infection, administration of drugs that block viral replication have limited effectiveness. However, some antiviral agents are useful as prophylactic agents. For example, *amantadine* [a MAN ta deen] and its congener, *rimantadine* [rih MAN ta deen] have been shown to be equally effective in preventing influenza A infections. [Note: *Amantadine* is also effective in the treatment of some cases of Parkinson's disease (see p. 87).]

1. **Mode of action:** The precise antiviral mechanism of *amantadine*

Lippincott's Illustrated Reviews: Pharmacology, Second Edition.
by Mary J. Mycek, Richard A. Harvey and Pamela C. Champe.
Lippincott Williams & Wilkins, Philadelphia, PA © 2000.

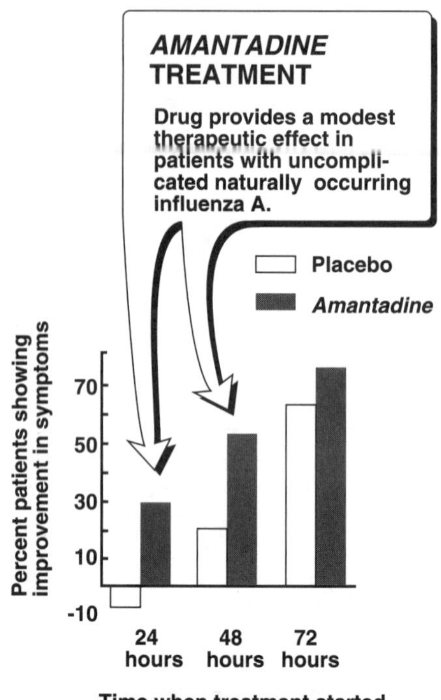

Figure 37.2
Improvement in symptoms of individuals with naturally occurring influenza infection treated with *amantadine*.

1. **Mode of action:** The precise antiviral mechanism of *amantadine* and *rimantadine* remains to be established. Recent evidence points to a blockade of the viral membrane matrix protein, M2, which functions as an ion channel. This channel is required for the fusion of the viral membrane with the cell membrane that ultimately forms the endosome (created when the virus is internalized by endocytosis). [Note: The acid environment of the endosome is required for viral uncoating.] These drugs may also interfere with the release of new virions.

2. **Resistance:** Influenza A resistance to *amantadine* and *rimantadine* is not a clinical problem as yet, although some viral isolates have shown a high incidence of resistance. Resistance has been shown to be due to a change in one amino acid of the M2 matrix protein. Cross-resistance occurs between the two drugs.

3. **Antiviral spectrum:** *Amantadine's* and *rimantadine's* therapeutic antiviral spectrum is limited to influenza A virus. Their effectiveness is directly related to their administration relative to infection, for example, these drugs are 70-90% effective in preventing infection if treatment is begun at the time of exposure to the virus. Neither impairs the immune response to influenza A vaccine, and either can be administered as a supplement to vaccination, thus providing protection until antibody response occurs (usually 2 weeks in healthy adults). Treatment is particularly useful in high-risk patients who have not been vaccinated, or during epidemics. In individuals with influenza A infection, both drugs reduce the duration and severity of systemic symptoms if started within the first 48 hours after exposure to the virus (Figure 37.2).

4. **Pharmacokinetics:** Both drugs are well absorbed orally. *Amantadine* distributes throughout the body and readily penetrates into the central nervous system (CNS), whereas *rimantadine* does not cross the blood-brain barrier to the same extent. *Amantadine* is not extensively metabolized. It is excreted into the urine and may accumulate to toxic levels in patients with renal failure. On the other hand, *rimantadine* is extensively metabolized by the liver. Metabolites and parent drug are eliminated by the kidney.

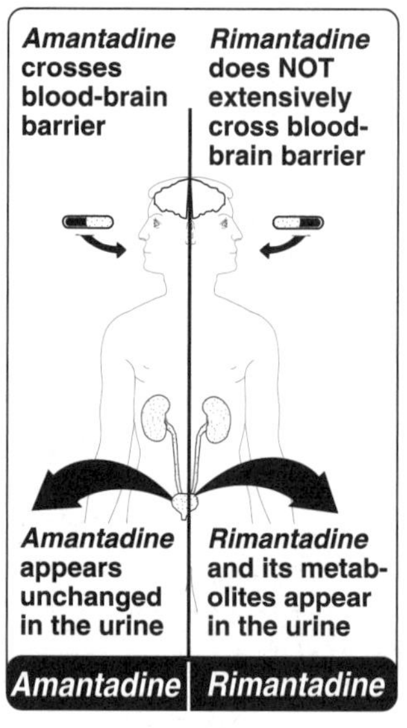

5. **Adverse effects:** *Amantadine's* side effects are mainly associated with the CNS. Minor neurologic symptoms include insomnia, dizziness, and ataxia. More serious side effects have been reported (for example, hallucinations, seizures). The drug should be employed cautiously in patients with psychiatric problems, cerebral atherosclerosis, renal impairment, or epilepsy. *Rimantadine* causes fewer CNS reactions since it does not efficiently cross the blood-brain barrier. *Amantadine* and *rimantadine* should be used with caution in pregnant and nursing mothers, because they have been found to be embryotoxic and teratogenic in rats.

B. Ribavirin

Ribavirin [rye ba VYE rin] is a synthetic guanosine analog. It is effective against a broad spectrum of RNA and DNA viruses.

1. **Mode of action:** The mode of action has been studied only for the influenza viruses. *Ribavirin* is first converted to the 5'-phosphate derivatives, the major product being the compound ribavirin-triphosphate (RTP), which has been postulated to exert its antiviral action by inhibiting viral mRNA synthesis. [Note: Rhinoviruses and enteroviruses, which contain preformed mRNA and do not need to synthesize mRNA in the host cell to initiate the infection, are relatively resistant to the action of *ribavirin*.]

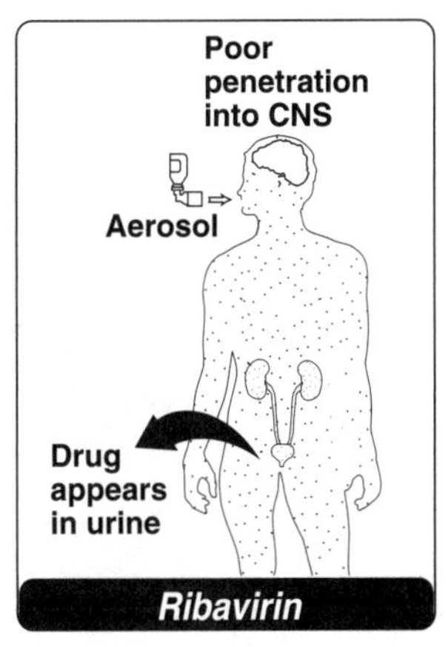
Poor penetration into CNS
Aerosol
Drug appears in urine
Ribavirin

2. **Antiviral spectrum:** *Ribavirin* is used in treating infants and young children infected with severe RSV infections. [Note: It is not indicated for use in adults.] Favorable responses of acute hepatitis A virus and influenza A and B infections have also been reported. *Ribavirin* may reduce the mortality and viremia of Lassa fever.

3. **Pharmacokinetics:** *Ribavirin* is effective orally and intravenously. Its current use is as an aerosol in certain respiratory viral conditions, such as the treatment of RSV infection. Studies of drug distribution in primates showed retention in all tissues, except brain. The drug and its metabolites are eliminated in the urine.

4. **Adverse effects:** Side effects reported for oral or parenteral use of *ribavirin* have included dose-dependent transient anemia in Lassa fever victims. Elevated bilirubin has been reported. The aerosol may be safer, although respiratory function in infants can deteriorate quickly after initiation of aerosol treatment and therefore, monitoring is essential. Because of teratogenic effects in experimental animals, *ribavirin* is contraindicated in pregnancy.

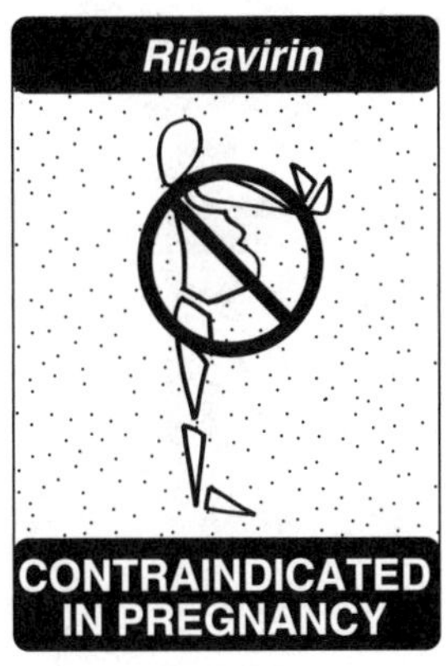
Ribavirin
CONTRAINDICATED IN PREGNANCY

III. TREATMENT OF HERPESVIRUS INFECTIONS

Herpesviruses are associated with a broad spectrum of diseases, e.g., cold sores, viral encephalitis, and genital infections, the latter being a hazard to the newborn during parturition. The drugs that are effective against these viruses exert their actions during the acute phase of viral infections and are without effect in the latent phase. Except for *foscarnet*, all are purine or pyrimidine analogs that inhibit viral DNA synthesis.

A. Acyclovir

Acyclovir [ay SYE kloe ver] (*acycloguanosine*) has become one of the most prescribed antiviral drugs because of its effectiveness against herpesviruses.

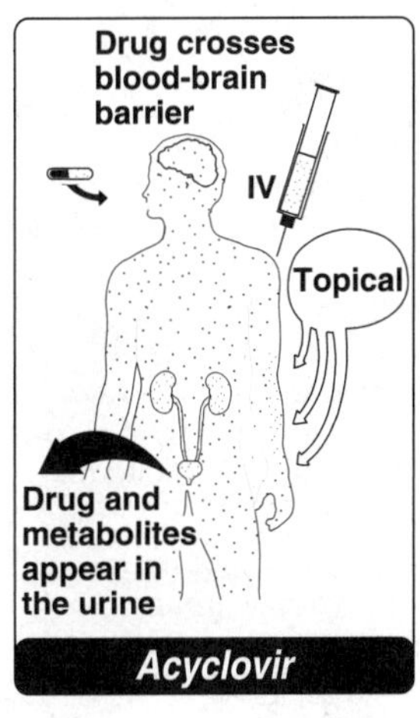
Drug crosses blood-brain barrier
IV
Topical
Drug and metabolites appear in the urine
Acyclovir

1. **Mode of action:** *Acyclovir*, a guanosine analog that lacks a true sugar moiety, is monophosphorylated in the cell by the herpes virus-encoded enzyme, thymidine kinase. Therefore virus-infected cells are most susceptible. The monophosphate analog is converted to the di- and triphosphate forms by the host cells (Figure 37.3). Acyclovir triphosphate competes with deoxyguanosine triphosphate (dGTP) as a substrate for viral DNA polymerase, and is itself incorporated into the viral DNA causing premature DNA-chain termination (see Figure 37.3). Irreversible binding of the *acyclovir*-containing template primer to viral DNA polymerase inactivates the enzyme. It is less effective against the host enzyme.

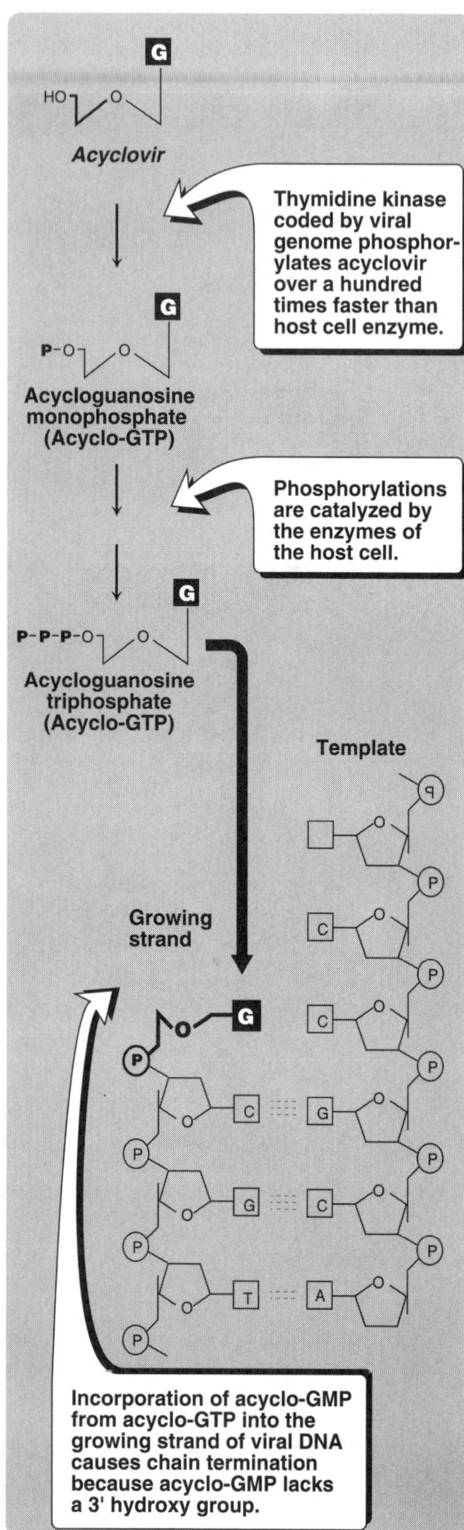

Figure 37.3
Incorporation into viral DNA, causing chain termination.

2. **Resistance:** Altered or deficient thymidine kinase and DNA polymerases have been found in some resistant viral strains. [Note: Cytomegalovirus (CMV) is resistant because it lacks a specific viral thymidine kinase.]

3. **Antiviral spectrum:** *Acyclovir* has a greater specificity than *vidarabine* against herpesviruses. Herpes simplex virus-1 (HSV-1), HSV-2, varicella-zoster virus, and some Epstein-Barr virus-mediated infections are sensitive to *acyclovir*, but CMV is resistant. *Acyclovir* is the treatment of choice in herpes simplex encephalitis, and is more efficacious than *vidarabine* in increasing the rate of survival (Figure 37.4). The most common use of *acyclovir* is in therapy of genital herpes infections. [Note: In all cases, *acyclovir* inhibits only actively replicating viruses and has no effect on latent viruses.] It is also given prophylactically to seropositive patients before bone marrow and after heart transplants to protect such individuals during posttransplant immunosuppressive treatments.

4. **Pharmacokinetics:** Administration can be by an intravenous, oral, or topical route. The efficacy of topical applications is doubtful. The drug distributes well throughout the body, including the cerebrospinal fluid. *Acyclovir* is partially metabolized to an inactive product. Excretion into the urine occurs both by glomerular filtration and tubular secretion. *Acyclovir* accumulates in patients with renal failure.

5. **Adverse effects:** Side effects depend on the route of administration. For example, local irritation may occur from topical application; headache, diarrhea, nausea, and vomiting may result after oral administration; transient renal dysfunction may occur at high doses or in a dehydrated patient receiving the drug intravenously.

B. Ganciclovir (DHPG)

The lack of effect of available nucleoside analogs on cytomegalovirus (CMV) infection led to the synthesis of the *acyclovir* analog, *ganciclovir* [gan SYE kloe ver] (*9-[(1,3-dihydroxy-2-propoxy)methyl]guanine, DHPG*). It is currently available for treatment of cytomegalic retinitis in immunocompromised patients.

1. **Mode of action:** Like *acyclovir*, *ganciclovir* is activated through conversion to the nucleoside triphosphate by viral and cellular enzymes, the actual pathway depending on the virus. Cytomegalovirus is deficient in thymidine kinase, and therefore forms the triphosphate by another route. The nucleotide competitively inhibits viral DNA polymerase and can be incorporated into the DNA to decrease the rate of chain elongation.

2. **Resistance:** Resistant CMV strains have been detected, but the mechanism of resistance is not yet known.

3. **Antiviral spectrum:** Its activity in vitro is the same as that of *acyclovir*, but *ganciclovir* is approved only for treatment of cytomegalic retinitis.

4. **Pharmacokinetics:** *Ganciclovir* is administered intravenously and distributed throughout the body, including the cerebrospinal fluid. Excretion into the urine occurs through glomerular filtration and tubular secretion. Like *acyclovir*, *ganciclovir* accumulates in patients with renal failure.

5. **Adverse effects:** Adverse effects include severe, dose-dependent neutropenia. [Note: Combined treatment with *zidovudine* can result in additive neutropenia.] *Ganciclovir* is carcinogenic as well as embryotoxic and teratogenic in experimental animals.

C. Famciclovir

Famciclovir [fam SYE kloe ver], another acyclic analog of 2'-deoxyguanosine, is a prodrug that is metabolized to the active *penciclovir* (pen SYE kloe ver). The antiviral spectrum is similar to that of *ganciclovir* but it is presently approved only for treatment of acute herpes zoster. The drug is effective orally. Adverse effects include headaches and nausea. Studies in experimental animals have shown an increased incidence in mammary adenocarcinomas and testicular toxicity.

O
||
Na^+O^-–P–COO^-Na^+
|
Na^+O^-

Foscarnet sodium

D. Foscarnet

Unlike most of the antiviral agents, *foscarnet* [FOS car ney] is not a purine or pyrimidine analog; it is phosphonoformate, a pyrophosphate derivative. Despite its broad antiviral activity in vitro, it is approved only as a treatment for cytomegalic retinitis in immunocompromised HIV-infected patients, especially if the infection is resistant to *ganciclovir*. *Foscarnet* works by reversibly inhibiting viral DNA and RNA polymerases, thereby terminating chain elongation. Mutation of the polymerase structure is responsible for resistant viruses. [Note: Cross-resistance between *foscarnet* and *ganciclovir* or *acyclovir* is uncommon.] *Foscarnet* is poorly absorbed orally and must be injected intravenously, and must be given frequently to avoid relapse when levels fall. It is dispersed throughout the body, Greater than 10% enters the bone matrix from which it slowly leaves. The parent drug is eliminated by glomerular filtration and tubular secretion into the urine. Adverse effects include nephrotoxicity, anemia, nausea, and fever. Due to chelation with divalent cations, hypocalcemia, and hypomagnesemia are also seen. In addition, hypokalemia, hypophosphatemia, seizures, and arrhythmias have been reported.

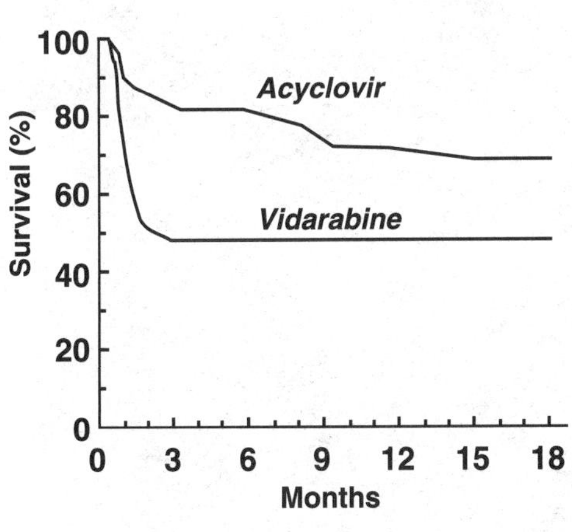

Figure 37.4
Comparison of survival in patients with biopsy-proved herpes simplex encephalitis treated with *vidarabine* or *acyclovir*.

E. Vidarabine (ara-A)

Vidarabine [vye DARE a been] (*arabinofuranosyl adenine, ara-A, adenine arabinoside*) is one of the most effective of the nucleoside analogs and is also the least toxic. However, it has been supplanted clinically by *acyclovir*, which is more efficacious and safe. Although *vidarabine* is active against herpes simplex virus type 1 (HSV-1), HSV-2, and varicella-zoster virus (VZV), its use is limited to treatment of immunocompromised patients with herpes simplex keratitis or encephalitis, or VZV infections. *Vidarabine*, an adenosine analog, is converted in the cell to its 5'-triphosphate analog (ara-ATP), which is postulated to inhibit viral DNA synthesis. Some resistant herpes virus

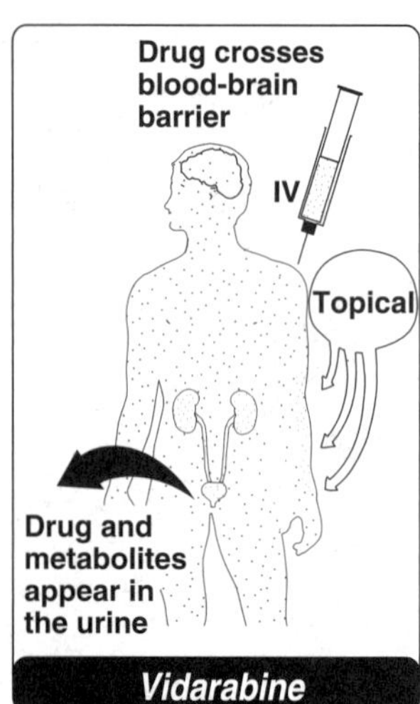
Drug crosses blood-brain barrier
IV
Topical
Drug and metabolites appear in the urine
Vidarabine

mutants have been detected that have altered DNA polymerase. To be effective systemically, poorly soluble *vidarabine* must be administered intravenously in large volumes over a prolonged time, usually 12 hours. *Vidarabine* penetrates into the brain and thus is effective in the treatment of herpes simplex encephalitis. *Vidarabine* ointment is effective in the treatment of herpetic and vaccinial keratitis and in herpes simplex keratoconjunctivitis. *Vidarabine* and its metabolites are found in the urine. Adverse effects during short-term use are not serious. CNS disturbances and fluid overload, however, can be a problem in patients with impaired hepatic or renal function.

F. Trifluridine

Trifluridine [try FLOO ri deen] has replaced the earlier drug, *idoxuridine* [eye dox Yoor i deen], in the topical treatment of keratoconjunctivitis due to herpes simplex viruses. Like *idoxuridine*, this pyrimidine analog is incorporated into the viral DNA to disrupt its function.

See p. 457 for a description of newly approved drugs, *penciclovir* and *cidofovir*.

IV. TREATMENT FOR AIDS

Presently six drugs are approved to fight human immunodeficiency virus (HIV) infection. Five are either pyrimidine or purine nucleoside analogs, and must be converted to their nucleotide forms to exert their antiviral effect. [Note: The 3' position of their deoxyribose moiety either lacks a hydroxyl group or is blocked by an azide substituent (Figure 37.5) thus preventing chain elongation.] The sixth drug is an HIV protease inhibitor. Although not curative, these agents interfere in the multiplication of the virus and slow progression of the disease to possibly prolong survival.

A. Zidovudine (3'-Azido-3'-Deoxythymidine, AZT)

One of the most effective drugs currently approved for treatment of HIV infection and AIDS is the pyrimidine analog, *3'-azido-3'-deoxythymidine* (*AZT*). *AZT* has the generic name of *zidovudine* [zye DOE vyoo deen]. *AZT* is presently employed in patients shown to have documented HIV infection. Improvement in immunologic status (increase in absolute number of helper-induced T cells) has been reported. Most encouraging is the protection of fetuses from becoming infected by the virus when HIV-infected pregnant mothers have been maintained on the drug.

1. **Mode of action:** *AZT* must be converted to the corresponding nucleoside triphosphate by mammallan thymidine kinase in order for it to exert its antiviral activity. AZT-triphosphate is then incorporated into the growing chain of viral (but not mammalian nuclear) DNA by reverse transcriptase[1]. Because *AZT* lacks a hydroxyl at the 3' position, another 5'-3' phosphodiester linkage cannot be formed. Thus, synthesis of the DNA chain is terminated, and replication of the virus cannot take place. The relative lack of discrimination of the viral reverse transcriptase is believed to favor the introduction of the *AZT* into the viral-catalyzed process; the cellular DNA polymerase is more selective. In addition, the phosphory-

[1]See p. 372 for Infolink references to other books in this series.

lation of deoxythymidylic acid (dTMP) to the corresponding diphosphate (dTDP) is inhibited by the azido-thymidine monophosphate (AZT-MP).

2. **Resistance:** Effectiveness decreases with time. Some resistant isolates have mutated reverse transcriptase, which has a lower affinity for the AZT-triphosphate.

3. **Antiviral spectrum:** Presently the only clinical use for *AZT* is in the treatment of patients infected with HIV.

4. **Pharmacokinetics:** The drug is well absorbed after oral administration. If taken with food, peak levels may be lower but total drug absorbed is not affected. Penetration across the blood-brain barrier is excellent, and the drug has a half-life of 1 hour. Most of the *AZT* is glucuronidated by the liver and then excreted in the urine.

5. **Adverse effects:** In spite of its seeming specificity, *AZT* is toxic to bone marrow. For example, severe anemia and leukopenia occur in patients receiving high doses. Headaches are also common. Seizures have been reported in patients with advanced AIDS. *AZT's* toxicity is potentiated if glucuronidation is decreased by co-administration of drugs like *probenecid*, *acetaminophen*, *lorazepam*, *indomethacin*, and *cimetidine*. [Note: These drugs are themselves glucuronidated and thus can interfere with the glucuronidation of *AZT*. They should be avoided or used with caution in patients receiving *AZT*.]

B. Didanosine (ddI)

The second drug approved to treat HIV-1 infection was *didanosine* [dye DAH no seen] (*dideoxyinosine*, *ddI*), which is also missing the 3' hydroxyl. It is not recommended for initial treatment of HIV disease, but rather is used for *AZT*-resistant HIV infections.

1. **Mechanism of action:** Upon entry into the host cell, *didanosine* is biotransformed into *ddATP* through a series of reactions that involve phosphorylation of the *ddI*, amination to ddAMP and further phosphorylation. The resulting *ddATP* is incorporated into the DNA chain like *AZT*, causing termination of chain elongation.

2. **Resistance:** Viral isolates from patients who have undergone prolonged therapy with *ddI* contain reverse transcriptase with amino acid substitutions. Cross-resistance with the other nucleoside agents has not been reported.

3. **Antiviral spectrum:** Its activity is confined to retroviruses, specifically HIV-1.

4. **Pharmacokinetics:** Due to its acid lability, *didanosine* is administered as either chewable, buffered tablets or in a buffered solution. Absorption is good if taken in the fasting state; food causes decreased absorption. The drug penetrates into the CSF but to a lesser extent than *AZT*. About 55% of the parent drug appears in the urine.

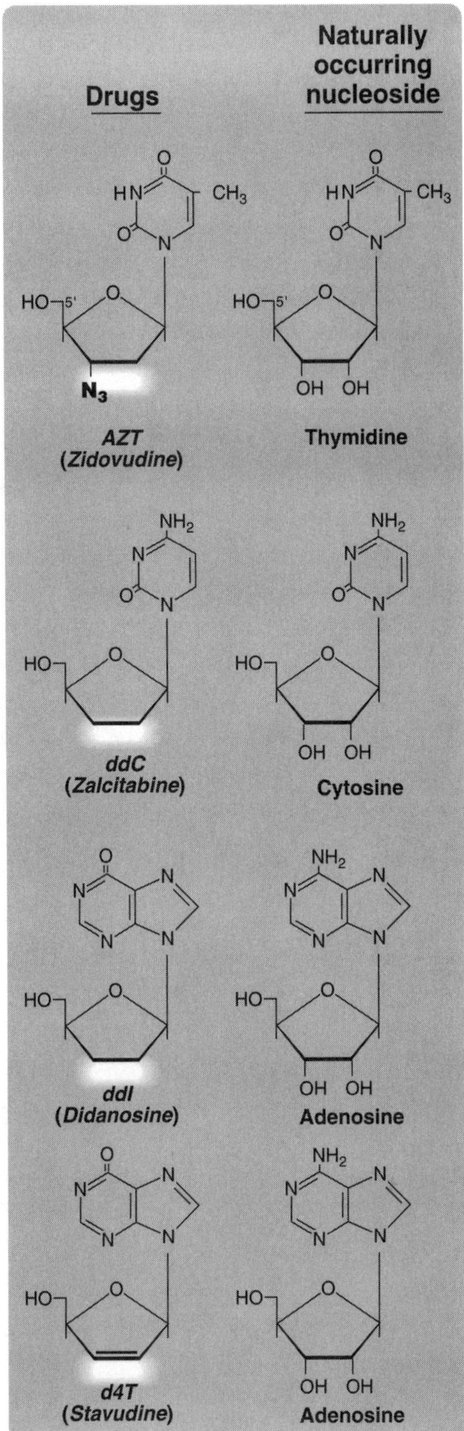

Figure 37.5
Nucleoside analogues used in HIV therapy.

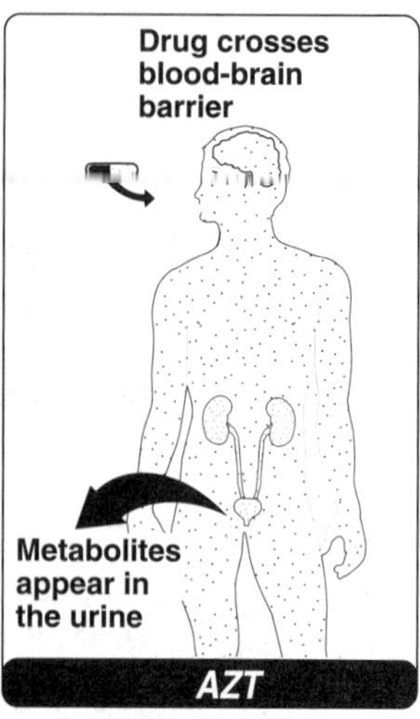
Drug crosses blood-brain barrier
Metabolites appear in the urine
AZT

5. **Adverse effects:** Pancreatitis, which may be fatal, is a major toxicity of *ddI* treatment, and requires monitoring of serum amylase. The dose-limiting toxicity of *didanosine* is peripheral neuropathy. [Note: The buffering of stomach contents may interfere in the absorption of other drugs that require an acidic milieu for absorption, such as *ketoconazole*.]

C. Zalcitabine (ddC)

An analog of deoxycytidine, *zalcitabine* [zal SIT a been] (*dideoxycytidine*, *ddC*) is used either in conjunction with *AZT* or as monotherapy in patients who cannot tolerate *AZT*. Like other drugs in this group, it is converted to the active triphosphate (ddCTP), which terminates chain elongation when incorporated into viral DNA and also inhibits viral reverse transcriptase. Point mutations in the reverse transcriptase lead to resistance. *Zalcitabine* is very well absorbed orally, but food or MAALOX TC reduces absorption. The drug is distributed throughout the body but penetration into the CSF is lower than that obtained with *AZT*. Some of the drug is metabolized to the inactive dideoxyuridine (ddU). The urine is the main route of excretion of *ddC,* although fecal elimination of *ddC*, along with its metabolite ddU, occurs. Rash and stomatitis are common but resolve on continued treatment. Peripheral neuropathy is the major toxicity and is probably a consequence of the inhibition of the mammalian mitochondrial DNA polymerase γ. Pancreatitis resulting in death has occurred, especially if *ddC* is given with *pentamidine* (see p. 354).

D. Stavudine (d4T)

Stavudine [STAY vue deen] is an analog of thymidine in which a double bond joins the 2' and 3' carbon of the sugar (see Figure 37.5. Like the others in this group *stavudine* must be converted by the intracellular kinases to the triphosphate (d4TTP) which inhibits the reverse-transcriptase to cause DNA chain termination. In addition it inhibits cellular enzymes such as the β and γ DNA polymerases thus reducing mitochondrial DNA synthesis. It is too early to assess the clinical advantage or resistance to *stavudine*. The drug is almost completely absorbed on oral ingestion and is not affected by food. *Stavudine* penetrates the blood brain barrier. About half the parent drug can be accounted for in the urine. Renal impairment interferes with clearance. The major and most common clinical toxicity is peripheral neuropathy.

E. Lamivudine (3TC)

Recently, *lamivudine* [LAM ih vue deen] or (-)-2'-deoxy-3'-thiacytidine (3TC) has been approved for treatment of HIV in combination with zidovudine. This dideoxynucleoside terminates the synthesis of the proviral DNA chain and also inhibits reverse-transcriptase of both HIV and hepatitis B virus (HBV). However, it does not affect mitochondrial DNA synthesis or bone marrow precursor cells. Resistance to *zidovudine* develops more slowly with the combination. *Lamivudine* has good bioavailability on oral administration and depends on the kidney for excretion. Though generally well tolerated, pancreatitis develops in a significant number of pediatric patients, requiring stoppage of the drug. Administration with trimethoprim/sulfamethoxazole increases the area under the curve (AUC) of *lamivudine*.

F. HIV Protease Inhibitors

Development of toxicity of and resistance to the reverse-transcriptase inhibitors led to the targeting of the HIV protease. This aspartate proteinase is essential for the final step of viral proliferation. It is encoded in the HIV genome, and thus is absent in uninfected CD4 cells. It is translated as part of the large viral precursor protein, and undergoes autocatlytic cleavage from this precursor. The active enzyme then hydrolytically attacks the precursor protein, generating proteins that are necessary to the virus. The HIV protease inhibitors interfere with this process, and lead to the assembly of nonfunctional virions (Figure 37.6). Four protease inhibitors have been approved for treatment of HIV-1 infections, and several more are in development. These potent drugs have revolutionized HIV therapy, reducing infections by opportunistic organisms, and prolonging and improving the lives of most patients. As with all antiretroviral therapy, surrogate markers are used to evaluate the efficacy of these agents. These markers are 1) the number of viral RNA copies in the plasma, and 2) the number of CD4+ cells.

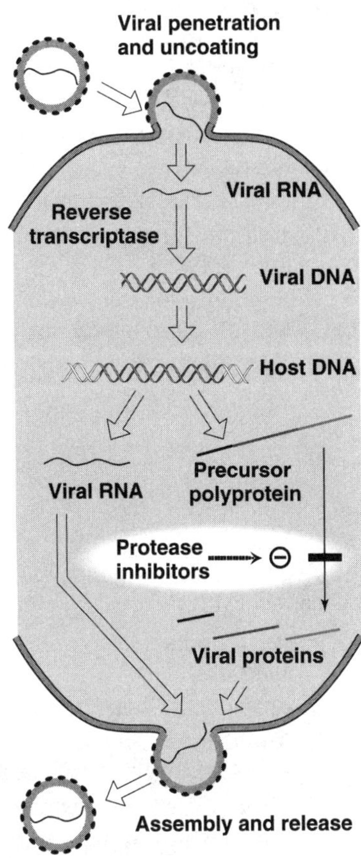

Figure 37.6
Role of HIV protease in viral replication.

Five HIV protease inhibitors have been approved— *saquinavir* [sah KWIN a veer], *ritonavir* [rih TONE a veer], *indinavir* [in DIN a veer], *nelfinavir* [nel FIN a veer] and *amprenavir* [am PREN a veer]. These drugs are described in detail on p. 461. It is critical that these drugs be given in dosages high enough to completely suppress viral replication, otherwise resistant virus can emerge. They are frequently given in combination with *zidovudine* and *lamivudine*. Some cross-resistance occurs with the protease inhibitors. Cessation of treatment results in reemergence of the virus. .

See p. 458-463 for a description of newly approved protease inhibitors and non-nucleoside reverse transcriptase inhibitors.

V. INTERFERON

Interferon [in ter FEER on] is a family of naturally occurring inducible glycoproteins that interfere with the ability of viruses to infect cells. Although *interferon* inhibits the growth of many viruses in vitro, its activity in vivo against viruses has been disappointing. At present the interferons are synthesized by recombinant DNA technology. At least three types of *interferon* exist, α, β, and γ (Figure 37.7). One of the 15 α-interferons, α-2b has been approved for treatment of hepatitis B and C, as well as against cancers such as hairy cell leukemia and Kaposi's sarcoma (see p. 398). Its antiviral mechanism is incompletely understood but appears to involve the induction of host cell enzymes (e.g., a protein kinase, 2',5'-oligoadenylate synthase, and a phosphodiesterase) that inhibit viral RNA translation, and ultimately lead to the degradation of viral mRNA and tRNA. *Interferon* is given intravenously and crosses into the CSF. Adverse effects include fever, lethargy, bone marrow depression, cardiovascular problems such as congestive heart failure, and acute hypersensitivity reactions. Hepatic failure and pulmonary infiltrates are rare.

Interferon-α	*Interferon-β*	*Interferon-γ*
Chronic hepatitis B and C	**Relapsing-remitting multiple sclerosis**	**Chronic granulo-matous disease**
Genital warts caused by papilloma-virus		
Hairy-cell leukemia		
Kaposi's sarcoma		

Figure 37.7
Some approved indications for *interferons*.

Choose the ONE best answer.

37.1 All of the following statements about acyclovir are correct EXCEPT:

A. It is the treatment of choice for influenza infections.
B. It is incorporated into the viral DNA causing premature DNA chain termination.
C. It is the treatment of choice in herpes simplex encephalitis.
D. It reduces the duration of lesions associated with genital herpes infections.
E. It inhibits only actively replicating viruses, not latent ones.

Correct choice = A. Amantadine is the drug of choice for influenza infections.

37.2 All of the following statements about amantadine are correct EXCEPT:

A. It is effective in the prophylaxis of influenza A infections.
B. It causes CNS disturbances at high doses.
C. It reduces the duration and severity of systemic symptoms of active influenza A.
D. It is extensively metabolized.
E. It is effective in the treatment of some cases of Parkinson's disease.

Correct choice = D. Amantadine is effective in the prophylaxis of influenza A infections only if administered before exposure to the virus. If amantadine is started within 48 hr after the onset of the disease, the drug will reduce the duration and severity of systemic symptoms of influenza A infection.

37.3 Which one of the following antiviral agents exhibits the greatest selective toxicity for the invading virus?

A. Interferon
B. Amantadine.
C. Acyclovir.
D. Zidovudine.
E. Ribavirin.

Correct answer = C. Acyclovir is monophosphorylated in the cell by the herpesvirus-coded enzyme, thymidine kinase. Thus, uninfected cells show little activation of the drug, and the toxicity is therefore highly selective for herpesvirus-infected cells

37.4 All of the following statements about zidovudine (AZT) are correct EXCEPT:

A. It must be converted to the nucleotide form to express its antiviral activity.
B. It is incorporated into growing viral but not mammalian nuclear DNA.
C. It is currently used to treat severe herpesvirus and respiratory syncytial virus infections as well as AIDS.
D. It is toxic to bone marrow and causes adverse hematologic effects.
E. It penetrates the CNS.

Correct choice = C. AZT is currently used only in the treatment of HIV infections. It is converted to the nucleotide (active) form by mammalian thymidine kinase. The viral reverse transcriptase then favors introduction of the drug into viral DNA; cellular DNA polymerases are more selective.

Questions 37.5 - 37.7: For each numbered phrase, select the ONE drug (A-E) that is most closely associated with it. Each drug (A-E) may be selected once, more than once, or not at all.

A. Amantadine
B. Zidovudine (AZT)
C. Ribavirin
D. Vidarabine
E. Ganciclovir

37.5 It is used solely in the treatment of influenza A infections.

Correct answer = A (amantadine).

37.6 It is an adenosine analog that is active against all members of the herpesvirus group that infects humans.

Correct answer = D (vidarabine).

37.7 It is used in the treatment of cytomegalovirus infections in immunocompromised patients

Correct answer = E (ganciclovir).

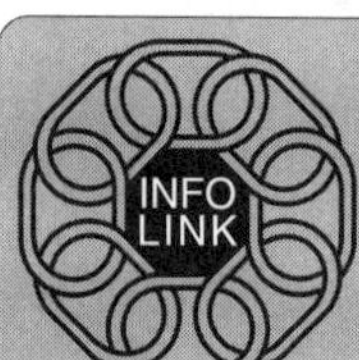

[1]See p. 407 in **Biochemistry** (2nd ed.) for a discussion of reverse transcriptase.

Anticancer Drugs

38

I. OVERVIEW

It is estimated that 25% of the population of the United States will face a cancer diagnosis during their lifetime, with 1 million new cancer patients diagnosed each year. Less than a quarter of these patients will be cured solely by surgery and/or local radiation. Most of the remainder will receive systemic chemotherapy at some time during their illness. (See Figure 38.1 for a summary of anticancer agents.) In a small fraction (approximately 10%) of cancer patients representing selected neoplasms, the chemotherapy will result in a cure or a prolonged remission. However, in most cases, the drug therapy will produce only a regression of the disease, and complications and/or relapse may eventually lead to death. Thus, the overall 5-year survival for cancer patients is about 40%, ranking cancer second only to cardiovascular disease as a cause of mortality.

II. PRINCIPLES OF CANCER CHEMOTHERAPY

Cancer chemotherapy strives to cause a lethal cytotoxic lesion that can arrest a tumor's progression. The attack is generally directed against metabolic sites essential to cell replication, for example, the availability of purine and pyrimidine precursors for DNA or RNA synthesis (Figure 38.2). Ideally these drugs should interfere only with cellular processes unique to the malignant cells. However, currently available anticancer drugs do not specifically recognize neoplastic cells, but rather affect all proliferating cells—both normal and abnormal. Therefore, almost all antitumor agents have a steep dose-response curve for both toxic and therapeutic effects; thus it is important to tailor the drug doses to the physical state of the patient.

A. Treatment strategies

1. **Goal of treatment:** The ultimate goal of chemotherapy is a cure, that is, long-term, disease-free survival. Cure requires the eradication of every neoplastic cell. If a cure is not attainable, then the goal becomes palliation (that is, alleviation of symptoms and avoidance of life-threatening toxicity), which allows the individual to maintain a "normal" existence. In either case, the neoplastic cell burden is initially reduced (debulking) either by surgery and/or radiation, followed

ANTICANCER DRUGS

- **ANTIMETABOLITES**
  - *Cytarabine*
  - *Fludarabine*
  - *5-Fluorouracil*
  - *6-Mercaptopurine*
  - *Methotrexate*
  - *6-Thioguanine*
- **ANTIBIOTICS**
  - *Bleomycin*
  - *Dactinomycin*
  - *Daunorubicin*
  - *Doxorubicin*
  - *Idarubicin*
  - *Plicamycin*
- **ALKYLATING AGENTS**
  - *Carmustine & lomustine*
  - *Cyclophosphamide & Ifosfamide*
  - *Mechlorethamine*
  - *Streptozotocin*
- **MICROTUBULE INHIBITORS**
  - *Navelbine*
  - *Paclitaxel (Taxol)*
  - *Vinblastine*
  - *Vincristine*
- **STEROID HORMONES AND THEIR ANTAGONISTS**
  - *Aminoglutethimides*
  - Estrogens
  - *Flutamide*
  - *Goserelin*
  - *Leuprolide*
  - *Prednisone*
  - *Tamoxifen*
- **OTHERS**
  - *Asparaginase*
  - *Cisplatin & Carboplatin*
  - *Etoposide*
  - *Interferons*
  - *Procarbazine*

Figure 38.1
Summary of cancer chemotherapy agents. See Pharmacology update, p. 463, for additional drugs.

Lippincott's Illustrated Reviews: Pharmacology, Second Edition.
by Mary J. Mycek, Richard A. Harvey and Pamela C. Champe.
Lippincott Williams & Wilkins, Philadelphia, PA © 2000.

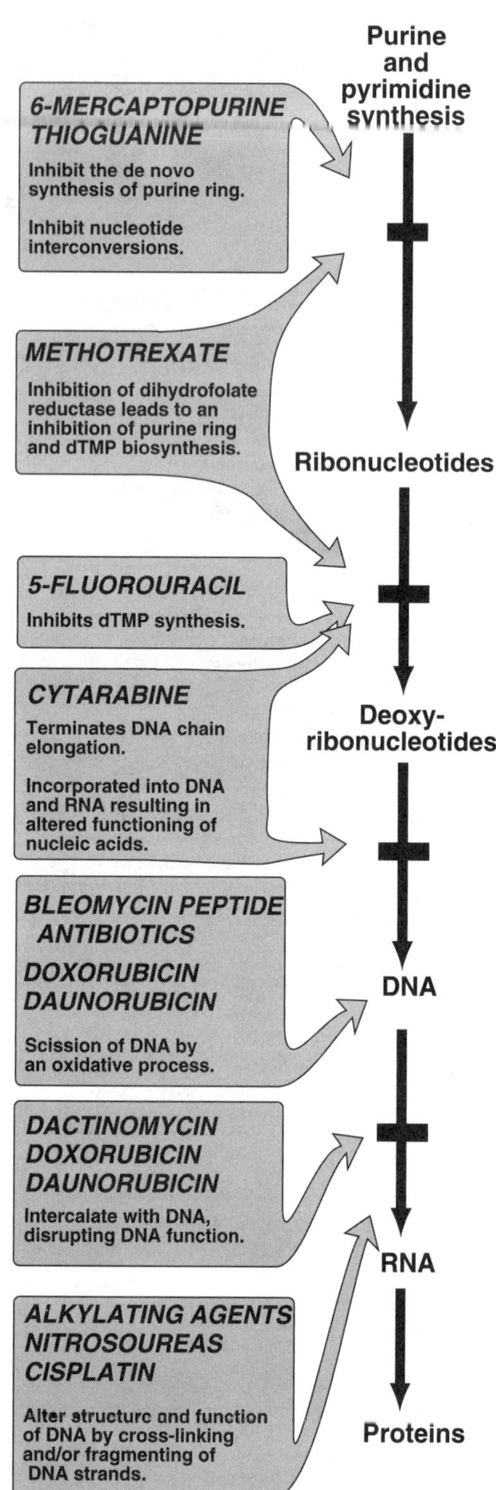

Figure 38.2
Examples of chemotherapeutic agents affecting the availability of RNA and DNA precursors.

by chemotherapy, immunotherapy, or a combination of these treatment modalities (Figure 38.3).

2. **Indications for treatment:** Chemotherapy is indicated when neoplasms are disseminated and not amenable to surgery. Chemotherapy is also used as a supplement to surgery and radiation treatment to attack micrometastases. [Note: Tumors most susceptible to current chemotherapy are undifferentiated and have high growth fractions.]

3. **Tumor susceptibility and the growth cycle:** The fraction of tumor cells that are in the replicative cycle ("growth fraction") influences their susceptibility to most cancer chemotherapeutic agents. Rapidly dividing cells are generally more sensitive to anticancer drugs, whereas nonproliferating cells (those in the G_0 phase) usually survive the toxic effects of these agents.

   a. **Cell-cycle specificity of drugs:** Both normal cells and tumor cells go through a growth cycle (Figure 38.4). However, normal and neoplastic tissue may differ in the number of cells that are in the various stages of the cycle. Chemotherapeutic agents that are effective only in replicating cells, that is those cells that are cycling, are said to be cell-cycle specific (see Figure 38.4), whereas other agents are cell-cycle nonspecific. The nonspecific drugs such as the alkylating agents, although generally more toxic in cycling cells, are also useful against tumors with a low percentage of replicating cells.

   b. **Tumor growth rate:** The growth rate of most tumors in vivo is initially rapid, but decreases as the tumor size increases because of the unavailability of nutrients and oxygen due to inadequate vascularization (see Figure 38.3). Reducing the tumor burden through surgery or radiation promotes the recruitment of the remaining cells into active proliferation and increases their susceptibility to chemotherapeutic agents.

B. Treatment regimens and scheduling

1. **Log kill:** Destruction of cancer cells by chemotherapeutic agents follows first-order kinetics, that is, a given dose of drug destroys a constant fraction of cells. The term "log kill" is used to describe this phenomenon. For example, a diagnosis of leukemia is generally made when there are about 10^9 (total) leukemic cells. Consequently if treatment leads to a 99.999% kill, then 0.001% of 10^9 cells (or 10^4 cells) would remain; this is equivalent to a 5-log kill. At this point the patient appears asymptomatic, that is, the patient is in remission (see Figure 38.3). For most bacterial infections, a 5-log (100,000-fold) reduction in the number of microorganisms results in a cure, since the immune system can eradicate the residual bacterial cells. However, tumor cells are not as readily eliminated, and additional treatment is required to totally eradicate the leukemic cell population.

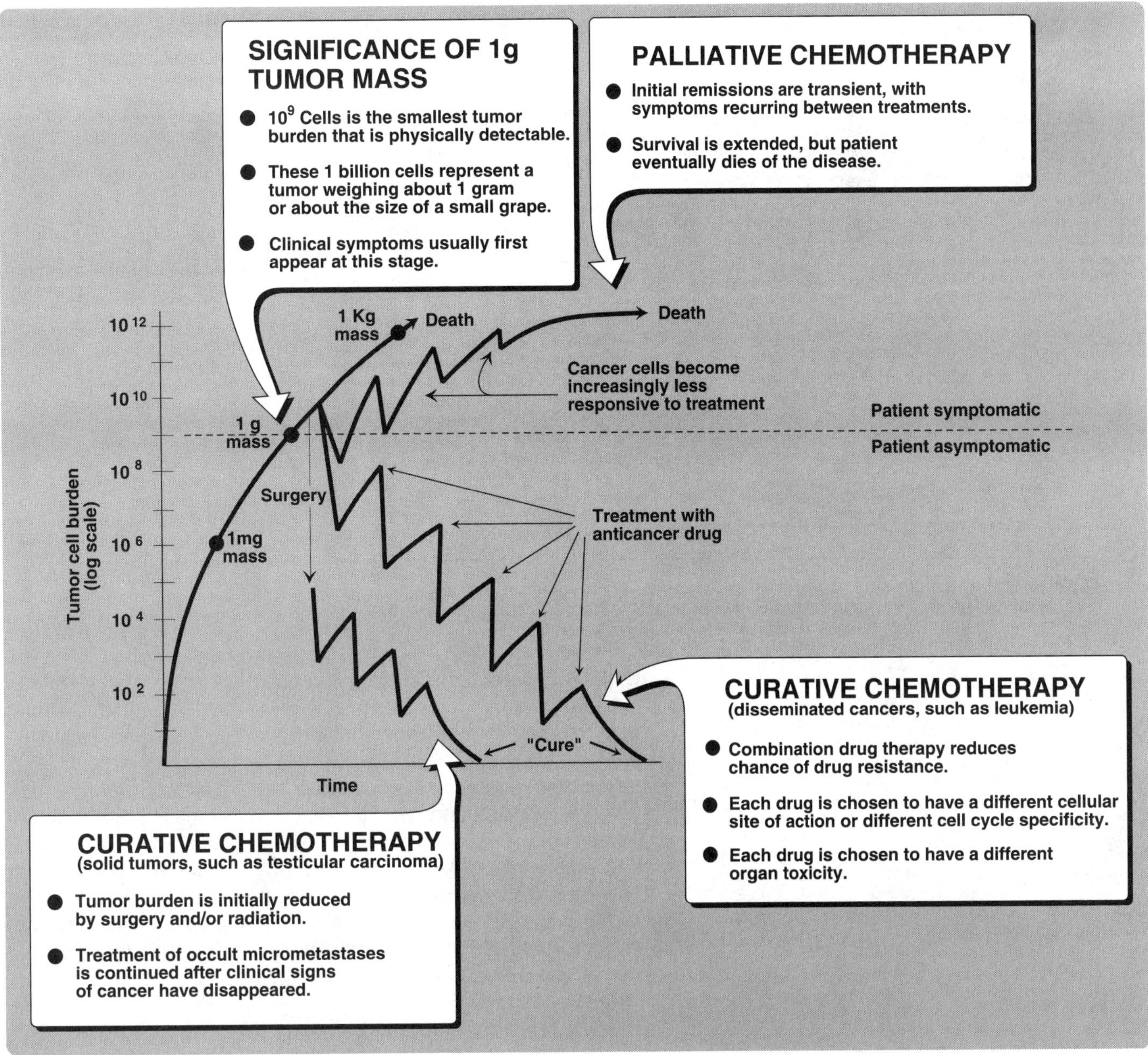

Figure 38.3
Effects of various treatments on the cancer cell burden in a hypothetical cancer patient.

2. **Pharmacologic sanctuaries:** Leukemic or other tumor cells find sanctuary in tissues, for example, the central nervous system (CNS), into which certain chemotherapeutic agents cannot enter because of transport constraints. Therefore, a patient may require irradiation of the craniospinal axis or intrathecal administration of drugs to eliminate the leukemic cells at that site. Similarly, drugs may be unable to penetrate certain areas of solid tumors.

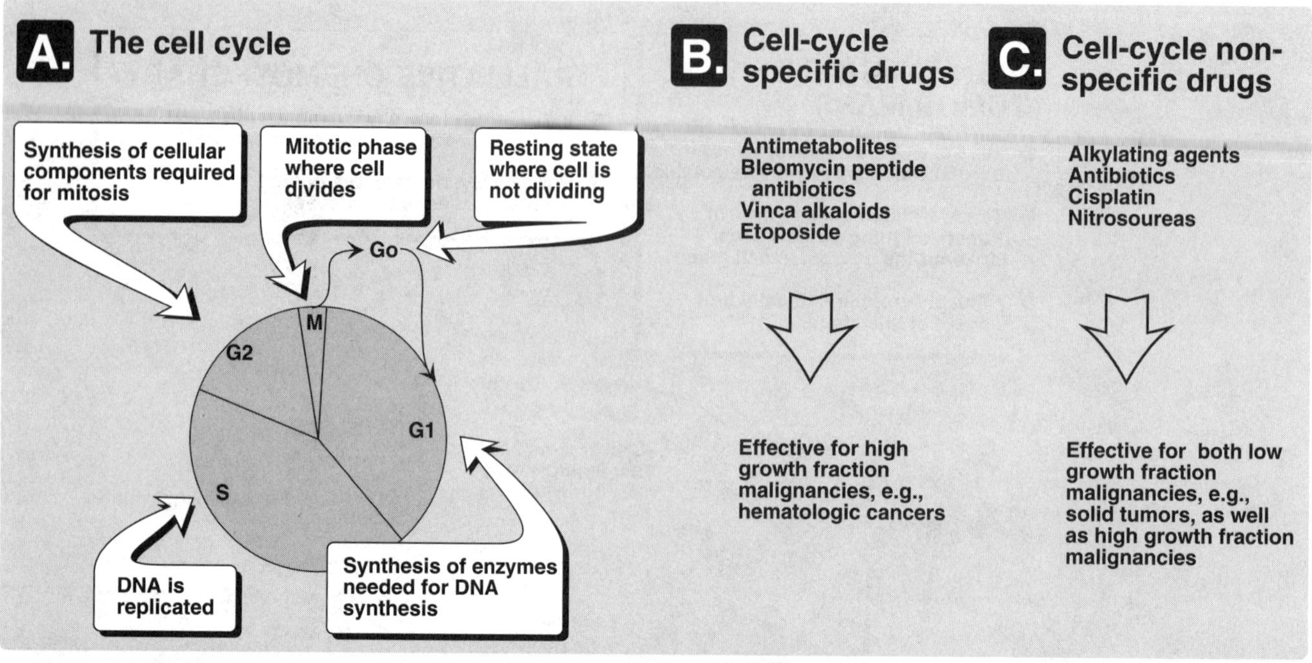

Figure 38.4
Effects of chemotherapeutic agents on the growth cycle of mammalian cells.

3. **Treatment protocols:** Combination chemotherapy is more effective than single-drug treatment in most cancers for which chemotherapy is effective.

   a. **Combinations of drugs:** Cytotoxic agents with qualitatively different toxicities and with different molecular sites and mechanisms of action are usually combined at full doses. This results in higher response rates due to both additive or potentiated cytotoxic effects and non-overlapping host toxicities. In contrast, agents with similar dose-limiting toxicities, such as myelosuppression, can be combined safely only by reducing the doses of each.

   b. **Advantages of drug combinations:** The advantages of such combinations are: 1) they provide maximal cell kill within the range of tolerated toxicity; 2) they are effective against a broader range of cell lines in the heterogeneous tumor population; and 3) they may slow or prevent the development of resistant cell lines.

   c. **Treatment protocols:** Many cancer treatment protocols have been developed; each one is applicable to a particular neoplastic state. They are usually identified by an acronym. For example, a common regimen called POMP, for the treatment of acute lymphocytic leukemia (ALL) consists of **P***rednisone* (see p. 393), **O***ncovin* (*vincristine*, p. 390), **M***ethotrexate* (see p. 378) and **P***urinethol* (*mercaptopurine*, p. 381). Therapy is scheduled intermittently to allow recovery of normal tissue, such as the patient's immune system, that has been affected by the drugs, thereby reducing the risk of serious infection.

C. Problems associated with chemotherapy

Cancer drugs are toxins that present a lethal threat to the cell. It is therefore not surprising that cells have evolved elaborate defense mechanisms to protect themselves from chemical toxins, including chemotherapeutic agents.

1. **Resistance:** Some neoplastic cells, for example, melanoma, are inherently resistant to most anticancer drugs. Other tumor types may be selected for or acquire resistance to the cytotoxic effects of the medication, particularly after prolonged administration of low drug doses. The development of drug resistance is minimized by short-term, intensive, intermittent therapy with combinations of drugs. Drug combinations are also effective against a broader range of resistant cell lines in the tumor population. A variety of mechanisms are responsible for drug resistance; each is considered separately under the particular drug.

2. **Multidrug Resistance:** Stepwise selection of an amplified gene that codes for a transmembrane protein (P-glycoprotein for "permeability" glycoprotein, Figure 38.5) is responsible for multidrug resistance (MDR). The resistance is due to ATP-dependent pumping of the drug out of the cell, associated with the presence of P-glycoprotein. Cross-resistance among structurally unrelated agents occurs. For example, cells resistant to the cytotoxic effects of the vinca alkaloids (see p. 390) are also resistant to *dactinomycin* (see p. 384) and the anthracycline antibiotics (see p.385) as well as to *colchicine* (see p. 416), and vice versa. These drugs are all naturally occurring substances, have a hydrophobic aromatic ring, and carry a positive charge at neutral pH. [Note: P-glycoprotein is normally expressed at low levels in most cell types, but higher levels are found in kidney, liver, pancreas, small intestine, colon, and adrenal gland. It has been suggested that its presence may account for the intrinsic resistance to chemotherapy observed in adenocarcinomas in these tissues.] Certain drugs (for example, *verapamil*, p. 187) can inhibit the pump and thus interfere with the efflux of the anticancer agent. However, these drugs are undesirable because of adverse pharmacological actions of their own. Pharmacologically inert pump blockers are being sought.

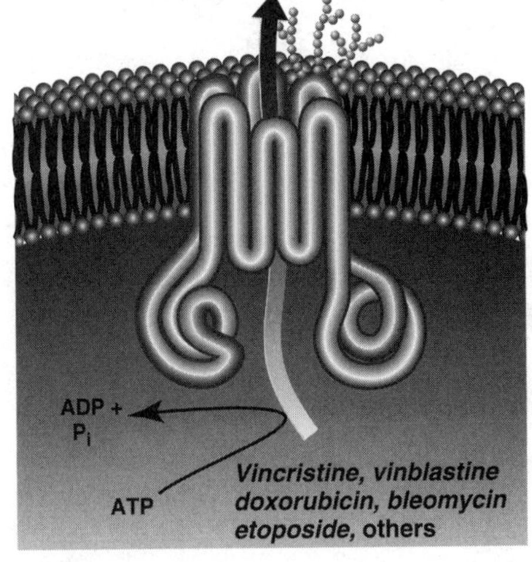

Figure 38.5
The six membrane-spanning loops of the P-glycoprotein form a central channel for the ATP-dependent pumping of drugs from the cell.

3. **Toxicity:** Therapy aimed at killing rapidly proliferating cells also affects normal cells undergoing rapid proliferation—for example, buccal mucosa, bone marrow, gastrointestinal (GI) mucosa, and hair cells—contributing to the toxic manifestations of chemotherapy.

   a. **Common adverse effects:** Most chemotherapeutic agents have a narrow therapeutic index. Severe vomiting, stomatitis, and alopecia occur to a lesser or greater extent during therapy with all antineoplastic agents. Vomiting can sometimes be controlled by administration of antiemetic drugs (see p. 241). Some toxicities such as myelosuppression, which predisposes to infection, are common to many chemotherapeutic agents (Figure 38.6), whereas other adverse reactions are confined to specific agents, for example, cardiotoxicity with *doxorubicin* (see p. 385) and pulmonary fibrosis with *bleomycin* (see p. 386).

b. **Duration of adverse effects:** The duration of the side effects varies widely. For example, alopecia is transient, but the cardiac, pulmonary, and bladder toxicities are irreversible.

c. **Minimizing adverse effects:** Some toxic reactions may be ameliorated by interventions, such as perfusing the tumor locally (for example, a sarcoma of the arm), removing some of the patient's marrow prior to intensive treatment then reimplanting it, or promoting intensive diuresis to prevent bladder toxicities. The megaloblastic anemia that occurs with *methotrexate* (see below) can be effectively counteracted by administering *folinic acid* (*leucovorin, 5-formyltetrahydrofolic acid*, p. 379). With the availability of human granulocyte colony stimulating factor (*filgrastim*), the neutropenia associated with treatment of cancer by many drugs can be partially reversed.

3. **Treatment-induced tumors:** Since most antineoplastic agents are mutagens, neoplasms (for example, acute nonlymphocytic leukemia) may arise 10 or more years after the original cancer was cured. Treatment-induced neoplasms are especially a problem after therapy with alkylating agents (see p. 387).

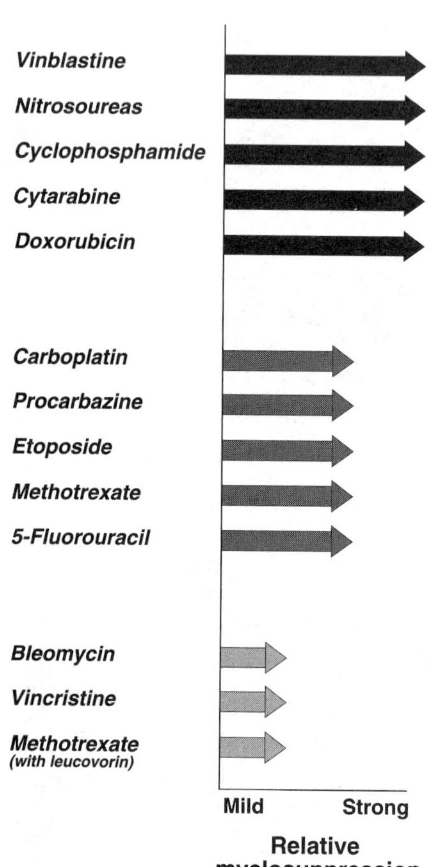

Figure 38.6
Comparison of myelosuppressive potential of anticancer drugs.

III. ANTIMETABOLITES

Antimetabolites are structurally related to normal cellular components. They generally interfere with the availability of normal purine or pyrimidine nucleotide precursors by inhibiting their synthesis or by competing with them in DNA or RNA synthesis. Their maximal cytotoxic effects are S-phase (and therefore cell-cycle) specific.

A. Methotrexate

Methotrexate [meth oh TREX ate] (*MTX*) is structurally related to folic acid and acts as an antagonist of that vitamin by inhibiting dihydrofolate reductase[1], the enzyme that converts folic acid to its active, coenzyme form, tetrahydrofolic acid (FH_4); it therefore acts as an antagonist of that vitamin. Folate plays a central role in a variety of metabolic reactions involving the transfer of one-carbon units. (Figure 38.7)[2].

1. **Site of action**

a. **Inhibition of dihydrofolate reductase:** After absorption of folic acid from dietary sources or from that produced by intestinal flora, the vitamin undergoes reduction to the tetrahydrofolate form (FH4) by the intracellular NADPH-dependent dihydrofolate reductase. *Methotrexate* enters the cell by an active transport process, which normally mediates the entry of N5-methyl FH4. At high MTX concentrations, the drug can diffuse into the

[1,2]See p. 400 for Infolink references to other books in this series.

cell. *MTX* has an unusually strong affinity for dihydrofolate reductase, and effectively inhibits the enzyme. Its inhibition can only be reversed by a thousand-fold excess of the natural substrate, dihydrofolate (FH_2, see Figure 38.7) or by administration of *leucovorin*, which bypasses the blocked enzyme and replenishes the folate pool. [Note: *Leucovorin*, or *folinic acid*, is the N^5-formyl group-carrying form of FH_4.]

b. **Consequences of decreased FH4:** Inhibition of dihydrofolate reductase deprives the cell of the various folate coenzymes and leads to decreased biosynthesis of thymidylic acid, methionine and serine, and the purines (adenine and guanine), and thus eventually to depressed DNA, RNA and protein synthesis and to cell death (see Figure 38.7).

c. **Polyglutamated MTX:** Like tetrahydrofolate itself, MTX becomes polyglutamated within the cell, a process that favors intracellular retention of the compound due to its larger size and increased negative charge (see below).

2. **Resistance:** Nonproliferating cells are resistant to *methotrexate*. Resistance in neoplastic cells can be due to amplification (production of additional copies) of the gene that codes for dihydrofolate reductase resulting in increased levels of this enzyme. The enzyme affinity for MTX may also be diminished. Resistance can also occur from a reduced influx of *MTX*, apparently caused by a change in the carrier-mediated transport responsible for pumping *methotrexate* into the cell.

3. **Therapeutic applications:** *Methotrexate,* often in combination with other drugs, is effective against acute lymphocytic leukemia, choriocarcinoma, Burkitt's lymphoma in children, breast cancer, and head and neck carcinomas. High-dose *MTX* is curative for osteogenic sarcoma and choriocarcinoma; treatment is followed by administration of *leucovorin* ("citrovorum factor") to rescue the bone marrow (see Figure 38.7, and the discussion of adverse effects, p. 380). In addition, low-dose *MTX* is effective as a single agent against certain inflammatory diseases, such as severe psoriasis and rheumatoid arthritis. These patients require close monitoring for possible toxic sequelae.

4. **Pharmacokinetics:**

a. **Administration and distribution:** *Methotrexate* is readily absorbed at low doses from the GI tract, but it can also be administered by intramuscular (IM), intravenous (IV), and intrathecal routes. [Note: Because *MTX* does not penetrate the blood-brain barrier, it is administered intrathecally to destroy neoplastic cells in the central sanctuary sites.] High concentrations of the drug are found in the intestinal epithelium, liver and kidney, as well as in ascites and pleural effusions. *MTX* is also distributed to the skin.

b. **Fate:** Although folates found in the blood have a single terminal glutamate, most intracellular folates are converted to

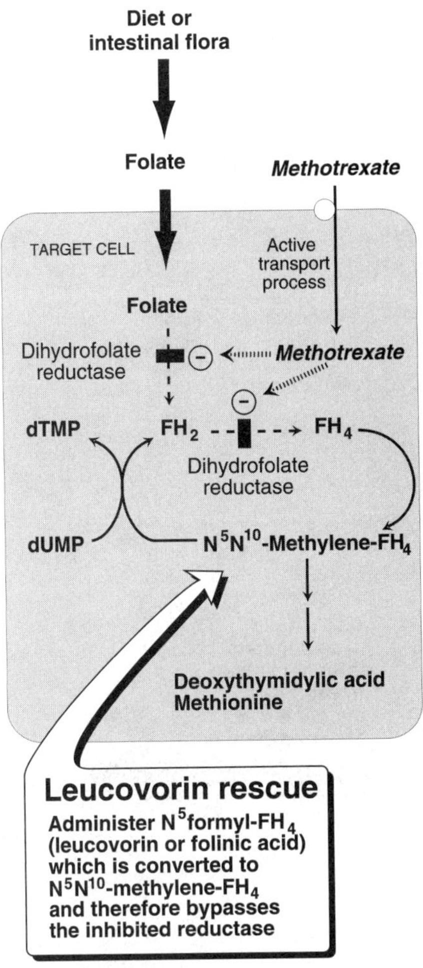

Figure 38.7
Mechanism of action of *methotrexate* and the effect of administration of leucovorin [FH_2 = dihydrofolate; FH_4 = tetrahydrofolate].

polyglutamates. These are preferentially retained inside the cells and are usually more efficient cofactors than are the monoglutamates. *Methotrexate* is also metabolized to poly-glutamate derivatives. This property is important, because the polyglutamates, which also inhibit dihydrofolate reductase, remain within the cell even in the absence of extracellular drug. This is in contrast to *MTX* per se, which rapidly leaves the cell as the extracellular drug levels fall. High doses of *methotrexate* undergo hydroxylation at the 7 position. This derivative is less water soluble, and may lead to crystalluria. Therefore, it is important to keep the urine alkaline and the patient well hydrated to avoid renal toxicity. Excretion of the parent drug and the 7-OH metabolite occurs via the urine.

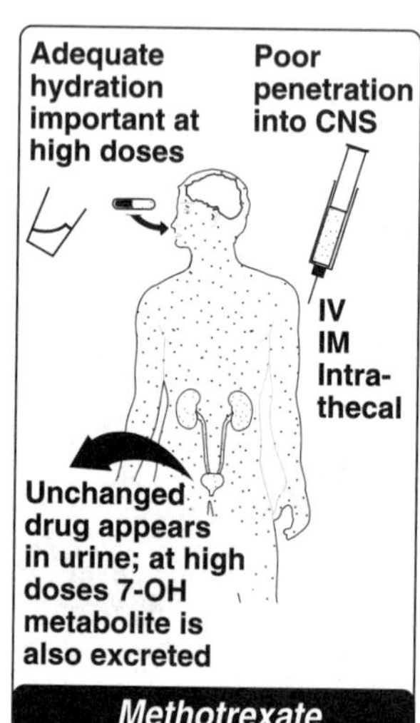
Adequate hydration important at high doses
Poor penetration into CNS
IV
IM
Intra-thecal
Unchanged drug appears in urine; at high doses 7-OH metabolite is also excreted
Methotrexate

5. **Adverse effects:**

a. **Commonly observed toxicities:** Most frequent toxicities are stomatitis, myelosuppression, erythema, rash, urticaria, alopecia, nausea, vomiting, and diarrhea. Some of these can be prevented or reversed by administering *leucovorin* (see Figure 38.7), which is taken up more readily by normal cells than by tumor cells. Doses of *leucovorin* must be kept minimal to avoid interference with the antitumor action of the *methotrexate*.

b. **Renal damage:** Although uncommon during conventional therapy, renal damage is a complication of high-dose *methotrexate*.

c. **Hepatic function:** Hepatic function should be monitored. Long-term use may lead to fibrosis.

d. **Pulmonary toxicity:** Children being maintained on *methotrexate* may develop cough, dyspnea, fever, and cyanosis. Infiltrates are seen on x-ray. This toxicity is reversible on suspension of the drug.

e. **Neurologic toxicities:** These are associated with intrathecal administration, and include subacute meningeal irritation, stiff neck, headache, and fever. Seizures, encephalopathy, or paraplegia occur rarely. Long-lasting effects, such as learning disabilities, have been seen in children who received the drug by this route.

f. **Contraindications:** Because *methotrexate* is teratogenic and an abortifacient it should be avoided in pregnancy. [Note: It is used with *misoprostol* (see p. 419) to induce abortion.]

B. 6-Mercaptopurine

The drug *6-mercaptopurine* [mer kap toe PYOOR een] (*6-MP*) is the thiol analog of hypoxanthine. It and *thioguanine* (*6-TG*) were the first purine analogs to prove beneficial for treating neoplastic disease. *Azathioprine*, an immunosuppressant, exerts its effects after conversion to *6-MP*.

1. **Site of action:**

a. **Formation of nucleotide:** To exert its antileukemic effect, *6-mercaptopurine* must penetrate target cells and be converted to the corresponding nucleotide, 6-mercaptopurine ribose phosphate (6-MPRP better known as 6-thioinosinic acid, or thio-IMP, Figure 38.8). The addition of the ribose phosphate is catalyzed by the salvage pathway enzyme, hypoxanthine-guanine phosphoribosyl transferase (HGPRT).[3]

b. **Inhibition of purine synthesis:** Although the nature of the exact cytotoxic step is not known, the unnatural nucleotide, thio-IMP, like AMP, can feedback to inhibit the first step of de novo purine ring biosynthesis as well as formation of AMP and xanthinylic acid (XMP) from inosinic acid (IMP).[4]

c. **Incorporation into nucleic acids:** Dysfunctional RNA and DNA result from incorporation of guanylate analogs generated from the unnatural nucleotides. Thio-IMP is dehydrogenated to thio-GMP, which after phosphorylation to di- and triphosphates, can be incorporated into RNA. The deoxyribonucleotide analogs that are also formed are incorporated into DNA.

2. **Resistance:** Resistance is associated with (1) an inability to biotransform *6-MP* to the corresponding nucleotide because of decreased levels of HGPRT (for example, in Lesch-Nyhan syndrome in which patients lack this enzyme); (2) an increased dephosphorylation; or (3) increased metabolism of the drug to thiouric acid.

3. **Therapeutic applications:** *6-MP* is used principally in the maintenance of remission in acute lymphoblastic leukemia (ALL).

4. **Pharmacokinetics**

a. **Administration and metabolism:** Absorption by the oral route is erratic. The drug is widely distributed throughout the body except for the cerebrospinal fluid. *6-MP* undergoes metabolism in the liver to the 6-methylmercaptopurine ($S\text{-}CH_3$) derivative or to thiouric acid. The latter reaction is catalyzed by xanthine oxidase. Because *allopurinol* (see p. 417), a xanthine oxidase[5] inhibitor, is frequently administered to cancer patients receiving chemotherapy to reduce hyperuricemia, it is important to decrease the dose of *6-MP* in these individuals to avoid accumulation of the drug and exacerbation of toxicities.

b. **Excretion:** The parent drug and its metabolites are excreted by the kidney.

5. **Adverse effects:** Side effects include nausea, vomiting, and diarrhea. Bone marrow depression is the chief toxicity. Hepatotoxicity has also been reported.

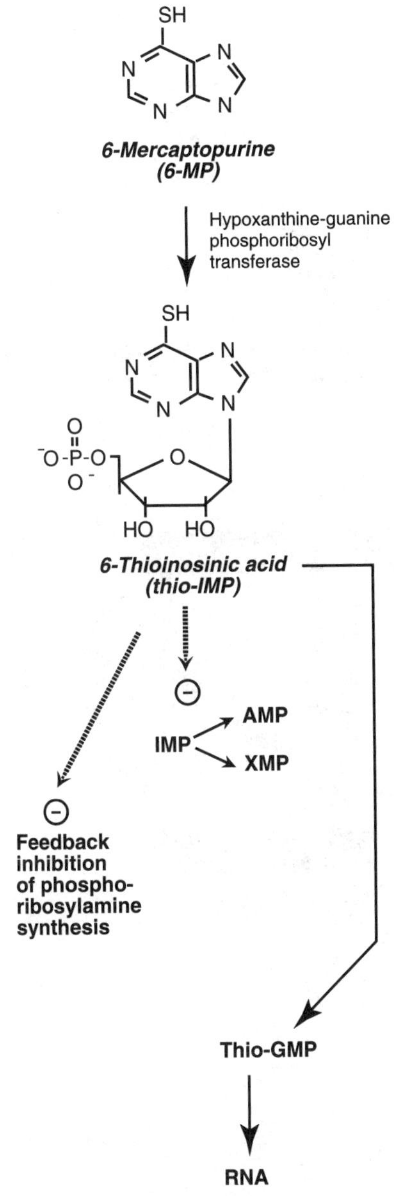

SH
N N N N
6-Mercaptopurine (6-MP)
Hypoxanthine-guanine phosphoribosyl transferase
SH
N N N N
O
⁻O-P-O
O⁻
O
HO HO
6-Thioinosinic acid (thio-IMP)
⊖
IMP
AMP
XMP
⊖
Feedback inhibition of phosphoribosylamine synthesis
Thio-GMP
RNA

Figure 38.8
Actions of *6-mercaptopurine.*

[3,4,5]See p. 400 for Infolink references to other books in this series.

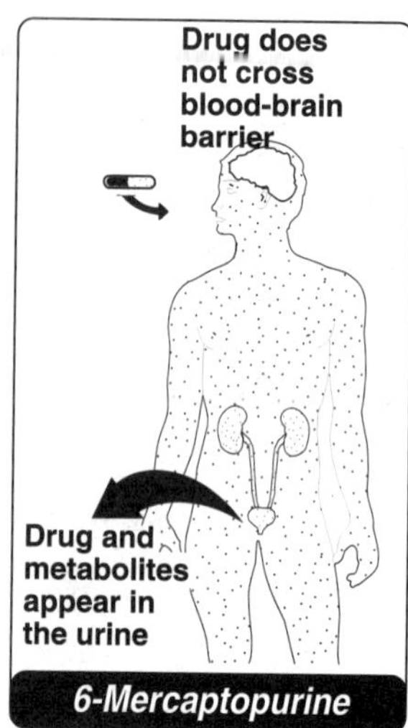
Drug does not cross blood-brain barrier
Drug and metabolites appear in the urine
6-Mercaptopurine

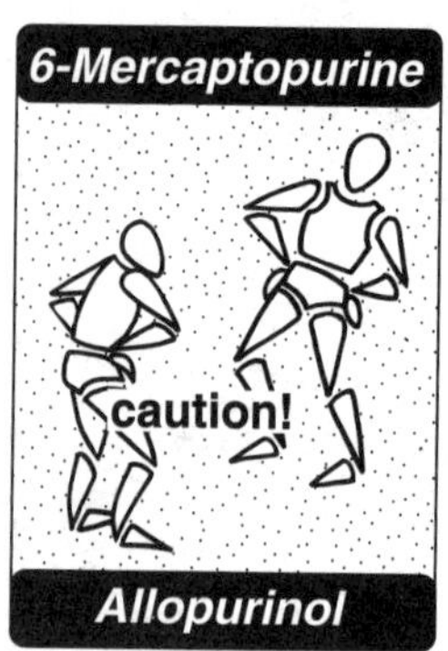
6-Mercaptopurine
caution!
Allopurinol

C. 6-Thioguanine

6-Thioguanine [thye oh GWAH neen] (*6-TG*), another purine analog, is primarily used in the treatment of acute nonlymphocytic leukemia in combination with *daunorubicin* (see p. 385) and *cytarabine* (see p. 383). Like *6-MP*, *6-TG* must first be converted to the nucleotide form, which then inhibits the biosynthesis of the purine ring and the phosphorylation of GMP to GDP. *6-TG* can also be incorporated into RNA and DNA. Cross-resistance occurs between 6-MP and 6-TG. Unlike *6-MP*, *allopurinol* does not potentiate *6-TG* action because very little of the drug is metabolized to thiouric acid. Otherwise, toxicities are the same as those for *6-MP*.

D. 5-Fluorouracil

5-Fluorouracil [flure oh YOOR a sil] (*5-FU*), a pyrimidine analog, has a stable fluorine atom in place of a hydrogen atom at position 5 of the uracil ring. The fluorine interferes with the conversion of deoxyuridylic acid to thymidylic acid, thus depriving the cell of one of the essential precursors for DNA synthesis.

1. **Site of action:** *5-FU* per se is devoid of antineoplastic activity and must be converted to the corresponding deoxynucleotide (5-FdUMP, Figure 38.9), which competes with deoxyuridine monophosphate (dUMP) for thymidylate synthetase. 5-FdUMP acts as a pseudosubstrate and is entrapped with the enzyme and its N^5,N^{10}-methylene tetrahydrofolic acid coenzyme in a ternary complex that cannot proceed to products. DNA synthesis decreases due to lack of thymidine, leading to imbalanced cell growth and cell death. [Note: *Leucovorin* is given with *5-FU* because the reduced folate coenzyme is required in the thymidylate synthetase reaction. Lack of sufficient coenzyme reduces the effectiveness of the antipyrimidine.] 5-FU is also incorporated into RNA and low levels have been detected in DNA.

2. **Resistance:** Resistant cells are encountered that have lost the ability to convert *5-FU* into its active form or have altered or increased thymidylate synthetase or have an increased rate of *5-FU* catabolism.

3. **Therapeutic applications:** *Fluorouracil* is employed primarily in the treatment of slowly growing, solid tumors (for example, colorectal, breast, ovarian, pancreatic, and gastric carcinomas). Adjuvant therapy with *levamisole*, a veterinary anthelmintic agent, improves the survival of patients with colonic cancer. *5-FU* is also effective for the treatment of superficial basal cell carcinomas when applied topically.

4. **Pharmacokinetics:** Because of its severe toxicity to the GI tract, *5-FU* is given intravenously or, in the case of skin cancer, topically. The drug penetrates well into all tissues including the CNS. *5-FU* is metabolized in the liver, largely to CO_2, which is expired. The dose must be adjusted in the case of impaired hepatic function.

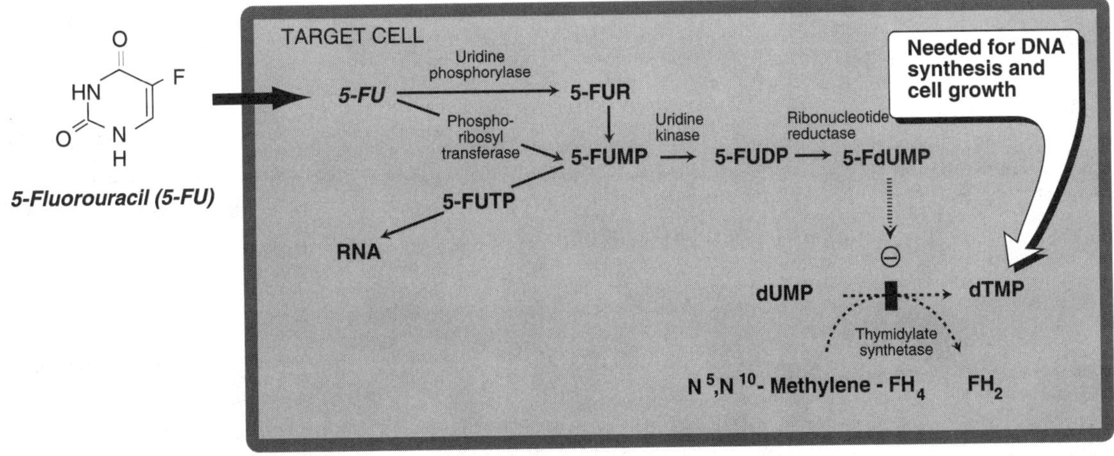

Figure 38.9
Mechanism of 5-fluorouracil's cytotoxic action. *5-Fluorouracil* is converted to 5-FdUMP, which competes with deoxyuridine monophosphate (dUMP) for the enzyme thymidylate synthetase.

5. **Toxicities:** In addition to nausea, vomiting, diarrhea, and alopecia, severe ulceration of the oral and GI mucosa, bone marrow depression (with bolus injection), and anorexia are frequently encountered. A dermopathy (erythematous desquamation of the palms and soles) called the "hand-foot syndrome" is seen after extended infusions.

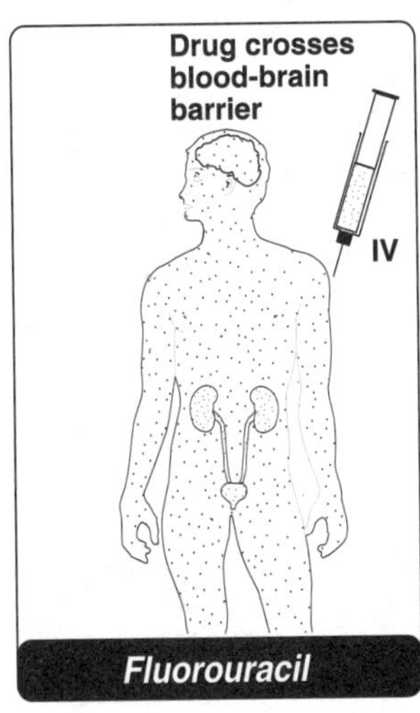

E. Cytarabine

Cytarabine [sye TARE a been] (*cytosine arabinoside, ara-C*) is an analog of 2'-deoxycytidine in which the natural ribose residue is replaced by D-arabinose. It acts as a pyrimidine antagonist.

1. **Site of action:** Like the other purine and pyrimidine antagonists, *ara-C* must be sequentially phosphorylated to the corresponding nucleotide, cytosine arabinoside triphosphate (ara-CTP), in order to be cytotoxic. It is S-phase (hence cell-cycle) specific. *Ara-C* is also incorporated into DNA and can terminate chain elongation. It can also inhibit the reduction of CDP to dCDP.

2. **Resistance:** Resistance to *ara-C* may result from a defect in the transport process, a change in phosphorylating enzymes, or an increased pool of the natural dCTP nucleotide. Increased deamination to uracil arabinoside, ara-U, a pharmacologically inactive metabolite, can also cause resistance.

3. **Therapeutic indications:** The major clinical use is in acute non-lymphocytic (myelogenous) leukemia in combination with *6-TG* (see p. 382) and *daunorubicin* (see p. 385).

4. **Pharmacokinetics:** *Ara-C* is not effective when given orally because of its deamination to the noncytotoxic uracil arabinoside (ara-U) by cytidine deaminase in the intestinal mucosa. Given IV, it distributes throughout the body, but does not penetrate the CNS in sufficient amounts to be effective against meningeal leukemia. However, it may be injected intrathecally. *Ara-C* undergoes exten-

sive oxidative deamination in the body to ara-U. Both *ara-C* and ara-U are excreted by the kidney.

5. **Adverse effects:** Nausea, vomiting, diarrhea, and severe myelosuppression (primarily granulocytopenia) are the major toxicities. Hepatic dysfunction is also occasionally encountered. At high doses or intrathecal injection, *ara-C* may cause seizures or altered mental states.

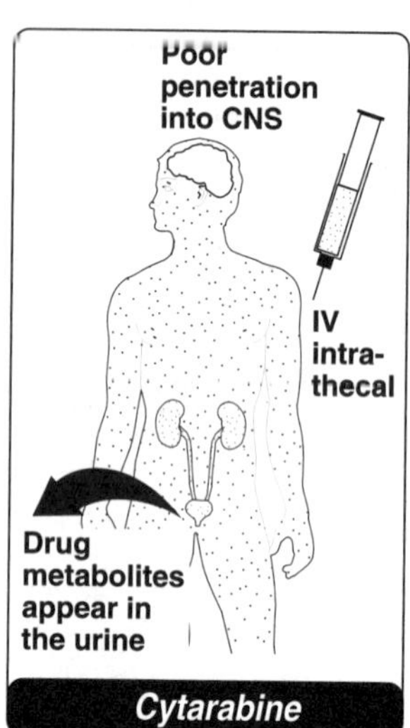
Poor penetration into CNS
IV intra-thecal
Drug metabolites appear in the urine
Cytarabine

F. Fludarabine

Fludarabine [flu DARE a been] is the 5' phosphate of 2-fluoro-adenine arabinoside, an unnatural purine nucleotide. Although the exact cytoxic lesion is uncertain, the triphosphate is incorporated into both DNA and RNA to decrease their synthesis and alter their function. *Fludarabine* is useful in the treatment of chronic lymphocytic leukemia. It may replace *chlorambucil*, the present drug of choice. *Fludarabine* is also effective against hairy-cell leukemia. It is administered intravenously rather than orally because intestinal bacteria split off the sugar to yield the very toxic metabolite, fluoroadenine. Urinary excretion accounts for partial elimination. In addition to nausea, vomiting and diarrhea, myelosuppression is the dose-limiting toxicity. Fever, edema, and severe neurologic toxicity also occur. At high doses, progressive encephalopathy, blindness, and death have been reported.

See p. 463 for a description of newly approved drug, *capecitabine*.

IV. ANTIBIOTICS

These drugs owe their cytotoxic action to their interactions with DNA, leading to disruption of DNA function. They are cell-cycle specific.

A. Dactinomycin

Dactinomycin [dak ti noe MYE sin], known to biochemists as *actinomycin D*, was the first antibiotic to find therapeutic application in tumor chemotherapy.

1. **Site of action:** The drug intercalates into the small groove of the double helix between guanine-cytosine base pairs of DNA, forming a stable *dactinomycin*-DNA complex. The complex interferes primarily with DNA-dependent RNA polymerase, although at high doses, *dactinomycin* also hinders DNA synthesis. The drug may also cause strand breaks. Evidence exists that *dactinomycin* stabilizes the DNA-topoisomerase II complex (see p. 397).

2. **Resistance:** Resistance is due to an increased efflux of the antibiotic from the cell via P-glycoprotein (see p. 377). DNA repair may also play a role.

3. **Therapeutic applications:** *Dactinomycin* is used in combination with surgery and *vincristine* (see p. 390) for the treatment of Wilm's tumor. With *methotrexate* (see p. 378) it is effective in the treatment of gestational choriocarcinoma. Some soft-tissue sarcomas also respond.

4. **Pharmacokinetics:** The drug, administered intravenously, is concentrated in the liver where it is partially metabolized. *Dactinomycin* does not enter the cerebrospinal fluid. Most of the parent drug and its metabolites are slowly excreted via the bile, and the remainder via the urine.

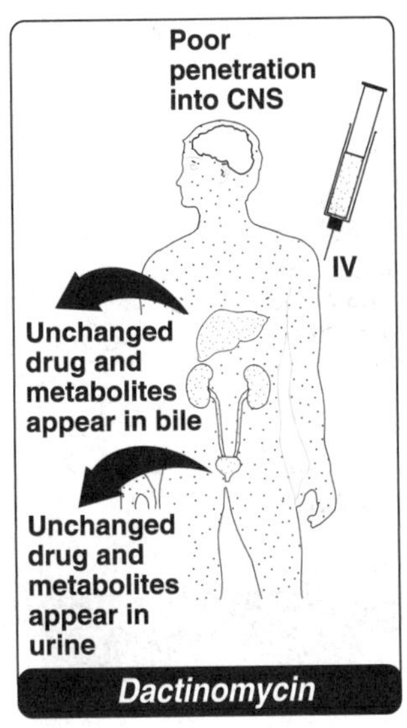

5. **Adverse effects:** The major dose-limiting toxicity is bone marrow depression, and the drug is immunosuppressive. Other adverse reactions include nausea, vomiting, diarrhea, stomatitis, and alopecia. Extravasation during injection produces serious problems. *Dactinomycin* sensitizes to radiation; inflammation at sites of prior radiation therapy may occur.

B. Doxorubicin and daunorubicin

Doxorubicin [dox oh ROO bi sin] and *daunorubicin* [daw noe ROO bi sin] are classified as anthracycline antibiotics. *Doxorubicin*, often referred to by its trade name *adriamycin*, is the hydroxylated analog of *daunorubicin*. *Idarubicin*, the 4-demethoxy analog of *daunorubicin* is also available.

1. **Site of action:** The anthracyclines have three major activities that may vary with the type of cell; all are maximal in the S and G_2 phases:

   a. **Intercalation in the DNA:** The drugs insert nonspecifically between adjacent base pairs and bind to the sugar-phosphate backbone of DNA causing a local uncoiling, thus blocking DNA and RNA synthesis. Intercalation can interfere with the topoisomerase II-catalyzed breakage-reunion reaction of DNA strands to cause unreparable breaks.

   b. **Binding to cell membranes:** This action alters the function of transport processes coupled to phosphatidylinositol activation.

   c. **Generation of oxygen radicals through lipid peroxidation:** Cytochrome P-450 reductase (present in cell nuclear membranes) catalyzes reduction of the anthracyclines to semiquinone free radicals. These in turn reduce molecular O_2, producing superoxide ions and hydrogen peroxide that mediate single strand scission of DNA (Figure 38.10). Tissues with ample superoxide dismutase (SOD) or glutathione peroxidase activity are protected.[6] Tumors and the heart are generally low in SOD. In addition, cardiac tissue lacks catalase and thus cannot dispose of hydrogen peroxide. This may explain the cardiotoxicity of anthracyclines.

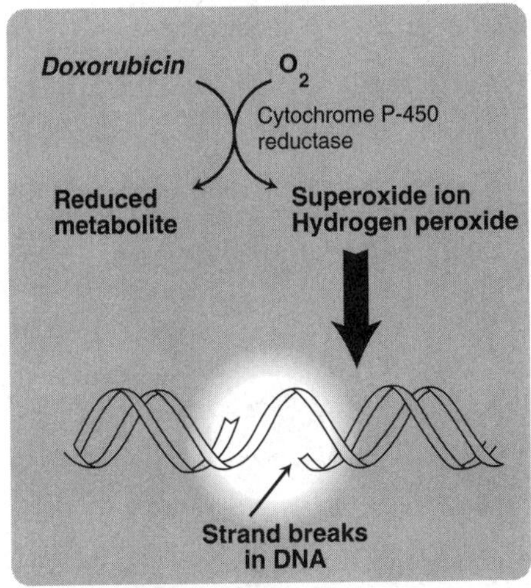

Figure 38.10
Doxorubicin interacts with molecular oxygen producing superoxide ions and hydrogen peroxide which cause single strand breaks in DNA.

2. **Resistance:** Resistance has been ascribed to increased efflux via the amplified transport P-glycoprotein (see p. 377). Cells rich in glutathione peroxidase are also resistant. Decreased cytochrome P-450 reductase, topoisomerase II and DNA repair may also play a role.

[6]See p. 400 for Infolink references to other books in this series.

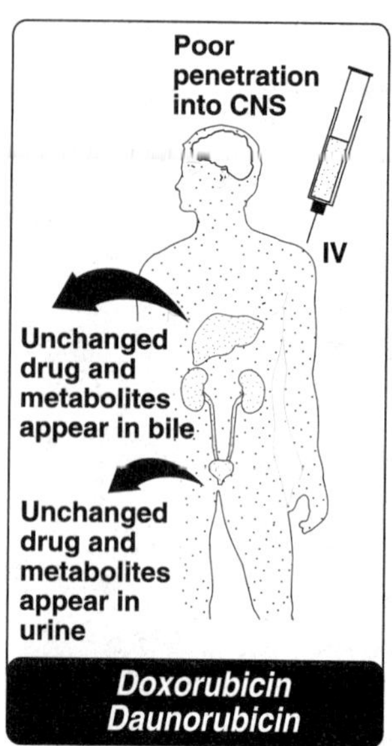
Poor penetration into CNS
IV
Unchanged drug and metabolites appear in bile
Unchanged drug and metabolites appear in urine
Doxorubicin
Daunorubicin

3. **Therapeutic applications:** Applications for these two agents differ despite their structural similarity and their apparently similar mechanisms of action. *Doxorubicin* is one of the most important and widely used anticancer drugs. It is used for treatment of sarcomas and a variety of carcinomas, including breast and lung, as well as acute lymphocytic leukemia and lymphomas. *Daunorubicin* is used in the treatment of acute lymphocytic and myelocytic leukemias.

4. **Pharmacokinetics**

   a. **Absorption and distribution:** Both drugs must be administered intravenously since they are inactivated in the gastrointestinal tract. Extravasation is a serious problem that can lead to tissue necrosis. These drugs bind to plasma proteins as well as to tissues where they are widely distributed. They do not penetrate into the central nervous system.

   b. **Fate:** Both drugs undergo extensive metabolism. The bile is the major route of excretion, and the drug dose must be modified in patients with impaired hepatic function. Some renal excretion also occurs, but the dose generally need not be adjusted in patients with renal failure. The drugs impart a red color to the urine.

5. **Adverse effects:** Irreversible, dose-dependent cardiotoxicity, apparently a result of the generation of free radicals, is the most serious adverse reaction. Irradiation of the thorax increases the risk of cardiotoxicity. There has been some success with the iron chelator, *dexrazone*, in protecting against the cardiotoxicity of *doxorubicin*. As with *dactinomycin*, both *doxorubicin* and *daunorubicin* also cause a transient bone marrow suppression, stomatitis, and GI tract disturbances. Alopecia is usually severe.

C. Bleomycin

Bleomycin [blee oh MYE sin] is a mixture of different copper chelating glycopeptides that, like the anthracycline antibiotics, cause scission of DNA by an oxidative process.

1. **Site of action:** A DNA-*bleomycin*-Fe(II) complex appears to undergo oxidation to *bleomycin*-Fe(III); the liberated electrons react with oxygen to form superoxide or hydroxide radicals, which in turn attack the phosphodiester bonds of the DNA, resulting in strand breakage and chromosomal aberrations (Figure 38.11). Redox recycling regenerates the Fe(II) form. *Bleomycin* is cell-cycle specific, and causes cells to accumulate in the G_2 phase.

2. **Resistance:** These mechanism(s) have not been elucidated, although experimental systems have implicated increased levels of *bleomycin* hydrolase (or deamidase), glutathione-S-transferase, and possibly increased efflux of the drug. DNA repair also may contribute.

3. **Therapeutic applications:** *Bleomycin* is primarily employed in the treatment of testicular tumors in combination with *vinblastine* (see p. 390) or *etoposide* (see p. 397). Response rates are close to

[8,9]See p. 400 for Infolink references to other books in this series.

100% if *cisplatin* (see p. 395) is added to the regimen. *Bleomycin* is also effective, although not curative, for squamous cell carcinomas and lymphomas.

4. **Pharmacokinetics:** *Bleomycin* is administered by a number of routes, including subcutaneous, intramuscular, intravenous, and intracavitary. The *bleomycin* inactivating enzyme (hydrolase) is high in a number of tissues (liver, spleen), but low in lung and absent in skin, accounting for its toxicity in those tissues. Most of the parent drug is excreted unchanged into the urine by glomerular filtration, necessitating dose adjustment in patients with renal failure.

5. **Adverse effects:** Pulmonary toxicity is the most serious adverse effect, progressing from rales, cough, and infiltrate to potentially fatal fibrosis. Mucocutaneous reactions and alopecia are common. Hypertrophic skin changes and hyperpigmentation of the hands are prevalent. There is a high incidence of fever and chills and a low incidence of serious anaphylactoid reactions. *Bleomycin* is unusual in that myelosuppression is rare.

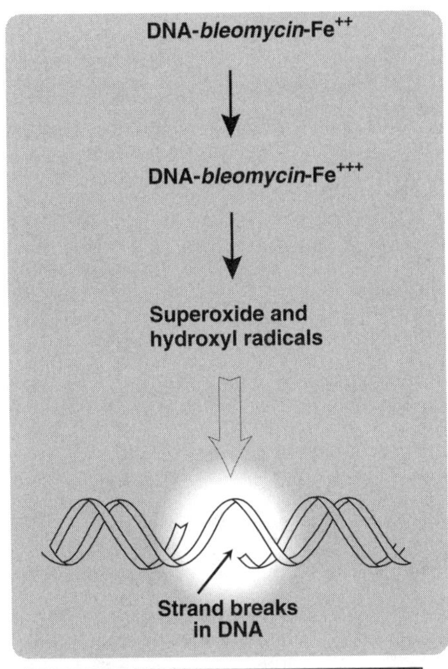

Figure 38.11
Bleomycin causes breaks in DNA by an oxidative process

D. Plicamycin

Plicamycin [plick a MYE sin] (*mithramycin*) also exerts its cytotoxicity through restriction of DNA-directed RNA synthesis. Resistance is due to P-glycoprotein efflux. *Plicamycin* has a relative toxic specificity for osteoclasts preventing their resorption, and lowers plasma calcium concentration in hypercalcemic patients—especially those with bone tumors. Toxicities include hemorrhage as well as effects on the bone marrow, liver, and kidneys.

V. ALKYLATING AGENTS

Alkylating agents exert their cytotoxic effects by covalently binding to nucleophilic groups on various cell constituents. Alkylation of DNA is probably the crucial cytotoxic reaction that is lethal to the tumor cell. Alkylating agents do not discriminate between cycling and resting cells, but are most toxic for rapidly dividing cells. They are used to treat a wide variety of lymphatic and solid cancers in combination with other agents. In addition to being cytotoxic, all are mutagenic and carcinogenic and can lead to a second malignancy such as acute leukemia.

A. Mechlorethamine

Mechlorethamine [me klor ETH a meen] was developed as a vesicant (nitrogen mustard) during World War I. Its ability to cause lymphocytopenia led to its use in lymphatic cancers. Because it can bind and react at two separate sites, it is called a "bifunctional agent."

1. **Mechanism of action:** *Mechlorethamine* is transported into the cell by a choline uptake process. The drug loses a chloride ion and forms a reactive intermediate that alkylates the N^7 nitrogen of a

guanine residue in one or both strands of a DNA molecule (Figure 38.12). This alkylation leads to cross-linkages between guanine residues in the DNA chains, and/or depurination that facilitates DNA strand breakage. Alkylation can also cause miscoding mutations. Although alkylation can occur in both cycling and resting cells (therefore cell-cycle nonspecific), proliferating cells are more sensitive to the drug, especially those in G_1 and S phases.

2. **Resistance:** Resistance has been ascribed to decreased permeability of the drug, increased conjugation with thiols such as glutathione, and possibly increased DNA repair.

3. **Therapeutic applications:** *Mechlorethamine* is used primarily in the treatment of Hodgkin's disease as part of the **MOPP** regimen (**M**echlorethamine, **O**ncovin, **P**rednisone, **P**rocarbazine), and is also useful in the treatment of some solid tumors.

4. **Pharmacokinetics:** *Mechlorethamine* is very unstable, and solutions must be made up just prior to administration. *Mechlorethamine* is also a powerful vesicant (blistering agent), and is administered only IV, because it can cause severe tissue damage if extravasation occurs. Because of its reactivity, hardly any drug is excreted.

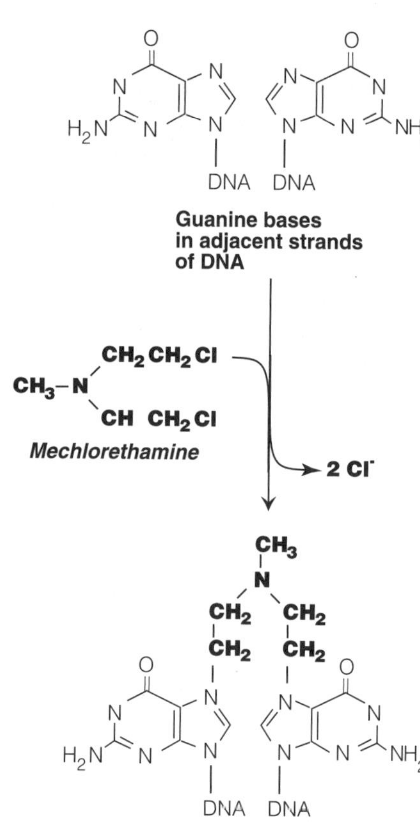

Figure 38.12
Alkylation of guanine bases in DNA is responsible for the cytotoxic effect of *mechlorethamine.*

5. **Adverse effects:** Its adverse effects include severe nausea and vomiting (centrally mediated). [Note: These effects can be diminished by pretreatment with *cannabinoids* (see p. 243) or *phenothiazine* (see p. 242).] Severe bone marrow depression limits extensive use. Latent viral infections (for example, Herpes zoster) may appear because of immunosuppression. Extravasation is a serious problem. If it occurs, the area should be infiltrated with isotonic sodium thiosulfite to inactivate the drug.

B. Cyclophosphamide and ifosfamide

These drugs are very closely related mustard agents that share most of the same toxicities. They are unique in that (1) they can be taken orally, and (2) they are cytotoxic only after generation of their alkylating species, following their hydroxylation by cytochrome P-450.

1. **Mechanism of action:** *Cyclophosphamide* [sye kloe FOSS fa mide] is the most commonly used alkylating agent. Both *cyclophosphamide* and *ifosfamide* [eye FOSS fa mide] are first biotransformed to hydroxylated intermediates by the cytochrome P-450 system (Figure 38.13). The hydroxylated intermediates undergo breakdown to form the active compounds, phosphoramide mustard and acrolein. Reaction of the phosphoramide mustard with DNA is considered to be the cytotoxic step. [Note: The therapeutic effect of these drugs is independent of the level of activity of the cytochrome P-450 system.]

2. **Resistance:** Resistance results from increased DNA repair, decreased drug permeability, and reaction of the drug with thiols (for example, glutathione). Cross-resistance, however, does not always occur.

3. **Therapeutic applications:** These agents have a broad clinical spectrum, being used either singly or as part of a regimen in treatment of a wide variety of neoplastic diseases, for example, Burkitt's lymphoma and breast cancer. Non-neoplastic disease entities, such as nephrotic syndrome and intractable rheumatoid arthritis, are also effectively treated with *cyclophosphamide*.

4. **Pharmacokinetics:** Unlike most of the alkylating agents, *cyclophosphamide* and *ifosfamide* are preferentially administered by the oral route. Minimal amounts of the parent drug are excreted into the feces (after biliary transport), or into the urine by glomerular filtration.

5. **Adverse effects:** The most prominent toxicities of both drugs (after alopecia, nausea, vomiting, and diarrhea) are bone marrow depression, especially leukocytosis, and hemorrhagic cystitis, which can lead to fibrosis of the bladder. The latter toxicity has been attributed to acrolein in the urine in the case of *cyclophosphamide* and toxic metabolites of *ifosfamide*. [Note: Adequate hydration as well as intravenous injection of *MESNA* (*sodium 2-mercaptoethane sulfonate*), which inactivates the toxic compounds, minimizes this problem. Other toxicities include effects on the germ cells resulting in amenorrhea, testicular atrophy, and sterility. A fairly high incidence of neurotoxicity has been reported in patients on high-dose *ifosfamide,* probably due to the metabolite, chloroacetaldehyde. Secondary malignancies may appear years after therapy.

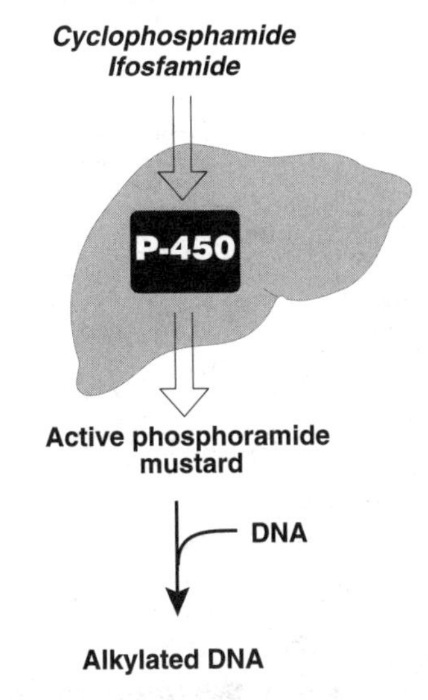

Figure 38.13
Activation of *cyclophosphamide* and *ifosfamide* by hepatic cytochrome P-450.

C. Nitrosoureas

Carmustine [kar MUS teen] and *lomustine* [loe MUSteen] are closely related nitrosoureas. [Note: *Streptozotocin* [strep toe ZOE toe sin] is another nitrosourea that is specifically toxic to the β-cells of the islets of Langerhans. Its use is in the treatment of insulinomas. It is diabetogenic and can cause reversible renal damage.]

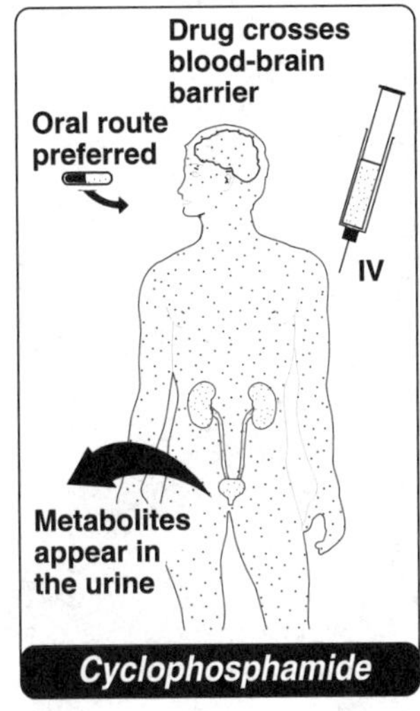

1. **Mechanism of action:** The nitrosoureas exert cytotoxic effects by an alkylation that cross-links strands of DNA to inhibit its replication and, eventually, RNA and protein synthesis. Although they alkylate DNA in resting cells, cytotoxicity is expressed only on cell division; therefore nondividing cells can escape death if DNA repair occurs.

2. **Resistance:** Although the true nature of resistance to nitrosoureas is unknown, it probably results from DNA repair and reaction of the drugs with thiols.

3. **Therapeutic applications:** Because of their ability to penetrate into the CNS, the nitrosoureas are primarily employed in the treatment of brain tumors. They find limited use in the treatment of other cancers.

4. **Pharmacokinetics:** In spite of the similarities in their structures, *carmustine* is administered intravenously, whereas *lomustine* is

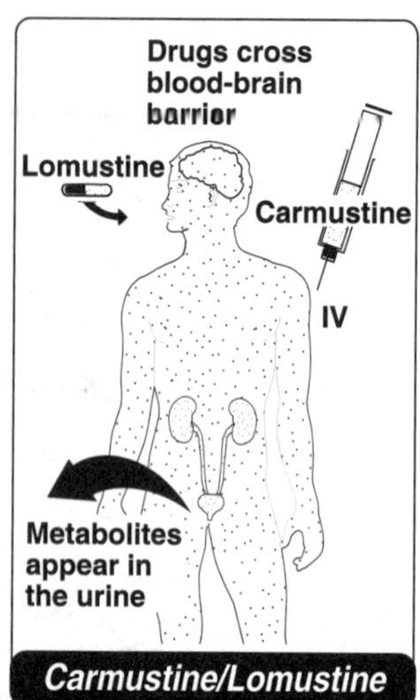

given orally. Because of their lipophilicity, they distribute to many tissues, but their most striking property is their ability to readily penetrate into the CNS. The drugs undergo extensive metabolism. *Lomustine* is metabolized to active products. The kidney is the major excretory route for the nitrosoureas.

5. **Adverse effects:** These include delayed hematopoietic depression, which may be due to metabolic products. An aplastic marrow may develop on prolonged use. Renal toxicity and pulmonary fibrosis related to duration of therapy is also encountered.

VI. MICROTUBULE INHIBITORS

The mitotic spindle is part of a larger intracellular skeleton (cytoskeleton) that is essential for the internal movements occurring in the cytoplasm of all eukaryotic cells. The mitotic spindle consists of chromatin, and a system of microtubules composed of the protein tubulin. The mitotic spindle is essential for the equal partitioning of DNA into the two daughter cells formed when a eukaryotic cell divides. Several plant-derived substances used as anticancer drugs disrupt this process by affecting the equilibrium between the polymerized and depolymerized forms of the microtubules, thereby causing cytotoxicity.

A. Vincristine and vinblastine

Vincristine [vin KRIS teen] and *vinblastine* [vin BLAST een] are structurally-related compounds derived from the periwinkle plant, Vinca rosea. They are therefore referred to as the vinca alkaloids. A structurally related new (and less toxic) agent, *vinorelbine* [vye NO rel been] shows promise in the treatment of advanced non-small cell lung cancer.

1. **Mechanism of action:** *Vincristine* and *vinblastine* are both cycle-specific and phase-specific, because they block mitosis in metaphase. Their binding to the microtubular protein, tubulin, is GTP-dependent and blocks the ability of tubulin to polymerize to form microtubules. Instead, paracrystalline aggregates consisting of tubulin dimers and the alkaloid drug are formed. The resulting dysfunctional spindle apparatus, frozen in metaphase, prevents chromosomal segregation and cell proliferation (Figure 38.14).

2. **Resistance:** Resistant cells have been shown to have enhanced binding of *vinblastine* to the P-glycoprotein, which is responsible for the efflux of *vincristine* and *vinblastine* and several other drugs. Alterations in tubulin structure may also affect binding of the vinca alkaloids.

3. **Therapeutic applications:** Although *vincristine* and *vinblastine* are structurally very similar, their therapeutic indications are different. They are generally administered in combination with other drugs. *Vincristine* is used in the treatment of acute lymphoblastic leukemia in children, Wilm's tumor, Ewing's soft-tissue sarcoma, and Hodgkin's and non-Hodgkin's lymphomas, as well as some

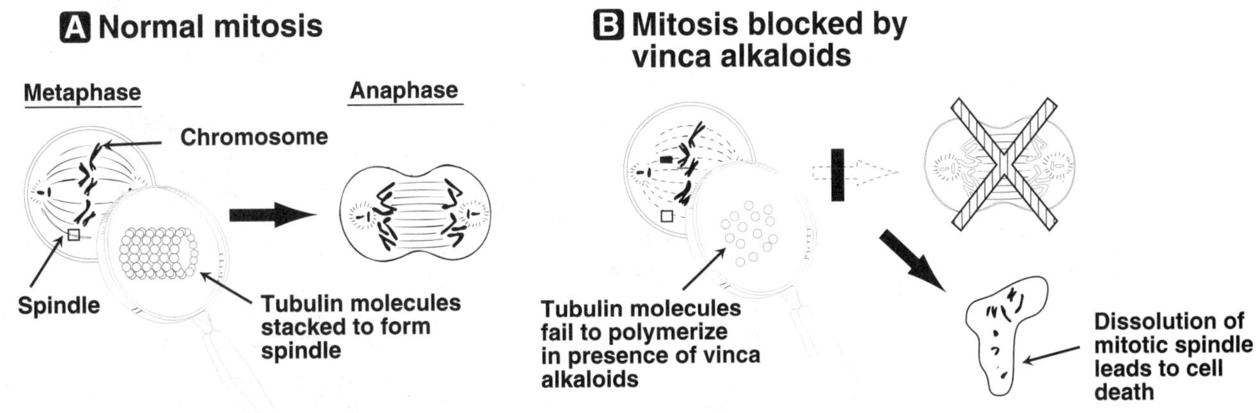

Figure 38.14
Mechanism of action of the microtubule inhibitors.

other rapidly proliferating neoplasms. [Note: *Vincristine* (trade name is ONCOVIN) is the "O" in the MOPP regimen (see p. 388) for Hodgkin's disease and a number of other protocols.] *Vinblastine* is administered with *bleomycin* (see p. 386) and *cisplatin* (see p. 395) for the treatment of metastatic testicular carcinoma. It is also used in the treatment of systemic Hodgkin's and non-Hodgkin's lymphomas.

4. **Pharmacokinetics:** Intravenous injection of *vincristine* or *vinblastine* leads to rapid cytotoxic effects and cell destruction. This in turn can cause hyperuricemia due to the oxidation of purines to uric acid. The hyperuricemia is ameliorated by administration of the xanthine oxidase inhibitor, *allopurinol* (see p. 417). The agents are concentrated and metabolized in the liver and are excreted into bile and feces. Doses must be modified in patients with impaired hepatic function or biliary obstruction.

5. **Adverse effects:**

   a. **Shared toxicities:** *Vincristine* and *vinblastine* have certain toxicities in common. These include phlebitis or cellulitis, if the drugs extravasate during injection, as well as nausea, vomiting, diarrhea, and alopecia.

   b. **Unique toxicities:** The adverse effects of *vincristine* and *vinblastine* are not identical. *Vinblastine* is a more potent myelosuppressant, whereas peripheral neuropathy (paresthesias, loss of reflexes, footdrop, and ataxia) is associated with *vincristine*. Gastrointestinal problems are also more frequently encountered with *vincristine*.

B. Paclitaxel

Better known as *taxol*, *paclitaxel* (pak lih tax el) is the first member of the taxane family used in cancer chemotherapy. A semi-synthetic *paclitaxel* is now available through chemical modification of a precursor found in the needles of yew species.

1. **Site of action:** *Paclitaxel* binds reversibly to tubulin, but unlike the vinca alkaloids, it promotes polymerization and stabilization of the polymer rather than disassembly (Figure 38.15). Thus it shifts the depolymerization-polymerization to favor the formation of microtubules. The overly stable microtubules formed in the presence of *paclitaxel* are dysfunctional, thereby causing the death of the cell.

2. **Resistance:** Like the vinca alkaloids, resistance has been associated with the presence of amplified P-glycoprotein, or a mutation in tubulin structure.

3. **Therapeutic indications:** *Paclitaxel* has shown good activity against advanced ovarian cancer and metastatic breast cancer. Early trials indicate favorable results in small-cell lung cancer, squamous-cell carcinoma of the head and neck, and several other cancers. Combination therapy with other anticancer drugs is being evaluated.

4. **Pharmacokinetics:** *Paclitaxel* is infused over 3-4 hours. Hepatic metabolism and biliary excretion are responsible for elimination of *paclitaxel*. Thus dose modification is not required in patients with renal impairment, but doses should be reduced in patients with hepatic dysfunction.

5. **Adverse effects**

   a. **Hypersensitivity:** Because of serious hypersensitivity reactions (dyspnea, urticaria, and hypotension), the patient to be treated with *paclitaxel* is currently premedicated with *dexamethasone* (see p. 275), and *diphenhydramine* (see p. 422), as well as with an H_2 blocker (see p. 236).

   b. **Neutropenia:** The dose-limiting toxicity of *paclitaxel* is neutropenia. Treatment with granulocyte colony-stimulating factor (*filgrastim*) prevents the problems associated with this condition.

   c. **Other toxicities:** Peripheral neuropathy and a transient asymptomatic bradycardia are sometimes observed. Alopecia occurs, but vomiting and diarrhea are uncommon.

A Normal mitosis

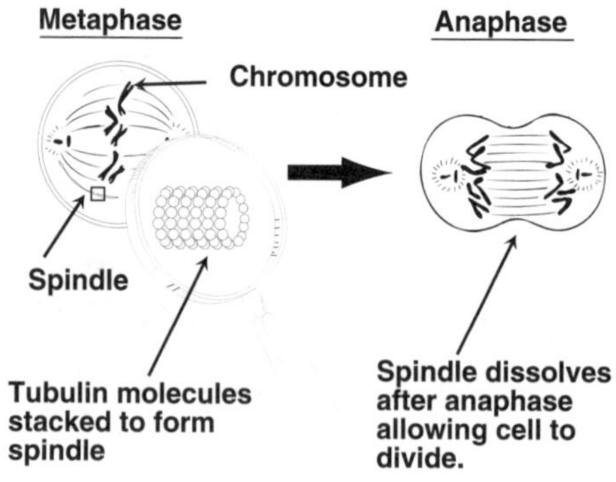

Metaphase
Anaphase
Chromosome
Spindle
Tubulin molecules stacked to form spindle
Spindle dissolves after anaphase allowing cell to divide.

B Mitosis blocked by *paclitaxel*

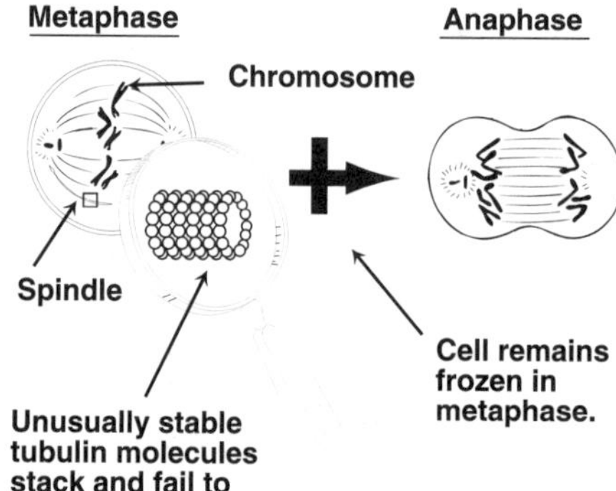

Metaphase
Anaphase
Chromosome
Spindle
Unusually stable tubulin molecules stack and fail to depolymerize.
Cell remains frozen in metaphase.

Figure 38.15
Paclitaxel stabilizes microtubules, rendering them nonfunctional.

VII. STEROID HORMONES AND THEIR ANTAGONISTS

Tumors that are steroid hormone-sensitive may be either (1) hormone-responsive, where the tumor regresses following treatment with a specific hormone; (2) hormone-dependent, where removal of a hormonal stimulus causes tumor regression; or (3) both. Hormone treatment of responsive tumors is usually only palliative, except in the case of the cytotoxic effect of glucocorticoids (for example, *prednisone*) on lymphomas. Removal of hormonal stimuli from hormone-dependent tumors can be accomplished by surgery, for example, in the case of orchiectomy for patients with advanced prostate cancer, or by drugs, for example in the case of breast cancer, treatment with the antiestrogen *tamoxifen* is used to prevent estrogen stimulation of breast cancer cells. For a steroid hormone to have an influence on a cell, that cell must have cytosolic receptors that are specific for that hormone (Figure 38.16A).

A. Prednisone

Prednisone [PRED ni sone] is a potent synthetic anti-inflammatory corticosteroid with less mineralocorticoid activity than cortisol (see p. 272). The use of this compound in the treatment of lymphomas arose when it was observed that patients with Cushing's syndrome (a syndrome associated with hypersecretion of cortisol) have lymphocytopenia and decreased lymphoid mass. These result from corticosteroid action on lymphocyte formation and distribution, that is, movement of these cells from the circulation to lymphoid tissue.

1. **Mechanism of action:** *Prednisone* itself is inactive and must first be reduced to *prednisolone* by 11-β-hydroxysteroid dehydrogenase[7]. The steroid binds to a receptor that triggers the production of specific proteins (see Figure 38.16A). The specific mechanism for its lymphocytopenic action after interaction with DNA remains to be elucidated.

2. **Resistance:** Resistance is associated with an absence of the receptor protein or a mutation that lowers receptor affinity for the hormone. However, some resistant cells appear to have functional receptors, but some subsequent step(s) is affected.

3. **Therapeutic applications:** *Prednisone* is primarily employed to induce remission in patients with acute lymphocytic leukemia, and in the treatment of both Hodgkin's and non-Hodgkin's lymphomas.

4. **Pharmacokinetics:** See p. 272 for a discussion of the pharmacologic aspects of *prednisone* and its toxic actions.

B. Tamoxifen

Tamoxifen [ta MOX i fen] is an estrogen antagonist, structurally related to the synthetic estrogen, *diethylstilbestrol*, and is active in the treatment of estrogen receptor-positive breast cancer. *Tamoxifen* has weak estrogenic activity.

1. **Mechanism of action:** *Tamoxifen* binds to the estrogen receptor but the complex is not productive, that is, the complex fails to induce estrogen-responsive genes and RNA synthesis does not ensue (Figure 38.16B). The result is a depletion of estrogen receptors, and the growth-promoting effects of the natural hormone and other growth factors are suppressed. [Note: Estrogen competes with *tamoxifen*; therefore, the drug is not effective in pre-menopausal women.] *Tamoxifen's* action is not related to any specific phase of the cell cycle.

2. **Resistance:** Resistance is associated either with a decreased affinity for the receptor, a decreased number of receptors, or the presence of a dysfunctional receptor.

[7] See p. 400 for Infolink references to other books in this series.

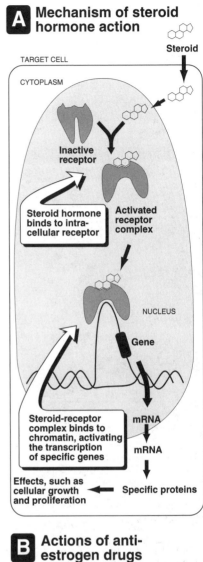

A Mechanism of steroid hormone action

Steroid
TARGET CELL
CYTOPLASM
Inactive receptor
Activated receptor complex
Steroid hormone binds to intracellular receptor
NUCLEUS
Gene
Steroid-receptor complex binds to chromatin, activating the transcription of specific genes
mRNA
mRNA
Effects, such as cellular growth and proliferation
Specific proteins

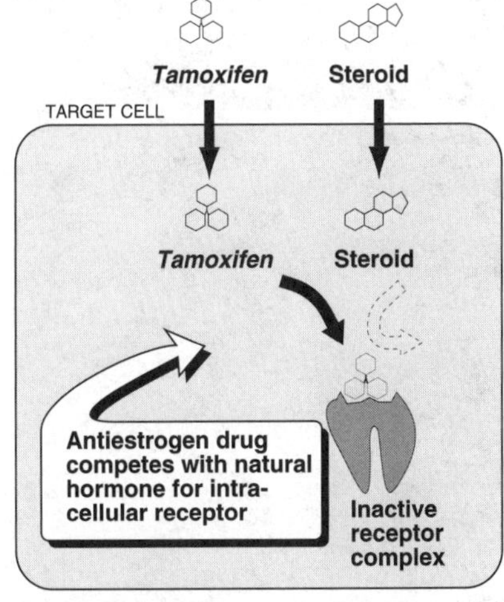

Figure 38.16
Action of steroid hormones and antiestrogen agents.

3. **Therapeutic applications:** Its clinical use is confined to the treatment of estrogen-dependent breast cancers.

4. **Pharmacokinetics:** *Tamoxifen* is effective on oral administration. It is partially metabolized by the liver. Some metabolites possess antagonist activity while others have agonist activity. Unchanged drug and its metabolites are excreted predominantly through the bile into feces.

5. **Adverse effects:** Side effects are similar to those of natural estrogen, that is, hot flashes, nausea, vomiting, skin rash, vaginal bleeding and discharge (due to some slight estrogenic activity of the drug and some of its metabolites). Hypercalcemia requiring cessation of the drug may also occur. *Tamoxifen* can also lead to increased pain if the tumor has metastasized to bone. *Tamoxifen* has the potential to cause endometrial cancer.

6. **Potential benefits:** *Tamoxifen* is being evaluated for possible protective activity against heart disease and osteoporosis due to its ability to decrease LDL cholesterol and increase bone mineralization.

C. Estrogens

Estrogens, such as *ethinyl estradiol* or *diethylstilbestrol*, are used in the treatment of prostatic cancer. Estrogens inhibit the growth of prostatic tissue by blocking the production of luteinizing hormone and thus decreasing the synthesis of androgens in the testis. Thus, tumors dependent on androgens are affected. Estrogen treatment can cause serious complications, such as thromboemboli, myocardial infarction, strokes, and hypercalcemia. In women, loss of libido may accompany menstrual changes. Men taking estrogens may experience gynecomastia and impotence.

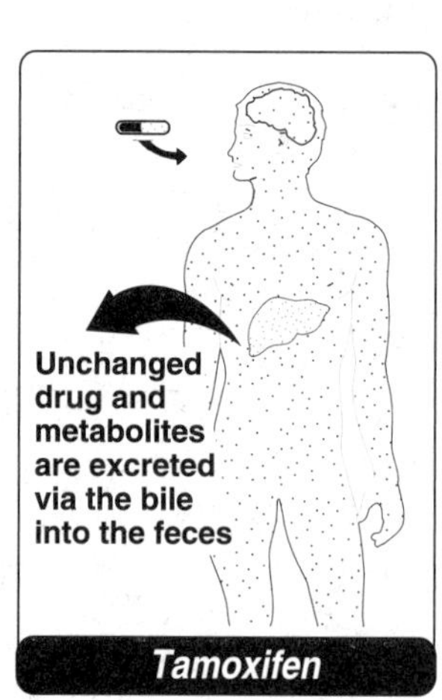
Unchanged drug and metabolites are excreted via the bile into the feces
Tamoxifen

D. Leuprolide and goserelin

The synthetic nonapeptides, *leuprolide* [loo PROE lide] and *goserelin* [gah SER e lin] are analogs of gonadotropin-releasing hormone (GnRH, LHRH). As LHRH agonists, they occupy the LHRH receptor in the pituitary, which leads to its desensitization and consequently inhibition of release of FSH and LH. Thus, androgen and estrogen synthesis are reduced (Figure 38.17). Response to *leuprolide* in prostatic cancer is equivalent to that of orchiectomy (surgical removal of one or both testes), with 40% regression of tumor and relief of bone pain. *Leuprolide* is effective either as a daily (SC) or depot (IM) injection against metastatic carcinoma of the prostate. *Goserelin acetate* is implanted intramuscularly. [Note: Depot forms are administered monthly.] Levels of androgen may initially rise, but then fall to castration levels. The adverse effects of these drugs, including impotence, hot flashes and tumor flare, are minimal compared to those experienced with estrogen treatment.

E. Flutamide

Flutamide [FLEW tah mide] is a synthetic nonsteroidal antiandrogen used in the treatment of prostate cancer. It is metabolized to an active hydroxy derivative that binds to the androgen receptor.

Flutamide blocks the inhibitory effects of testosterone on gonadotropin secretion causing an increase in serum LH and testosterone levels. *Flutamide* is always administered in combination with *leuprolide* or *goserelin*. It is administered orally and cleared through the kidney. Side effects include gynecomastia and gastrointestinal distress.

F. Aminoglutethimide

Aminoglutethimide [ah me no glue TETH i mide] is useful in second line therapy for the treatment of metastatic breast cancer. It inhibits the adrenal synthesis of pregnenolone from cholesterol, and the extra-adrenal aromatase reaction responsible for the synthesis of estrogen from androstenedione. *Aminoglutethimide* is administered orally, and is metabolized by the hepatic cytochrome P-450 system to inactive products. Because of its ability to induce this system, its own metabolism is accelerated, and interactions that increase the metabolism of *dexamethasone* (see p. 275), *theophylline* (see p. 220) and *digoxin* (see p. 158) can occur. *Aminoglutethimide* causes transient CNS depression and a maculopapular rash.

VIII. OTHER CHEMOTHERAPEUTIC AGENTS

A. Cisplatin and carboplatin

Cisplatin [SIS pla tin] is a member of the platinum coordination complex class of anticancer drugs. Because of *cisplatin's* severe toxicity, *carboplatin* [KAR bow pla tin] was developed. The therapeutic effectiveness of the two drugs is similar but their pharmacokinetics, patterns of distribution and dose-limiting toxicities differ. *Cisplatin* has synergistic cytotoxicity with radiation and other chemotherapeutic agents.

1. **Mechanism of action:** Their mechanism of action is similar to that of the alkylating agents. In the high chloride milieu of the plasma, *cisplatin* persists as the neutral species, which enters the cell and binds to the N^7 of guanine of DNA, forming inter- and intra-strand crosslinks. The resulting cytotoxic lesion inhibits both DNA and RNA synthesis. Both drugs can also bind to proteins and other compounds containing SH groups. Cytotoxicity can occur at any stage of the cell cycle, but the cell is most vulnerable to the actions of these drugs in G_1 and S.

2. **Resistance:** Sensitivity to these agents is decreased if cells have elevated glutathione levels or increased DNA repair, or if metallothionein (a protein rich in SH groups) is induced.

3. **Therapeutic applications:** *Cisplatin* has found wide application in the treatment of solid tumors such as metastatic testicular carcinoma in combination with *vinblastine* (see p. 390) and *bleomycin* (see p. 386), ovarian carcinoma in combination with *cyclophosphamide* (see p. 388), or alone for bladder carcinoma. *Carboplatin* is employed when patients cannot be vigorously hydrated as is required for *cisplatin* treatment, or if they suffer from kidney dysfunction or are prone to neuro- or ototoxicity.

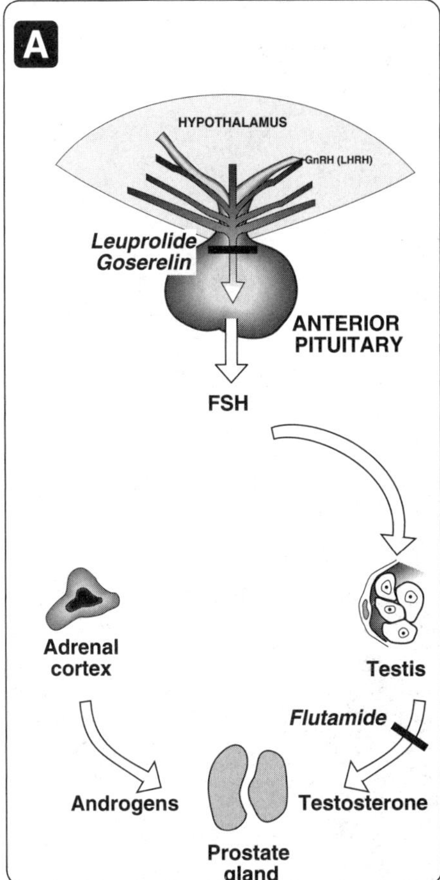

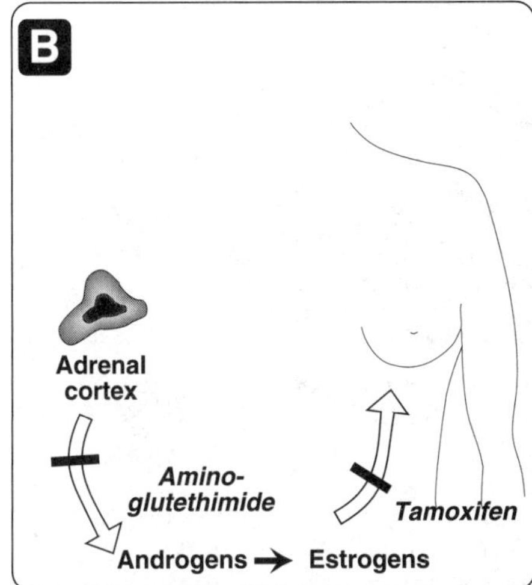

Figure 38.17
Effects of some anticancer drugs on the endocrine system. A. In therapy of prostatic cancer. B. In therapy of postmenopausal breast cancer.

4. **Pharmacokinetics:** *Cisplatin* and *carboplatin* are administered IV in saline solution; they can also be given intraperitoneally for ovarian cancer. Over 90% of *cisplatin* is bound to serum proteins. Highest concentrations are found in liver, kidney, intestinal, testicular and ovarian cells, but little penetrates into the cerebral spinal fluid (CSF). The renal route is the main avenue for excretion.

5. **Adverse effects:** Severe, persistent vomiting occurs 1 hour after administration of *cisplatin* and may continue for as long as 5 days. Premedication with antiemetic agents is usually helpful (see p. 241 for a discussion of antiemetic drugs). The major limiting toxicity is dose-related nephrotoxicity, involving the distal convoluted tubule and collecting ducts. This can be ameliorated by aggressive hydration and diuresis. Hypomagnesemia and hypocalcemia usually occur concurrently; it is important to correct calcium levels before correcting magnesium levels. Other toxicities include ototoxicity, with high frequency hearing loss and tinnitus; mild bone marrow suppression; some neurotoxicity characterized by paresthesia and loss of proprioception; and hypersensitivity reactions, ranging from skin rashes to anaphylaxis. Patients receiving aminoglycosides (see p. 314) concomitantly are at a greater risk for nephrotoxicity and ototoxicity. Unlike *cisplatin*, *carboplatin* causes only mild nausea and vomiting and is not nephro- neuro- or ototoxic. Its dose-limiting toxicity is myelosuppression.

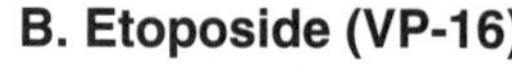

B. Etoposide (VP-16)

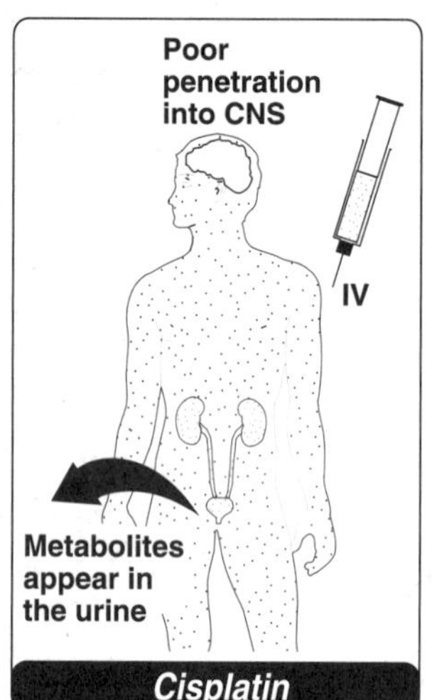

Cisplatin

Etoposide [e toe POE side] and its analog, *teniposide* [TEN ih poe side] are semisynthetic derivatives of the plant alkaloid, podophyllotoxin. They block cells in the late S-G_2 phase of the cell cycle. Their major target is topoisomerase II[8]. Binding of the drugs to the enzyme-DNA complex results in the persistence of the transient cleavable form of the complex and thus renders it susceptible to irreversible double-strand breaks (Figure 38.18). Resistance to topoisomerase inhibitors is conferred by either the presence of the multi-drug resistant P-glycoprotein, or mutation of the enzyme. *Etoposide* finds its major clinical use in the treatment of oat cell carcinoma of the lung and refractory testicular carcinoma. It is currently being tested in other therapeutic protocols. *Etoposide* may be administered either IV or orally. It is highly bound to plasma proteins and distributes throughout the body, but it enters the CSF poorly. Metabolites are converted to glucuronide and sulfate conjugates and are excreted in the urine. Dose-limiting myelosuppression (primarily leukopenia) is the major toxicity for both drugs. Other toxicities are alopecia, anaphylactic reactions, nausea, and vomiting. Hypotension may occur if the drug is injected rapidly.

C. Procarbazine

Procarbazine [proe KAR ba zeen] inhibits DNA and RNA sythesis. *Procarbazine* is used in the treatment of Hodgkin's disease as part of the "MOPP" regimen (see p. 388), and also other cancers. *Procarbazine* rapidly equilibrates between the plasma and the CSF after oral or parenteral administration. Metabolites and the parent

[8]See p. 400 for Infolink references to other books in this series.

drug are excreted through the kidney. Bone marrow depression is the major toxicity. Nausea, vomiting, and diarrhea are common. The drug is also neurotoxic, causing symptoms ranging from drowsiness to hallucinations to paresthesias. Because it inhibits monoamine oxidase, patients should be warned against ingesting foods that contain tyramine (for example, aged cheeses, beer, and wine). Ingestion of alcohol leads to a *disulfiram*-type reaction, see p. 96). *Procarbazine* is both mutagenic and teratogenic. Nonlymphocytic leukemia has developed in patients treated with the drug.

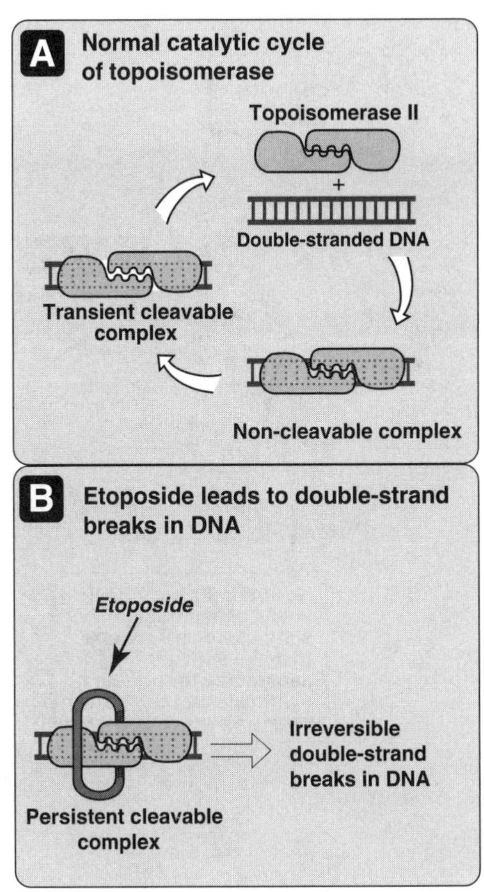

Figure 38.18
Mechanism of action of *etoposide*.

D. L-Asparaginase

L-Asparaginase [a SPAR a gi nase] catalyzes the deamination of asparagine to aspartic acid and ammonia. The form of the enzyme used chemotherapeutically is derived from bacteria.

1. **Mechanism of action:** Some neoplastic cells require an external source of asparagine, because of their limited capacity to make sufficient L-asparagine to support growth and function. *L-Asparaginase* hydrolyzes blood asparagine and thus deprives the tumor cells of this nutrient required for protein synthesis (Figure 38.19).

2. **Resistance:** Resistance is due to increased capacity of tumor cells to synthesize asparagine.

3. **Therapeutic application:** *L-Asparaginase* is used to treat childhood acute lymphocytic leukemia in combination with *vincristine* (see p. 390) and *prednisone* (see p. 393).

4. **Pharmacokinetics:** The enzyme must be administered either IV or IM because it is destroyed by gastric enzymes. Disposition remains undefined.

5. **Adverse effects:** Toxicities include a range of hypersensitivity reactions (since it is a foreign protein), a decrease in clotting factors, and liver abnormalities, as well as pancreatitis, seizures, and coma due to ammonia toxicity.

E. Interferons

1. **Classification:** Human interferons have been classified into three type's, α, β, and γ, on the basis of their antigenicity. The α interferons are primarily leukocytic, whereas the β and γ interferons are produced by connective tissue fibroblasts and T lymphocytes, respectively. Recombinant DNA techniques in bacteria have made available large quantities of α *interferon/species A*—designated *α2(A) interferon*—which has the advantage of being purer than previous preparations derived from leukocytes. Currently the other interferons have also been obtained by recombinant techniques.

2. **Site of action:** The exact mechanism by which the interferons are cytotoxic is unknown, but they have the capacity to stimulate natural killer (NK) cells. γ Interferon is also a potent activator of tumoricidal macrophages. Interferon secreted from producing cells interacts with surface receptors on other cells, at which site they

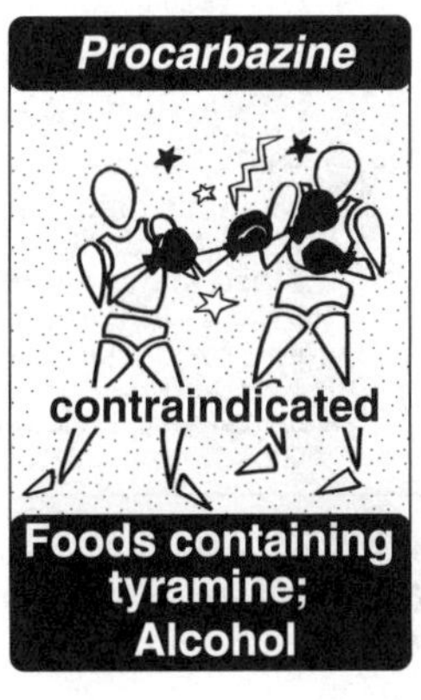

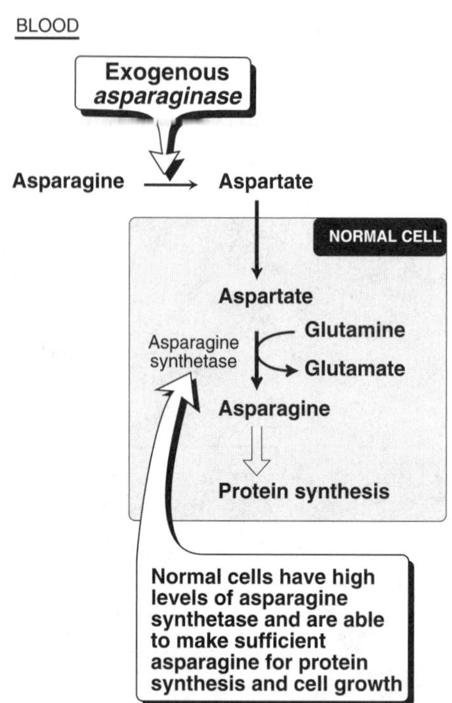

BLOOD

Exogenous *asparaginase*

Asparagine → Aspartate

NEOPLASTIC CELL

Aspartate

Asparagine synthetase

Glutamine

Glutamate

Asparagine

Protein synthesis

Neoplastic cells have low levels of asparagine synthetase and are unable to make sufficient asparagine for protein synthesis and cell growth

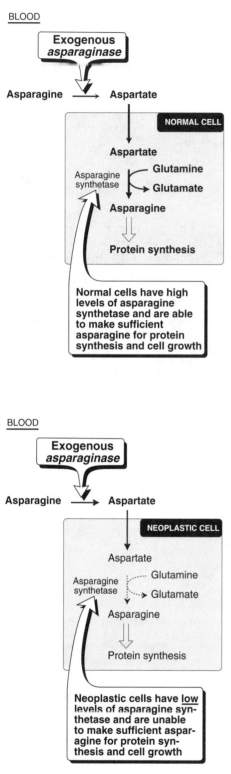

Figure 38.19
Mechanism of action of *L-asparaginase.*

exert their effects. Bound interferons are not internalized nor degraded. The α and β interferons compete for binding and presumably bind at the same receptor or in close proximity; γ interferons bind at different receptors.

3. **Therapeutic indications:** α2(A)*Interferon* is presently approved for the management of hairy cell leukemia. More than 90% of patients treated with α *interferon* have shown resolution of cytopenia, reduction in the incidence of serious infection, and reduction in the need for transfusions. Other interferons are being tested in the treatment of various tumors, including squamous cell carcinoma, melanoma, and multiple myeloma, among others.

4. **Pharmacokinetics:** Interferons are well absorbed after intramuscular injections. Being proteins, they are probably degraded by proteases.

5. **Adverse effects:** Fever with chills occurs during the first few days of treatment. Dose-related toxicity includes leukopenia and possibly thrombocytopenia. Fatigue, malaise, anorexia, weight loss, alopecia, and transient elevation of liver enzymes have also been reported. Transient and reversible nephrotoxicity with proteinuria have been seen at high doses.

The anticancer agents are summarized in Figure 38.20

See pp. 464-466 for a description of newly approved drugs, *topotecan*, *trastuzumab* and *rituxmab.*

Study Questions

Choose the ONE best answer.

38.1 Which one of the following agents shows cytotoxicity that is cell-cycle specific?

A. Methotrexate.
B. Dactinomycin.
C. Cisplatin.
D. Mechlorethamine.
E. Doxorubicin.

The correct answer = A. Methotrexate shows maximal cytotoxic effects in the S phase. With the exception of bleomycin, all the antibiotic anticancer agents, including dactinomycin and doxorubin, are cell-cycle nonspecific, but they tend to have a greater effect in cycling cells. Cisplatin and the alkylating agents, such as mechlorethamine, are toxic in both cycling and resting cells.

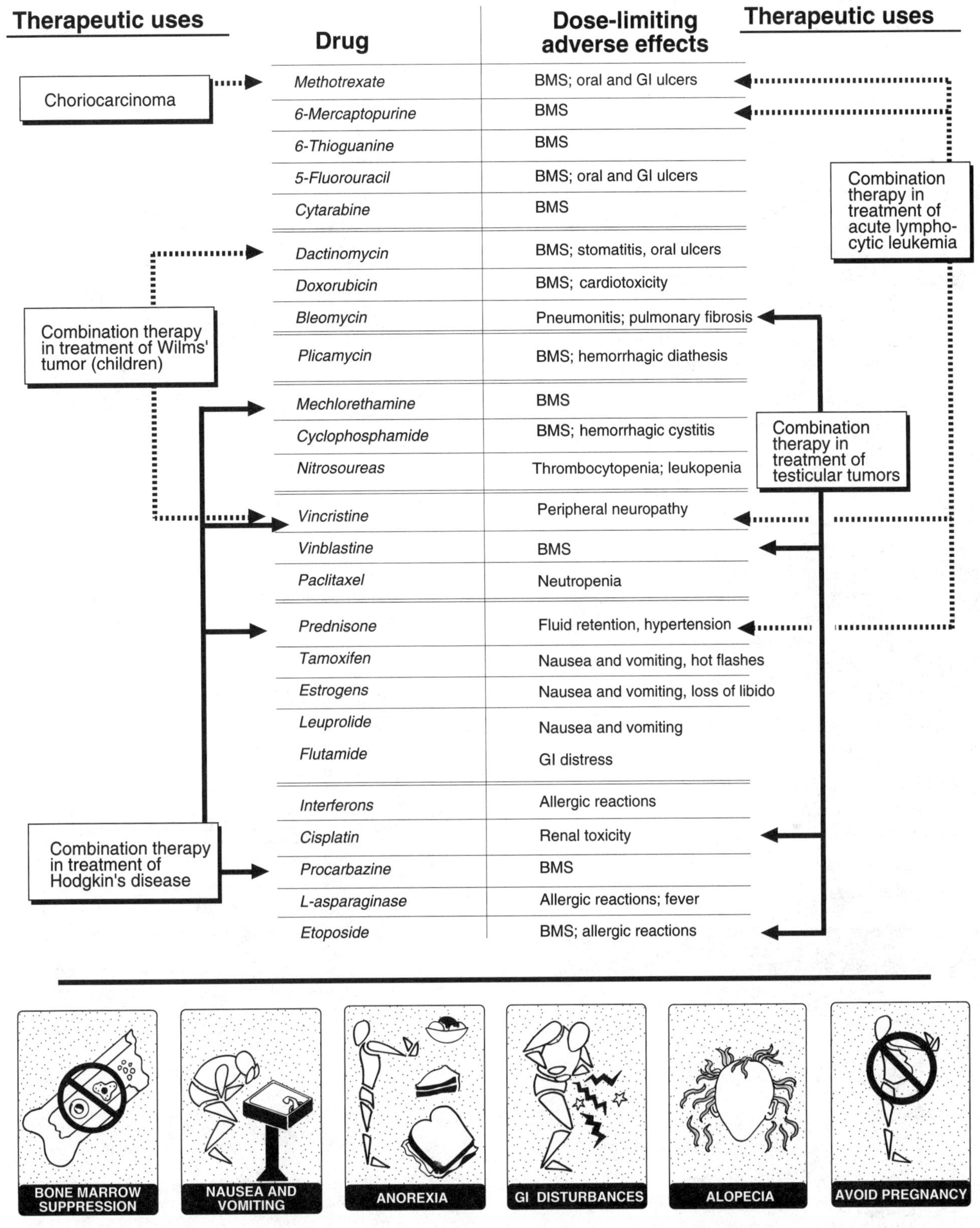

Therapeutic uses
Drug
Dose-limiting adverse effects
Therapeutic uses
Choriocarcinoma
Combination therapy in treatment of acute lymphocytic leukemia
Combination therapy in treatment of Wilms' tumor (children)
Combination therapy in treatment of testicular tumors
Combination therapy in treatment of Hodgkin's disease
Methotrexate — BMS; oral and GI ulcers
6-Mercaptopurine — BMS
6-Thioguanine — BMS
5-Fluorouracil — BMS; oral and GI ulcers
Cytarabine — BMS
Dactinomycin — BMS; stomatitis, oral ulcers
Doxorubicin — BMS; cardiotoxicity
Bleomycin — Pneumonitis; pulmonary fibrosis
Plicamycin — BMS; hemorrhagic diathesis
Mechlorethamine — BMS
Cyclophosphamide — BMS; hemorrhagic cystitis
Nitrosoureas — Thrombocytopenia; leukopenia
Vincristine — Peripheral neuropathy
Vinblastine — BMS
Paclitaxel — Neutropenia
Prednisone — Fluid retention, hypertension
Tamoxifen — Nausea and vomiting, hot flashes
Estrogens — Nausea and vomiting, loss of libido
Leuprolide — Nausea and vomiting
Flutamide — GI distress
Interferons — Allergic reactions
Cisplatin — Renal toxicity
Procarbazine — BMS
L-asparaginase — Allergic reactions; fever
Etoposide — BMS; allergic reactions
BONE MARROW SUPPRESSION
NAUSEA AND VOMITING
ANOREXIA
GI DISTURBANCES
ALOPECIA
AVOID PREGNANCY
Adverse effects and precautions commonly observed with anticancer drugs

Figure 38.20
Summary of cancer chemotherapy agents. BMS= bone marrow suppression.

38.2 Which one of the following drugs is metabolized to a cytotoxic product?

A. Vincristine.

B. Dactinomycin.

C. 5-Fluorouracil.

D. Lomustine.

E. Paclitaxel.

The correct answer = C. 5-Fluorouracil is devoid of antineoplastic activity and must be converted to the corresponding deoxynucleotide. The other agents exert their cytotoxic effects directly.

38.3 All of the following agents cause their cytotoxic effects by interference in DNA transcription EXCEPT:

A. Doxorubicin.

B. Tamoxifen.

C. Cyclophosphamide.

D. Mechlorethamine.

E. Cisplatin.

The correct choice = B. Tamoxifen binds to the estrogen receptor and acts as an antagonist. Doxorubicin intercalates in DNA and thus interferes in transcription. Cyclophosphamide, mechlorethamine and cisplatin can cross-link with DNA strands to inhibit its function.

38.4 Myelosuppression is a particularly serious toxicity with all of the following EXCEPT:

A. Vinblastine.

B. Cyclophosphamide.

C. Cytarabine.

D. Mechlorethamine.

E. L-Asparaginase.

The correct choice = E. L-Asparaginase is a foreign protein and causes hypersensitivity reactions.

38.5 Cells resistant to methotrexate may

A. have higher than normal levels of dihydrofolate reductase.

B. have higher levels of formyltetrahydrofolate.

C. metabolize the drug to inactive products.

D. have a decreased metabolic need for folate.

E. show an increased uptake of methotrexate.

The correct answer = A. Resistant cells may have elevated levels of dihydrofolate reductase. Methotrexate inhibits dihydrofolate reductase and, therefore, leads to lower than normal levels of the reduced tetrahydrofolate derivatives. Methotrexate does undergo metabolism by the host, but this is not a factor in resistance. The metabolic need for folate is high in all rapidly dividing cells. A decrease in influx may be associated with resistance.

38.6 All of the following statements are true EXCEPT:

A. Patients with Hodgkin's disease being treated with procarbazine should be cautioned against ingesting food derived from fermentative sources.

B. Vincristine is effective in inducing remission in childhood acute lymphocytic leukemia.

C. X-irradiation of the cranio-spinal axis is an effective adjuvant therapy in the treatment of acute lymphocytic leukemia.

D. Treatment with alkylating agents can induce secondary tumors.

E. Tamoxifen complexes with DNA to inhibit RNA synthesis.

The correct choice = E. Tamoxifen forms a complex with the estrogen receptor. Procarbazine inhibits monoamine oxidase, an enzyme required to metabolize tyramine found in fermentative sources, such as cheese and some wines. X-irradiation is effective in eradicating leukemic cells which have found sanctuary in the CNS. Many anticancer drugs are mutagenic and carcinogenic, particularly the alkylating agents.

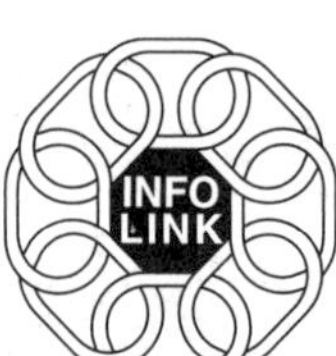

[1]See p. 325 in **Biochemistry** (2nd ed.)for role of methotrexate in preventing cell division.

[2]See p. 250 in **Biochemistry** (2nd ed.) for a more detailed discussion of tetrahydrofolate metabolism.

[3]See p. 349 in **Biochemistry** (2nd ed.) for a discussion of the salvage pathway of purine metabolism.

[4]See p. 247 in **Biochemistry** (2nd ed.) for a discussion of the feed-back inhibition of purine synthesis.

[5]See p. 350 in **Biochemistry** (2nd ed.) for role of xanthine oxidase in purine degradation.

[6]See p. 114 in **Biochemistry** (2nd ed.) for role of reactive oxygen intermediates.

[7]See p. 224 in **Biochemistry** (2nd ed.) for role of 11-β-hydroxysteroid dehydrogenase in steroid synthesis.

[8]See p. 365 in **Biochemistry** (2nd ed.) for role of topoisomerase in DNA synthesis.

Anti-inflammatory Drugs

39

I. OVERVIEW

Inflammation is a normal, protective response to tissue injury caused by physical trauma, noxious chemicals, or microbiologic agents. Inflammation is the body's effort to inactivate or destroy invading organisms, remove irritants, and set the stage for tissue repair. When healing is complete, the inflammatory process usually subsides. However, inflammation is sometimes inappropriately triggered by an innocuous agent, such as pollen, or by an autoimmune response, as in asthma or rheumatoid arthritis. In such cases, the defense reactions themselves may cause progressive tissue injury, and anti-inflammatory or immunosuppressive drugs may be required to modulate the inflammatory process. Inflammation is triggered by the release of chemical mediators from injured tissues and migrating cells. The specific chemical mediators vary with the type of inflammatory process and include amines, such as histamine and 5-hydroxytryptamine; lipids, such as the prostaglandins; small peptides, such as bradykinin; and larger peptides, such as interleukin-1. Discovery of the wide variation among chemical mediators has clarified the apparent paradox that an anti-inflammatory drug may interfere with the action of a particular mediator important in one type of inflammation but be without effect in inflammatory processes not involving the drug's target mediator. The drugs described in this chapter are summarized in Figure 39.1. [Note: The use of corticosteroids in the treatment of inflammation is discussed on p. 276.]

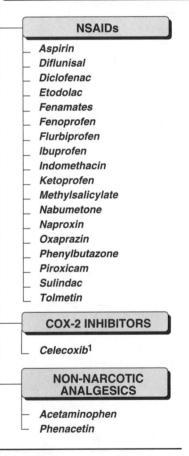

ANTI-INFLAMMATORY DRUGS

NSAIDs
- *Aspirin*
- *Diflunisal*
- *Diclofenac*
- *Etodolac*
- *Fenamates*
- *Fenoprofen*
- *Flurbiprofen*
- *Ibuprofen*
- *Indomethacin*
- *Ketoprofen*
- *Methylsalicylate*
- *Nabumetone*
- *Naproxin*
- *Oxaprazin*
- *Phenylbutazone*
- *Piroxicam*
- *Sulindac*
- *Tolmetin*

COX-2 INHIBITORS
- *Celecoxib*[1]

NON-NARCOTIC ANALGESICS
- *Acetaminophen*
- *Phenacetin*

Figure 39.1
Summary of nonsteroidal anti-inflammatory drugs. [1]Described in Pharmacology update, p. 466. (Continued on next page.)

II. PROSTAGLANDINS

Many of the nonsteroidal anti-inflammatory drugs (NSAIDs) act by inhibiting the synthesis of prostaglandins. Thus, an understanding of NSAIDs requires a comprehension of the actions and biosynthesis of prostaglandins—unsaturated fatty acid derivatives containing 20 carbons that include a cyclic ring structure. [Note: These compounds are sometimes referred to as eicosanoids; "eicosa" refers to the 20 carbon atoms.] Figure 39.2 illustrates the important structural features of the prostaglandins.

Lippincott's Illustrated Reviews: Pharmacology, Second Edition.
by Mary J. Mycek, Richard A. Harvey and Pamela C. Champe.
Lippincott Williams & Wilkins, Philadelphia, PA © 2000.

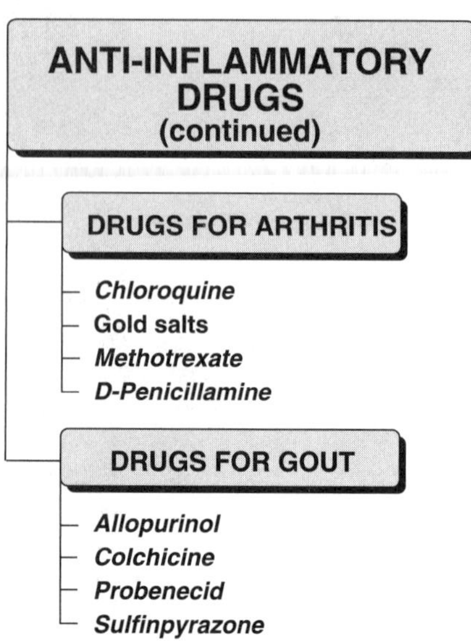
ANTI-INFLAMMATORY DRUGS (continued)
DRUGS FOR ARTHRITIS
Chloroquine
Gold salts
Methotrexate
D-Penicillamine
DRUGS FOR GOUT
Allopurinol
Colchicine
Probenecid
Sulfinpyrazone

Figure 39.1 (continued)
Summary of nonsteroidal anti-inflammatory drugs.

A. Role of prostaglandins as local mediators

Prostaglandins and related compounds are produced in minute quantities by virtually all tissues. They generally act locally on the tissues in which they are synthesized, and are rapidly metabolized to inactive products at their sites of action. Therefore, the prostaglandins do not circulate in the blood in significant concentrations. Thromboxanes, leukotrienes, and the hydroperoxyeicosatetraenoic and hydroxyeicosatetraenoic acids (HPETEs and HETEs) are related lipids, synthesized from the same precursors as are the prostaglandins, using interrelated pathways (Figure 39.3).

B. Synthesis of prostaglandins

Arachidonic acid, a 20-carbon fatty acid, is the primary precursor of the prostaglandins and related compounds (see Figure 39.3). Arachidonic acid is present as a component of the phospholipids of cell membranes, primarily phosphatidyl inositol and other complex lipids.[1] Free arachidonic acid is released from tissue phospholipids by the action of phospholipase A_2 and other acyl hydrolases, via a process controlled by hormones and other stimuli (see Figure 39.3). There are two major pathways in the synthesis of the eicosanoids from arachidonic acid (see Figure 39.3).

1. **Cyclooxygenase pathway:** All eicosanoids with ring structures, that is, the prostaglandins, thromboxanes, and prostacyclins, are synthesized via the cyclooxygenase pathway. Two cyclooxygenases have been identified: COX-1 and COX-2. The former is ubiquitous and constitutive, whereas the latter is induced in response to inflammatory stimuli. The products of these and subsequent reactions in this pathway are summarized in Figure 39.3.

2. **Lipoxygenase pathway:** Alternatively, several lipoxygenases can act on arachidonic acid to form 5-HPETE, 12-HPETE and 15-HPETE, which are unstable peroxidated derivatives that are converted to the corresponding hydroxylated derivatives (the HETES), or to leukotrienes or lipoxins, depending on the tissue (Figure 39.3).[2]

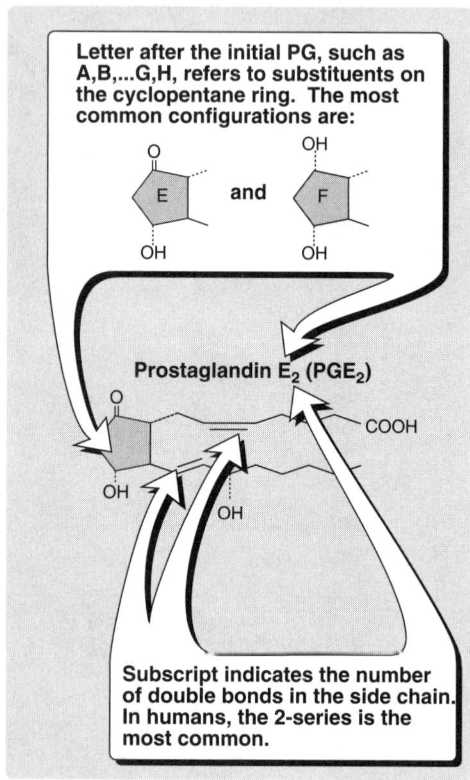
Letter after the initial PG, such as A,B,...G,H, refers to substituents on the cyclopentane ring. The most common configurations are:
O
OH
E
and
F
OH
OH
Prostaglandin E_2 (PGE_2)
O
COOH
OH
OH
Subscript indicates the number of double bonds in the side chain. In humans, the 2-series is the most common.

Figure 39.2
Structural features of prostaglandins.

C. Actions of prostaglandins

Many of the actions of prostaglandins are mediated by their binding to a wide variety of distinct membrane receptors that operate via G proteins, which subsequently activate or inhibit adenylyl cyclase or stimulate phospholipase C. This causes an enhanced formation of diacylglycerol and inositol-1,4,5-trisphosphate (IP_3). $PGF_{2\alpha}$, the leukotrienes, and thromboxane A_2 (TXA_2) mediate certain actions by activating phosphatidylinositol metabolism and causing an increase of intracellular Ca^{++}. [Note: Some prostaglandin receptor antagonists have been developed but they have no clinical use.]

D. Functions in the body

Prostaglandins and their metabolites produced endogenously in tissues act as local signals that fine-tune the response of a specific cell type. Their functions vary widely depending on the tissue. For example, the release of TXA_2 from platelets triggers the recruitment of new

[1,2]See p. 418 for Infolink references to other books in this series.

platelets for aggregation (the first step in clot formation). However, in other tissues, elevated levels of TXA_2 convey a different signal; for example, in certain smooth muscle, this compound induces contraction. Prostaglandins are one of the chemical mediators that are released in allergic and inflammatory processes (see p. 221).

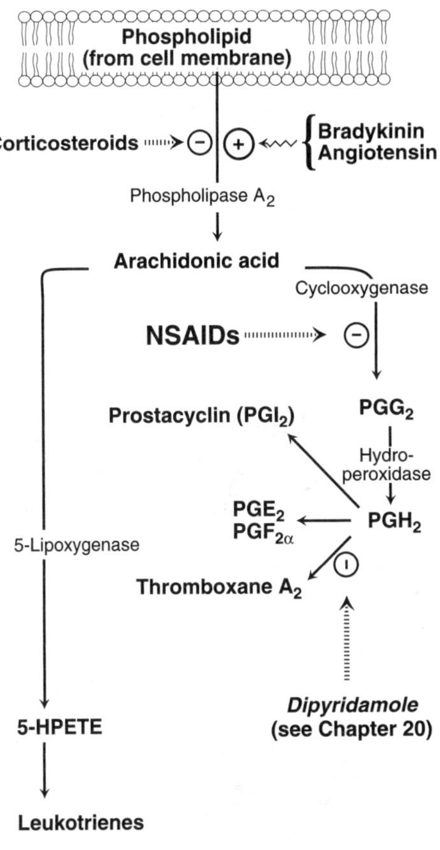

Figure 39.3
Synthesis of prostaglandins and leukotrienes.

III. NONSTEROIDAL ANTI-INFLAMMATORY DRUGS

The nonsteroidal anti-inflammatory drugs (NSAIDs) are a group of chemically dissimilar agents that differ in their antipyretic, analgesic and anti-inflammatory activities. They act primarily by inhibiting the cyclooxygenase enzymes but not the lipoxygenase enzymes. *Aspirin* is the prototype of this group; it is the most commonly used and the drug to which all other anti-inflammatory agents are compared. However, about 15% of patients show an intolerance to *aspirin*. Therefore, these individuals may benefit from other NSAIDs. In addition, some of the newer NSAIDs are marginally superior to *aspirin* in certain patients, because they have greater anti-inflammatory activity and/or cause less gastric irritation, or can be taken less frequently. However, the newer NSAIDs are considerably more expensive than *aspirin*, and some have proved to be more toxic in other ways.

A. Aspirin and other salicylates

Aspirin [AS pir in] is a weak organic acid that is unique among the NSAIDs in irreversibly acetylating (and thus inactivating) cyclooxygenase (Figure 39.4). The other NSAIDs, including salicylate, are all reversible inhibitors of cyclooxygenase. [Note: The NSAIDs do not appear to be strictly selective for either of the cyclooxygenase isozymes. Theoretically, selective inhibition of COX-2 might be advantageous because it would be confined to inflamed tissues.] *Aspirin* is rapidly deacetylated by esterases in the body, producing salicylate, which has anti-inflammatory, antipyretic, and analgesic effects. [Note: *Diflunisal* [dye FLOO ni sal], a difluorophenyl derivative of salicylic acid, is not metabolized to salicylate and therefore cannot cause salicylate intoxication (see p. 406). *Diflunisal* is 3 to 4 times more potent than *aspirin* as an analgesic and an anti-inflammatory agent, but it has no antipyretic properties. *Diflunisal* does not enter the CNS and therefore cannot relieve fever.]

1. **Mechanism of action:** The antipyretic and anti-inflammatory effects of the salicylates are due primarily to the blockade of prostaglandin synthesis at the thermoregulatory centers in the hypothalamus and at peripheral target sites. Furthermore, by decreasing prostaglandin synthesis, the salicylates also prevent the sensitization of pain receptors to both mechanical and chemical stimuli. *Aspirin* may also depress pain stimuli at subcortical sites (that is, the thalamus and hypothalamus).

2. **Actions**

The NSAIDs, including *aspirin*, have three major therapeutic actions, namely they reduce inflammation (antiinflammation), pain (analgesia), and fever (antipyrexia, see Figure 39.5). However, as described later in this section, not all of the NSAIDs are equally potent in each of these actions.

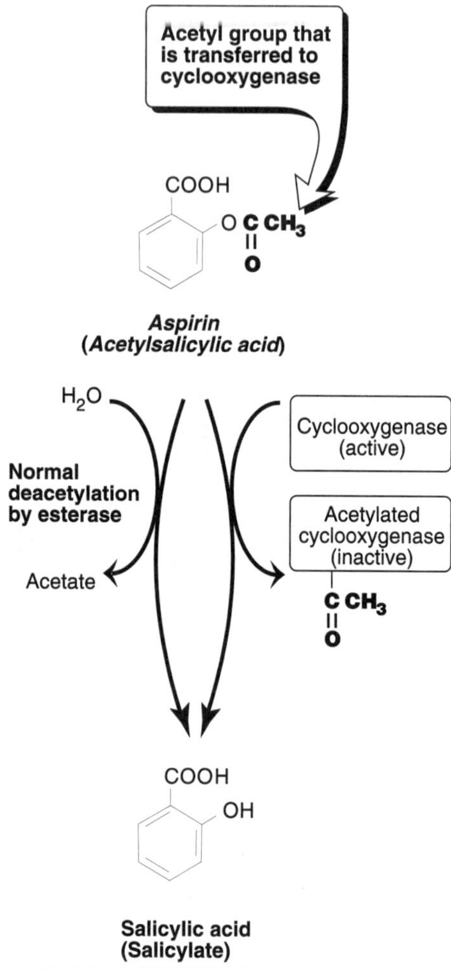

Figure 39.4
Metabolism of *aspirin* and acetylation of cyclooxygenase by *aspirin*.

a. **Anti-inflammatory actions:** Because *aspirin* inhibits cyclooxygenase activity, it diminishes the formation of prostaglandins and thus modulates those aspects of inflammation in which prostaglandins act as mediators (see Figure 39.3). *Aspirin* inhibits inflammation in arthritis, but it neither arrests the progress of the disease nor does it induce remission. [Note: *Acetaminophen*, although a useful analgesic and antipyretic, has weak anti-inflammatory activity and is therefore not useful in the treatment of inflammation such as that seen with rheumatoid arthritis (see Figure 39.5). *Acetaminophen* is therefore discussed separately (see p. 412).]

b. **Analgesic action:** Prostaglandin E_2 (PGE_2) is thought to sensitize the nerve endings to the action of bradykinin, histamine, and other chemical mediators released locally by the inflammatory process. Thus, by decreasing PGE_2 synthesis, *aspirin* and other NSAIDs repress the sensation of pain. The salicylates are used mainly for the management of pain of low to moderate intensity arising from integumental structures rather than that arising from the viscera. NSAIDs are superior to opioids in the management of pain in which inflammation is involved; combinations of opioids and NSAIDs are effective in treating pain in malignancy.

c. **Antipyretic action:** Fever occurs when the set-point of the anterior hypothalamic thermoregulatory center is elevated. This can be caused by PGE_2 synthesis, stimulated when an endogenous fever-producing agent (pyrogen) such as a cytokine is released from white cells that are activated by infection, hypersensitivity, malignancy, or inflammation. The salicylates lower body temperature in patients with fever by impeding PGE_2 synthesis and release. *Aspirin* resets the "thermostat" toward normal and rapidly lowers the body temperature of febrile patients by increasing heat dissipation as a result of peripheral vasodilation and sweating. *Aspirin* has no effect on normal body temperature.

d. **Respiratory actions:** At therapeutic doses, *aspirin* increases alveolar ventilation. [Note: Salicylates uncouple oxidative phosphorylation, which leads to elevated CO_2 and increased respiration.] Higher doses work directly on the respiratory center in the medulla, resulting in hyperventilation and respiratory alkalosis that is usually adequately compensated for by the kidney. At toxic levels, central respiratory paralysis occurs and respiratory acidosis ensues due to continued production of CO_2.

e. **Gastrointestinal effects:** Normally, prostacyclin (PGI_2) inhibits gastric acid secretion, whereas PGE_2 and $PGF_{2\alpha}$ stimulate synthesis of protective mucus in both the stomach and small intestine. In the presence of *aspirin*, these prostanoids are not formed, resulting in increased gastric acid secretion and diminished mucus protection. This may cause epigastric distress, ulceration, and/or hemorrhage. At ordinary *aspirin* doses, as much as 3 to 8 ml of blood may be lost in the feces per day. [Note: Buffered and enteric-coated preparations are only marginally helpful in dealing with this problem. The PGE_1 derivative, *misoprostol*, is used in the treatment of gastric damage induced by NSAIDs (see p. 238).]

f. **Effect on platelets:** TXA_2 enhances platelet aggregation, whereas PGI_2 decreases it. Low doses (60 to 80 mg daily) of *aspirin* can irreversibly inhibit thromboxane production in platelets without markedly affecting TXA_2 production in the endothelial cells of the blood vessel. [Note: The acetylation of cyclooxygenase is irreversible. Because platelets lack nuclei, they cannot synthesize new enzyme, and the lack of thromboxane persists for the lifetime of the platelet (3 to 7 days). This contrasts with the endothelial cells, which have nuclei and therefore can produce new cyclooxygenase.] As a result of the decrease in TXA_2, platelet aggregation (the first step in thrombus formation) is reduced, producing an anticoagulant effect with a prolonged bleeding time. [Note: The actions of *aspirin* as an antithrombotic drug are described on p. 197.]

g. **Actions on the kidney:** Cyclooxygenase inhibitors prevent the synthesis of PGE_2 and PGI_2–prostaglandins that are responsible for maintaining renal blood flow, particularly in the presence of circulating vasoconstrictors (Figure 39.6). Decreased synthesis of prostaglandins can result in retention of sodium and water and may cause edema and hyperkalemia in some patients. Interstitial nephritis can also occur with all of the NSAIDs except *aspirin*.

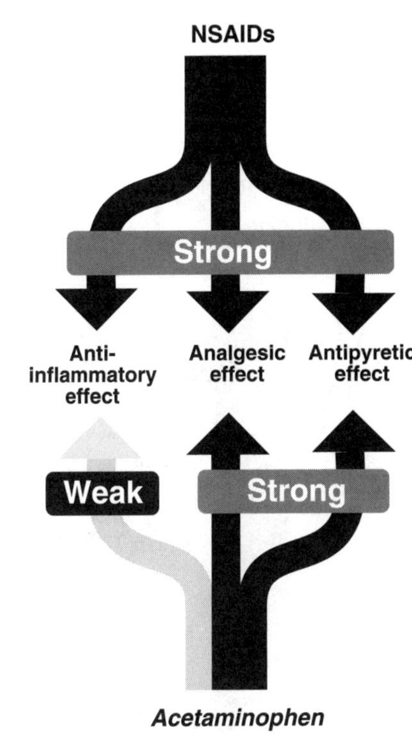

Figure 39.5
Actions of NSAIDs and *acetaminophen*.

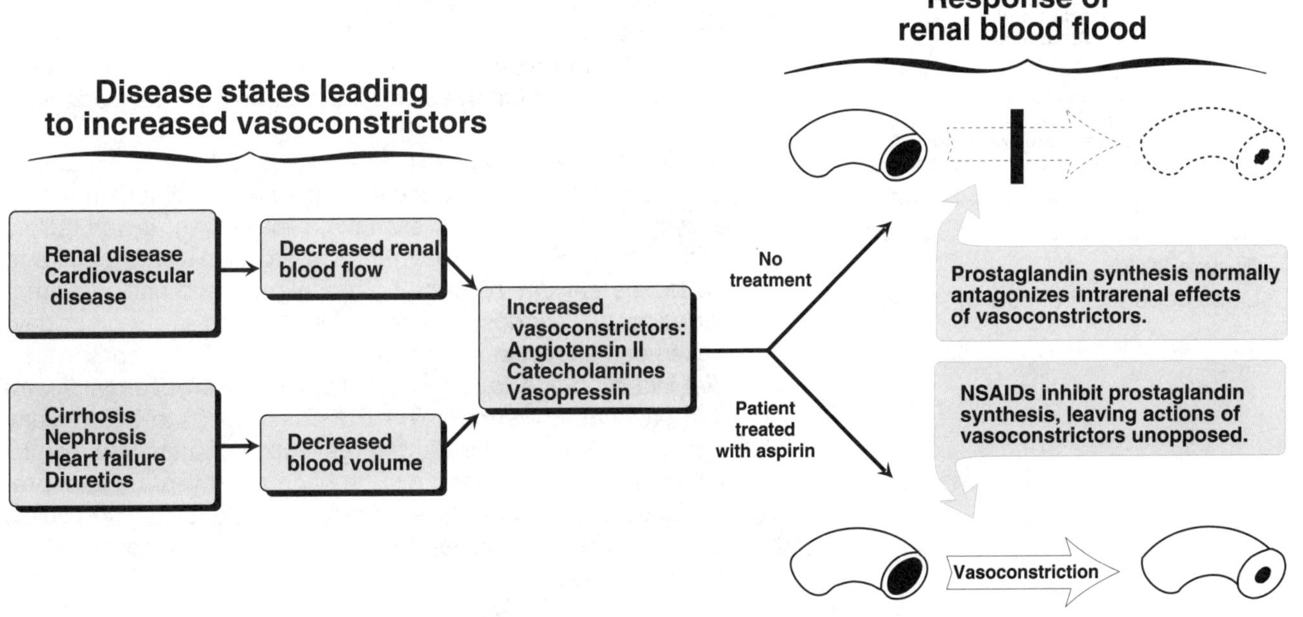

Figure 39.6
Renal effect of *aspirin* inhibition of prostaglandin synthesis.

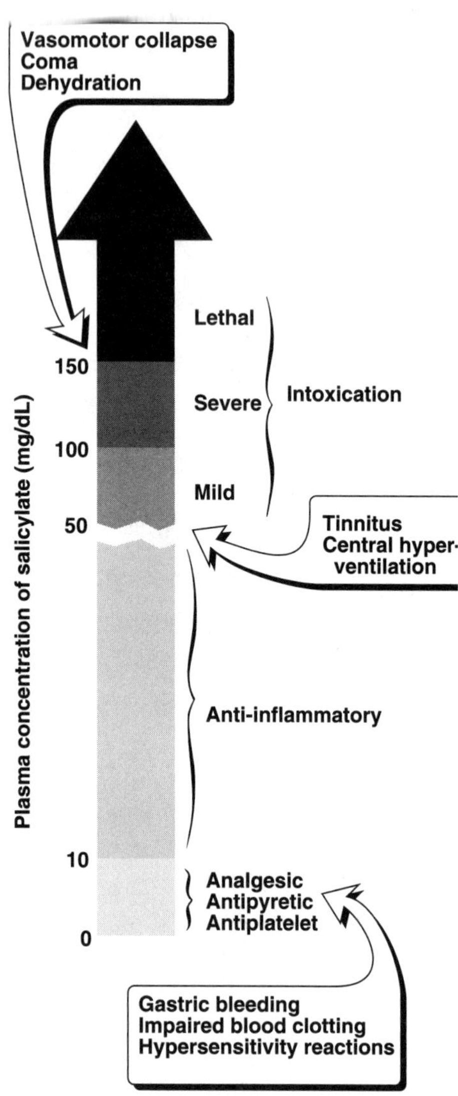

Figure 39.7
Dose-dependent effects of salicylate.

3. Therapeutic uses

a. **Antipyretics and analgesics:** *Sodium salicylate*, *choline salicylate* (in the liquid formulation), *choline magnesium salicylate*, and *aspirin* are used as antipyretics and analgesics in the treatment of gout, rheumatic fever, and rheumatoid arthritis. [Note: Salicylates are the drugs of choice in the treatment of rheumatoid arthritis.] Commonly treated conditions requiring analgesia include headache, arthralgia, and myalgia.

b. **External applications:** *Salicylic acid* is used topically to treat corns, calluses, and epidermophytosis (an eruption caused by fungi). *Methyl salicylate* ("oil of wintergreen") is used externally as a cutaneous counterirritant in liniments.

c. **Cardiovascular applications:** Salicylates are used to inhibit platelet aggregation (see above). Low doses of *aspirin* are used prophylactically to decrease the incidence of transient ischemic attack and unstable angina in men as well as that of coronary artery thrombosis. (See p. 197 for a further discussion of this phenomenon). *Aspirin* also facilitates closure of a patent ductus arteriosus (PGE_2 is responsible for keeping the ductus arteriosus open).

d. **Colon cancer:** There is evidence that chronic use of *aspirin* reduces the incidence of colorectal cancer.

4. Pharmacokinetics

a. **Administration and distribution:** Salicylates, especially *methyl salicylate*, are absorbed through intact skin. After oral administration, the unionized salicylates are passively absorbed from the stomach and the small intestine (dissolution of the tablets is favored at the higher pH of the gut). Rectal absorption of the salicylates is slow and unreliable, but it is a useful route for administration to vomiting children. Salicylates (except for *diflunisal*) cross both the blood-brain barrier and the placenta.

b. **Dosage:** The salicylates exhibit analgesic activity at low doses; only at higher doses do these drugs show anti-inflammatory activity (Figure 39.7). For example, two 300 mg *aspirin* tablets administered 4 times a day produce analgesia, whereas 12 to 20 tablets per day produce both analgesic and anti-inflammatory activity. Low dosages of *aspirin* (160 mg every other day) have been shown to reduce the incidence of recurrent myocardial infarction and to reduce mortality in postmyocardial infarction patients. Further, *aspirin* in a dose of 160 to 325 mg/day appears to be beneficial in the prevention of a first myocardial infarction, at least in men over the age of 50 years. Thus, prophylactic *aspirin* therapy is advocated in patients with clinical manifestations of coronary disease if no specific contraindications are present.

c. **Fate:** At normal low dosages (600 mg/day), *aspirin* is hydrolyzed to salicylate and acetic acid by esterases present in tissues and blood (see Figure 39.4). Salicylate is converted by the liver to water-soluble conjugates that are rapidly cleared by the kidney, resulting in elimination with first-order kinetics and a serum half-life of 3.5 hours. At anti-inflammatory dosages (>4 g/day), the hepatic metabolic pathway becomes saturated, and zero-order kinetics are observed, with the drug having a half-life of 15 hours or more (Figure 39.8). Saturation of the hepatic enzymes requires treatment for several days to 1 week. Being an organic acid, salicylate is secreted into the urine and can affect uric acid excretion. At low doses of *aspirin,* uric acid secretion is decreased; at high doses, it is increased. [Note: Alkalinization of the urine promotes excretion.]

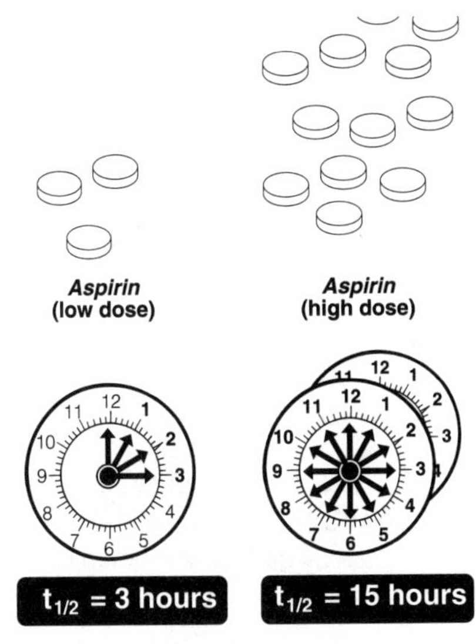

Figure 39.8
Effect of dose on the half-life of *aspirin.*

5. Adverse effects

a. GI: The most common GI effects of the salicylates are epigastric distress, nausea, and vomiting. Microscopic GI bleeding is almost universal in patients treated with salicylates. [Note: *Aspirin* is an acid. At stomach pH, *aspirin* is uncharged; consequently it readily crosses into the mucosal cells where it ionizes (becomes negatively charged) and becomes trapped (see p. 23 for discussion of ion trapping), thus potentially causing direct damage to the cells. *Aspirin* should be taken with food and large volumes of fluids to diminish GI disturbances. Alternatively, *misoprostol* (see p. 238) may be taken concurrently.]

b. Blood: The irreversible acetylation of platelet cyclooxygenase reduces the level of platelet TXA_2, resulting in inhibition of platelet aggregation and a prolonged bleeding time. For this reason *aspirin* should not be taken for at least 1 week prior to surgery. When salicylates are administered, anticoagulants may have to be given in reduced dosage.

c. Respiration: In toxic doses, salicylates cause respiratory depression and a combination of uncompensated respiratory and metabolic acidosis.

d. Metabolic processes: Large doses of salicylates uncouple oxidative phosphorylation. The energy normally used for the production of ATP is dissipated as heat, which explains the hyperthermia caused by salicylates when taken in toxic quantities.

e. Hypersensitivity: Approximately 15% of patients taking *aspirin* experience hypersensitivity reactions. Symptoms of true allergy include urticaria, bronchoconstriction, or angioneurotic edema. Fatal anaphylactic shock is rare.

f. Reye's syndrome: *Aspirin* given during viral infections has been associated with an increased incidence of Reye's syndrome, an often fatal, fulminating hepatitis with cerebral edema. This is especially encountered in children, who therefore should be given *acetaminophen* instead of *aspirin* when such medication is required.

g. Drug interactions: Concomitant administration of salicylates with many classes of drugs may produce undesirable side effects (Figure 39.9).

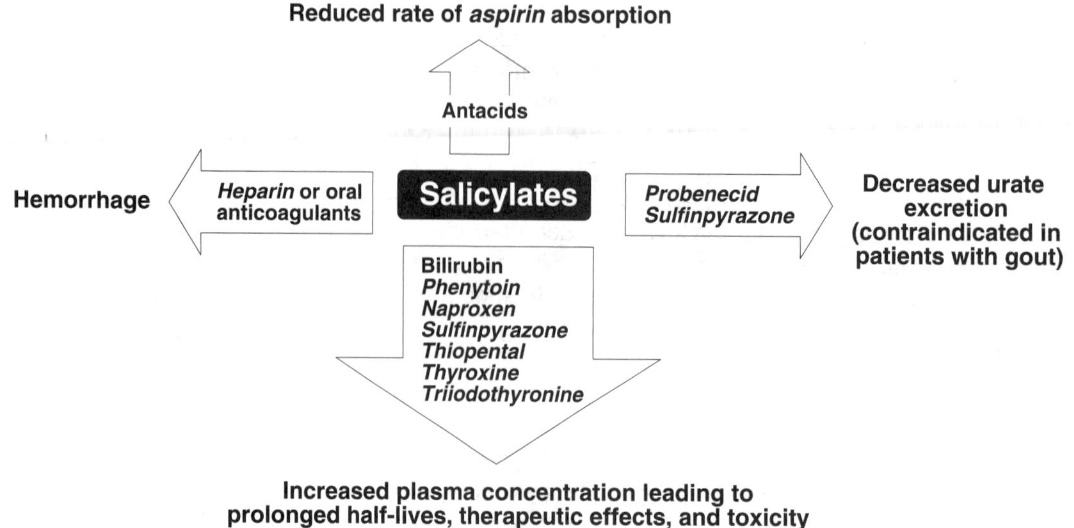

Figure 39.9
Drugs interacting with salicylates.

6. **Toxicity:** Salicylate intoxication may be mild or severe. The mild form is called salicylism and is characterized by nausea, vomiting, marked hyperventilation, headache, mental confusion, dizziness, and tinnitus (ringing or roaring in the ears). When large doses of salicylate are administered, severe salicylate intoxication may result (see Figure 39.7). The symptoms listed above are followed by restlessness, delirium, hallucinations, convulsions, coma, respiratory and metabolic acidosis, and death from respiratory failure. Children are particularly prone to salicylate intoxication. Ingestion of as little as 10 g of *aspirin* (or 5 g of *methyl salicylate*, the latter being used as a counterirritant in liniments) can cause death in children. Treatment of salicylism should include measurement of serum salicylate concentrations and of pH to determine the best form of therapy. In mild cases, symptomatic treatment is usually sufficient. Increasing the urinary pH enhances the elimination of salicylate. In serious cases, mandatory measures include the intravenous administration of fluid, dialysis (hemodialysis or peritoneal dialysis), and the frequent assessment and correction of acid-base and electrolyte balances. [Note: *Diflunisal* does not cause salicylism.]

B. Propionic acid derivatives.

Ibuprofen [eye byoo proe fen] was the first in this class of agents to become available in the United States. It has been joined by *naproxen* [nah PROX en], *fenoprofen* [fen oh proe fen], *ketoprofen* [key toe proe fen], *flurbiprofen* [flur bye proe fen]. and *oxaprozin* [ox ah PROE zin]. All of these drugs possess anti-inflammatory, analgesic and antipyretic activity and have gained wide acceptance in the chronic treatment of rheumatoid and osteoarthritis because their gastrointestinal effects are generally less intense than that of *aspirin*. These drugs are reversible inhibitors of the cyclooxygenases and thus, like *aspirin*, inhibit the synthesis of prostaglandins but not that of leukotrienes. All are well absorbed on oral administration and are almost totally bound to serum albumin. [Note: *Oxaprozin* has the longest half-life and is administered once daily.] They undergo hepatic metabolism and are excreted by the kidney. The most common adverse effect is gastrointestinal, ranging from dyspepsia to bleeding. Side effects involving the CNS, such as headache, tinnitus and dizziness, have also been reported.

C. Indoleacetic acids

This group of drugs includes *indomethacin* [in doe METH a sin], *sulindac* [sul IN dak] and *etodolac* [eh TOE doh lak]. All have anti-inflammatory, analgesic and antipyretic activity. They act by reversibly inhibiting cyclooxygenase. They are generally not used to lower fever.

1. **Indomethacin:** This NSAID is more potent than *aspirin* as an anti-inflammatory agent, but it is inferior to the salicylates at doses tolerated by rheumatoid arthritic patients. In certain instances, however (for example, with acute gouty arthritis, ankylosing spondylitis, and osteoarthritis of the hip), *indomethacin* is more effective in relieving inflammation than is *aspirin* or any of the other NSAIDs.

    a. **Therapeutic uses:** Despite its potency as an anti-inflammatory agent, *indomethacin's* toxicity limits its use to the treatment of the conditions described above. *Indomethacin* is also beneficial in the control of pain associated with uveitis and postoperative ophthalmic procedures, and as an antipyretic for Hodgkin's disease, when the fever is refractory to other agents. Like *aspirin*, *indomethacin* can delay labor by suppressing uterine contractions. It is also effective in treating patent ductus arteriosus.

    b. **Pharmacokinetics:** *Indomethacin* is rapidly and almost completely absorbed from the upper GI tract after oral administration. It is metabolized by the liver. Unchanged drug and metabolites are excreted in bile and urine.

    c. **Adverse effects:** Adverse effects with *indomethacin* occur in up to 50% of patients treated; approximately 20% find the adverse effects to be intolerable (Figure 39.10) and discontinue use of the drug. Most adverse effects are dose-related. GI complaints consist of nausea, vomiting, anorexia, diarrhea, and abdominal pain. Ulceration of the upper GI tract can occur, sometimes with perforation and hemorrhage. The most severe and frequent CNS effect is frontal headache, which occurs in 25 to 50% of patients who chronically use *indomethacin*. Other frequent CNS effects are dizziness, vertigo, light-headedness, and mental confusion. Acute pancreatitis has been known to occur. Hepatic effects are rare, but some fatal cases of hepatitis and jaundice have been reported. Hematopoietic reactions reported with *indomethacin* include neutropenia, thrombocytopenia, and (rarely) aplastic anemia. Hypersensitivity reactions include rashes, urticaria, itching, acute attacks of asthma, and 100% cross-reactivity with *aspirin*. Concurrent administration of *indomethacin* may decrease the antihypertensive effects of *furosemide*, the thiazide diuretics, β-blocking drugs and ACE inhibitors.

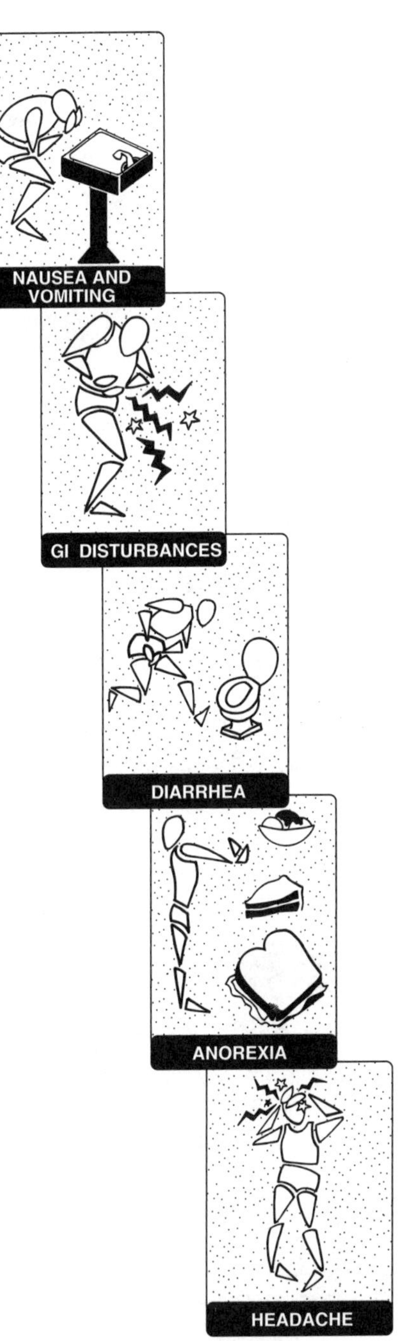

Figure 39.10
Some adverse effects of *indomethacin*.

2. **Sulindac:** This inactive pro-drug is closely related to *indomethacin*. Metabolism by hepatic microsomal enzymes produces the active form (a sulfide) of the drug, which has a long duration of action. Although the drug is less potent than *indomethacin*, it is useful in the treatment of rheumatoid arthritis, ankylosing spondylitis, osteoarthritis, and acute gout. The adverse reactions are similar to but less severe than those of the other NSAIDs, including *indomethacin*.

3. **Etodolac:** This drug has effects similar to those of the other NSAIDs. Gastrointestinal problems may be less common. However, other adverse effects such as fluid retention and abnormal kidney and liver function have been reported. *Etodolac* may increase the serum levels and thus raise the risk of adverse reactions caused by *digoxin, lithium*, *methotrexate*, and enhance the nephrotoxicity of *cyclosporine*.

D. Oxicam derivatives

Presently, only *piroxicam* [peer OX i kam] is available in the United States. Other members of this group are being tested and may become available. Its mechanism of action has not been established, but *piroxicam* is used to treat rheumatoid arthritis, ankylosing spondylitis, and osteoarthritis. Its mean half-life of 50 hours permits administration once a day. GI disturbances are encountered in approximately 20% of patients. The drug and its metabolites are excreted in the urine. *Piroxicam* can interfere with the renal excretion of *lithium*.

E. Fenamates

Mefenamic acid [meh FEN a mick] and *meclofenamate* [meh KLO fen a mate] have no advantages over the other NSAIDs as anti-inflammatory agents. Their side effects, such as diarrhea, can be severe and associated with inflammation of the bowel. Cases of hemolytic anemia have been reported.

F. Phenylbutazone

Phenylbutazone [fen ill BYOO ta zone] has powerful anti-inflammatory effects but weak analgesic and antipyretic activities. It is not a first line drug.

1. **Therapeutic uses:** *Phenylbutazone* is prescribed chiefly in short-term therapy of acute gout and in acute rheumatoid arthritis when other NSAID agents have failed. The usefulness of *phenylbutazone* is limited by its toxicity. *Aspirin* and newer NSAIDs are superior to *phenylbutazone* in most applications.

2. **Pharmacokinetics:** *Phenylbutazone* is rapidly and completely absorbed after oral or rectal administration. Oxyphenbutazone is an active metabolite and contributes to the activity of the parent drug. Like most of the other NSAIDs, *phenylbutazone* is extensively bound to plasma proteins. This property causes displace-

ment of *warfarin*, oral hypoglycemics and sulfonamides from binding sites on plasma proteins, causing transient elevations in the free fraction of these drugs.

3. **Adverse effects:** *Phenylbutazone* is poorly tolerated by many patients; adverse effects occur in nearly one half of those treated. The most serious adverse effects are agranulocytosis and aplastic anemia. However, the most common adverse effects of *phenylbutazone* are nausea, vomiting, skin rashes, and epigastric discomfort (Figure 39.11). Other side effects include fluid and electrolyte (sodium and chloride) retention, with resulting edema and decreased urine volume. Also, diarrhea, vertigo, insomnia, blurred vision, euphoria, nervousness, and hematuria may occur. *Phenylbutazone* reduces the uptake of iodine by the thyroid gland, sometimes resulting in goiter and myxedema. *Phenylbutazone* can also displace other drugs from plasma proteins, resulting in serious consequences (see above). Because of all these potential side-effects, the drug should be given for short periods of time—up to 1 week only. Patients should be observed closely, and frequent blood tests should be taken.

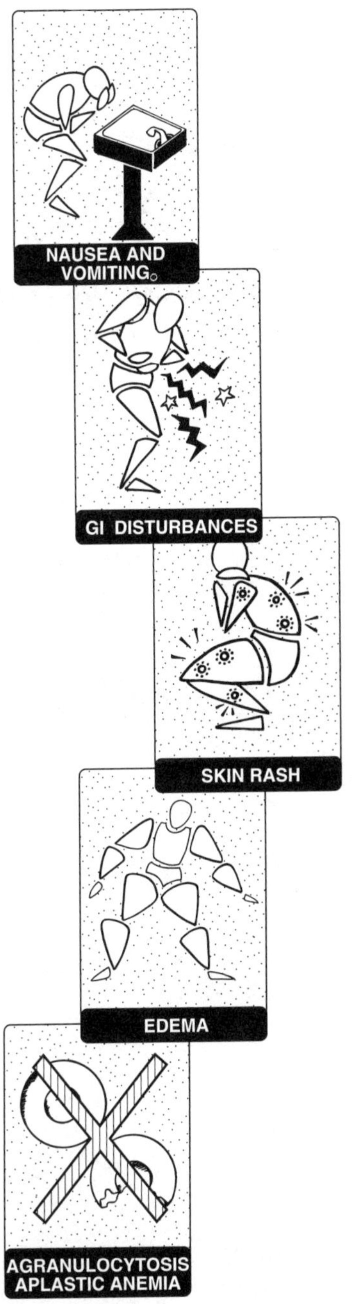

Figure 39.11
Some adverse effects of *phenylbutazone*.

G. Other agents

1. **Diclofenac:** A cyclooxygenase inhibitor, *diclofenac* [dye KLO fe nak] is approved for long-term use in the treatment of rheumatoid arthritis, osteoarthritis and ankylosing spondilitis. It is more potent than *indomethacin* or *naproxen*. An ophthalmic preparation is also available. *Diclofenac* accumulates in synovial fluid. The urine is the primary route of excretion for the drug and its metabolites. Its toxicities are similar to those of the other NSAIDs, for example, gastrointestinal problems are common, and the drug can also give rise to elevated hepatic enzyme levels.

2. **Ketorolac:** This drug acts like the other NSAIDs. In addition to the oral route, *ketorolac* [key TOE row lak] can be administered intramuscularly in the treatment of postoperative pain, and topically for allergic conjunctivitis. *Ketorolac* undergoes hepatic metabolism; the drug and its metabolites are eliminated via the urine. It causes the same side effects as the other NSAIDs.

3. **Tolmetin and nabumetone:** *Tolmetin* [TOLL me tin] and *nabumetone* [na BYOO me tone] are as potent as *aspirin* in treating adult or juvenile rheumatoid arthritis or osteoarthritis, but may have fewer adverse effects.

(See Figure 39.12 for a summary of the therapeutic advantages and disadvantages of members of the NSAID family.)

See pp. 466-467 for a description of newly approved COX-2 inhibitor, *celecoxib*.

IV. NON-NARCOTIC ANALGESICS

Non-narcotic analgesics, unlike the NSAIDs, have little or no anti-inflammatory activity. They have a therapeutic advantage over narcotic analgesics in that they do not cause physical dependence or tolerance.

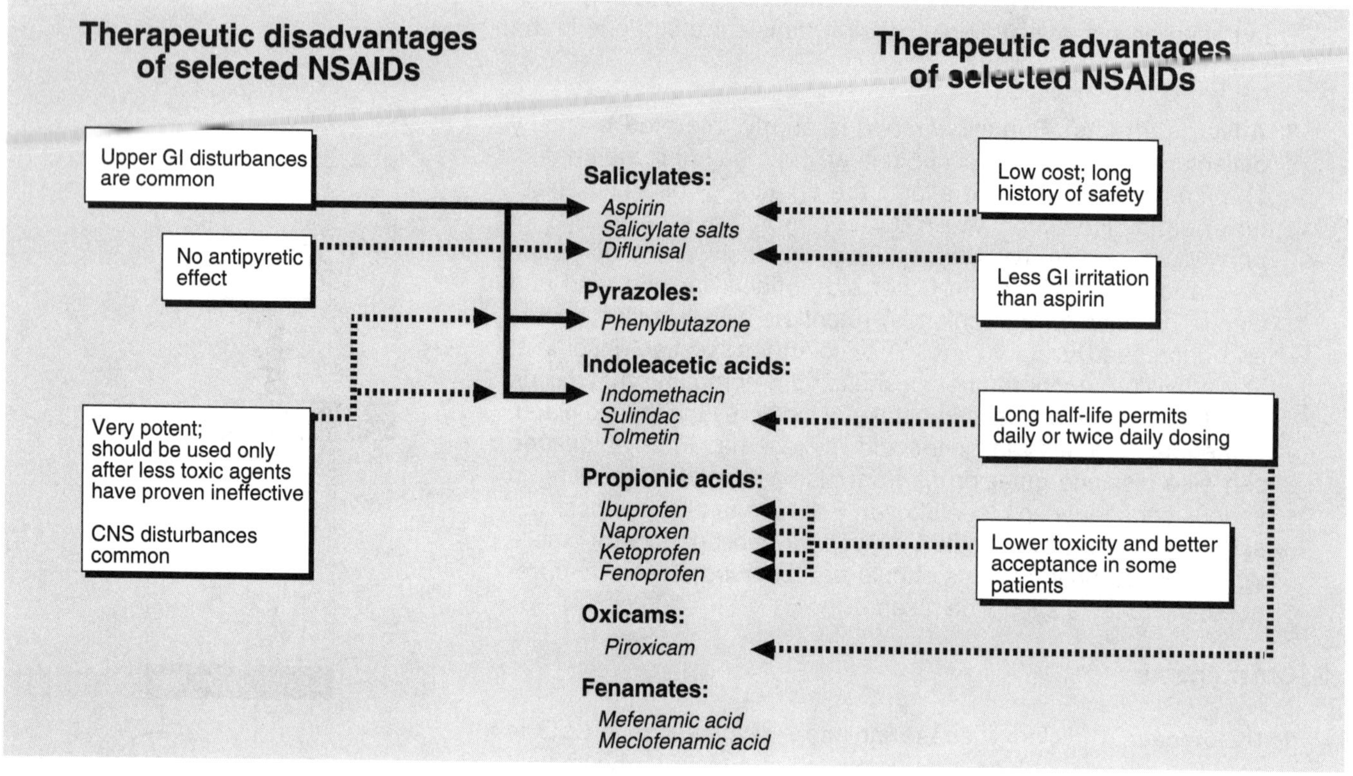

Figure 39.12
Summary of nonsteroidal anti-inflammatory agents (NSAIDs).

A. Acetaminophen and phenacetin

Acetaminophen [a seat a MIN oh fen] and *phenacetin* [fe NASS e tin] act by inhibiting prostaglandin synthesis in the CNS. This explains their antipyretic and analgesic properties. They have less effect on cyclooxygenase in peripheral tissues, which accounts for their weak anti-inflammatory activity. *Acetaminophen* and *phenacetin* do not affect platelet function or increase blood clotting time, and they lack many of the side-effects of *aspirin*. [Note: *Phenacetin* can no longer be prescribed in the United States because of its potential for renal toxicity. However, it is present in some proprietary preparations.]

1. **Therapeutic uses:** *Acetaminophen* is a suitable substitute for the analgesic and antipyretic effects of *aspirin* in those patients with gastric complaints and in those for whom prolongation of bleeding time would be a disadvantage or who do not require the anti-inflammatory action of *aspirin*. [Note: Because of its lower toxicity, *acetaminophen* has replaced *phenacetin* in virtually all headache products.] *Acetaminophen* is the analgesic-antipyretic of choice for children with viral infections or chicken pox (recall that *aspirin* increases the risk of Reye's syndrome, see p. 407). *Acetaminophen* does not antagonize the uricosuric agent *probenecid* and therefore may be used in patients with gout taking that drug.

2. **Pharmacokinetics:** *Acetaminophen* is rapidly absorbed from the GI tract. A significant first-pass metabolism occurs in the luminal cells of the intestine and in the hepatocytes. *Phenacetin* is largely converted to *acetaminophen* within 3 hours of administration. Under normal circumstances, *acetaminophen* is conjugated in the liver to form inactive glucuronidated or sulfated metabolites. A portion of *acetaminophen* is hydroxylated to form N-acetyl-benzoquinoneimine—a highly reactive and potentially dangerous metabolite that reacts with sulfhydryl groups. At normal doses of *acetaminophen*, the N-acetyl-benzoquinoneimine reacts with the sulfhydryl group of glutathione, forming a nontoxic substance (see Figure 39.13). *Acetaminophen* and its metabolites are excreted in the urine.

3. **Adverse effects:** With normal therapeutic doses, *acetaminophen* is virtually free of any significant adverse effects. Skin rash and minor allergic reactions occur infrequently. There may be minor alterations in leukocyte count, but these are generally transient. Renal tubular necrosis and hypoglycemic coma are rare complications of prolonged large-dose therapy. With large doses of *acetaminophen,* the available glutathione in the liver becomes depleted and N-acetyl-benzoquinoneimine reacts with the sulfhydryl groups of hepatic proteins, forming covalent bonds (Figure 39.13). Hepatic necrosis, a very serious and potentially life-threatening condition, can result. Renal tubular necrosis may also occur. [Note: Administration of N-acetylcysteine, which contains sulfhydryl groups to which the toxic metabolite can bind, can be life-saving if administered within 10 hours of the overdose.]

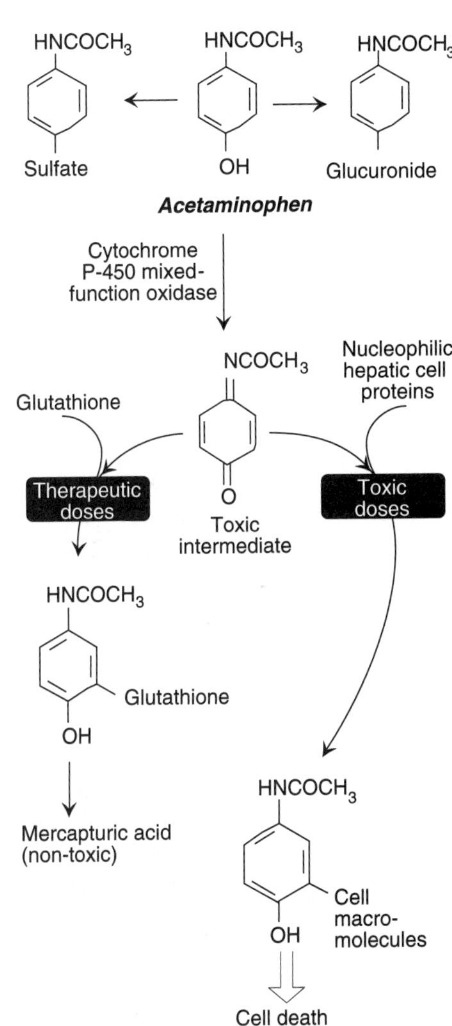

Figure 39.13
Metabolism of *acetaminophen.*

V. DISEASE-MODIFYING ANTI-RHEUMATIC AGENTS

In contrast to the NSAID drugs described earlier, remittive remission-inducing arthritis drugs are slow-acting. They do not act by inhibiting cyclooxygenases and may have no little analgesic or anti-inflammatory activity. These drugs are used primarily for rheumatic disorders, especially in cases where the inflammation disease does not respond to cyclooxygenase inhibitors NSAIDs. They disease-modifying anti-rheumatic agents (DMARDs) slow the course of the disease and may can induce remission, preventing further destruction of the joints and involved tissue. They have a long onset of action, sometimes taking 3 to 4 months. Their onset of action may be up to several months.

A. Gold salts

Gold compounds, like the other drugs in this group, cannot repair existing damage. Rather, they can only prevent further injury. The currently available gold preparations are *gold sodium thiomalate, aurothioglucose*, and *auranofin.* It is believed that gold salts are taken up by macrophages and suppress phagocytosis and lysosomal enzyme activity. This mechanism retards the progression of bone and articular destruction. Other mechanisms have also been proposed.

1. **Therapeutic uses:** The major use of gold salts is in the treatment of rheumatoid arthritis that does not respond to salicylates or

other nonsteroidal anti-inflammatory therapy. They are the most effective agents for the rapidly progressive types of the disease, particularly if given in its early stages.

2. **Pharmacokinetics:** *Gold sodium thiomalate* and *aurothioglucose* are water-soluble salts that are administered intramuscularly. *Auranofin* is taken by mouth. If a favorable response is achieved without serious toxic reaction, the drug can be continued indefinitely. The half-life of the drug lengthens with continued use. The gold concentrates in synovial fluid and in macrophages in a number of tissues including liver, kidney, spleen and adrenal cortex. Elimination is largely through the urine but some is also excreted in the feces. Sulfhydryl compounds such as *dimercaprol*, *penicillamine* or *N-acetylcysteine* hasten excretion.

3. **Adverse effects:** *Auranofin* is better tolerated than the injectable compounds. About one third of those patients receiving treatment with gold salts experience some adverse effects, the most common of which is dermatitis of the skin or of the mucous membranes (especially in the mouth), occuring in up to 20% of patients. Other possible adverse effects include proteinuria and nephrosis (5 to 8% of patients) and rare, severe blood disorders, such as agranulocytosis and aplastic anemia. Gold salts should be avoided in patients suffering from hepatic or renal disease, who have a history of toxicity to these agents, are pregnant, or are taking other drugs with a potential for blood dyscrasias. In the event of a serious toxicity, *dimercaprol* is administered.

B. Chloroquine and hydroxychloroquine

The pharmacology of these drugs, which are also used in the treatment of malaria, is presented on p. 351. The mechanism of their anti-inflammatory activity is uncertain. Besides inhibiting nucleic acid synthesis, they are known to stabilize lysosomal membranes and trap free radicals. In treating inflammatory disorders, they are reserved for rheumatoid arthritis that has been unresponsive to the NSAIDs or else they are used in conjunction with an NSAID, which allows a lower dose of *chloroquine* or *hydroxychloroquine* to be administered. These drugs have been shown to slow progression of erosive bone lesions and may induce remission. They do cause serious adverse effects (see p. 351).

C. D-Penicillamine

D-Penicillamine [pen i SILL a meen], an analog of the amino acid cysteine, slows the progress of bone destruction and rheumatoid arthritis. Its mechanism of action is unknown, but rheumatoid factor levels fall with administration. Prolonged treatment with *penicillamine* has serious side effects ranging from dermatologic problems to nephritis and aplastic anemia; therefore it is used primarily in the treatment of rheumatoid arthritis after use of gold salts has failed but before use of corticosteroids has been attempted. [Note: *Penicillamine* is used as a chelating agent in the treatment of poisoning by heavy metals. It is also of benefit in treating cystinuria.]

D. Methotrexate

Methotrexate [meth oh TREX ate] is used for the treatment of patients with severe rheumatoid arthritis who have not responded adequately to NSAIDs and at least one other slow-acting agent. Response to *methotrexate* occurs sooner than is usual for other slow-acting agents—often within 3 to 6 weeks of starting treatment. It is an immunosuppressant, and this may account for its effectiveness in arthritis–an autoimmune disease. Doses of *methotrexate* required for this treatment are much lower than those needed in cancer chemotherapy and are given once a week; therefore the adverse effects (see p. 380) are minimized. The most common side effects observed after *methotrexate* treatment of rheumatoid arthritis are mucosal ulceration and nausea. Cytopenias (particularly depression of the white blood cell count), cirrhosis of the liver, and an acute pneumonia-like syndrome may occur on chronic administration. [Note: Taking *leucovorin* a day after *methotrexate* reduces the severity of the adverse effects (see p. 379).] Other immunosuppressants such as *azathioprine* and *cyclosporine* are being investigated as possible anti-inflammatory agents.

See p. 467 for a description of newly approved drugs used in treating rheumatoid disease

VI. DRUGS EMPLOYED IN THE TREATMENT OF GOUT

Gout is a metabolic disorder characterized by high levels of uric acid in the blood. This hyperuricemia results in the deposition of crystals of sodium urate in tissues, especially the kidney and joints. Hyperuricemia does not always lead to gout, but gout is always preceded by hyperuricemia. In humans, sodium urate is the endproduct of purine metabolism.[3] The deposition of urate crystals initiates an inflammatory process involving the infiltration of granulocytes that phagocytize the urate crystals. This process generates oxygen metabolites, which damage tissue, resulting in the release of lysosomal enzymes that evoke an inflammatory response. In addition, lactate production in the synovial tissues increases. The resulting local decrease in pH fosters further deposition of urate crystals. (See Figure 39.14 for a summary of this process.) The cause of hyperuricemia is an overproduction of uric acid relative to the patient's ability to excrete it. Most therapeutic strategies for gout involve lowering the uric acid level below the saturation point, thus preventing the deposition of urate crystals. This can be accomplished by (1) interfering with uric acid synthesis with *allopurinol*, (2) increasing uric acid excretion with *probenecid* or *sulfinpyrazone*, (3) inhibiting leukocyte entry into the affected joint with *colchicine*, or (4) administration of NSAIDs.

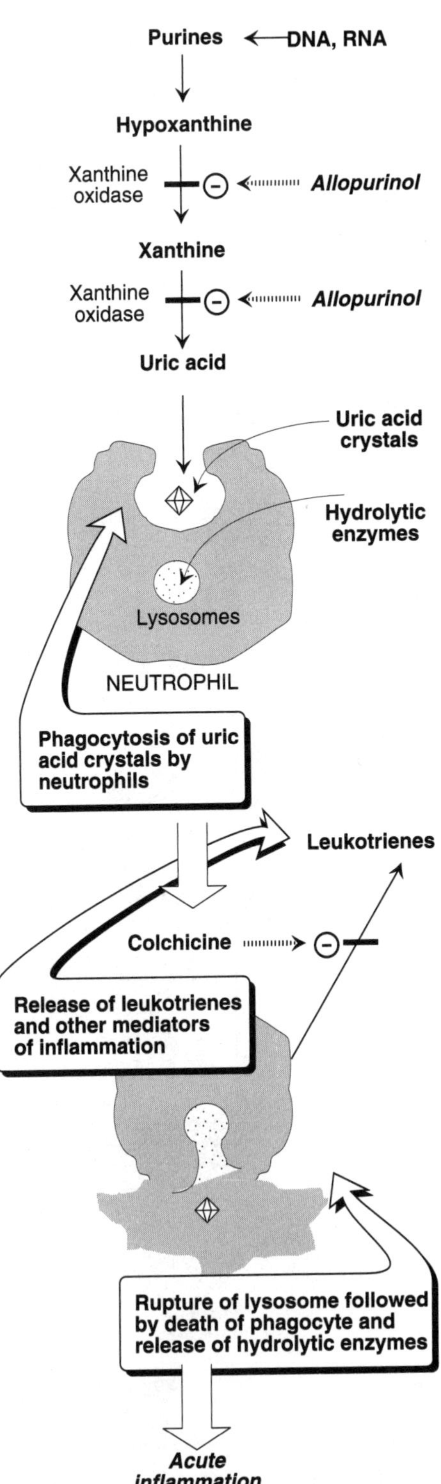

Figure 39.14
Role of uric acid in the inflammation of gout.

A. Treating acute gout

Acute gouty attacks can result from a number of conditions, including excessive alcohol consumption, a diet rich in purines, or kidney disease. Acute attacks are treated with *colchicine* to decrease movement of granulocytes into the affected area, and with NSAIDs to decrease pain and inflammation. [Note: *Aspirin* is contraindicated, because it competes with uric acid for the organic acid secretion mechanism in the proximal tubule of the kidney.]

[3]See p. 418 for Infolink references to other books in this series.

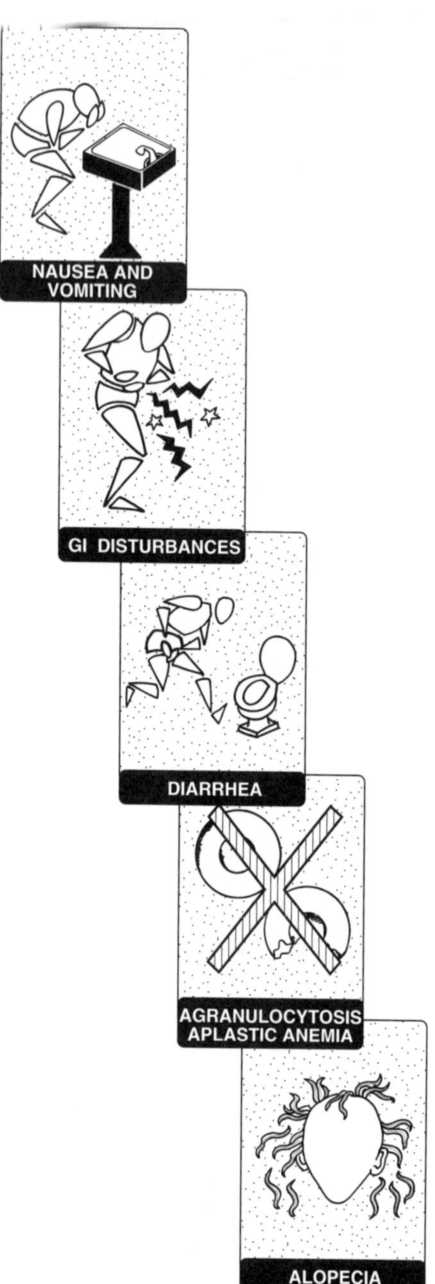

Figure 39.15
Some adverse effects of *colchicine.*

B. Treating chronic gout

Chronic gout can be caused by (1) a genetic defect, for example, one resulting in an increase in the rate of purine synthesis, (2) renal deficiency, (3) Lesch-Nyhan Syndrome,[4] or (4) excessive synthesis of uric acid associated with cancer chemotherapy. Treatment strategies for chronic gout include the use of uricosuric drugs that increase the excretion of uric acid, thereby reducing its concentration in plasma, and the use of *allopurinol*, which is a selective inhibitor of the terminal steps in the biosynthesis of uric acid.

C. Colchicine

Colchicine [KOL chi seen], a plant alkaloid, is reserved for the treatment of acute gouty attacks when they occur. It is not a uricosuric nor an analgesic agent, although it relieves pain in acute attacks of gout. *Colchicine* does not prevent the progression of gout to acute gouty arthritis, but it does have a suppressive, prophylactic effect that reduces the frequency of acute attacks and relieves pain.

1. **Mechanism of action:** *Colchicine* binds to tubulin, a microtubular protein, causing its depolymerization. This disrupts cellular functions, such as the mobility of granulocytes, thus decreasing their migration into the affected area. Furthermore, *colchicine* blocks cell division by binding to mitotic spindles. *Colchicine* also inhibits the synthesis and release of the leukotrienes (see Figure 39.14).

2. **Therapeutic uses:** The anti-inflammatory activity of *colchicine* is specific for gout, usually alleviating the pain of acute gout within 12 hours. It is only rarely effective in other kinds of arthritis.

3. **Pharmacokinetics:** *Colchicine* is administered orally, followed by rapid absorption from the GI tract. It is also available combined with *probenecid* (see below). *Colchicine* is recycled in the bile and is excreted unchanged in the feces or urine.

4. **Adverse effects:** *Colchicine* treatment may cause nausea, vomiting, abdominal pain, and diarrhea (Figure 39.15). Chronic administration may lead to myopathy, agranulocytosis, aplastic anemia, and alopecia. The drug should not be used in pregnancy, and should be used with caution in patients with hepatic, renal or cardiovascular disease.

D. Allopurinol

Allopurinol [al oh PURE i nole] is a purine analog. It reduces the production of uric acid by competitively inhibiting the last two steps in uric acid biosynthesis, which are catalyzed by xanthine oxidase (see Figure 39.14). [Note: Uric acid is less water-soluble than its precursors. When xanthine oxidase is inhibited, the circulating purine derivatives (xanthine and hypoxanthine) are more soluble and therefore are less likely to precipitate].

[4] See p. 418 for Infolink references to other books in this series.

1. **Therapeutic uses:** *Allopurinol* is effective in the treatment of primary hyperuricemia of gout and hyperuricemia secondary to other conditions, such as that associated with certain malignancies (those in which large amounts of purines are produced) or in renal disease.

2. **Pharmacokinetics:** *Allopurinol* is completely absorbed after oral administration. The primary metabolite is alloxanthine (oxypurinol) which is also a xanthine oxidase inhibitor. The pharmacologic effect of administered *allopurinol* results from the combined activity of these two compounds. The plasma half-life of *allopurinol* is short (2 hours), whereas the half-life of oxypurinol is long (15 hours). Thus, effective inhibition of xanthine oxidase can be maintained with once daily dosage. The drug and its metabolite are excreted in the feces and urine.

3. **Adverse effects:** *Allopurinol* is well tolerated by most patients. Hypersensitivity reactions, especially skin rashes, are the most common adverse reactions, occurring among approximately 3% of patients. The reactions may occur even after months or years of chronic administration. Acute attacks of gout may occur more frequently during the first several weeks of therapy; therefore *colchicine* and NSAIDs should be administered concurrently. Gastrointestinal side effects such as nausea and diarrhea are common. *Allopurinol* interferes with the metabolism of the anticancer agent, *6-mercaptopurine* (see p. 381) and the immunosuppressant, *azathioprine*, requiring a reduction in dosage of these drugs.

E. Uricosuric agents: probenecid and sulfinpyrazone

Probenecid [proe BEN e sid], a general inhibitor of the tubular secretion of organic acids, and *sulfinpyrazone* [sul fin PEER a zone], a derivative of *phenylbutazone* (see p. 411), are the two most commonly used uricosuric agents. At therapeutic doses, they block proximal tubular resorption of uric acid. [Note: At low dosage, these agents block proximal tubular secretion of uric acid.] These drugs have few adverse effects although gastric distress may force discontinuance of *sulfinpyrazone*. *Probenecid* blocks the tubular secretion of *penicillin* and is sometimes used to increase levels of the antibiotic. It also inhibits excretion of *naproxen*, *ketoprofen*, and *indomethacin*.

Choose the ONE best answer.

39.1 In which one of the following conditions would aspirin be contraindicated?

A. Myalgia
B. Fever
C. Peptic ulcer
D. Rheumatoid arthritis
E. Unstable angina

Correct answer = C. Among the NSAIDs, aspirin is among the worst for causing gastric irritation. Aspirin is an effective analgesic and is used to reduce muscle pain. It also has antipyretic actions so that it can be used to treat fever. Because of its anti-inflammatory properties, aspirin is used to treat pain related to the inflammatory process, for example, in the treatment of rheumatoid arthritis. Low doses of aspirin also decrease the incidence of transient ischemic attacks.

39.2 Overdoses of salicylates lead to all of the following EXCEPT:

A. Nausea and vomiting.
B. Tinnitus (ringing or roaring in the ears).
C. Marked hyperventilation.
D. Increased metabolic rate.
E. Increase in blood pH.

Correct choice = E. An overdose of salicylates causes acidosis.

39.3 Acetaminophen has all of the following properties EXCEPT:

A. It is a weaker anti-inflammatory agent than aspirin.
B. It reduces fever of viral infections in children.
C. It is an aspirin substitute in patients with peptic ulcer.
D. It exacerbates gout.
E. It causes hepatotoxic effects at high doses.

Correct choice = D. Acetaminophen does not antagonize the uricosuric agent probenecid and therefore may be used in patients with gout. Acetaminophen has little anti-inflammatory effect, but has analgesic and antipyretic activities equal to those of aspirin. It is the analgesic-antipyretic of choice for children with viral infections; aspirin can increase the risk for Reye's syndrome in children. Acetaminophen is a suitable substitute for the analgesic and antipyretic effects of aspirin in those patients with gastric complaints.

39.4 Which of the following statements concerning gold salts is CORRECT?

A. They may provide immediate relief of arthritic pain.
B. They act by inhibiting prostaglandin synthesis.
C. They frequently cause dermatitis of the skin or mucous membranes.
D. They are drugs of first choice in treating arthritis.
E. They must all be given intramuscularly.

Correct answer = C. Gold salts may not provide clinical improvement until after several weeks of administration. They are thought to suppress phagocytosis and lysosomal enzyme activity in macrophages. Gold salts are used in rheumatoid arthritis that does not respond to NSAIDs. Auranofin can be taken by mouth.

39.5 Which of the following is INCORRECTLY paired?

A. Indomethacin:	Causes frontal headaches
B. Sulindac:	Long half-life permits daily or twice daily dosing
C. Naproxen:	Better tolerated than aspirin in some patients
D. Phenylbutazone:	Less toxic than aspirin
E. Aspirin:	Can cause GI symptoms

Correct choice = D. Phenylbutazone is more toxic than aspirin and should be used only after less toxic agents have proven ineffective.

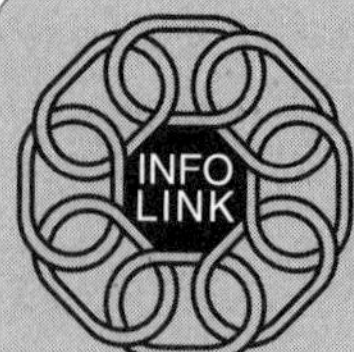

[1]See p. 172 in **Biochemistry** (2nd ed.) for a discussion of the chemistry of arachidonic acid.

[2]See p. 185 in **Biochemistry** (2nd ed.) for a discussion of prostaglandin synthesis.

[3]See p. 350 in **Biochemistry** (2nd ed.) for a discussion of purine metabolism.

[4]See p. 348 in **Biochemistry** (2nd ed.) for a discussion Lesch-Nyhan syndrome.

Autacoids and Autacoid Antagonists

40

I. OVERVIEW

Prostaglandins, histamine, and serotonin belong to a group of compounds called autacoids. These heterogenous substances have widely differing structures and pharmacologic activities. They all have the common feature of being formed by the tissues on which they act; thus, they function as local hormones. [Note: The word autacoid comes from the Greek: autos (self) and akos (medicinal agent, or remedy).] The autacoids also differ from circulating hormones in that they are produced by many tissues rather than in specific endocrine glands. The drugs described in this chapter (Figure 40.1) are either autacoids (both naturally occurring and synthetic analogs) or autacoid antagonists (that is, compounds that inhibit the synthesis of certain autacoids, or interfere with their interactions with receptors).

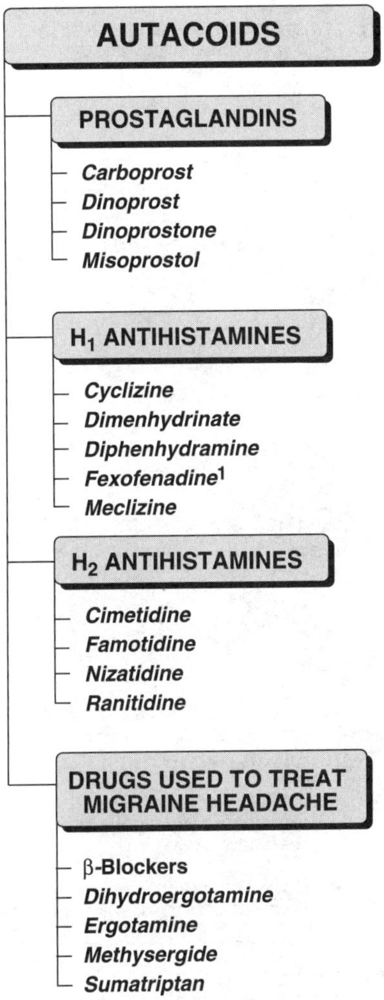

AUTACOIDS

PROSTAGLANDINS
- *Carboprost*
- *Dinoprost*
- *Dinoprostone*
- *Misoprostol*

H_1 ANTIHISTAMINES
- *Cyclizine*
- *Dimenhydrinate*
- *Diphenhydramine*
- *Fexofenadine*[1]
- *Meclizine*

H_2 ANTIHISTAMINES
- *Cimetidine*
- *Famotidine*
- *Nizatidine*
- *Ranitidine*

DRUGS USED TO TREAT MIGRAINE HEADACHE
- β-Blockers
- *Dihydroergotamine*
- *Ergotamine*
- *Methysergide*
- *Sumatriptan*

Figure 40.1
Summary of drugs affecting the autacoids. [1]Described in Pharmacology update, p. 470.

II. PROSTAGLANDINS

Prostaglandins are unsaturated fatty acid derivatives that act on the tissues in which they are synthesized and are rapidly metabolized to inactive products at the site of action. The biosynthesis and actions of the prostaglandins are presented on p. 402 and Figure 39.3.

A. Therapeutic uses of prostaglandins

Systemic administration of prostaglandins evokes a bewildering array of effects, a fact that limits the therapeutic usefulness of these agents.

1. **Abortion:** Several of the naturally occurring prostaglandins, such as *dinoprost* [DYE noe prost], *dinoprostone* [dye noe PROST one], and *carboprost* [KAR boe prost], find use as abortifacients (that is, agents causing abortions, Figure 40.2). *Misoprostol* in combination with *methotrexate* is particularly effective in terminating pregancy in the first trimester.

2. **Peptic ulcers:** *Misoprostol* [MIZ o prost ol] is a synthetic prostaglandin E_1 analog used to inhibit the secretion of hydrochloric acid in the stomach. It produces inhibition of gastric acid and pepsin secretion and enhances mucosal resistance to injury. *Misoprostol* is particularly useful in patients with gastric ulcer who are chronically taking nonsteroidal anti-inflammatory agents (see p. 238 for a more complete discussion of this drug).

3. **Erectile dysfunction:** *Alprostadil* injected into the corpus cavernosum of the penis provides effective treatment of some forms of male impotence. The drug increases arterial inflow through vasodilation and decreases venous outflow by causing relaxation of the corporal smooth muscle that occludes draining venules. Possible side effects include pain at the site of injection and, rarely, prolonged erection.

Dinoprost, dinoprostone, carboprost, misoprostol

- Act directly on myometrium to induce contractions and labor.
- Administration is by intraamnionic or intravaginal instillation from the 12th week through the second trimesterof pregnancy.
- *Misoprostol* in combination with *methotrexate* is effective in terminating pregnancy in the first trimester.

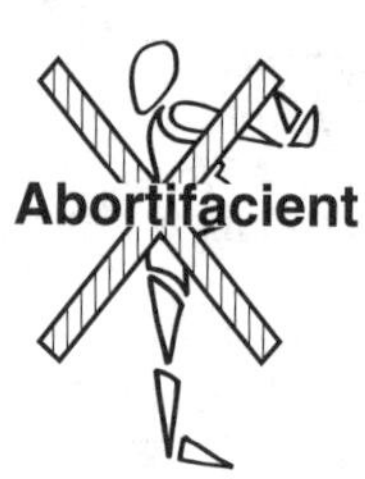

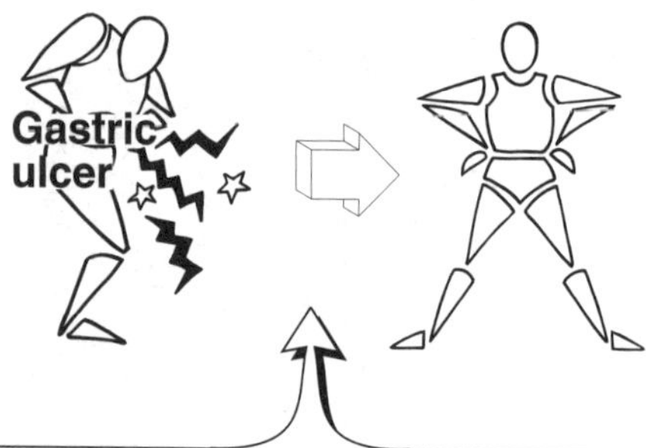

Misoprostol

- Inhibits secretion of HCl and pepsin and enhances mucosal resistance.
- Useful in patients with gastric ulcer who chronically take *aspirin*.

Figure 40.2
Therapeutic applications of prostaglandin derivatives.

III. ANTIHISTAMINES

Histamine is a chemical messenger that mediates a wide range of cellular responses, including allergic and inflammatory reactions, gastric acid secretion, and possibly neurotransmission in parts of the brain. Histamine has no clinical applications, but agents that interfere with the action of histamine (antihistamines) have important therapeutic applications.

A. Location, synthesis, and release of histamine

1. **Location:** Histamine occurs in practically all tissues, but it is unevenly distributed, with high amounts found in lung, skin, and the gastrointestinal tract (sites where the "inside" of the body meets the "outside"). It is found in high concentration in mast cells or basophils. Histamine also occurs as a component of venoms and in secretions from insect stings.

2. **Synthesis:** Histamine is an amine formed by the decarboxylation of the amino acid histidine (Figure 40.3). This process occurs primarily in the mast cells, basophils, and in the lungs, skin, and gastrointestinal mucosa—the same tissues in which histamine is stored. In mast cells, histamine is stored in granules as an inactive complex composed of histamine and the polysulfated anion, heparin, along with an anionic protein. If histamine is not stored, it is rapidly inactivated by amine oxidase enzymes.

3. **Release of histamine:** The release of histamine may be the primary response to some stimuli, but most often, histamine is just one of several chemical mediators released. Stimuli causing the release of histamine from tissues include the destruction of cells as a result of cold, bacterial toxins, bee sting venoms, or trauma. Allergies and anaphylaxis can also trigger release of histamine.

B. Mechanism of action of histamine

Histamine released in response to the stimuli just described exerts its effects by binding to two types of receptors, designated H_1 and

H_2, located on the surfaces of cells. Some of histamine's wide range of pharmacologic effects are mediated by both H_1 and H_2 receptors, whereas others are mediated by only one class (Figure 40.4). For example, the H_1 receptors are important in producing smooth muscle contraction and increasing capillary permeability. Histamine promotes vasodilation by causing vascular endothelium to release nitric oxide; this chemical signal diffuses to the vascular smooth muscle where it stimulates cGMP production, causing vasodilation. Histamine H_2 receptors mediate gastric acid secretion. The two histamine receptors exert their effects by different second messenger pathways; for example, binding of an agonist to the H_1 receptor stimulates the intracellular activity of the polyphosphatidylinositol pathway, whereas stimulation of H_2 receptors enhances the production of cAMP by adenylyl cyclase (see p. 33).

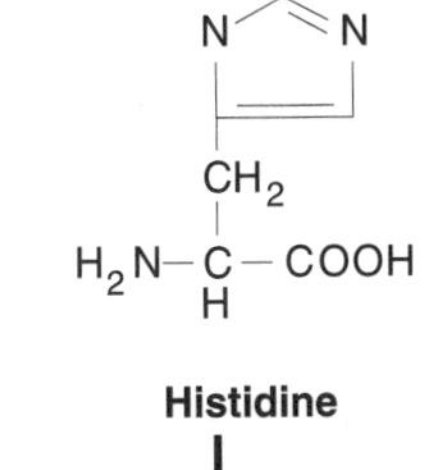

Histidine

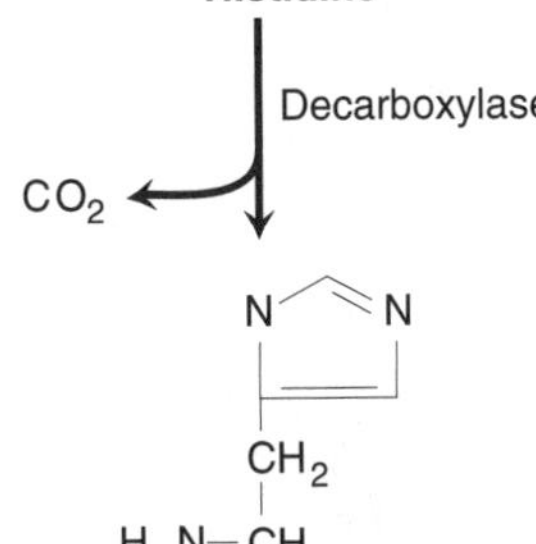

Histamine

Figure 40.3
Biosynthesis of histamine.

C. Role of histamine in allergy and anaphylaxis

There is a similarity between the symptoms resulting from intravenous (IV) injection of histamine and those associated with anaphylactic shock and allergic reactions. These include contraction of smooth muscle, stimulation of secretions, dilation and increased permeability of the capillaries, and stimulation of sensory nerve endings.

H_1-Receptors

EXOCRINE EXCRETION

Increased production of nasal and bronchial mucus, resulting in respiratory symptoms.

BRONCHIAL SMOOTH MUSCLE

Constriction of bronchioles results in symptoms of asthma, decreased lung capacity.

INTESTINAL SMOOTH MUSCLE

Constriction results in intestinal cramps and diarrhea.

SENSORY NERVE ENDINGS

Cause itch and pain

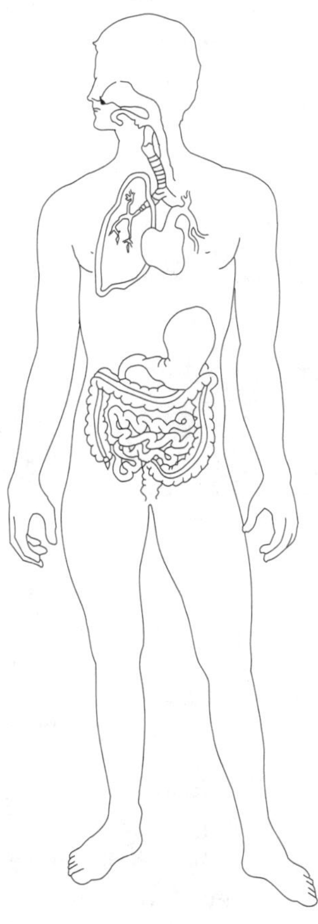

H_1-and H_2-Receptors

CARDIOVASCULAR SYSTEM

Lowers systemic blood pressure by reducing peripheral resistance, Causes positive chronotropism (mediated by H_2 receptors) and a positive inotropism (mediated by both H_1 and H_2 receptors).

SKIN

Dilation and increased permeability of the capillaries results in leakage of proteins and fluid into the tissues.
In the skin this results in the classical "triple response" - wheal formation, reddening due to local vasodilation, and flare ("halo").

H_2-Receptors

Stomach

Stimulation of gastric hydrochloric acid secretion.

Figure 40.4
Actions of histamine.

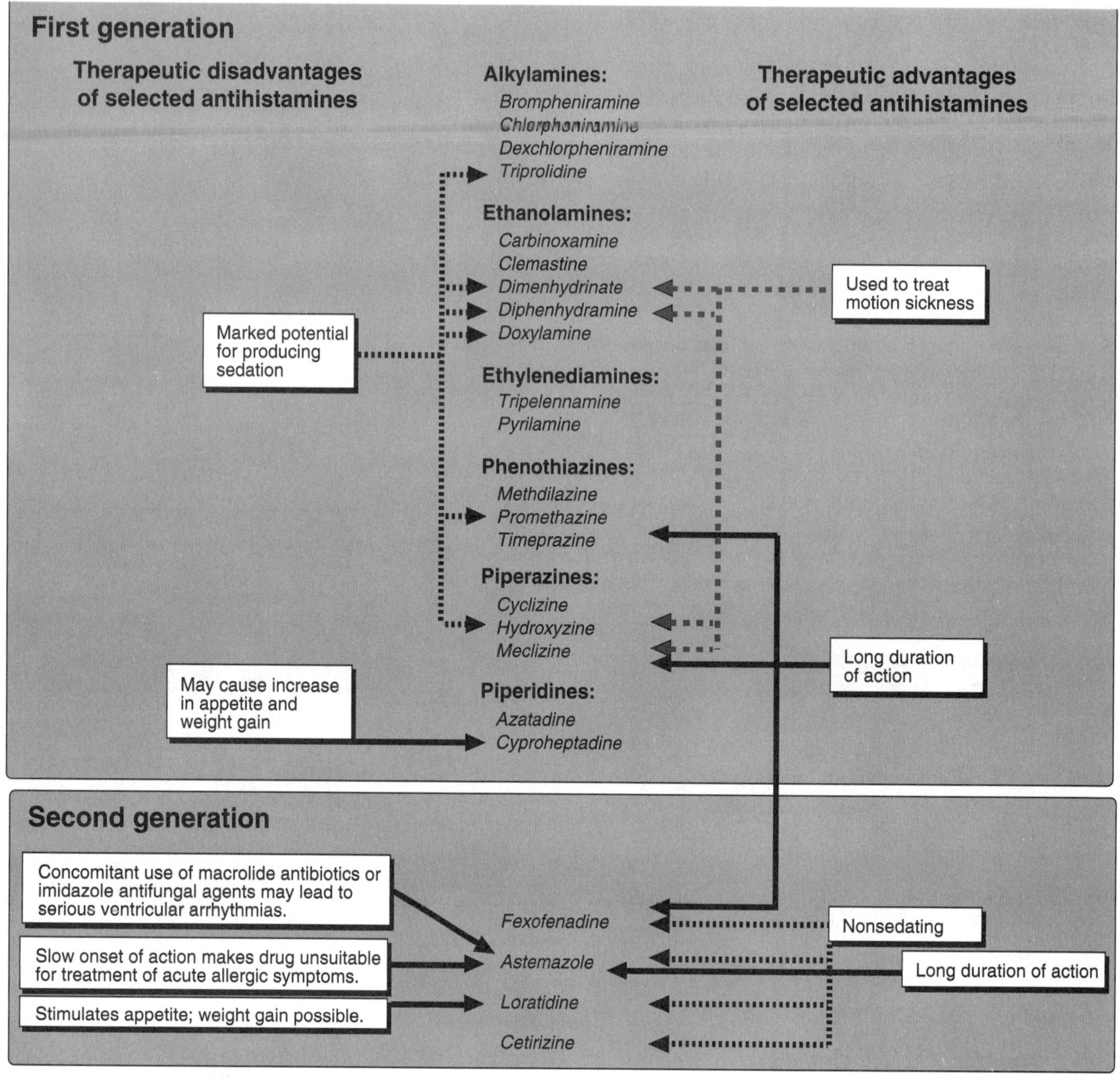

Figure 40.5
Summary of therapeutic advantages and disadvantages of the H_1-histamine receptor blocking agents.

1. **Role of mediators:** Symptoms associated with allergy and anaphylactic shock result from the release of certain mediators from their storage sites. Such mediators include histamine, serotonin leukotrienes and the eosinophil chemotactic factor of anaphylaxis. In some cases, these cause a localized allergic reaction, producing, for example, actions on the skin or respiratory tract. Under other conditions, these mediators may cause a full-blown anaphylactic response. It is thought that the difference between these two situations results from differences in the sites from which mediators are released and their rates of release. For example, if the release of histamine is slow enough to permit its inactivation before it enters the bloodstream, a local allergic reaction results.

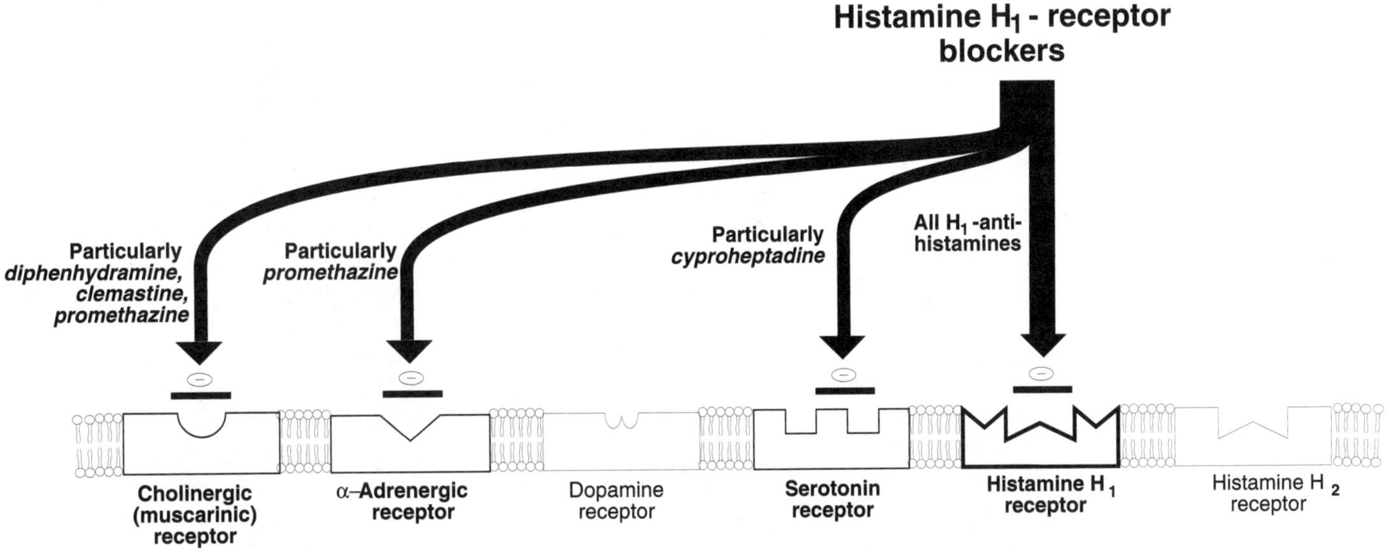

Figure 40.6
H_1-antihistamines block at histamine receptors as well as at adrenergic, cholinergic, and serotonin-binding receptors.

However, if histamine release is too fast for inactivation to be efficient, a full-blown anaphylactic reaction occurs. (See p. 221 for a more complete discussion of allergic reactions.)

D. Histamine H_1 receptor blockers

The term "antihistamine," without a modifying adjective, refers to the classic H_1 receptor blockers. These compounds do not influence the formation or release of histamine, but rather they competitively block the receptor-mediated response of a target tissue. [Note: This contrasts with the action of *cromolyn* (see p. 220), which inhibits the release of histamine from mast cells and is useful in the treatment of asthma.] The H_1 receptor blockers can be divided into first- and second generation drugs.(Figure 40.5). The first generation drugs are still widely used because they are effective and inexpensive. However, the second generation agents, because they do not penetrate the blood-brain barrier, show less CNS toxicity than the older drugs. [Note: The histamine receptors are distinct from those that bind serotonin, acetylcholine, and the catecholamines.]

1. **Actions:** H_1 antihistamines antagonize all actions of histamine except for those mediated solely by H_2 receptors. The action of all of the H_1 receptor blockers is qualitatively similar. However, most of these blockers have additional effects unrelated to their blocking of H_1 receptors; these effects probably reflect binding of the H_1 antagonists to cholinergic, adrenergic, or serotonin receptors (Figure 40.6). Some H_1 blockers, such as *diphenhydramine*, have good local anesthetic activity.

2. **Therapeutic uses**

   a. **Allergic conditions:** H_1 Blockers are useful in treating allergies caused by antigens acting on IgE-antibody sensitized mast cells. For example, antihistamines are the drugs of choice in controlling the symptoms of allergic rhinitis and urticaria because histamine is the principal mediator. However, the H_1 receptor blockers are ineffective in treating bronchial asthma (see p. 217), because histamine is only one of several mediators. [Note: *Epinephrine* (see p. 61) has actions on smooth muscle that are opposite to those of histamine and it acts at different receptors. Therefore, *epinephrine* is the drug of choice in treating systemic anaphylaxis and other conditions that involve massive release of histamine.]

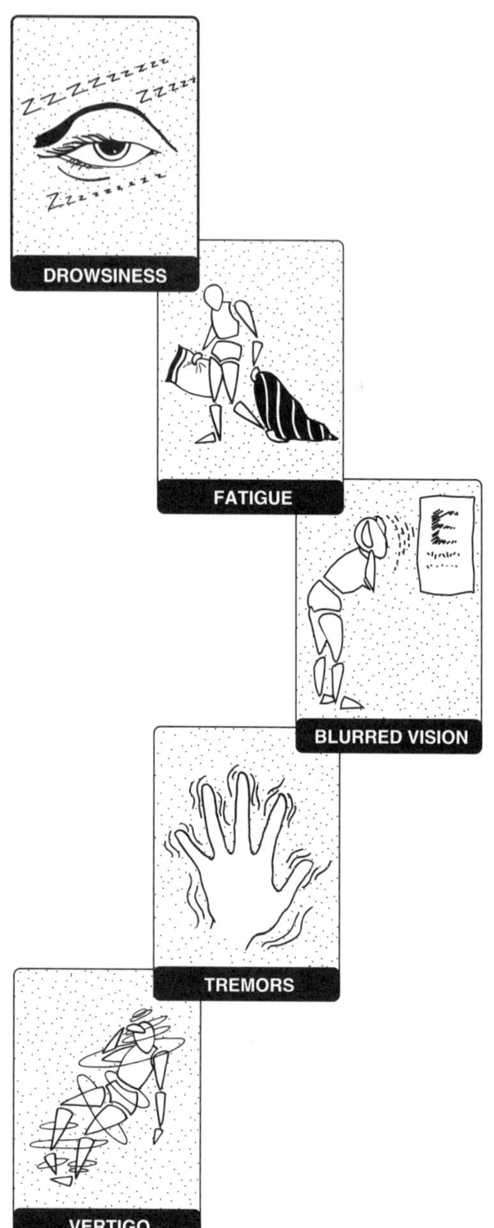

Figure 40.7
Some adverse effect observed with first generation H_1-histamine blockers.

b. Motion sickness and nausea: Along with the antimuscarinic agent *scopolamine* (see p. 48), certain H_1 receptor blockers, such as *diphenhydramine* [dye fen HYE dra meen], *dimenhydrinate* [dye men HYE dri nate], *cyclizine* [SYE kli zeen], and *meclizine* [MEK li zeen] (see Figure 40.5), are the most effective agents for the prevention of the symptoms of motion sickness. The antihistamines prevent or diminish vomiting and nausea mediated by both the chemoreceptor and vestibular pathways. The antiemetic action of these substances seems to be independent of their antihistaminic and other actions. (Other antiemetic agents are summarized in Figure 24.6, p. 243.).

c. Somnifacients: Some of the antihistamines, such as *diphenhydramine*, have strong sedative properties and are used in the treatment of insomnia.

3. Pharmacokinetics: H_1 receptor blockers are well absorbed after oral administration, with maximum serum levels occurring at 1 to 2 hours. The average plasma half-life is 4 to 6 hours, except for *meclizine*, which has a half-life of 12 to 24 hours. H_1 receptor blockers have high bioavailability; they are distributed in all tissues, including the CNS.The major site of biotransformation is the liver. Minute amounts of unchanged drug and most of the metabolites are excreted in the urine.

4. Adverse effects: H_1 receptor blockers have a low specificity, that is, they interact not only with histamine receptors but also with muscarinic cholinergic receptors, α-adrenergic receptors, and serotonin receptors (see Figure 40.6). The extent of interaction with these receptors and, as a result, the nature of the side effects, vary with the structure of the drug. Some side effects may be undesirable, and others may have therapeutic value. Furthermore, the incidence and severity of adverse reactions varies between individual subjects.

a. Sedation: The most frequently observed adverse reaction is sedation (Figure 40.7). Other central actions include tinnitus, fatigue, dizziness, lassitude, incoordination, blurred vision, and tremors. Sedation is less common with the second generation drugs that do not readily enter the CNS.

b. Dry mouth: Oral antihistamines also exert weak anticholinergic effects, leading not only to a drying of the nasal passage but also to a tendency to dry the oral cavity. Blurred vision can also occur with some drugs.

c. Drug interactions: Interaction of H_1 receptor blockers with other drugs can cause serious consequences, such as the potentiation of the effects of all other CNS depressants, including alcohol. Persons taking MAO inhibitors (see p. 123) should not take antihistamines, since the MAO inhibitors can exacerbate the anticholinergic effects of the antihistamines. *Erythromycin* and *clarithromycin* interfere in the metabolism of *terfenadine* and *astemizole* and may cause serious cardiac arrhythmias.

d. Overdoses: Although the margin of safety of H_1 receptor blockers is relatively high and chronic toxicity is rare, acute poisoning is relatively common, especially in young children. The most common and dangerous effects of acute poisoning are those on the CNS, including hallucinations, excitement, ataxia, and convulsions. If untreated, the patient may experience a deepening coma and collapse of the cardiorespiratory system.

See p. 470 for a description of *fexofenadine*.

E. Histamine H_2 receptor blockers

Histamine H_2 receptor blockers have little if any affinity for H_1 receptors. Although antagonists of the histamine H_2 receptor (H_2 antagonists) block the actions of histamine at all H_2 receptors, their chief clinical use is as inhibitors of gastric acid secretion in the treatment of ulcers. (see p. 236). By competitively blocking the binding of histamine to H_2 receptors, these agents reduce intracellular concentrations of cyclic AMP and thereby, secretion of gastric acid. The four drugs used in the United States, *cimetidine, ranitidine, famotidine* and *nizatidine*, are discussed in Chapter 24.

IV. DRUGS USED TO TREAT MIGRAINE HEADACHE

It has been estimated that 18 million women and 6 million men in the United States suffer from severe migraine headaches. Migraine can usu-

	Migraine	Cluster	Tension type
Family history	**Yes**	**No**	**Yes**
Sex	**Females more often than males**	**Males more often than females**	**Females more than males**
Onset	**Variable**	**During sleep**	**Under stress**
Location	**Usually unilateral**	**Behind or around one eye**	**Bilateral in band around head**
Character, severity	**Pulsating, throbbing**	**Excruciating, sharp, steady**	**Dull, persistent, tightening/pressing**
Duration	**Two to 72 hours per episode;**	**15 to 90 minutes per attack**	**30 minutes to 7 days per episode**
Associated symptoms	**Visual auras, sensitivity to light and sound, pale facial appearance, nausea and vomiting**	**Unilateral or bilateral sweating, facial flushing, nasal congestion, ptosis, lacrimation, pupillary changes**	**Mild intolerance to light and noise, anorexia**

Figure 40.8
Characteristics of migraine, cluster and tension-type headaches.

ally be distinguished clinically from the two other common types of headaches—the cluster headache and tension-type headache—by its characteristics (Figure 40.8). For example, migraines present as a pulsatile, throbbing pain; cluster headaches as excruciating, sharp, steady pain; whereas tension-type headaches show dull pain with a persistent tightening feeling in the head. Migraine headaches typically affect patients for a major part of their lives, and result in considerable health costs.

A. Types of migraine

There are two main types of migraine headaches. The first, migraine without aura (previously called common migraine), is a severe, unilateral, pulsating headache that typically lasts from 2 to 72 hours. These headaches are often aggravated by physical activity and are accompanied by nausea, vomiting, photophobia (hypersensitivity to light), and phonophobia (hypersensitivity to sound). Approximately 85% of patients with migraine do not have aura. In the second type, migraine with aura (previously called classic migraine), the headache is preceded by neurologic symptoms called aura, which can be visual, sensory, and/or cause speech or motor disturbances. Most commonly these prodromal symptoms are visual, occurring 20 to 40 minutes before headache pain begins. In the 15% of migraine patients whose headache is preceded by an aura, the aura itself allows diagnosis. The headache itself in migraine with or without aura is similar. For both types of migraines, women are three times more likely to experience either type of migraine than are men.

B. Biologic basis of migraine headaches

The first manifestation of migraine with aura is a spreading depression of neuronal activity accompanied by reduced blood flow in the most posterior part of the cerebral hemisphere. This hypoperfusion gradually spreads forward over the surface of the cortex to other contiguous areas of the brain. The vascular alteration is accompanied by functional changes, for example, the hypoperfused regions show an abnormal response to changes in arterial pCO_2. The hypoperfusion persists throughout the aura and well into the headache phase, after which hyperperfusion occurs. Patients with migraine without aura do not show hypoperfusion. However, the pain of both types of migraine may be due to extracranial and intracranial arterial dilation leading to release of neuroactive molecules such as substance P.

C. Symptomatic treatment of acute migraine

A migraine can usually be aborted if therapy is initiated at the onset of symptoms—either during the aura or at the first hint of migraine pain without aura. The most useful drugs for averting an acute attack are *sumatriptan*, *ergotamine*, and nonsteroidal antiinflammatory drugs .

1. **Sumatriptan:** *Sumatriptan* [sew mah TRIP tan] rapidly and effectively aborts or markedly reduces the severity of migraine headaches in about 80 % of patients. *Sumatriptan* is a serotonin agonist, acting at 5-HT_{1D} receptors, a subgroup of serotonin

receptors found on small, peripheral nerves that innervate the intracranial vasculature. Their activation probably suppresses release of sensory neuropeptides, such as substance P. The nausea that occurs with *dihydroergotamine* and the vasoconstriction caused by *ergotamine* (see next sections) are much less pronounced with *sumatriptan*. *Sumatriptan* is given subcutaneously or orally. The onset of the parenteral drug is about 20 minutes compared to 1 to 2 hours for drug adminisatered orally. The drug has a short duration of action, with an elimination half-life of two hours. Headache commonly recurs within 24 to 48 hours after a single dose of *sumatriptan*; in most patients a second dose is effective in aborting the headache. Because of its high cost, *sumitriptan* should be reserved for patients for whom other drugs have been ineffective, or were not well-tolerated.

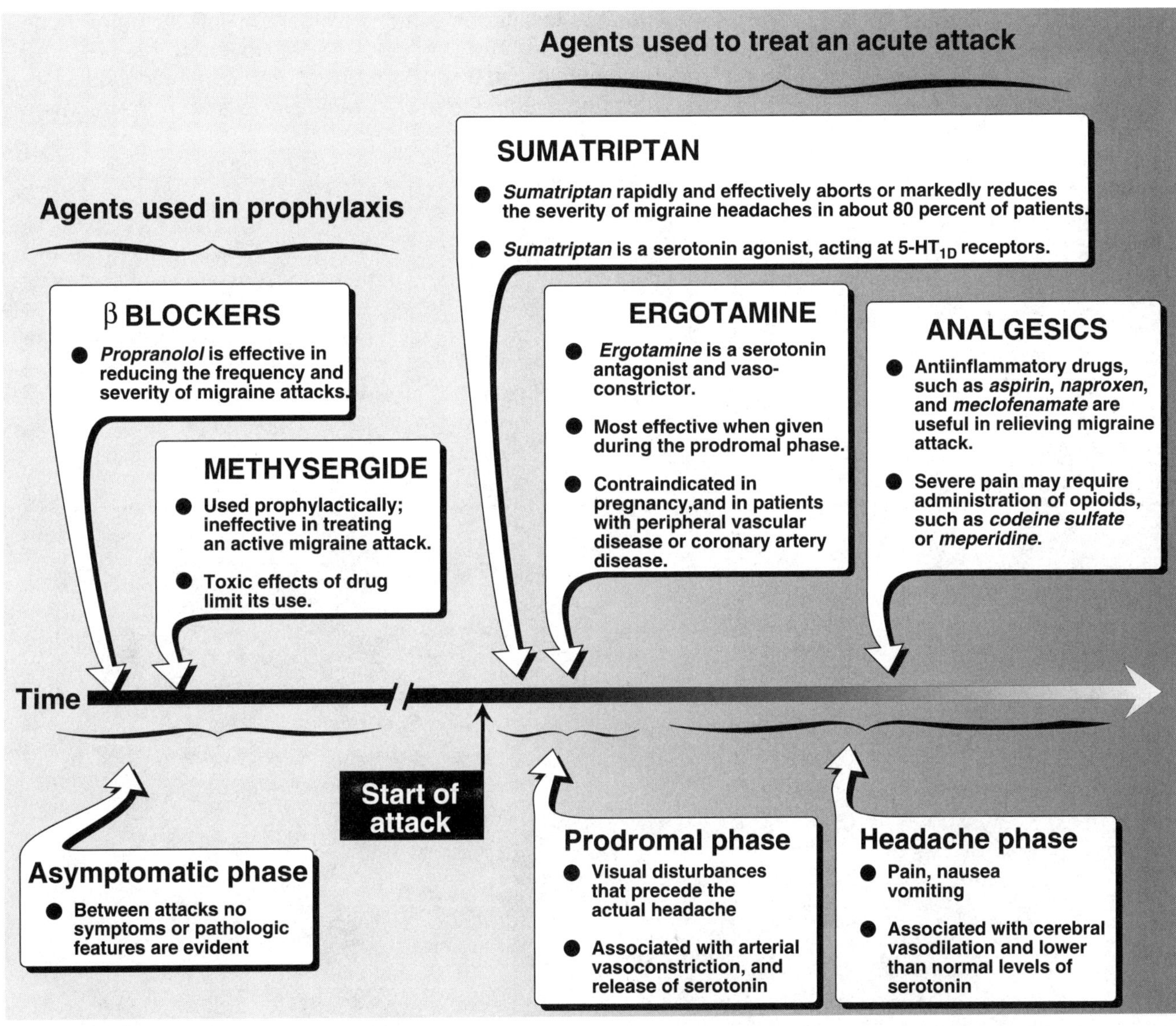

Figure 40.9
Drugs useful in the treatment and prophylaxis of migraine headaches.

2. **Ergotamine:** *Ergotamine* [er GOT a meen] has in the past been the drug of choice for treatment of moderate-to-severe migraine. *Ergotamine* and *dihydroergotamine* (see below) have similar actions to *sumatriptan*, but they have less selectivity for the 5-HT receptors. *Ergotamine* can be given orally, sublingually, rectally or nasally, and is effective in about 50% of patients. The gastrointestinal absorption of the ergot alkaloids is variable, but it can be increased by *caffeine* (that is, coffee increases effectiveness of ergot alkaloids). The drug is most effective when administered during the early phase of an attack. The most common side effects are diarrhea, nausea, and vomiting.

3. **Dihydroergotamine:** *Dihydroergotamine* [dye hye droe er GOT a meen], a derivative of *ergotamine*, is administered intravenously and has an efficacy similar to that of *sumatriptan*, but nausea is a common adverse effect.

4. **Analgesics:** Analgesics or nonsteroidal anti-inflammatory drugs are often effective in mild-to-moderate migraine. *Aspirin*, *acetaminophen*, *naproxen*, *propoxyphene*, *acetaminophen* with *butalbital*, and *caffeine* are all effective in treating a migraine attack.

D. Prophylaxis

Therapy to prevent migraine is indicated if the attacks occur two times or more a month, and if the headaches are severe or complicated by serious neurologic signs. *Propranolol* (see p. 74) is the drug of choice, but other β-blockers, particularly *nadolol* (see p. 76), have been shown to be effective. *Methysergide* [meth i SER jide], another ergot alkaloid, is effective for prevention of recurrent, refractory, severe migraine (Figure 40.9).

Study Questions

Choose the ONE best answer.

40.1 Ergot alkaloids:

A. cause vasodilation.
B. exert their actions by binding to specific ergotamine receptors.
C. are useful in treating acute migraine headache.
D. are useful to maintain uterine muscle tone during pregnancy.
E. have actions similar to those of nitroprusside.

Correct answer = C. Ergotamine acts to counteract cerebral vasodilation that plays a role in migraine headaches. Vasoconstriction leading to tissue ischemia is one of the toxic complications associated with an overdose of these drugs. The ergot alkaloids interact with adrenergic, dopaminergic, and serotonin receptors. They are contraindicated in pregnancy because of their ability to cause uterine contraction and abortion. Nitroprusside is a powerful vasodilator used to treat vasoconstriction that is characteristic of an overdose with ergot alkaloids.

40.2 Histamine H_1 receptor blockers are useful in the treatment of all of the following EXCEPT:

A. urticaria.
B. seasonal rhinitis.
C. drug reactions.
D. bronchial asthma.
E. insomnia.

Correct choice = D. H_1 histamine receptor blockers are not effective in bronchial asthma.

Appendix: Illustrated Case Studies

I. OVERVIEW

These extended case studies complement the basic information presented in Chapters 1 to 40. They reinforce basic principles of pharmacology, such as the role of patient factors in empiric antimicrobial therapy. Most of the cases provide clinical information obtained from a single patient; some cases describe a composite of typical features derived from several patients. These cases illustrate simple pharmacologic principles, such as consideration of kidney function in drug dosing—concepts useful in answering examination questions, and in the clinics.

CASE 1

A 53-year-old man was admitted into a hospital with fever, a cough that produced purulent sputum, and shortness of breath that had been present for several days.

Two years earlier he had developed Kaposi's sarcoma and was human immunodeficiency virus (HIV) positive. In the interim, therapy with anti-HIV drugs had been discontinued because of his inability to tolerate them. However, the Kaposi's sarcoma was treated with anticancer drugs, including *doxorubicin*. He was being maintained with *cotrimoxazole*, *fluconazole*, and *rifabutin* (a rifamycin antibiotic similar to *rifampin*) and receiving weekly treatments with *filgramstin* (*granulocyte stimulating factor*) and *erythropoietin*. At the time of admission for the cough his helper-induced T-cell (CD4) count was 13/μL.

A chest X-ray revealed a cavitary lesion of the right upper lobe. Cultures obtained from bronchoscopic biopsy and broncho-alveolar lavage specimens yielded methicillin-resistant Staphylococcus aureus (MRSA) with no evidence of fungal or acid-fast organisms. Treatment with the normal therapeutic dose of *vancomycin*, 1 gram intravenously (IV) every 12 hours, was begun. Because he insisted on receiving his treatment at home, he was discharged with a peripherally-inserted central venous catheter in place. Though his fevers abated initially, he again experienced frequent chills, fever, cough producing white-to-yellow sputum, and progressively disabling weakness 48 hours after the *vancomycin* had been started.

Several days later he was admitted to the hospital, where it was noted that he was alert, fully oriented, and extremely weak. His temperature was 103.6°F, his pulse 130 beats per minute (BPM), his blood pressure (BP) 80/60 mm Hg, and his respirations labored at a rate of 28 per minute. He was extremely cachetic at 6'4" in height and weighing 135 pounds (61 kg). There were purple tumorous plaques covering parts of his body. His chest revealed dullness and coarse crackles throughout the right upper and midlung fields, suggesting pneumonia. A chest X-ray confirmed the diagnosis (Figure A.1).

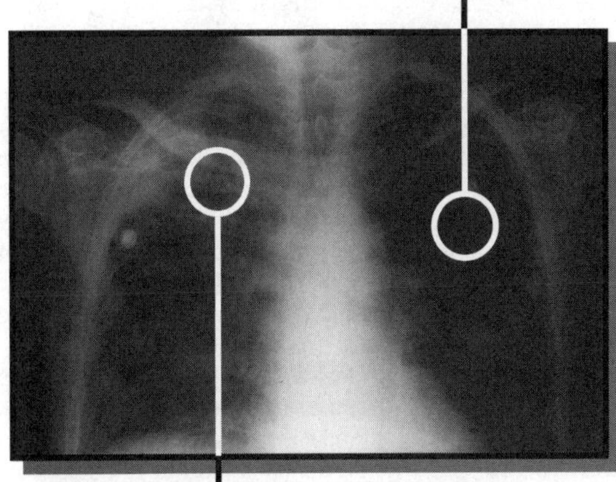
Dark areas in lung are normal and show expected presence of air which has little ability to absorb X-rays.
This lighter area in the lung is abnormal and shows the presence of cells and pus rather than air. This indicates the possible presence of infection.

Figure A.1
Chest X-ray of patient.

The patient was profoundly leukopenic with a white blood cell count of 700/µL–28% polymorphonuclear leukocytes (PMN's), 53% band forms, 3% metamyelocytes, 11% lymphocytes, 5% monocytes. [Normally, the total white blood cell count should be between about 4000 and 10,000 per mL.] The serum creatinine was 3.6 mg/dL (indicating significant renal dysfunction, normal creatinine ordinarily should not exceed about 1 mg/dL). A random plasma *vancomycin* level was 48.8 µg/mL. (Therapeutic range for "peak" level is 18 to 30 µg/mL.)

Question A.1: Was *vancomycin* the appropriate drug for treating this patient?

Answer: Yes. *Vancomycin* is the drug of choice (in fact, the only effective drug currently available) for the treatment of methicillin-resistant Staphylococcus aureus (MRSA) infections. It is bactericidal and thus important for treatment of a leukopenic individual.

Question A.2 : The best explanation for this extremely high plasma level of *vancomycin* is:

A. The very low CD4-positive lymphocyte count

B. The excessively high dose of *vancomycin* for this patient's weight

C. The impaired renal function

D. The leukopenia

E. Inhibition of *vancomycin* metabolism by *fluconazole*

The correct answer is **C** (impaired renal function). *Vancomycin* is excreted almost exclusively by the kidneys, with renal clearance linearly related to that of creatinine. Hence, even in patients with modest renal impairment, *vancomycin* regimens must be modified. This patient, presumably because of septic shock, developed renal failure while receiving vancomycin. Because his physicians were not aware of his clinical deterioration, his *vancomycin* regimen was not altered and he began to retain it significantly. **A** (very low CD4-positive lymphocyte count) is unrelated to *vancomycin* kinetics. **B** (excessive dose for weight) is not the best answer because, with a recommended dose of 15 mg/kg every 12 hours in adults with normal renal function, this patient's weight of 61 kg called for about 900 mg per dose, only slightly less than the dose that he was receiving. **D** (leukopenia) does not of itself result in changes in *vancomycin* kinetics. **E** (inhibition of *vancomycin* metabolism by *fluconzaole*).The azole antifungal agents interfere with the metabolism of many drugs, by inhibiting the hepatic microsomal enzymes. However, *vancomycin* is not one of the the drugs that is metabolized by microsomal enzymes.

The *vancomycin* regimen was suspended, and blood, sputum, and urine cultures were obtained. A gram stain of the patient's sputum revealed many polymorphonuclear leukocytes and many gram-negative rods (Figure A.2).

Urine gram stain showed no organisms. The patient was treated with IV fluids, and, based on the gram stain and other data, *ceftazidime* (one gram IV every 12 hours) was begun. In addition, the *granulocyte colony-stimulating factor* was increased to daily doses, in an effort to improve his quantitative leukocyte defenses. The patient's temperature came down and his renal function improved to nearly normal levels over the next 5 days, allowing resumption of regularly scheduled *vancomycin* doses. Cultures of sputum and blood yielded Pseudomonas aeruginosa.

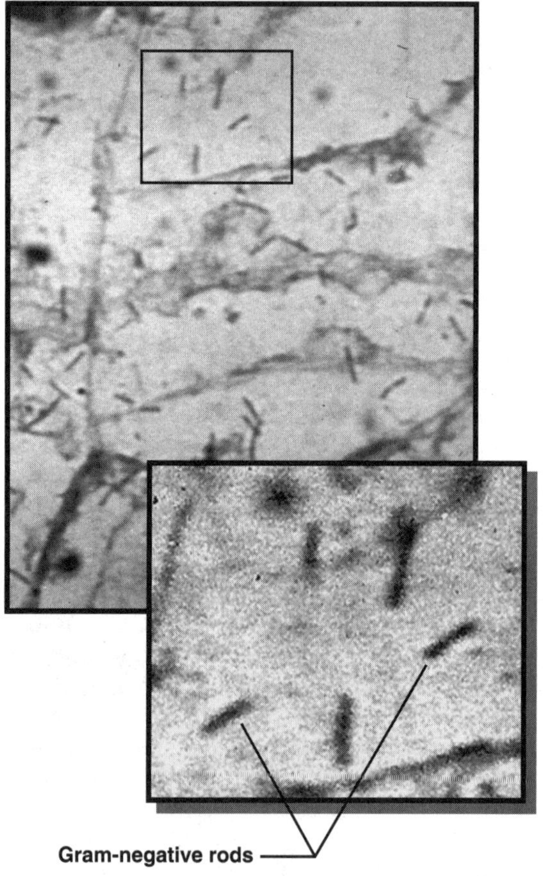

Figure A.2
Gram stain of patient's sputum.

Question A.3: Was the selection of *ceftazidime* a rational choice?

Answer: Yes. Patients with a profound leukopenia have very low numbers of neutrophils and are predisposed to severe infections with gram-negative rods, especially Pseudomonas aeruginosa. The patient's sputum gram stain is in accord with such an infection. *Ceftazidime* is a third generation cephalosporin, which covers many gram-negative organisms including Pseudomonas aeruginosa. It is also bactericidal.

Question A.4: Why was the patient not treated concurrently with an aminoglycoside, such as *tobramycin*?

Answer: The patient's high serum creatinine indicates compromised renal function. The aminoglycosides can be nephrotoxic and thus the drug was not employed. However, *tobramycin* might have been used together with *ceftazidime* if the dose were adjusted for renal function.

Question A.5: Which one of the following statements are true for *ceftazidime*?

A. Effective on oral administration.
B. Excretion depends on the kidney.
C. Interferes in vitamin K function to cause an anticoagulant effect.
D. Causes ototoxicity at high serum levels.
E. Ceftazidime is administered orally

The correct answer is **B** (excretion depends on the kidney). Most of the β-lactam antibiotics depend on the kidney for excretion. *Ceftazidime* is predominantly eliminated by glomerular filtration. Thus in this patient the dose of *ceftazidime* would have to be modified due to the patient's renal status. **A** (effective on oral administration) is incorrect. *Ceftazidime* is only given parenterally. **C** (interferes in vitamin K function to cause an anticoagulant effect) is incorrect. This property is peculiar to *cefoperazone* and *cefamandole*. **D** (causes ototoxicity at high serum levels) is not correct. **E**. *Ceftazidine* is administered IV or intramuscularly (IM).

This case illustrates the importance of considering patient-related information in selecting empiric antimicrobial therapy. Impaired renal function caused him to retain *vancomycin* to very high levels, requiring substantial modification of the dosage (that is, waiting while the drug was very slowly excreted). The renal failure also influenced on the dosage of *ceftazidime* that was initially given. An adult with normal renal function requires 2 grams of *ceftazidime* every 8 hours. The other important patient-related information that guided the antibiotic choice was his profound neutropenia, which led his physicians to suspect Pseudomonas on the first day. Had he not been treated with the right drug from the very beginning, the outcome would not have been good.

CASE 2

A 27-year-old woman with a history of asthma accidently inhaled a small nut from a candy bar she was eating. The presence of this foreign body in the airway triggered an explosive series of coughs, which ultimately expelled the food fragment from her lungs. After several minutes the airway was fully cleared, but she experienced progressive tightness in her chest. Her breathing became difficult and soon she was gasping for breath. She removed a canister from her purse and inhaled several puffs of medication. Her symptoms resolved over the next 20 minutes.

Question A.6: Which one of the following aerosolized medications would proved relief from the acute bonchoconstriction described for this woman?

A. *Salmeterol*
B. *Cromolyn*
C. *Beclomethasone*
D. *Albuterol*
E. *Nedocromil*

Correct answer is **D**. *Albuterol* is one of several of β_2 agonists available as an aerosol for treatment of bronchoconstrictive episodes associated with asthma. Its onset of action is rapid (5 to 10 minutes) and its effects on alveolar smooth muscle last several hours. **A** *Salmeterol*, also a β_2 agonist, has a slow onset of action and is not used in acute asthmatic attacks. **B**, **E** *Cromolyn* and *nedocromil* are used prophylacticlly, but are not effective in acute asthma. **C** *Beclomethasone* is an anti-inflamatory agent indicated for moderate to severe asthma. Inhaled *beclomethasone* reduces airway inflammation but its actions are not immediate; the drug is administered chronically, but it is not effective in the treatment of an acute asthmatic attack.

Simple spirometric testing with a bronchodilator challenge can identify patients with reversible airway obstruction, such as asthma (Figure A.3). The patient fills his or her lungs maximally and then expels the air as rapidly as possible. First a baseline reading is taken for this forced expiratory volume in the first second (FEV_1). Next, an aerosol bronchodilator, such as *albuterol*, is administered and the test is repeated after 15 minutes. Airway obstruction is considered to be reversible when the FEV_1 improves by more than

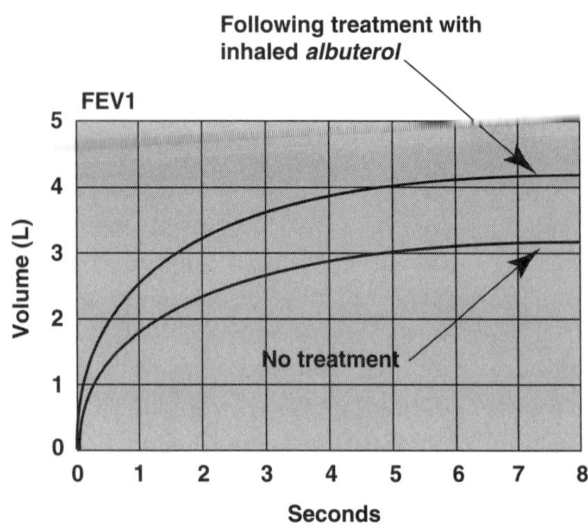

Figure A.3
Effect of bronchodilators (β_2 agonists) on pulmonary air flow.

15% following bronchodilator use. Figure A.3 shows results with an asthmatic patient in which the FEV_1 increased by 50% following administration of *albuterol*.

CASE 3

A 21-year-old woman was seen in consultation because of intermittent fever of 6 days' duration.

She had been in good health and, at the time of onset of the current complaint, she was in the twelfth week of her first pregnancy. Seven days prior to admission she developed a fever as high as 101°F, with chills. These symptoms occurred on alternate days, beginning about noon and lasting for several hours. On the days that she didn't have a fever she felt relatively well. The day after the onset of fever and chills she began to feel pain in her left side. Two days later she developed dysuria, but had no urinary urgency or frequency. Because of persistence of the symptoms, she was admitted to the hospital the day before the consultant's visit, for presumed sepsis of urinary tract origin. At that time it was determined that she had gone back to visit her family in India. Her illness began 6 months after she had returned to the United States.

Upon admission, her temperature was 97°F, her pulse 80 BPM, and her BP was 100/65 mm Hg. Remarkable physical findings were confined to the abdomen, which contained an obviously enlarged uterus. The spleen tip could be felt 3 cm below the left costal margin at the end of deep inspiration (definitely enlarged).

Her hemoglobin level was 10.9 g/dL (moderately anemic), white blood cell count was 5200/μL (normal), and her platelet count was 103,000/μL (the lower limit of normal for platelet count is 140,000/μL). Examination of a peripheral blood smear revealed clear evidence of malaria due to Plasmodium vivax (Figure A.4).

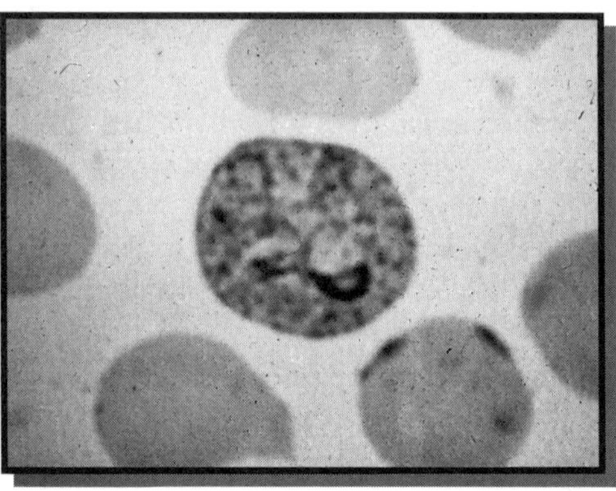

Figure A.4
Peripheral blood smear.

Question A.7: In general, what are the drugs of choice for the treatment of malaria due to Plasmodium vivax?

Answer: For a "radical cure", patients are treated with a 14-day course of *primaquine*. It usually follows a course of *chloroquine* or other blood schizontocide. *Primaquine* is active against the exoerythrocytic forms of P. vivax. It is also strongly gametocidal against all four plasmodial species.

Question A.8: What are the usual toxicities associated with *primaquine*?

Answer: At the usual doses it is generally well tolerated though patients may complain of gastrointestinal problems, such as abdominal cramps, nausea, and epigastric pain, as well as of headache. In patients with glucose 6-phosphate dehydrogenase deficiency, *primaquine* is contraindicated because it can induce hemolysis

The patient was treated with *chloroquine phosphate*

(1 gram by mouth, followed by 500 mg 6 hours later and 500 mg once on each of the subsequent 2 days). She was advised to take *chloroquine phosphate* 500 mg orally once weekly for approximately the next six months.

Question A.9: Will *chloroquine phosphate* effect a "radical cure"?

Answer: No. This drug is a blood schizonticide and acts as a malarial suppressant for P. vivax.

Question A.10: The reason that "radical cure" with *primaquine* was not undertaken for this patient is:

A. Vivax malaria cannot be eradicated, only suppressed.
B. *Chloroquine* alone is adequate for the cure of vivax malaria.
C. *Primaquine* is contraindicated in pregnancy.
D. The patient's hemoglobin level was too low to allow use of *primaquine*.
E. With only 7 days of fever, the malaria was not established enough to require radical cure.

The correct answer is **C** (*primaquine* is contraindicated in pregnancy). *Primaquine* is toxic to the fetus and should not be given to pregnant women. **A** (vivax malaria can't be eradicated) is incorrect: the exoerythrocytic phase of P. vivax escapes destruction by *chloroquine*, but is eradicated by *primaquine*. **B** (adequacy of *chloroquine* in eradicating P. vivax) is wrong for the reasons just stated. **D** (the extent of the patient's anemia) is incorrect because a hemoglobin level of 10.9 g/dL is not unusual, especially in pregnancy, and is to be expected in a patient with malaria that has been ongoing for six months, because disruption of red blood cells is part of the pathology of malaria. **E** (relatively short duration of symptoms) is incorrect because naturally-acquired vivax malaria always requires radical cure with *primaquine*. The only form of vivax malaria that does not require this second phase of therapy is that which is acquired by transfusion of blood from an individual infected with P. vivax, since there is no exoerythrocytic phase in transfusion-associated malaria.

This patient illustrates the importance of pregnancy in guiding the choice of an any drug! Adverse effects of drugs are not only exerted on the patient, but also the fetus, which cannot avoid exposure to drugs that are taken by the mother, and which cross the placenta. With this patient, radical cure had to be delayed until the delivery of her baby (who was born perfectly healthy), 6 months after her malaria was diagnosed. At that time she was given another course of chloroquine, followed by 14 days of *primaquine*, and she remained asymptomatic. Malarial forms disappeared from smears of her peripheral blood.

This patient also illustrates the importance of a travel history in clinical medicine. Her "intermittent" fevers came with striking regularity on alternate days, a history that suggests malaria in an individual who has been in an area in which malaria is known to exist. Her flank pain was not due to a urinary tract infection, but was actually related to the splenic enlargement that is so characteristic of malaria.

CASE 4

A woman, age 36, entered the clinic complaining of fatigue, muscle weakness and difficulty in breathing. A physical exam revealed pneumonia. A sputum sample was taken and she was placed on oral *clarithromycin*. Two days later, the laboratory finding indicated that the organism was Klebsiella pneumoniae and she was switched to *amikacin* and *cefoxitin*. While the respiratory infection began to resolve the patient continued to complain of fatigue and muscle weakness. Ptosis (drooping of the upper eyelid), diplopia (perception of two images of a single object—"double vision") and difficulty in chewing and swallowing developed. A provisional diagnosis of myasthenia gravis was made.

Question A.11: Intravenous injection of which one of the following agents could be used to confirm this diagnosis.

A. *Atropine*
B. *Acetylcholine*
C. *Edrophonium*
D. *Bethanechol*
E. *Pilocarpine*

Correct answer is **C**. A diagnosis of myasthenia gravis can be confirmed by the response of the patient to a short-acting anticholinesterase, such as *edrophonium*. Two mg of the drug is given IV. If there is no response, or no serious side effects appear within 30 seconds, an additional 8 mg is administered. In the myasthenic patient shown on p. 434, there is an obvious improvement in the strength of weak muscles following treatment with *edrophonium* (Figure A.5).

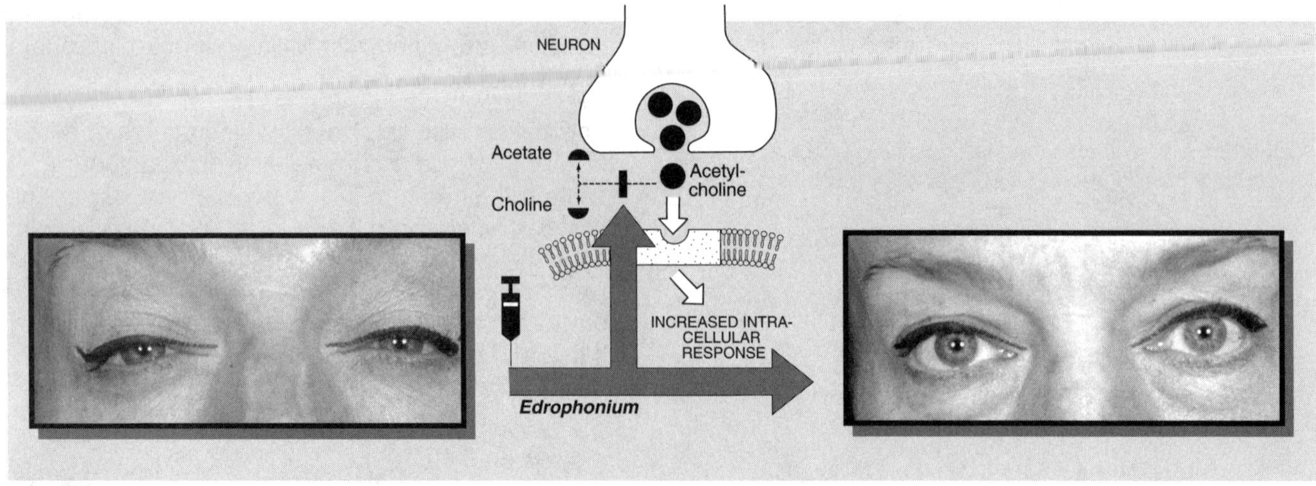

Figure A.5
Efffect of *edrophonium* in a patient showing symptoms of myasthenia gravis.

Question A.12: What antibiotic medication may have contributed to the unmasking of the myasthenia?

The aminoglycoside, *amikacin*. The aminoglycosides can inhibit Ca^{++} uptake which is required for the release of acetylcholine at the neuromuscular junction, and can cause neuromuscular blockade. This is rare at usual doses of the drug, but patients with myasthenia gravis are particularly susceptible.

CASE 5

A 36-year-old man was admitted to the hospital with fever and chills, which began 3 weeks earlier. Until that time he was well except for a heart murmur which was asymptomatic. Three months prior to admission, he developed a dental abscess which was treated with surgical drainage of the abscess and *erythromycin ethylsuccinate* (400 mg orally three times daily for 10 days). He felt well until 3 weeks prior to admission, when he began to have fever as high as 101°F every evening, sometimes accompanied by low back pain. He saw his physician ten days after the onset of the fever and was again given *erythromycin ethylsuccinate* (400 mg orally three times daily). When his symptoms did not improve, he was admitted to the hospital.

Upon admission, the patient's temperature was 100.4°F, his pulse 100 BPM, and his BP 135/70 mm Hg. An oral examination revealed several carious teeth. There was a soft systolic murmur consistent with mitral insufficiency. His spleen was palpable 2 centimeters below the left costal margin. The remainder of the physical examination was unremarkable. His past history included an episode of wheezing and shortness of breath when he had received *penicillin* for a sore throat at age 10.

Question A.13: What tentative diagnosis would you make?

Answer: Because of the patient's dental history, that is, an abscess and several carious teeth, and the presence of heart murmurs and low grade fever at night, the possibility of subacute bacterial endocarditis is likely. Streptococcus of the viridans group is a common etiological agent for this condition in patients with dental problems.

Question A.14: Assuming that the patient is suffering from endocarditis due to Streptococci, what antibiotic would be appropriate to employ empirically before the etiological organism was identified?

Answer: The patient's history suggests a hypersensitivity to *penicillin* (wheezing and shortness of breath indicative of bronchospasm). Therefore, ß-lactam antibiotics would carry a risk of a serious allergic attack and be inappropriate despite their known efficacy against this organism. *Vancomycin* is effective against this organism and has no cross-allergenicity with penicillin. In addition, like *penicillin*, it is bactericidal. Rapid treatment is indicated for this life-threatening condition .

This patient was treated empirically with *vancomycin* alone because his physicians suspected that he had endocarditis, caused by Streptococcus of the viridans group. The history indicated that the origin of the infection was the patient's mouth. Three days later the results from the clinical microbiology laboratory showed that three blood cultures, taken at the time of admission, grew Enterococcus faecalis, susceptible to *ampicillin*, *vancomycin*, *gentamicin*, and *streptomycin*.

Question A.15: The appropriate regimen for this patient's enterococcal endocarditis is:

A. *Ampicillin* and *gentamicin*
B. *Ceftriaxone* and *gentamicin*
C. *Vancomycin*
D. *Vancomycin* and *gentamicin*
E. *Clindamycin* and *gentamicin*

The correct answer is **D** . Ordinarily one would treat enterococcal endocarditis with regimen **A** (*ampicillin* and *gentamicin*), but this patient's history of bronchospasm (wheezing and shortness of breath) when he received *penicillin*, even many years before, makes any penicillin derivative unacceptable in him, unless there is no alternative. **B** is not a correct answer because the cephalosporins do not have activity against Enterococcus species and the fact that *ceftriaxone* is a β-lactam places the patient at risk of an allergic attack. **C** is incorrect specifically because the infection to be treated is endocarditis. *Vancomycin* is effective against most strains of Enterococcus, but in endocarditis it is adequately bactericidal only when it is used in combination with an aminoglycoside such as gentamicin. The combination is synergistic because vancomycin's effect on cell wall synthesis facilitates the entry of the aminoglycoside. Both drugs are bactericidal. **E** is incorrect for two reasons: *clindamycin* is ineffective against Enterococcus and, even in patients with endocarditis due to an organism susceptible to *clindamycin*, such as many strains of Staphylococcus aureus, *clindamycin* should not be used, because it is bacteriostatic. Endocarditis must be treated with a bactericidal drug, since the valvular lesion of endocarditis, called a "vegetation," contains only fibrin, platelets, and bacteria. Thus it has no cells that intrinsically kill bacteria. Cure requires that all the killing be done by antibiotics. The only correct answer, therefore, is **D**. Because the etiology turned out to be Enterococcus, a combination of *vancomycin* and *gentamicin* was employed with beneficial results.

Many principles of antibiotic selection are illustrated by this patient. (1) His history of serious allergy to penicillin eliminated this entire family of antibiotics from consideration. Thus, when his dental abscess had to be treated, he had to be given a "second-line" drug, *erythromycin*, when his dentist really would have preferred to give him *penicillin*. [Note: *Erythromycin* has the benefit of being able to penetrate abscesses.] (2) A cephalosporin would not have been safe enough, because a small percentage of patients who are allergic to *penicillin* also manifest allergy to cephalosporins. The reaction (bronchospasm) that this patient had could be so life-threatening that the dentist correctly chose not to take the risk, however small, that this patient might be allergic to both β-lactam categories. (3) That the patient had endocarditis required that the drug(s) with which he was to be treated must be bactericidal. (4) Finally, the role of Enterococcus in his endocarditis made it necessary to treat him with two antibiotics which act synergistically on this organism. [Note: The treatment of Enterococcal faecalis is becoming a problem due to resistant strains.]

CASE 6

A 41-year-old female presented to her primary medical doctor with a chief complaint of insomnia and nervousness worsening over the past several months. Since her last gynocologic exam, which was normal, she has experienced irregular menstrual cycles. She described her job as stressful and attributed some of the nervousness to her job.

BP 135/80 (120/80); pulse 135 bpm (60-80) and regular; respiratory rate of 20(12-18) and temperature of 99.5°F.

Physical exam reveals exophthalmos (abnormal protrusion of the eyeball) with weakened extraocular muscles (Figure A.6). Her skin was warm and moist

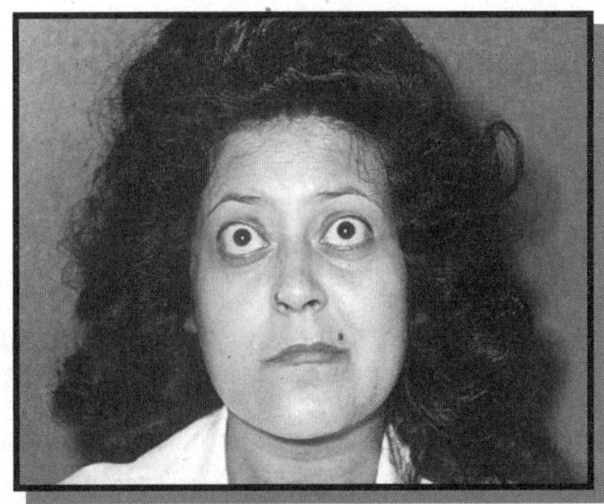

Figure A.6
Patient with exophthalmos.

and her hair was fine. Upon palpation the thyroid gland appeared slightly enlarged, uniform and without palpable nodules or masses. Pulses were strong bilaterally. Heart sounds were normal. Hand tremors presented as well as slight hyperreflexia.

Laboratory Tests reveal elevated thyroxine (T_4) and slightly decreased thyroid-stimulating hormone (TSH). All other tests were within normal limits.

The woman was treated with *propylthiouracil* 100mg every 8 hours, and *propranolol* 40 mg twice daily.

Question A.16: Which one of the following best describes the mechanism of action of *propylthiouracil*?

A. blocking the thyroid hormone receptor.
B. inhibiting the formation of thyroid hormone.
C. attenuation of the sympathetic excess seen in hyperthyroidism.
D. inhibition of iodine uptake into the thyroid gland.
E. inhibition of TSH release from pituitary

Correct answer is **B**. *Propylthiouracil* inhibits the formation of thyroid hormone.

Questions A.17: When using a thioamide, either *methimazole* or *propylthiouracil*, the most serious adverse drug reaction to monitor for is?

A. Agranulocytosis
B. Fatigue
C. Myalgias
D. Gastrointestinal (GI) upset
E. Edema

Correct a answer is **A**. The other side effects may occur, but the primary concern is agranulocytosis ,because this can be life threatening. The edema may be managed with diuretics and the diarrhea with antidiarrheal agents.

Question A.18: Why are β adrenergic blocking agents needed in addition to thioamides at the onset of treatment of hyperthyroidism?

Because thioamides inhibit the synthesis of new thyroid hormone and do little to inhibit the activity of circulating thyroid hormone, β blockers are needed to control the hypertension and tachycardia of hyperthyroidism in the first few weeks of therapy. In addition, adrenergic receptors are upregulated (there is a higher population in the vasculature) in the hyperthyroid patient, this it is important to block these β receptors and thereby reduce the blood pressure. With return to euthryroid condition, the receptor number decreases.

CASE 7

A 32 year-old homeless, HIV-negative man arrived at the clinic complaining of general malaise and a chronic productive cough.

The patient stated that he had been feeling poorly for about 5 weeks and thought he was losing weight. Upon physical examination, a slightly elevated temperature and chest congestion were noted; no other apparent irregularities were present. Lab tests were ordered, including a complete blood count (CBC), sputum culture, and an acid-fast bacilli (AFB) stain. A chest X-ray (Figure A.7) was obtained and a purified protein derivative (PPD) was administered. The patient was told to return in 2 days for a follow-up visit.

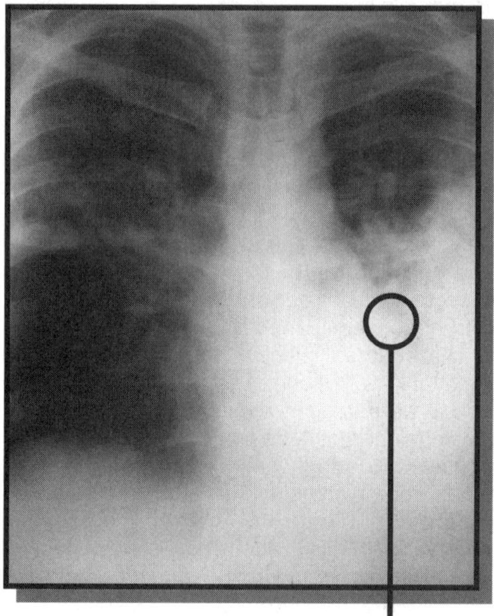

This lighter area in the lung is abnormal and shows the presence of cells and pus rather than air. This indicates the possible presence of infection.

Figure A.7
Chest X-ray of patient.

Question A.19: Based on these findings, the patient is suspected of having:

A. Streptococcal pneumonia
B. Mycobacterium infection
C. Pneumocystis carinii pneumonia (PCP)
D. Pseudomonas infection
E. Autoimmune deficiency syndrome (AIDS)

The correct answer is **B**. The chest X-ray with lung infiltrates could indicate lung cancer, pneumonia or other lung diseases. However, in conjunction with a positive AFB stain, the tests indicate a mycobacterium infection. [Note: A positive AFB stain does not identify the species of mycobacterium, only the genus. A diagnosis of Mycobacterium tuberculosis at this time is not confirmed but should be suspected.] **A** is incorrect. Streptococcal pneumonia might have been a possibility given the appearance of the chest X-ray, but this diagnosis is not definitive without an identification of the microbe in the sputum or blood cultures. The presence of AFB bacteria points strongly toward tuberculosis (TB). **C** is incorrect. PCP is seen primarily in individuals with AIDS who have a CD4 count (a measure of cell-mediated immunity) less than 200. This patient has no history of HIV or AIDS and therefore this diagnosis is unlikely. **D** is incorrect because Pseudomonas was not observed in the sputum. **C** is incorrect because the patient has no history of HIV infection.

Two days later the patient returned to the clinic for a follow-up examination. The lab results indicated that his sputum culture was negative for growth, and the CBC showed a slight leukocytosis (increase in white blood cells).

[Note: The PPD is a purified protein derivative of Mycobacterium tuberculosis that is injected subcutaneously into the volar surface of the forearm to stimulate a hypersensitivity reaction. If, within 24 to 48 hours there is an area of induration greater than 10 mm in diameter, it is a positive PPD test and indicates that the patient had been exposed to and infected with Mycobacterium tuberculosis.] The patient's test was positive. Due to his homeless status, it is likely that he came in contact with TB-infected individuals.

Based on the patient's history and lab information, he was started on a regimen of isoniazid, rifampin, pyrazinamide, and ethambutol while waiting for definitive cultures. (Six weeks later, definitive culture results demonstrated growth of Mycobacterium tuberculosis.) The patient returned to the clinic complaining of blurred vision and an inability to differentiate between green and red colors.

Question A.20: Which of the drugs he is taking could be causing these adverse visual symptoms?

A. *Isoniazid*
B. *Rifampin*
C. *Ethambutol*
D. *Pyrazinamide*

The correct answer is **C**. *Ethambutol* is a bacteriostatic agent used in conjunction with other drugs to treat Mycobacterium tuberculosis infections. A major side effect of *ethambutol* therapy is optic neuritis, which could be the cause of the patient's blurred vision and red/green color blindness. A baseline vision test is recommended prior to starting *ethambutol* therapy and should be conducted periodically throughout the regimen. **A** is incorrect. *Isoniazid* is a bactericidal agent used to treat TB, but its side-effects profile does not include visual disturbances. **B** is incorrect. Side effects of *rifampin* therapy include hepatitis, thrombocytopenia, acute renal failure, and a red/orange discoloration of body fluids, but does not affect the vision. **D** is incorrect. *Pyrazinamide* has been known to cause hepatotoxicity and hyperuricemia, but it does not cause visual disturbances.

CASE 8

A 47-year-old woman complained of recurrent headaches. She described the pain as unilateral, located in the temple, and having a rhythmic or pulsating quality. The headaches arise spontaneously—often awakening her in the middle of the night. The headaches are accompanied by nausea, abdominal pain, and spots before the eyes.

Question A.21: Which one of the following agents is most likely to provide symptomatic relief for this patient?

A. Oral *sumatriptan*
B. Oral *acetaminophen* plus *butalbital*
C. *Propranolol*
D. Oral *ergotamine*
E. *Sumatriptan* subcutaneously

Correct answer is **E**; *Sumatriptan* administered subcutaneously is rapidly absorbed and provides pain relief within 20 minutes. However, the half-life of the the drug administered subcutaneoulsy is only about 2 hours, so that the headache my be of longer duration than the drug's effect. The drug is approved for two doses per 24 hours. **A** Oral *sumatriptan* is appropriate in patients whose headaches slowly increase in severity. Taken at the start of the headache, oral *sumatripan* provides relief within 1 to 2 hours. The headaches described by this patient peak rapidly and *sumatriptan* administered orally would not act rapidly enough to provide relief for the acute pain of her migraine attacks. The bioavailability of the oral form is only about 15% due to poor absorption and presystemic metabolism. **B** Oral *acetominophen* plus *butalbital* has a slow onset of action and is unlikely to be effective in treating headaches that develop so rapidly as to awaken a sleeping patient. These moderately effective agents are used in mild to moderate headaches. **C** *Propranolol* is used as a prophylactic agent. **D** Oral *ergotamine* is a possible treatment option. However, the agent is most effective when give before the headache is established.

CASE 9

A 9 year-old boy was brought to the clinic by his mother. He was complaining of severe pruritus (itching) and bubbles on his arm.

Viewing the child's arm, the doctor noticed erythema (a red rash) and small vesicles (fluid-filled sacs) arranged linearly on the child's arm (Figure A.8). The doctor checked the child's profile and noticed no prior history of allergies to medication or foods, and no prior history of skin eruptions. The mother stated her son had not been wearing new clothing or taking any over the-counter-medications (OTC).

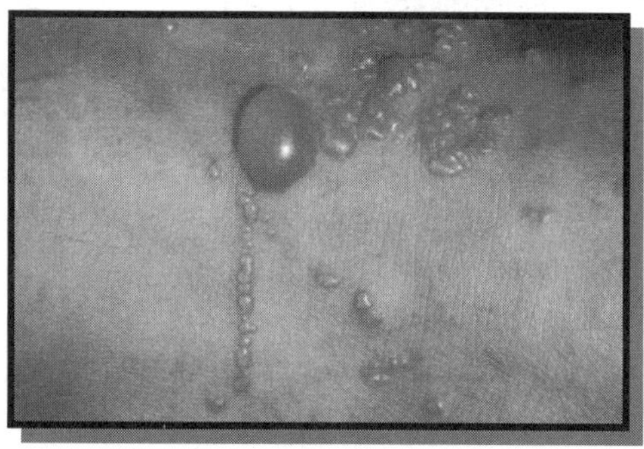

Figure A.8
Rash and vesicles on patient's arm.

The boy had recently been playing more outside in the yard, due to the hot weather, and his mother asked if the rash could have been caused by chiggers (larvae of mites that attached to the skin). With the patient's history of playing outdoors, and the characteristic linear vesicles, the doctor believed that the child had an allergic contact hypersensitivity reaction to poison ivy, and instructed the mother to apply cloths soaked in Burow's solution (aluminum acetate) until the vesicles crusted over. The mother was also told to thinly apply1% hydrocortisone cream (a low potency steroid) twice per day.

Question A.22: The hypersensitivity reaction was not serious enough to warrant stronger pharmacologic therapy, but the patient requests some remedy to stop the pruritus (itching). Which of the following drugs should be recommended?

A. *Ranitidine*
B. *Alprazolam*
C. *Diphenhydramine* (oral)
D. *Scopolamine*
E. *Phenobarbital*

The correct answer is **C**. *Diphenhydramine* is an antihistamine that is a competitive inhibitor of the H_1 receptor. It is used to treat various hypersensitivity reactions that are mediated by histamine such as allergic contact dermatitis. It will decrease the pruritus (itching) and some of the erythema produced by the release of histamine. [Note: Topical *diphenhydramine* should be used with caution in treating allergic contact dermatitis because it can act as an allergen itself and stimulate further irritation.] **A** is incorrect. *Ranitidine* is an H_2 histamine antagonist that is used to treat gastric ulcers. H_2 antagonists are not effective against hypersensitivity reactions except in rare instances when they are used in combination with H_1 antagonists. **B** is incorrect. *Alprazolam* is a benzodiazepine drug that is used in the treatment of anxiety and panic attacks. It is not indicated for the treatment of pruritus. **D** is incorrect. *Scopolamine* is a cholinergic antagonist used primarily to treat motion sickness, and has no antipruritic effect. **E** is incorrect. *Phenobarbital* is a sedative without antihistaminic (and thus without antipruritic) activity.

Five days later the child returned to the clinic. His hands, forearms, and chest are erythematous, swollen, and covered with blisters. His mother explained the poison ivy was starting to clear up, but then her son disobeyed her and went into the woods to play.

Question A.23: Which one of the following pharmacologic therapies should have been prescribed next to attenuate the inflammatory response.?

A. Apply the *hydrocortisone* cream more frequently
B. Oral *prednisone* therapy, tapered down over 2 weeks
C. Hospitalization
D. *Betamethasone* ointment with occlusion
E. Apply ice frequently

The correct answer is **B**. Due to the increased severity of this allergic reaction secondary to re-exposure, the next step in therapy is oral steroids. *Prednisone*, a glucocorticoid, is commonly used to treat conditions such as skin inflammation, asthma, and arthritis. *Prednisone* acts by decreasing the production of the mediators of inflammation, thereby resulting in its antiinflammatory action. **A** is incorrect. *Hydrocortisone* is a low potency glucocorticoid that is indicated for mild inflammation and irritation of the skin. The child's inflammation is severe enough to require systemic steroid therapy.

Spreading a cream over such a large area is not very practical and may lead to a decrease in patient compliance. **C** is incorrect. Hospitalization might be required if the child's inflammation compromised respiration in some way or if it were severely debilitating. This child is ambulatory and in no severe distress, and so can be treated on an outpatient basis. **D** is incorrect. *Betamethasone* is a strong topical steroid that should be avoided in this patient. Applying this steroid over large areas and possibly broken skin could lead to excessive absorption and thus toxicity. **E** is incorrect. Ice may decrease some of the itching but it has limited use in such a severe skin eruption.

Question A.24: What are some of the problems associated with glucocorticoid therapy?

Answer: *Prednisone* therapy given over a long period is associated with a multitude of side effects which include hyperglycemia, increased susceptibility to infection, osteoporosis, Cushing's syndrome, central nervous systme (CNS) effects, electrolyte disturbances and adrenal insufficiency. To avoid these adverse effects, prednisone is given for a short period and is tapered down throughout the regimen.

CASE 10

A 50-year-old female visited the clinic for the first time. Her chief complaint was stomach pain and recent swelling in her legs.

The woman described her pain as sharp and localized, and stated that it had occurred frequently during the previous 2 weeks. One week prior to the clinic visit she had started taking MAALOX (aluminum/magnesium hydroxide antacid) and it seemed to help at first, but the pain persisted and shortly thereafter the leg swelling appeared. Her past medical history included a prior diagnosis of congestive heart failure (CHF) and rheumatoid arthritis. A physical examination of the patient was insignificant except for noted arthritic joints in the hands and obvious ankle edema (Figure A.9). Further questioning revealed recent episodes of shortness of breath and increased fatigue. Her current medications included digoxin, ibuprofen, Maalox, and furosemide (LASIX). She also stated that she had heard on the news that aspirin might be good for the heart, so she had begun to take two tablets a day for her heart condition. The physician ordered a CBC, electrolyte panel, digoxin level, and a hemoccult test (to test the stool for signs of gastrointestinal bleeding).

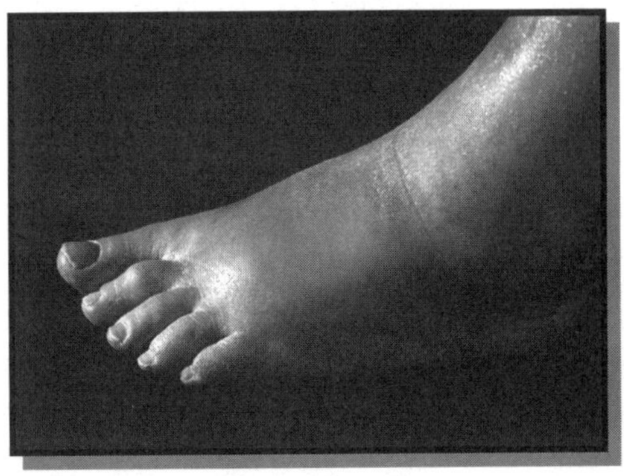

Figure A.9
Patient's ankle showing edema.

Question A.25: Based on the information presented above, what could be precipitating the stomach pain?

A. *Digoxin*
B. H. pylori
C. Nonsteroidal anti-inflammatory drugs (NSAIDs)
D. *Furosemide*
E. *Aluminum/magnesium hydroxide* combination antacid (Maalox®)

The correct answer is **C**. NSAIDs are used to decrease pain, inflammation, and fever. NSAIDs work by inhibiting the enzyme cyclooxygenase, which is responsible for producing prostaglandins, the body's mediators of pain and inflammation. Certain prostaglandins also have a protective effect on the stomach, causing a reduction in the production of stomach acid and maintaining the protective mucous barrier of the GI wall. Prolonged NSAID therapy leads to decreased quantities of prostaglandins and thus can result in GI erosion. The patient was prescribed the NSAID, *ibuprofen*, to decrease the symptoms associated with her rheumatoid arthritis. She was also taking a second NSAID, *aspirin*, which could result in additive stomach irritation and possible ulceration. This combination is probably responsible for the pain. **A** is incorrect. *Digoxin* belongs to the class of drugs called the cardiac glycosides, used to treat CHF by increasing the strength of the heart contraction and improving cardiac output. Side effects include nausea and vomiting, arrhythmias, and CNS effects including blurred vision and headache, but not sharp stomach pain. **B** is incorrect. Helicobacter pylori has been shown to be associated with stomach ulcers. From the patient history, there is no way to know without further investigation if she was colonized with H. pylori. **D** is incorrect. *Furosemide* is a loop diuretic used to eliminate fluid in patients with fluid overload such as in CHF or patients experiencing pulmonary edema. *Furosemide* is a fast acting diuretic with side effects that include: hypokalemia (low potassium), ototoxicity , and hypovolemia (dehydration). Side effects do not include excessive stomach pain. **E** is incorrect.

MAALOX is an *aluminum/magnesium hydroxide* combination antacid that is used to treat heartburn and sour stomach. The combination antacid has been known to cause constipation, diarrhea, and even CNS effects when used in renally compromised patients for extended periods, but does not cause sharp stomach pain.

The doctor hypothesized that the woman might have gastric or duodenal ulcers from NSAID therapy, and told her to collect three stool samples to be analyzed for the presence of blood. The doctor instructed the patient to discontinue using *ibuprofen* and *aspirin* until the actual reason for her pain could be diagnosed. She was to return for a follow-up visit in a few days. The doctor started treatment with an H_2 receptor antagonist to prevent any further GI irritation.

Question A.26: Why has the doctor prescribed the H_2 receptor antagonist?

Answer: All H_2 receptor antagonists work by preventing histamine from interacting with the H_2 receptor, thus decreasing the production of hydrochloric acid by the stomach. This decrease in acid production allows the stomach ulcer to heal. They also interfere in gastrin-mediated acid secretion. Basal and nocturnal acid secretion is also reduced. In addition, pepsin output also declines. Figure A.10 shows data obtained in a 24-week, double-blind, comparison of placebo with the H_2 receptor antagonist, *famotidine*. *Famotidine* significantly reduces the cumulative incidence of both gastric and duodenal ulcers in patients with arthritis receiving long-term NSAID therapy.

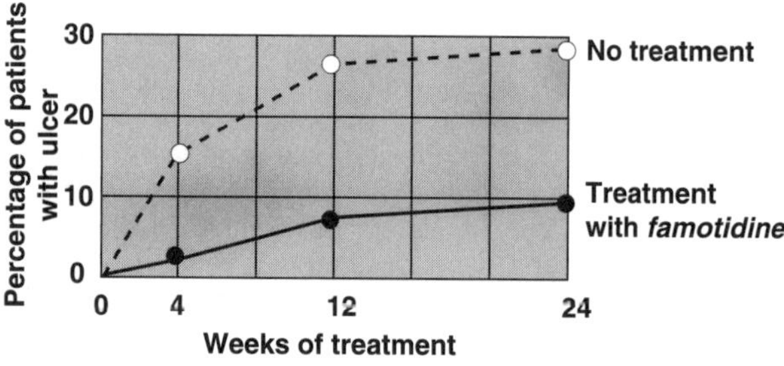

Figure A.10
Cumulative incidence of gastric or duodenal ulcers in patients receiving long-term NSAID therapy.

Question A.27: Which of the following drugs is NOT an H_2 receptor antagonist?

A. *Cimetidine*
B. *Famotidine*
C. *Omeprazole*
D. *Nizatidine*
E. *Ranitidine*

The correct answer is **C**. *Omeprazole* is an irreversible inhibitor of the H^+,K^+-ATPase (the "proton pump" of the parietal cell). It is used as an alternative to the H_2 receptor antagonists when the latter agents cannot control peptic ulcers. All of the other drugs are H_2 receptor antagonists. They vary in their side effect profile and to some extent in their pharmacokinetics. *Cimetidine* has the most side effects, which include confusion, dizziness, diarrhea, muscle pain, and gynecomastia (breast enlargement). In addition, *cimetidine* is a cytochrome P-450 enzyme inhibitor that decreases the metabolism of other drugs and can lead to drug toxicity. *Famotidine* has few side effects associated with its use.

Question A.28: Would you have recommended that she continue to take the MAALOX?

Answer: Probably not since she was placed on the H_2 receptor antagonist therapy and the antacid could have caused problems such as constipation and diarrhea.

The doctor next addressed the problem of edema. The patient's blood *digoxin* level was found to be in a subtherapeutic range, probably accounting for the ankle edema. The patient was questioned about being noncompliant (not taking her medication), but she insisted that she took her *digoxin* every day and that the swelling in the ankles appeared after she started taking MAALOX.

Question A.29: If the patient was being truthful about taking her medication every day, what could have caused the subtherapeutic blood levels of digoxin?

A. The *furosemide* was increasing her urine output and thereby increasing the elimination of digoxin from the blood.
B. *Aspirin* was competing for protein binding with *digoxin*, leading to increased concentrations of free *digoxin* and thus more free *digoxin* eliminated by the kidneys.
C. The patient is simply forgetful, and believes she takes her medication regularly, but frequently misses a dose.

D. The antacid she had been taking had been binding the *digoxin* in the GI tract and decreasing its absorption into systemic circulation.

E. The CHF is progressing and the patient is starting to deteriorate.

The correct answer is **D**. Combination *aluminum/magnesium hydroxide* antacids have been known to bind certain drugs such as *digoxin* in the GI tract and prevent them from being absorbed and distributed into systemic circulation. The patient had no edema prior to taking MAALOX, but developed it shortly after she started taking it. It is very likely that much of her *digoxin* dose was never absorbed by the body. If this is true then suspension of antacid intake should restore digoxin levels to the therapeutic range. If it does not, then the dose of digoxin must be increased. **A** is incorrect. *Furosemide* is a loop diuretic that increases urine output by inhibiting a carrier system in the ascending loop of Henle. It does not increase blood clearance of drugs by the kidney. **B** is incorrect. *Aspirin* is approximately 80% protein-bound. *Digoxin* is less than 25% protein-bound. Even if aspirin did displace *digoxin* from blood proteins, the increase in the free fraction of *digoxin* would not be significant and it is unlikely that there would be any increase in elimination of *digoxin* from the body. **C** is incorrect. It is certainly possible that the patient was noncompliant. However, the leg edema developed shortly after the stomach pain, but was absent prior to taking the antacid. This suggests possible drug interactions with concurrent patient medications. **E** is incorrect. It is a possibility that the patient's CHF was becoming worse and the disease was progressing. However, it would be wise to rule out the smaller problems (such as drug interactions) as a cause of edema before increasing the dose of *digoxin* or taking any drastic therapeutic measures.

CASE 11

A 57-year-old obese male with a history of mild asthma and hypertension arrived at the clinic for a flu shot and annual physical examination.

The doctor noticed that the patient had been placed on hydrochlorothiazide 8 months earlier for treatment of his high blood pressure. Through the course of the examination, the patient complained of cramps and fatigue that had been continuous over the previous month. The patient's baseline lab tests, performed 8 months prior to this visit, had all been within the normal ranges.

The doctor performed a physical examination that revealed a BP of 143/92 mm Hg with no other abnormal signs. The patient was questioned about his diet and any other medications he had been taking, and he responded that he usually ate a lot of meat and potatoes, but few vegetables. His other medications included an *albuterol* inhaler, metamucil, and a daily multivitamin tablet. The doctor ordered serum electrolyte levels and a CBC with differential from the lab. Recognizing that the patient had a couple of problems, the doctor decided to deal first with the cramps and fatigue.

Question A.30: What could be causing the patient's fatigue and muscle cramps?

A. He has come down with the flu, which is responsible for the fatigue and cramps.

B. The *albuterol* is responsible for the symptoms, commonly seen in asthmatics on *albuterol* therapy.

C. Continued high blood pressure is responsible for the symptoms (that is, the patient's blood pressure is not controlled with the thiazide therapy).

D. Thiazide therapy is causing potassium depletion and resulting in the cramps and fatigue.

E. *Metamucil*, a bulk forming laxative, is leading to dehydration, which gives rise to fatigue and cramps.

The correct answer is **D**. *Hydrochlorothiazide* is a thiazide diuretic that exerts its action at the distal tubule of the kidney. It works by inhibiting a sodium/chloride transporter, which leads to increased sodium and water excretion into the urine and diuresis. When the elimination of sodium is increased, the kidney exchanges potassium for sodium in the transporter (both are monovalent cations), which over an extended period can lead to potassium depletion. If sufficient quantities of potassium are not obtained through the diet or by exogenous supplements, an individual may experience cramps, fatigue, and possibly arrhythmias. **A** is incorrect. The patient does not have a fever, chills or the muscle aches and pains that are characteristic of the flu. Also, the flu usually lasts no more than 2 weeks, whereas the patient had been having these symptoms for over a month with no fever. **B** is incorrect. *Albuterol* is a β_2-specific agonist that is used in the treatment of mild asthma. *Albuterol* promotes bronchodilation that counteracts the bronchoconstriction experienced by asthma sufferers during an attack. The most common side effects of *albuterol* therapy are tachycardia, tremor, and increased blood pressure. The patient had presumably been on this medication for quite a while, with no previous symptoms of cramps and fatigue. **C** is incorrect. Symptoms of high blood pressure are usually only seen when the pressure is extremely high. Under these circumstances, the patient will be in obvious distress, and rapid medical treatment is imperative. The patient's continued hypertension might result in future disease, but his current symptoms are not indicators of hypertension. **E** is incorrect. *Metamucil* is an OTC bulk forming laxative which, when taken with water, forms a bulky mass that stimulates GI motility. It has been known to adhere to some medications in the GI tract and prevent them from being absorbed into systemic circulation. Adverse side effects include nausea, vomiting and stomach pain. *Metamucil* does not cause dehydration, and it is doubtful that this agent was causing the patient's symptoms of cramping and fatigue.

The lab test results were returned, and the doctor noted that there were no leukocytosis or abnormalities on the CBC, but that the serum electrolyte results showed a marked hypokalemia, as was expected. This provided an explanation for the patient's cramping and the fatigue. The doctor prescribed a potassium supplement for the patient, due to the extent of his hypokalemia.

Next, the doctor began to address the patient's uncontrolled hypertension. Believing him to be reasonably dependable and compliant with his diuretic therapy, the doctor realized that the patient's current hypertension medication was not working. Instead of increasing the dose of hydrochlorothiazide, he felt that the patient would benefit from an additional antihypertensive medication in combination with his present therapy.

Question A.31: Which additional antihypertensive medication will most benefit the patient?

A. An angiotensin converting enzyme (ACE) inhibitor
B. *Nitroglycerin*
C. A β-blocker
D. *Clonidine*
E. *Hydralazine*

The correct answer is **A**. ACE inhibitors are an effective group of antihypertension medications with a favorable side-effect profile. In addition to preventing vasoconstriction, ACE inhibitors also decrease aldosterone secretion, resulting in less sodium and water reabsorption and less potassium wasting. ACE inhibitors also decrease the breakdown of bradykinins, which are potent vasodilators. Since ACE inhibitors do not block β-receptors, they are a good choice for the treatment of asthma patients. ACE inhibitors are generally well tolerated, and are the best choice for this patient. **B** is incorrect. *Nitroglycerin* is an organic nitrate used for its vasodilator action to treat angina. It is not indicated for the treatment of hypertension. **C** is incorrect. β-Blockers are a group of medications used to treat hypertension, angina, glaucoma, and refractory migraine headaches. Although many β-blockers are β_1-specific blockers, they may also have β_2 blocking action. Use of β-blockers should be avoided in asthma patients, because they may experience bronchoconstriction and an asthma attack if their β_2 receptors are blocked. Also, β-blockers may complicate treatment of bronchospasm by decreasing the effectiveness of β_2 agonists such as *albuterol*. The patient suffered from mild asthma and, therefore, β-blockers are a poor choice for treating his hypertension. **D** is incorrect. *Clonidine* is a central-acting α_2 receptor agonist used to treat moderate hypertension. *Clonidine* works by decreasing sympathetic outflow to the periphery and thus decreases cardiac output. *Clonidine* does not decrease renal blood flow like other antihypertensive agents, which makes it a good agent for treatment of hypertensive patients with renal disease. The patient is suffering from mild hypertension. *Clonidine* could be used, but it has a larger side-effect profile and should probably be reserved for patients with more severe hypertension. **E** is incorrect. *Hydralazine* is a direct acting vasodilator used to treat moderately severe hypertension. *Hydralazine* is not a first line agent, due to its many side effects, and is used in combination with other agents. Since the patient suffers only from mild hypertension, strong antihypertensive therapy with *hydralazine* is not warranted.

Pharmacology Update

This addendum provides a current update on important drugs that have been added to the clinical arsenal since the second edition of *Lippincott's Illustrated Reviews: Pharmacology* was published. The addendum is organized by chapter, and each drug is presented either as a continuation of a preexisting section covering similar-acting drugs (for example, additions to the list of drugs used to treat Parkinson's disease, below), or as totally new types of drugs (see the section on thrombin inhibitors, p. 448). Extensive cross-references to relevant pages in the body of the text allow the reader to place these recently approved drugs in their proper clinical context.

Treatment of Parkinson's Disease 8

V. DRUGS USED IN PARKINSON'S DISEASE (continued from p. 88)

The following are new, **non-ergot dopamine agonists** that have been approved for the treatment of Parkinson's disease. *Pramipexole* and *ropinirole* are effective as first-line and adjunctive therapy, whereas *tolcapone* should only be used as an adjunct in patients on *levodopa/carbidopa*.

F. Pramipexole and ropinirole

Pramipexole [pram i PECKS ole] and *ropinirole* [ROH pin i role] are non-ergot agonists at dopamine receptors. They alleviate the motor deficits in both *levodopa*-naïve patients (patients that have never been treated with *levodopa*), and patients with advanced Parkinson's disease taking *levodopa*. These dopamine agonists may delay the need to employ *levodopa* therapy in early Parkinson's, and may decrease the dose of *levodopa* in advanced Parkinson's. Unlike *bromocriptine* (an ergotamine derivative, see p. 87), *pramipexole* and *ropinirole* do not exacerbate peripheral vasospasm. Nausea, hallucinations, insomnia, dizziness, constipation, and orthostatic hypotension are among the more distressing side-effects of these drugs; dyskinesias are less frequent than with *levodopa*. The dependence of *pramipexole* on renal function for its elimination cannot be overly stressed. For example, *cimetidine* (see p. 236), which inhibits renal tubular secretion of organic bases, increases the half-life of *pramipexole* by forty percent. The fluoroquinolone antibiotics (see p. 323) have been shown to inhibit the metabolism of *ropinirole*, and enhance the AUC (area under the concentration vs. time curve, see p. 7) by some eighty percent. Figures 8.9 and 8.10 summarize some properties of *pramipexole* and *ropinirole.*

	Pramipexole	*Ropinirole*
Bioavailability	> 90%	55 %
V_d	7 L/kg	7.5 L/kg
Half-life	8 hours[1]	6 hours
Metabolism	Negligible	Extensive
Elimination	Renal	Renal[2]

[1]Increases to 12 hours in patients greater than 65 years old
[2]Less than 10 % excreted unchanged

Figure 8.9
Pharmacokinetic properties of dopamine agonists of *pramipexole* and *ropinirole*.

	Pramipexole	Ropinirole
Somnolence	+++	++
Insomnia	++++	+
Dizziness or lightheadedness	+++	++
Hallucinations or confusion	++	++
Headache		++
Orthostasis	++	+++
Nausea	++++	++
Constipation	++	
Others		
Arthralgia		++
Blurred vision	+	
Dry mouth	++	
Upper respiratory infection		++

+ = Incidence of 1 to 5 percent;
++ = incidence of 6 to 15 percent;
+++ = incidence of 16 to 25 percent;
++++ = incidence of greater than 25 percent.

Figure 8.10
Side effects of dopamine agonists *pramipexole* and *ropinirole.*

G. Tolcapone

Tolcapone [TOLE ka pone] is a nitrocatechol derivative that represents a new class of anti-Parkinson's drugs. It selectively and reversibly inhibits both peripheral and central catechol-O-methyltransferase (COMT) (Figure 8.11). Normally, the methylation of *levodopa* by COMT to 3-O-methyldopa is a minor pathway for *levodopa* metabolism. However, when peripheral dopamine decarboxylase activity is inhibited by *carbidopa*, a significant concentration of 3-O-methyldopa is formed that competes with *levodopa* for active transport into the CNS. Inhibition of COMT by *tolcapone* leads to decreased plasma concentrations of 3-O-methyldopa, increased central uptake of *levodopa*, and greater concentrations of brain dopamine. *Tolcapone* has been demonstrated to reduce the frequency of the "on-off" phenomenon.

1. **Pharmacokinetics:** *Tolcapone*, taken orally, is readily absorbed, and its absorption is not influenced by food. It is extensively bound to plasma albumin (>99 percent), and has a small volume of distribution (0.13 L/kg). The plasma half-life is approximately two hours, although inhibition of COMT may last considerably longer due to its affinity for the enzyme. *Tolcapone* is extensively metabolized, and its metabolites are eliminated in both the urine and feces. Dosage may need to be adjusted in individuals with moderate or severe cirrhosis.

2. **Adverse effects:** Diarrhea is the most common side effect of *tolcapone*. As expected, *levodopa*-related adverse effects increase when *tolcapone* is added. These include postural hypotension, nausea, sleep disorders, anorexia, dyskinesias, and hallucinations. Most seriously, fulminating hepatic necrosis is associated with *tolcapone* use. Baseline and frequent, regular determinations of hepatic serum enzymes are suggested by the manufacturer. Any elevations above normal are cause for discontinuation. Because of the hepatotoxicity, *tolcapone* should only be used as an adjunct in patients on *levodopa/carbidopa* who are experiencing symptom fluctuations.

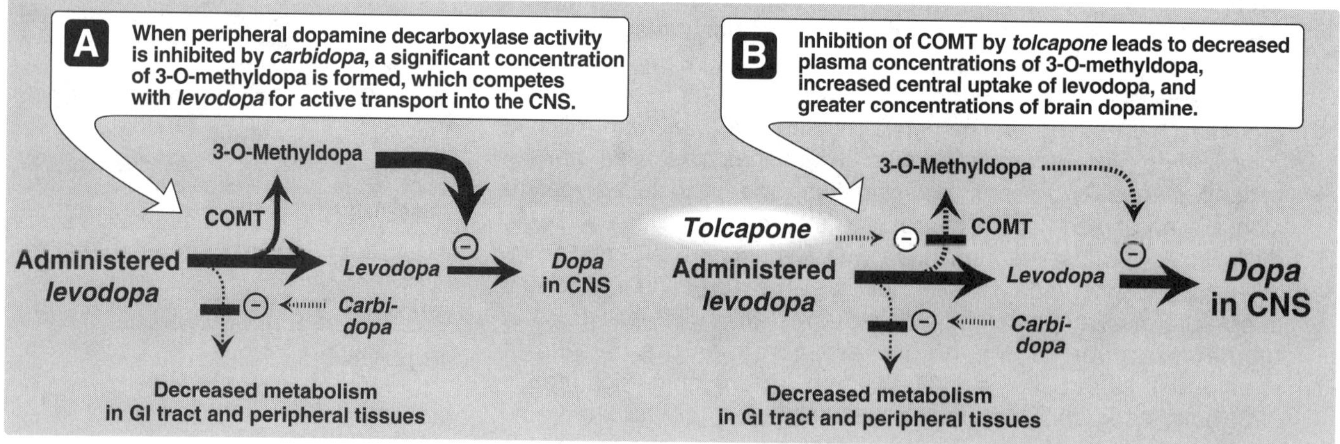

Figure 8.11
Effect of *tolcapone* on dopa concentration in the central nervous system (CNS). COMT = catechol-O-methyltransferase.

Drugs Used to Treat Epilepsy 15

II. ANTIEPILEPTIC DRUGS (continued from page 150)

Partial seizures account for the majority of refractory convulsant disorders in adults, often requiring more than one drug to achieve adequate therapeutic control. Three new compounds with unique mechanisms of action have been approved for use in **partial seizures** and, secondarily, **generalized seizures**. Figure 15.9 summarizes some therapeutic advantages and disadvantages of selected antiepileptic drugs.

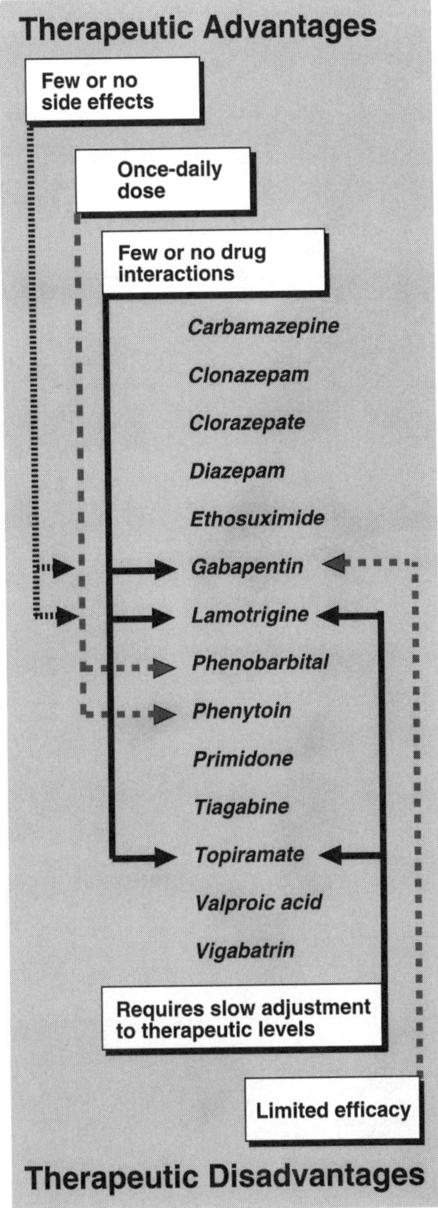

Figure 15.9
Summary of therapeutic advantages and disadvantages of antiepileptic drugs.

I. Tiagabine

Tiagabine [tye aga been] blocks GABA uptake into presynaptic neurons, permitting more GABA to be available for receptor binding, thus causing enhanced inhibitory activity. In clinical trials, *tiagabine* was effective in decreasing the number of seizures in refractory patients with focal epileptic disorders.

1. **Pharmacokinetics:** *Tiagabine* is well absorbed orally (bioavailability is 90 percent), although food slows the rate but not extent of absorption. Binding to plasma proteins is 96 percent. *Tiagabine* undergoes two major metabolic pathways: 1) oxidation of the thiophene ring, and 2) glucuronidation. Only two percent is excreted unchanged. The majority of the excretion is biliary (65 percent), with some urinary excretion (25 percent). The half-life in healthy volunteers is seven to nine hours.

2. **Adverse effects:** Decreased maintenance doses may be necessary in individuals with hepatic impairment. Adverse effects include tiredness, dizziness and gastrointestinal upset.

J. Topiramate

Topiramate [to PYRE a mate], a chemical relative of fructose, has several actions at therapeutic concentrations that contribute to its anticonvulsant activity. These actions include blockade of Na^+–channels, increased GABA activity at GABA receptors, and blockade of some glutamate receptors. When added to conventional therapy in refractory patients, *topiramate* causes a 50 percent or greater reduction in the number of partial seizures in approximately 50 percent of the patients.

1. **Pharmacokinetics:** *Topiramate* is well absorbed, with an oral bioavailability of 80 percent. Peak concentrations occur in about two hours. Some 30 percent of each dose is metabolized, the remainder is excreted unchanged in the urine. The half-life of *topiramate* is about 20 to 25 hours.

2. **Adverse effects:** These are primarily related to CNS and GI disturbances. They include impaired concentration, dizziness, ataxia, diplopia, somnolence, nervousness, and confusion, as well as nausea and weight loss. Renal stones have been reported in 1.5 percent of patients. *Topiramate* is teratogenic in animals, and should be avoided during pregnancy. Inducers of drug metabolism such as *phenytoin* and *carbamazepine* decrease *topiramate* serum concentrations by approximately 50 percent. *Topiramate* decreases *ethinyl estradiol* concentrations of oral contraceptive preparations, and individuals should supplement the amount of *ethinyl estradiol*.

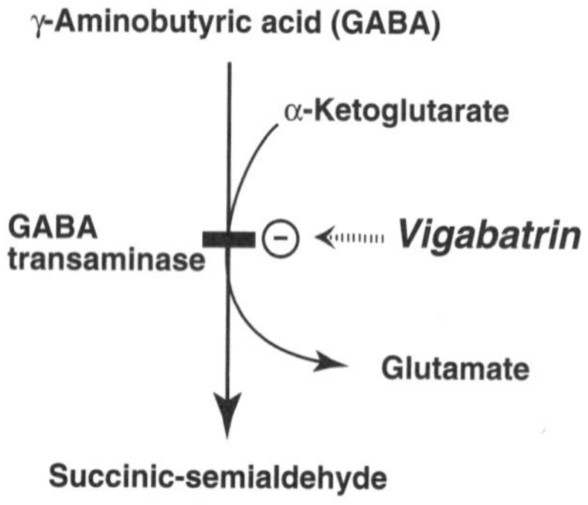

γ-Aminobutyric acid (GABA)

α-Ketoglutarate

GABA transaminase

⊖ ← *Vigabatrin*

Glutamate

Succinic-semialdehyde

Figure 15.10
Mechanism of action of *vigabatrin.*

K. Vigabatrin

Vigabatrin [vig a BAT rin] was designed specifically to irreversibly inhibit the enzyme GABA transaminase (Figure 15.10). Inhibition results in increased levels of GABA in the brain. Numerous studies have established its effectiveness in reducing the number of partial seizures in refractory patients. *Vigabatrin* is rapidly absorbed orally, and its bioavailability is greater than 60 percent. The plasma half-life is six to eight hours. GABA transaminase requires three days to be resynthesized. Elimination is primarily of unchanged drug in the urine. Adverse effects include the usual drowsiness and dizziness. Some patients experience weight gain. Less frequent but significant toxicities include confusion, agitation and psychoses. *Vigabatrin*, unlike other anticonvulsants, has minimal drug interactions.

20 Drugs Affecting Blood

V. PLATELET AGGREGATION INHIBITORS

(continued from p. 197)

Platelets respond to vascular trauma by "activation" processes, which involve three steps: adhesion to the site of injury, release of intracellular granules and signaling molecules, followed by aggregation of the platelets. The last step, aggregation, is mediated by a family of membrane glycoprotein receptors that can bind adhesive proteins, such as fibrinogen, von Willebrand factor, and fibronectin. The most important is the GP IIb/IIIa receptor, which ultimately regulates platelet-platelet interaction and thrombus formation. Thus, platelet activation agents, such as thromboxane A_2, ADP, thrombin, serotonin, and collagen all promote the conformational change necessary for the GP IIb/IIIa receptor to bind ligands, particularly fibrinogen. Fibrinogen simultaneously binds to GP IIb/IIIa receptors on two separate platelets, resulting in platelet crosslinking and aggregation (Figure 20.14). Platelet aggregation inhibitors described here block GP IIb/IIIa or ADP receptors, thereby decreasing chemical signals that promote platelet aggregation.

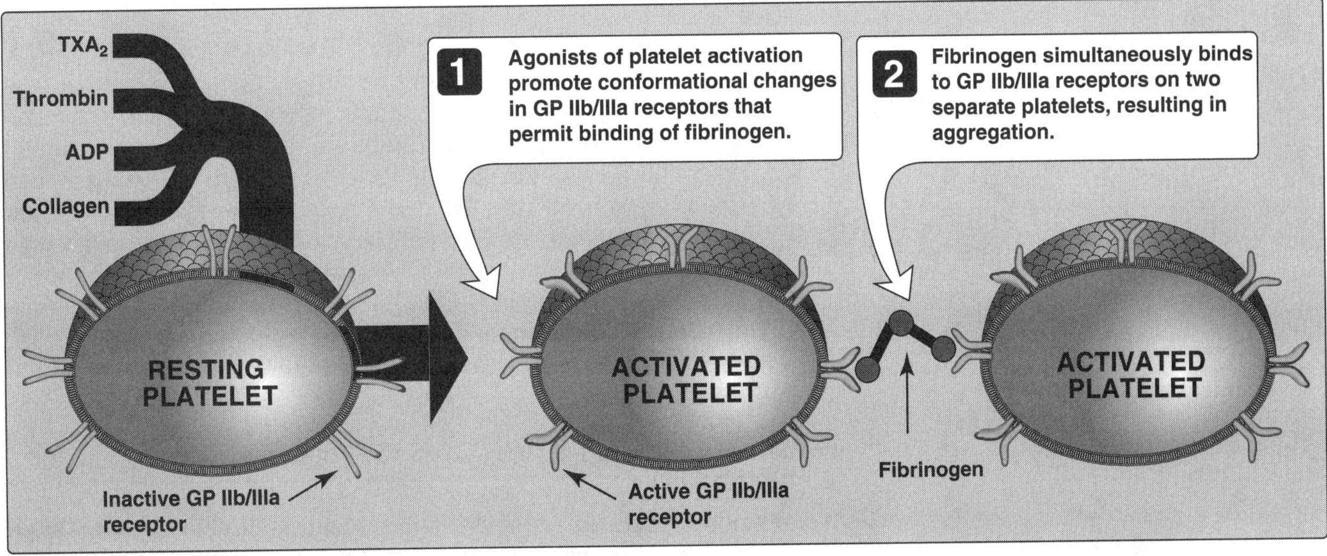

Figure 20.14
Summary of antiplatelet and antithrombin agents.

D. Abciximab

Realization of the key role of the platelet GP IIb/IIIa receptor in stimulating platelet aggregation directed attempts to block this receptor on activated platelets. This led to the development of a chimeric monoclonal antibody, *abciximab* (ab SIH ksih mab), which is composed of Fab fragments of a murine monoclonal antibody directed against the glycoprotein GP IIb/IIIa complex joined to the constant regions of human immunoglobulin. By binding to GP IIb/IIIa, the antibody blocks the binding of fibrinogen (see p. 194) and von Willebrand factor, and consequently, aggregation does not occur (see Figure 20.16). *Abciximab* is given intravenously as an adjunct to percutaneous coronary intervention for the prevention of cardiac ischemic complications. *Heparin* or *aspirin* is given with *abciximab*. After cessation of infusion, platelet function gradually returns towards normal, the antiplatelet effect persisting for 24 to 48 hours. Optimal duration of treatment has not been determined. The major adverse effect is potential for bleeding, especially if *abciximab* is used with anticoagulants, or if the patient has a clinical hemorrhagic condition.

E. Eptifibatide and tirofiban

These two antiplatelet drugs act similarly to *abciximab*, blocking the GP IIb/IIIa receptor. *Eptifibatide* [ep tee FIH ba tyde] and *tirofiban* [tye roe FYE ban] mimic the arginine-glycine-aspartic acid sequence of fibrinogen, which accounts for their specific antagonism at this receptor. These compounds, like *abciximab*, can decrease the incidence of thrombotic complications associated with acute coronary syndromes. When intravenous infusion is stopped, these agents are rapidly cleared from the plasma, but their effect can persist for four hours. *Eptifibatide* and its metabolites are excreted by the kidney. *Tirofiban* is excreted unchanged by the kidney. The major adverse effect of both drugs is bleeding. Figure 20.15 summarizes some clinical effects of the GP IIb/IIIa receptor antagonists.

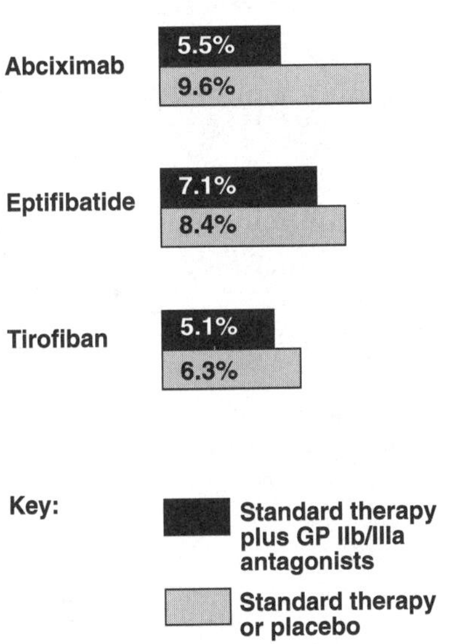

Figure 20.15
Effects of glycoprotein IIb/IIIa receptor antagonists on the incidence of death or nonfatal myocardial infarction following percutaneous transluminal coronary angioplasty. [Note: Data are from several studies; thus reported incidence of complications with standard therapy is not the same for each drug.]

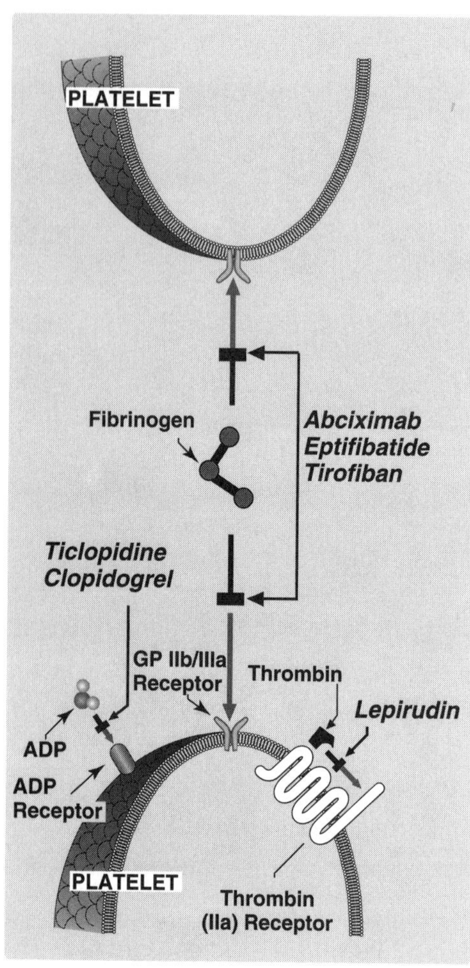

Figure 20.16
Summary of antiplatelet and antithrombin agents.

F. Clopidogrel

Clopidogrel [clo PIH doh grel] is an analog of *ticlopidine* (see p. 197). Like that drug, *clopidogrel* selectively and irreversibly blocks ADP binding to platelets. It thus prevents ADP-mediated activation of the glycoprotein complex GPIIb/IIIa, thereby inhibiting platelet aggregation (Figure 20.16). *Clopidogrel* is extensively metabolized by the liver, and its action is due to one of these metabolites that has yet to be identified. Elimination of the drug and its metabolites occurs by both the renal and fecal routes. Its primary adverse effect is bleeding. Since *clopidogrel* can inhibit cytochrome P-450 (see p. 14), it may interfere with the metabolism of *phenytoin, tolbutamide, warfarin, fluvastatin* and *tamoxifen* if taken concomitantly.

XI. THROMBIN INHIBITORS (continued from p. 206)

Thrombocytopenia (a condition in which circulating blood contains an abnormally small number of platelets) is a common abnormality among hospital patients, and can be caused by a variety of factors. One of these is associated with the use of *heparin*, and is called either *heparin*-induced thrombocytopenia (HIT) or *heparin*-associated thrombocytopenia (HAT). Two types of this abnormality have been identified: HIT type I is a mild decrease of platelets due to nonimmunologic mechanisms, and is not serious. HIT type II, on the other hand, involves immunologic mechanisms, and can cause clinical sequelae that range from mild to life-threatening. Platelet counts can drop 50 percent or more, and thromboembolic complications can develop. Although HIT is relatively rare, the wide use of *heparin* has resulted in a greater recognition of its role in thrombocytopenia. The treatment of HIT requires anticoagulation and, up until recently, low molecular weight heparins (which appear to lead to fewer clinical problems) have been employed with variable results. Recently, a new agent, *lepirudin*, has been approved for the specific treatment of this condition.

A. Lepirudin

Lepirudin [le pee RUE din] is a polypeptide that is a highly specific thrombin antagonist. One molecule of *lepirudin* binds to one molecule of thrombin, resulting in the blockade of the thrombogenic activity of thrombin (Figure 20.16). The drug is produced in yeast cells by recombinant DNA technology. Administered intravenously, *lepirudin* is effective in the treatment of *heparin*-induced thrombocytopenia and other thromboembolic disorders, and can prevent further thromboembolic complications. *Lepirudin* has a half-life of about one hour, and is believed to undergo hydrolysis. The parent drug and its fragments are eliminated in the urine. Bleeding is the major adverse effect of treatment with *lepirudin*, and can be exacerbated by concommitant thrombolytic therapy, for example, treatment with *streptokinase* or *tissue-type plasminogen activator* (*tPA,* see p. 202*)*.

Antihyperlipidemic Drugs 21

F. HMG-CoA reductase inhibitors (continued from p. 214)

These antihyperlipidemic agents inhibit de novo cholesterol synthesis, and deplete the intracellular supply of cholesterol. This prompts the cell to increase the number of specific cell-surface LDL receptors that can bind and internalize circulating LDLs. Thus the end result is a reduction in plasma cholesterol, both by lowered cholesterol synthesis and by increased catabolism of LDL.

1. Atorvastatin

Atorvastatin (a TOR va stah tin) limits cholesterol formation by competitively inhibiting the conversion of HMG-CoA to mevalonate by HMG-CoA reductase. Dose-dependent reductions in total cholesterol, low density lipoprotein (LDL)-cholesterol, and triglyceride levels have been observed with *atorvastatin* in patients with hypercholesterolemia and in patients with hypertriglyceridemia. In large trials involving patients with hypercholesterolemia, *atorvastatin* produced greater reductions in total cholesterol, LDL cholesterol, apolipoprotein B, and triglyceride levels than did *lovastatin*, *pravastatin,* and *simvastatin* (Figure 21.12). As with other HMG-CoA reductase inhibitors, the most frequently reported adverse event associated with *atorvastatin* is gastrointestinal upset.

Characteristic	*Lovastatin*	*Pravastatin*	*Simvastatin*	*Atorvastatin*	*Fluvastatin*	*Cerivastatin*
Serum LDL cholesterol reduction produced (%)*	34	34	41	50	24	28
Serum triglyceride reduction produced (%)*	16	24	18	29	10	13
Serum HDL cholesterol increase produced (%)*	8.6	12	12	6	8	10
Plasma half-life (hr)	2	1-2	1-2	14	1-2	2-3
Penetration of central nervous system	Yes	No	Yes	No	No	Yes
Renal excretion of absorbed dose (%)	10	20	13	2	<6	33

*This effect was elicited by a daily dose of 40 mg of *lovastatin, pravastatin, simvastatin, atorvastatin,* and *fluvastatin,* and by a daily dose of 0.3 mg of *cerivastatin* in patients with hypercholesterolemia. Reductions in LDL cholesterol of 30 to 32 percent are more typical of once-daily treatment with *lovastatin* and twice-daily treatment with *pravastatin.*

Figure 21.12
Summary of HMG-CoA reductase inhibitors.

22 Drugs Affecting the Respiratory System

II. Drugs Used to Treat Asthma (continued from p. 220)

A new class of antiasthma drugs has recently been developed that targets the formation or function of leukotrienes (Figure 22.7). These drugs include *zileuton* [ZYE loo ton], *zafirlukast* [zah FUR loo kast], and *montelukast* [mon TEE loo kast].

F. Anti-leukotriene Drugs

Leukotriene B_4 (LTB_4) and the cysteinyl leukotrienes, LTC_4, LTD_4, and LTE_4, are products of the 5-lipoxygenase pathway of arachidonic acid metabolism. 5-Lipoxygenase is found in cells of myeloid origin, such as mast cells, basophils, eosinophils, and neutrophils. LTB_4 is a potent chemoattractant to neutrophils and eosinophils,

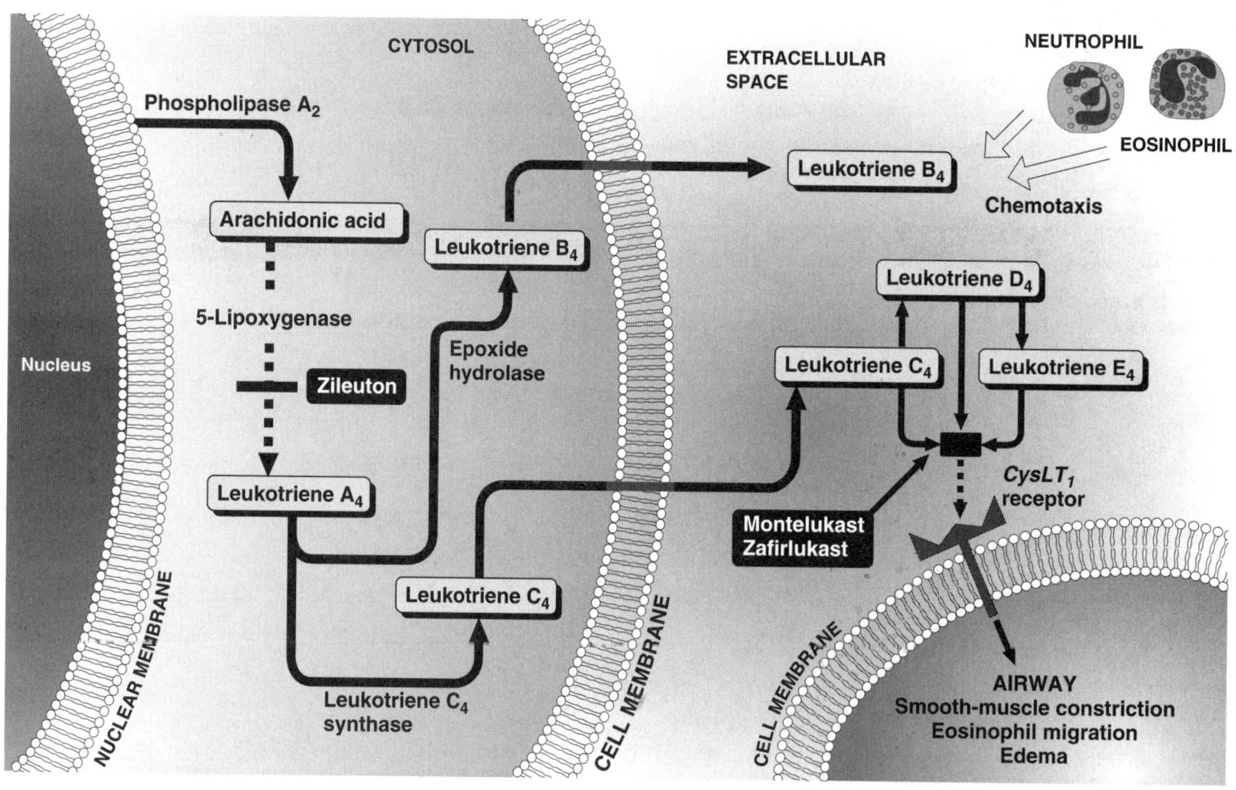

Figure 22.7
Biochemical pathways of the formation and action of leukotrienes and sites of action of leukotriene-modifying drugs.

whereas the cysteinyl leukotrienes constrict bronchiolar smooth muscle, increase endothelial permeability, and promote mucus secretion. [Note: Cysteinyl leukotrienes are the components of "slow-reacting substance" (SRS) of anaphylaxis and allergy.] *Zileuton* is a selective and specific inhibitor of 5-lipoxygenase, preventing the formation of both LTB_4 and the cysteinyl leukotrienes. *Zafirlukast* and *montelukast* are selective, reversible inhibitors of the cysteinyl leukotriene-1 receptor, thereby blocking the effects of cysteinyl leukotrienes (Figure 22.7). All three drugs are approved for the prophylaxis of asthma. They are not effective in situations where immediate bronchodilation is required. Reductions in the doses of β-adrenergic agonists and corticosteroids, and improved respiratory function, are among the therapeutic benefits. *Montelukast* is approved for use in children six years old, and older.

1. **Pharmacokinetics:** All three drugs are orally active, although food impairs the absorption of *zafirlukast.* Greater than 90 percent of each drug is bound to plasma protein. The drugs are extensively metabolized; *zileuton* and its metabolites are excreted in the urine, whereas *zafirlukast* and *montelukast* and their metabolites undergo biliary excretion.

2. **Adverse Effects:** Elevations in serum hepatic enzymes have occurred with all three agents, requiring periodic monitoring and discontinuation when enzyme levels exceed three times the normal. Although rare, eosinophilic vasculitis (Churg-Strass syndrome) has been reported with all agents, particularly when the dose of concurrent glucocorticoid is reduced. Other effects include headache and dyspepsia. Both *zafirlukast* and *zileuton* are inhibitors of cytochrome P-450. Both drugs can increase serum levels of *warfarin. Montelukast* has not been shown to inhibit cytochrome P-450 (see p. 14). The chewable tablet form of *montelukast* contains 0.8 mg of phenylalanine; patients with phenylketonuria should be so informed. Figure 22.8 summarizes the drugs that modify the action of leukotrienes.

	Zafirlukast	Montelukast	Zileuton
Oral dose	40 mg twice daily	10 mg daily	600 mg 4 times daily
Reduction in β-adrenergic agonist use - %	31	27	30
Improvement in morning PEFR - %	6	6.1	7.1
Treatment failure or glucocorticoid rescue therapy, treatment vs. placebo - %	2 vs. 10	6.9 vs. 9.6	8.3 vs 21.5
Decrease in symptoms - %	28	20	36

Figure 22.8
Effects of leukotriene modifiers in patients with chronic persistent asthma. PEFR = peak expiratory flow rate.

26 Insulin and Oral Hypoglycemic Drugs

IV. INSULIN PREPARATIONS (continued from p. 260)

Most of the *insulins* derived from beef and pork have been largely replaced by the human form, synthesized utilizing recombinant DNA technology. For example, *lispro insulin* is synthesized by recombinant DNA technology, using a non-pathogenic strain of E. coli.

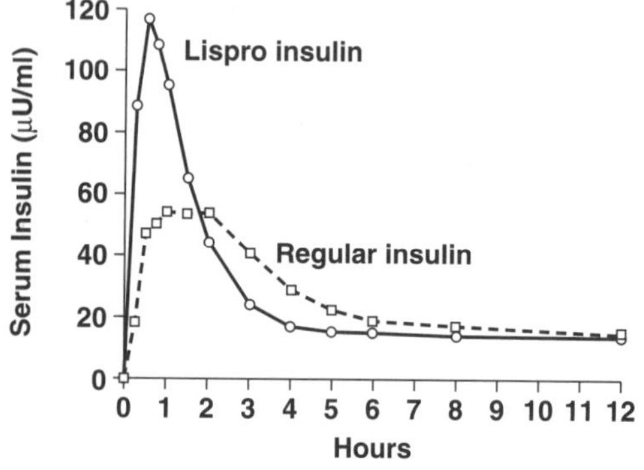

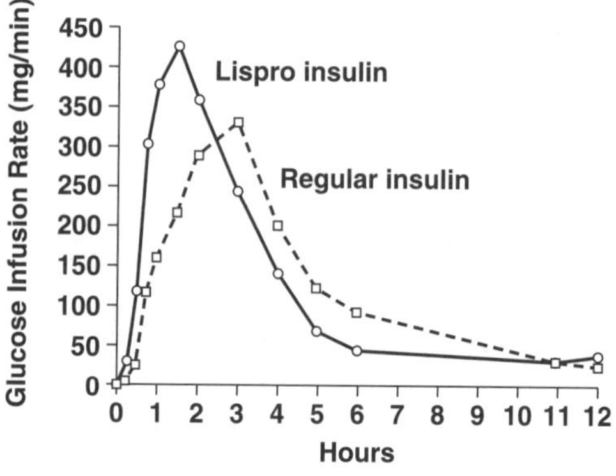

Figure 26.10
Effect of subcutaneous administration of lispro insulin and regular insulin on (A) serum insulin concentrations, and (B) the rate of glucose infusion necessary to maintain normal blood glucose levels in 10 normal subjects.

E. Lispro insulin

Lispro [LIS pro] *insulin* differs from regular *insulin* in that lysine and proline at positions 28 and 29 in the B chain are reversed. This results in more rapid absorption after subcutaneous injection than is seen with regular *insulin*; as a consequence, *lispro insulin* is more rapidly-acting (Figure 26.10). When used before mealtime, *lispro insulin* should be administered 15 minutes prior to the meal. Peak levels of *lispro insulin* are seen at 30 to 90 minutes after injection, as compared to 50 to 120 minutes for regular *insulin. Lispro insulin* also has a shorter duration of activity. *Lispro insulin* is usually not used alone, but requires a longer acting *insulin* to assure proper glucose control. Otherwise no differences exist between *lispro insulin* and regular *insulin*. Adverse effects are those reported for other *insulin* preparations, the most important being hypoglycemia.

V. ORAL HYPOGLYCEMIC AGENTS (continued from p. 261)

These agents are useful in the treatment of patients who have non-insulin-dependent diabetes, but cannot be managed by diet alone. Oral hypoglycemic agents should not be given to patient's with Type 1 diabetes. Figure 26.11 summarizes the oral antidiabetic drugs.

A. Sulfonylureas

Glimepiride [gly MEH pih ride] is a new, second generation sulfonylurea. It was the first sulfonylurea to be approved for concurrent use with *insulin*, but has no additional advantage over the other sulfonylureas. Elimination is through the urine and feces. Like all sulfonyl ureas, it can cause hypoglycemia, hyperinsulinemia, and weight gain.

D. Repaglinide

Although *repaglinide* [reh PAG lih nide] is not a sulfonylurea, it has actions in common with this group of drugs. *Repaglinide* binds to the ATP-sensitive potassium channels of the pancreatic β cells, causing the release of *insulin*. *Repaglinide* is well absorbed orally, and is taken three times a day before meals (its $t_{1/2}$ = 1 hr).

Combined therapy with *metformin* (see p. 261) is better than monotherapy with either agent in improving glycemic control. *Repaglinide* is metabolized to inactive products by the liver, and excretion takes place through the bile. Although the drug can cause hypoglycemia, the incidence of this adverse effect appears to be lower than that reported for the sulfonylureas. Drug interactions have not been reported. Its future role in the treatment of type 2 diabetes remains to be determined.

E. Troglitazone and Rosiglitazone

Troglitazone [troh GLI tah zone] is the first thiazolidinedione approved for the treatment of Type 2 diabetic patients—particularly those whose hyperglycemia is not controlled despite *insulin* therapy. Unlike the sulfonylureas, *troglitazone* acts as an *insulin* sensitizer, enhancing *insulin's* actions in the liver and skeletal muscle. *Troglitazone* treatment reduces the increased hepatic output of glucose common in Type 2 diabetics with hyperglycemia. It also promotes *insulin*-dependent glucose utilization in skeletal muscle. Hyperglycemia, hyperinsulinemia, hypertriglyceridemia, and elevated glycosylated hemoglobin (HbA_{1c}) levels are improved. The drug can also counteract *insulin* resistance. Although *insulin* is required for its action, *troglitazone* does not promote its release from the pancreatic β cells, and thus does not result in hyperinsulinemia. It is usually administered with *insulin*, and may lower the dose of this hormone required for adequate glucose control.

Generic Name	Duration of Action (hours)	Comments
First Generation Sulfonylureas		
Tolbutamide	6-12	Metabolized by liver to inactive product; excreted by kidneys; taken 2 to 3 times a day
Chlorpropamide	60	Metabolized by liver (~70%) to less active metabolites and excreted intact (~30%) by kidneys; can potentiate antidiuretic hormone action; taken once a day
Tolazamide	12-24	Metabolized by liver to both active and inactive products; excreted by kidneys; taken 1 to 2 times a day
Second-Generation Sulfonylureas		
Glipizide	12-24	Metabolized by liver to inert products; excreted by kidneys; taken 1 to 2 times a day
Glipizide (Controlled Release)	24	Controlled-release preparation produces sustained plasma levels
Glyburide (Diabeta, Micronase)	16-24	Metabolized by liver to mostly inert products; excreted in bile and by kidneys; taken 1 to 2 times a day
Glyburide (Glynase, PresTab)	12-24	Small particle size facilitates rapid absorption
Biguanides		
Metformin	~5.5	Not metabolized; excreted by kidneys; may be used alone or in combination with sulfonylureas
α-Glucosidase Inhibitors		
Acarbose	~2	Slows absorption of nutrients from jejunum by inhibiting α-glucosidase; taken with meals
Thiazolidinediones		
Troglitazone	24	Decreases insulin resistance

Figure 26.11
Summary of oral antidiabetic agents.

1. **Pharmacokinetics:** Oral absorption of the drug increases when taken with food. It is extensively bound to serum albumin, and has a plasma half-life of 16 to 34 hours. *Troglitazone* is metabolized to several inactive metabolites, and can induce cytochrome P-450. The primary excretory route is in the feces. The drug is contraindicated in breast-feeding women.

2. **Adverse effects:** There have been deaths due to hepatotoxicity in patients taking *troglitazone*. [NOTE: The FDA and the manufacturer have restricted the use of *troglitazone* to patients in hospitals and convalescent homes.] It is strongly recommended that liver enzymes and bilirubin levels of patients on the medication be measured initially and periodically thereafter. [Note: A related, less hepatotoxic thiazolidinedione, *rosiglitazone*, has recently been approved by the FDA.] Adverse effects that have been reported include: upper respiratory infections, headache, anemia and edema as well as weight gain. *Troglitazone* increases metabolism of oral contraceptives, which may result in ovulation and pregnancy. Levels of other drugs such as *cyclosporine*, which is metabolized by cytochrome P-450, may also be affected.

27 Steroid Hormones

II. Estrogens (continued from p. 266)

E. Anitestrogens (selective estrogen receptor modulators)

Selective estrogen receptor modulators (SERMs) act as estrogen agonists in some tissues, but block the action of estrogen in others. The first widely used SERM, *tamoxifen* (see p. 266), has the antiestrogenic effect of reducing the risk for breast cancer as well as the beneficial estrogen effects on serum lipids and bone density in women (Figure 27.14). However, *tamoxifen* also has the undesirable antiestrogen effect of causing hot flashes, and the undesirable estrogen effect of increasing the risk for endometrial cancer and venous thromboembolism in women. *Raloxifene*, a second-generation SERM, increases women's bone density without increasing the risk for endometrial cancer. .

3. **Raloxifene:** Like *tamoxifen*, which is also a SERM (see p 266), *raloxifene's* [ra LOCKS ih feen] actions are mediated through the estrogen receptors, and it has both estrogenic and antiestrogenic effects. Its clinical use is based on its ability to decrease bone resorption and overall bone turnover. However, unlike *estrogen* and *tamoxifen*, it apparently has little to no effect on the endometrium, and therefore may not predispose to uterine cancer. *Raloxifene* lowers total cholesterol and LDL in the serum, but has no effect on HDL or triglycerides. [Note: Whether the latter

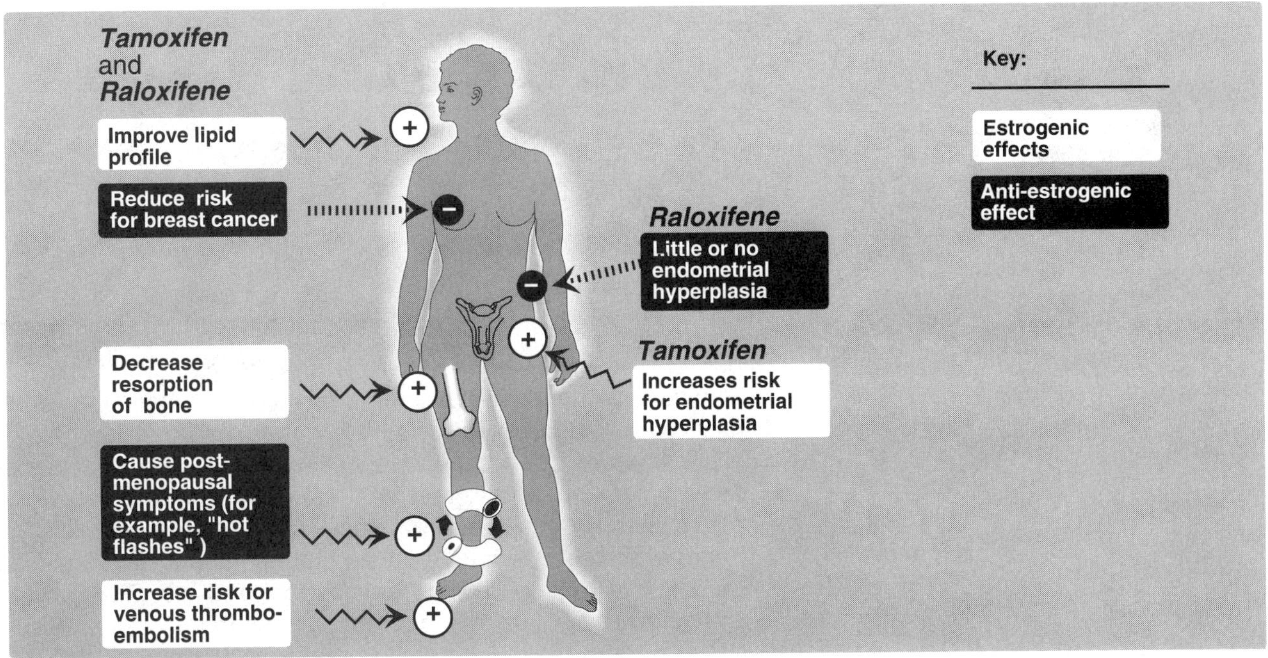

Figure 27.14
Comparison of the estrogenic and antiestrogenic effects of *raloxifene* and *tamoxifen* .

protects against cardiovascular problems remains to be ascertained.] *Raloxifene* has been reported to increase the risk of thromboembolic episodes. The drug is currently approved only for the preventive treatment of osteoporosis in postmenopausal women. *Raloxifene* decreases the risk of estrogen receptor-positive breast cancer (Figure 27.15).

a. **Pharmacokinetics:** *Raloxifene*, taken orally, is readily absorbed, and is rapidly converted to glucuronide conjugates through first-pass metabolism. More than 95 percent of *raloxifene* is bound to plasma proteins, but no resulting drug–drug interactions have been reported. Both the parent drug and conjugates undergo enterohepatic cycling. The primary route of excretion is through the bile into the feces.

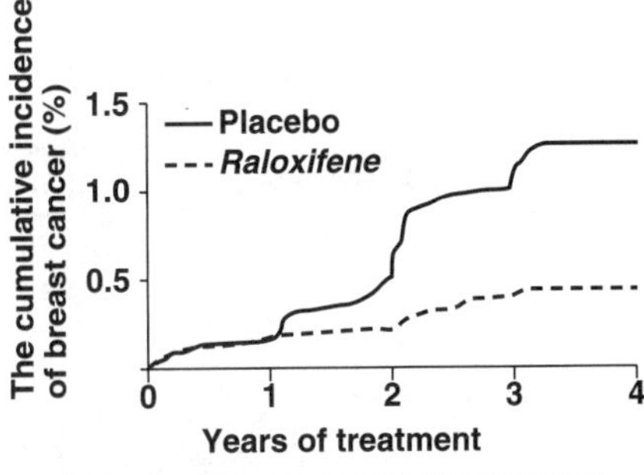

Figure 27.15
Effect of *raloxifene* on cumulative incidence of breast cancer in 7,705 postmenopausal women.

b. **Adverse effects:** Like *estrogen* and *tamoxifen*, the use of *raloxifene* has an increased risk of deep vein thrombosis, pulmonary embolism and retinal vein thrombosis. However, the benefits of the drug are believed to generally outweigh the risks. *Raloxifene* should be avoided in women who are or may become pregnant. In addition, women who have a past or active history of venous thromboembolic events should not take the drug. Coadministration of *raloxifene* with *cholestyramine* can reduce the absorption of *raloxifene* by 60 percent. Therefore they should not be taken together. Also, in one study, *raloxifene* caused a 10 percent drop in prothrombin time in patients taking *warfarin* Thus, it is prudent to monitor prothrombin time in these individuals.

32 Quinolones and Urinary Tract Antiseptics

II. FLUOROQUINOLONES (continued from page 327)

Four recently approved fluoroquinolones—*levofloxacin*, *trovaflaxacin*, *grepafloxacin* and *sparfloxacin*—offer greater potency, a broader spectrum of antimicrobial activity, greater in vitro efficacy against resistant organisms, and in some cases, a better safety profile than older quinolones. Compared with *ciprofloxacin*, these new compounds show increased activity against gram-positive organisms, and retain the favorable activity against gram-negative microorganisms. *Gatifloxacin*, *clinafloxacin*, *trovafloxacin* and *moxifloxacin* show increased activity against anaerobes, compared with *ciprofloxacin*. Clinical evidence, although preliminary, suggests the enhanced efficacy of these drug in the treatment of community-acquired and nosocomial infections, for example, respiratory, urinary tract and skin infections, and sexually transmitted diseases. Adverse effects observed with most quinolones are mild. Serious toxicities include phototoxicity (particularly with *sparfloxacin*), and prolongation of the QT_c interval (seen with *sparfloxacin* and *grepafloxacin*). Drugs that prolong the QT_c interval should not be coadministered with *sparfloxacin* and *grepafloxacin*. Drug interactions can occur between quinolones and compounds containing multivalent cations (Mg^{++}, Al^{+++}, Ca^{++}). Because of its clinical advantages, yet serious side effects, *trovafloxacin* is described in detail below. Figure 32.7 shows some therapeutic advantages and adverse effects of quinolones.

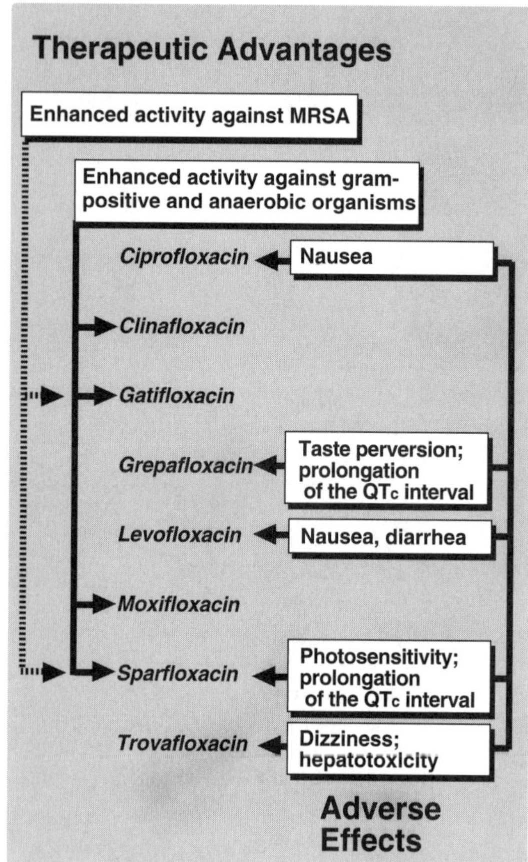

Figure 32.7
Summary of therapeutic advantages and adverse effects of quinolones.

F. Trovafloxacin

Trovafloxacin [TRO vah flocks a sin] is a new fluoroquinolone, which has several properties that give it some clinical advantages. These properties include a long half-life of about 10 hours, which permits once-a-day dosing, and an extended spectrum of antimicrobial activity that includes most anaerobes. However, *trovafloxin* is associated with serious liver injury, and use of the drug is restricted to infections that are life-threatening (for example, pneumonia, intra-abdominal infections, gynecologic and pelvic infections). Therapy with *trovafloxin* should not continue for longer than 14 days, and should only be used in hospital and long-term nursing care facilities. Unlike other fluoroquinolones, *trovafloxacin* is extensively metabolized—23 percent of the dose is converted to the glucuronide, which is excreted in the urine. Sixty-three percent of the dose is excreted in the feces as a mixture of parent drug and metabolites. Dosage adjustments are not necessary in patients with renal impairment. *Trovafloxacin* has a similar adverse effect profile as other quinolones, including dizziness, insomnia and GI disturbances.

Antiviral Drugs 37

III. DRUGS FOR THE TREATMENT OF HERPESVIRUS INFECTIONS (continued from p. 368)

Herpesviruses are associated with a broad spectrum of diseases, for example, cold sores, viral encephalitis, and genital infections, the latter being a hazard to the newborn during parturition. The drugs that are effective against these viruses exert their actions during the acute phase of viral infections, and are without effect in the latent phase. Two new anti-herpes agents are *penciclovir* and *cidofovir*.

G. Penciclovir

Penciclovir [pen SIK lo veer] is an acyclic guanosine nucleoside derivative that is active against herpes simplex virus Types I and II, and against varicella-zoster virus. *Penciclovir* is only administered topically (Figure 37.8). *Penciclovir* is monophosphorylated by viral thymidine kinase, and cellular enzymes form the nucleoside triphosphate, which inhibits herpes DNA polymerase. *Penciclovir triphosphate* has an intracellular half-life 20 to 30 times longer than does *acyclovir triphosphate* (see p. 365). *Penciclovir* is negligibly absorbed from topical application, and is well tolerated. Both healing and pain are shortened approximately one-half day in duration, compared to placebo-treated subjects.

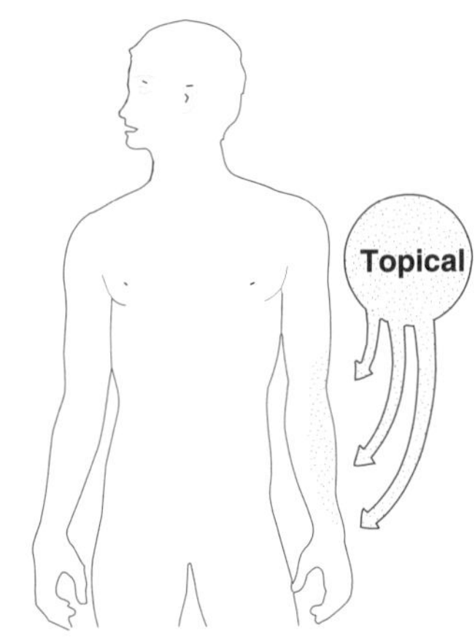

Figure 37.8
Penciclovir is only administered topically.

H. Cidofovir

Cidofovir [si DOF o veer] is approved for treatment of cytomegalovirus-induced retinitis in patients with AIDS. *Cidofovir* is a nucleotide analog of cytosine, whose phosphorylation is not dependent on viral enzymes. Slow elimination of the active intracellular metabolite permits prolonged dosage intervals, and eliminates the permanent venous access used for *ganciclovir* therapy. *Cidofovir* produces significant toxicity to the kidney (Figure 37.9), and is contraindicated in patients with preexisting renal impairment, or in those who are taking concurrent nephrotoxic drugs including NSAIDs. Neutropenia, metabolic acidosis, and ocular hypotony also occurs. *Probenecid* is coadministered with *cidofovir* to reduce the risk of nephrotoxicity, but *probenecid* itself causes rash, headache, fever and nausea. Figure 37.10 summarizes some antiviral agents.

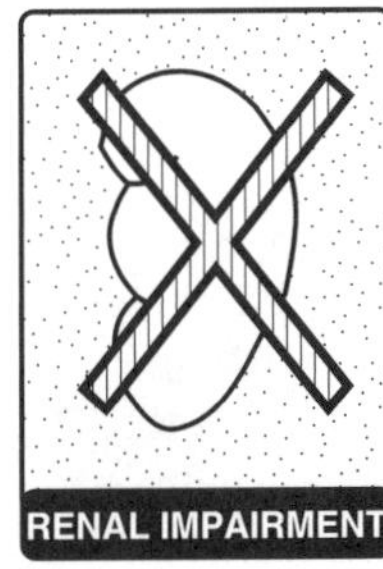

Figure 37.9
Renal impairment is the the major toxicity of *cidofovir*.

Antiviral Drug	Mechanism of Action	Viruses Affected†	Plasma Half-life (hours)
Acyclovir	Metabolized to acyclovir triphosphate, which inhibits viral DNA polymerase	Herpes simplex, varicella-zoster, cytomegalovirus	2-3
Valacyclovir	Same as acyclovir	Herpes simplex, varicella-zoster, cytomegalovirus	2-3
Ganciclovir	Metabolized to ganciclovir triphosphate, which inhibits viral DNA polymerase	Cytomegalovirus	2.5
Penciclovir	Metabolized to penciclovir triphosphate, which inhibits viral DNA polymerase	Herpes simplex	Topical
Famciclovir	Same as penciclovir	Herpes simplex, varicella-zoster	2
Cidofovir	Inhibition of viral DNA polymerase	Cytomegalovirus; indicated only for virus-induced retinitis	2-3*
Foscarnet	Inhibition of viral DNA polymerase and reverse transcriptase at the pyrophosphate-binding site	Cytomegalovirus, acyclovir-resistant herpes simplex, acyclovir-resistant varicella-zoster	6
Ribavirin	Interference with viral messenger RNA	Lassa fever, hantavirus (hemorrhagic fever renal syndrome), hepatitis C (in chronic cases in combination with interferon α)	30 – 60
Lamivudine	Inhibition of viral DNA polymerase and reverse transcriptase	Hepatitis B (chronic cases), human immunodeficiency virus type 1	5 – 7
Amantadine	Blockage of the M2 protein ion channel and its ability to modulate intracellular pH	Influenza A	10 – 30
Rimantadine	Blockage of the M2 protein ion channel and its ability to modulate intracellular pH	Influenza A	25 – 36
Interferon α	Induction of cellular enzymes that interfere with viral protein synthesis	Hepatitis B and C, human herpesvirus 8, papilloma-virus	2 – 3

*Intracellular half-life of cidofovir diphosphate is 17-30 hours.

Figure 37.10
Summary of selected antiviral agents.

IV. TREATMENT OF ACQUIRED IMMUNODEFICIENCY DISEASE (AIDS) (continued from p. 371)

Treatment of human immunodeficiency virus (HIV) infections has been radically modified during the past two years by the introduction of powerful antiretroviral drugs, and by the development of methods to determine the viral burden in plasma. The introduction of HIV protease inhibitors and non-nucleoside reverse transcriptase inhibitors has made this breakthrough possible. However, the long-term therapeutic benefits and safety profiles of these agents are still being evaluated.

F. HIV protease inhibitors (continued from p. 371)

These drugs are peptidyl analogs that reversibly inhibit the proteinase that is essential for the final step of viral proliferation. Protease inhibitors have revolutionized HIV therapy, reducing infections by opportunistic organisms, and prolonging and improving the lives of most patients.

1. **Saquinavir** [sa KWIN a veer]**:** This drug is taken orally. It has been recently reformulated in a soft-gel capsule form that improves its bioavailability, although the amount absorbed remains the lowest of all the protease inhibitors at approximately 12 percent of the oral dose. In order to maximize absorption, *saquinavir* needs to be taken with high fat meals. Distribution into tissues is good as evidenced by a large volume of distribution. Elimination of *saquinavir* is primarily by metabolism followed by biliary excretion; its half-life is 5 hours. Plasma levels can be significantly increased when *saquinavir* is combined with other antiretroviral agents that inhibit its metabolism, such as *delavirdine* (see p.xxx). On the other hand, drugs that enhance the metabolism of *saquinavir*, such as *rifampin* (see p. 333), *rifabutin* (see p. 333), and other enzyme inducers should be avoided if possible. The most common adverse effects of *saquinavir* treatment (5 to 10 percent of patients) include headache, fatigue, diarrhea, nausea, and other gastrointestinal disturbances (Figure 37.11). Increased levels of hepatic aminotransferases have been noted.

2. **Ritonavir** [ri TON a veer]**:** This drug favorably alters the surrogate markers for HIV infection in both antiretroviral naïve (patients who have never had HIV therapy) and experienced patients (those who have had previous HIV therapy). Bioavailability following oral administration is at least 60 percent, and is unaffected by food. However, *ritonavir* is unpalatable, and is taken with chocolate milk or nutritional supplements to improve palatability. Metabolism and biliary excretion are the primary methods of elimination. *Ritonavir* has a half-life of 3 to 5 hours. One of its metabolites has equal antiviral activity, but its plasma level is low. *Ritonavir* is primarily an inhibitor of cytochrome P-450 isozymes, resulting in numerous drug interactions (see p. 14). Nausea, vomiting, diarrhea, and asthenia are among the more common adverse effects). Titration to the standard dose is effective in diminishing the gastrointestinal side effects. [Note: This maneuver is not effective with other protease inhibitors.] Circumoral paresthesia and headache frequently occur. Elevated aminotransferase and triglyceride levels are also seen.

3. **Indinavir** [in DIN a veer] **:** Clinical trials have demonstrated the efficacy of *indinavir* in both antiretroviral naïve and experienced patients by using the surrogate markers. When used in combination with reverse transcriptase inhibitors, sustained effects have been demonstrated for as long as 100 weeks. *Indinavir* is well absorbed orally, and, of all the protease inhibitors, is the least protein-bound at 60 percent. [Note: Whether this accounts for its ability to reduce HIV RNA in tissue and fluids such as lymph nodes, vaginal secretions or semen is unknown.] Acidic gastric conditions are necessary for absorption. Absorption is decreased when administered with meals, although a light, low-fat snack is permissible. Metabolism and hepatic clearance account for elimination of *indinavir*; the dosage should therefore be reduced in the presence of hepatic insufficiency. *Indinavir* has the shortest half-life of the protease inhibitors at 1.8 hours. It is well tolerated, with the usual gastrointestinal symptoms and headache predominating. There is a risk of

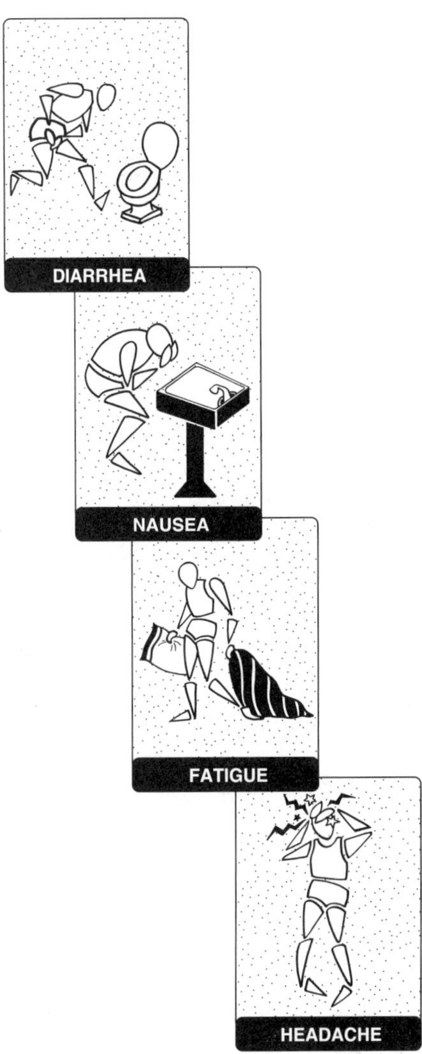

Figure 37.11
Some adverse effects of the HIV protease inhibitors.

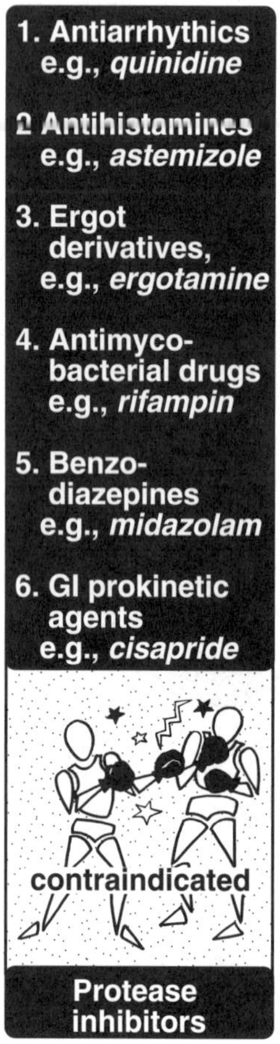

nephrolithiasis and reversible hyperbilirubinemia. Adequate hydration is important to reduce the incidence of kidney stone formation; patients should drink at least 1.5 liters of water per day.

4. **Nelfinavir [nel FIN a veer]:** This drug, when used in combination with *zidovudine* (*AZT*, see p. 368) and *lamivudine* (*3TC*, see p. 370), decreases viral load by at least 100-fold, and increases CD4+ counts. These effects have been sustained for as long as 21 months. *Nelfinavir* is well absorbed and does not require strict food or fluid conditions; however, it is usually given with food. A hydroxylated metabolite appears to be the active agent. The half-life of *nelfinavir* is 5 hours. Diarrhea is the most common side effect, and can be controlled by *loperamide* (see p. 244). Like other members of the class, *nelfinavir* can inhibit the metabolism of other drugs, resulting in required alterations of drug dosages, or the prohibition of combined use.

5. **Amprenavir [am PREN a veer]:** Like other protease inhibitors, *amprenavir* is used in combination with a least two nucleoside reverse transcriptase inhibitors. Its long plasma half-life permits twice daily dosing, but the large size and number of capsules per day (16) day may reduce patient compliance. The drug may be less well tolerated than some other protease inhibitors and it is unclear whether *amprenavir* offers any clinical advantages over other protease inhibitors.

6. **Common adverse effects of protease inhibitors:** As experience with the protease inhibitors has grown, two important adverse reactions that are common to all of them have been uncovered.

   a. **Inhibition of cytochrome P-450-dependent oxidations:** All of the protease inhibitors inhibit cytochrome P-450-dependent oxidations. The following drugs should not be coadministered with any protease inhibitor: 1) antiarrhythmics such as *amiodarone* or *quinidine*; 2) antihistamines such as *astemizole* or *terfenadine*; 3) antimigraine-ergot derivatives; 4) antimycobacterial drugs such as *rifampin* (it decreases protease inhibitor levels); 5) benzodiazepines such as *midazolam* or *triazolam*; or 6) GI prokinetic agents such as *cisapride* (Figure 37.12).

   b. **Lipodystrophy and hyperglycemia:** The protease inhibitors can cause these two disorders. These effects are primarily associated with *indinavir* and *ritonavir*, but *nelfinavir* and *saquinavir* have also been reported to have these effects. The lipodystrophy is characterized by a redistribution of fat, so that the limbs become skinny, and the fat is deposited along the abdomen and the upper back. The hyperglycemia is associated with either the exacerbation of existing diabetes, or the initiation of a diabetic condition; the mechanism is not known. Fortunately, hyperglycemica is a rare occurrence. Additionally, significant elevations in triglyceride and cholesterol levels have been reported. The long-term implications of these effects are not known. Figure 37.13 shows some of the precautions in using the protease inhibitors.

Figure 37.12
Drugs that should not be coadministered with any protease inhibitor.

Drugs	Major toxicities and concerns	Monitoring
Saquinavir	Diarrhea, nausea, abdominal discomfort, elevated transaminase levels Take with high-fat meal or within 2 hours of a full meal	Periodic chemistry profile
Ritonavir	Diarrhea, nausea, taste perversion, vomiting, anemia, increased hepatic enzymes, increased triglycerides. Requires refrigeration; take with meals; chocolate milk improves the taste	Periodic liver function tests
Indinavir	Benign hyperbilirubinemia, nephrolithiasis; Take 1 hour before or 2 hours after food; may take with skim milk or a low-fat meal; drink > 1.5 L of liquid daily	—
Nelfinavir	Diarrhea (16 to 32%), nausea, flatulence, rash	
Amprenavir	Nausea, diarrhea, vomiting, oral and perioral paresthesia and rash	

Figure 37.13
Summary of protease inhibitors.

G. Non-nucleoside reverse transcriptase inhibitors:

These drugs are highly selective, noncompetitive inhibitors of HIV-1 reverse transcriptase. They do not interfere with the binding of primer, template, or nucleoside triphosphates. They have no effect on human DNA polymerases. Their major advantage is their lack of effect on the host blood-forming elements, and lack of cross-resistance with nucleoside reverse transcriptase inhibitors.

1. Nevirapine

Nevirapine is more effective than a placebo in reducing the number of copies of viral RNA, and increasing the CD4+ count in individuals who have had previous antiretroviral therapy.

a. **Pharmacokinetics:** *Nevirapine* [ne VYE ra peen] is well absorbed orally, and its absorption is not affected by food and antacids. The lipophilic nature of *nevirapine* accounts for its entrance into the fetus and mother's milk, and wide tissue distribution, including the central nervous system. *Nevirapine* is dependent upon metabolism for elimination; most of the drug is excreted in the urine as the glucuronides of hydroxylated metabolites.

b. **Adverse effects:** The most frequently observed side effects are rash, fever, headache, and elevated serum transaminases. Severe dermatologic effects have been encountered, including Stevens-Johnson syndrome, and toxic epidermal necrolysis. A 14 day titration period at one-half the dose is mandatory in order to reduce the risk of serious epidermal reactions. Fatal hepatotoxicity has occurred, and serum transaminase activity should be monitored closely during the first six months of therapy. *Nevirapine* is an inducer of CYP3A4 family of cytochrome P-450 drug metabolizing enzymes (see p. 14). Interactions with antiretroviral and other drugs have been determined. No dosage adjustments are necessary when *nevirapine* is given concomitantly with nucleoside reverse transcriptase inhibitors, such as *didanosine* (*ddl*, see p. 369) or *zidovudine* (*AZT*, see p. 368). Since *nevirapine* can increases the metabolism of protease inhibitors, dose adjustment of concurrent protease inhibitor therapy is as follows: *ritonavir*—none; *indinavir* and *nelfinavir*—increase dosage; and do not use *nevirapine* with *saquinavir* because of *saquinavir's* low bioavailability. *Nevirapine* increases the metabolism of a number of drugs, such as oral contraceptives, *ketoconazole*, *methadone*, *metronidazole*, *quinidine*, *theophylline*, and *warfarin*.

2. Delavirdine

Delavirdine [de la VUR deen] has not undergone as extensive clinical trials as did *nevirapine*, but in one study, *delavirdine* added to *AZT* and *ddl* was more effective than the nucleoside reverse transcriptase inhibitors alone. As with other members of the class, resistance develops rapidly with monotherapy.

a. Pharmacokinetics: *Delavirdine* is rapidly absorbed after oral administration, and is unaffected by the presence of food. It is extensively bound to plasma albumin (98 percent). *Delavirdine* is extensively metabolized, and very little is excreted as the parent compound. Fecal and urinary excretion each account for approximately one-half the elimination.

b. Adverse effects: Rash is the most common side effect of delavirdine; it may occur in up to 44 percent of the patients. Nausea, dizziness, and headache have also been reported. *Delavirdine* is an inhibitor of drug metabolism, including that of protease inhibitors. Although *ritonavir* levels are not altered significantly by the presence of *delavirdine*, the levels of *saquinavir* and *indinavir* are significantly increased. *Fluoxetine* and *ketoconazole* increase *delavirdine* plasma levels, whereas *phenytoin*, *phenobarbital*, and *carbamazepine* result in substantial decreases in plasma levels of *delavirdine*.

3. Efavirenz

Efavirenz [ef FA ver enz] treatment results in increases in CD4+ cell counts, and a decrease in viral load, comparable to that achieved by protease inhibitors when used in combination with nucleoside reverse transcriptase inhibitors. Following oral administration, *efavirenz* is well distributed, including to the CNS. Most of the drug is bound to plasma albumin (99 percent) at therapeutic doses. A half-life of over 40 hours accounts for its recommended once-a-day dosing. Most adverse effects are tolerable, and are associated with the CNS, including dizziness, headache, vivid dreams, and loss of concentration. Nearly half of the patients experience these complaints. Rash is the other most common side effect, with an incidence of approximately 25 percent. Severe, life-threatening reactions are rare. *Efavirenz* is a modest inducer of cytochrome P-450. The dose of *indinavir* may need to be increased when given with *efavirenz*.

H. Other reverse transcriptase inhibitors

Abacavir [a BAK a veer] is a nucleoside analog available for children and adults with AIDS who cannot tolerate or who are failing current regimens. There may be some cross-resistance with strains resistant to *AZT* and *3TC*. Approximately 3 percent of patients exhibit drug fever, GI symptoms, malaise, and sometimes a rash. Once the individual is sensitized, repeated exposure results in more rapidly appearing and severe reactions, including hypotension and respiratory distress. ***Adefovir*** [a DEF o veer] is a nucleotide reverse transcriptase inhibitor reserved for those who have failed current regimens, including a protease inhibitor. *Adefovir* exhibits in vitro activity against HIV, herpes, and hepatitis B viruses. Some 30 percent of patients exhibit mild to moderate nephrotoxicity. Nausea, diarrhea, asthenia, and increased hepatic enzymes also occur with some frequency. Both *abacavir* and *adefovir* appear to be free of adverse interactions with other drugs commonly employed in HIV therapy.

Anticancer Drugs 38

III. Antimetabolites (continued from p. 384)

Antimetabolites are structurally related to normal cellular components. They generally interfere with the availability of normal purine or pyrimidine nucleotide precursors by inhibiting their synthesis, or by competing with them in DNA or RNA synthesis. Their maximal cytotoxic effects are S-phase—and therefore cell-cycle—specific.

G. Capecitabine

Capecitabine [cape SITE ah bean] is a novel oral fluoropyrimidine carbamate. It was approved in 1999 for the treatment of metastatic breast cancer that is resistant to first line drugs [for example, *paclitaxel* (see p. 391) and anthracyclines], and is currently also used for treatment of colorectal cancer.

1. **Mechanism of action:** *Capecitabine* per se is non-toxic; it must undergo bioactivation to *5-FU* in vivo. After being absorbed, the drug undergoes a series of enzymic steps, the last of which is hydrolysis to *5-FU* by thymidine phosphorylase—an enzyme that is concentrated primarily in tumors (Figure 38.21). Thus, *capecitabine's* cytotoxic activity is the same as that of *5-FU*, and is tumor-specific. The most important reaction inhibited by *5-FU* (and thus *capecitabine*) is thymidylate synthetase (see page 382). Resistance to *capecitabine* has not been reported at this time, although it will probably be the same as to *5-FU*.

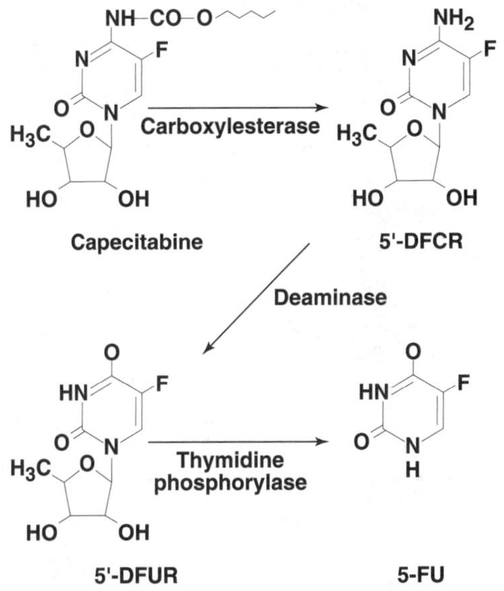

Figure 38.21
Metabolic pathway of *capecitabine* to 5-FU. 5'-DFCR = 5'-deoxy-5-fluorocytidine; 5'-DFUR = 5'-deoxy-5-fluorouridine

2. **Pharmacokinetics:** *Capecitabine* is well absorbed following oral administration. It is extensively metabolized to *5-FU* (as described above), but also, like uracil, is eventually biotransformed into α-fluoro-β-alanine. Metabolites are primarily eliminated in the urine.

3. **Adverse effects:** These are similar to those with *5-FU* (see p. 383), with the toxicity occurring primarily in the gastrointestinal tract. They include diarrhea that can be severe, necrotizing enterocolitis, nausea, vomiting, and hyperbilirubinemia. Dermatologic toxicity includes palmar-plantar erythrodysesthesia (numbness, painful swelling, dysesthesia/paresthesia, and erythema of the palms of the hands and soles of the feet.) *Capecitabine* should be used cautiously in patients with hepatic or renal impairment. The drug is contraindicated in individuals who are hypersensitive to *5-FU*, are pregnant, or are lactating.

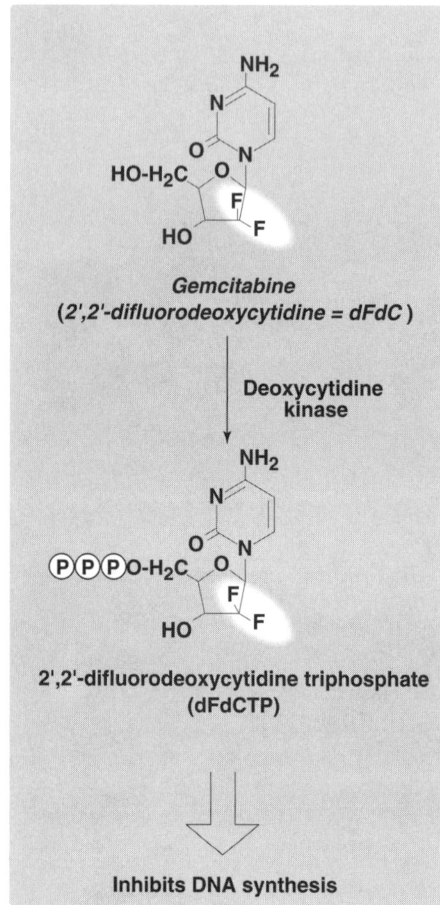

Figure 38.22
Mechanis of action of *gemcitabine*. dFdC = 2',2'-difluoro-deoxycytidine; dFdCTP = 2',2'-difluorodeoxycytidine triphosphate

H. Gemcitabine

Gemcitabine [gem SITE ah bean] is an analog of the nucleoside deoxycytidine; its chemical structure is 2'2'-difluorodeoxycytidine (dFdC). Its use is indicated in the first-line treatment of locally advanced or metastatic adenocarcinoma of the pancreas. It has also shown some activity against other tumors.

1. **Mechanism of action:** *Gemcitabine* is a substrate for dexoxycytidine kinase, which phosphorylates it to dFdCTP (Figure 38.22). The latter compound inhibits DNA synthesis by incorporating into sites that would ordinarily have cytosine in the growing strand. Evidence suggests that DNA repair does not readily occur. Levels of the natural nucleotide, dCTP, are lowered, because *gemcitabine* competes with the normal nucleoside substrate for deoxycytidine kinase. *Gemcitabine* may also inhibit ribonucleotide reductase.

2. **Pharmacokinetics:** *Gemcitabine* is administered intravenously. It is deaminated to difluorodeoxyuridine, which is not cytotoxic, and is excreted in the urine.

3. **Adverse effects:** Myelosuppression is the dose-limiting toxicity of *gemcitabine*. Other toxicities are nausea, vomiting, alopecia, and rash. Transient elevations of serum transaminases, proteinuria, and hematuria are common. Resistance to the drug is probably due to its inability to be converted to a nucleotide: the tumor cell produces increased levels of endogenous deoxycytidine that compete for the kinase, thereby by-passing the inhibition.

VIII. OTHER CHEMOTHERAPEUTIC AGENTS (continued from p. 398)

F. Topotecan

Topotecan (toe poe TEA can) has recently been approved for the treatment of metastic ovarian cancer. It is a semi-synthetic derivative of an earlier drug, *camptothecin*. *Topotecan* has a complicated multiring structure containing a lactone ring that is essential for activity. The drug inhibits topoisomerase I, which is essential in the replication of DNA in human cells (Figure 38.23). Unlike *etoposide*, which inhibits the related enzyme, topoisomerase II, *topotecan* is the first clinically useful toposisomerase I inhibitor. The topoisomerases relieve torsional strain in DNA by causing reversible, single strand breaks. *Topotecan* binds to the enzyme-DNA complex, and prevents reannealing of the single strand breaks. It is thought that *topotecan* can also cause double-stranded DNA damage during DNA synthesis; such breaks do not readily undergo repair, resulting in cytotoxicity.

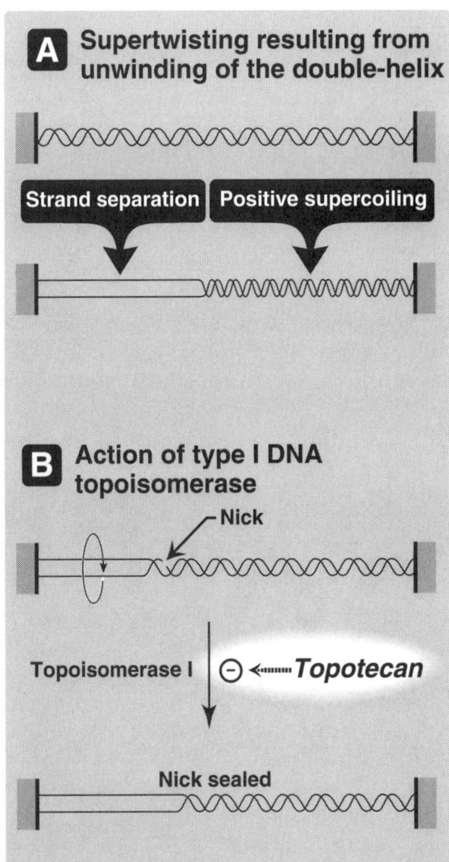

Figure 38.23
Mechanism of action of *topotecan*.

1. **Pharmacokinetics:** *Topotecan* is given by IV infusion over 30 minutes for five consecutive days. Responses may not be seen for three weeks. Hydrolysis of the lactone ring destroys the drug's activity. About 30 percent of the drug and its metabolites is eliminated in the urine; hence, the dose may have to be modified with impaired kidney function.

2. **Adverse effects:** The most important of these effects are hematologic, including bone marrow suppression—particularly neutropenia—which is the dose-limiting toxicity. Frequent peripheral blood counts should be performed on patients taking this drug. [Note: *Topotecan* should not be used in patients with a baseline neutrophil count of less than 1500 cells/mm^3. Doing so could result in infection and death.] Other hematologic complications including thrombocytopenia and anemia may also occur. Nonhematologic effects include diarrhea, nausea, vomiting, alopecia, and headache. Resistance has not yet been described, but in accord with other agents, *topotecan* may amplify the P-glycoprotein (see p. 377). The topoisomerase may also mutate.

G. Monoclonal antibodies

Monoclonal antibodies are produced by hybrid cells created from B lymphocytes fused with "immortal" B lymphocyte tumor cells. The resulting hybrids can be individually cloned, and each clone will produce antibodies directed against a single antigen type. Two new monoclonal antibody types have been created that are useful in the treatment of cancer.

1. **Trastuzumab:** In metastatic breast cancer patients, overexpression of human epidermal growth factor receptor protein 2 (HER2) is seen in 25 to 30 percent of patients. *Trastuzumab* [tra STEW zoo mab] is a monoclonal antibody that binds to HER2 sites in breast cancer tissue, and inhibits the proliferation of cells that overexpress the HER2 protein. Thus, *trastuzumab* specifically targets the underlying genetic defect that causes the cancer. The drug can cause regression of breast cancer and metastases in these individuals. *Trastuzumab* is administered intravenously; its metabolism and elimination have not been described. The most serious toxicity associated with *trastuzumab* use is congestive heart failure. Other adverse effects include headache, dizziness, nausea, vomiting, abdominal pain and back pain. Cautious use of the drug is recommended in patients who are hypersensitive to it, to Chinese hamster ovary cell proteins, or to benzyl alcohol (in which case sterile water can be used for preparation of the injection). Extreme caution should be exercised in patients with a preexisting cardiac dysfunction.

2. **Rituximab:** *Rituximab* (rih TUCKS ih mab) is a genetically engineered, chimeric monoclonal antibody directed against the CD20 antigen found on the surfaces of normal and malignant B lymphocytes. CD20 plays a role in the activation process for cell cycle initiation and differentiation. The CD20 antigen is expressed on nearly all of the B cell non-Hodgkin's lymphomas, but not in other bone marrow cells. The Fab domain of *rituximab* binds to the CD20 antigen on the B-lymphocytes, while the Fc domain recruits immune effector functions that cause the lysis of the B cells. *Rituximab* is infused intravenously, and causes a rapid depletion of B-cells (both normal and malignant). The fate of the antibody has not been described. It is important to infuse *rituximab* slowly. Hypotension, bronchospasm, and angioedema may occur, and must be treated with *diphenhydramine*, *acetaminophen*, and bronchodilators if necessary. Chills and fever frequently accompany the first infusion. Leukopenia, thrombocytopenia and neutropenia have been reported in less than 10 percent of patients.

39 Anti-inflammatory Drugs

III. NONSTEROIDAL ANTI-INFLAMMATORY DRUGS (continued from p. 411)

The nonsteroidal anti-inflammatory drugs (NSAIDs) are a group of chemically dissimilar agents that differ in their antipyretic, analgesic, and anti-inflammatory activities. They act primarily by inhibiting the cyclooxygenase enzymes, but not the lipoxygenase enzymes (see Figure 39.3, p. 403). Cyclooxygenase 2 (COX-2) is a close structural analog of COX-1 and, like the latter, catalyzes the conversion of arachidonic acid to prostaglandin PGH_2 via PGG_2 (see p. 402). These isozymes are encoded by two different genes. COX-1 is generally regarded to be constitutive and COX-2 inducible. However, this is an oversimplification, since COX-2 is constitutive in the kidney and brain, but is inducible in other sites, including those that are inflamed, such as joints. Nearly all NSAIDs have greater a selectivity for COX-1. They are used primarily for conditions not considered inflammatory (for example, headache and analgesia). Their unwanted side effect of causing gastric damage is ascribed to inhibition of COX-1, resulting in an inability to form protective prostaglandins (see p. 404). This led to the search for a COX-2 inhibitor, commonly referred to as a "safe *aspirin*", reasoning that if COX-1 in the stomach is unaffected by the new drug, then the gastrointestinal effects would be minimized. The first COX-2 inhibitor, *celecoxib*, was approved in the United States in 1998, and *rofecoxib* approved in 1999. Interest in this area continues high because COX-2 expression is associated with the development of colon cancer, and also with inflammatory processes in the brain that appear to be involved in the development of Alzheimer's disease.

H. Celecoxib

Celecoxib [sel eh COCKS ib] is significantly more selective for inhibition of COX-2 than of COX-1 (Figure 39.16). In fact, at concentrations achieved in vivo, *celecoxib* does not block COX-1. Unlike the inhibition of COX-1 by *aspirin* (which is rapid and irreversible), the inhibition of COX-2 is time-dependent and ireversible. *Celecoxib* was approved for treatment of osteoarthritis and rheumatoid arthritis, but not for analgesia. [Note: In some trials, *celecoxib* had analgesic activity; in others it was no more effective than the placebo. Its ability to reduce acute pain is poor.] Unlike aspirin, *celecoxib* does not inhibit platelet aggregation, and does not increase bleeding time.

1. **Pharmacokinetics:** *Celecoxib* is readily absorbed, reaching a peak concentration in about three hours. It is extensively metabolized in the liver by cytochrome P-450 (CYP2C9), and is excreted in the feces and urine. Its half-life is about eleven hours, thus the drug is usually taken once a day.

2. **Adverse effects:** Abdominal pain, diarrhea and dyspepsia are the most common adverse effects. Over a 12 week period the incidence of gastroduodenal ulcers in patients taking *celecoxib* was about double that found in patients on placebo, and only one-third and one-fifth that found in patients taking *ibuprofen* and *naproxen*, respectively. *Celecoxib* is contraindicated in patients allergic to sulfonamides. As with other NSAIDs, kidney toxicity has occurred. [Note: COX-2 is expressed constitutively in the kidney, and is inducible in the macula densa in response to salt restriction.] Inhibitors of CYP2C9, such as *fluconazole*, *fluvastatin*, and *zafirlukast*, may increase serum levels of *celecoxib*. *Celecoxib* has the ability to inhibit CYP2D6, and thus could lead to elevated levels of some beta-blockers, antidepressants and antipsychotic drugs (see p. 14)

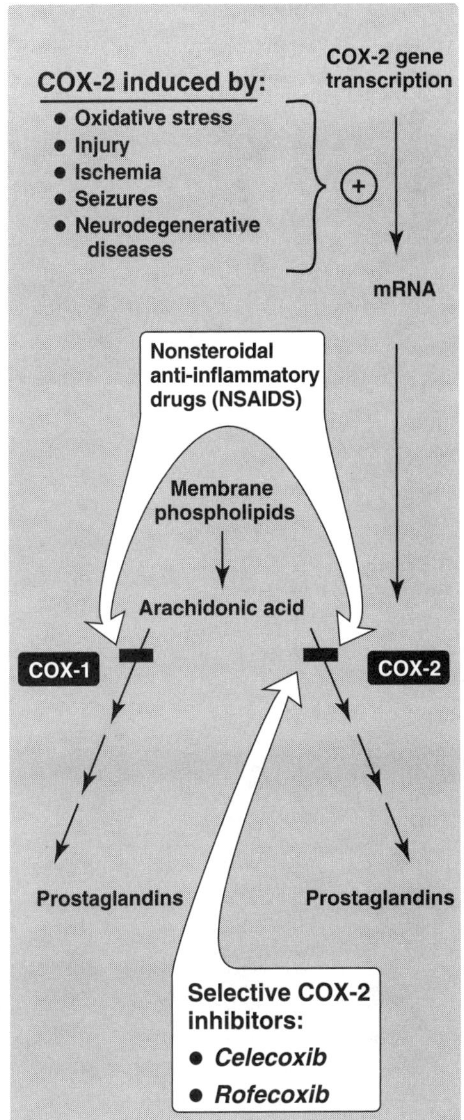

Figure 39.16
Action of cyclooxygenase-2 (COX-2) inhibitors.

V. SLOW-ACTING, ANTI-INFLAMMATORY AGENTS (continued from p. 415)

In contrast to the NSAID drugs, remittive (remission-inducing) arthritis drugs are slow-acting. These drugs are used primarily for rheumatic disorders, especially in cases where the inflammation does not respond to cyclooxygenase inhibitors. They slow the course of the disease, and may also induce a remission, preventing further destruction of the joints and involved tissues. Three new disease-modifiying anti-rheumatic drugs are described below.

E. Leflunomide

Leflunomide (le FLEW nom eyed) is an isoxazole immunomodulatory agent that preferentially causes cell arrest of the autoimmune lymphocytes through its action on dihydroorotate dehydrogenase (DHODH). Stimulation of a T cell by an antigen-presenting cell drives the lymphocyte into its replicative cycle. Many enzymes, including those required for de novo purine, pyrimidine, RNA, and membrane synthesis, are upregulated in the G1 phase of the cycle.

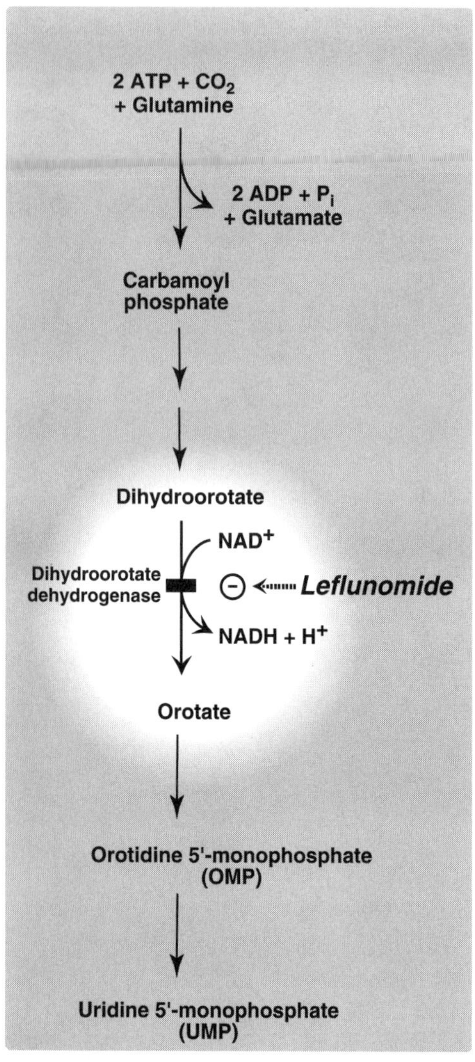

Figure 39.17
Site of action of *leflunomide.*

Dihydroorotate dehydrogenase (DHODH), which catalyzes the formation of orotate (a precursor of the pyrimidines) from dihydroorotate in the mitochondria, is among these (Figure 39.17). [Note: Resting lymphocytes can meet their requirements for ribonucleotides through the salvage pathway, but cell division requires an 8 to 16-fold expansion of the ribonucleotide pool]. Inhibition of DHODH deprives the cell of the precursor for uridine monophosphate (UMP)—a necessary component for RNA synthesis, and a precursor of the thymidine-containing nucleotide required for DNA synthesis. After biotransformation, *leflunomide* is a reversible inhibitor of DHODH. [Note: *Leflunomide* has also been reported to inhibit tyrosine kinases, but it is not known how this might influence the anti-inflammatory action of the drug.] *Leflunomide* has been approved for the treatment of rheumatoid arthritis. It not only reduces pain and inflammation associated with the disease, but also appears to slow the progression of structural damage.

1. **Pharmacokinetics:** *Leflunomide* is well absorbed after oral administration. It is extensively bound to albumin (>90 percent), and has a half-life of 14 to 18 days. [Note: Because of its long half-life, loading doses are necessary (see p. 19).] *Leflunomide* is rapidly converted to the active metabolite. The metabolites are excreted in the urine and the feces. The active metabolite undergoes biliary recycling.

2. **Adverse effects:** The most common of these are headache, diarrhea, and nausea. Other untoward effects are weight loss, allergic reactions including a flu-like syndrome, skin rash, alopecia, and hypokalemia. *Leflunomide* is teratogenic in experimental animals, and is therefore contraindicated in pregnancy, and in women of childbearing potential. It should be used with caution in patients with liver disease, because it is cleared by both biliary and renal excretion. *Cholestyramine* increases the clearance of *leflunomide.*

F. Etanercept

Tumor necrosis factor (TNF) plays a key role in the host's immune system. Its inflammatory and immune regulating activities are myriad. For example, TNF causes local activation of the vascular endothelium, and also release of nitric oxide, which causes vasodilatation and increased vascular permeability. Platelet activation and adhesion are also increased by TNF, causing local blood vessel occlusion. These actions of TNF result after its binding to two different receptors that are found on neutrophils, vascular endothelial cells, and fibroblasts. These receptors also exist in the serum and synovial fluid in a soluble form. The targeting of TNF-α rests on the observation that cytokines produced by macrophages (TNF-α, IL-1, IL-6, IL-8) predominate in the rheumatoid synovium. *Etanercept* and *infliximab* decrease the activity of tumor necrosis factor. The former is a fusion protein composed of TNF receptors; the latter is a chimeric antibody directed against TNF-α. *Etanercept* has been approved for the treatment of rheumatoid arthritis. A recent trial showed that the combination of *etanercept* and *methotrexate* provided greater clinical benefit than *methotrexate* alone. [Note: Upon discontinuation of *etanercept*, the symptoms of arthritis generally return within a month.]

1. **Mechanism of action:** *Etanercept* [ee TAN er sept] is a genetically engineered fusion protein composed of two identical chains of the recombinant human TNF-receptor p75 monomer fused with the Fc domain of human IgG_1. This soluble fusion protein binds two molecules of TNF, and prevents them from binding to cellular receptors. The protein does not discriminate between TNF-α and TNF-β (lymphotoxin). [Note: Because TNF is important in modulating cellular immune responses to infection and tumors, there is some concern about the long-term use of *etanercept.*]

2. **Pharmacokinetics:** *Etanercept* is given subcutaneously twice a week. The time to maximum serum concentration after a single injection is about 72 hours. Its median half-life is 115 hours. Data on elimination is not available.

3. **Adverse effects:** *Etanercept* is well-tolerated. No toxicities or antibodies have been reported. However, it can produce local inflammation at the site of injection. Patients with life-threatening infection such as sepsis should not receive therapy with *etanercept.*

G. Infliximab

Infliximab (in FLICKS ih mab) is a chimeric IgGκ monoclonal antibody composed of human and murine regions. The antibody binds specifically to human TNF-α, thereby neutralizing that cytokine. *Infliximab* has been approved for Crohn's disease for both fistulizing and non-fistula disease. [Note: Increased levels of TNF-α are found in fecal samples of patients with Crohn's disease.] It is not approved for maintenance therapy beyond six weeks. Approval for the treatment of rheumatic arthritis in combination with *methotrexate* is anticipated in the near future.

1. **Pharmacokinetics:** *Infliximab* is infused intravenously over at least two hours. It distributes in the vascular compartment, and has a half-life of 9.5 days. Its metabolism and elimination have not been described.

2. **Adverse effects:** Long-term use of *infliximab* is associated with development of anti-*infliximab* antibodies unless the drug is used in combination with *methotrexate*. Infusion reactions such as fever, chill, pruritus, or urticaria have occurred. Infections leading to pneumonia, cellulitis, and other conditions have also been reported. Whether treatment with *infliximab* predisposes to lymphoma, a condition that occurs with immunosuppressive or immune-altering drugs, remains to be established.

40 Autacoid and Autacoid Antagonists

III. ANTIHISTAMINES (continued from p. 425)

Readers should be aware that *terfenadine* (Seldane®), the once widely-used, selective H_1 histamine receptor antagonist, has been voluntarily withdrawn from the market by the manufacturer. The withdrawal was instituted because of the risk of life-threatening cardiac arrhythmias when *terfenadine* was taken concomitantly with drugs such as *ketoconazole* that inhibit the CYP3A4 isozyme of cytochrome P-450. The active metabolite of *terfenadine* is currently being marketed as *fexofenadine* [fecks o FEN a deen] (carboxylated *terfenadine*), which lacks the cardiac toxicity of *terfenadine*.

F. Fexofenadine

Fexofenadine is indicated for the relief of the symptoms of allergic rhinitis in adults and children 12 years of age and older. *Fexofenadine* is a selective antagonist of the H_1 histamine receptor in the periphery of the body. Experimental studies demonstrated that the drug does not cross the blood-brain barrier. *Fexofenadine* is rapidly absorbed following oral administration. Very little of the drug is metabolized, with 80 percent excreted in the feces, and 11 percent in the urine. Its half-life is about 15 hours. In patients older than 65 years, the peak concentration was twice that of normal volunteers less than 65 years old. Renal impairment also results in increased plasma levels. Adverse effects are mild and infrequent, and include drowsiness, dyspepsia and fatigue.

41 Immunosuppressants

I. IMMUNOSUPPRESSANTS

Organ transplantation has become a routine procedure due to improved surgical techniques, better tissue typing, and the availability of drugs that more selectively inhibit rejection of transplanted tissues, and prevent the patient from becoming immunologically compromised. Earlier drugs were non-selective, and suppressed both the expansion of activated T cells and the formation of antibodies through interference of B cell conversion to plasma cells. These drugs included the anticancer agents *methotrexate* and *cyclophosphamide*, the related drug *azathio-*

prine, and the glucocorticoid pro-drug, *prednisone*. Patients frequently succumbed to infection. Generally, a combination of immunosuppressant agents are used to prevent rejection.

A. Non-selective immunosuppressants

1. Azathioprine

Azathioprine [a zah THIO preen] has been the cornerstone of immunosuppressive therapy over the last several decades. It has a nitroimidazoloyl side chain attached to the sulfur of 6-mercaptopurine, which is removed by non-enzymatic reduction in the body by glutathione to yield *6-mercaptopurine* (*6-MP*). The latter is then converted to the corresponding nucleotide, thioinosinic acid (TIMP), by the salvage pathway enzyme, hypoxanthine-guanine phosphoribosyl transferase. The immunosuppressant effects of *azathioprine* are due to this fraudulent nucleotide. (See pp. 380–381 for a discussion of *6-MP's* mechanism of action, resistance, pharmacokinetics, and adverse effects.) Because of their rapid proliferation in the immune response, and their dependence on de novo synthesis of purines required for cell division, lymphocytes are predominantly affected by the cytotoxic effects of *azathioprine*. The drug has little effect on suppressing a secondary immune response.

2. Mycophenolate mofetil

In many centers, *azathioprine* is being replaced by *mycophenolate mofetil* [my koh FEN oh late MOW fe till]. An ester, it is rapidly hydrolyzed in the gastrointestinal tract to mycophenolic acid, which is quickly and almost completely absorbed. It is a potent, reversible, uncompetitive inhibitor of inosine monophosphate dehydrogenase, blocking the de novo formation of guanosine phosphate (GMP), and thus, like *6-MP*, it deprives the rapidly proliferating T and B cells of a key component of nucleic acids (Figure 41.1). Mycophenolic acid is glucuronidated and excreted predominantly in the urine. Adverse effects include pain, diarrhea, leukopenia, sepsis, and lymphoma. Concomittant administration with antacids containing magnesium or aluminum, or with *cholestyramine*, can decrease the absorption of the drug.

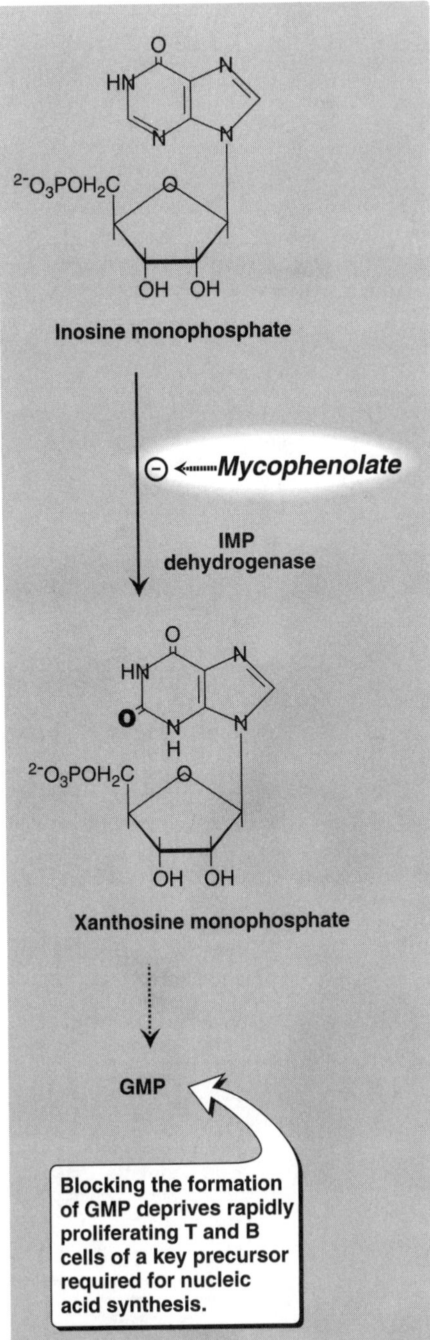

Figure 41.1
Mechanism of action of *mycophenolate*

B. Antibodies

1. Antilymphocyte and antithymocyte globulin

These antibodies are prepared either by immunization of large animals with human lymphoid cells (polyclonal), or by hybridoma technology, producing monoclonal antibodies. The antibodies bind to the surface of circulating T lymphocytes. The antibody-bound cells are then opsonized and phagocytosed in the liver and spleen, resulting in lymphopenia and impaired T-cell responses. They are primarily employed to treat the acute phase of allograft rejection. The antibodies are administered intramuscularly, or infused intravenously, and their half-life extends from three to nine days. Since the humoral antibody mechanism remains active, antibodies can be formed against these foreign proteins. Other adverse affects are chills and fever, leukopenia and thrombocytopenia, and skin rashes.

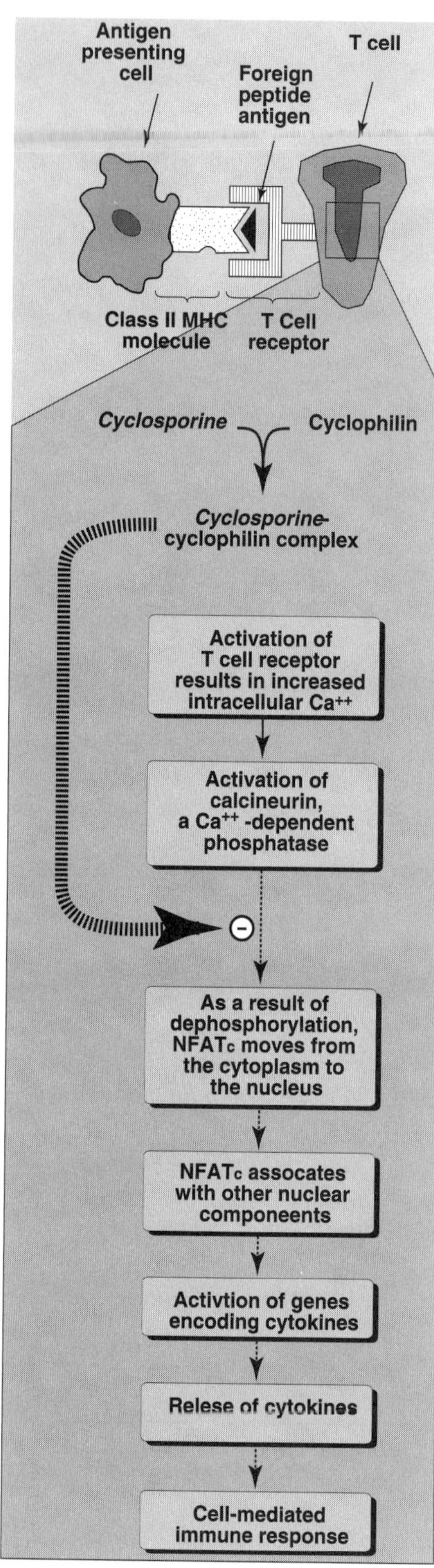

Figure 41.2
Mechanism of action of *cyclosporine*.

2. Muromonab-CD3 (OKT3)

Muromonab-CD3 [myour oh MOW nab] is a murine monoclonal antibody directed against the glycoprotein CD3 antigen of human T cells. Binding to the CD3 protein results in a disruption of T lymphocyte function, because access of antigen to the recognition site is blocked. Thus T lymphocyte participation in the immune response is decreased. Circulating T cells are depleted. *Muromonab-CD3* is indicated for treatment of acute rejection of renal allografts as well as for steroid-resistant acute allograft rejection in cardiac and hepatic transplant patients. It is also used to deplete T cells from donor bone marrow prior to transplantation.

a. **Pharmacokinetics:** The antibody is administered intravenously. Since initial binding of the *muromonab-CD3* to the antigen results in cytokine release due to activation of the T lymphocyte, it is customary to premedicate the patient with *methylprednisolone*, *diphenhydramine*, and *acetaminophen* to alleviate the cytokine release syndrome. The antibody is extensively metabolized, and eliminated predominantly in the bile.

b. **Adverse effects:** Anaphylactoid reactions may occur. Cytokine release syndrome may occur on the first dose. The symptoms can range from a mild, flu-like illness, to a life-threatening, shock-like reaction. High fever is common. CNS effects such as seizures, encephalopathy, cerebral edema, aseptic meningitis, and headache may occur. Infections can increase, including some due to cytomegalovirus. *Muromonab-CD3* is contraindicated in patients with a history of seizures, in those with uncompensated heart failure, as well as in pregnant women, or those who are breast feeding.

C. Selective immunosuppressants

The advent of *cyclosporine* revolutionized organ transplantation by prolonging organ survival.

1. **Cyclosporine:** *Cyclosporine* [SIGH klo spore inn] is a cyclic peptide composed of 11 amino acids (several are methylated on the peptidyl nitrogen) extracted from a soil fungus. *Cyclosporine* preferentially suppresses cell-mediated immune reactions, whereas humoral immunity is affected to a far lesser extent. After diffusing into the T cell, *cyclosporine* binds to a cyclophilin to form a complex which binds to calcineurin (Figure 41.2). The latter is responsible for dephosphorylating NFATc (cytosolic Nuclear Factor of Activated T cells). The *cyclosporine*/calcineurin complex cannot carry out this reaction and thus the subsequent reactions required for the synthesis of a number of cytokines, including IL-2, cannot occur. The end result of *cyclosporine* action is to decrease IL-2, the main stimulus for increase in the number of the T lymphocytes. *Cyclosporine* is used to prevent rejection of kidney, liver, and cardiac allogeneic transplants (Figure 41.3). Although it can be used alone, it is more effective if glucocorticoids are also administered, and this is the usual practice. *Cyclosporine* is an alternative to *methotrexate* for the treatment of severe, active, rheumatoid arthritis. It can also be used for patients with recalcitrant psoriasis that does not respond to other therapies.

a. **Pharmacokinetics:** *Cyclosporine* may be given either orally or by intravenous infusion. Oral absorption is variable, although a new preparation is more reliable. Interpatient variability may be due to metabolism by a cytochrome P-450 (CYP3A4) present in the gastrointestinal tract, which metabolizes the drug. [Note: Grapefruit juice, which lowers the levels of this enzyme, increases the amount of *cyclosporine* absorbed.] About 50 per cent of the drug is associated with the blood fraction. Half of this is in the erythrocytes, and less than one-tenth is bound to the lymphocytes. *Cyclosporine* is extensively metabolized, primarily by hepatic CYP3A4. [Note: When other drug substrates for this enzyme are given concomittantly, many drug interactions have been reported.] It is not clear whether any of the 25 or more metabolites have any activity. Excretion of the metabolites is through the biliary route, with only a small amount of the parent drug appearing in the urine.

b. **Adverse effects:** Many of the adverse effects caused by *cyclosporine* are dose-dependent, and therefore it is important to monitor levels of the drug, although a direct correlation between drug level and toxicity doesn't pertain. Nephrotoxicity is the most common and important adverse effect of *cyclosporine*. It is therefore critical to monitor kidney function. Reduction of *cyclosporine* dosage can result in reversal of nephrotoxicity. Hepatotoxicity can also occur, and therefore liver function should be periodically assessed. Infections in patients taking *cyclosporine* are common, and may be life-threatening. Viral infections due to herpes group and cytomegalovirus are prevalent. Lymphoma may occur, presumably due to immunosuppression, although recent evidence has raised a question as to whether *cyclosporine* itself may promote lymphoma formation. Anaphylactic reactions can occur on parenteral administration. Other toxicities include: hypertension, hyperkalemia (it is important not to use K^+–sparing diuretics in these patients), tremor, hirsutism, glucose intolerance, and gum hyperplasia.

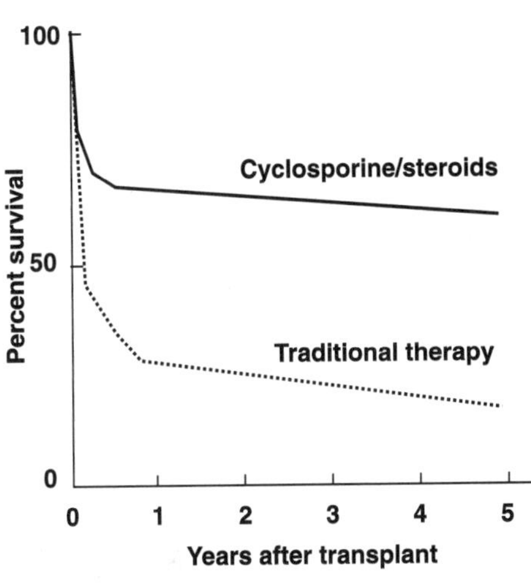

Figure 41.3
Effect of cyclosporine on liver transplant survival.

2. **Tacrolimus (FK506):** *Tacrolimus* (TACK row lee muss) is a macrolide that is isolated from a soil fungus. Its mechanism of action is the same as that of *cyclosporine*, except that it binds to a different immunophilin, FKBP (FK binding protein). *Tacrolimus* is approved for the prevention of rejection of liver and kidney transplants, and is given with a glucocorticoid. This drug has found favor over *cyclosporine*, not only because episodes of rejection have been decreased, but also because lower doses of glucocorticoid can be used, reducing the likelihood of infections.

a. **Pharmacokinetics:** The oral route is preferable, but, like *cyclosporine*, oral absorption is incomplete and variable, requiring tailoring of doses. *Tacrolimus* is from 10 to 100 times more potent than *cyclosporine*. It is highly bound to serum proteins. It is also concentrated in erythrocytes. Like *cyclosporine*, *tacrolimus* undergoes hepatic metabolism by the CYP3A4 isozyme and thus the same drug interactions occur. Renal excretion is very low; most of the drug and its metabolites are found in the feces.

b. **Adverse effects:** *Tacrolimus* is more toxic than *cyclosporine*. For example, nephrotoxicity and neurotoxicity (tremor, seizures, hallucinations) tend to be more severe in patients treated with *tacrolimus*. Other toxicities are the same as those for *cyclosporine*, except that *tacrolimus* does not cause hirsutism or gingival hyperplasia. Anaphylactoid reactions to the injection vehicle have been reported. The drug interactions are the same as those described above for *cyclosporine*.

42 Drugs Used to Treat Obesity

I. ANOREXIC AGENTS

Obesity refers to presence of excess body fat. The amount of body fat is difficult to measure directly, and is usually determined from body measures that have been shown to correlate with body fat in most people. The body mass index (BMI) is a useful clinical calculation for diagnosing obesity because it correlates with total body fat, and is relatively unaffected by height. It can be calculated

$$\text{BMI} = (\text{weight in kg}) / (\text{height in meters})^2$$

or determined from tables. The normal range for BMI is between 19.8 and 26.0. Individuals with BMI between 26.1 and 29.0 are overweight, those who have a BMI greater than 30 are obese by definition. Obesity is a serious health problem, and its treatment is difficult, because individuals find it hard to adhere to a program of dieting and exercise. Currently, two new anorexiants (appetite suppressants) are available. They are *phentermine* [FEN tur meen] and *sibutramine* [SI byoo tra meen], both amphetamine-like agents (see p. 103).

A. Phentermine and sibutramine

These agents have many properties in common. Both are sympathomimetic amines that exert their pharmacologic action by interfering in the reuptake of serotonin and norepinephrine into the presynaptic nerve terminal, thereby increasing their brain levels. In the case of *phentermine*, there is an increased release of dopamine, whereas with *sibutramine*, the reuptake into the presynaptic nerve terminal of serotonin, norepinephrine, and to a lesser extent dopamine, is hindered.

1. **Pharmacokinetics:** *Sibutramine* undergoes first pass demethylation to active metabolites, which are further biotransformed in the liver and excreted primarily in the urine. The half-life is about 15 hours.

2. **Adverse effects and contraindications:** These are similar for both drugs. For example, they are both controlled as Schedule IV agents (they have a low liability for dependence or abuse). Heart rate and blood pressure may be increased, and dry mouth, headache, insomnia, and constipation are common problems. Pulmonary hypertension has occurred (rarely) with *phentermine*, especially when it is in combination with *fenfluramine*. [Note: This combination, referred to as "fen-phen", was widely used as a diet aid. It was not only reported to cause pulmonary hypertension, but also heart valve abnormalities. *Fenfluramine* has since been withdrawn from the market.] These adverse effects have not been reported for *sibutramine*. *Sibutramine* should be avoided in patients taking monoamine oxidase inhibitors, selective serotonin inhibitors such as *fluoxetine*, or serotonin agonists for migraine, such as *sumatriptan*, as well as *lithium*, *dextromethorphan*, and *pentazocine*. Drug interactions can occur when *sibutramine* is administered with drugs that inhibit CYP3A4, such as *ketoconazole*, *erythromycin* and *cimetidine*. The increases in *sibutramine* are small, and no untoward consequences have been reported.

II. LIPASE INHIBITORS

Orlistat [OR li stat] is the first drug in a new class of nonsystemically acting antiobesity drugs know as lipase inhibitors. *Orlistat* is a pentanoic acid ester that inhibits gastric and pancreatic lipases, thus decreasing the breakdown of dietary fat into smaller molecules. Fat absorption is decreased by about 30 percent. The loss of calories is the main cause of weight loss, but adverse gastrointestinal effects associated with the drug may also contribute to a decreased food intake. *Orlistat* is indicated in inviduals with a body mass index of 30 or more, or in persons with a BMI of 27 or more who have other risk factors, such as high blood pressure, high cholesterol levels and diabetes. In clinical trials, individuals treated with *orlistat* lost an average of 10 percent of their body weight (compared to 6 percent for the placebo group) within one year (Figure 42.1). Total and low-density lipoprotein (LDL) decreased more in the treatment group than the placebo group. The most common side effects associated with *orlistat* are gastrointestnal symptoms, such as oily spotting, flatulence with discharge, fecal urgency, and increased defecation. *Orlistat* interferes with the absorption of the fat-soluble vitamins, β carotene and carotenoids. *Orlistat* is contraindicated in patients with chronic malabsorption syndrome or cholestasis.

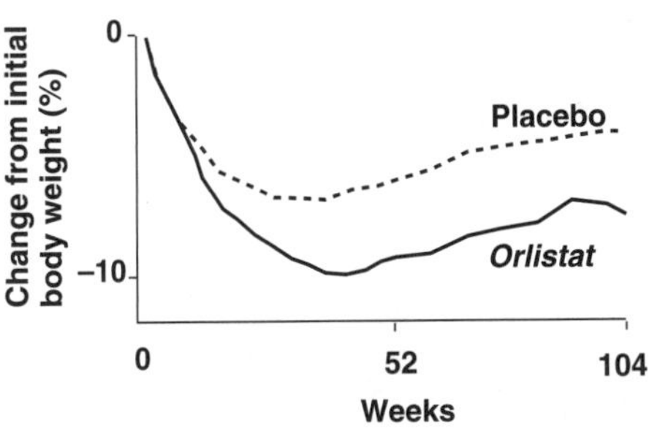

Figure 42.1
Effect of *orlistat* treatment on body weight.

43 Drug Used to Treat Osteoporosis

I. OVERVIEW

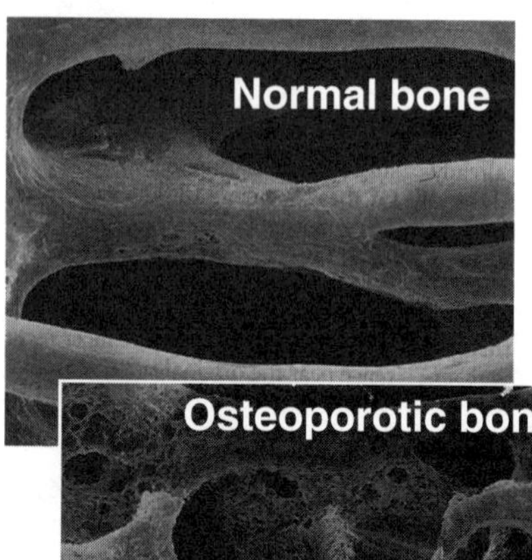

Figure 43.1
Changes in bone morphology seen in osteoporosis.

Osteoporosis is a condition of skeletal fragiity due to progressive loss of bone mass. It occurs in the elderly of both sexes, but is most pronounced in postmenopausal women. Osteoporosis is characterized by frequent bone fractures, which are a major cause of disability among the elderly. Figure 43.1 showns changes in bone morphology seen in osteoporosis.

II. BISPHOSPHONATES

These analogs of pyrophosphate, including *etidronate* [e ti DROE nate], *risedronate* [ris ED roe nate], *alendronate* [a LEN droe nate] , and *pamidronate* [pa MID roe nate], comprise an important drug group used for the treatment of disorders of bone remodeling, such as osteoporosis and Paget's disease, as well as metastatic bone cancers. The bisphosphonates decrease osteoclastic bone resorption via several mechanisms, including: 1) inhibition of the osteoclastic proton pump necessary for dissolution of hydroxyapatite; 2) decrease in osteoclastic formation/activation; and 3) increased osteoclastic apoptosis (programmed cell death). The relative importance of the mechanisms may differ among the individual bisphosphonates, and it is not known if they are due to a single molecular activity. The decrease in osteoclastic bone resorption results in a small but significant net gain in bone mass in osteoporotic patients, because the bone-forming osteoblasts are not inhibited (Figure 43.2). In Paget's disease, the bisphosphonates result in the return to normal of bone remodeling rates, since the disorder is characterized by excessive activity of osteoclasts. Decreased rates of bone fracture have been reported in both osteoporostic and Paget's disease patients treated with bisphosphonates. In addition, bisphosphonates have been shown to decrease the number of bone and visceral metastases in patients with breast cancer.

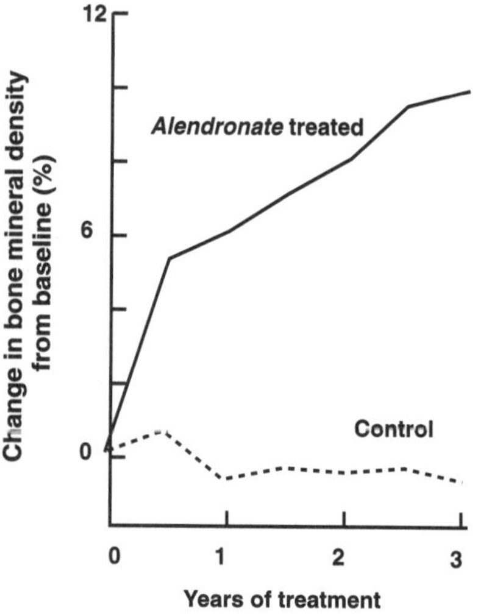

Figure 43.2
Effect of *alendronate* therapy on the bone mineral density of lumbar spine.

A. **Pharmacokinetics:** *Pamidronate* is administered intravenously. All of the other bisphosphonates are orally active, although less than ten percent of the administered dose is absorbed. Food significantly interferes with absorption. Bisphosphonates should be administered with six to eight ounces of water at least one hour before eating breakfast. The bisphosphonates are rapidly cleared from the plasma, primarily because they avidly bind to hydroxyapatite mineral of bone. Once bound to bone they are cleared over a period of months to years. Elimination from the body is solely through renal clearance, and the bisphosphonates should not be given to individuals with severe renal impairment.

B. **Adverse effects:** These include diarrhea, nausea, and abdominal pain. *Alendronate*, *etidronate*, and *risedronate* are associated with

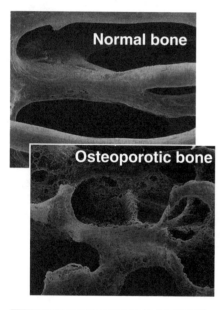

esophageal ulcers. *Etidronate* is the only member of the class that causes osteomalacia following long-term, continuous administration. Figure 43.3 shows the relative potencies of the bisphosphonates.

Bisphosphonate	Antiresorptive activity
Etidronate	1
Pamidronate	100
Alendronate	100-1,000
Risedronate	1,000-10.000

Figure 43.3
Structure and antiresorptive activity of some bisphosphonates.

III. OTHER THERAPIES

A. Estrogen therapy

Estrogen replacement (see p. 264) is the most effective therapy for the prevention of postmenopausal bone loss. When initiated in the immediate postmenopausal period, estrogen prevents osteoporosis and reduces the risk of hip fracture. *Raloxifene*, a second-generation selective estrogen receptor modulator (see p. xxx), increases women's bone density without increasing the risk for endometrial cancer. In addition, *raloxifene* has recently been reported to decrease the risk of estrogen receptor-positive breast cancer.

B. Calcitonin

In clinical trials, salmon *calcitonin*, administered intranasally, has been effective and well tolerated in postmenopausal women at risk of developing osteoporosis. In trials lasting several years the drug reduced bone resorption and improved bone architecture, relieved pain, and increased function.

C. Calcium

Calcium intake through diet and, if necessary, use of supplement, should total 1,000 mg/day. In postmenopausal women not taking estrogen, total calcium intake should be 1,500 mg/day. In men and women over 65 years of age, calcium and vitamin D supplementation have been shown to reduce the risk of fracture from 13% to 6% over a three year period. This suggests that the benefits of calcium and vitamin D supplementation is clinically import for prevention of fractures due to bone loss, particularly in elderly patients .

Miscellaneous Drugs 44

I. DRUGS FOR ERECTILE DYSFUNCTION

Erectile dysfunction, that is, the inability to maintain penile erection for the successful performance of sexual activity, has both organic and psychogenic causes, including as a sequelae to prostatic surgery. Erectile dysfunction is estimated to affect up to 30 million men in the United States. Previous therapies have included penile implants, and intrapenile injections of *alprostadil* (see p. 420). *Sildenafil* [sil DEN a fil], the first oral drug approved for the treatment of erectile dysfunction in males, was introduced in early 1998.

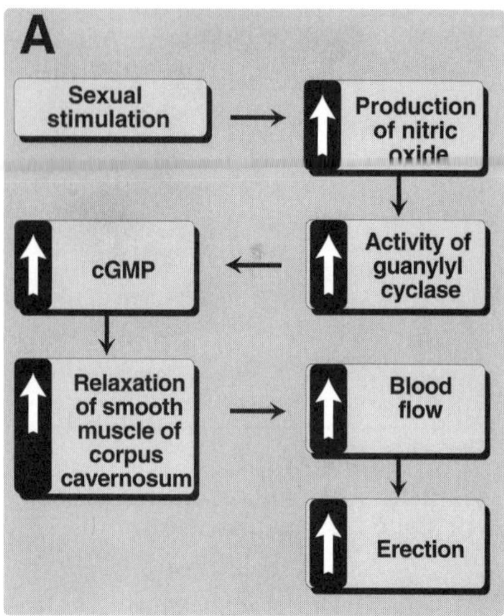

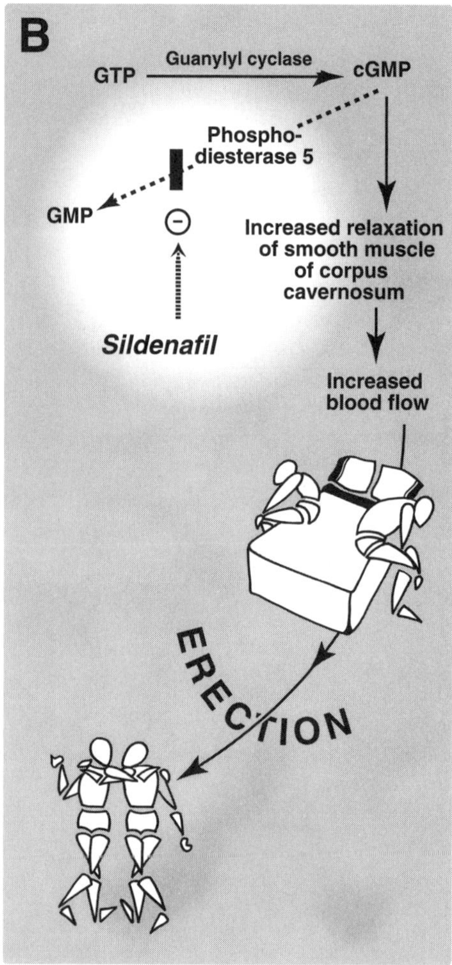

Figure 44.1
A. Chemical mediators leading to erection. B. Effect of *sildenafil* on cGMP levels in the smooth muscle of the corpus cavernosum.

A. Sildenafil

Sexual stimulation results in smooth muscle relaxation of the corpus cavernosum, increasing the inflow of blood (Figure 44.1). The mediator of this response is nitric oxide (NO). NO activates guanylyl cyclase, which forms cGMP from GTP. Cyclic-GMP produces smooth muscle relaxation. The duration of action of cyclic nucleotides is controlled by the action of phosphodiesterase (PDE). At least six isozymes of PDE have been characterized. *Sildenafil* inhibits PDE-5, the isozyme responsible for termination of cGMP in the corpus cavernosum. The result of the presence of *sildenafil* is an increased duration of blood flow into the corpus cavernosum at any given level of sexual stimulation. At recommended doses, *sildenafil* has no effect in the absence of sexual stimulation. *Sildenafil* is indicated for the treatment of erectile dysfunction in men due to organic or psychogenic causes. *Sildenafil* should be taken approximately one hour prior to anticipated sexual activity, although its benefit is observed up to four hours after administration. It should not be used more than once per day. The tissue distribution of PDE5 accounts for some of the side effects of sildenafil since low concentrations of the isozyme are found in vascular smooth muscle and platelets.

1. **Pharmacokinetics:** *Sildenafil* is rapidly absorbed after oral administration, and peak plasma levels are achieved within one hour. Bioavailability is about 40 percent of the oral dose. *Sildenafil* enters tissues, and has an apparent volume of distribution of 1.5 L/kg. Both *sildenafil* and its major N-desmethylated metabolite are > 95 percent bound to plasma proteins. Both CYP3A4 (major route) and CYP2C9 (minor route) are responsible for the metabolism of *sildenafil*. The major metabolite, N-desmethyl sildenafil, is approximately 50 percent as potent as *sildenafil* in inhibiting PDE5. The major route of elimination for *sildenafil* and its metabolites is via the bile. Clearance is decreased in older individuals; free plasma concentrations are 40 percent higher in healthy volunteers > 65 years old. Severe renal impairment (< 30 mL/min) increases the AUC (see p. 7) by two-fold. Similarly, cirrhosis of the liver also significantly increases the AUC.

2. **Adverse Effects:** The most frequent adverse effects reported for *sildenafil* are headache, flushing, dyspepsia, and nasal congestion. Disturbances in color vision (loss of blue/green discrimination) also occur, probably because of inhibition of PDE-6 (a phosphodiesterase found in the retina that is important in color vision). The incidence of these reactions appears to be dose-dependent. Diarrhea, rash, and dizziness have also been reported. *Sildenafil* results in mild decreases in blood pressure. Because of its ability to potentiate the activity of NO, however, there is an absolute contraindication against the use of concurrent organic nitrates in any form. *Sildenafil* was negative in several experimental models for mutagenicity and carcinogenicity. In vivo studies in normal volunteers demonstrated that general and specific inhibitors of CYP3A4 such as *cimetidine* and *erythromycin* significantly elevate plasma levels of *sildenafil*. Stronger inhibitors such as *itraconazole* would be expected to cause even greater increases. Inducers such as *rifampin* may significantly decrease *sildenafil* plasma concentrations.

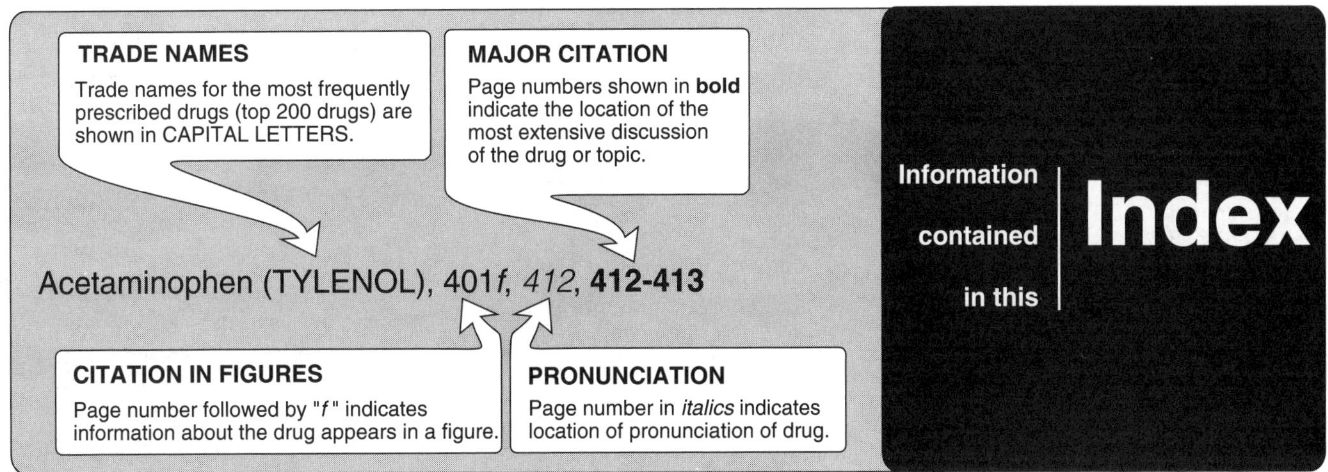

"*See*" cross-references direct the reader to the synonymous term. "*See also*" cross-references direct the reader to related topics. [Note: Positional and configurational designations in chemical names (for example, "3-", "α-", "N-", "D-") are ignored in alphabetizing.]

Abacavir, 463
Abciximab, 447
Abortion, drugs for, 419
Absence seizures, **144,** 144*f*-145*f*
  treatment, 149
Absorption, drug, 1, 1*f*, **4-6**
Abstinence, percent use, 268*f*
Acarbose, **261,** *261*
ACCOLATE see Zafirlukast
ACCUPRIL. *See* Ramipril
Acebutolol, 71*f*, **77,** *77,* 79*f*
  actions, 75*f*
  clinical applications, 78*f*
  contraindication, 177
  drug elimination, 74*f*
Acetaminophen (TYLENOL), 401*f*, *412,* **412-413**
  actions, 405*f*
  drug interactions, 140
  metabolism, 413*f*
  for migraine, 428
  for Reye's syndrome, 407
Acetazolamide, 223*f*, **226-227**
  and changes in urine composition, 226*f*, 233*f*
  drug interactions, 292
  for glaucoma, 41
  site of action, 224*f*
Acetohexamide, 255*f*, 260, *260*
  properties, 261*f*
Acetylcholine, 35*f*, *39,* **39-40**
  binding, 36-37, 37*f*
  degradation, 37, 37*f*
  drug interactions, 236
  interaction with membrane receptors, 21
  and muscarinic receptor, 46*f*
  as neurotransmitter, 32*f*, 33
  release, 36, 37*f*
  sites of action, 36*f*
  storage, 35, 37*f*
  structure, 39*f*
  synthesis, 35, 37*f*
Acquired immunodeficiency syndrome (AIDS), treatment, **368-371**
ACTH. *See* Corticotropin
Actinomycetes, 290*f*
Actinomycin D. *See* Dactinomycin
Activated attapulgite, 244, 244*f*
ACTONEL see Risedronate
Acycloguanosine. *See* Acyclovir
Acyclovir (ZOVIRAX), 363*f*, *365,* **365-366,** 458
  mechanism of action, 365, 366*f*
  survival rate with, 367*f*
Acylureido penicillins, 301
  drug elimination, 303
ADALAT. *See* Nifedipine
Addison's disease, treatment, 274
Adenosine, 163*f*, **174**
  antiarrhythmic effects, 164*f*
Administration routes, drug, **1-4,** 2*f*
Adrenal androgens, production, 272
Adrenal corticosteroids, **272-277**
  drug interactions, 270
  inhibitors, 277
  therapeutic uses, 274-276
β-Adrenergic agents, for chronic obstructive pulmonary disease, 222
Adrenergic agonists, **55-70**
  adverse effects, 68*f*
  for asthma, 218, 218*f*
  characteristics, 59-61
  direct-acting, **61-67**
    mechanism of action, 61
    sites of action, 62*f*
  indirect-acting, **67-68**
    mechanism of action, 61
    sites of action, 62*f*
  mechanism of action, 61
  mixed-action, **68-69**
    mechanism of action, 61
    sites of action, 62*f*
  sites of action, 56*f*, 62*f*
  specific agents, 55*f*
  structures, 61*f*
  summary, 69*f*
β-Adrenergic agonists, 151*f*
  for asthma, 217*f*
  for chronic obstructive pulmonary disease, 217*f*
  for congestive heart failure, 161
  sites of action, 161*f*
α-Adrenergic agonists, for rhinitis, 221
  specific agents, 217*f*
Adrenergic agonists, specific agents
  albuterol, 55*f*, 67*f*, 69*f*, 218, 431-432, 441
  clonidine, 55*f*, **67,** *67,* 69*f*, 180*f*, *189,* **189-190,** 442
  dobutamine, 55*f*, **66,** *66,* 69*f*, 151*f*, 159, 161, 161*f*
  dopamine, 55*f*, 56, 61*f*, *65,* **65-66,** 66*f*, 69*f*, 161*f*, 248*f*

Lippincott's Illustrated Reviews: Pharmacology, Second Edition.
by Mary J. Mycek, Richard A. Harvey and Pamela C. Champe.
Lippincott–Raven Publishers, Philadelphia, PA © 1997.

epinephrine, 3, 32*f*, **33,** 40-41, 55*f*, 58*f*, 58-59, 60*f*, 61, *61,* 61*f*, **61-63,** 63*f*, 67*f*, 69*f*, 72, 72*f*, 118, 164*f*, 218, 424
isoproterenol, 55*f*, 58, 58*f*, 61, 61*f*, *64,* **64-65,** 65*f*-67*f*, 69*f*, 72*f*, 75
metaproterenol, 55*f*, **67,** *67,* 67*f*, 69*f*
methoxamine, 55*f*, *66,* **66-67,** 69*f*
norepinephrine, 32*f*, **33,** 36*f*, 55, 55*f*, 56, 57*f*-58*f*, 58-59, 61, 61*f*, *64,* **64,** 64*f*, 69*f*, 72*f*, 78-79
phenylephrine, 47, 55*f*, 58, 60, 60*f*, 61, *66,* **66,** 69*f*, 113, 221
ritodrine, 55*f*, 69*f*
terbutaline, 55*f*, 62-63, *67,* **67,** 67*f*, 69*f*, 218
Adrenergic blockers, **71-80**
α-Adrenergic blockers, 58, 58*f*-59*f*, **71-73**
adverse effects, 73*f*
blood pressure and, 72*f*
effects, 60*f*
for hypertension, **189**
specific agents, 71*f*, 180*f*
β-Adrenergic blockers, 58*f*, 58-59, **73-78,** 163*f*, 419*f*, 436, 442
actions, 60*f*, 75*f*
adverse effects, 79*f*
for angina, 176-177
specific agents, 175*f*
treatment with concomitant diseases, 178*f*
clinical applications, 78*f*
contraindications, 185
drug interactions, 188*f*, 409
elimination, 74*f*
for hypertension, **184-187**
actions, 184*f*
adverse effects, 185, 185*f*
with concomitant diseases, 182*f*
specific agents, 179*f*
for migraine, 427*f*, 428
summary, 79*f*
Adrenergic blockers, specific agents, 71*f*
acebutolol, 71*f*, 74*f*-75*f*, *77,* **77,** 78*f*-79*f*, 177
atenolol, 71*f*, 75*f*, *77,* **77,** 79*f*, 176, 179*f*, 185
doxazosin, 71*f*, **73,** *73,* 180*f*
labetalol, 71*f*, 74*f*, *78,* **78,** 79*f*, 179*f*, 191
metoprolol, 71*f*, 74*f*-75*f*, *77,* **77,** 78*f*-79*f*, 171, 176, 179*f*, 185
nadolol, 71*f*, 74*f*, *76,* **76,** 78*f*, 179*f*, 428
phenoxybenzamine, *71,* 71*f*, **71-72,** 72*f*
phentolamine, 71*f*, **72,** *72,* 124
pindolol, 71*f*, 74*f*, *77,* **77,** 79*f*, 171, 177
prazosin, 71*f*, **73,** *73,* 124, 180*f*, 189
propranolol, 7, 71*f*, *74,* 74*f*, **74-76,** 75*f*-76*f*, 78*f*-79*f*, 163*f*-164*f*, 171, 175*f*, 176, 179*f*, 185, 190, 334*f*, 427*f*, 428, 436-437
terazosin, 71*f*, **73,** *73,* 180*f*, 189
timolol, 71*f*, 74*f*, *70,* **70,** 70*f*-79*f*, 179*f*
β-Adrenergic blockers, specific agents, 71*f*
Adrenergic, definition, **33**
Adrenergic neuron, **55-59**
Adrenergic receptors (adrenoceptors), **57-59**
types, 58*f*
Adrenocortical insufficiency
primary, treatment, 274
secondary, treatment, 274
tertiary, treatment, 274
treatment, 274
Adrenocorticotropic hormone. *See* Corticotropin
ADRIAMYCIN. *See* Doxorubicin
Adsorbent agents, 244
ADVIL. *See* Ibuprofen
Afferent neuron, **28**
African sleeping sickness, 353
Agar, 245
AGGRASTAT see Tirofiban
Agonists. *See also* β-Adrenergic agonists; Adrenergic agonists; α-Adrenergic agonists
cholinergic, **35-44,** 36*f*. *See also* **Cholinergic agonists, specific agents**
adverse effects, 49*f*
antidote for, 47
indirect, 41, 42*f*
reversible, 41, 42*f*
sites of action, 36*f*
structures, 39*f*
indirect-acting, 61
opioid
actions, 134*f*
adverse effects, 137*f*
moderate, **140**
onset and duration of action, 139*f*
strong, **135-140**
AIDS. *See* Acquired immunodeficiency syndrome
Albumin
binding capacity, 11
drug binding to, 11-12, 12*f*
Albuterol (VENTOLIN, PROVENTIL), 55*f*, 69*f*, 431-432, 441
for asthma, 218
and bronchodilation, 67*f*
ALDOMET. *See* Methyldopa
Aldosterone, production, 272, 272*f*
Alendronate, 476
Alkylamines, therapeutic advantages and disadvantages, 422*f*
Alkylating agents
actions, 374*f*
in cancer therapy, **387-390**
specific agents, 373*f*
ALLEGRA see Fexofenadine
Allergic conjunctivitis, treatment, 411
Allergic rhinitis, treatment, 276, 424
Allergies, treatment, 276, 423-424, 438-439
Allopurinol, 402*f*, *416,* **416-417**
drug interactions, 260*f*, 382
for hyperuricemia, 415
for leishmaniasis, 356
Aloe, 244, 244*f*
Alprazolam (XANAX), *90,* 242*f*, 438
adverse effects of, 94*f*
for chemotherapy-induced nausea and vomiting, 243
duration of action, 92*f*
for panic disorders, 90
therapeutic advantages and disadvantages, 97*f*
withdrawal reactions, 93*f*
Alprostadil, for erectile dysfunction, 420
ALTACE. *See* Ramipril
Alteplase (tPA), 193*f*, 201, *202,* **202**
activation of plasminogen, 202*f*
properties, 202*f*
Aluminum acetate, 438
Aluminum hydroxide, 236*f*, 240, 439-441
Alveolar wash-in, 111
Amantadine, 81*f*, **87,** *87,* *363,* 363*f*, **363-364,** 364*f*, 458
AMARYL see Glimepiride
AMBIEN. *See* Zolpidem
Amebiasis
chemotherapy, 345*f*, **345-348**
extraintestinal, treatment, 351
Amebic dysentery. *See* Amebiasis
Amebicides
luminal, 346, **348**
sites of action, 346*f*
mixed, 346, **347-348**
sites of action, 346*f*
systemic, 346, **348**
sites of action, 346*f*
American sleeping sickness. *See* Chagas' disease
Amikacin, 311*f*, 315, *315,* 433
adverse effects, 316
therapeutic applications, 315*f*

Amiloride, 223*f*, **233,** *233*
  site of action, 224*f*
Amine nitrogen, substitution on, 61
γ-Aminobutyric acid, binding, 89-90, 91*f*
Aminocaproic acid, 193*f*, **204,** *204*
Aminoglutethimide, **277,** *277,* 373*f*
  in cancer therapy, 395, *395*
Aminoglycosides, **314-317**
  adverse effects, 316-317, 317*f*
  classification, 287*f*
  drug interactions, 51, 338
  penicillins and, 301
  resistance to, 285*f*
  for urinary tract infections, 328*f*
Aminoglycosides, specific agents, 311*f*
  amikacin, 311*f*, 315, *315,* 315*f*, 316, 433
  gentamicin, 51, 311*f*, 315, *315,* 315*f*, 316, 435
  neomycin, 311*f*, 316, *316,* 317
  netilmicin, 311*f*, 316, *316*
  streptomycin, 311*f*, 314, *314,* 315, 315*f*, 331
  tobramycin (TOBREX), 51, 311*f*, 315, *315,* 315*f*, 316, 316*f*, 431
p-Aminomethylbenzensulfonamide, for burns, 291
5-Aminosalicylate, in inflammatory bowel disease, 291
Aminosalicylic acid, 331*f*, **335,** *335*
Amiodarone, 163*f*, **172,** *172*
  antiarrhythmic effects, 164*f*
  drug interactions, 160*f*
Amitriptyline (ELAVIL), 96, 119, *119,* 119*f*
  therapeutic advantages and disadvantages, 125*f*
Amlodipine (NORVASC), 180*f*, 188, *188*
  for angina, 188*f*
  for congestive heart failure, **157,** 188*f*
  drug interactions, 188*f*
  for hypertension, 188*f*
Amobarbital, 90*f*, *94*
  duration of action, 95
  therapeutic advantages and disadvantages, 97*f*
Amoxapine, 119, *119,* 119*f*
  therapeutic advantages and disadvantages, 125*f*
Amoxicillin (AMOXIL, POLYMOX, TRIMOX, WYMOX), 235*f*, 298*f*, 300, *300*
  absorption, 302
  administration route, 302
  cost, 282, 282*f*
  drug interactions, 308, 308*f*
  to eliminate Helicobacter pylori, 236
  stability
    to acid, 300*f*
    to penicillinase, 300*f*
  for urinary tract infections, 328*f*
AMOXIL. *See* Amoxicillin
Amphetamines, 55*f*, *67,* **67-68,** 69*f*, 99*f*, **103-104**
  adverse effects, 105
  dependence potential, 100*f*
  drug interactions, 138
  as indirect-acting agonist, 61
  mechanism of action, 104*f*
  non-catecholamine, 60
Amphotericin B, *337,* 337*f*, **337-339,** 338*f*
  for cryptococcal meningitis, 284*f*
  drug interactions, 339-340
  for leishmaniasis, 356
Ampicillin (PRINCIPEN), 298*f*, 300, *300,* 435
  administration route, 302
  as chemotherapeutic agent, 283
  for listeriosis, 299*f*
  stability
    to acid, 300*f*
    to penicillinase, 300*f*
  therapeutic applications, 290, 301
  for urinary tract infections, 328*f*
Amprenavir, 460
Amrinone, 151*f*, 161, *161,* 161*f*
Anabolic steroids, 270
  adverse effects, 271
Analgesic(s)
  for migraine, 427*f*, 428
  morphine as, 137
  non-narcotic, **411-413**
    specific agents, 401*f*
  salicylates as, 404, 406
Anaphylactic shock, treatment, 62-63
Anaphylaxis, acute, treatment, 218
ANAPROX. *See* Naproxen
Ancylostoma duodenale infection, 361*f*
  treatment, 359
Androgenic steroids, 270
Androgens, **269-272**
Androgens, specific agents, 263*f*
  danazol, 263*f*, 270, *270,* 271
  fluoxymesterone, 263*f*, 271, *271*
  nandrolone, 263*f*, 271, *271*
  stanozolol, 263*f*, 271, *271*
  testosterone cypionate, 263*f*, 271, *271*
Anemia
  megaloblastic, and folate deficiency, 205
  treatment, 205-206
    specific agents, 193*f*
Anesthesia, **107-118**
  adjuncts to, specific agents, 107*f*
  components, 109*f*
  induction, 109
  maintenance, 109
  patient selection for, 107-108
  recovery, 109
  stages, 110, 110*f*
Anesthetics
  barbiturates as, 95
  cocaine as, 102
  epinephrine in, 63
  inhalation, **110-115**
    changes in alveolar blood concentrations, 112*f*
    therapeutic advantages and disadvantages, 116*f*
  intravenous, **115-117**
    therapeutic advantages and disadvantages, 116*f*
  uptake, 111-112
  uptake curves, 112, 112*f*
  vapor (gas), minimal alveolar concentrations (MAC), 111, 111*f*
Anesthetics, specific agents, 107*f*-108*f*
Angina pectoris
  with concomitant diseases, treatment, 178*f*
  with hypertension, 182*f*-183*f*, 185
  treatment, 73, 75, 77, 78*f*, 173, **175-178,** 187, 188*f*, 189, 196, 204-206, 406
Angiotensin converting enzyme inhibitors, 151*f*, **156-157,** 442
  drug interactions, 409
  effects, 156*f*
  for hypertension, 186-187
    actions, 186, 186*f*
    adverse effects, 186*f*, 186-187
    with concomitant diseases, 182*f*
    specific agents, 179*f*
Angiotensin II antagonists, for hypertension, 187
  specific agents, 179*f*
Anisoylated plasminogen streptokinase activator complex. *See* Anistreplase
Anistreplase, 193*f*, **203,** *203*
  properties, 202*f*
Ankylosing spondylitis, treatment, 409-411
Anorexia nervosa, treatment, 122
Anorexic agents, 474
ANSAID. *See* Flurbiprofen
Antacids
  drug interactions, 408*f*

    - for peptic ulcer disease, 236f, 240
- Antagonists, 22f
    - angiotensin II, for hypertension, 187
        - specific agents, 179f
    - benzodiazepine, 94
        - specific agents, 90f
    - cholinergic, **45-54**
        - for asthma, 220
        - sites of action, 46f
        - specific agents, 45f
        - summary, 49f
    - folate, **289-296**
        - specific agents, 289f
    - histamine H_2-receptor, 440
    - opioid, **133-142, 141-142**
        - actions, 134f
        - specific agents, 133f
    - reversible, 22
    - serotonin, antiemetic potency, 243f
    - steroid, for cancer, 392-395
        - specific agents, 373f
- Anterior pituitary hormones, 247f, **247-250**
    - actions, 248f
- Anthelmintic drugs, **359-362**
    - specific agents, 359f
- Antiandrogens, **272**
- **Antiandrogens, specific agents**
    - cyproterone acetate, 272, *272*
    - finasteride, 73, 272, *272*
    - flutamide, 272, *272,* 373f, *394,* 394-395, 399f
- Antianginal drugs, **175-178**
- **Antianginal drugs, specific agents,** 175f
    - diltiazem (CARDIZEM CD, DILACOR XR), 163f, **173,** *173,* 173f, 175f, *177,* **177,** 180f, 187, *187,* 187f-188f
    - isosorbide dinitrate, **157,** 175f, **176,** *176,* 177f
    - nifedipine (ADALAT, PROCARDIA XL), 173, 173f, 175f, *177,* **177,** *187,* 187f, 187-188, 188f
    - nitroglycerin (NITROSTAT), 2, 4, 175f, **175-176,** *176,* 177f, 442
    - propranolol (INDERAL), 7, 71f, *74,* 74f, **74-76,** 75f-76f, 78f-79f, 163f-164f, 171, 175f, 176, 179f, 185, 190, 334f, 427f, 428, 436-437
    - verapamil (ISOPTIN, VERELAN), 160f, 163f-164f, 167, 169, **173,** *173,* 173f, 175f, *177,* **177,** 180f, 187, *187,* 187f-188f, 189, 377
- **Antianxiety drugs, specific agents**
    - alprazolam (XANAX), 90, *90,* 92f-94f, 97f, 242f, 243, 438
    - buspirone (BUSPAR), **93,** *93,* 94f, 97f
    - chlordiazepoxide, *91,* 92f, 97f
    - clonazepam (KLONOPIN), 91, *91,* 97f, 143f, 145f, 149
    - clorazepate (TRANXENE), 91, *91,* 92f, 97f, 143f, 149
    - diazepam (VALIUM), 50, 90, *90,* 90f, 91, *91,* 92f-93f, 97f, 103, 108, 108f, 116, 143f, 145f, 149, 239
    - estazolam, 92f
    - flurazepam, 91, *91,* 92, 92f-93f, 97f, 137
    - hydroxyzine, **93,** *93,* 97f, 138, 422f
    - lorazepam (ATIVAN), 92f-93f, 97f, 108f, 116, 242f, 243, 243f
    - midazolam, 97f, 108f, 116
    - quazepam, 92f-93f, 97f
    - temazepam (RESTORIL), *91,* 92, 92f-93f, 97f
    - triazolam (HALCION), *91,* 92, 92f-93f, 97f
    - zolpidem (AMBIEN), **93,** *93,* 97f
- **Antiarrhythmic drugs, specific agents**
    - adenosine, 163f-164f, **174**
    - amiodarone, 160f, 163f-164f, *172,* **172**
    - bretylium, 163f-164f, *172,* **172**
    - digoxin (LANOXIN), 151f, 156, 158, *158,* 159, 160f, 163f-164f, 169, 174, 177, 188, 213, 320, 352, 395, 410, 439-441
    - diltiazem (CARDIZEM CD, DILACOR XR), 163f, **173,** *173,* 173f, 175f, *177,* **177,** 180f, 187, *187,* 187f-188f
    - disopyramide, 167f, **169,** *169*
    - disopyramide (IA), 163f
    - esmolol, 74f, **77,** *77,* 78f, 163f, *171,* **171**
    - flecainide, **170,** *170,* 170f
    - flecainide (IC), 163f
    - lidocaine, 3, 7, 108f, 117f, 164f, *169,* **169,** 169f, 174
    - lidocaine (IB), 163f
    - metoprolol and pindolol, 163f
    - mexiletine, 147, 169f, **170,** *170,* 171, 172f
    - mexiletine (IB), 163f
    - procainamide, 167f, **168,** *168,* 171, 172f
    - procainamide (IA), 163f
    - propafenone, **170,** *170,* 170f, 171, 172f
    - propafenone (IC), 163f
    - propranolol (INDERAL), 7, 71f, *74,* 74f, **74-76,** 75f-76f, 78f-79f, 163f-164f, 171, 175f, 176, 179f, 185, 190, 334f, 427f, 428, 436-437
    - quinidine, 147, 160f, 164f, *167,* 167f, **167-168,** 169, 171, 172f, 214, 334f, 345f
    - quinidine (IA), 163f
    - quinidine sulfate, 168
    - sotalol, 163f-164f, *171,* **171-172,** 214
    - tocainide, 169f, **170,** *170*
    - tocainide (IB), 163f
    - verapamil (ISOPTIN, VERELAN), 160f, 163f-164f, 167, 169, **173,** *173,* 173f, 175f, *177,* **177,** 180f, 187, *187,* 187f-188f, 189, 377
- Antiarrhythmics, **163-174,** 164f
    - class I, 163f, **166-170**
    - class II, 163f, **170-171**
    - class III, 163f, 171f, **171-172**
    - class IV, 163f, **173**
        - effects, 173f
    - long-term effects, 166, 166f
- **Antiarrhythmics, specific agents,** 163f
- **Antiarthritis drugs, specific agents,** 402f
    - chloroquine, 345f-346f, 350, 350f, *351,* **351-352,** 352, 352f, 402f, 414
    - chloroquine phosphate, 432-433
    - gold salts, 402f, **413-414**
    - methotrexate, 205, 241f, 292-293, 295, 373f-374f, 378, *378,* 378f, **378-380,** 379f, 384, 399f, 402f, 410, 415, *415,* 419
    - D-Penicillamine, 402f, **414,** *414*
- Antibiotics. *See also* Antimicrobial agents; *specific agent*
    - for cancer, **384-387**
        - specific agents, 373f
    - complications, 286
- Anticancer drugs, **373-400**
    - adverse effects, 399f
    - emetic potential, 241f
- **Anticancer drugs, specific agents,** 373f
    - asparaginase, 241f
    - bleomycin, 241f, 373f, 378, 378f, *386,* **386-387,** 387f, 395, 399f
    - carboplatin, 241f, 373f, 378f, *395,* 395-396
    - carmustine, 241f, 373f, *389,* **389-390**
    - cisplatin, 241f, 242-243, 316, 373f-374f, 387, *395,* 395-396, 399f
    - cyclophosphamide, 241f, 373f, 378f, *388,* **388-389,** 389f, 395, 399f
    - cytarabine, 373f-374f, 378f, *383,* **383-384,** 399f
    - dactinomycin, 21, 241f, 373f-374f, 377, *384,* **384-385,** 399f
    - daunorubicin, 373f-374f, 382, *385,* **385-386**
    - doxorubicin, 241f, 242, 373f-374f, 378, 378f, *385,* 385f, **385-386,** 399f, 429
    - estrogens (PREMARIN), 263, **263-266,** 266, 266f, 268, 268f, 373f, 394, 399f
    - etoposide, 241f, 373f, 378f, 386, *396,* **396,** 397f, 399f
    - fludarabine, 373f, **384,** *384*
    - 5-fluorouracil, 373f-374f, 378f, *382,* **382-383,** 383f, 399f

flutamide, 272, *272,* 373*f*, *394,* 394-395, 399*f*
goserelin, 247*f*, 250, *250,* 373*f*, 394, *394,* 395, 395*f*
goserelin acetate, 394
idarubicin, 373*f*, 385
ifosfamide, 373*f*, *388,* **388-389,** 389*f*
interferons, 363*f*, **371,** *371,* 371*f*, 373*f*, **397-398,** 399*f*
leuprolide, 247*f*, 250, *250,* 373*f*, 394, *394,* 395, 395*f*, 399*f*
mechlorethamine, 241*f*, 373*f*, *387,* **387-388,** 388*f*, 399*f*
6-mercaptopurine, 373*f*-374*f*, *380,* **380-381,** 381*f*, 399*f*, 417
navelbine, 373*f*
paclitaxel, 373*f*, *391,* **391-392,** 392*f*, 399*f*
plicamycin, 373*f*, *387,* **387,** 399*f*
prednisone (DELTASONE, ORASONE), 219, 275*f*, 276, 334*f*, 373*f*, **393,** *393,* 397, 399*f*, 438-439
procarbazine, 373*f*, 378*f*, *396,* **396-397,** 399*f*
streptozocin, 241*f*
tamoxifen (NOLVADEX), 263*f*, **266,** *266,* 373*f*, *393,* **393-394,** 399*f*
6-thioguanine, 373*f*, *382,* **382,** 399*f*
vinblastine, 373*f*, 378*f*, 386, *390,* **390-391,** 395, 399*f*
vincristine, 241*f*, 373*f*, 378*f*, 384, *390,* **390-391,** 397, 399*f*
Anticholinergics, 107*f*
antiemetic potency, 243*f*
for chronic obstructive pulmonary disease, 222
preanesthetic, 108
Anticholinergics, specific agents
atropine (DONNATAL), 4, 40-41, 41*f*, 42-43, *45,* 45*f*, **45-48,** 46*f*, 49*f*, 64, 220, 220*f*
ipratropium (ATROVENT), 45*f*, **48,** *48,* 49*f*, 217*f*, 220, *220,* 220*f*, 222
scopolamine, 45*f*-46*f*, *48,* **48,** *48,* 48*f*-49*f*, 108, 129*f*, 130, 242, 438
Anticholinesterases
irreversible, **43**
reversible, **41-43**
Anticoagulants, **197-201**
for atrial fibrillation, 164*f*
drug interactions, 147
Anticoagulants, specific agents, 193*f*
enoxaprin, 193*f*, 198-199, *199*
heparin, 193*f*, **197-199,** 198, 198*f*, *199,* 204, 339, 408*f*
warfarin (COUMADIN), 22*f*, 22-23, 188, 193*f*, 196, *199,* **199-201,** 200, 200*f*-201*f*, 213, 239, 292, 295, 320, 326, 334*f*, 341, 411
Anticonvulsive drugs. *See also* Antiepileptic drugs
barbiturates as, 95
therapeutic indications, 145*f*
Antidepressants, 90*f*, 96, **119-126**
onset, 121*f*
polycyclic. *See* Polycyclic antidepressants
receptor specificity, 121*f*
therapeutic advantages and disadvantages, 125*f*
tricyclic. *See* Tricyclic antidepressants
Antidepressants, specific agents, 119*f*
amitriptyline (ELAVIL), 96, 119, *119,* 119*f*, 125*f*
amoxapine, 119, *119,* 119*f*, 125*f*
desipramine, 119, *119,* 119*f*, 125*f*
doxepin, 96, 119, *119,* 119*f*, 125*f*
fluoxetine (PROZAC), 119*f*, 121*f*, *122,* 122*f*, **122-123,** 123*f*, 125*f*
fluvoxamine, 119*f*, 123, *123,* 125*f*
imipramine, 56, 119, *119,* 119*f*, 120-121, 121*f*, 125*f*, 171, 172*f*
isocarboxazid, 119*f*, 123, *123,* 125*f*
lithium salts, **125**
maprotiline, 119, *119,* 119*f*, 125*f*
nefazodone, 119*f*, 123, *123,* 125*f*
nortriptyline (PAMELOR), 119, *119,* 119*f*, 125*f*
paroxetine (PAXIL), 119*f*, 123, *123,* 125*f*
phenelzine, 86, 119*f*, 123, *123,* 125*f*
protriptyline, 119, *119,* 119*f*, 125*f*
sertraline (ZOLOFT), 119*f*, 123, *123,* 125*f*
tranylcypromine, 119*f*, 123, *123,* 125*f*
trazodone, 96, 119*f*, 123, *123,* 125*f*
trimipramine, 119*f*, 125*f*
venlafaxine, 119*f*, 123, *123,* 125*f*
Antidiarrheal agents, **243-244**
specific agents, 244*f*
Antidiuretic hormone, **251**
Antiemetic agents, 107*f*, 129*f*, 242-243
administration route, 2
potency, 243*f*
preanesthetic, 108
Antiemetic drugs, specific agents
alprazolam (XANAX), 90, *90,* 92*f*-94*f*, 97*f*, 242*f*, 243, 438
dexamethasone, 235, 242*f*, 243, 243*f*, 275*f*-276*f*, 277, 362, 392, 395
domperidone, 129*f*, 242*f*, 242-243
dronabinol, **105,** *105,* 242*f*, 243, *243*
droperidol, 108, 117, 129*f*, 130, *130,* 139, 242*f*, 242-243, 243*f*
granisetron, 242*f*, 243, *243*
haloperidol, 84, 105, 127, *127,* 127*f*-129*f*, 130-131, 131*f*-132*f*, 242*f*, 242-243
haloperidol decanoate, 3, 130
lorazepam (ATIVAN), 92*f*-93*f*, 97*f*, 108*f*, 116, 242*f*, 243, 243*f*
methylprednisolone, 219, 242*f*, 243, 275*f*-276*f*
metoclopramide (REGLAN), 129*f*, 242, *242,* 242*f*, 242-243, 243*f*
nabilone, 242*f*, 243
ondansetron, 242*f*, 243, *243,* 243*f*
prochlorperazine (COMPAZINE), 127*f*, 129, 129*f*, 242, *242,* 242*f*, 243
Antiepileptic drugs, **145-150.** *See also* Anticonvulsive drugs
drug interactions, 147
mechanism of action, 145
Antiepileptic drugs, specific agents, 143*f*
carbamazepine (TEGRETOL), 143*f*, 145*f*, 147, *147,* **147,** 147*f*-148*f*, 150, 319-320, 362
clonazepam (KLONOPIN), 91, *91,* 97*f*, 143*f*, 145*f*, 149
clorazepate (TRANXENE), 91, *91,* 92*f*, 97*f*, 143*f*, 149
diazepam (VALIUM), 50, 90, *90,* 90*f*, 91, *91,* 92*f*-93*f*, 97*f*, 103, 108, 108*f*, 116, 143*f*, 145*f*, 149, 239
ethosuximide, 143*f*, 145*f*, *149,* **149**
gabapentin, 143*f*, *149,* **149-150**
lamotrigine, 143*f*, *149,* **149-150**
phenobarbital, 23-24, 90*f*, *94,* 95, 97*f*, 143*f*, 145*f*, 148, 148*f*, 213, 253, 343, 347, 438
phenytoin (DILANTIN), 13, 143*f*, 145*f*, 146, *146,* 146*f*, **146-147,** 147*f*, 150, 174, 239, 253, 295, 333, 341, 362, 408*f*
primidone, 143*f*, 145*f*, *148,* **148,** 148*f*
tiagabine, 445
topiramate, 445
valproic acid (DEPAKOTE), 143*f*, 145*f*, *148,* **148-149,** 149*f*, 150
vigabatrin, 446
Antiestrogens, **266**
mechanism of action, 393*f*
Antiestrogens, specific agents, 263*f*
clomiphene, 263*f*, **266,** *266*
tamoxifen (NOLVADEX), 263*f*, **266,** *266,* 373*f*, *393,* **393-394,** 399*f*
Antifungal drugs, **337-344**
Antifungal drugs, specific agents, 337*f*

- amphotericin B, 284*f*, *337,* 337*f*, **337-339,** 338*f*, 339-340, 356
- clotrimazole, 3-4, 337*f*, **343,** *343*
- econazole, 337*f*, **343,** *343*
- fluconazole, 337*f*, **341-342,** *342,* 342*f*, 429
- flucytosine, 284*f*, 337, 337*f*, 339, *339,* 339*f*, **339-340,** 340
- griseofulvin, 201*f*, 337*f*, *342,* **342-343,** 343*f*
- itraconazole, 215, 337*f*, **342,** *342,* 342*f*
- ketoconazole (NIZORAL), 272, 277, *277,* 334*f*, 337*f*, *340,* 340*f*, **340-341,** 342*f*
- miconazole (MONISTAT), 337*f*, **343,** *343*
- nystatin, 337*f*, **343,** *343*

Antigout drugs, specific agents
- allopurinol, 260*f*, 356, 382, 402*f*, 415, *416,* **416-417**
- colchicine, 377, 402*f*, 415, *416,* **416,** 416*f*
- probenecid, 260*f*, 303, 402*f*, 408*f*, 415, *417,* **417**
- sulfinpyrazone, 402*f*, 408*f*, 415, *417,* **417**

Antihelminthic drugs, specific agents
- ivermectin, 359*f*, **360,** *360*
- mebendazole, *359,* **359,** 359*f*, 361*f*
- niclosamide, 359*f*, **362,** *362*
- praziquantel, 359*f*, **360-362,** 362, *362*
- pyrantel pamoate, *359,* 359*f*, **359-360,** 361*f*
- thiabendazole, 359*f*, **360,** *360,* 361*f*

Antihistamines, 90*f*, 96, **96,** 107*f*
- antiemetic potency, 243*f*
- as autacoids, 420-425
- in combination therapy, 243
- preanesthetic, 108
- for rhinitis, 221
  - specific agents, 217*f*

Antihistamines, specific agents
- astemizole (HISMANAL), 214, 221, 341, 422*f*
- azatadine, 422*f*
- brompheniramine, 422*f*
- carbinoxamine, 422*f*
- cetirizine, 422*f*
- chlorpheniramine, 221, 422*f*
- cimetidine (TAGAMET), 108, 147, 147*f*, 201*f*, 235*f*, *236,* **236-238,** 237*f*, 326, 340, 347, 362, 419*f*, 440
- clemastine (TAVIST), 422*f*
- cyclizine, 242, 419*f*, 422*f*, 424, *424*
- cyproheptadine, 422*f*
- dexchlorpheniramine, 422*f*
- dimenhydrinate, 129*f*, 242, 419*f*, 422*f*, 424, *424*
- diphenhydramine, 96, 108, 221, 243, 243*f*, 392, 419*f*, 422*f*, 423-424, *424,* 438
- doxylamine, 96, 422*f*
- famotidine (PEPCID), 235*f*, *236,* **236-238,** 419*f*, 440, 440*f*
- hydroxyzine, **93,** *93,* 97*f*, 138, 422*f*
- loratidine (CLARITIN), 221, 422*f*
- meclizine, 129*f*, 242, 419*f*, 422*f*, 424, *424*
- methdilazine, 422*f*
- nizatidine (AXID), 235*f*, *236,* **236-238,** 419*f*, 440
- promethazine (PHENERGAN), 127*f*-129*f*, 130, *130,* 422*f*
- pyrilamine, 422*f*
- ranitidine (ZANTAC), 235*f*, *236,* **236-238,** 419*f*, 438, 440
- terfenadine (SELDANE), 214, 221, 320, 341, 422*f*
- timeprazine, 422*f*
- tripelennamine, 422*f*
- triprolidine, 422*f*

Antihyperlipidemic drugs, **207-216**

Antihyperlipidemic drugs, specific agents, 207*f*
- atorvastatin, 449
- cholestyramine (QUESTRAN), 207*f*, 212, *212,* 212*f*, **212-213,** 215
- cerivastatin, 449*f*
- clofibrate, 207*f*, *211,* 211*f*, **211-212,** 260*f*, 334*f*
- colestipol, 207*f*, 212, *212,* 212*f*, **212-213**
- fluvastatin, 207*f*, 213, *214,* **214-215,** 449*f*
- gemfibrozil (LOPID), 207*f*, 211, *211,* 211*f*, **211-212,** 215
- lovastatin (MEVACOR), 207*f*, *214,* **214-215,** 449*f*
- niacin, 207*f*, 210, 210*f*, **210-211,** *211,* 212, 215
- pravastatin (PRAVACHOL), 207*f*, 213, *214,* 214*f*, **214-215,** 449*f*
- probucol, 207*f*, 213, *213,* 213*f*, **213-214**
- simvastatin (ZOCOR), 207*f*, *214,* **214-215,** 449*f*

Antihypertensive drugs, **179-192**

Antihypertensive drugs, specific agents, 179*f*-180*f*
- amlodipine (NORVASC), **157,** 180*f*, 188, *188,* 188*f*
- atenolol (TENORMIN), 71*f*, 75*f*, *77,* **77,** 79*f*, 176, 179*f*, 185
- benazepril, 179*f*
- bumetanide (BUMEX), 151*f*, 179*f*, 223*f*-224*f*, *227,* **227-228,** 292, 316
- captopril (CAPOTEN), 151*f*, 179*f*
- clonidine (CATAPRES), 55*f*, **67,** *67,* 69*f*, 180*f*, *189,* **189-190,** 442
- diazoxide, 180*f*, **191,** *191,* 292
- diltiazem (CARDIZEM CD, DILACOR XR), 163*f*, **173,** *173,* 173*f*, 175*f*, *177,* **177,** 180*f*, 187, *187,* 187*f*-188*f*
- doxazosin (CARDURA), 71*f*, **73,** *73,* 180*f*
- enalapril (VASOTEC), 151*f*, 156, *156,* 157*f*, 179*f*
- felodipine, **157,** 180*f*, 188, *188,* 188*f*
- fosinopril, 151*f*
- furosemide (LASIX), 151*f*, 179*f*, 223*f*, 224, 224*f*, *227,* **227-228,** 292, 316, 409, 439-441
- hydrochlorothiazide, 151*f*, 179*f*, 183, *183,* 223*f*, 229, **231,** 441
- isradipine (DYNACIRC), 180*f*, 188, *188,* 188*f*
- labetalol (NORMODYNE), 71*f*, 74*f*, *78,* **78,** 79*f*, 179*f*, 191
- lisinopril (ZESTRIL, PRINIVIL), 151*f*, 179*f*
- losartan, 179*f*, **187,** *187*
- α-Methyldopa, 180*f*, **190,** *190*
- metoprolol (LOPRESSOR), 71*f*, 74*f*-75*f*, *77,* **77,** 78*f*-79*f*, 171, 176, 179*f*, 185
- minoxidil (ROGAINE), 151*f*, 180*f*, *190,* **190-191**
- moexipril, 179*f*
- nadolol (CORGARD), 71*f*, 74*f*, *76,* **76,** 78*f*, 179*f*, 428
- nicardipine, 180*f*, 188, *188,* 188*f*
- nifedipine (ADALAT, PROCARDIA XL), 173, 173*f*, 175*f*, *177,* **177,** *187,* 187*f*, 187-188, 188*f*
- nisoldipine, 180*f*, 188, *188*
- prazosin (MINIPRESS), 71*f*, **73,** *73,* 124, 180*f*, 189
- propranolol, 7, 71*f*, *74,* 74*f*, **74-76,** 75*f*-76*f*, 78*f*-79*f*, 163*f*-164*f*, 171, 175*f*, 176, 179*f*, 185, 190, 334*f*, 427*f*, 428, 436-437
- propranolol (INDERAL), 190
- quinapril (LOTENSIN), 151*f*, 179*f*
- ramipril (ACCUPRIL, ALTACE), 179*f*
- sodium nitroprusside, 151*f*, 180*f*, **191,** *191*
- spironolactone, 179*f*, 183, *183,* 223*f*-224*f*, **232-233,** *233,* 274, 277
- terazosin (HYTRIN), 71*f*, **73,** *73,* 180*f*, 189
- timolol (TIMOPTOL, TIMOPTIC), 71*f*, 74*f*, *76,* **76,** 78*f*-79*f*, 179*f*
- triamterene (DYAZIDE), 179*f*, 223*f*-224*f*, *233,* **233**
- verapamil (ISOPTIN, VERELAN), 160*f*, 163*f*-164*f*, 167, 169, **173,** *173,* 173*f*,

175*f*, *177*, **177**, 180*f*, 187, *187*, 187*f*-188*f*, 189, 377

Antiinflammatory agents, **401-418.** *See also* Nonsteroidal antiinflammatory drugs
- slow-acting, **413-415**
- specific agents, 401*f*-402*f*

Antileukotriene drugs, 450

Antilymphocyte and antithymocyte globulin, 471

Antimetabolites, for cancer, **378-384**
- specific agents, 373*f*

Antimicrobial agents
- classification, 287, 287*f*
- combinations, 284, 284*f*
- for peptic ulcer disease, 235*f*, 235-236
- resistance to, 284-286
- selection, 279*f*, **279-282**
- therapy with, principles, **279-288**

Antimigraine drugs, specific agents
- β-Adrenergic blockers, 58*f*, 58-59, 60*f*, **73-78,** 74*f*-75*f*, 78*f*-79*f*, 163*f*, 176-177, 178*f*, 182*f*, 184*f*, **184-187,** 185, 185*f*, 188*f*, 409, 419*f*, 427*f*, 428, 436, 442
- dihydroergotamine, 419*f*, **428,** *428*
- ergotamine, 419*f*, 427*f*, *428*, **428,** 437
- methysergide, 419*f*, 427*f*, 428, *428*
- sumatriptan (IMITREX), 419*f*, *426*, **426-427,** 427*f*, 437

Antimotility agents, 244

Antimuscarinic agents, **45-48,** 81*f*
- for Parkinson's disease, 87-88
- for peptic ulcer disease, 236*f*, 239-240

Antimycobacterial agents, **331-336**
- specific agents, 331*f*

Antiparkinson's drugs, specific agents, 81*f*
- amantadine, 81*f*, **87,** *87*, *363*, 363*f*, **363-364,** 364*f*
- antimuscarinic agents, **45-48,** 81*f*, 87-88, 236*f*, 239-240
- bromocriptine, 81*f*, **87,** *87*, 87*f*
- carbidopa (SINEMET), 81*f*, 84-86, 85*f*
- deprenyl, 81*f*, **87,** *87*, 87*f*
- levodopa, 8, 81*f*, 84-86, 85*f*-86*f*, 147, 240
- pramipexole, 443
- ropinirole, 443
- tolcapone, 444
- selegiline, 81*f*

Antiprogestin, 263*f*, **267**

Antiprogestin, specific agent, mifepristone, 263*f*, 267-268, 277

Antiprotozoal drugs, **345-358**

Antiprotozoal drugs, specific agents, 345*f*
- dehydroemetine, 345*f*-346*f*, *348*, **348**
- diloxanide furoate, 345*f*-346*f*, 347, *348*, **348**
- emetine, 345*f*-346*f*, *348*, **348**
- mefloquine, 345*f*, 350*f*, *352*, **352-353**
- melarsoprol, 345*f*, *353*, 353*f*, **353-354**
- metronidazole, 201*f*, 235*f*, 236, 282, 282*f*, 345*f*-346*f*, *347*, **347-348,** 357
- nifurtimox, 345*f*, 353*f*, **355,** *355*
- paromomycin, 345*f*-346*f*, *348*, **348**
- pentamidine, 339, 345*f*, 353*f*, 356, 370
- pentamidine isethionate, *354*, **354-355**
- primaquine, 345*f*, *349*, **349-350,** 350, 350*f*-351*f*, 432-433
- quinacrine, 345*f*, 357
- quinidine, 147, 160*f*, 163*f*-164*f*, *167*, 167*f*, **167-168,** 169, 171, 172*f*, 214, 334*f*, 345*f*
- quinidine sulfate, 168
- quinine, 345*f*, 350*f*, **352,** *352*
- sodium stibogluconate, 345*f*, *356*, **356-357**
- suramin, 345*f*, 353*f*, **356,** *356*

Antipseudomonal penicillins, 300*f*, **301**
- adverse reactions, 303

Antipsychotic drugs, **127-132**
- actions, 128*f*
- adverse effects, 130*f*
- antiemetic uses, 129*f*
- dopamine-blocking agents, 128*f*
- and LSD, 105
- summary, 132*f*

Antipsychotic drugs, specific agents
- chlorpromazine, 90*f*, 127, *127*, 127*f*-128*f*, 129-131, 131*f*-132*f*
- clozapine, 127*f*, 128, *128*, 128*f*, 130-131, 131*f*-132*f*
- fluphenazine, 127, *127*, 127*f*-128*f*, 130, 131*f*-132*f*
- haloperidol, 84, 105, 127, *127*, 127*f*-129*f*, 130-131, 131*f*-132*f*, 242*f*, 242-243
- haloperidol decanoate, 3, 130
- prochlorperazine (COMPAZINE), 127*f*, 129, 129*f*, 242, *242*, 242*f*, 243
- promethazine (PHENERGAN), 127*f*-129*f*, 130, *130*, 422*f*
- risperidone, 127*f*, 128, *128*, 128*f*, 130-131, 132*f*
- thioridazine, 127*f*-128*f*, 129, *129*, 130, 132*f*
- thiothixene, 127, *127*, 127*f*-128*f*, 132*f*

Antipyretic agents, salicylates as, 404, 406

Antischizophrenic drugs. *See* Antipsychotic drugs

Antisecretory agent, atropine as, 47

Antispasmodic agent, atropine as, 47

Antistaphylococcal penicillins, **300,** 300*f*

Antithyroid drugs, specific agents
- iodide, 247*f*, 254
- levothyroxine (LEVOXYL), 247*f*, 253
- methimazole, 247*f*, *253*, 253-254, 436
- propylthiouracil, 247*f*, *253*, 253-254, 436
- thyroxine, 247*f*, 251, 252*f*, 408*f*
- triiodothyronine, 247*f*, 251, 252*f*, 408*f*

Antituberculosis drugs, specific agents
- aminosalicylic acid, 331*f*, **335,** *335*
- cycloserine, 331*f*, **335,** *335*
- ethambutol, 331, 331*f*, *334*, **334-335,** 335*f*, 437
- ethionamide, 331*f*, **335,** *335*
- isoniazid, 147, 147*f*-148*f*, 283, 283*f*-284*f*, 331, 331*f*, 332, *332*, 332*f*, **332-333,** 333*f*, 334, 335*f*, 437
- pyrazinamide, *f*, 284*f*, 331, 334, **334,** *334*, 335, 437
- rifampin, 201*f*, 253, 284*f*, 285, 285*f*, 287*f*, 300, 331, 331*f*, *333*, **333-334,** 334, 340-341, 437

Antiviral drugs, **363-372**

Antiviral drugs, specific agents, 363*f*
- acyclovir (ZOVIRAX), 363*f*, 365, *365*, **365-366,** 366*f*-367*f*
- amantadine, 81*f*, **87,** *87*, *363*, 363*f*, **363-364,** 364*f*
- cidofovir, 457
- didanosine (ddl), 363*f*, *369*, 369*f*, **369-370**
- famciclovir, 363*f*, **367,** *367*
- foscarnet, 363*f*, **367,** *367*
- ganciclovir (DHPG), 363*f*, *366*, **366-367**
- interferons, 363*f*, **371,** *371*, 371*f*, 373*f*, **397-398,** 399*f*
- penciclovir, 457
- ribavirin, 363*f*, *364*, **364-365**
- rimantadine, *363*, 363*f*, **363-364**
- stavudine (d4T), 363*f*, 369*f*, **370,** *370*
- trifluridine, 363*f*, **368,** *368*
- vidarabine (ara-A), 363*f*, *367*, 367*f*, **367-368**
- zalcitabine (ddC), 363*f*, 369*f*, *370*, **370**
- zidovudine (AZT), 339, 363*f*, 367, *368*, **368-369,** 369*f*

Anxiety disorders
- benzodiazepines and, 90
- treatment, 90, 95, 148

Anxiolytic agents, **89-98**
- specific agents, 89*f*-90*f*
- therapeutic advantages and disadvantages, 97*f*

APSAC. *See* Anistreplase

Ara-A. *See* Vidarabine
Arabinofuranosyl adenine. *See* Vidarabine
Ara-C. *See* Cytarabine
ARAVA see Leflunomide
Arrhythmias, **163-166.** *See also specific arrhythmia*
  atrial, treatment, 164*f*, 168, 173
  atrioventricular, treatment, 168
  causes, 165
  treatment, 73, 78*f*, 169, 171, 172*f*
  types, 164*f*
Arterial thrombosis, treatment, 203
Arthralgia, treatment, 406
Arthritis
  rheumatoid, treatment, 351, 406, 408, 411, 413-415
  treatment. *See* **Antiarthritis drugs, specific agents**
Ascaris lumbricoides infection, 361*f*-362*f*
  treatment, 359, 361*f*
L-Asparaginase, 373*f*, *397*, **397,** 399*f*
  mechanism of action, 398*f*
Asparaginase, emetic potential, 241*f*
Aspergillosis, treatment, 342
Aspirin, 193*f*, 196, **196,** *196,* 401*f*, *403,* **403-408,** 439-440
  for diarrhea, 244, 244*f*
  dose, 407*f*
  drug interactions, 140, 201*f*, 211, 213
  half-life, 407*f*
  metabolism, 13, 404*f*
  for migraine, 427*f*, 428
  and prostaglandin synthesis inhibition, 405*f*
  therapeutic advantages and disadvantages, 412*f*
Astemizole (HISMANAL)
  drug interactions, 214, 341
  for rhinitis, 221
  therapeutic advantages and disadvantages, 422*f*
Asthma, 431, **450**
  and angina, 178*f*
  and hypertension, 182*f*-183*f*
  treatment, 3, 48, 62-63, 67-68, 189, **217-220,** 218*f*, 276
    specific agents, 217*f*
Atenolol (TENORMIN), 71*f*, **77,** *77,* 79*f*, 179*f*
  actions, 75*f*
  for angina, 176
  for hypertension, 185
ATIVAN. *See* Lorazepam
Atorvastatin, 449
Atracurium, 45*f*, 107*f*
  with anesthesia, 109
  onset and duration of action, 52*f*
  therapeutic advantages, 52*f*
Atrial fibrillation, treatment, 164*f*, 173-174
Atrial flutter, treatment, 164*f*, 173-174
Atrioventricular nodal reentry, treatment, 164*f*
Atropine (DONNATAL), *45,* 45*f*, **45-48,** 49*f*
  and acetylcholine, 40
  actions, 41, 41*f*
  administration route, 4
  dose-dependent effects, 47
  drug interactions, 42-43, 64
  and muscarinic receptor, 46*f*
  structure, 220, 220*f*
ATROVENT. *See* Ipratropium
Attention deficit syndrome, treatment, 104
Atypical depression, treatment, 124
Auranofin, 413-414
Aurothioglucose, 413-414
Autacoids, **419-428**
  specific agents, 419*f*
Autolysins, 299
Autonomic hyperreflexia, treatment, 72
Autonomic nervous system, 27*f*, **27-34,** 32*f*
  cholinergic agonists in, **35-44,** 36*f*
AXID. *See* Nizatidine
Azacytidine, emetic potential, 241*f*
Azatadine, therapeutic advantages and disadvantages, 422*f*
Azathioprine, 380, 471
  drug interactions, 417
3'-Azido-3'-Deoxythymidine. *See* Zidovudine
Azithromycin (ZITHROMAX), 311*f*, 317-320
  antimicrobial activity, 318, 319*f*
Azlocillin, 298*f*, 301, *301*
  administration route, 302
  stability to acid, 300*f*
AZMACORT. *See* Triamcinolone
AZT. *See* Zidovudine
Aztreonam, 298*f*, **307,** *307*
  structure, 307*f*
Bacilli
  gram-negative, 283*f*
  gram-positive, 283*f*
Bacillus anthracis infection, treatment, 299*f*
Bacitracin, 298*f*, **309,** *309*
Baclofen, 50
Bacterial prostatitis, treatment, 281
Bactericidal drugs, 282*f*, 283
Bacteriostatic drugs, 282*f*, 283
Bacteroides fragilis infection, treatment, 304, 305*f*, 321
BACTRIM. *See* Trimethoprim
Barbiturates, **94-96,** 107*f*, 115-116
  dependence potential, 100*f*
  drug interactions, 201*f*
  duration of action, 95
  preanesthetic, 108
  specific agents, 90*f*
  therapeutic advantages and disadvantages, 97*f*
  toxicity (poisoning), 96
Barbiturates, specific agents
  amobarbital, 90*f*, *94,* 95, 97*f*
  pentobarbital, 90*f*, *94,* 95, 97*f*, 108
  phenobarbital, 23-24, 90*f*, *94,* 95, 97*f*, 143*f*, 145*f*, 148, 148*f*, 213, 253, 343, 347, 438
  secobarbital, 90*f*, *94,* 95, 97*f*
BAYCOL Cerivastatin
Beclomethasone (BECONASE, VANCENASE, VANCERIL), 431
  administration route, 276*f*
  for asthma, 219
  drug elimination, 276*f*
  for rhinitis, 221
Beclomethasone dipropionate, 276, *276*
BECONASE. *See* Beclomethasone
Benazepril, 179*f*
Benign prostatic hyperplasia, treatment, 73, 272
Benzathine penicillin G, administration route, 302
Benzisoxazoles, 127*f*
Benzodiazepine receptor antagonists, 94
Benzodiazepine receptor antagonists, specific agents, 90*f*
  flumazenil, 90*f*, **94,** *94*
Benzodiazepines, **89-93,** 107*f*, 116
  antiemetic potency, 243*f*
  antiepileptics effects, 149
  for chemotherapy-induced nausea and vomiting, 242*f*, 243
  in combination therapy, 243
  duration of action, 92*f*
  preanesthetic, 108
  therapeutic advantages and disadvantages, 97*f*
  withdrawal reactions, 93*f*
Benzodiazepines, specific agents, 89*f*
  alprazolam (XANAX), 90, *90,* 92*f*-94*f*, 97*f*, 242*f*, 243, 438
  buspirone (BUSPAR), **93,** *93,* 94*f*, 97*f*
  chlordiazepoxide, *91,* 92*f*, 97*f*
  clonazepam (KLONOPIN), 91, *91,* 97*f*, 143*f*, 145*f*, 149
  clorazepate (TRANXENE), 91, *91,* 92*f*, 97*f*, 143*f*, 149
  diazepam (VALIUM), 50, 90, *90,* 90*f*, 91, *91,* 92*f*-93*f*, 97*f*, 103, 108, 108*f*, 116, 143*f*, 145*f*, 149, 239

estazolam, 92*f*
flurazepam, 91, *91,* 92, 92*f*-93*f*, 97*f*, 137
hydroxyzine, **93,** *93,* 97*f*, 138, 422*f*
lorazepam (ATIVAN), 92*f*-93*f*, 97*f*, 108*f*, 116, 242*f*, 243, 243*f*
midazolam, 97*f*, 108*f*, 116
quazepam, 92*f*-93*f*, 97*f*
temazepam (RESTORIL), *91,* 92, 92*f*-93*f*, 97*f*
triazolam (HALCION), *91,* 92, 92*f*-93*f*, 97*f*
zolpidem (AMBIEN), **93,** *93,* 97*f*
Benzothiazepines, 187, *187*
Benztropine
and neuroleptic drugs, 130
for Parkinson's disease, 88
Benzylpenicillin. *See* Penicillin G
Betamethasone, 438-439
properties, 275*f*
BETAPEN VK. *See* Penicillin V
Bethanechol, 35*f*, **40,** *40*
drug interactions, 236
structure, 39*f*
BIAXIN. *See* Clarithromycin
Biguanides, **261**
Bile acid binding resins, **212-213**
Bilirubin, drug interactions, 408*f*
Bioavailability, **6-7**
determination, 7*f*
Bioequivalence, 7
Biotransformation, of epinephrine, 62
Biperiden, for Parkinson's disease, 87-88
Bisacodyl, as laxative, 244, 244*f*
Bishydroxycoumarin. *See also* Dicumarol
adverse effects, 292
Bismuth (compounds), 235*f*
to eliminate Helicobacter pylori, 236
Bismuth subsalicylate, 244, 244*f*
cost, 282, 282*f*
Bisphosphonates, 476
Bladder carcinoma, treatment, 395
Blastomyces dermatitidis infection, treatment, 338
Blastomycosis, systemic, treatment, 355
Bleeding, drug treatment, **204**
Bleomycin, 373*f*, *386,* **386-387,** 387*f*, 399*f*
adverse effects, 378
drug interactions, 395
emetic potential, 241*f*
myelosuppressive potential, 378*f*
Bleomycin peptide antibiotics, actions, 374*f*
Blood
anesthetic solubility in, 111, 111*f*
coagulation, **196,** 196*f*
drugs affecting, **193-206**
specific agents, 193*f*
Blood-brain barrier, 8
and antibiotics, 281
Blood flow, and drug distribution, 8
Blood pressure
acetylcholine and, 39-40
factors affecting, 180*f*
mechanisms for controlling, 180-181
phenylephrine and, 66
Borrelia burgdorferi infection, treatment, 312*f*
Brain tumors, treatment, 389
Bran, 244*f*, 245
Breast cancer
metastatic, treatment, 392, 395
treatment, 277, 379, 382, 386, 389, 393, 395
effect on endocrine system, 395*f*
Bretylium, 163*f*, **172,** *172*
as antiarrhythmic, 164*f*
Bromocriptine, 81*f*, **87,** *87*
adverse effects, 87*f*
Brompheniramine, therapeutic advantages and disadvantages, 422*f*
Bronchitis, treatment, 324
Bronchodilators, 431-432, 432*f*
adrenergic agonists as, 67*f*
Bronchospasm, treatment, 62-63, 67
Brugia malayi, 361*f*
Bulimia nervosa, treatment, 122
Bulking agents, 244-245
Bumetanide (BUMEX), 151*f*, 179*f*, 223*f*, *227,* **227-228**
drug interactions, 292, 316
site of action, 224*f*
BUMEX. *See* Bumetanide
Bupivacaine, 108*f*
pharmacokinetic properties, 117*f*
Buprenorphine, 133*f*, **141,** *141*
Burkitt's lymphoma, treatment, 379, 389
Burns, treatment, 270, 291
BUSPAR. *See* Buspirone
Buspirone (BUSPAR), **93,** *93*
adverse effects, 94*f*
therapeutic advantages and disadvantages, 97*f*
Butalbital (FIORINAL), 437
for migraine, 428
Butyrophenones, 127*f*
antiemetic potency, 243*f*
for chemotherapy-induced nausea and vomiting, 242*f*, 242-243
in combination therapy, 243
Caffeine, *99,* 99*f*, **99-100**
dependence potential, 100*f*
drug interactions, 326, 428
for migraine, 428
CALAN SR. *See* Verapamil
Calcitonin, 477
administration route, 3
Calcium carbonate, 236*f*, 240, 477
Calcium channel blockers, 163*f*
adverse effects, 189*f*
for angina, 177
specific agents, 175*f*
treatment with concomitant diseases, 178*f*
classes, 187-188
drug interactions, 51
for hypertension, 187-189
actions, 187*f*
with concomitant diseases, 182*f*
therapeutic applications, 188*f*
Calcium channel blockers, specific agents, 180*f*
Calcium gluconate, drug interactions, 317
Calluses, treatment, 406
Cancer
anemia with, treatment, 206
bladder, treatment, 395
breast
metastatic, treatment, 392, 395
treatment, 277, 379, 382, 386, 389, 393, 395, 395*f*
chemotherapy. *See also* Anticancer drugs
principles, **373-378**
choriocarcinoma
gestational, treatment, 384
treatment, 379, 399*f*
colorectal, treatment, 382, 406
gastric, treatment, 382
head and neck, 379
lung
oat cell carcinoma, treatment, 396
small-cell, treatment, 392
treatment, 386, 396
ovarian, treatment, 382, 392, 395
pancreatic, treatment, 382
prostatic, treatment, 272, 394
effect on endocrine system, 395*f*
treatment, 386
Candida infection, 314
candidemia, treatment, 342
drug interactions, 340
treatment, 338-339, 343
Candidiasis. *See* Candida infection
Cannabinoids

  antiemetic potency, 243f
  for chemotherapy-induced nausea and vomiting, 242f, 243
  in combination therapy, 243
Cannabis, dependence potential, 100f
Canrenone, 232, *232*
Capecitabine, 463
Capillary
  permeability, 8, 8f
  structure, 8, 8f
CAPOTEN. *See* Captopril
Captopril (CAPOTEN), 151f, 179f
CARAFATE. *See* Sucralfate
Carbachol, 35f, *40*, **40-41**
  structure, 39f
Carbamazepine (TEGRETOL), 143f, **147**, *147*
  drug interactions, 147, 147f-148f, 150, 319-320, 362
  for seizures, 145f
Carbamylcholine. *See* Carbachol
Carbapenems, **306-307**
  specific agents, 298f
Carbenicillin, 298f, 301, *301*
  administration route, 302
  adverse reactions, 303
  stability to acid, 300f
  therapeutic applications, 301f
Carbidopa (SINEMET), 81f
  dopamine synthesis with, 85f
  for Parkinson's disease, 84-86
Carbinoxamine, therapeutic advantages and disadvantages, 422f
Carbonic anhydrase inhibitors, 223f
  diuretic effects, **226-227**
    and sodium retention, 226, 226f
Carboplatin, 373f, *395*
  in cancer therapy, 395-396
  emetic potential, 241f
  myelosuppressive potential, 378f
Carboprost, *419*, **419**, 419f-420f
Cardiac glycosides, 151f. *See also* Digitalis
Cardiac muscle, contraction, 153-154, 154f
Cardiac output, acetylcholine and, 39
CARDIZEM CD. *See* Diltiazem
CARDURA. *See* Doxazosin
Carmustine, 373f, *389*, **389-390**
  emetic potential, 241f
Cascara, 244
Case studies, **429-442**
Castor oil, 244, 244f
CATAPRES. *See* Clonidine
Catecholamines, 69f
Catechol, structure, 61f
Catechol-O-methyltransferase, 444
CECLOR. *See* Cefaclor
CEDAX see Ceftibuten
Cefaclor (CECLOR), 298f
  therapeutic advantages and disadvantages, 305f
Cefadroxil (DURICEF), 298f
  therapeutic advantages and disadvantages, 305f
Cefamandole, 298f, 306, *306*
  adverse effects, 306
  therapeutic advantages and disadvantages, 305f
  vitamin K with, 204
Cefazolin, 298f, 306, *306*
  therapeutic advantages and disadvantages, 305f
Cefepime, 304
Cefixime (SUPRAX), 298f
  therapeutic advantages and disadvantages, 305f
Cefmetazole, 298f, 304, *304*
  therapeutic advantages and disadvantages, 305f
Cefonicid, 298f
  therapeutic advantages and disadvantages, 305f
Cefoperazone, 298f, 306, *306*
  adverse effects, 306
  therapeutic advantages and disadvantages, 305f
  vitamin K with, 204
Ceforanide, therapeutic advantages and disadvantages, 305f
Cefotaxime, 298f, 304, *304*
  for meningitis, 306
  therapeutic advantages and disadvantages, 305f
Cefotetan, 298f, 304, *304*
  therapeutic advantages and disadvantages, 305f
Cefoxitin, 298f, 304, *304*, 433
  for bacteroides fragilis infection, 304
  therapeutic advantages and disadvantages, 305f
Ceftazidime, 298f, 304, *304*, 430-431
  therapeutic advantages and disadvantages, 305f
CEFTIN. *See* Cefuroxime axetil
Ceftizoxime, 298f
  therapeutic advantages and disadvantages, 305f
Ceftriaxone, 298f, 304, *304*, 435
  for gonorrhea, 299f
  for meningitis, 306
  therapeutic advantages and disadvantages, 305f
  for urinary tract infections, 328f
Cefuroxime, 298f
  therapeutic advantages and disadvantages, 305f
Cefuroxime axetil (CEFTIN), therapeutic advantages and disadvantages, 305f
CELEBREX see Celecoxib
Celecoxib, 466-467
CELLCEPT see Mycophenolate mofetil
Cell-cycle specificity, in anticancer drugs, 374, 376f
Cell wall synthesis inhibitors, **297-310**
  specific agents, 298f
Centrally-acting adrenergic drugs, for hypertension, **189-190**
Central nervous system (CNS), 27, 27f
  in autonomic control of viscera, 30, 31f
  infections, 281
  neurotransmission in, 81-82
  stimulation by ephedrine, 68
Central nervous system depressants, dependence potential, 100f
Central nervous system stimulants, **99-106**
  dependence potential, 100f
Central nervous system stimulants, specific agents, 99f
  amphetamines, 55f, 60-61, *67*, **67-68,** 69f, 99f-100f, **103-104,** 104f, 105, 138
  caffeine, *99*, 99f, **99-100,** 100f, 326, 428
  cocaine, 3, 56, 63, 71f, **79,** *79*, 99f-100f, *101*, **101-103,** 102f-103f
  methylphenidate (RITALIN HYDROCHLORIDE), 99f, *104*
  nicotine, 45f, *49*, **49,** 49f, 99f, *100*, 100f, **100-101,** 101, 101f
  nicotine gum, 101f
  theobromine, *99*, 99f
  theophylline (SLO-BID, THEO-DUR), *99*, 99f, 100, **220,** 222, 319-320, 326, 395
    specific agents, 217f
Cephadrine, 298f
Cephalexin (KEFLEX, KEFTAB), 298f
  therapeutic advantages and disadvantages, 305f
Cephalosporins, **304-305**
  first generation, 304
    specific agents, 298f
    therapeutic advantages and disadvantages, 305f
  fourth generation, 304
  second generation, 304
    specific agents, 298f

therapeutic advantages and disadvantages, 305*f*
third generation, 304
specific agents, 298*f*
therapeutic advantages and disadvantages, 305*f*
structure, 304*f*
therapeutic advantages and disadvantages, 305*f*
for urinary tract infections, 328*f*
vitamin K with, 204
Cephalosporins, specific agents, 298*f*
first generation
cefadroxil (DURICEF), 298*f*, 305*f*
cefazolin, 298*f*, 305*f*, 306, *306*
cephadrine, 298*f*
cephalexin (KEFLEX, KEFTAB), 298*f*, 305*f*
cephalothin, 298*f*, 305*f*
cephapirin, 298*f*, 305*f*
second generation
cefaclor (CECLOR), 298*f*, 305*f*
cefamandole, 204, 298*f*, 305*f*, 306, *306*
cefmetazole, 298*f*, 304, *304,* 305*f*
cefonicid, 298*f*, 305*f*
cefotetan, 298*f*, 304, *304,* 305*f*
cefoxitin, 298*f*, 304, *304,* 305*f*, 433
cefuroxime, 298*f*, 305*f*
cefuroxime axetil (CEFTIN), 305*f*
third generation
cefixime (SUPRAX), 298*f*, 305*f*
cefoperazone, 204, 298*f*, 305*f*, 306, *306*
cefotaxime, 298*f*, 304, *304,* 305*f*, 306
ceftazidime, 298*f*, 304, *304,* 305*f*, 430-431
ceftizoxime, 298*f*, 305*f*
ceftriaxone, 298*f*-299*f*, 304, *304,* 305*f*, 306, 328*f*, 435
moxalactam, 204, 298*f*
fourth geeneration
cefepime, 304, 305*f*
Cephalothin, 298*f*
therapeutic advantages and disadvantages, 305*f*
Cephapirin, 298*f*
therapeutic advantages and disadvantages, 305*f*
Cephradine, therapeutic advantages and disadvantages, 305*f*
Cerebral palsy, treatment, 90
Cerebrospinal fluid, drug penetration, 281
Cerivastatin, 449
Cestodes, chemotherapy, 359*f*, **362**
Cetirizine, therapeutic advantages and disadvantages, 422*f*
Chagas' disease, 353, 353*f*
Chemotherapeutic agents, emetic actions/potential, 241*f*, 242
Chemotherapy
for amebiasis, 345*f*, **345-348**
cancer. *See also* Anticancer drugs
curative, 375*f*
nausea and vomiting with, 241*f*, 242
treatment, 241-243, 242*f*
palliative, 375*f*
principles, **373-378**
problems with, 377-378
for cestodes, 359*f*, **362**
for giardiasis, 345*f*, **357**
for helminthic infections, 359*f*
for leishmaniasis, 345*f*, **356-357**
for leprosy, **335-336**
for malaria, 345*f*, **349-353**
for nematodes, 359*f*, **359-360**
for toxoplasmosis, 345*f*, **357**
for trematodes, 359*f*, **360-362**
for trypanosomiasis, 345*f*, **353-356**
for tuberculosis, **332-335**
Chicken pox, treatment, 412
Chlamydia infection, 283*f*, 290*f*
lymphogranuloma venereum, 290*f*
treatment, 290, 312*f*, 317-318, 318*f*, 324, 328*f*
Chloral hydrate, 90*f*, **96,** *96*
Chloramphenicol, 282*f*, 283, 311*f*, *320,* **320-321**
classification, 287*f*
drug interactions, 147, 147*f*, 201*f*, 260*f*
effect on neonates, 282
metabolism, 15
resistance to, 285*f*
safety, 282
Chlordiazepoxide, *91*
for alcohol withdrawal, *91*
duration of action, 92*f*
therapeutic advantages and disadvantages, 97*f*
Chloroform, 107
Chloroguanide, 350*f*
Chloroquine, 345*f*, 350*f*, *351,* **351-352,** 402*f*
adverse effects, 352, 352*f*
antiinflammatory effects, 414
drug interactions, 350
sites of action, 346*f*
Chloroquine phosphate, 432-433
Chlorothiazide, 223*f*, **229-231,** *231*
hyperuricemia with, 224
Chlorotrianisene, 263, *263,* 263*f*
Chlorpheniramine
for rhinitis, 221
therapeutic advantages and disadvantages, 422*f*
Chlorpromazine, 127, *127,* 127*f*, 129, 132*f*
actions, 128*f*
affinities at dopaminergic receptors, 131*f*
for hiccups, 130
ratio of lethal to effective dose, 90*f*
for schizophrenia, 131
Chlorpropamide, 255*f*, *260,* 260-261
properties, 261*f*
Chlorthalidone, 223*f*, 229, **231,** *231*
Cholera, treatment, 312*f*
Cholesterol, niacin for, 210
Cholestyramine (QUESTRAN), 207*f*, *212,* **212-213**
in combination drug therapy, 215
mechanism of action, 212, 212*f*
Choline magnesium salicylate, 406
Choline, recycling, 37, 37*f*
Cholinergic agents, adverse effects, 40*f*
Cholinergic agonists, **35-44**
adverse effects, 49*f*
antidote for, 47
indirect, mechanisms of action, 41, 42*f*
reversible, mechanisms of action, 41, 42*f*
sites of action, 36*f*
structures, 39*f*
Cholinergic agonists, specific agents, 35*f*
acetylcholine, 21, 32*f*, 33, 35*f*, 36-37, 37*f*, *39,* 39*f*, **39-40,** 46*f*, 236
bethanechol, 35*f*, 39*f*, *40,* **40,** 236
carbachol, 35*f*, 39*f*, *40,* **40-41**
pilocarpine, 35*f*, **41,** *41,* 41*f*, 75, 227
Cholinergic antagonists, **45-54**
for asthma, 220
sites of action, 46*f*
specific agents, 45*f*
summary, 49*f*
Cholinergic, definition, 33
Cholinergic neurons, **35-37**
Cholinergic receptors, **38-39**
types, 38*f*
Choline salicylate, 406
Cholinesterase inhibitors, drug interactions, 51
Cholinesterase inhibitors, specific agents
echothiophate, 35*f*, **43,** *43*
edrophonium, 35*f*, **43,** *43,* 50-51, 433,

434*f*
isoflurophate, 35*f*, **43,** *43*
neostigmine, 35*f*, **42,** *42,* 50-51, 317
physostigmine, 35*f*, **42,** *42,* 47, 51
pyridostigmine, 35*f*, **42,** *42*
Cholinoceptors. *See* Cholinergic receptors
Choriocarcinoma
gestational, treatment, 384
treatment, 379, 399*f*
Chromoblastomycosis, treatment, 339
Chronic obstructive pulmonary disease
and angina, 178*f*
and hypertension, 182*f*
treatment, 3, 48, 221-222
specific agents, 217*f*
Cidofovir, 457
Cigarettes, nicotine concentration, 101*f*
Cilastatin, 298*f*
with imipenem, 306-307
Cimetidine (TAGAMET), 235*f*, *236,* **236-238,** 419*f*, 440
drug interactions, 147, 147*f*, 201*f*, 326, 340, 347, 362
and gastric acid regulation, 237*f*
preanesthetic, 108
CIPRO. *See* Ciprofloxacin
Ciprofloxacin (CIPRO), 323, *323,* **324,** 325-326
for methicillin-resistant staphylococcus aureus, 300
therapeutic applications, 325*f*
Cirrhosis, 226
edema with, treatment, 229
Cisplatin, 373*f*, *395,* 399*f*
actions, 374*f*
in cancer therapy, 395-396
drug interactions, 242-243, 316, 387
emetic potential, 241*f*
Clarithromycin (BIAXIN), 235*f*, 311*f*, 317-320, 433
antimicrobial activity, 317, 319*f*
cost, 282, 282*f*
to eliminate Helicobacter pylori, 236
CLARITIN. *See* Loratidine
Class I drugs, 12, 12*f*
Class II drugs, 12, 12*f*
Clavulanic acid, 298*f*, *307,* **307-308,** 308*f*
administration route, 302
drug interactions, 300-301
stability to penicillinase, 300*f*
Clemastine (TAVIST), therapeutic advantages and disadvantages, 422*f*
CLEOCIN-T. *See* Clindamycin
Clinafloxacin, 456*f*
Clindamycin (CLEOCIN-T), 311*f*, **321,** *321,* 435
classification, 287*f*
resistance to, 285*f*
CLINORIL. *See* Sulindac
Clofazimine, 331*f*, **336,** *336*
Clofibrate, 207*f*, *211,* **211-212**
drug interactions, 260*f*, 334*f*
mechanism of action, 211*f*
Clomiphene, 263*f*, **266,** *266*
Clonazepam (KLONOPIN), *91,* 143*f*
antiepileptic effects, 149
for seizures, 91, 145*f*
therapeutic advantages and disadvantages, 97*f*
Clonidine (CATAPRES), 55*f*, **67,** *67,* 69*f*, 180*f*, *189,* **189-190,** 442
Clopidogrel, 448
Clorazepate (TRANXENE), *91,* 143*f*
for alcohol withdrawal, 91
as antiepileptic, 149
duration of action, 92*f*
therapeutic advantages and disadvantages, 97*f*
Clostridia infection, treatment, 347
Clostridium difficile infection
resistance, 304, 321
treatment, 308
Clostridium perfringens infection, treatment, 299*f*
Clot, formation, 193-194
Clotrimazole, 337*f*, **343,** *343*
administration route, 3-4
Cloxacillin, 298*f*, 300, *300*
stability to penicillinase, 300*f*
Clozapine, 127*f*, 128, *128,* 130-131, 132*f*
actions, 128*f*
affinities at dopaminergic receptors, 131*f*
Cluster headache, characteristics, 425*f*
Cocaine, 71*f*, **79,** *79,* 99*f*, *101,* **101-103**
administration route, 3
dependence potential, 100*f*
drug interactions, 63
effects, 103*f*
mechanism of action, 102*f*
and norepinephrine removal, 56
Cocci
gram-negative, 283*f*
gram-positive, 283*f*
Coccidioides immitis infection (coccidioidomycosis), treatment, 338, 342
Codeine, 133*f*, **140,** *140*
absorption, 137
actions, 134*f*, 140*f*
for cough, 137, 222
efficacy and addiction/abuse liability, 135*f*
Codeine sulfate, for migraine, 427*f*
Colchicine, 402*f*, **416,** *416*
adverse effects, 416*f*
for hyperuricemia, 415
resistance to, 377
Colestipol, 207*f*, *212,* **212-213**
mechanism of action, 212, 212*f*
Colloidal bismuth, 236*f*, 241
Colorectal cancer, treatment, 382, 406
COMPAZINE. *See* Prochlorperazine
Condom
failure rate, 268*f*
percent use, 268*f*
Congenital adrenal hyperplasia (CAH), treatment, 274-275
Congestive heart failure
edema with, treatment, 229
and hypertension, 182*f*-183*f*
kidney function during, 225
physiological responses, 154-155, 155*f*
treatment, 66, **151-162,** 188*f*, 228, 230
specific agents, 151*f*
ventricular function curves, 159*f*
Congestive heart failure drugs, specific agents, 151*f*
amrinone, 151*f*, 161, *161,* 161*f*
bumetanide (BUMEX), 151*f*, 179*f*, 223*f*-224*f*, *227,* **227-228,** 292, 316
captopril (CAPOTEN), 151*f*, 179*f*
digitoxin, 151*f*, 158, *158,* 160*f*, 334*f*
digoxin (LANOXIN), 151*f*, 156, 158, *158,* 159, 160*f*, 163*f*-164*f*, 169, 174, 177, 188, 213, 320, 352, 395, 410, 439-441
dobutamine, 55*f*, **66,** *66,* 69*f*, 151*f*, 159, 161, 161*f*
enalapril (VASOTEC), 151*f*, 156, *156,* 157*f*, 179*f*
fosinopril, 151*f*
furosemide (LASIX), 151*f*, 179*f*, 223*f*, 224, 224*f*, *227,* **227-228,** 292, 316, 409, 439-441
hydralazine, 151*f*, 157, 180*f*, *190,* **190,** 442
hydrochlorothiazide, 151*f*, 179*f*, 183, *183,* 223*f*, 229, **231,** 441
isosorbide (ISORDIL), 151*f*
isosorbide dinitrate, **157,** 175*f*, **176,** *176,* 177*f*
isosorbide mononitrate, 176
lisinopril (ZESTRIL, PRINIVIL), 151*f*, 179*f*
metolazone, 151*f*, 223*f*, **231,** *231*
milrinone, 151*f*, 161, *161*

- minoxidil (ROGAINE), 151*f*, 180*f*, *190*, **190-191**
- quinapril (LOTENSIN), 151*f*, 179*f*
- sodium nitroprusside, 151*f*, 180*f*, **191**, *191*

Constipation, treatment, specific agents, 244*f*

Contraception, **267-269**
- failure rate, 268*f*
- implantable, **267-269**
- oral, **267-269**
- percent use, 268*f*

CORGARD. *See* Nadolol

Corns, treatment, 406

Coronary artery disease, 207

Coronary artery thrombosis, treatment, 406

Corticosteroids
- administration route, 276*f*
- adverse effets, 277*f*
- antiemetic potency, 243*f*
- for asthma, 218-220
  - specific agents, 217*f*
- for chemotherapy-induced nausea and vomiting, 242*f*, 243
- for chronic obstructive pulmonary disease, specific agents, 217*f*
- in combination therapy, 243
- drug interactions, 160*f*
- elimination, 276*f*
- properties, 275*f*
- for rhinitis, 221
  - specific agents, 217*f*
- secretion, regulation, 272*f*

Corticosteroids, specific agents
- beclomethasone (BECONASE, VANCENASE, VANCERIL), 219, 221, 276*f*, 431
- beclomethasone dipropionate, 276, *276*
- betamethasone, 275*f*, 438-439
- cortisone, 275*f*, 276*f*
- desoxycorticosterone, 276*f*
- dexamethasone, 235, 242*f*, 243, 243*f*, 275*f*-276*f*, 276*f*, 277, 362, 392, 395
- fludrocortisone, 274, *274*, 275*f*
- hydrocortisone, 274, *274*, 275*f*-276*f*, 438-439
- methylprednisolone, 219, 242*f*, 243, 275*f*-276*f*
- paramethasone, 275*f*
- prednisolone, 275*f*, 393
- prednisone (DELTASONE, ORASONE), 219, 275*f*, 276, 334*f*, 373*f*, *393*, **393**, 397, 399*f*, 438-439
- triamcinolone (AZMACORT), 219, 221, 275*f*, 276, *276*, 276*f*

Corticotropin (ACTH), 247*f*, **249**, *249*, 249*f*

Corticotropin-releasing hormone, 249*f*
- actions, 248*f*

Cortisol, *272*, 274
- production, 272, 272*f*
- suppression of synthesis, 340

Cortisone
- administration route, 276*f*
- elimination, 276*f*
- properties, 275*f*

Corynebacterium diphtheriae infection, treatment, 299*f*, 318*f*

Cosyntropin, 249, *249*

COTRIM. *See* Co-trimoxazole

Cotrimoxazole (COTRIM), 289, *289*, 289*f*, 290, **293-295**
- drug interactions, 201*f*
- for gonorrhea, 299*f*
- for Kaposi's sarcoma, 429
- therapeutic application, 290

Cough, treatment, 137, 140, 222
- specific agents, 217*f*

COUMADIN. *See* Warfarin

Coumarin, drug interactions, 215

Cramps, treatment, 441-442

CRIXIVAN see Indinavir

Cromolyn (INTAL), 423, 431
- for asthma, 218*f*, **220**, *220*
  - specific agents, 217*f*
- for rhinitis, 221
  - specific agents, 217*f*

Cryptococcal meningitis, treatment, 284*f*

Cryptococcus neoformans infection (cryptococcosis), treatment, 338-339, 341-342

Crystalline zinc suspension, 258-259

Cushing's syndrome
- diagnosis, 274
- treatment, 277

Cutaneous larva migrans, treatment, 360

Cutaneous leishmaniasis, 356

Cyanide, nitroprusside and, 191*f*

Cyanocobalamin (B_{12}), 193*f*, **205**. *See also* Vitamin B_{12}

Cyclizine, 419*f*, *424*
- for motion sickness, 242, 424
- therapeutic advantages and disadvantages, 422*f*

Cyclophosphamide, 373*f*, *388*, **388-389**, 389*f*, 399*f*
- drug interactions, 395
- emetic potential, 241*f*
- myelosuppressive potential, 378*f*

Cycloserine, 331*f*, **335**, *335*

Cyclosporine, **472**
- drug interactions, 147, 215, 239, 320, 326, 339, 341, 410

Cyproheptadine, therapeutic advantages and disadvantages, 422*f*

Cyproterone acetate, 272, *272*

Cystinuria, treatment, 414

Cystitis, treatment, 328*f*

Cytarabine, 373*f*, *383*, **383-384**, 399*f*
- actions, 374*f*
- myelosuppressive potential, 378*f*

Cytochrome P-450, **14**, 14*f*
- thyroid hormones and, 253

Cytomegalic retinitis, treatment, 366-367

Cytomegalovirus infection
- resistance, 366
- treatment, specific agents, 363*f*

Cytopenia, treatment, 398

Cytosine arabinoside. *See* Cytarabine

Dacarbazine, emetic potential, 241*f*

Dactinomycin, 373*f*, *384*, **384-385**, 399*f*
- actions, 374*f*
- emetic potential, 241*f*
- interaction with nucleic acids, 21
- resistance to, 377

Danazol, 263*f*, 270, *270*, 271

Dantrolene, 50
- with anesthesia, 113
- for hyperthermia, 53

Dapsone, 331*f*, *335*, **335-336**

DARVOCET-N. *See* Propoxyphene

DARVON. *See* Propoxyphene

Daunorubicin, 373*f*, 382, *385*, **385-386**
- actions, 374*f*

DAYPRO. *See* Oxaprozin

ddC. *See* Zalcitabine

ddI. *See* Didanosine

Deep-vein thrombosis, treatment, 198, 201, 203

Dehydroemetine, 345*f*, **348**, *348*
- sites of action, 346*f*

Dehydroepiandrosterone, production, 272

Delavirdine, 462

DELTASONE. *See* Prednisone

Demeclocycline, 311*f*, 314, *314*

DEMULEN. *See* Ethinyl estradiol

DENAVIR see Penciclovir

Deoxycorticosterone, properties, 275*f*

DEPAKOTE. *See* Valproic acid

Deprenyl, 81*f*, **87**, *87*

in dopamine metabolism, 87*f*
Depression, treatment, 120, 122-124
Dermatophytosis, treatment, 4
Desipramine, 119, *119,* 119*f*
therapeutic advantages and disadvantages, 125*f*
Desmopressin, 247*f*, **251,** *251*
administration route, 3
DESOGEN. *See* Ethinyl estradiol
Desoxycorticosterone
administration route, 276*f*
elimination, 276*f*
Dexamethasone, 242*f*
administration route, 276*f*
antiemetic effects, 235
for chemotherapy-induced nausea and vomiting, 243
in combination therapy, 243, 243*f*
drug interactions, 277, 362, 392, 395
elimination, 276*f*
properties, 275*f*
Dexamethasone suppression test, 274
Dexchlorpheniramine, therapeutic advantages and disadvantages, 422*f*
Dextromethorphan, 140, *222*
for cough, 137, 222
specific agents, 217*f*
DFP. *See* Isoflurophate
DHPG. *See* Ganciclovir
DIABETA. *See* Glyburide
Diabetes insipidus, treatment, 3, 230
Diabetes mellitus, **255-257**
and angina, 178*f*
insulin-dependent, 255, **256,** 256*f*
and hypertension, 182*f*-183*f*
insulin release, 256*f*
non-insulin-dependent, 255, 256*f*, **256-257**
insulin release, 256*f*
treatment, 257*f*, 261
treatment, 77, 189
Diabetic neuropathy, treatment, 122
Diaphragm (contraceptive)
failure rate, 268*f*
percent use, 268*f*
Diarrhea, treatment, 137, 235
specific agents, 244*f*
Diazepam (VALIUM), 50, *90,* 108*f*, 116, 143*f*
for alcohol withdrawal, *91*
antiepileptic effects, 149
for anxiety disorders, 90
and cocaine, 103
drug interactions, 239
duration of action, 92*f*
for epilepsy, 91
preanesthetic, 108
ratio of lethal to effective dose, 90*f*
for seizures, 145*f*
therapeutic advantages and disadvantages, 97*f*
withdrawal reactions, 93*f*
Diazoxide, 180*f*, **191,** *191*
drug interactions, 292
Dibenzodiazepines, 127*f*
Diclofenac (VOLTAREN), 401*f*, **411,** *411*
Dicloxacillin, 298*f*, 300, *300*
stability to penicillinase, 300*f*
Dicumarol, *199,* **199-201**
drug interactions, 147, 147*f*, 260*f*
Didanosine (ddl), 363*f*, *369,* 369*f*, **369-370**
Dideoxycytidine. *See* Zalcitabine
Dideoxyinosine. *See* Didanosine
DIDRONEL see Etidronate
Diethylcarbamazine, 361*f*
Diethyl ether, 107
Diethylstilbestrol, 263, *263,* 263*f*, 268
adverse effects, 266
in cancer therapy, 394
Diflunisal (DOLOBID), 401*f*, 403, *403,* 406, 408
therapeutic advantages and disadvantages, 412*f*
Digitalis, **157-161**
distribution, 11
drug interactions, 160*f*, 184, 214, 339
epinephrine and, 63
mechanism of action, 158*f*
ventricular function curves, 159*f*
Digitoxin, 151*f*, 158, *158*
drug interactions, 334*f*
properties, 160*f*
Digoxin (LANOXIN), 151*f*, 158, *158,* 163*f*, 439-441
antiarrhythmic effects, 164*f*, 174
for congestive heart failure, 159
drug interactions, 156, 160*f*, 169, 188, 213, 320, 352, 395, 410
properties, 160*f*
verapamil and, 177
Dihydroergotamine, 419*f*, **428,** *428*
Dihydropyridines, 187-188
5-α-Dihydrotestosterone (DHT), 270
Dihydroxyphenylalanine, in norepinephrine synthesis, 55
Diisopropylflurophosphate. *See* Isoflurophate
DILACOR. *See* Diltiazem
DILANTIN. *See* Phenytoin
Diloxanide furoate, 345*f*, **348,** *348*
drug interactions, 347
sites of action, 346*f*
Diltiazem (CARDIZEM CD, DILACOR XR), 163*f*, **173,** *173,* 175*f*, **177,** *177,* 180*f*, 187, *187*
actions, 187*f*
for angina, 188*f*
drug interactions, 188*f*
effects, 173*f*
for hypertension, 188*f*
for supraventricular tachyarrhythmia, 188*f*
Dimenhydrinate, 419*f*, *424*
antiemetic effects, 129*f*
for motion sickness, 242, 424
therapeutic advantages and disadvantages, 422*f*
Dimercaprol, drug interactions, 414
Dinoprost, *419,* **419,** 419*f*-420*f*
Dinoprostone, *419,* **419,** 419*f*-420*f*
Diphenhydramine, 96, 419*f*, 423, *424,* 438
in combination therapy, 243, 243*f*
drug interactions, 392
for motion sickness, 424
preanesthetic, 108
for rhinitis, 221
therapeutic advantages and disadvantages, 422*f*
Diphenhydrinate, therapeutic advantages and disadvantages, 422*f*
Diphenoxylate, 244, *244,* 244*f*
for diarrhea, 235
Diphenylalkalines, 187
Diphenylhydantoin. *See* Phenytoin
Dipyridamole (PERSANTINE), 193*f*, **196,** *196*
Discoid lupus erythematosus, treatment, 351
Disease modifying antirheumatic drugs, 467
Disopyramide, 163*f*, **169,** *169*
effects, 167*f*
Distribution, drug, 1, 1*f*, 7-9, **7-9**
with elimination, 10*f*
volume, 9*f*, **9-11**
and elimination, 25
without elimination, 10*f*
Disulfiram, **96**
drug interactions, 201*f*
Dithromycin, 317, *317*
Diuretics, **157**
and changes in urine composition, 233*f*
for hypertension, with concomitant diseases, 182*f*
sites of action, 224*f*

Diuretics, specific agents, 151*f*, 179*f*, 223*f*
acetazolamide, 41, 223*f*-224*f*, 226*f*, **226-227,** 233*f*, 292
amiloride, 223*f*-224*f*, *233,* **233**
bumetanide (BUMEX), 151*f*, 179*f*, 223*f*-224*f*, *227,* **227-228,** 292, 316
chlorothiazide, 223*f*, 224, **229-231,** *231*
chlorthalidone, 223*f*, 229, **231,** *231*
ethacrynic acid, 224*f*, *227,* **227-228,** 316
furosemide (LASIX), 151*f*, 179*f*, 223*f*, 224, 224*f*, *227,* **227-228,** 292, 316, 409, 439-441
hydrochlorothiazide, 151*f*, 179*f*, 183, *183,* 223*f*, 229, **231,** 441
indapamide (LOZOL), 223*f*, **231,** *231*
mannitol, 223*f*, 233, *233*
metolazone, 151*f*, 223*f*, **231,** *231*
spironolactone, 179*f*, 183, *183,* 223*f*-224*f*, **232-233,** *233,* 274, 277
torsemide, 223*f*-224*f*, *227,* **227-228**
triamterene (DYAZIDE), 179*f*, 223*f*-224*f*, *233,* **233**
urea, 223*f*, 233, *233*
Dobutamine, 55*f*, **66,** *66,* 69*f*, 151*f*
for congestive heart failure, 159, 161, 161*f*
Docusate sodium, 244*f*, 245
DOLOBID. *See* Diflunisal
Domperidone, 242*f*
antiemetic effects, 129*f*
for chemotherapy-induced nausea and vomiting, 242-243
DONNATAL. *See* Atropine
DOPA. *See* Dihydroxyphenylalanine
L-Dopa. *See* Levodopa
Dopamine, 55*f*, *65,* **65-66,** 69*f*
actions, 66*f*, 248*f*
for congestive heart failure, 161*f*
and neurotransmission, 56
structure, 61*f*
Dopaminergic neurons, and Parkinson's disease, 84-85, 85*f*
Dose-response curve, **21,** 21*f*
Dose-response quantitation, 20-22
Douche, percent use, 268*f*
Doxacurium, 45*f*
onset and duration of action, 52*f*
pharmacokinetics, 51
Doxazosin (CARDURA), 71*f*, **73,** *73,* 180*f*
Doxepin, 96, 119, *119,* 119*f*
therapeutic advantages and disadvantages, 125*f*
Doxorubicin, 373*f*, *385,* 385*f*, **385-386,** 399*f*
actions, 374*f*
adverse effects, 378
drug interactions, 242
emetic potential, 241*f*
for Kaposi's sarcoma, 429
myelosuppressive potential, 378*f*
Doxycycline (VIBRAMYCIN), 311*f*, 313, *313*
for cholera, 312*f*
drug interactions, 147
phototoxicity, 314
for urinary tract infections, 328*f*
Doxylamine, 96
therapeutic advantages and disadvantages, 422*f*
Dronabinol, **105,** *105,* 242*f*, 243, *243*
Droperidol, 117, 130, *130,* 242*f*
antiemetic effects, 129*f*
for chemotherapy-induced nausea and vomiting, 242-243
in combination therapy, 243*f*
drug interactions, 139
plus fentanyl, 108*f*
preanesthetic, 108
Drug binding, to proteins, 8-9, **11-12**
Drug receptors, 17-26
Drug structure
chemical, 8
and distribution, 8
d4T. *See* Stavudine
Duodenal ulcers, treatment, 239-241
DURICEF. *See* Cefadroxil
DYAZIDE. *See* Triamterene
DYNACIRC. *See* Isradipine
Dysphoria, treatment, 243
Dysrhythmias. *See* Arrhythmias
Echothiophate, 35*f*, **43,** *43*
for glaucoma, 41
Eclampsia, treatment, 95
Econazole, 337*f*, **343,** *343*
Edema
kidney function during, 226
treatment, 223, 229, 440-441
Edrophonium, 35*f*, **43,** *43,* 433, 434*f*
drug interactions, 51
and neuromuscular blockers, 50
E.E.S. *See* Erythromycin
Efavirenz, 462
Efferent neurons, **28,** 28*f*
ELAVIL. *See* Amitriptyline
Elimination, drug, 1, 1*f*, **23-25**
by kidney, 23, 23*f*
Emboli, 194. *See also* Pulmonary embolism
treatment, 201
Emesis, chemotherapy-induced, 241*f*, 242
treatment, 241-243, 242*f*
Emetine, 345*f*, **348,** *348*
sites of action, 346*f*
Emodin, 244
Emodinmega, 244
E-MYCIN. *See* Erythromycin
Enalapril (VASOTEC), 151*f*, 156, *156,* 179*f*
success rate, 157*f*
Enanthate, 271
ENBREL see Etanercept
Endocarditis, treatment, 315
Endometriosis, treatment, 270
Enflurane, 107*f*, *113,* **113-114**
blood/gas partition coefficient, 111*f*
characteristics, 114*f*
minimal alveolar concentration, 111*f*
therapeutic advantages and disadvantages, 116*f*
uptake curve, 112, 112*f*
Enoxacin, **324,** *324,* 326-327
Enoxaprin, 193*f*, 198, *199*
adverse effects, 199
Entamoeba histolytica infection, 345-346
life cycle, 346
treatment, 347-348
Enteral administration, **2**
Enteric rods, gram-negative, 283*f*, 290*f*
Enterobacter infection, treatment, 290, 301*f*, 304, 315*f*, 325*f*, 361*f*
Enterobius vermicularis infection, 361*f*
treatment, 359
Enterococcal endocarditis, treatment, 284*f*
Enterococcus faecalis infection
resistance, 308
treatment, 435
Enterococcus faecium infection, resistance, 308
ENTEX LA. *See* Phenylephrine
Ephedrine, 55*f*, **68,** *68,* 69*f*
as mixed-action agonist, 61
non-catecholamine, 60
structure, 60*f*
Epidermophyton infection (epidermophytosis), treatment, 343, 406
Epilepsy
classification, 144*f*, **144-145**
drug treatment, **143-150, 445**
etiology, 143
primary, **143**

secondary, **143**
treatment, 90-91, 227
Epinephrine, **33,** 55*f*, *61,* **61-63,** 69*f*
for acute anaphylaxis, 218
administration route, 3
and adrenergic receptors, 58*f*, 58-59
and amine nitrogen, 61
with anesthesia, 118
antiarrhythmic effects, 164*f*
in autonomic nervous system, 32*f*
and bronchodilation, 67*f*
and carbachol, 40
cardiovascular effects, 63*f*
as direct-acting agonist, 61
effect on blood pressure, 72*f*
for glaucoma, 41
and histamines, 424
reversal, 72
structure, 60*f*-61*f*
Eptifibatide, 447
Equilin, 263
Erectile dysfunction, 477
treatment, 420, 477
Ergotamine, 419*f*, **428,** *428,* 437
for migraine, 427*f*
Erosive esophagitis, treatment, 239
ERYC. *See* Erythromycin
ERY-TAB. *See* Erythromycin
Erythromycin (E.E.S., ERYC, E-MYCIN, ERY-TAB), 311*f*, 317, *317,* 317-320, 435
antimicrobial activity, 317, 319*f*
contraindications, 282
drug interactions, 148*f*, 215
for mycoplasma pneumonia, 312*f*
therapeutic applications, 290, 318*f*
for urinary tract infections, 328*f*
Erythromycin base, drug interactions, 160*f*
Erythromycin ethylsuccinate, 434
Erythropoietin, 193*f*, **206,** *206*
for Kaposi's sarcoma, 429
Escherichia coli infection, 290*f*, 327
and insulin, 257
resistance, 300
treatment, 294*f*, 301*f*, 304, 308, 308*f*, 315*f*, 324, 325*f*, 329
Esmolol, **77,** *77,* 163*f*, **171,** *171*
clinical applications, 78*f*
drug elimination, 74*f*
Estazolam, duration of action, 92*f*
ESTRACE. *See* Estradiol
ESTRADERM. *See* Estradiol
Estradiol (ESTRACE, ESTRADERM), 263, *263,* 263*f*, 270
menstrual cycle and, 266, 267*f*
metabolism, 265
transdermal path for, 264
Estriol, 263, *263,* 263*f*
Estrogen replacement therapy, 264, 265*f*
Estrogens (PREMARIN), 263, **263-266,** 268, 373*f*, 399*f*
adverse effects, 266, 266*f*
in cancer therapy, 394
failure rate, 268*f*
Estrogens, specific agents, 263*f*
chlorotrianisene, 263, *263,* 263*f*
diethylstilbestrol, 263, *263,* 263*f*, 266, 268, 394
estradiol (ESTRACE, ESTRADERM), 263, *263,* 263*f*, 264-266, 267*f*, 270
estriol, 263, *263,* 263*f*
estrone, 263, *263,* 263*f*
ethinyl estradiol (TRI-LEVLIN, DEMULEN, LO/OVRAL, OVCON, TRI-NORINYL, TRIPHASIL, LOESTRIN-FE, DESOGEN), 263, **263,** 263*f*, 265, 268, 394
mestranol, 263*f*, *265,* 268
quinestrol, 263, *263,* 263*f*
Estrone, 263, *263,* 263*f*
Etanercept, 468
Ethacrynic acid, 223*f*, *227,* **227-228**
drug interactions, 316
site of action, 224*f*
Ethambutol, 331, 331*f*, *334,* **334-335,** 437
adverse effects, 335*f*
Ethanol
dependence potential, 100*f*
metabolism, 13
Ethanol, 96
Ethanolamines, therapeutic advantages and disadvantages, 422*f*
Ether, minimal alveolar concentration, 111*f*
Ethinyl estradiol (TRI-LEVLIN, DEMULEN, LO/OVRAL, OVCON, TRI-NORINYL, TRIPHASIL, LOESTRIN-FE, DESOGEN), 263, **263,** 263*f*, 265, 268
in cancer therapy, 394
pharmacokinetics, 268
Ethionamide, 331*f*, **335,** *335*
Ethosuximide, 143*f*, **149,** *149*
for seizures, 145*f*
Ethylenediamines, therapeutic advantages and disadvantages, 422*f*
Etidronate, 476
Etodolac (LODINE), 401*f*, *409,* **410**
Etomidate, 108*f*, 116, *116*
Etoposide, 373*f*, *396,* **396,** 399*f*
drug interactions, 386
emetic potential, 241*f*
mechanism of action, 397*f*
myelosuppressive potential, 378*f*
EVISTA see Raloxifene
Ewing's soft tissue sarcoma, 390
Excitatory postsynaptic potentials (EPSP), 82, 82*f*
Exophthalmos, treatment, 435*f*, 435-436
Famciclovir, 363*f*, **367,** *367,* 458
Familial combined (mixed) hyperlipidemia, 209*f*. *See also* Hyperlipoproteinemia, type IIB
Familial dysbetalipoproteinemia, 209*f*. *See also* Hyperlipoproteinemia, type III
treatment, 211
Familial hypercholesterolemia, 209*f*. *See also* Hyperlipoproteinemia, type IIA
combination drug therapy, 215, 215*f*
Familial hyperchylomicronemia, 209*f*. *See also* Hyperlipoproteinemia, type I
Familial hypertriglyceridemia, 209*f*. *See also* Hyperlipoproteinemia, type IV
Familial mixed hypertriglyceridemia, 209*f*. *See also* Hyperlipoproteinemia, type IV
Famotidine (PEPCID), 235*f*, *236,* **236-238,** 419*f*, 440, 440*f*
Fansidar, 352
FASTIN see Phentermine
Fatigue, treatment, 441-442
5-FC. *See* Flucytosine
Febrile seizures, **144,** 144*f*-145*f*
treatment, 148
FELDENE. *See* Piroxicam
Felodipine, 180*f*, 188, *188*
for congestive heart failure, **157,** 188*f*
drug interactions, 188*f*
for hypertension, 188*f*
Fenamates, 401*f*, **410**
therapeutic advantages and disadvantages, 412*f*
Fenoprofen, 401*f*, *408,* **408-409**
drug interactions, 327
therapeutic advantages and disadvantages, 412*f*
Fentanyl, 108*f*, 117, 133*f*, **139,** *139*
action, 134*f*
distribution, 137
efficacy and addiction/abuse liability, 135*f*
onset and duration of action, 139*f*
preanesthetic, 108
therapeutic advantages and disadvantages, 116*f*
Ferrous sulfate, for anemia, 205
Fetal distress, drug contraindications, 251
Fetal presentation, abnormal, drug

contraindications, 251
Fever, treatment, 432
Fexofenadine, 470
Fibrinolysis, 194
Fibrinogen, 446
Fibrin, role in clotting, 194
Filariasis, treatment, 361*f*
Filgrastim
drug interactions, 392
for Kaposi's sarcoma, 429
for neutropenia, 378
Finasteride, 272, *272*
for benign prostatic hypertrophy, 73
FIORINAL. *See* Butalbital
Flecainide, 163*f*, **170,** *170*
effects, 170*f*
FLOXIN. *See* Ofloxacin
Fluconazole, 337*f*, **341-342,** *342*
for Kaposi's sarcoma, 429
properties, 342*f*
Flucytosine, 337*f*, *339*, **339-340**
for cryptococcal meningitis, 284*f*
drug interactions, 337, 340
mode of action, 339, 339*f*
Fludarabine, 373*f*, **384,** *384*
Fludrocortisone, 274, *274*
properties, 275*f*
Flumazenil, 90*f*, **94,** *94*
Flunisolide (NASACORT), *219*
for asthma, 219
for rhinitis, 221
Fluoroquinolones, **323-327, 456**
classification, 287*f*
effect on children, 282
resistance to, 285*f*
Fluoroquinolones, specific agents, 323*f*
clinafloxacin, 456*f*
ciprofloxacin (CIPRO), 300, 323, *323*, **324,** 325, 325*f*, 326
enoxacin, **324,** *324*, 326-327
lomefloxacin, **324,** *324*, 325
norfloxacin (NOROXIN), 323, *323*, **324,** 325, 325*f*, 326
ofloxacin (FLOXIN), **324,** *324*, 325-326
sparfloxacin, 456
trovaflaxacin, 456
5-Fluorouracil, 373*f*, *382*, **382-383,** 399*f*
actions, 374*f*
drug interactions, 242
emetic potential, 241*f*
mechanism of action, 383*f*
myelosuppressive potential, 378*f*
Fluoxetine (PROZAC), 119*f*, *122*, **122-123**
adverse effects, 123*f*
and p-450 metabolism, 122*f*
receptor specificity, 121*f*
therapeutic advantages and disadvantages, 125*f*
Fluoxymesterone, 263*f*, 271, *271*
Fluphenazine, 127, *127*, 127*f*, 132*f*
actions, 128*f*
anticholinergic activity, 130
schizophrenia relapse after, 131*f*
Fluphenazine decanoate, metabolism, 130
Flurazepam, *91*
duration of action, 92*f*
for sleep disorders, 91
as sleep-inducer, 137
therapeutic advantages and disadvantages, 97*f*
withdrawal reactions, 92, 93*f*
Flurbiprofen (ANSAID), 401*f*, *408*, **408-409**
Flutamide, 373*f*, 399*f*
as antiandrogen, 272, *272*
in cancer therapy, *394*, 394-395
Fluticasone
administration route, 276*f*
elimination, 276*f*
for rhinitis, 221
Fluvastatin, 207*f*, *214*, **214-215,** 449
drug interactions, 213
Fluvoxamine, 119*f*, 123, *123*
therapeutic advantages and disadvantages, 125*f*
Folate antagonists, **289-296**
Folate antagonists, specific agents, 289*f*
cotrimoxazole (COTRIM), 201*f*, 289, *289*, 289*f*, 290, **293-295,** 299*f*, 429
mafenide, 289*f*, 290
mafenide acetate, 291
pyrimethamine, 289*f*, 290, *290*, 293, 345*f*, 350*f*, 352-353, 357, *357*
silver sulfadiazine, 289*f*, 290-291
succinylsulfathiazole, 289*f*, 291, *291*
sulfacetamide, 289*f*, 290
sulfadiazine, 290
sulfamethoxazole, 289, *289*, 289*f*, 290, 293, 293*f*, 294, 315*f*. *See also* Co-trimoxazole
sulfasalazine, 289*f*, 291, *291*
sulfisoxazole, 289*f*, 290, 292, *292*, 328*f*
trimethoprim (BACTRIM), 20, 205, 281, 281*f*, 285, 285*f*, 287*f*, 289, *289*, 289*f*, 290, 292*f*, 293, *293*, **293,** 293*f*, 294, 315*f*. *See also* Co-trimoxazole
Folate reduction inhibitors, 289*f*
Folate synthesis inhibitors, 289*f*
Folic acid, 193*f*, **205**
deficiency, 205*f*
with vitamin B_{12}, 205
Folinic acid, 379
for megaloblastic anemia, 378
Follicle-stimulating hormone, 250, **250**
secretion, 250, 250*f*
5-Formyltetrahydrofolic acid. *See* Folinic acid
FORTASE see Saquinavir
FOSAMAX see Alendronate
Foscarnet, 363*f*, **367,** *367*, 458
Fosinopril, 151*f*
5-Fu. *See* 5-Fluorouracil
Furosemide (LASIX), 151*f*, 179*f*, 223*f*, *227*, **227-228,** 439-441
drug interactions, 292, 316, 409
hyperuricemia with, 224
site of action, 224*f*
Gabapentin, 143*f*, *149*, **149-150**
GABITRIL see Tiagabine
Ganciclovir (DHPG), 363*f*, *366*, **366-367,** 458
Ganglionic blockers, **48-50,** 49*f*
Ganglionic blockers, specific agents
mecamylamine, 45*f*, 49*f*, **50,** *50*
trimethaphan, 45*f*, *49*, **49,** 49*f*
Gastric acid secretion, regulation, 236
Gastric cancer, treatment, 382
Gastroesophageal reflux disease, treatment, 237
Gastrointestinal drugs, **235-246**
Gastrointestinal tract
absorption in, 4
infections, treatment, 325*f*
Gatifloxacin, 456
Gemcitabine, 464
Gemfibrozil (LOPID), 207*f*, *211*, **211-212**
drug interactions, 215
mechanism of action, 211, 211*f*
GEMZAR see Gemcitabine
General anesthetics, 107*f*-108*f*
inhaled, 107*f*
intravenous, 108*f*
General anesthetics, specific agents
diazepam (VALIUM), 50, 90, *90*, 90*f*, 91, *91*, 92*f*-93*f*, 97*f*, 103, 108, 108*f*, 116, 143*f*, 145*f*, 149, 239
droperidol plus fentanyl, 108*f*
enflurane, 107*f*, 111*f*, 112, 112*f*, *113*, **113-114,** 114*f*, 116*f*
etomidate, 108*f*, 116, *116*
fentanyl, 108, 108*f*, 116*f*, 117, 133*f*-135*f*, 137, *139*, **139,** 139*f*
halothane, 51, 53, 67, 107*f*, 111, 111*f*, 112, 112*f*, *113*, **113,** 114*f*, 116*f*

isoflurane, 107*f*, 111*f*, 112, 112*f*, *114*, **114,** 114*f*, 116*f*
ketamine, 108*f*, 116*f*, *117*, **117**
lorazepam (ATIVAN), 92*f*-93*f*, 97*f*, 108*f*, 116, 242*f*, 243, 243*f*
methohexital, 108*f*, *115*
methoxyflurane, 107*f*, **114,** *114*
morphine, 90*f*, 100*f*, 108*f*, 117, 133*f*-135*f*, **135-138,** 139, 139*f*, 141, 141*f*, 142
nitrous oxide, 107*f*, 111, 111*f*, 112, 112*f*, 113, *114*, 114*f*, **114-115,** 116*f*, 117
propofol, 108*f*, 116*f*, *117*, **117**
sevoflurane, 107*f*, **115,** *115*
thiamylal, 108*f*, *115*
thiopental, 9, 90*f*, *94*, 95, 97*f*, 108*f*, 109, 115, 115*f*, 115-116, 116*f*, 408*f*
Genital infections, treatment, 294*f*
Gentamicin, 311*f*, 315, *315*, 435
adverse effects, 316
drug interactions, 51
therapeutic applications, 315*f*
Gestational choriocarcinoma, treatment, 384
GHRH. *See* Growth hormone releasing hormone
Giardia lamblia infection, 357
treatment, 347
Glaucoma
concomitant with hypertension, treatment, 185
treatment, 41-42, 63, 74-76, 78*f*, 227
Glimepiride, 452
Glipizide (GLOUCOTROL), 255*f*, 260, *260*
properties, 261*f*
Glucocorticoids, **272-273**
inhaled, for asthma, 218*f*-219*f*
production, 272
properties, 275*f*
α-Glucosidase inhibitor, **261**
GLUCOTROL. *See* Glipizide
Glutethimide, drug interactions, 201*f*
Glyburide (DIABETA, MICRONASE, GLYNASE PRESTAB), 255*f*, 260, *260*
properties, 261*f*
Glycerine suppositories, 244*f*, 245
GLYNASE. *See* Glyburide
Gold salts, 402*f*, **413-414**
Gold sodium thiomalate, 413-414
Gonadal hormone, 250
Gonadotropin-releasing hormone (GnRH), 247*f*, **250**
actions, 248*f*
and testosterone, 270
Gonadotropins, **250**
Gonococcal ophthalmia, treatment, 299*f*
Gonococcal urethritis, acute, treatment, 294*f*
Gonorrhea
oropharyngeal, treatment, 294*f*
treatment, 294*f*, 299*f*, 324, 325*f*
Goserelin, 247*f*, 250, *250*, 373*f*, *394*, 395*f*
in cancer therapy, 394
drug interactions, 395
Goserelin acetate, 394
Gout
chronic, 416
treatment, 406, 412, **415-417**
specific agents, 402*f*
Gouty arthritis, acute, treatment, 409
Gouty attacks, acute, treatment, 410, 415-416
GP IIb/IIIa receptor, 446
Gram-negative microorganisms
bacilli, 283*f*
cocci, 283*f*
enteric rods, 283*f*, 290*f*
identification, 279-280, 280*f*
resistance, 284
Gram-positive microorganisms
bacilli, 283*f*
cocci, 283*f*
identification, 279-280, 280*f*
Grand mal seizures. *See* Seizures, tonic-clonic
Granisetron, 242*f*, 243, *243*
Granulocyte stimulating factor, for Kaposi's sarcoma, 429-430
Grepafloxacin, 456
Griseofulvin, 337*f*, *342*, **342-343,** 343*f*
drug interactions, 201*f*
Group IA agents, 167
effects, 167*f*
Group IB agents, 167, 169
effects, 169*f*
Group IC agents, 167, 170
effects, 170*f*
Growth fractions, of tumors, 374
Growth hormone, **249**
Growth hormone-inhibiting hormone (GHIH), **250**
Growth hormone-releasing hormone (GHRH), 247*f*, 249
actions, 248*f*
Guanethidine, 71*f*, *78*, **78-79**
and norepinephrine release, 56
Haemophilus influenzae infection
resistance, 300
treatment, 294*f*, 301*f*, 304, 306, 317-318, 324, 325*f*
Hairy cell leukemia, treatment, 384, 398
HALCION. *See* Triazolam
Hallucinogens, **104-105**
dependence potential, 100*f*
Halogenated hydrocarbon anesthetics, drug interactions, 51
Haloperidol, 127, *127*, 127*f*, 132*f*, 242*f*
actions, 128*f*
affinities at dopaminergic receptors, 131*f*
anticholinergic activity, 130
antiemetic effects, 129*f*
for chemotherapy-induced nausea and vomiting, 242-243
and LSD, 105
and parkinsonian symptoms, 84
for schizophrenia, 131
schizophrenia relapse after, 131*f*
Haloperidol decanoate
administration route, 3
metabolism, 130
Halothane, 107*f*, **113,** *113*
blood/gas partition coefficient, 111, 111*f*
characteristics, 114*f*
drug interactions, 51, 53
elimination, 112
methoxamine and, 67
minimal alveolar concentration, 111, 111*f*
therapeutic advantages and disadvantages, 116*f*
uptake curve, 112, 112*f*
Hansen's disease. *See* Leprosy
Headache, treatment, 406, 412, 437-438
Heartburn, treatment, 237
Heart rate, and acetylcholine, 39
Heavy metal poisoning, treatment, 414
Helicobacter pylori infection, 439
elimination, 239-240
and peptic ulcer disease, 235-236, 236*f*
Helminthic infections
chemotherapy, 359*f*
incidence, 360*f*
Hemicholinium, and acetylcholine, 35
Heparin, 193*f*, **197-199,** *199*
binding to antithrombin III, 198, 198*f*
drug interactions, 204, 339, 408*f*
Hepatic ascites, kidney function with, 226
Hepatitis A virus, treatment, 365
Hepatitis, treatment, specific agents, 363*f*
HERCEPTIN see Trastuzumab
Heroin, 133*f*, **140,** *140*
action, 134*f*

dependence potential, 100*f*
distribution, 137
naloxone and, 141*f*, 142
naltrexone and, 142
Heroin withdrawal, treatment, 139
Herpesvirus, 457
Herpes simplex encephalitis, treatment, 367*f*
Herpes simplex virus type 1, treatment, 367
Herpes simplex virus type 2, treatment, 367
Herpes virus infection, treatment, **365-368**
specific agents, 363*f*
Hexamethonium, and nicotinic receptors, 39
H_1-Histamine receptor antagonists
adverse effects, 424*f*
sites of action, 423*f*
specific agents, 419*f*
therapeutic advantages and disadvantages, 422*f*
Hiccups, treatment, 130
High-ceiling diuretics. *See* Loop diuretics
Hirsutism, treatment, 272
HISMANAL. *See* Astemizole
Histamine, 420-425
actions, 421*f*
biosynthesis, 421*f*
Histamine H_1-receptor antagonists, 423-425. *See also* Antihistamines
Histamine H_2-receptor antagonists, **425,** 440. *See also* Antihistamines
as gastric acid inhibitors, 236-238
for peptic ulcer disease, 235*f*
specific agents, 419*f*
Histoplasma capsulatum infection (histoplasmosis), treatment, 338, 342
Histrelin, 247*f*, 250, *250*
HIV protease inhibitors, 458
HMG-CoA reductase inhibitors, 449
Hodgkin's disease, 390
treatment, 388, 393, 396, 399*f*, 409
Hookworm infection, treatment, 359, 361*f*
Hormones, **31**
Hormones, specific agents
androgens, 263*f*, 270, *270*, 271, *271*
danazol, 263*f*, 270, *270*, 271
fluoxymesterone, 263*f*, 271, *271*
nandrolone, 263*f*, 271, *271*
stanozolol, 263*f*, 271, *271*
testosterone cypionate, 263*f*, 271, *271*
antiandrogens, 73, 272, *272*, 373*f*, *394*, 394-395, 399*f*
cyproterone acetate, 272, *272*
finasteride, 73, 272, *272*
flutamide, 272, *272*, 373*f*, *394*, 394-395, 399*f*
antiestrogens, 263*f*, *266*, **266,** *266*, 373*f*, *393*, **393-394,** 399*f*
clomiphene, 263*f*, **266,** *266*
tamoxifen (NOLVADEX), 263*f*, **266,** *266*, 373*f*, *393*, **393-394,** 399*f*
antiprogestin, 263*f*, 267-268, 277
mifepristone, 263*f*, 267-268, 277
corticosteroids, 219, 221, 235, 242*f*, 243, 243*f*, 274, *274*, 275*f*, 275*f*, 276, *276*, 276*f*, 276*f*, 277, 334*f*, 362, 373*f*, 392-393, **393,** *393*, 395, 397, 399*f*, 431, 438-439
beclomethasone (BECONASE, VANCENASE, VANCERIL), 219, 221, 276*f*, 431
beclomethasone dipropionate, 276, *276*
betamethasone, 275*f*, 438-439
cortisone, 275*f*, 276*f*
desoxycorticosterone, 276*f*
dexamethasone, 235, 242*f*, 243, 243*f*, 275*f*-276*f*, 276*f*, 277, 362, 392, 395
fludrocortisone, 274, *274*, 275*f*
hydrocortisone, 274, *274*, 275*f*-276*f*, 438-439
methylprednisolone, 219, 242*f*, 243, 275*f*-276*f*
paramethasone, 275*f*
prednisolone, 275*f*, 393
prednisone (DELTASONE, ORASONE), 219, 275*f*, 276, 334*f*, 373*f*, *393*, **393,** 397, 399*f*, 438-439
triamcinolone (AZMACORT), 219, 221, 275*f*, 276, *276*, 276*f*
corticotropin (ACTH), 247*f*, **249,** *249*, 249*f*
desmopressin, 3, 247*f*, **251,** *251*
estrogens, 263, *263*, **263,** *263*, 263*f*, 263*f*, 264-266, *265*, 266, 267*f*, 268, 270, 394
chlorotrianisene, 263, *263*, 263*f*
diethylstilbestrol, 263, *263*, 263*f*, 266, 268, 394
estradiol (ESTRACE, ESTRADERM), 263, *263*, 263*f*, 264-266, 267*f*, 270
estriol, 263, *263*, 263*f*
estrone, 263, *263*, 263*f*
ethinyl estradiol (TRI-LEVLIN, DEMULEN, LO/OVRAL, OVCON, TRI-NORINYL, TRIPHASIL, LOESTRIN-FE, DESOGEN), 263, **263,** 263*f*, 265, 268, 394
mestranol, 263*f*, *265*, 268
quinestrol, 263, *263*, 263*f*
gonadotropin-releasing hormone (GnRH), 247*f*-248*f*, **250,** 270
goserelin, 247*f*, 250, *250*, 373*f*, 394, *394*, 395, 395*f*
growth hormone-releasing hormone (GHRH), 247*f*-248*f*, 249
histrelin, 247*f*, 250, *250*
leuprolide, 247*f*, 250, *250*, 373*f*, 394, *394*, 395, 395*f*, 399*f*
luteinizing hormone-releasing hormone (LHRH), 247*f*-248*f*
nafarelin, 247*f*, 250, *250*
octreotide, 247*f*, **250,** *250*
oxytocin, 247*f*, 250, **251,** *251*
progestins, 3, 263*f*, 267, *267*, 268, 268*f*-269*f*
hydroxyprogesterone, 263*f*, 267, *267*
levonorgestrel, 3, 268, 269*f*
medroxyprogesterone (PROVERA), 263*f*, 267, *267*
norethindrone, 263*f*, 267, *267*, 268
norgestrel, 263*f*, 267, *267*, 268, 268*f*
somatostatin, 247*f*-248*f*, **250**
somatotropin, 247*f*, **249,** *249*
vasopressin, 247*f*, 250, **251,** *251*
5-HT_3 Serotonin receptor blockers, for chemotherapy-induced nausea and vomiting, 242*f*, 243
Human chorionic gonadotropin (hCG), **250**
Human immunodeficiency virus
anemia with, treatment, 206
treatment, **368-371**
specific agents, 363*f*
Human immunodeficiency virus protease inhibitors, **371**
Human insulin (HUMULIN N), 257
Human menopausal gonadotropin (hMG), **250**
HUMULIN. *See* Human insulin
HYCAMTIN see Topotecan
Hydralazine, 151*f*, 180*f*, **190,** *190*, 442
for congestive heart failure, 157
Hydrochlorothiazide, 151*f*, 179*f*, 183, *183*, 223*f*, 229, **231,** 441
Hydrocodone, for cough, 222
Hydrocortisone, 274, *274*, 438-439
administration route, 276*f*
elimination, 276*f*
properties, 275*f*

Hydromorphone, for cough, 222
Hydrophilic colloids, 244*f*, 244-245
Hydroxychloroquine, as antiinflammatory agent, 414
Hydroxymethylglutaryl-CoA reductase inhibitors, 214*f*, **214-215, 440**
 adverse effects, 215*f*
Hydroxyprogesterone, 263*f*
Hydroxyprogesterone acetate, 267, *267*
Hydroxyurea, 193*f*
 for sickle cell disease, 193, 206
Hydroxyzine, **93,** *93*
 drug interactions, 138
 therapeutic advantages and disadvantages, 97*f*, 422*f*
Hyoscyamine, 236*f*
 for peptic ulcer disease, 239
Hyperaldosteronism
 secondary, 226
  treatment, 232
 treatment, 274, 277
Hypercalcemia, treatment, 228
Hypercalciuria, treatment, 230
Hypercholesterolemia
 type IIA, treatment, 213
 type IIB, treatment, 213
Hypercholesterolemias, treatment, 210
Hyperlipidemias, 207, 208*f*-209*f*
 and hypertension, 182*f*-183*f*
 primary, 207
 secondary, 207
 treatment, 214
 type I, 209*f*
 type IIA, 209*f*
 type IIB, 209*f*
 type III, 209*f*
 type II, treatment, 215
 type IV, 209*f*
 type V, 209*f*
Hyperlipoproteinemia
 treatment, 210
 type IIA, treatment, 212
 type IIB, treatment, 210, 212
 type III, treatment, 211
 type IV, treatment, 210-211
 type V, treatment, 211
Hypertension
 and angina, 178*f*
 concomitant disease with, 183*f*
 etiology, 179
 treatment, 73, 75-78, 78*f*, 173, 188*f*, 223, 230-231, 441-442
 treatment strategies, 181-183
  with concomitant diseases, 182*f*
Hypertensive emergency, **191**
Hyperthyroidism, 252
 and epinephrine, 63
 treatment, 75, 253-254
Hypertriglyceridemias, treatment, 211
Hyperuricemia, 415
 treatment, 417
Hypnotic drugs, **89-98**
 specific agents, 89*f*-90*f*
Hypoalbuminemia, and drug binding, 11
Hypochromic microcytic anemia, and folate deficiency, 205
Hypoglycemic drugs
 oral, 255*f*, **255-262, 260-261**
  adverse effects, 261*f*
  drug interactions, 260*f*
 oral, specific agents
  acetohexamide, 255*f*, 260, *260,* 261*f*
  chlorpropamide, 255*f*, *260,* 260-261, 261*f*
  glimepiride, 452
  glipizide (GLOUCOTROL), 255*f*, 260, *260,* 261*f*
  glyburide (DIABETA, MICRONASE, GLYNASE PRESTAB), 255*f*, 260, *260,* 261*f*
  metformin, 255*f*, **261,** *261,* 261*f*
  repaglinide, 452
  rosiglitazone, 453
  tolazamide, 255*f*, 260, *260,* 261*f*
  tolbutamide, 255*f*, 260, *260,* 261*f*, 292, 341
  troglitazone, 453
 properties, 261*f*
Hypoglycemic drugs, specific agents
 human insulin (HUMULIN N), 257
 insulin, 2-3, 7, 77, 255*f*, **255-262,** *257,* **257-258,** 258*f*-259*f*, 259-260, 260*f*
 insulin zinc suspension, 255*f*
 intermediate action insulin preparations, **258-259**
 isophane insulin suspension (ILETIN), 255*f*, **258-259**
 lente insulin, **259**
 prolonged action insulin preparations, **259**
 rapid action insulin preparations, **258**
 semilente insulin, 255*f*, 259*f*
 semilente insulin suspension, **258**
 ultralente insulin, 255*f*, **259**
 zinc insulin, 255*f*
Hypogonadism
 primary, treatment, 264
 treatment, 270
Hypomania, treatment, 125
Hypothalamic hormones, 247*f*, **247-250**
 actions, 248*f*
Hypothyroidism, 251
 treatment, 253
HYTRIN. *See* Terazosin
Ibuprofen (ADVIL, MOTRIN), 401*f*, *408,* **408-409,** 440
 therapeutic advantages and disadvantages, 412*f*
Idarubicin, 373*f*, 385
Idoxuridine, **368,** *368*
IFN. *See* Interferon
Ifosfamide, 373*f*, *388,* **388-389,** 389*f*
ILETIN. *See* Insulin; Isophane
Imipenem, 298*f*, *306,* **306-307**
 structure, 307*f*
Imipramine, 119, *119,* 119*f*
 for arrhythmias, 171, 172*f*
 half-life, 120
 and norepinephrine removal, 56
 precautions, 121
 receptor specificity, 121*f*
 therapeutic advantages and disadvantages, 125*f*
IMITREX. *See* Sumatriptan
Immunosuppressants, 470
IMODIUM. *See* Loperamide
IMURAN see Azathioprine
Indapamide (LOZOL), 223*f*, **231,** *231*
INDERAL. *See* Propranolol
Indinavir, **371,** *371,* 458
Indoleacetic acids, **409-410**
 therapeutic advantages and disadvantages, 412*f*
Indomethacin, 401*f*, **409,** *409*
 adverse effects, 409*f*
 for diarrhea, 244, 244*f*
 drug interactions, 417
 therapeutic advantages and disadvantages, 412*f*
Infertility, treatment, 250
Infliximab, 469
Inflammation, treatment, 275-276
Inflammatory bowel disease, treatment, 291
Influenza A infection, treatment, 363, 364*f*, 365
Influenza B infection, treatment, 365
Inhalation administration, **3**
Inhibitory postsynaptic potentials (IPSP), 82-83, 83*f*
INNOVAR, 117
Inotropic drugs, **157-161**
 specific agents, 151*f*
Insomnia, treatment, 424, 435-436
Insulin, 255*f*, **255-262,** *257,* **257-258**

administration route, 2-3
adverse effects, 258, 258*f*
bioavailability, 7
β-blockers and, 77
extent and duration of action, 259*f*
intermediate-acting preparations, **258-259**
in pregnancy, 260
lispro 452
preparations, **258-260**
prolonged action preparations, **259**
rapid action preparations, **258**
standard vs. intensive treatment, 259-260, 260*f*
Insulin zinc suspension, 255*f*
INTAL. *See* Cromolyn
INTEGRILIN see Eptifibatide
Interferons, 363*f*, **371,** *371,* 371*f*, 373*f*, **397-398,** 399*f*, 458
Intra-arterial injection, **3**
Intramuscular (IM) administration, **3**
Intranasal administration, **3**
Intrathecal administration, **3**
Intrauterine device (IUD)
failure rate, 268*f*
percent use, 268*f*
Intravascular administration, **2-3**
Intravenous (IV) injection, **2-3,** 3*f*
kinetics, **17-19**
multiple, kinetics, 20, 20*f*
single, kinetics, 19, 20*f*
Intraventricular administration, **3**
Invermectin, 361*f*
contraindications, 359*f*
INVIRASE see Saquinavir
Iodide, 247*f*, 254
Ipratropium (ATROVENT), 45*f*, **48,** *48,* 49*f*, *220*
for asthma, 217*f*, 220
for chronic obstructive pulmonary disease, 217*f*, 222
structure, 220*f*
Iron, 193*f*, **205**
erythropoietin and, 206
Isocarboxazid, 119*f*, 123, *123*
therapeutic advantages and disadvantages, 125*f*
Isoflurane, 107*f*, **114,** *114*
blood/gas partition coefficient, 111*f*
characteristics, 114*f*
minimal alveolar concentration, 111*f*
therapeutic advantages and disadvantages, 116*f*
uptake curve, 112, 112*f*
Isoflurophate, 35*f*, **43,** *43*
for glaucoma, 41
and reactivation of acetylcholinesterase, 43, 43*f*
Isoniazid, 283, 283*f*, 331, 331*f*, *332,* **332-333,** 437
adverse effects, 333*f*
distribution, 332, 332*f*
drug interactions, 147, 147*f*-148*f*, 334, 335*f*
for tuberculosis, 284*f*
Isophane insulin suspension (ILETIN), 255*f*, **258-259**
Isoproterenol, 55*f*, *64,* **64-65,** 69*f*
actions, 66*f*
and adrenergic receptors, 58, 58*f*
and amine nitrogen, 61
blockage by β-blockers, 75
and bronchodilation, 67*f*
cardiovascular effects, 65*f*
as direct-acting agonist, 61
effect on blood pressure, 72*f*
structure, 61*f*
ISOPTIN. *See* Verapamil
ISORDIL. *See* Isosorbide
Isosorbide (ISORDIL), 151*f*
Isosorbide dinitrate, 175*f*, **176,** *176*
for congestive heart failure, **157**
onset and duration of action, 177*f*
Isosorbide mononitrate, onset of action, 176
Isradipine (DYNACIRC), 180*f*, 188, *188*
for congestive heart failure, 188*f*
drug interactions, 188*f*
for hypertension, 188*f*
Itraconazole, 337*f*, **342,** *342*
drug interactions, 215
properties, 342*f*
Ivermectin, 359*f*, **360,** *360*
Kaolin, 244, 244*f*
Kaposi's sarcoma, treatment, specific agents, 363*f*
K-DUR. *See* Potassium
KEFLEX. *See* Cephalexin
KEFTAB. *See* Cephalexin
Ketamine, 108*f*, **117,** *117*
therapeutic advantages and disadvantages, 116*f*
Ketoconazole (NIZORAL), 337*f*, *340,* **340-341**
as adrenocorticoid inhibitor, 277, *277*
as antiandrogen, 272
drug interactions, 334*f*
mode of action, 340*f*
properties, 342*f*
Ketoprofen (ORUDIS), 401*f*, *408,* **408-409**
drug interactions, 417
therapeutic advantages and disadvantages, 412*f*
Ketorolac (TORADOL), **411,** *411*
Kidney
collecting ducts, 225, 225*f*
collecting tubules, 225, 225*f*
distal convoluted tubule, 225
drug elimination by, 23, 23*f*
function during disease, 225-226
loop of Henle, 223-224
proximal convoluted tubule, 223-224
regulation of fluid and electrolytes by, 223-225
Klebsiella infection, resistance, 301
Klebsiella pneumonia infection, 327
treatment, 304, 315*f*, 325*f*, 433
KLONOPIN. *See* Clonazepam
KLOR-CON. *See* Potassium
Labetalol (NORMODYNE), 71*f*, **78,** *78,* 79*f*, 179*f*
drug elimination, 74*f*
for hypertensive emergency, 191
Labor, premature, terbutaline in, 67
β-Lactam antibiotics
classification, 287*f*
resistance to, 285*f*
specific agents, 298*f*
structure, 297*f*
β-Lactamase, drug interactions, 300
β-Lactamase inhibitors, **307-308**
β-Lactamase inhibitors, specific agents, 298*f*
clavulanic acid, 298*f*, 300, 300*f*, 301-302, *307,* **307-308,** 308*f*
sulbactam, 298*f*, 300, 300*f*, 302, 307, *307*
tazobactam, 298*f*, 300*f*, 301-302, 307, *307*
Lactulose, 244*f*, 245
Lamivudine, **370-371,** *371,* 458
Lamotrigine, 143*f*, *149,* **149-150**
Lanoprazole, 235*f*, 239, *239*
LANOXIN. *See* Digoxin
LASIX. *See* Furosemide
Lassa fever, treatment, 365
Laxatives, **244-245**
specific agents, 244*f*
Leflunomide, 467
Legionella infection, treatment, 294*f*, 317, 324, 325*f*, 326
Legionellosis. *See* Legionnaires' disease
Legionnaires' disease, treatment, 318*f*
Leishmaniasis

chemotherapy, 345*f*, **356-357**
treatment, 355
Lente insulin, **259**
extent and duration of action, 259*f*
Lepirudin, 448
Leprosy, treatment, 331*f*, **335-336**
Leptotrichia buccalis infection, treatment, 299*f*
Leucovorin, 379, 379*f*, 380. *See also* Folinic acid
for anemia, 353
drug interactions, 382, 415
myelosuppressive potential, 378*f*
Leukemia
acute lymphoblastic, treatment, 381, 390
acute lymphocytic, treatment, 3, 376-377, 379, 386, 393, 397, 399*f*
acute myelocytic, treatment, 386
acute non-lymphocytic (myelogenous), treatment, 382-383
chronic lymphocytic, treatment, 384
chronic myelogenous, for sickle cell disease, 206
treatment, specific agents, 363*f*
Leuprolide, 247*f*, 250, *250,* 373*f*, *394,* 395*f*, 399*f*
in cancer therapy, 394
drug interactions, 395
Levamisole, drug interactions, 382
Levarterenol, 64, *64*
Levodopa, 81*f*
and blood-brain barrier, 8
distribution, 8
dopamine synthesis with, 85*f*
drug interactions, 86*f*, 147, 240
for Parkinson's disease, 84-86
Levofloxacin, 456
Levonorgestrel, 268, 269*f*
administration route, 3
Levothyroxine (LEVOXYL), 247*f*, 253
LEVOXYL. *See* Levothyroxine
Lidocaine, 108*f*, 163*f*, *169,* **169**
as antiarrhythmic, 164*f*
for arrhythmias, 174
effects, 169*f*
with epinephrine, 3
metabolism, 7
pharmacokinetic properties, 117*f*
Lipase inhibitors, 475
LIPITOR see Atorvastatin
Lisinopril (ZESTRIL, PRINIVIL), 151*f*, 179*f*
Lispro insulin, 452
Listeria monocytogenes infection
resistance, 304
treatment, 299*f*, 300
Listeriosis, treatment, 299*f*
Lithium, drug interactions, 410
Lithium salts, **125**
Local anesthesia, 108*f*, **117-118**
cocaine as, 102
epinephrine in, 63
Local anesthetics, specific agents
bupivacaine, 108*f*, 117*f*
lidocaine, 3, 7, 108*f*, 117*f*, 163*f*-164*f*, *169,* **169,** 169*f*, 174
procaine, 108*f*, 117*f*
procaine penicillin G, 302
tetracaine, 108*f*, 117*f*
LODINE. *See* Etodolac
LOESTRIN-FE. *See* Ethinyl estradiol
Log kill, 374
Lomefloxacin, **324,** *324,* 325
Lomustine, 373*f*, *389,* **389-390**
Loop diuretics, 223*f*, **227-228**
adverse effects, 228*f*
and changes in urine composition, 227*f*, 233*f*
drug interactions, 160, 160*f*
LO/OVRAL. *See* Ethinyl estradiol
Loperamide (IMODIUM), 244, *244,* 244*f*
LOPID. *See* Gemfibrozil
LOPRESSOR. *See* Metoprolol
Loratidine (CLARITIN)
for rhinitis, 221
therapeutic advantages and disadvantages, 422*f*
Lorazepam (ATIVAN), 108*f*, 116, 242*f*
for chemotherapy-induced nausea and vomiting, 243
in combination therapy, 243*f*
duration of action, 92*f*
therapeutic advantages and disadvantages, 97*f*
withdrawal reactions, 93*f*
Losartan, 179*f*, **187,** *187*
LOTENSIN. *See* Quinapril
Lovastatin (MEVACOR), 207*f*, *214,* **214-215,** 449
LOZOL. *See* Indapamide
Lung cancer
oat cell carcinoma, treatment, 396
small-cell, treatment, 392
treatment, 386, 396
Luteinizing hormone, 250
secretion, 250, 250*f*
Luteinizing hormone-releasing hormone (LHRH), 247*f*
actions, 248*f*
Lyme disease, treatment, 312*f*
Lymphogranuloma venereum, treatment, 312*f*
Lymphomas. *See also* Hodgkin's disease
non-Hodgkin's, 390
treatment, 393
squamous cell, treatment, 387
treatment, 386, 393
Lysergic acid diethylamide (LSD), 99*f*, **105**
dependence potential, 100*f*
Maalox TC, drug interactions, 370
MACRO-BID. *See* Nitrofurantoin
MACRODANTIN. *See* Nitrofurantoin
Macrolides, **317-329**
classification, 287*f*
resistance to, 285*f*
Macrolides, specific agents, 311*f*
azithromycin (ZITHROMAX), 311*f*, 317-320, 319*f*
clarithromycin (BIAXIN), 235*f*, 236, 282, 282*f*, 311*f*, 317-320, 319*f*, 433
erythromycin (E.E.S., ERYC, E-MYCIN, ERY-TAB), 148*f*, 215, 282, 290, 311*f*-312*f*, 317, *317,* 317-320, 318*f*, 319, 319*f*, 328*f*, 435
Mafenide, 289*f*
therapeutic application, 290
Mafenide acetate, for burns, 291
Magnesium aluminum silicate, 244
Magnesium hydroxide, 236*f*, 240, 244*f*, 245, 439-441
Magnesium sulfate, 244*f*, 245
Major tranquilizers. *See* Neuroleptic drugs
Malaria, treatment, 345*f*, **349-353,** 432
Mania, treatment, 119*f*, 125
Manic-depression, treatment, 125, 147
Mannitol, 223*f*, 233, *233*
Maprotiline, 119, *119,* 119*f*
therapeutic advantages and disadvantages, 125*f*
Marijuana. *See* Tetrahydrocannabinol
MAXIPIME see Cefepime
Mebendazole, *359,* **359,** 359*f*, 361*f*
contraindications, 359*f*
Mecamylamine, 45*f*, 49*f*, **50,** *50*
Mechlorethamine, 373*f*, *387,* **387-388,** 388*f*, 399*f*
emetic potential, 241*f*
Meclizine, 419*f*, *424*
antiemetic effects, 129*f*
for motion sickness, 242, 424
therapeutic advantages and disadvantages, 422*f*
Meclofenamate, **410,** *410*
for migraine, 427*f*
Meclofenamic acid, therapeutic

advantages and disadvantages, 412*f*
Medroxyprogesterone (PROVERA), 263*f*
Medroxyprogesterone acetate, 267, *267*
Mefenamic acid, **410,** *410*
therapeutic advantages and disadvantages, 412*f*
Mefloquine, 345*f*, 350*f*, *352,* **352-353**
Melarsoprol, 345*f*, *353,* 353*f*, **353-354**
Meningitis
cryptococcal, treatment, 284*f*
treatment, 281, 306, 333, 339
Menotropin, 250
Menstrual cycle
irregular, treatment, 435-436
progesterone in, 266, 267*f*
Mepenzolate, 236*f*
Meperidine, 133*f*, *138,* **138-139,** 244
drug interactions, 338
efficacy and addiction/abuse liability, 135*f*
for migraine, 427*f*
onset and duration of action, 139*f*
6-Mercaptopurine, 373*f*, *380,* **380-381,** 399*f*
actions, 374*f*, 381*f*
drug interactions, 417
MERIDIA see Sibutramine
Mersalyl oxide, 353
Mestranol, 263*f*, *265,* 268
pharmacokinetics, 265
Metabolism, drug, 1, 1*f*, 12-15, 14*f*
effect of drug dose on, 13*f*
elimination in, 24, 25*f*
hepatic, 7
Metamucil, 441-442
Metaproterenol, 55*f*, **67,** *67,* 69*f*
and bronchodilation, 67*f*
Metaraminol, 55*f*, **69,** *69*
as mixed-action agonist, 61
Metformin, 255*f*, **261,** *261*
properties, 261*f*
Methadone, **139,** *139*
drug interactions, 147
efficacy and addiction/abuse liability, 135*f*
Methdilazine, therapeutic advantages and disadvantages, 422*f*
Methenamine, *327,* 327*f*, **327-328**
drug interactions, 292
Methicillin, 298*f*, 300, *300*
administration route, 302
resistance to, 285
stability to penicillinase, 300*f*
Methimazole, 247*f*, *253,* 253-254, 436
Methohexital, 108*f*, *115*
Methotrexate, 373*f*, *378,* **378-380,** 399*f*, 402*f*, *415*
for abortion, 419
actions, 374*f*
adverse effects, 292, 378
as antiinflammatory, 415
drug interactions, 295, 384, 410
emetic potential, 241*f*
and folate deficiency, 205
as folate reductase inhibitor, 293
mechanism of action, 379*f*
myelosuppressive potential, 378*f*
Methoxamine, 55*f*, *66,* **66-67,** 69*f*
Methoxyflurane, 107*f*, **114,** *114*
Methylcellulose, 244, 244*f*, 245
α-Methyldopa, 180*f*, **190,** *190*
3-O-Methyldopa, 444
Methylphenidate (RITALIN HYDROCHLORIDE), 99*f*, *104*
for attention deficit syndromes, *104*
Methylprednisolone, 242*f*
administration route, 276*f*
for asthma, 219
for chemotherapy-induced nausea and vomiting, 243
elimination, 276*f*
properties, 275*f*
Methylsalicylate, 401*f*, 406, 408
Methylxanthines, **99-104**
Methysergide, 419*f*, *428*
for migraine, 427*f*, 428
Metoclopramide (REGLAN), 242, *242,* 242*f*
antiemetic effects, 129*f*
for chemotherapy-induced nausea and vomiting, 242-243
in combination therapy, 243, 243*f*
Metocurine, 45*f*
onset and duration of action, 52*f*
pharmacokinetics, 51
Metolazone, 151*f*, 223*f*, **231,** *231*
Metoprolol (LOPRESSOR), 71*f*, **77,** *77,* 79*f*, 179*f*
actions, 75*f*
for angina, 176
antiarrhythmic effects, 171
clinical applications, 78*f*
drug elimination, 74*f*
for hypertension, 185
Metoprolol and pindolol, 163*f*
Metronidazole, 235*f*, 345*f*, *347,* **347-348**
cost, 282, 282*f*
drug interactions, 201*f*
to eliminate Helicobacter pylori, 236
for giardiasis, 357
sites of action, 346*f*
Metyrapone, **277,** *277*
MEVACOR. *See* Lovastatin
Mexiletine, 163*f*, **170,** *170*
for arrhythmias, 171, 172*f*
drug interactions, 147
effects, 169*f*
Mezlocillin, 298*f*, 301, *301*
administration route, 302
stability to acid, 300*f*
Miconazole (MONISTAT), 337*f*, **343,** *343*
MICRO-K. *See* Potassium
Micromonospora, aminoglycosides from, 314
MICRONASE. *See* Glyburide
Microsporum infection, treatment, 343
Microtubule inhibitors, **390-392**
for cancer, specific agents, 373*f*
mechanism of action, 391*f*
Midazolam, 108*f*, 116
therapeutic advantages and disadvantages, 97*f*
Mifepristone, 263*f*, 267-268
as adrenocorticoid inhibitor, 277
Migraine headache
characteristics, 425*f*
concomitant with hypertension, treatment, 185
treatment, 75, 78*f*, 187, **425-428,** 427*f*
specific agents, 419*f*
Milrinone, 151*f*, 161, *161*
Mineralocorticoids, **273-274**
production, 272
properties, 275*f*
Mineral oil, 244*f*, 245
Minimal alveolar concentrations (MAC), for anesthetic gases, 111, 111*f*
MINIPRESS. *See* Prazosin
MINOCIN. *See* Minocycline
Minocycline (MINOCIN), 311*f*, 313, *313,* 314
Minoxidil (ROGAINE), 151*f*, 180*f*, *190,* **190-191**
MIRAPEX see Pramipexole
Misoprostol, 235*f*, *238,* 238-239, 267, *267,* 419*f*, 420, *420,* 420*f*
for abortion, 419
drug interactions, 380, 407
and gastric acid regulation, 237*f*
Mithramycin. *See* Plicamycin
Mitomycin, emetic potential, 241*f*
Mivacurium, 45*f*
onset and duration of action, 52*f*
pharmacokinetics, 51

therapeutic advantages, 52*f*
Moexipril, 179*f*
MONISTAT IV. *See* Miconazole
Monoamine oxidase, 123-125
Monoamine oxidase inhibitors, 119*f*, **123-125**
drug interactions, 86, 86*f*, 138, 260*f*, 425
mechanism of action, 124*f*
therapeutic advantages and disadvantages, 125*f*
Monobactams, **307**
specific agents, 298*f*
Monoclonal antibodies, 456
Montelukast , 450
MOPP regimen, 388
Moraxella catarrhalis infection, treatment, 318, 324
Morganella infection, treatment, 315*f*
Morning-after pill, 268
Morphine, 108*f*, 117, 133*f*, **135-138**
action, 134*f*
dependence potential, 100*f*
drug interactions, 141
efficacy and addiction/abuse liability, 135*f*
naloxone and, 141*f*, 142
onset and duration of action, 139*f*
ratio of lethal to effective dose, 90*f*
withdrawal, treatment, 139
Motion sickness, treatment, 48, 48*f*, 130, 242, 424
MOTRIN. *See* Ibuprofen
Mountain sickness, treatment, 227
Moxalactam, 298*f*
vitamin K with, 204
Moxifloxacin, 456
6-MP. *See* 6-Mercaptopurine
MTX. *See* Methotrexate
Mucocutaneous leishmaniasis, 356, 356*f*
Mucosal protective agents, for peptic ulcer disease, 236*f*, 241
Multidrug resistance gene, 377, 377*f*
Multiple sclerosis, treatment, 90
Muromonab-CD3, 472
Muscarinic blockers, 49*f*
Muscarinic receptors, 38*f*, **38-39**
Muscle contraction, physiology, 152*f*, **153-155**
Muscle relaxants. *See* Neuromuscular blockers
Muscular disorders, treatment, 90
Myalgia, treatment, 406
Myasthenia gravis, treatment, 68, 433, 434*f*
Mycobacterium avium intracellulare infection, treatment, 318, 333, 336
Mycobacterium infection, 436-437
Mycobacterium kansasii infection, treatment, 332, 334
Mycobacterium leprae infection, 335
treatment, 333
Mycobacterium tuberculosis infection, 331. *See also* Tuberculosis
resistance, 285
treatment, 332-334
Mycophenolate mofetil, 471
Mycoplasma, 283*f*
pneumonia, treatment, 312*f*, 318*f*
Mycoplasma pneumoniae infection, treatment, 312*f*
Mycoses
subcutaneous, treatment, **337-342**
specific agents, 337*f*
superficial, treatment, **342-343**
specific agents, 337*f*
systemic, treatment, **337-342**
specific agents, 337*f*
Myocardial infarction
acute, treatment, 171, 201, 203
and angina, 178*f*
and hypertension, 182*f*-183*f*
treatment, 185
treatment, 74-76, 186, 196, 198, 202
Nabilone, 242*f*, 243
Nabumetone (RELAFEN), 401*f*, **411,** *411*
Nadolol (CORGARD), 71*f*, **76,** *76,* 179*f*
clinical applications, 78*f*
drug elimination, 74*f*
for migraine, 428
Nafarelin, 247*f*, 250, *250*
Nafcillin, 298*f*, 300, *300*
elimination, 303
stability to penicillinase, 300*f*
Nalidixic acid, 323, *323,* **327**
Naloxone, 133*f*, *141,* **141-142**
action, 134*f*
and anesthesia, 117
competition with opioid agonists, 141*f*
drug interactions, 140
Naltrexone, 133*f*, **142,** *142*
action, 134*f*
Nandrolone, 263*f*, 271, *271*
NAPROSYN. *See* Naproxen
Naproxen (ANAPROX, NAPROSYN), 401*f*, *408,* **408-409**
drug interactions, 408*f*, 417
for migraine, 427*f*, 428
therapeutic advantages and disadvantages, 412*f*
Narcolepsy, treatment, 104
Narcotic analgesics, drug interactions, 138, 138*f*
Narcotics, dependence potential, 100*f*
NASACORT. *See* Flunisolide
Nasal decongestant
ephedrine as, 68
phenylephrine as, 66
Nausea. *See also* Emesis
treatment, 129-130, 424
Navelbine, 373*f*
Necator americanus infection, 361*f*
treatment, 359
Nedocromil, **220,** *220,* 431
for asthma, 217*f*
Nefazodone, 119*f*, 123, *123*
therapeutic advantages and disadvantages, 125*f*
Neisseria gonorrhoeae infection, treatment, 294*f*, 299*f*, 305*f*, 325*f*
Neisseria infection, treatment, 304
Neisseria meningitidis infection, treatment, 294*f*, 299*f*
Nelfinavir, 460
Nematode infections
characteristics, 361*f*
treatment, 359*f*, **359-360,** 361*f*
Neomycin, 311*f*, 316, *316*
adverse effects, 317
NEORAL see Cyclosporine
Neostigmine, 35*f*, **42,** *42*
drug interactions, 51, 317
and neuromuscular blockers, 50
Nephrotic syndrome
kidney function during, 226
treatment, 230, 389
Nervous system, organization, 27*f*, **27-31**
Netilmicin, 311*f*, 316, *316*
adverse effects, 316
Neuroleptanesthesia, **117**
Neuroleptic drugs, **127-132**
actions, 128*f*
adverse effects, 130*f*
antiemetic uses, 129*f*
dopamine-blocking agents, 128*f*
and LSD, 105
summary, 132*f*
Neuroleptic drugs, specific agents, 127*f*
chlorpromazine, 90*f*, 127, *127,* 127*f*-128*f*, 129-131, 131*f*-132*f*
clozapine, 127*f*, 128, *128,* 128*f*, 130-131, 131*f*-132*f*
fluphenazine, 127, *127,* 127*f*-128*f*, 130, 131*f*-132*f*

haloperidol, 84, 105, 127, *127*, 127*f*-129*f*, 130-131, 131*f*-132*f*, 242*f*, 242-243
haloperidol decanoate, 3, 130
prochlorperazine (COMPAZINE), 127*f*, 129, 129*f*, 242, *242*, 242*f*, 243
promethazine (PHENERGAN), 127*f*-129*f*, 130, *130*, 422*f*
risperidone, 127*f*, 128, *128*, 128*f*, 130-131, 132*f*
thioridazine, 127*f*-128*f*, 129, *129*, 130, 132*f*
thiothixene, 127, *127*, 127*f*-128*f*, 132*f*
Neuromuscular blockers, **50-53,** 107*f*
depolarizing, 53, 53*f*
duration of action, 52*f*
mechanism of action, 50*f*
nondepolarizing (competitive) agents, 50-51
onset of action, 52*f*
Neuromuscular blockers, specific agents
atracurium, 45*f*, 52*f*, 107*f*, 109
doxacurium, 45*f*, 51, 52*f*
metocurine, 45*f*, 51, 52*f*
mivacurium, 45*f*, 51, 52*f*
pancuronium, 45*f*, 51, 52*f*
pipecuronium, 45*f*, 52*f*
rocuronium, 45*f*, 51, 52*f*
succinylcholine, 45*f*, 52*f*, 53, *53*, **53,** 53*f*, 107*f*, 109
tubocurarine, 39, 42, 45*f*, 50, *50*, 50*f*, 51, 52*f*
vecuronium, 45*f*, 51, 52*f*, 107*f*, 109
Neurotransmission
at adrenergic neurons, 55
in central nervous system, 81-82
at cholinergic neurons, **35-37**
Neurotransmitters, **31-33**
cellular effects, 33*f*
summary, 32*f*, 32-33
types, 32
Neutral protamine Hagedorn. *See* Isophane insulin suspension
Nevirapine, 461
Niacin, 207*f*, **210-211,** *211*
cholesterol levels during, 210*f*
in combination drug therapy, 215
drug interactions, 212, 215
mechanism of action, 210, 210*f*
Nicardipine, 180*f*, 188, *188*
for angina, 188*f*
drug interactions, 188*f*
for hypertension, 188*f*
Niclosamide, 359*f*, **362,** *362*
NICORETTE. *See* Nicotine gum
Nicotine, 45*f*, *49*, **49,** 49*f*, 99*f*, *100*, **100-101**
actions, 100*f*
blood concentration, 101*f*
dependence potential, 100*f*
withdrawal from, 101
Nicotine gum, nicotine concentration, 101*f*
Nicotinic acid. *See* Niacin
Nicotinic receptors, 38*f*, 39
Nifedipine (ADALAT, PROCARDIA XL), 173, 175*f*, **177,** *177*, *187*, 187-188
actions, 187*f*
for angina, 188*f*
drug interactions, 188*f*
effects, 173*f*
for hypertension, 188*f*
Nifurtimox, 345*f*, 353*f*, **355,** *355*
Nisoldipine, 180*f*, 188, *188*
Nitrates
for angina, treatment with concomitant diseases, 178*f*
effects on smooth muscle, 176, 176*f*
Nitrites, effects on smooth muscle, 176, 176*f*
NITRO-DUR. *See* Nitroglycerin
Nitrofurantoin (MACRODANTIN, MACROBID), **329,** *329*
Nitroglycerin (NITROSTAT), 175*f*, **175-176,** *176*, 442
administration route, 2, 4
onset and duration of action, 177*f*
Nitroprusside, **191,** *191*
and cyanide, 191*f*
Nitrosoureas, 399*f*
actions, 374*f*
in cancer therapy, 389-390
myelosuppressive potential, 378*f*
NITROSTAT. *See* Nitroglycerin
Nitrous oxide, 107*f*, *114*, **114-115,** 117
blood/gas partition coefficient, 111, 111*f*
characteristics, 114*f*
elimination, 112
with halothane, 113
minimal alveolar concentration, 111, 111*f*
therapeutic advantages and disadvantages, 116*f*
uptake curve, 112, 112*f*
Nizatidine (AXID), 235*f*, *236*, **236-238,** 419*f*, 440
NIZORAL. *See* Ketoconazole
Nocardia asteroides, 290*f*
Nocardia infection, treatment, 290, 290*f*
NOLVADEX. *See* Tamoxifen
Nonbarbiturate sedatives, **96**
Nonbarbiturate sedatives, specific agents, 90*f*
antihistamines, 90*f*, 96, **96,** 107*f*, 108, 221, 243, 243*f*, 419*f*, 420-425
specific agents, 217*f*
chloral hydrate, 90*f*, **96,** *96*
polycyclic antidepressants, 119*f*, **119-121,** 120*f*, 125*f*
tricyclic antidepressants, 42, 119*f*, **119-121,** 120*f*-122*f*, 125*f*, 138
Non-catecholamines, 60, 69*f*
Non-Hodgkin's lymphomas, 390
treatment, 393
Non-narcotic analgesics, **411-413**
Non-narcotic analgesics, specific agents, 401*f*
acetaminophen (TYLENOL), 140, 401*f*, 405*f*, 407, *412*, **412-413,** 413*f*, 428
phenacetin, 401*f*, *412*, **412-413**
Nonsteroidal antiinflammatory drugs, **403-411,** 439, 440*f*
Actions, 405*f*
for diarrhea, 244
for migraine, 428
and prostaglandins, 401
summary, 412*f*
Nonsteroidal antiinflammatory drugs, specific agents, 401*f*
aspirin, 13, 140, 193*f*, 196, *196*, **196,** 201*f*, 211, 213, 244, 244*f*, 401*f*, *403*, **403-408,** 404*f*-405*f*, 407*f*, 412*f*, 427*f*, 428, 439-440
diclofenac (VOLTAREN), 401*f*, **411,** *411*
diflunisal (DOLOBID), 401*f*, 403, *403*, 406, 408, 412*f*
etodolac (LODINE), 401*f*, *409*, **410**
fenamates, 401*f*, **410,** 412*f*
fenoprofen, 327, 401*f*, *408*, **408-409,** 412*f*
flurbiprofen (ANSAID), 401*f*, *408*, **408-409**
ibuprofen (ADVIL, MOTRIN), 401*f*, *408*, **408-409,** 412*f*, 440
indomethacin, 244, 244*f*, 401*f*, **409,** *409*, 409*f*, 412*f*, 417
ketoprofen (ORUDIS), 401*f*, *408*, **408-409,** 412*f*, 417
methylsalicylate, 401*f*, 406, 408
nabumetone (RELAFEN), 401*f*, **411,** *411*
phenylbutazone, 201*f*, 260*f*, 401*f*, *410*, **410-411,** 411*f*-412*f*
piroxicam (FELDENE), 401*f*, **410,** *410*, 412*f*
sulindac (CLINORIL), 401*f*, *409*, **410,** 412*f*

tolmetin, 401*f*, **411,** *411,* 412*f*
NORDETTE. *See* Ethinyl estradiol
Norepinephrine, **33,** 55*f*, **64,** *64,* 69*f*
adrenergic neurons and, 55
and adrenergic receptors, 58*f*, 58-59
and amino nitrogen, 61
in autonomic nervous system, 32*f*
binding, 56, 57*f*
cardiovascular effects, 64*f*
as direct-acting agonist, 61
effect on blood pressure, 72*f*
guanethidine and, 79
indirect-acting agonists and, 61
metabolism, 57*f*
recapture, 56
release, 56, 57*f*
removal, 56, 57*f*
reserpine and, 78
sites of action, 36*f*
storage, 56, 57*f*
structure, 61*f*
synthesis, 55, 57*f*
Norethindrone, 263*f*, 267, *267,* 268
Norfloxacin (NOROXIN), 323, *323,* **324,** 325-326
for urinary tract infections, 325*f*
Norgestrel, 263*f*, 267, *267,* 268
implants, failure rate, 268*f*
NORMODYNE. *See* Labetalol
NOROXIN. *See* Norfloxacin
NORPLANT. *See* Levonorgestrel
Nortestosterone progestins, 267
Nortriptyline (PAMELOR), 119, *119,* 119*f*
therapeutic advantages and disadvantages, 125*f*
NORVASC. *See* Amlodipine
NORVIR see Ritonavir
Nystatin, 337*f*, **343,** *343*
Oat cell carcinoma, of lung, treatment, 396
Obesity, 474
Obsessive-compulsive disorder, treatment, 122
Octreotide, 247*f*, **250,** *250*
Ofloxacin (FLOXIN), **324,** *324,* 325-326
Oil of wintergreen, 406
Omeprazole (PRILOSEC), 235*f*, 239, *239,* 440
to eliminate Helicobacter pylori, 236
and gastric acid regulation, 237*f*
OMNICEF see Cefdinir
Onchocerca volvulus infection, treatment, 356, 360, 361*f*
Ondansetron, 242*f*, 243, *243*
in combination therapy, 243*f*
Opiates, for cough, specific agents, 217*f*
Opioid agonist-antagonist, **140-141**
Opioid agonists
actions, 134*f*
adverse effects, 137*f*
moderate, **140**
onset and duration of action, 139*f*
Opioid antagonists, **133-142, 141-142**
actions, 134*f*
Opioid antagonists, specific agents, 133*f*
naloxone, 117, 133*f*-134*f*, 140, *141,* 141*f*, **141-142**
naltrexone, 133*f*-134*f*, *142,* **142**
Opioid receptors, **133-135**
Opioids, 107*f*, 116-117, **133-142**
preanesthetic, 108
Opioids, specific agents, 133*f*
buprenorphine, 133*f*, **141,** *141*
codeine, 133*f*-135*f*, 137, *140,* **140,** 140*f*, 222, 427*f*
fentanyl, 108, 108*f*, 116*f*, 117, 133*f*-135*f*, 137, *139,* **139,** 139*f*
heroin, 100*f*, 133*f*-134*f*, 137, 139, *140,* **140,** 141*f*, 142
meperidine, 133*f*, 135*f*, *138,* **138-139,** 139*f*, 244, 338, 427*f*
methadone, 135*f*, **139,** *139,* 147
morphine, 90*f*, 100*f*, 108*f*, 117, 133*f*-135*f*, **135-138,** 139, 139*f*, 141, 141*f*, 142
pentazocine, 133*f*-134*f*, *141,* **141**
propoxyphene (DARVON COMP 65, DARVOCET-N-100), 133*f*, 135*f*, *140,* **140,** 148*f*, 428
sufentanil, 133*f*, 139, *139*
Oral administration, drug, **2,** 3*f*
kinetics, 20, 21*f*
Oral contraception
drug interactions, 147
failure rate, 268*f*
percent use, 268*f*
Oral surgery, antibiotics in, 300
ORASONE. *See* Prednisone
Organic nitrates, for angina, **175-176**
specific agents, 175*f*
Orlistat, 475
ORTHOCLONE OKT3 see Muromonab-CD3
ORUDIS. *See* Ketoprofen
Osmotic diuretics, 223*f*, **233**
Osteoarthritis
of hip, treatment, 409
treatment, 275, 408, 410-411
Osteogenic sarcoma, 379
Osteoporosis
senile, treatment, 270
treatment, 3
Ovarian cancer, treatment, 382, 392, 395
OVCON. *See* Ethinyl estradiol
Oxacillin, 298*f*, 300, *300*
stability to penicillinase, 300*f*
Oxaprozin (DAYPRO), 401*f*, *408,* **408-409**
Oxazepam, *91*
for alcohol withdrawal, 91
duration of action, 92*f*
therapeutic advantages and disadvantages, 97*f*
Oxazosin, for hypertension, 189
Oxicam derivatives, **410**
therapeutic advantages and disadvantages, 412*f*
Oxymetazoline, *221*
for rhinitis, 221
Oxytocin, 247*f*, 250, **251,** *251*
Paclitaxel, 373*f*, *391,* **391-392,** 392*f*, 399*f*
PAMELOR. *See* Nortriptyline
Pamidronate , 476
Pancreatic cancer, treatment, 382
Pancuronium, 45*f*
onset and duration of action, 52*f*
pharmacokinetics, 51
therapeutic disadvantages, 52*f*
Panic disorders, treatment, 120, 122
Para-aminobenzoic acid (PABA), 289
structure, 290*f*
Paramethasone, properties, 275*f*
Parasympathetic nervous system, 27*f*, 29*f*, 30, 30*f*
Parasympathetic neurons, **28**
Parenteral administration, **2-3**
Parkinsonism, secondary, 84
Parkinson's disease
etiology, 83-84
treatment, 81-88, 443
Paromomycin, 345*f*, **348,** *348*
sites of action, 346*f*
Paroxetine (PAXIL), 119*f*, 123, *123*
therapeutic advantages and disadvantages, 125*f*
Patent ductus arteriosus, treatment, 406, 409
PAXIL. *See* Paroxetine
Pectin, 244, 244*f*
Pencyclovir, **367,** *367,* 457-458
D-Penicillamine, 402*f*, **414,** *414*
Penicillinases, drug interactions, 300
Penicillin-binding proteins, **298,** 302
Penicillin G, 298*f*, **300**
absorption, 302

adverse reactions, 303
bioavailability, 7
metabolism, 302
stability to acid, 300*f*
substitutes for, 304
Penicillins, 282*f*, *297*, **297-303**, 318*f*, 434-435
administration route, 2
antipseudomonal, 300*f*, **301**
adverse reactions, 303
antistaphylococcal, **300**, 300*f*
diffusion, 281*f*
distribution, 302, 303*f*
drug interactions, 315, 417
for enterococcal endocarditis, 284*f*
extended spectrum, **300**, 300*f*
for listeriosis, 299*f*
natural, **300**, 300*f*
resistance to, 301-302
safety, 282
therapeutic index, 22-23, 23*f*
Penicillins, specific agents, 298*f*
amoxicillin (AMOXIL, POLYMOX, TRIMOX, WYMOX), 235*f*, 236, 282, 282*f*, 298*f*, 300, *300*, 300*f*, 302, 308, 308*f*, 328*f*
ampicillin (PRINCIPEN), 283, 290, 298*f*-299*f*, 300, *300*, 300*f*, 301-302, 328*f*, 435
azlocillin, 298*f*, 300*f*, 301, *301*, 302
carbenicillin, 298*f*, 300*f*, 301, *301*, 301*f*, 302-303
cloxacillin, 298*f*, 300, *300*, 300*f*
dicloxacillin, 298*f*, 300, *300*, 300*f*
methicillin, 285, 298*f*, 300, *300*, 300*f*, 302
mezlocillin, 298*f*, 300*f*, 301, *301*, 302
nafcillin, 298*f*, 300, *300*, 300*f*, 303
oxacillin, 298*f*, 300, *300*, 300*f*
penicillin G, 7, 298*f*, **300**, 300*f*, 302-304
penicillin V (PEN-VEE K, VEETIDS, BETAPEN VK), 298*f*, **300**, 300*f*, 302
piperacillin, 298*f*, 300*f*, 301, *301*, 301*f*, 302
ticarcillin, 298*f*, 300*f*, 301, *301*, 301*f*, 302-303
Penicillin V (PEN-VEE K, VEETIDS, BETAPEN VK), 298*f*, **300**
administration route, 302
stability to acid, 300*f*
Penicillium chrysogenum, and penicillin formation, 300
Pentamidine, 345*f*, 353*f*
drug interactions, 339, 370
for leishmaniasis, 356
Pentamidine isethionate, *354*, **354-355**
Pentazocine, 133*f*, **141,** *141*
action, 134*f*
Pentobarbital, 90*f*, *94*
duration of action, 95
preanesthetic, 108
therapeutic advantages and disadvantages, 97*f*
PEN-VEE K. *See* Penicillin V
PEPCID. *See* Famotidine
Peptic ulcers, treatment, **235-241,** 241, 282, 282*f*, 420
specific agents, 235*f*-236*f*
Pepto-Bismol. *See* Bismuth subsalicylate
Peripheral arterial thrombosis, treatment, 201
Peripheral nervous system, 27, 27*f*
afferent division, 27, 27*f*
efferent division, 27, 27*f*
Peripheral vascular disease, treatment, 189
Pernicious anemia, treatment, 205
PERSANTINE. *See* Dipyridamole
Petit mal seizures. *See* Absence seizures
pH, and drug absorption, 4-5, 6*f*
Pharmacokinetics, 17-26
Phase I reactions, **13-14,** 14*f*
Phase II reactions, 14*f*, **14-15**
Phenacetin, 401*f*, *412*, **412-413**
Phencyclidine (PCP), 99*f*, **105,** *105*
dependence potential, 100*f*
opioid receptors and, 133
Phenelzine, 119*f*, 123, *123*
drug interactions, 86
therapeutic advantages and disadvantages, 125*f*
PHENERGAN. *See* Promethazine
Phenformin, 261
Phenobarbital, 90*f*, *94*, 143*f*, 438
as anticonvulsant, 95
drug interactions, 213, 343, 347
duration of action, 95
overdose, 23-24
primidone and, 148, 148*f*
ratio of lethal to effective dose, 90*f*
for seizures, 145*f*
therapeutic advantages and disadvantages, 97*f*
and thyroid hormone metabolism, 253
Phenolphthalein, as laxative, 244, 244*f*
Phenothiazines, 127*f*
antiemetic potency, 243*f*
for chemotherapy-induced nausea and vomiting, 242, 242*f*
in combination therapy, 243
drug interactions, 138
and parkinsoniam symptoms, 84
and physostigmine, 42
therapeutic advantages and disadvantages, 422*f*
Phenoxybenzamine, *71*, 71*f*, **71-72,** 72*f*
Phentermine, 474
Phentolamine, 71*f*, **72,** *72*
for hypertension, 124
Phenylbutazone, 401*f*, *410*, **410-411**
adverse effects, 411*f*
drug interactions, 201*f*, 260*f*
therapeutic advantages and disadvantages, 412*f*
Phenylephrine (ENTEX LA), 55*f*, **66,** *66*, 69*f*
and adrenergic receptors, 58
with anesthesia, 113
as direct-acting agonist, 61
as non-catecholamine, 60
in ophthalmic therapy, 47
for rhinitis, 221
structure, 60*f*
β-Phenylethylamine, structure, 61*f*
Phenylethylmalonamide, primidone and, 148, 148*f*
Phenytoin (DILANTIN), 143*f*, *146*, **146-147**
for arrhythmias, 174
drug interactions, 147*f*, 150, 239, 295, 333, 341, 362, 408*f*
metabolism, 13
and plasma concentration, 146, 146*f*
for seizures, 145*f*
and thyroid hormone metabolism, 253
Pheochromocytoma
diagnosis, 72
treatment, 72
Phosphodiesterase inhibitors, 151*f*
for congestive heart failure, 161, 161*f*
Physostigmine, 35*f*, **42,** *42*
and atropine, 47
drug interactions, 51
Phytonadione. *See* Vitamin K
Pilocarpine, 35*f*, **41,** *41*
actions, 41*f*
for glaucoma, 75, 227
structure, 39*f*
Pindolol, 71*f*, **77,** *77*, 79*f*
as antiarrhythmic, 171
contraindication, 177
drug elimination, 74*f*
Pinworm infection, 360*f*
treatment, 359, 361*f*
Pipecuronium, 45*f*
onset and duration of action, 52*f*
Piperacillin, 298*f*, 301, *301*

administration route, 302
stability
to acid, 300*f*
to penicillinase, 300*f*
therapeutic applications, 301*f*
Piperazines, therapeutic advantages and disadvantages, 422*f*
Piperidines, therapeutic advantages and disadvantages, 422*f*
Pirbuterol, for asthma, 218
Pirenzepine, 236*f*, 240
and gastric acid regulation, 237*f*
and gastrointestinal problems, 46
and muscarinic receptors, 38
Piroxicam (FELDENE), 401*f*, **410,** *410*
therapeutic advantages and disadvantages, 412*f*
Pituitary dwarfism, treatment, 270
Pituitary hormones, **247-254**
Plague, treatment, 315
Plasma lipoproteins, metabolism, 208*f*
Plasma proteins, binding of drugs to, **11-12**
Plasmodium falciparum infection, 349
chloroquine-resistant, 351
treatment, 349, 351-353
Plasmodium, life cycle, 350*f*
Plasmodium malariae infection, 349
treatment, 353
Plasmodium ovale infection, 349
treatment, 349
Plasmodium vivax infection, 349, 432, 432*f*
treatment, 349, 351
Platelet activation, 194-196, 195*f*
Platelet aggregation, 195-196
inhibitors, 446
Platelet inhibitors, **196-197**
Platelet inhibitors, specific agents, 193*f*
abciximab, 447
aspirin, 13, 140, 193*f*, 196, *196*, **196,** 201*f*, 211, 213, 244, 244*f*, 401*f*, *403*, **403-408,** 404*f*-405*f*, 407*f*, 412*f*, 427*f*, 428, 439-440
clopidogrel, 448
dipyridamole (PERSANTINE), 193*f*, **196,** *196*
eptifibatide, 447
ticlopidine, 193*f*, **196,** *196*
tirofiban, 447
Platelets, role in clotting, 193, 194*f*
PLAVIX see Clopidogrel
Plicamycin, 373*f*, *387*, **387,** 399*f*
Pneumococcal pneumonia, treatment, 299*f*
Pneumocystis carinii pneumonia, 294*f*
treatment, 289-290, 335, 354-355
Pneumonia
mycoplasmal, treatment, 312*f*, 318*f*
pneumococcal, treatment, 299*f*
Pneumocystis carinii, 294*f*
treatment, 289-290, 335, 354-355
treatment, 315*f*, 433
Poisoning, heavy metal, treatment, 414
Polycyclic antidepressants, 119*f*, **119-121**
mechanism of action, 120*f*
therapeutic advantages and disadvantages, 125*f*
Polycythemia vera, for sickle cell disease, 206
Polyethylene glycol, 244*f*, 245
POLYMOX. *See* Amoxicillin
Pork insulin, 257
Postcoital contraception, 268
Posterior pituitary hormones, 247*f*, **250-251**
Postganglionic neuron, **28**
Postmenopausal hormone therapy, **264,** 265*f*
Potassium channel blockers, 163*f*
Potassium-sparing diuretics, 223*f*, **232-233**
and changes in urine composition, 232*f*-233*f*
Pralidoxime, 35*f*
and reactivation of acetylcholinesterase, 43, 43*f*
Pramipexole, 443
PRANDIN see Repaglinide
PRAVACHOL. *See* Pravastatin
Pravastatin (PRAVACHOL), 207*f*, *214*, **214-215,** 449
cardiac death rate with, 214*f*
drug interactions, 213
Praziquantel, 359*f*, **360-362,** *362*
drug interactions, 362
Prazosin (MINIPRESS), 71*f*, **73,** *73*, 180*f*
for hypertension, 124, 189
Prednisolone, 393
properties, 275*f*
Prednisone (DELTASONE, ORASONE), 373*f*, 399*f*, 438-439
for asthma, 219
in cancer therapy, **393,** *393*
in chemotherapy, 276
drug interactions, 334*f*, 397
properties, 275*f*
Preganglionic neuron, **28**
Pregnancy-induced hypertension, treatment, 78
PREMARIN. *See* Estrogens
Premature births, drug contraindications, 251
Premenstrual edema, kidney function during, 226
Premenstrual syndrome, treatment, 122
PREVEON see Adefovir
PRILOSEC. *See* Omeprazole
Primaquine, 345*f*, *349*, **349-350,** 350*f*, 432-433
adverse effects, 350, 351*f*
Primidone, 143*f*, **148,** *148*
metabolism, 148*f*
for seizures, 145*f*
PRINCIPEN. *See* Ampicillin
PRINIVIL. *See* Lisinopril
Probenecid, 402*f*, **417,** *417*
drug interactions, 260*f*, 303, 408*f*
for hyperuricemia, 415
Probucol, 207*f*, *213*, **213-214**
mechanism of action, 213, 213*f*
Procainamide, 163*f*, **168,** *168*
for arrhythmias, 171, 172*f*
effects, 167*f*
Procaine, 108*f*
pharmacokinetic properties, 117*f*
structure, 117*f*
Procaine penicillin G, administration route, 302
Procarbazine, 373*f*, *396*, **396-397,** 399*f*
myelosuppressive potential, 378*f*
PROCARDIA XL. *See* Nifedipine
Prochlorperazine (COMPAZINE), 127*f*, 242, *242*, 242*f*
antiemetic effects, 129*f*
in combination therapy, 243
for nausea, 129
Progesterone, 266-267
menstrual cycle and, 266, 267*f*
Progestin implants, 268
Progestins, **266-267,** 268
failure rate, 268*f*
Progestins, specific agents, 263*f*
hydroxyprogesterone, 263*f*, 267, *267*
levonorgestrel, 3, 268, 269*f*
medroxyprogesterone (PROVERA), 263*f*, 267, *267*
norethindrone, 263*f*, 267, *267*, 268
norgestrel, 263*f*, 267, *267*, 268, 268*f*
PROGRAFT see Tacrolimus
Pro-insulin, 257
Prolactin-inhibiting hormone, actions, 248*f*
Prolactin-releasing hormone, actions, 248*f*
Promethazine (PHENERGAN), 127*f*, 130, *130*

actions, 128*f*
antiemetic effects, 129*f*
therapeutic advantages and disadvantages, 422*f*
Propafenone, 163*f*, **170,** *170*
for arrhythmias, 171, 172*f*
effects, 170*f*
Prophylactic antibiotics, 286, 286*f*
Propionic acid
derivatives, **408-409**
therapeutic advantages and disadvantages, 412*f*
Propofol, 108*f*, **117,** *117*
therapeutic advantages and disadvantages, 116*f*
Propoxyphene (DARVON COMP 65, DARVOCET-N-100), 133*f*, **140,** *140*
drug interactions, 148*f*
efficacy and addiction/abuse liability, 135*f*
for migraine, 428
Propranolol (INDERAL), 71*f*, *74,* **74-76,** 79*f*, 163*f*, 175*f*, 179*f*, 436-437
actions, 75*f*
adverse effects, 76*f*
for angina, 176
as antiarrhythmic, 164*f*, 171
clinical applications, 78*f*
drug interactions, 334*f*
elimination, 74*f*
with hydralazine, 190
for hypertension, 185
metabolism, 7
for migraine, 427*f*, 428
Propylthiouracil, 247*f*, *253,* 253-254, 436
Prostaglandin E1, 267
Prostaglandins, **401-403**
as autacoids, 419-420
for peptic ulcer disease, 235*f*, 238-239
specific agents, 419*f*
structure, 402*f*
synthesis, 403*f*
therapeutic applications, 420*f*
Prostaglandins, specific agents
carboprost, *419,* **419,** 419*f*-420*f*
dinoprost, *419,* **419,** 419*f*-420*f*
dinoprostone, *419,* **419,** 419*f*-420*f*
misoprostol, 235*f*, 237*f*, *238,* 238-239, 267, *267,* 380, 407, 419, 419*f*, 420, *420,* 420*f*
Prostate
cancer
metastatic, treatment, 394
treatment, 272, 394
effect on endocrine system, 395*f*
infections, 281
treatment, 294*f*, 328*f*
Prostatic hyperplasia, benign, treatment, 73, 272
Prostatitis. *See* Prostate, infections
Protamine sulfate, 193*f*, **204,** *204*
for excessive bleeding, 199
Protamine zinc suspension, 255*f*
Proteins
binding of drugs to, 8-9
drugs binding to, 8-9
Protein synthesis inhibitors, **311-321**
specific agents, 311*f*
Proteus
infection (iodide positive), treatment, 301*f*, 315*f*
resistance, 328
Proteus mirabilis infection, 327
treatment, 294*f*, 301*f*, 304, 325*f*
Proton pump inhibitors, for peptic ulcer disease, 235*f*, 239
Proton pump inhibitors, specific agents
lansoprazole, 235*f*, 239, *239*
omeprazole (PRILOSEC), 235*f*, 236, 237*f*, 239, *239,* 440
Protriptyline, 119, *119,* 119*f*
therapeutic advantages and disadvantages, 125*f*
PROVENTIL. *See* Albuterol
PROVERA. *See* Medroxyprogesterone
PROZAC. *See* Fluoxetine
Pruritus, treatment, 130, 212
Pseudomonas aeruginosa infection, 430-431
treatment, 301, 301*f*, 304, 305*f*, 307, 315*f*, 324, 325*f*
Pseudomonas infection, treatment, 324
Psittacosis, treatment, 312*f*
Psychomotor stimulants, **99-104**
specific agents, 99*f*
Psychotomimetic drugs, specific agents, 99*f*
lysergic acid diethylamide (LSD), 99*f*-100*f*, **105**
phencyclidine (PCP), 99*f*-100*f*, *105,* **105,** 133
tetrahydrocannabinol (THC), 99*f*, **105,** *105,* 243
Psyllium seeds, 244*f*, 245
PTU. *See* Propylthiouracil
Pulmonary edema, acute, treatment, 228
Pulmonary embolism
acute, treatment, 203
massive, treatment, 202
treatment, 198, 201, 203
Purkinje fiber, action potential, 152*f*
Pyelonephritis, acute, treatment, 328*f*
Pyrantel pamoate, *359,* 359*f*, **359-360,** 361*f*
Pyrazinamide, 331, **334,** *334,* 437
adverse effects, *f*, 335
drug interactions, 334
for tuberculosis, 284*f*
Pyrazoles, therapeutic advantages and disadvantages, 412*f*
Pyridostigmine, 35*f*, **42,** *42*
Pyridoxine, drug interactions, 86*f*
Pyrilamine, therapeutic advantages and disadvantages, 422*f*
Pyrimethamine, 289*f*, 290, *290,* 345*f*, 350*f*, *357*
as folate reductase inhibitor, 293
for malaria, 352-353
for toxoplasmosis, 357
Quazepam
duration of action, 92*f*
therapeutic advantages and disadvantages, 97*f*
withdrawal reactions, 93*f*
QUESTRAN. *See* Cholestyramine
Quinacrine, 345*f*
for giardiasis, 357
Quinapril (LOTENSIN), 151*f*, 179*f*
Quinestrol, 263, *263,* 263*f*
Quinidine, 163*f*, *167,* **167-168,** 169, 345*f*
antiarrhythmic effects, 164*f*, 171, 172*f*
drug interactions, 147, 160*f*, 169, 214, 334*f*
effects, 167*f*
Quinidine sulfate, 168
Quinine, 345*f*, 350*f*, **352,** *352*
Quinolones, **323-330**
specific agents, 323*f*
Raloxifene, 454, 477
Ramipril (ACCUPRIL, ALTACE), 179*f*
Ranitidine (ZANTAC), 235*f*, *236,* **236-238,** 419*f*, 438, 440
Raynaud's disease, treatment, 72
Rectal administration, **2**
Reentry, 165, 165*f*
REFLUDAN see Lepirudin
REGLAN. *See* Metoclopramide
Regulation, with second messenger molecules, 34
RELAFEN. *See* Nabumetone
REMICAN see Infliximab
Renal disease
anemia with, treatment, 206
chronic
and angina, 178*f*

and hypertension, 182*f*-183*f*
Renal elimination, **23-24,** 24*f*
Renal failure, acute, treatment, 233
Renin-angiotensisn-aldosterone system, and blood pressure, 180-181, 181*f*
REOPRO see Abciximab
Repaglinide, 452
REQUIP see Ropinirole
RESCRIPTOR see Delavirdine
Reserpine, 71*f*, **78,** *78*
and norepinephrine storage, 56
Respiratory infections, 294*f*
lower, treatment, 324
treatment, 300, 325*f*
specific agents, 363*f*
viral, treatment, **363-365**
Respiratory syncytial virus, treatment, 365
Respiratory system, drugs affecting, **217-222**
specific agents, 217*f*
RESTORIL. *See* Temazepam
REZULIN see Troglitazone
Rheumatic fever, treatment, 406
Rheumatoid arthritis
acute, treatment, 410
intractable, treatment, 389
treatment, 351, 406, 408, 410-411, 413-415
Rheumatoid inflammations, treatment, 275
Rhinitis
causes, 220, 221*f*
drug treatment, specific agents, 217*f*
treatment, **220-221**
Rhythm method, of contraception, failure rate, 268*f*
Ribavirin, 363*f*, *364,* **364-365,** 458
Rifabutin, 333
for Kaposi's sarcoma, 429
Rifampin, 331, 331*f*, *333,* **333-334,** 437
classification, 287*f*
drug interactions, 201*f*, 334, 340-341
for methicillin-resistant staphylococcus aureus, 300
resistance to, 285, 285*f*
and thyroid hormone metabolism, 253
for tuberculosis, 284*f*
Rimantadine, *363,* 363*f*, **363-364,** 458
Risedronate, 467
Risperidone, 127*f*, 128, *128,* 130-131, 132*f*
actions, 128*f*
RITALIN HYDROCHLORIDE. *See* Methylphenidate
Ritodrine, 55*f*, 69*f*
Ritonavir, **371,** *371,* 459
RITUXAN see Rituximab
Rituximab, 466
River blindness, treatment, 360, 361*f*
Rocky Mountain spotted fever, treatment, 312*f*
Rocuronium, 45*f*
onset and duration of action, 52*f*
pharmacokinetics, 51
therapeutic advantages, 52*f*
Rofecoxib, 466
ROGAINE. *See* Minoxidil
Rolaids. *See* Calcium carbonate
Ropinirole, 443
Rosiglitazone, 453
Roundworm infection, treatment, 359, 361*f*
RU 486. *See* Mifepristone
Salicylates, **403-408**
dose-dependent effects, 406*f*
drug interactions, 260*f*, 408*f*
therapeutic advantages and disadvantages, 412*f*
Salicylate salts, therapeutic advantages and disadvantages, 412*f*
Salicylic acid, 406
Salmeterol xinatoate
for asthma, 218, *218*
and bronchodilation, 67*f*
Salmonella infection
non-typhoid, treatment, 294*f*
treatment, 289, 291
Salmonella typhi infection, treatment, 294*f*
SANDIMMUNE see Cyclosporine
Saquinavir, **371,** *371,* 459
Sarcoma. *See also* Kaposi's sarcoma
Ewing's soft tissue, 390
osteogenic, 379
soft tissue, treatment, 384
treatment, 386
Schizonticides
blood, for malaria, 351-353
tissue, for malaria, 349-350
Schizophrenia, **127**
rates of relapse, 131*f*
treatment, 129, 131
Scopolamine, 45*f*, **48,** *48,* 48*f*-49*f*, 438
antiemetic effects, 129*f*
for motion sickness, 130, 242
and muscarinic receptor, 46*f*
preanesthetic, 108
Secobarbital, 90*f*, *94*
duration of action, 95
therapeutic advantages and disadvantages, 97*f*
Second messenger systems, **33-34**
Seizures
absence, **144,** 144*f*-145*f*
treatment, 149
classification, 144*f*, **144-145**
complex partial, **144,** 144*f*-145*f*
treatment, 146-147, 150
febrile, **144,** 144*f*-145*f*
treatment, 148
generalized, 144*f*, **144-145,** 145*f*
grand mal. *See* Seizures, tonic-clonic
myoclonic, **144,** 144*f*-145*f*
treatment, 149
partial, **144,** 144*f*-145*f*
treatment, 146-150
petit mal. *See* Seizures, absence
simple partial, **144,** 144*f*-145*f*
treatment, 146-148, 150
tonic-clonic, **144,** 144*f*-145*f*, 148
treatment, 91, 146-150
treatment, 90-91, 95
SELDANE. *See* Terfenadine
Selective estrogen receptor modulators, 454
Selegiline, 81*f*
Semilente insulin, 255*f*
extent and duration of action, 259*f*
Semilente insulin suspension, **258**
Senna, 244, 244*f*
SERM, 454
Sermorelin, 247*f*, 249, *249*
Serotonin antagonists, antiemetic potency, 243*f*
Serotonin reuptake inhibitors, 119*f*, **122-123**
receptor specificity, 121*f*
therapeutic advantages and disadvantages, 125*f*
Serratia marcescens infection, treatment, 304, 315*f*, 325*f*
Sertraline (ZOLOFT), 119*f*, 123, *123*
therapeutic advantages and disadvantages, 125*f*
Serum lipoprotein, 207, 208*f*
drugs that lower concentration, **210-215**
Sevoflurane, 107*f*, **115,** *115*
Shigella infection (shigellosis), treatment, 291, 294*f*, 325*f*
Shock
blood flow with, 5-6
treatment, 64-66, 69
Sibutramine, 474
Sickle cell disease (anemia)
specific agent for, 193*f*
treatment, 206

Sildenafil, 478
Silver sulfadiazine, 289*f*
  for burns, 291
  therapeutic application, 290
Simvastatin (ZOCOR), 207*f*, *214*, **214-215,** 449
SINEMET. *See* Carbidopa
SINGULAIR see Montelukast
Skin infections, treatment, 324
Sleep disorders, treatment, 91
SLO-BID. *See* Theophylline
SLOW-K. *See* Potassium
Smooth muscle
  effects of nitrites and nitrates on, 176, 176*f*
  relaxants, direct, **157**
Sodium bicarbonate, 236*f*, 240
Sodium channel blockers, 163*f*
Sodium nitroprusside, 151*f*, 180*f*, **191,** *191*
Sodium pentothal, with anesthesia, 110
Sodium salicylate, 406
Sodium stibogluconate, 345*f*, *356*, **356-357**
Soft tissue sarcomas, treatment, 384
Solid tumors, treatment, 388
Somatic nervous system, 27*f*, **31,** 32*f*
  cholinergic agonists in, 36*f*
Somatostatin, 247*f*, **250**
  actions, 248*f*
Somatotropin, 247*f*, **249,** *249*
Somatrem, 247*f*, 249, *249*
Sotalol, 163*f*, *171*, **171-172**
  antiarrhythmic effects, 164*f*
  drug interactions, 214
Spacer, for asthma, 219, 220*f*
Sparfloxacin, 456
Spectinomycin, 311*f*
  for gonorrhea, 299*f*
Spermicide
  failure rate, 268*f*
  percent use, 268*f*
Spirochetes, 283*f*
Spironolactone, 179*f*, 183, *183*, 223*f*, **232-233,** *233*
  as adrenocorticoid inhibitor, 277
  for hyperaldosteronism, 274
  site of action, 224*f*
Sporontocide, blood, 353
Squamous cell carcinoma
  of head and neck, treatment, 392
  treatment, 387
Stanozolol, 263*f*, 271, *271*
Staphylococcal infections, treatment, 308
Staphylococcus aureus infection, 435
  methicillin-resistant, 298, 300, 304, 308, 429-430
  resistance, 285
  treatment, 299*f*, 306
Staphylococcus epidermiditis infection, methicillin-resistant, 308
Staphylococcus saprophyticus infection, 327
Status epilepticus, 144*f*, **145,** 145*f*
  treatment, 91, 95, 146, 149
Stavudine (d4T), 363*f*, 369*f*, **370,** *370*
Steady-state, 17*f*, **17-19,** 18*f*-19*f*
Sterilization, contraceptive
  failure rate, 268*f*
  percent use, 268*f*
Steroid antagonists, in cancer therapy, 392-395
  specific agents, 373*f*
Steroid hormones, **263-278, 454**
  for cancer, 392-395
    specific agents, 373*f*
  mechanism of action, 393*f*
  specific agents, 263*f*-264*f*
Stool softeners, 245
Streptococcus pneumoniae infection, treatment, 294*f*, 299*f*
Streptococcus pyogenes infection, treatment, 299*f*
Streptococcus viridans infection, 434
  treatment, 299*f*
Streptokinase, 193*f*, 201, *202*, **202-203,** 204*f*
  activation of plasminogen, 202*f*
  mechanism of action, 202, 203*f*
  properties, 202*f*
Streptomyces, aminoglycosides from, 314
Streptomycin, 311*f*, 314, *314*, 331
  antibacterial spectrum, 315
  therapeutic applications, 315*f*
Streptozocin, emetic potential, 241*f*
Streptozotocin, 373*f*
Stress ulcers, acute, treatment, 237
Stroke, treatment, 72
Strongyloides stercoralis infection (strongyloidiasis), 361*f*
  treatment, 360, 361*f*
Subcutaneous (SC) administration, **3**
Sublingual administration, **2**
Substance abuse, potential for, 100*f*
Substituted benzamides
  antiemetic potency, 243*f*
  for chemotherapy-induced nausea and vomiting, 242*f*
Substituted benzodiazepines, for chemotherapy-induced nausea and vomiting, 242
Succinylcholine, 45*f*, *53*, **53,** 53*f*, 107*f*
  adverse effects, 53
  with anesthesia, 109
  onset and duration of action, 52*f*
  therapeutic disadvantages, 52*f*
Succinylsulfathiazole, 289*f*, *291*
  administration, 291
Sucralfate (CARAFATE), 236*f*, **241,** *241*
  drug interactions, 341
Sufentanil, 133*f*, 139, *139*
Sulbactam, 298*f*, 307, *307*
  administration route, 302
  drug interactions, 300
  stability to penicillinase, 300*f*
Sulfacetamide, 289*f*
  therapeutic application, 290
Sulfadiazine, 289*f*, 290, *290*, 292
  therapeutic application, 290
Sulfadoxine, for malaria, 352
Sulfamethoxazole, 289, *289*, 289*f*, 290. *See also* Co-trimoxazole
  antimicrobial activity rate, 293*f*
  drug interactions, 293
  mechanism of action, 294
  for urinary tract infection, 315*f*
Sulfanilamide, 289, *289*
  mechanism of action, 292*f*
Sulfapyridine
  in inflammatory bowel disease, 291
  metabolism, 291
Sulfasalazine, 289*f*, *291*
  administration, 291
  metabolism, 291
Sulfinpyrazone, 402*f*, **417,** *417*
  drug interactions, 408*f*
  for hyperuricemia, 415
Sulfisoxazole, 289*f*, 292, *292*
  therapeutic application, 290
  for urinary tract infections, 328*f*
Sulfonamides
  classification, 287*f*
  drug interactions, 147, 147*f*, 260*f*
  effect on neonates, 282
  and folate inhibition, 290
  inactivation, 291
  for malaria, 352
  mechanism of action, 292*f*
  resistance to, 285*f*
Sulfonamides, specific agents
  mafenide, 289*f*, 290
  mafenide acetate, 291
  silver sulfadiazine, 289*f*, 290-291
  succinylsulfathiazole, 289*f*, 291, *291*
  sulfacetamide, 289*f*, 290

sulfadiazine, 290
sulfamethoxazole, 289, *289*, 289*f*, 290, 293, 293*f*, 294, 315*f*. *See also* Co-trimoxazole
sulfasalazine, 289*f*, 291, *291*
sulfisoxazole, 289*f*, 290, 292, *292*, 328*f*
Sulfonylureas, **260-261**
drug interactions, 260*f*, 292, 334*f*
Sulindac (CLINORIL), 401*f*, *409*, **410**
therapeutic advantages and disadvantages, 412*f*
Sumatriptan (IMITREX), 419*f*, *426*, **426-427,** 437
for migraine, 427*f*
SUMYCIN. *See* Tetracycline
Supraventricular tachyarrhythmia
concomitant with hypertension, treatment, 185
treatment, 187, 188*f*
Supraventricular tachycardia
acute, treatment, 164*f*
treatment, 66, 78*f*, 164*f*, 172-173
SUPRAX. *See* Cefixime
Suramin, 345*f*, 353*f*, **356,** *356*
SUSTIVA see Efavirenz
Sympathetic nervous system, 27*f*, 29*f*, 29-30, 30*f*
and blood pressure, 180, 181*f*
Sympathetic neurons, **28**
SYNTHROID. *See* Levothyroxine
Syphilis, treatment, 299*f*, 318*f*
Tacrolimus, 473
TAGAMET. *See* Cimetidine
Tamoxifen (NOLVADEX), 263*f*, **266,** *266*, 373*f*, 399*f*, 458
in cancer therapy, *393*, **393-394**
Tapeworm infection, treatment, 362
TASMAR see Tolcapone
TAVIST. *See* Clemastine
Taxol, 373*f*
Tazobactam, 298*f*, 307, *307*
administration route, 302
drug interactions, 301
stability to penicillinase, 300*f*
3TC. *See* Lamivudine
TEGRETOL. *See* Carbamazepine
Temazepam (RESTORIL), *91*
duration of action, 92*f*
for sleep disorders, 92
therapeutic advantages and disadvantages, 97*f*
withdrawal reactions, 93*f*
Teniposide, **396,** *396*
TENORMIN. *See* Atenolol
Tension headache, characteristics, 425*f*
Terazosin (HYTRIN), 71*f*, **73,** *73*, 180*f*
for hypertension, 189
Terbutaline, 55*f*, **67,** *67*, 69*f*
for asthma, 62-63, 218
and bronchodilation, 67*f*
Terfenadine (SELDANE)
drug interactions, 214, 320, 341
for rhinitis, 221
withdrawn from market, 470
Testicular carcinoma
metastatic, treatment, 395
refractory, treatment, 396
Testicular tumors, treatment, 386, 399*f*
Testosterone, *269*, 269-271
production, 272*f*
secretion, regulation, 270*f*
synthesis, suppression, 340
Testosterone cypionate, 263*f*, 271, *271*
Tetracaine, 108*f*
pharmacokinetic properties, 117*f*
Tetracycline (SUMYCIN), 235*f*, 283, 283*f*, 311*f*, 345-346
classification, 287*f*
contraindications, 282
cost, 282, 282*f*
drug interactions, 160*f*, 213, 240
to eliminate Helicobacter pylori, 236
phototoxicity, 314
resistance to, 285*f*
sites of action, 346*f*
Tetracyclines, *311*, **311-314**
absorption, 313, 313*f*
adverse effects, 314*f*
effect on children, 282
for listeriosis, 299*f*
therapeutic applications, 290, 312*f*
for urinary tract infections, 328*f*
Tetracyclines, specific agents, 311*f*
demeclocycline, 311*f*, 314, *314*
doxycycline (VIBRAMYCIN), 147, 311*f*-312*f*, 313, *313*, 314, 328*f*
minocycline (MINOCIN), 311*f*, 313, *313*, 314
tetracycline (SUMYCIN), 160*f*, 213, 235*f*, 236, 240, 282, 282*f*, 283, 283*f*, 285*f*, 287*f*, 311*f*, 314, 345-346, 346*f*
Tetrahydrocannabinol (THC), 99*f*, **105,** *105*
for chemotherapy-induced nausea and vomiting, 243
6-TG. *See* 6-Thioguanine
Theobromine, *99*, 99*f*
THEO-DUR. *See* Theophylline
Theophylline (SLO-BID, THEO-DUR), *99*, 99*f*, **220**
for asthma, 100, 217*f*
for chronic obstructive pulmonary disease, 222
drug interactions, 319-320, 326, 395
Therapeutic equivalence, 7
Therapeutic index, 22*f*, 22-23
Thiabendazole, 359*f*, **360,** *360*, 361*f*
Thiamylal, 108*f*, *115*
Thiazide diuretics, 157, 223*f*, 228-231
adverse effects, 230*f*, 230-231
for angina, **183-184**
actions, 183*f*
and changes in urine composition, 229*f*, 233*f*
drug interactions, 160, 160*f*, 213, 292, 409
site of action, 224*f*
therapy with, 441
Thiethylperazine, antiemetic effects, 129*f*
Thioamides, 253-254
6-Thioguanine, 373*f*, 380, **382,** *382*, 399*f*
actions, 374*f*
Thiopental, 90*f*, *94*, 108*f*, 109
as anesthetic, 95, 115-116
distribution, 9
drug interactions, 408*f*
duration of action, 95
redistribution, 115, 115*f*
therapeutic advantages and disadvantages, 97*f*, 116*f*
Thioridazine, 127*f*, 129, *129*, 132*f*
actions, 128*f*
anticholinergic activity, 130
Thiothixene, 127, *127*, 127*f*, 132*f*
actions, 128*f*
Thioxanthenes, 127*f*
Threadworm infection, treatment, 360, 361*f*
Thrombin inhibitors, 448
Thrombolytic agents, **201-204**
adverse effects, 202, 203*f*
comparison, 202*f*
specific agents, 193*f*
Thrombus, 194
Thyroid
drugs affecting, 247*f*
removal, 253
Thyroid hormones, **251-254**
biosynthesis, 252*f*
Thyroid-stimulating hormone, 252-253
Thyroid storm, treatment, 254
Thyrotoxicosis, treatment, 78*f*, 253-254
Thyrotropin, 252-253
Thyrotropin-releasing hormone, 252-253

actions, 248*f*
Thyroxine, 247*f*, 251
biosynthesis, 252*f*
drug interactions, 408*f*
Tiagabine, 445
Ticarcillin, 298*f*, 301, *301*
administration route, 302
adverse reactions, 303
stability
to acid, 300*f*
to penicillinase, 300*f*
therapeutic applications, 301*f*
Ticlopidine, 193*f*, **196,** *196*
Timolol (TIMOPTOL, TIMOPTIC), 71*f*, **76,** *76*, 79*f*, 179*f*
clinical applications, 78*f*
drug elimination, 74*f*
TIMOPTIC. *See* Timolol
TIMOPTOL. *See* Timolol
Tirofiban, 447
Tissue-type plasminogen activator (tPA). *See* Alteplase
Tobramycin (TOBREX), 311*f*, 315, *315*, 431
adverse effects, 316
concentration, 316*f*
drug interactions, 51
therapeutic applications, 315*f*
TOBREX. *See* Tobramycin
Tocainide, 163*f*, **170,** *170*
effects, 169*f*
Tolazamide, 255*f*, 260, *260*
properties, 261*f*
Tolbutamide, 255*f*, 260, *260*
adverse effects, 292
drug interactions, 341
properties, 261*f*
Tolcapone, 444
Tolmetin, 401*f*, **411,** *411*
therapeutic advantages and disadvantages, 412*f*
TOPAMAX see Topiramate
Topical administration, **3-4**
Topiramate, 445
Topoisomerase, 323, 324*f*
Topotecan, 464
TORADOL. *See* Ketorolac
Torsemide, 223*f*, *227*, **227-228**
site of action, 224*f*
Total body clearance, 24-25
Toxoplasma gondii infection (toxoplasmosis), 357
treatment, 290, 345*f*, 353, **357**
Trachoma infections, 290*f*
Tranexamic acid, 193*f*, **204,** *204*
Transdermal patch, nicotine concentration, 101*f*
TRANSDERM-NITRO. *See* Nitroglycerin
Transient ischemic attacks, treatment, 196, 406
TRANXENE. *See* Clorazepate
Tranylcypromine, 119*f*, 123, *123*
therapeutic advantages and disadvantages, 125*f*
Trastuzumab, 465
Trazodone, 96, 119*f*, 123, *123*
therapeutic advantages and disadvantages, 125*f*
Trematodes, chemotherapy, 359*f*, **360-362**
Treponema pallidum infection, treatment, 299*f*, 312*f*
Treponema pertenue infection, treatment, 299*f*
Triacylglycerol, niacin for, 210
Triamcinolone (AZMACORT), 276, *276*
administration route, 276*f*
for asthma, 219
elimination, 276*f*
properties, 275*f*
for rhinitis, 221
Triamterene (DYAZIDE), 179*f*, 223*f*, **233,** *233*
site of action, 224*f*
Triazolam (HALCION), *91*
duration of action, 92*f*
for sleep disorders, 92
therapeutic advantages and disadvantages, 97*f*
withdrawal reactions, 92, 93*f*
Trichinella spiralis infection, 361*f*
treatment, 360
Trichinosis, treatment, 360, 361*f*
Trichomonas vaginalis infection, treatment, 347
Trichophyton infection, treatment, 343
Trichuris trichiura infection (trichuriasis), 361*f*
treatment, 359, 361*f*
Tricyclic antidepressants, 119*f*, **119-121**
drug interactions, 122*f*, 138
mechanism of action, 120*f*
and physostigmine, 42
receptor specificity, 121*f*
therapeutic advantages and disadvantages, 125*f*
Trifluridine, 363*f*, **368,** *368*
Trigeminal neuralgia, treatment, 147
Trihexyphenidyl, for Parkinson's disease, 87-88
Triiodothyronine, 247*f*, 251
biosynthesis, 252*f*
drug interactions, 408*f*
TRI-LEVLIN. *See* Ethinyl estradiol
Trimeprazine, therapeutic advantages and disadvantages, 422*f*
Trimethaphan, 45*f*, *49*, **49,** 49*f*
Trimethoprim (BACTRIM), 289, *289*, 289*f*, 290, **293,** *293*. *See also* Co-trimoxazole
antimicrobial activity rate, 293*f*
for bacterial prostatitis, 281, 281*f*
classification, 287*f*
drug interactions, 289
and folate deficiency, 205
interaction with enzymes, 20
mechanism of action, 292*f*, 293-294
resistance to, 285, 285*f*
for urinary tract infection, 315*f*
Trimethoprim-sulfmethoxazole, for urinary tract infections, 328*f*
Trimipramine, 119*f*
therapeutic advantages and disadvantages, 125*f*
TRIMOX. *See* Amoxicillin
TRI-NORINYL. *See* Ethinyl estradiol
Tripelennamine, therapeutic advantages and disadvantages, 422*f*
TRIPHASIL. *See* Ethinyl estradiol
Triprolidine, therapeutic advantages and disadvantages, 422*f*
Troglitazone, 453
Trovaflaxacin, 456
TROVAN see Trovafloxacin
Trypanosoma brucei gambiense infection, 353, 353*f*
treatment, 354
Trypanosoma brucei rhodesiense infection, 353, 353*f*
treatment, 354
Trypanosoma cruzi infection, 353, 353*f*
resistance, 355
treatment, 355
Trypanosomiasis
chemotherapy, 345*f*, **353-356**
summary, 353*f*
Tuberculosis, 436-437. *See also* Mycobacterium tuberculosis infection
chemotherapy, **332-335**
incidence, 332*f*
treatment, 284, 284*f*, 315, 331*f*
Tubocurarine, 45*f*, 50, *50*, 50*f*
drug interactions, 51
and neostigmine, 42
and nicotinic receptors, 39
onset and duration of action, 52*f*

pharmacokinetics, 51
therapeutic disadvantages, 52*f*
Tularemia, treatment, 315, 315*f*
Tumors. *See also* Cancer; Testicular tumors
growth rate, 374
mass, 375*f*
treatment-induced, 378
Tums. *See* Calcium carbonate
TYLENOL. *See* Acetaminophen
Type I diabetes. *See* Diabetes mellitus, insulin-dependent
Type II diabetes. *See* Diabetes mellitus, non-insulin-dependent
Tyramine, 55*f*, **68,** *68*
as indirect-acting agonist, 61
Tyrosine, in norepinephrine synthesis, 55
Ultralente insulin, 255*f*, **259**
extent and duration of action, 259*f*
Urea, 223*f*, 233, *233*
Ureaplasma infection, 318*f*
treatment, 317
Ureaplasma urealyticum infection, treatment, 318*f*, 328*f*
Urethral syndrome, acute, treatment, 328*f*
Urethritis, treatment, 318
Uric acid, in gout, 415, 415*f*
Uricosuric agents, **417**
Urinary tract antiseptics, **323-330, 327-329**
Urinary tract antiseptics, specific agents, 323*f*
methenamine, 292, *327,* 327*f*, **327-328**
nitrofurantoin (MACRODANTIN, MACRO-BID), **329,** *329*
Urinary tract infections, 290*f*
treatment, 294*f*, 315*f*, 324, 328*f*
Urofolitropin, **250**
Urokinase, 193*f*, 201, **203,** *203,* 204*f*
activation of plasminogen, 202*f*
properties, 202*f*
Urticaria, treatment, 424
Uveitis, treatment, 409
Vaginal infections, treatment, 294*f*
Valacyclovir, 458
VALIUM. *See* Diazepam
Valproic acid (DEPAKOTE), 143*f*, *148,* **148-149**
adverse effects, 149*f*
drug interactions, 150
for seizures, 145*f*
VANCENASE. *See* Beclomethasone
VANCERIL. *See* Beclomethasone
Vancomycin, 298*f*, *308,* **308-309,** 429-431, 434-435
classification, 287*f*
for methicillin-resistant staphylococcus aureus, 300
resistance to, 284, 285*f*
Varicella-zoster virus, treatment, 367
Vascular trauma, normal response to, 193-194
Vasodilators, **155-157**
for hypertension, 190-191
Vasodilators, specific agents, 151*f*
Vasopressin, 247*f*, 250, **251,** *251*
VASOTEC. *See* Enalapril
Vecuronium, 45*f*, 107*f*
with anesthesia, 109
onset and duration of action, 52*f*
pharmacokinetics, 51
therapeutic advantages, 52*f*
VEETIDS. *See* Penicillin V
Venlafaxine, 119*f*, 123, *123*
therapeutic advantages and disadvantages, 125*f*
Venous thromboembolism, treatment, 198
Venous thrombosis, treatment, 198
VENTOLIN. *See* Albuterol
Ventricular arrhythmias, treatment, 169-170, 172
Ventricular fibrillation, treatment, 164*f*, 172
Ventricular tachyarrhythmia, treatment, 168, 170, 172
Ventricular tachycardia
acute, treatment, 164*f*
treatment, 164*f*, 171-172
Verapamil (ISOPTIN, VERELAN), 163*f*, 167, **173,** *173,* 175*f*, **177,** *177,* 180*f*, 187, *187*
actions, 187*f*
adverse effects, 189
for angina, 188*f*
as antiarrhythmic, 164*f*
drug interactions, 160*f*, 169, 377
effects, 173*f*
for hypertension, 188*f*
for supraventricular tachyarrhythmia, 188*f*
VERELAN. *See* Verapamil
VIAGRA see Sildenafil
VIBRAMYCIN. *See* Doxycycline
Vibrio cholerae infection, treatment, 312*f*, 315*f*
Vidarabine (ara-A), 363*f*, *367,* 367*f*, **367-368**
Vigabatrin, 446
Vinblastine, 373*f*, *390,* **390-391,** 399*f*
drug interactions, 386, 395
myelosuppressive potential, 378*f*
Vincristine, 373*f*, *390,* **390-391,** 399*f*
drug interactions, 384, 397
emetic potential, 241*f*
myelosuppressive potential, 378*f*
Vinorelbine, 390, *390*
VIRACEPT see Nelfinavir
Viral infections, treatment, 412
VIRAMUNE see Nevirapine
Visceral leishmaniasis, 356
VISTIDE see Cidofovir
Vitamin B_{12}. *See also* Cyanocobalamin
deficiency, as similar to folate deficiency, 205
Vitamin K, 193*f*, **204**
for bleeding, 204
and warfarin, 200
VOLTAREN. *See* Diclofenac
Vomiting. *See also* Emesis
mechanisms that trigger, 241-242
treatment, 129-130
Warfarin (COUMADIN), 193*f*, *199,* **199-201**
adverse effects, 292
drug interactions, 188, 196, 201*f*, 213, 239, 295, 320, 326, 334*f*, 341, 411
mechanism of action, 200, 200*f*
therapeutic index, 22*f*, 22-23
Whipworm infection, treatment, 359, 361*f*
Wilm's tumor, 390
treatment, 384, 399*f*
Withdrawal method, of contraception
failure rate, 268*f*
percent use, 268*f*
Wucheria bancrofti, 361*f*
WYMOX. *See* Amoxicillin
XANAX. *See* Alprazolam
XELODA see Capecitabine
Yaws, treatment, 299*f*
Yersinia pestis infection, treatment, 315*f*
Zafirlukast, 450
Zalcitabine (ddC), 363*f*, 369*f*, *370,* **370**
ZANTAC. *See* Ranitidine
ZESTRIL. *See* Lisinopril
ZIAGEN see Abacavir
Zidovudine (AZT), 363*f*, *368,* **368-369,** 369*f*
drug interactions, 339, 367
Zileuton, 450
Zinc insulin, 255*f*
ZITHROMAX. *See* Azithromycin
ZOCOR. *See* Simvastatin
Zollinger-Ellison syndrome, treatment, 237, 239
ZOLOFT. *See* Sertraline
Zolpidem (AMBIEN), **93,** *93*
therapeutic advantages and disadvantages, 97*f*
ZOVIRAX. *See* Acyclovir
ZYFLO see Zileuton

Figure Sources

Figure 2.5 modified from H. P. Range and M. M. Dale, Pharmacology, Churchill Livingstone (1987).
Figures 6.9, 6.10 and 6.11 modified from Allwood, Cobbold and Ginsburg, British Medical Bulletin 19:132 (1963).
Figure 8.10, modified from R. Young, American Family Physician, 59:2155 (1999)
Figure 9.5 modified from A. Kales, Excertpa Medical Congress Series 899:149 (1989).
Figure 9.6 from data of E. C. Dimitrion, A. J. Parashos, J. S. Giouzepas, Drug Invest. 4:316 (1992).
Figure 10.4 modified from N. L. Benowitz, Science 319:1318 (1988).
Figure 16.6 data from Results of the Cooperative North Scandinavian Enalapril Survival Study, N. Engl. J. Med. 316:80 (1988).
Figure 17.3 modified from J. A. Beven and J. H. Thompson, Essentials of Pharmacology, Harper and Row (1983).
Figure 17.11 modified from J. W. Mason, N. Engl. J. Med., 329:452 (1993).
Figure 19.5 modified from B. J. Materson, Drug Therapy, November p. 157 (1985).
Figure 20.14, modified from D. J. Schneider, P. B. Tracy, and B. E. Sobel, Hospital Practice, May 15, (1998), p. 107
Figure 20.15, data from D.A. Vorchheimer, J. J. Badimon, and V. Fuster, Journal American Medical Association 281: 1407 (1999)
Figure 21.12, modified from Knopp, R. H., N. Engl. J. Med. 341:498 (1999)
Figure 22.7, modified from J. M. Drazen, E. Israel, and P. M. O'Bryne, N. Engl. J. Med., 340: 197 (1999).
Figure 22. 8, modified from Drazen, J. M., Israel, E., and O'Byrne, P. M., N. Engl. J. Med., 340:197 (1999)
Figures 21.4 and 21.10 modified from R. H. Knopp, Hospital Practice 23:22 (1988).
Figure 24.2 modified from D. Cave, Hospital Practice, Sept 30, 1992.
Figure 24.4 modified from S. M. Grunberg and P. J. Hesketh, N. Engl. J. Med. 329: 1790 (1993).
Figures 24.6, 24.7 from data of S. Bilgrami and B. G. Fallon, Postgraduate Medicine, 94:55 (1993).
Figures 25.2 and 26.6 modified from B. G. Katzung, Basic and Clinical Pharmacology, Appleton and Lange (1987).
Figure 26.4 modified from M. C. Riddle, Postgraduate Med. 92:89 (1992).
Figure 26.7 modified from O. B Crofford, Ann. Rev. Medicine 46:267 (1995).
Figure 26.10, from F. Holleman and J. B. L. Hoekstra, N. Engl. J. Med. 337:179 (1997)
Figure 26.11 modified from A. E. Kitabchi and M. Bryer-Ash, Hospital Practice, March 15, 1997, p. 135.
Figures 27.6 and 27.7 modified from D. R. Mishell, Jr.., N. Engl. J. Med. 320:777 (1989).
Figure 27.8 modified from M. Polaneczky, G. S. Slap, C.F. Forke, A. R. Rappaport, and S. Sondheimer, N. Engl. J. Med 331:1201 (1994).
Figure 27.15 modified from Cummings, S. R., et al, J.A.M.A 281:2189 (1999)
Figure 31.6 modified from J. Inter. Med Res 2:100 (1974)
Figure 32.2 from data of U. S. Public Health Service.
Figure 33.3 modified from data of D. A. Evans, K. A. Maley and V. A. McRusick, British Medical Journal 2:485 (1960).
Figure 35.3 from W. Peters and H. R. Folmer, Malaria, Royal Tropical Institute.
Figure 35.8 from G. Mandel, J. Bennett, R. Dolin, Principles and Practices of Infectious Diseases, Churchill Livingstone (1995).
Figure 36.3 from M. Weber, N. Engl. J. Med., 328:927 (1993) .
Figure 36.5 from R. Bratton, R. E. Nesse, Postgraduate Medicine, 93: 177 (1993).
Figure 37.2 modified from R. Dolin, Science 227:1296 (1985).
Figure 37.10 modified from Balfour, H. H., N. Engl. J. Med. 340:1255 (1999)
Figure 37.13 modified from Flexner, C., N. Engl. J. Med. 338:1281 (1998)
Figure 38.5 modified from N. Kartner and V. Ling. Scientific American, March (1989).

Figure 40.8 modified from D. D. Dubose, A. C. Cutlip, and W. D. Cutlip. American Family Medicine 51:1498 (1995).
Figure 43.1 photo from Jordan, V. C., Scientific American, October, p. 60 (1998)
Figure 43.2 data from Tucci, J. R., Tonino, R. P. and Emkey, R.D, et al., Am. J. Med 101:488 (1996)
Figure A.2 H. Lambert, and F. W. Edmund, Slide Atlas of Infectious Disease, Gower Medical Publishing (1982).
Figure A.3 modified from G. S. Rachelefsky, Hospital Practice, Nov. 15, 1995.
Figure A.4 from W. Peters and H. R. Folmer, Malaria, Royal Tropical Institute.
Figure A.6 modified from H. Kupperman and I. S. Young, MedCom Famous Teaching in Modern Medicine: Endocrinology, MedCom (1970).
Figure A.8 from T. P. Habif, Clinical Dermatology, 2nd ed., Mosby (1990).
Figure A.9 modified from M. J. Jamieson, K.K. McHardy, H. M. A. Towler, G. Chessell, K. P. Duguid, T. M. MacDonald, and J. C. Petrie, Essential Clinical Signs, Churchill Livingstone (1990).
Figure A.10 modified from A.S. Taha, N. Hudson, C.J. Hawkey, A.J. Swannell, P.N. Trye, J. Cottrell, S.G. Mann, T.J. Simon, R.D. Sturrock, and R.I. Russell, N. Engl. J. Med 334:1435 (1996).